D.W. Bainbridge

Misprinting → Kirk VII pg 1240

consulting editors

DR. WILLIAM C. WAGNER	Principles of Hormone Therapy
DR. THOMAS POWERS	Clinical Pharmacology
DR. K. J. BETTERIDGE	Embryo Transfer
DR. W. C. D. HARE	Cytogenetics
DR. DAVID MORROW	Bovine
DR. VICTOR SHILLE	Canine and Population Control in Urban Pets
DR. EDWARD MATHER	Equine
DR. DOUGLAS MITCHELL	Equine
DR. EMERSON COLBY	Feline
DR. NICKOLAS SOJKA	Feline
DR. E. D. FIELDEN	Ovine
DR. A. N. BRUERE	Ovine
DR. MARY SMITH	Caprine
DR. A. D. LEMAN	Porcine
DR. S. W. J. SEAGER	Laboratory and Zoo Animals
DR. RICHARD MILLER	Diagnostic Procedures
DR. KARIN L. HARTER	Appendix C

Current Therapy in Theriogenology:

diagnosis, treatment and prevention of reproductive diseases in animals

DAVID A. MORROW, *D.V.M., Ph.D.*

*Professor of Large Animal Surgery and Medicine,
Michigan State University, College of Veterinary Medicine,
East Lansing, Michigan; Charter Diplomate, American
College Theriogenologists*

W. B. SAUNDERS COMPANY
Philadelphia   London   Toronto   Mexico City   Rio de Janeiro   Sydney   Tokyo

W. B. Saunders Company: West Washington Square
                             Philadelphia, PA   19105

                             1 St. Anne's Road
                             Eastbourne, East Sussex BN21 3UN, England

                             1 Goldthorne Avenue
                             Toronto, Ontario M8Z 5T9, Canada

                             Apartado 26370 — Cedro 512
                             Mexico 4, D. F., Mexico

                             Rua Coronel Cabrita, 8
                             Sao Cristovao Caixa Postal 21176
                             Rio de Janeiro, Brazil

                             9 Waltham Street
                             Artarmon, N.S.W. 2064, Australia

                             Ichibancho, Central Bldg., 22-1 Ichibancho
                             Chiyoda-Ku, Tokyo 102, Japan

Library of Congress Cataloging in Publication Data

Main entry under title:

Current therapy in theriogenology.

Includes bibliographical references.

1. Generative organs–Diseases.   2. Veterinary obstetrics.
   3. Reproduction.   I. Morrow, David A.   II. Title:
   Theriogenology. [DNLM: 1. Reproduction–Periodicals.
   2. Veterinary medicine–Periodicals. W1 CU819T]

SF871.C84   636.089′66   77–84675

ISBN 0–7216–6564–0

CURRENT THERAPY IN THERIOGENOLOGY: ISBN   0-7216-6564-0
Diagnosis, Treatment and Prevention
of Reproductive Diseases in Animals

Last digit is the print number: 9   8   7

Contributors

BRUCE ABBITT, D.V.M., M.S., Diplomate, American College of Theriogenologists, Texas Veterinary Medical Diagnostic Laboratory, College Station, Texas.

C. E. ADAMS, Ph.D., Agricultural Research Council, Institute of Animal Physiology, Cambridge, England.

KJELL ANDERSEN, D.V.M., Associate Professor, Department of Reproductive Physiology and Pathology, Veterinary College of Norway, Oslo, Norway.

C. BEN BAKER, D.V.M., Resident Veterinarian, Lana Labell Farms, Montgomery, New York.

LESLIE BALL, D.V.M., M.S., Diplomate, American College of Theriogenologists, Professor, Departments of Clinical Science and Physiology and Biophysics, Colorado State University, Fort Collins, Colorado.

DAVID E. BARTLETT, D.V.M., Ph.D., Diplomate, American College of Theriogenologists, Consultant in Veterinary Medicine, Madison, Wisconsin.

PARVATHI K. BASRUR, B.Sc., M.Sc., Ph.D., Professor, Department of Biomedical Sciences, Ontario Veterinary College, University of Guelph, Guelph, Ontario, Canada.

DAVID BENNETT, B.Sc., B.Vet.Med., M.R.C.V.S., Lecturer, Veterinary Surgery, University of Glasgow, Glasgow, Scotland.

EZRA BERMAN, D.V.M., Veterinary Practitioner, Research Triangle Park, North Carolina.

WILLIAM EVERETT BERNDTSON, Ph.D., Assistant Professor, Department of Animal Sciences, University of New Hampshire, Durham, New Hampshire.

KEITH JAMES BETTERIDGE, M.V.Sc., Ph.D., M.R.C.V.S., Agriculture Canada, Animal Diseases Research Institute (Eastern), Ottawa, Ontario, Canada.

NILS BILLE, D.V.M., Associate Professor, Department of Pathology, Royal Veterinary and Agricultural University, Copenhagen, Denmark.

PAUL E. BLACKMER, D.V.M., Veterinary Practitioner, Partner, Chino Valley Veterinary Group, Ontario, California.

WILLIAM J. BOEVER, D.V.M., Adjunct Assistant Professor, Department of Veterinary Pathology, College of Veterinary Medicine, University of Missouri, Columbia, Missouri; Senior Staff Veterinarian, St. Louis Zoological Park, St. Louis, Missouri.

WILHELM BOLLWAHN, D.V.M., Professor of Swine Diseases, Klinik für kleine Klauentiere, Tierärztliche Hochschule, Hanover, Germany.

ARIFFEN T. BONGSO, B.V.Sc., M.Sc., Ph.D., Assistant Professor, Department of Veterinary Clinical Studies, Veterinary School, University of Sri Lanka, Peradeniya, Sri Lanka.

J. M. BOWEN, B.Vet.Med., F.R.C.V.S., Associate Professor, Large Animal Medicine, Texas A&M University, College Station, Texas.

RICHARD A. BOWEN, D.V.M., M.S., Postdoctoral Fellow, College of Veterinary Medicine and Biomedical Sciences, Colorado State University, Fort Collins, Colorado.

ARIE BRAND, D.V.M., Ph.D., Professor, Chairman of Herd Health and Ambulatory Clinic, State University of Utrecht, Utrecht, The Netherlands.

JACK H. BRITT, Ph.D., Associate Professor of Reproductive Physiology, North Carolina State University, Raleigh, North Carolina.

A. NEIL BRUERE, B.V.Sc., Ph.D., M.R.C.V.S., F.A.C.V.Sc., Professor of Veterinary Medicine and Clinical Pharmacology, Massey University, Palmerston North, New Zealand.

RON E. BUFFINGTON, Ph.D., Sales Coordinator, Select Sires, Plains City, Ohio.

THOMAS J. BURKE, D.V.M., M.S., Associate Professor of Medicine, College of Veterinary Medicine, University of Illinois, Urbana, Illinois; Consultant in Medicine, Capital Illini Veterinary Hospitals, Springfield, Illinois.

C. J. CALLAHAN, D.V.M., Diplomate, American College of Theriogenologists, Professor of Bovine Theriogenology, School of Veterinary Medicine, Purdue University, Lafayette, Indiana.

LELAND E. CARMICHAEL, D.V.M., Ph.D., Professor of Virology, New York State College of Veterinary Medicine, Cornell University, Ithaca, New York.

HELEN M. CHAPMAN, B.V.Sc., Ph.D., Lecturer in Sheep Medicine and Production, School of Veterinary Studies, Murdoch University, Murdoch Western Australia.

PETER J. CHENOWETH, B.V.Sc., Diplomate, American College of Theriogenologists, Associate Professor (Theriogenology), Texas A & M University, College Station, Texas.

CHARLES J. CHRISTIANS, Ph.D., Professor of Animal Science, University of Minnesota, St. Paul, Minnesota.

EMERSON D. COLBY, M.S., D.V.M., Associate in Physiology, Director of Animal Research Facilities, Dartmouth Medical School, Hanover, New Hampshire.

GABEL H. CONNER, D.V.M., Ph.D., Professor Emeritus, Large Animal Surgery and Medicine, Michigan State University; Presently, Professor and Senior Clinician, Food Animal Medicine, University of Idaho, Caldwell Branch, Caldwell, Idaho.

M. D. COPLAND, B.V.Sc., M.A.C.V.Sc., M.R.C.V.S., Regional Veterinary Officer, Department of Agriculture and Fisheries, Naracoorte, South Australia.

STEVEN E. CROW, D.V.M., Diplomate, American College of Veterinary Medicine, Assistant Professor of Internal Medicine, College of Veterinary Medicine, Michigan State University; Clinical Oncologist, Veterinary Clinical Center, Michigan State University, East Lansing, Michigan.

STANLEY E. CURTIS, B.S.A., M.S., Ph.D., Professor of Animal Science, College of Agriculture, University of Illinois, Urbana, Illinois.

LLOYD E. DAVIS, D.V.M., Ph.D., Professor of Clinical Pharmacology, College of Veterinary Medicine, University of Illinois, Urbana, Illinois.

BILLY N. DAY, B.S., M.S., Ph.D., Professor of Animal Husbandry, University of Missouri–Columbia, Columbia, Missouri.

STANLEY M. DENNIS, B.V.Sc., Ph.D., F.R.C.V.S., F.R.C.Path., Diplomate, American College of Theriogenologists, Professor and Head of Pathology, College of Veterinary Medicine, Kansas State University, Manhattan, Kansas.

JOHN R. DIEHL, B.S., Ph.D., Associate Professor of Reproductive Physiology, Department of Agriculture Sciences, Tuskegee Institute, Tuskegee, Alabama.

PAUL A. DOIG, D.V.M., M.Sc., Associate Professor (Theriogenology), Ontario Veterinary College, University of Guelph, Guelph, Ontario, Canada.

MAARTEN DROST, D.V.M., Diplomate, American College of Theriogenologists, Chairman and Professor (of Reproduction), Department of Reproduction, College of Veterinary Medicine, University of Florida, Gainesville, Florida.

W. RICHARD DUKELOW, Ph.D., Director and Professor, Endocrine Research Unit, Michigan State University, East Lansing, Michigan.

THOMAS G. DUNN, B.S., M.S., Ph.D., Professor of Animal Physiology, Division of Animal Science, University of Wyoming, Laramie, Wyoming.

GERALD W. DYCK, B.S.A., M.Sc., Ph.D., Research Scientist II, Reproductive Physiology, Agriculture Canada Research Station, Brandon, Manitoba, Canada.

PHILIP F. DZUIK, Ph.D., Professor of Animal Science, University of Illinois, Urbana, Illinois.

STIG G. EINARSSON, D.V.M., Ph.D., Professor of Obstetrics and Gynecology, College of Veterinary Medicine, Swedish University of Agricultural Sciences, Uppsala, Sweden.

ALLEN R. ELLICOTT, Ph.D., Assistant Professor, Clemson University, Clemson, South Carolina.

RONNIE G. ELMORE, D.V.M., M.S., Diplomate, American College of Theriogenologists, Assistant Professor (Theriogenology), University of Missouri, Columbia, Missouri.

R. PETER ELSDEN, M.V.Sc., Assistant Professor, College of Veterinary Medicine and Biomedical Sciences, Colorado State University, Fort Collins, Colorado.

R. E. ERB, Ph.D., Professor Emeritus, Purdue University, Lafayette, Indiana.

LAWRENCE E. EVANS, D.V.M., Ph.D., Diplomate, American College of Theriogenologists, Professor of Theriogenology, College of Veterinary Medicine, Iowa State University, Ames, Iowa.

LLOYD C. FAULKNER, D.V.M., Ph.D., Diplomate, American College of Theriogenologists, Professor and Associate Dean for Research and Graduate Studies, College of Veterinary Medicine, University of Missouri, Columbia, Missouri.

E. D. FIELDEN, B.Agr.Sci., B.V.Sc., F.R.C.V.S., F.A.C.V.Sc., Professor of Veterinary Clinical Sciences, Massey University, Palmerston North, New Zealand.

DELMAR R. FINCO, D.V.M., Ph.D., Professor, University of Georgia, Faculty Member, University of Georgia, Veterinary Medical Teaching Hospital, Athens, Georgia.

REGINALD J. FITZPATRICK, B.Sc., Ph.D., M.R.C.V.S., Professor of Clinical Studies, Faculty of Veterinary Science, University of Liverpool, Liverpool, England.

B. FLOW, D.V.M., Ph.D., Austin, Texas.

RAMESH C. GARG, B.V.Sc. & A.H. (Hons), M.V.Sc., Ph.D., Visiting Assistant Professor, Department of Veterinary Physiology and Pharmacology, College of Veterinary Medicine, The Ohio State University, Columbus, Ohio.

BRIAN GERLOFF, D.V.M., Woodstock, Illinois.

CHARLES D. GIBSON, D.V.M., Ph.D., Diplomate, American College of Theriogenologists, Associate Professor, College of Veterinary Medicine, Michigan State University, East Lansing, Michigan.

THOMAS PAUL GREINER, D.V.M., Staff Surgeon, Animal Medical Center, New York, New York.

EBERHARD GRUNERT, M.D., Ph.D., Professor of Veterinary Obstetrics and Gynecology, Veterinary College of Hanover; Director of the Clinic of Obstetrics and Gynecology, Hanover, Germany.

BORJE K. GUSTAFSSON, D.V.M., Ph.D., Professor and Head, Department of Veterinary Clinical Medicine, College of Veterinary Medicine, University of Illinois, Urbana, Illinois.

LYLE E. HANSON, Ph.B., D.V.M., M.S., Ph.D., Professor and Head, Department of Pathology and Hygiene, College of Veterinary Medicine, University of Illinois, Urbana, Illinois.

ROBERT M. HARDY, D.V.M., M.S., Associate Professor, University of Minnesota, St. Paul, Minnesota.

W. C. DOUGLAS HARE, M.A. (h.c.), B.Sc. (vet.), Ph.D., D.V.M. & S, M.R.C.V.S., Research Scientist and Head, Diseases of Cattle Section, Animal Pathology Division, Health of Animals Branch, Agriculture Canada, Animal Diseases Research Institute, Ottawa, Ontario, Canada.

BENJAMIN L. HART, D.V.M., Ph.D., Professor, Department of Physiological Sciences, School of Veterinary Medicine, University of California, Davis, California.

KARIN L. HARTER, D.V.M., Private practice, Detroit, Michigan.

KEVIN G. HAUGHEY, B.V.Sc., M.A.C.V.Sc., Senior Lecturer in Veterinary Medicine, Department of Veterinary Clinical Studies, The University of Sydney, Camden, N.S.W., Australia.

LAWRENCE E. HEIDER, D.V.M., Professor, Veterinary Preventive Medicine, The Ohio State University, Columbus, Ohio.

HARVEY D. HILLEY, D.V.M., Associate Professor, Large Animal Surgery and Medicine, University of Minnesota, St. Paul, Minnesota.

ROBERT B. HILLMAN, D.V.M., M.S., Diplomate, American College of Theriogenologists, Senior Clinician, New York State College of Veterinary Medicine, Cornell University, Ithaca, New York.

H. F. HINTZ, Ph.D., Associate Professor of Nutrition, Cornell University, Ithaca, New York.

HAROLD H. HODSON, JR., Ph.D., Professor, Animal Industries Department, Southern Illinois University, Carbondale, Illinois.

ALVIN B. HOERLEIN, D.V.M., Ph.D., Professor Emeritus, Microbiology, Colorado State University, Fort Collins, Colorado.

R. J. HOLMES, B.V.M.S., Ph.D., M.R.C.V.S., Lecturer in Animal Behaviour, Department of Veterinary Clinical Sciences, Massey University, Palmerston North, New Zealand.

THOMAS H. HOWARD, D.V.M., Animal Reproduction Laboratory, Colorado State University, Fort Collins, Colorado.

ROBERT S. HUDSON, D.V.M., M.S., Diplomate, American College of Theriogenologists, Professor, Large Animal Surgery and Medicine, School of Veterinary Medicine, Auburn University, Auburn, Alabama.

JOHN P. HUGHES, D.V.M., Diplomate, American College of Theriogenologists, Professor and Chairman, Department of Reproduction, School of Veterinary Medicine, University of California–Davis; Clinician, Veterinary Medical Teaching Hospital, University of California–Davis, Davis, California.

JOHN B. HURTGEN, D.V.M., M.S., Ph.D., Diplomate, American College of Theriogenologists, Assistant Professor of Animal Reproduction, School of Veterinary Medicine, University of Pennsylvania, New Bolton Center, Kennett Square, Pennsylvania.

ALDON H. JENSEN, Ph.D., Professor of Animal Nutrition, Department of Animal Science, University of Illinois, Urbana, Illinois.

DAVID R. JOHNSON, Ph.D., B.Sc., Lecturer in Anatomy, School of Medicine, University of Leeds, Leeds, United Kingdom.

DONALD W. JOHNSON, D.V.M., Ph.D., Professor of Large Animal Clinical Sciences, College of Veterinary Medicine, University of Minnesota, St. Paul, Minnesota.

RODNEY G. JOHNSON, D.V.M., Lake Region Veterinary Center, Elbow Lake, Minnesota.

SHIRLEY D. JOHNSTON, D.V.M., M.S., Veterinary Medical Associate, Theriogenology, College of Veterinary Medicine, University of Minnesota, St. Paul, Minnesota.

ROBERT F. KAHRS, D.V.M., Ph.D., Professor and Chairman, Department of Preventive Medicine, College of Veterinary Medicine, University of Florida, Gainesville, Florida.

C. COLIN KALTENBACH, Ph.D., Professor of Animal Physiology, University of Wyoming, Laramie, Wyoming.

RICHARD DEAN KEALY, B.S., M.S., Ph.D., Research Associate, Ralston Purina Company, St. Louis, Missouri.

KEITH W. KELLEY, B.S., M.S., Ph.D., Assistant Professor of Animal Sciences, College of Agriculture, Washington State University, Pullman, Washington.

ROBERT M. KENNEY, D.V.M., Ph.D., Diplomate, American College of Theriogenologists, Professor of Animal Reproduction, School of Veterinary Medicine, University of Pennsylvania, New Bolton Center, Kennett Square, Pennsylvania.

D. C. KRAEMER, D.V.M., Ph.D., Professor of Veterinary Physiology and Pharmacology, Texas A & M University, College Station, Texas.

T. J. KUEHL, Ph.D., Associate Foundation Scientist, Southwest Foundation for Research and Education, San Antonio, Texas; Visiting Professor, Department of Veterinary Physiology and Pharmacology, Texas A & M University, College Station, Texas.

PHILIP W. LADDS, M.V.Sc., Ph.D., Senior Lecturer in Veterinary Pathology, Department of Tropical Veterinary Science, James Cook University, Queensland, Australia.

JAN LADEWIG, D.V.M., Post-doctoral Research Associate, School of Veterinary Medicine, University of California–Davis, Davis, California.

ELDEN G. LAMPRECHT, D.V.M., Ph.D., Diplomate, American College of Theriogenologists, Research Veterinary Pathologist, 3M Company, St. Paul, Minnesota.

KEITH ROBERT LAPWOOD, B.V.Sc., Ph.D., Senior Lecturer in Physiology, Faculty of Veterinary Science, Massey University, Palmerston North, New Zealand.

ROLF E. LARSEN, D.V.M., Ph.D., Assistant Professor of Reproduction, College of Veterinary Medicine, University of Florida, Gainesville, Florida.

LESTER L. LARSON, D.V.M., Ph.D., Diplomate, American College of Theriogenologists, Head, Veterinary Department, American Breeders Service, De Forest, Wisconsin.

HORST W. LEIPOLD, D.V.M., Ph.D., Professor of Pathology, Kansas State University, Manhattan, Kansas.

A. D. LEMAN, D.V.M., Ph.D., Associate Professor, Large Animal Clinical Sciences, University of Minnesota, St. Paul, Minnesota.

ALAN D. McCAULEY, D.V.M., Veterinary Practitioner, Elizabethtown, Pennsylvania.

KEITH D. McSPORRAN, B.V.Sc., Ph.D., Scientist, Wallaceville Animal Research Centre, Private Bag, Upper Hutt, New Zealand.

C. A. MARTIN, Director, International Advisory Services, New Zealand Romney Sheep Breeders' Association, Feilding, New Zealand.

CHARLES E. MARTIN, D.V.M., M.S., Diplomate, American College of Theriogenologists, Professor (Theriogenology), and Chairman, Department of Veterinary Medicine and Surgery, University of Missouri, Columbia, Missouri.

EDWARD C. MATHER, D.V.M., Ph.D., Diplomate, American College of Theriogenologists, Professor and Chairman, Department of Large Animal Surgery and Medicine, Michigan State University; Staff, Veterinary Clinical Center, Michigan State University, East Lansing, Michigan.

WILLIAM L. MENGELING, D.V.M., M.S., Ph.D., Chief, Virological Research Laboratory, USDA, SEA-AR, National Animal Disease Center, Ames, Iowa.

RICHARD B. MILLER, B.Sc., D.V.M., Associate Professor of Pathology, Ontario Veterinary College, University of Guelph, Guelph, Ontario, Canada.

S. J. MILLER, M.V.Sc., F.A.C.V.Sc., Private Practitioner, Warwick, Queensland, Australia.

DOUGLAS MITCHELL, B.Sc., M.R.C.V.S., Diplomate, American College of Theriogenologists, Director, Animal Diseases Research Institute (West), Agriculture Canada, Lethbridge, Alberta, Canada.

N. W. MOORE, M.Agric.Sci., Ph.D., Associate Professor in Animal Husbandry, Department of Animal Husbandry, University of Sydney, N.S.W., Australia.

DAVID A. MORROW, D.V.M., Ph.D., Diplomate, American College of Theriogenologists, Associate Professor of Large Animal Surgery and Medicine, College of Veterinary Medicine, Michigan State University, East Lansing, Michigan.

JACOB E. MOSIER, D.V.M., M.S., Professor of Veterinary Medicine, College of Veterinary Medicine, Kansas State University; Director, Kansas State University Veterinary Hospital, Manhattan, Kansas.

JOHN B. MULDER, D.V.M., M.S., M.Ed., Professor of Physiology and Cell Biology, University of Kansas; University Veterinarian and Director, Animal Care Unit, University of Kansas, Lawrence, Kansas.

R. F. NACHREINER, D.V.M., Ph.D., Associate Professor, Animal Health Diagnostic Laboratory, Michigan State University, East Lansing, Michigan.

DEAN P. NEELY, V.M.D., Diplomate, American College of Theriogenologists, Maryland Equine Center, Cockeysville, Maryland.

PATRICIA SCHULTZ OLSON, D.V.M., M.S., Diplomate, American College of Theriogenologists, Department of Clinical Sciences and Department of Physiology and Biophysics, Colorado State University, Fort Collins, Colorado.

RICHARD S. PATTON, Ph.D., Dext Company, Los Angeles, California.

RICHARD H. C. PENNY, D.V.Sc., Ph.D., F.R.C.V.S., M.A.C.V.Sc., Professor of Clinical Veterinary Medicine, Royal Veterinary College, University of London, London, England.

ROBERT D. PHEMISTER, D.V.M., Ph.D., Dean and Professor of Pathology, College of Veterinary Medicine and Biomedical Sciences, Colorado State University, Fort Collins, Colorado.

BILL WAYNE PICKETT, M.S., Ph.D., Professor, Department of Physiology and Biophysics, Colorado State University, Fort Collins, Colorado.

DAVID GWYNNE POWELL, B.V.Sc., F.R.C.V.S., Epidemiologist, Equine Research Station, Newmarket, Suffolk, England.

THOMAS E. POWERS, D.V.M., M.Sc., Ph.D., Professor and Chairman, Department of Veterinary Physiology and Pharmacology, College of Veterinary Medicine, The Ohio State University, Columbus, Ohio.

W. J. PRYOR, M.V.Sc., Ph.D., F.A.C.V.Sc., Faculty of Veterinary Science, Massey University, Palmerston North, New Zealand.

T. D. QUINLIVAN, M.V.Sc., Ph.D., F.A.C.V.Sc., Veterinary Practitioner, Waipukurau, New Zealand.

A. L. RAE, M.Agr.Sc., Ph.D., Professor of Sheep Husbandry, Massey University, Palmerston North, New Zealand.

DAVID E. REED, M.D., Ph.D., Associate Professor, Veterinary Medical Research Institute, Iowa State University, Ames, Iowa.

ADRIAN PAUL RHODES, B.V.S., Ph.D., Superintendent, New Zealand Dairy Board, A. B. Service, Hamilton, New Zealand.

LAWRENCE E. RICE, D.V.M., M.S., Diplomate, American College of Theriogenologists, Associate Professor, Department of Medicine and Surgery, Oklahoma State University, Stillwater, Oklahoma.

STEPHEN J. ROBERTS, D.V.M., M.S., Diplomate, American College of Theriogenologists, Professor Emeritus, New York State College of Veterinary Medicine, Cornell University, Ithaca, New York; Presently, Woodstock Veterinary Clinic, Woodstock, Vermont.

HERIBERTO ROMAN-PONCE, Ph.D., D.V.M., M.S., Researcher, Instituto Nacional de Investigaciones, Mexico City, Mexico.

PETER DANIEL ROSSDALE, M.A., F.R.C.V.S., Senior Partner in Practice of Rossdale, Hunt, Peace, Hopes, Ricketts and Wingfield Digby, M's.R.C.V.S., Newmarket, England.

ROBERT F. ROWE, D.V.M., Ph.D., Veterinary Reproductive Specialties, Middleton, Wisconsin.

LEWIS J. RUNNELS, D.V.M., Professor of Large Animal Medicine, School of Veterinary Medicine, Purdue University, West Lafayette, Indiana.

RUTH SAISON, Assistant Professor, Department of Biomedical Sciences, University of Guelph, Guelph, Ontario, Canada.

ROBERT SCHNEIDER, D.V.M., M.S., Associate Adjunct Professor, School of Veterinary Medicine, University of California–Davis; Director, Animal Neoplasm Registry, Davis, California.

H. F. SCHRYVER, D.V.M., Ph.D., Associate Professor of Pathology, Cornell University, Ithaca, New York.

GERRIT SCHUIJT, D.V.M., State University of Utrecht, Utrecht, The Netherlands.

RONALD D. SCHULTZ, Ph.D., Professor, School of Veterinary Medicine, Auburn University, Auburn, Alabama.

STEPHEN W. J. SEAGER, M.R.C.V.S., Associate Professor, Department of Veterinary Pathology and Pharmacology, College of Veterinary Medicine, Texas A&M University, College Station, Texas.

BRADLEY E. SEGUIN, D.V.M., M.S., Ph.D., Diplomate, American College of Theriogenologists, Associate Professor of Theriogenology, College of Veterinary Medicine, University of Minnesota, St. Paul, Minnesota.

INGEMAR SETTERGREN, D.V.M., Ph.D., Professor of Animal Reproduction, Department of Obstetrics and Gynecology, College of Veterinary Medicine, Uppsala; Director, FAO/SIDA International Postgraduate Programme on Animal Reproduction, Uppsala, Sweden.

BEN E. SHEFFY, Ph.D., Professor, J. A. Baker Institute, New York State College of Veterinary Medicine, Cornell University, Ithaca, New York.

VICTOR M. SHILLE, D.V.M., Ph.D., Associate Professor, Department of Reproduction, College of Veterinary Medicine, University of Florida, Gainesville, Florida.

WAYNE L. SINGLETON, M.S., Ph.D., Associate Professor of Animal Science, Department of Animal Sciences, Purdue University, West Lafayette, Indiana.

KENNETH LARRY SMITH, B.Sc., M.Sc., Ph.D., Associate Professor, Department of Dairy Science and Department of Veterinary Science, Ohio Agricultural Research and Development Center, Wooster, Ohio, and The Ohio State University, Columbus, Ohio.

MARY C. SMITH, D.V.M., Assistant Professor of Medicine, Department of Clinical Sciences, New York State College of Veterinary Medicine, Cornell University, Ithaca, New York.

NICKOLAS J. SOJKA, D.V.M., M.S., Associate Professor of Surgery and Director of the Vivarium, School of Medicine, University of Virginia, Charlottesville, Virginia.

JAMES H. SOKOLOWSKI, D.V.M., Ph.D., Formerly, Research Head, Reproduction Research, Agricultural Division, The Upjohn Company, Kalamazoo, Michigan.

ALLEN G. SQUIRE, D.V.M., Practicing Veterinarian, Chino Valley Veterinary Group, Ontario, California.

GEORGE H. STABENFELDT, D.V.M., Ph.D., Professor, School of Veterinary Medicine, University of California–Davis, Davis, California.

HUBERT C. STANTON, Ph.D., Affiliate Professor of Pharmacology, College of Veterinary Medicine, University of Illinois, Urbana, Illinois.

BARBARA SYDNEY STEIN, D.V.M., Director, Chicago Cat Clinic, Chicago, Illinois.

ERICH STUDER, D.V.M., Head Resident Veterinarian, Carnation Research Farm, Carnation, Washington.

JØRGEN SVENDSEN, D.V.M., M.Sc., Research Officer, Department of Farm Buildings, The Swedish University of Agricultural Sciences, Lund, Sweden.

RICHARD H. TESKE, D.V.M., M.S., Acting Director, Division of Veterinary Medical Research, Bureau of Veterinary Medicine, Food and Drug Administration, Beltsville, Maryland.

WILLIAM W. THATCHER, M.S., Ph.D., Professor (Physiologist), Institute of Food and Agricultural Sciences, University of Florida, Gainesville, Florida.

STEPHEN D. VAN CAMP, D.V.M., Diplomate, American College of Theriogenologists, Assistant Professor, College of Veterinary Medicine, Mississippi State University, Jackson, Mississippi.

J. T. VAUGHAN, D.V.M., M.S., Diplomate, American College of Veterinary Surgeons, Dean, School of Veterinary Medicine, Professor, Department of Large Animal Surgery and Medicine, Auburn University, Auburn, Alabama.

VICTORIA LEA VOITH, D.V.M., M.Sc., Veterinarian Behaviorist, School of Veterinary Medicine, University of Pennsylvania, Philadelphia, Pennsylvania.

WILLIAM C. WAGNER, D.V.M., Ph.D., Diplomate, American College of Theriogenologists, Professor of Physiology and Head, Department of Veterinary Biosciences, College of Veterinary Medicine, University of Illinois, Urbana, Illinois.

DONALD F. WALKER, D.V.M., Diplomate, American College of Theriogenologists, Professor and Head, Department of Large Animal Surgery and Medicine, Auburn University, Auburn, Alabama.

W. ROBERT WARD, Ph.D., B.V.Sc., M.R.C.V.S., Lecturer, Faculty of Veterinary Science, University of Liverpool; Charge of Clinical Farm Practice, Liverpool University Veterinary Field Station, Liverpool, England.

CORNELIS J. G. WENSING, D.V.M., Ph.D., Professor of Anatomy and Embryology, School of Veterinary Medicine, State University of Utrecht, Utrecht, The Netherlands.

DAVID M. WEST, Lecturer, Department of Veterinary Clinical Sciences, Massey University, Palmerston North, New Zealand.

HOWARD L. WHITMORE, D.V.M., Ph.D., Diplomate, American College of Theriogenologists, Professor and Chief, Food Animal Medicine and Surgery, College of Veterinary Medicine, University of Illinois, Urbana, Illinois.

DAVID E. WILDT, Ph.D., Instructor of Comparative Medicine, Baylor College of Medicine, Texas A & M University, Houston, Texas.

MICHAEL ROBERT WILSON, B.V.Sc., Ph.D., M.R.C.V.S., Professor and Department Chairman, Ontario Veterinary College, University of Guelph, Guelph, Ontario, Canada.

JOHN M. WOODS, D.V.M., Deceased.

RAYMOND ZEMJANIS, D.V.M., Ph.D., Diplomate, American College of Theriogenologists, Professor and Head of Theriogenology, College of Veterinary Medicine, University of Minnesota, St. Paul, Minnesota.

GIDEON ZIV, M.R.C.V.S., M.P.H., Ministry of Agriculture, Kimron Veterinary Institute, Bet Dagan, Israel.

GREGORY M. ZOLTON, V.M.D., Head Surgeon, Animal Hospitals of New Jersey, Inc., Readington, New Jersey.

Preface

The objective of *Current Therapy in Theriogenology* is to provide the practicing veterinarian and veterinary student with a concise source of current information documented by controlled research on the diagnosis, treatment and prevention of reproductive conditions in animals. This book is designed to supplement existing publications on theriogenology.

The information is presented in a problem-oriented manner by species in an effort to help the reader solve the reproductive problem and also to provide rational, scientific reasons for the solution. The first part of the book includes information on principles of hormone and antibiotic therapy, embryo transfer and cytogenetics. In subsequent sections reproductive problems are discussed by animal species. The concluding section on diagnostic procedures is designed to aid the clinician and student in establishing a laboratory diagnosis.

While the authors have tried to present information documented by controlled research, the reader is referred to existing publications in theriogenology for additional information. The references at the end of each chapter are designed to provide the reader with access to the literature.

The impetus for *Current Therapy in Theriogenology* came from conversations with Doctors L. Ball, L. Faulkner and R. Phemister during my sabbatical leave at Colorado State University. Doctors S. Roberts and R. Kirk, former instructors at Cornell, also provided encouragement and valuable advice. Members of the American College of Theriogenologists indicated strong support for the project and many subsequently served as consulting editors, authors and reviewers.

The editor would like to express his appreciation for the cooperation and support provided by the consulting editors, authors, reviewers, colleagues and publisher in completing this book. Doctors D. Ellis, R. Phemister, W. Sack and J. Sokolowski read and commented on various chapters of the manuscript. The editorial assistance provided by Dr. Karin Harter is gratefully acknowledged.

The editor would like to thank his wife Linda and children David, Laurie and Melanie for being understanding and providing sympathetic support during the preparation of *Current Therapy in Theriogenology.*

East Lansing, Michigan   DAVID MORROW

Contents

Section XI

NOTICE

Each country may at a specific time approve or disapprove usage of an individual drug and define withdrawal times for milk and meat in food-producing animals. Therefore, the clinician is responsible for knowing current regulations and observing the manufacturer's instructions on the label with regard to approved animals, recommended dosage and withdrawal times for the specific drug.

The authors, editors and publisher have made every effort possible to assure the accuracy of information provided in this book; however, they cannot assume responsibility for changing local regulations.

THE EDITORS

PRINCIPLES OF HORMONE THERAPY

Consulting Editor

WILLIAM C. WAGNER

Principles of Hormone Therapy

WILLIAM C. WAGNER
University of Illinois, Urbana, Illinois

INTRODUCTION

Since this book is designed to assist the veterinarian with therapeutic problems in theriogenology, it is important that the reader be aware of some types of pharmacological information. This chapter attempts to discuss several general questions of hormone therapy, such as residues, half-life and dosage versus blood level, and also presents some average hormone values for the common species. More specific information on particular clinical problems and individual therapy will be found in the appropriate locations under each species in other sections.

RESIDUE PROBLEMS

As most veterinarians are well aware, the problems associated with hormone residues have become increasingly more critical. The widespread use of hormone therapy not only for therapeutic purposes but also for growth promotion has led to widespread abuses and the occurrence of hormone residues in materials being sold for human consumption. Because of this, one should be extremely careful in the use of these steroid preparations and should be sure to indicate the appropriate withdrawal period for each compound that is used. It is also important to remember that the use of these hormone preparations for purposes or in species for which they have not yet been cleared by federal agencies can also lead to difficulties with residue problems. The amount of a given hormone treatment that may remain as a tissue residue after a standard time period is dependent on factors such as route of administration, formulation and metabolic clearance rate, as well as the animal's individual biological variation. Furthermore, the actual tissue content of such materials is usually highest in the liver and kidney, since these organs are actively involved in the excretion of these substances.

It is also important to be aware of species differences in the metabolic clearance rate or rate of removal from the body for compounds that may be used in more than one species. A good example of the differences that one might see occurs with the use of the synthetic glucocorticoid flumethasone. Studies in pigs and in cattle by Karg, Hoffmann and colleagues demonstrated that the steroid was much more slowly absorbed in the cow and therefore took a longer period of time to be cleared from the body when compared with steroid absorption and clearance in the pig. Therefore, identical treatment dosages based on body weight in these two species would result in entirely different periods of retention before they were completely cleared from the body.

SPECIES VARIATION IN PROTEIN/HORMONE STRUCTURE

Although the steroid hormones have an identical molecular structure regardless of the species in which they occur, there may be significant problems with variations in structure of the protein hormones. One example would be growth hormone, which demonstrates a different structure for most of the major species that have been studied. This means that the growth hormone isolated from one species may be relatively ineffective when used in some other animal. The hormones that we will commonly be concerned with in theriogenology do not present this degree of variation. Generally the luteinizing hormone (LH) preparations are one of two types. Human chorionic gonadotropin, a compound isolated from the urine of pregnant women, is effective as a luteinizing preparation in virtually all common animal species. The other luteinizing preparation frequently used is natural luteinizing hormone, which is isolated and purified primarily from sheep pituitary glands. This also seems to be effective when used in cattle and therefore suggests that the naturally occurring LH from sheep may be useful in a number of other species. For use as a follicle-stimulating hormone (FSH) preparation, most clinicians utilize the material known as pregnant mare serum gonadotropin (PMSG), which has a predominantly FSH-like activity in nearly all species. An exception to this would be use in the mare, in which PMSG does not seem to be effective in stimulating ovarian activity and the growth of follicles.

DOSAGE VERSUS BLOOD CONCENTRATION

Speaking first about the steroid hormones, it is evident that the amount of material required to generate a particular effective plasma concentration will differ from one species to another. The existing evidence would suggest that most steroid hormones have two distinct disappearance rates or half-lives. To illustrate, the data for progesterone have indicated that during the initial phase after intravenous administration the half-life is approximately 5 minutes, while the half-life determined 20 to 30 minutes or more after the initial administration will be in the vicinity of 20 to 30 minutes. Ganjam *et al.*[11] reported on studies in the mare that indicated three phases of progesterone clearance. The first phase had a half-life (t½) of 2.5 minutes and the second had a t½ of 20 minutes. The third phase was much slower, although not specifically determined. Using these data the investigators commented on the apparent uselessness of current therapy for aborter mares and suggested a re-evaluation of both this procedure and the dosage of progesterone being used.

In studies done in this laboratory we have demonstrated an apparent half-life of about 3 minutes during the early phase in cattle, with a later half-life of approximately 25 minutes. This extremely rapid clearance in the early period after administration means that one must increase the dosage rather significantly in order to provide an effective blood level that will exert a significant effect on a target organ.

In recent studies by Fathalla[10] a single intramuscular injection of 1 gm of progesterone in oil resulted in a plasma concentration of approximately 6 or 7 ng/ml on the following day. This level declined continuously, reaching a basal level of approximately 0.5 ng/ml within 5 to 6 days after the initial administration. Administration of a smaller quantity of material, e.g., 200 mg, would presumably have resulted in an initial concentration of approximately 1 to 2 ng with a disappearance to a basal level somewhat earlier.

Similar evidence can be cited for other steroids such as estrogens, in which there appears to be two separate disappearance rates, one of approximately 7 minutes and a second one of 20 minutes. The reason for these varied clearance rates is probably related to the protein binding of these steroids. Thus the early, rapid disappearance results from those steroid molecules that do not have an opportunity to become bound to some protein carrier in the plasma, while the secondary, slower clearance rate is related to molecules that do become protein-attached and therefore are less easy to remove by the liver or the kidney.

PHYSIOLOGICAL VERSUS PHARMACOLOGICAL THERAPY

One must always be careful to distinguish between the use of drugs for physiological purposes, as compared with pharmacological purposes. The use of small amounts of estrogen to generate an increased uterine tone and perhaps some dilation of the cervix in instances in which a mild uterine infection is present might be considered a physiological therapy. On the other hand, the use of massive amounts of estrogens for regression of a corpus luteum, for expulsion of the exudate in a pyometra case or for the purpose of initiating an abortion during early pregnancy in the cow would probably be considered a pharmacological usage. The difference lies in the relative amount of material administered and the plasma concentration produced when considering the differences between physiological and pharmacological applications. One should remember, as will be pointed out in the next part of this section, that the natural hormone levels are usually quite small, being expressed in nanograms (10^{-9} gram) or picograms (10^{-12} gram). Thus, although it may take rather large amounts to effectively sustain the blood levels observed in physiological states, it is possible to overwhelm the system and produce pharmacological results by the use of altered steroids that give a greatly prolonged half-life or an abnormally exaggerated biological effect.

NORMAL HORMONAL PROFILES

The material in this part of the section has been organized by species. For each species we will attempt to demonstrate a range of values, as obtained from the available literature, for the more important hormones related to the reproductive cycle. Whenever possible, we will demonstrate plasma concentrations of these hormones during the estrous cycle and during pregnancy and parturition. We will not be able to do this in all cases because the data may be lacking or are considered inappropriate for this particular presentation.

Bovine

The hormone levels for the nonpregnant cow are presented in Figures 1 and 2. Figure 1 shows the values for follicle-stimulating hormone (FSH) and for estradiol. There is a small increase in FSH near the end of the cycle, as the time of ovulation is approached, which will have an effect on the growth of the follicle during this period. Along the time sequence this is followed by an increase in the estradiol concentrations on days 19 to 21. Figure 2 presents the pattern of hormone concentrations for progesterone and luteiniz-

ing hormone (LH) during the estrous cycle. There is a peak of LH on day 0, which would represent the day of estrus, and the level remains low with some fluctuations during the middle of the cycle. Near the end of the cycle there is another increase as the next estrus approaches. The precise time of the rise in the LH concentration is very specific relative to the next estrous period, but as we have presented the data timed from the preceding estrus and ovulation, this LH peak will vary between 19 and 22 days, depending upon the precise length of the individual estrous cycle.

The progesterone values in Figure 2 represent the extreme variations found in the literature, with average values generally about 5 to 7 ng/ml during midcycle. The values, as depicted, simply show the outside range that is possible. Note that the progesterone decline in the latter part of the cycle begins before there is a significant increase in luteinizing hormone.

The data for the pregnant cow are shown in Figures 3 and 4. We have presented only the data for the terminal portion of pregnancy, particularly the last week, as parturition approaches. The data for steroid hormone concentrations in early pregnancy can be summarized by stating that there is a gradual slow increase in estrogen concentrations

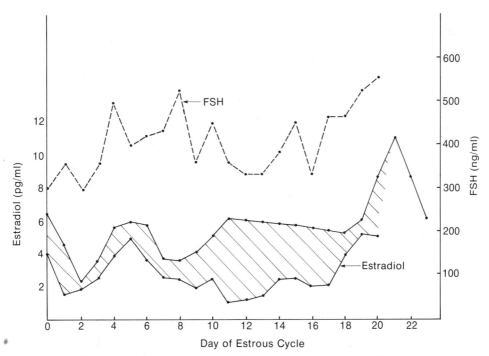

Figure 1. Nonpregnant cow — FSH and estrogen concentrations.

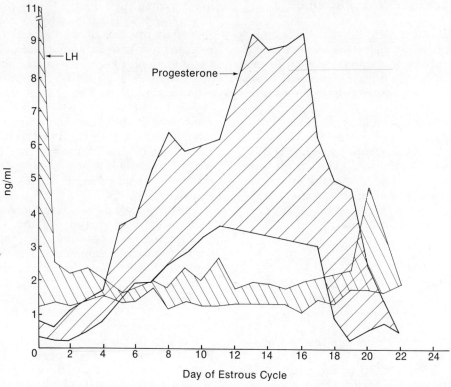

Figure 2. Nonpregnant cow — LH and progesterone concentrations.

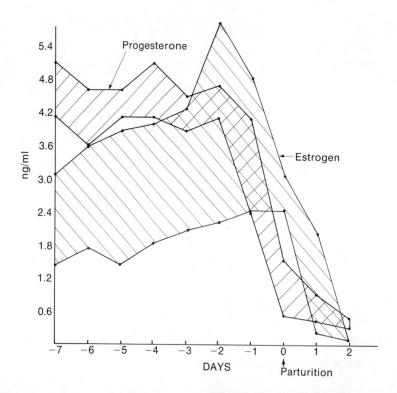

Figure 3. Pregnant cow — estrogen and progesterone concentrations.

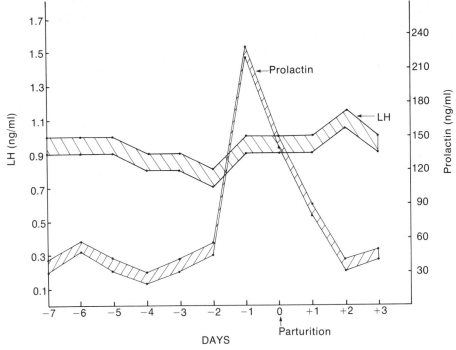

Figure 4. Pregnant cow — LH and prolactin concentrations.

from the level seen in the midluteal phase of the estrous cycle to the level seen in Figure 3. Then there is a further pronounced rise in estrogen values until the last 24 or 48 hours prior to parturition. After that time the decrease begins and is accelerated as the process of parturition is completed and the placenta is expelled. The estrogen levels seen at parturition, i.e., 3000 to 5000 pg of total estrogen, should be compared with the peak values seen during estrus, which will be about 10 to 20 pg. Clearly the concentrations of estrogen found in late pregnancy just prior to parturition are much higher than those found in the nonpregnant animal.

The levels of progesterone that are seen during the major part of pregnancy in the cow are not significantly different from those seen in the middle of the estrous cycle. Since the cow is primarily dependent upon luteal progesterone, there is no significant increase in this secretory rate, and the plasma concentration, reflecting production, remains fairly constant. During the last 1 or 2 days before parturition there is a rapid decrease in progesterone concentration in peripheral plasma, and most authors have indicated that the progesterone concentration in jugular plasma will be at or below 1.0 ng/ml at the time that labor commences.

Figure 4 presents the data for prolactin and LH. There is a pronounced rise in prolactin levels at the time of parturition, while luteinizing hormone concentrations do not change to any appreciable extent at this time. The change in prolactin concentration may be the result of the changes in estrogen/progesterone ratios occurring at this time as well as of the effect of the stress of labor, since stress has been shown to cause the release of prolactin in a number of situations.

Canine

The hormone concentrations for the dog are illustrated in Figures 5 and 6. Figure 5 presents the data for progesterone concentrations in the pregnant and the nonpregnant bitch. Note that even in the nonpregnant animal there is a significant secretion of progesterone, which gradually declines and reaches basal levels at about the time that one would expect whelping to occur if the animal were pregnant. The pregnant bitch, on the other hand, exhibits a substantially increased circulating level of progesterone with peak values in the range of 25 to 30 ng/ml and with the decline in progesterone

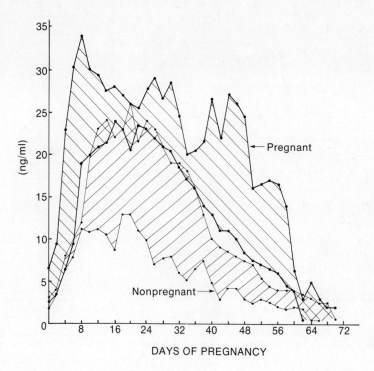

Figure 5. Pregnant and nonpregnant dogs — progesterone concentrations.

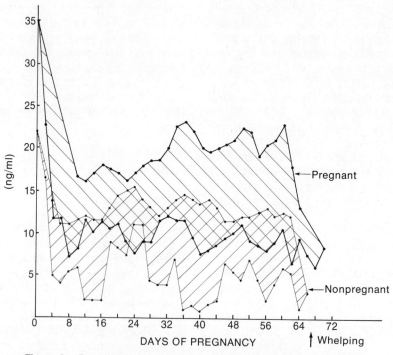

Figure 6. Pregnant and nonpregnant dogs — estrogen concentrations.

approaching basal levels at the time of whelping. Figure 6 presents the data for estrogen concentrations, comparing the pregnant and the nonpregnant female. Again the pregnant animal exhibits the higher levels of estrogens throughout the 60 days of pregnancy, although even in the nonpregnant animal there appears to be a significant amount of estrogen produced throughout this time period, with the values reported in the literature showing some overlap. In both cases there appears to be a decline in estrogen levels near the time of parturition.

Data on the concentration of LH in the nonpregnant dog indicate that the peak of LH (7 to 8 ng/ml) occurs at the beginning of estrus and lasts for approximately 1 to 2 days before reaching a basal level (1.0 ng/ml) at which it remains thereafter.

Equine

The hormone concentrations for the nonpregnant mare are shown in Figure 7 (LH, FSH, progesterone) and Figure 8 (estradiol). The estrous cycle, as depicted in Figure 7, utilizes day 0 as the initial LH peak. The

concentration of LH then gradually declines over a 4 to 6 day period, is at a low level for approximately 6 or 7 days in midcycle and then begins to increase again at approximately day 17 or 18. In contrast, the one study that reports measurement of FSH concentrations suggests that there is an FSH peak in the middle of the cycle during the luteal phase, a slight decline and then a second elevation just preceding the rise in LH. The increase in progesterone is noticeable by the second day after ovulation, reaches its peak value on the fifth or sixth day and begins to decline by approximately day 13, reaching basal levels again by day 16 to 18. Figure 8 demonstrates a pronounced peak in estradiol values approximately 48 hours prior to the LH peak that occurs just before ovulation. It is of interest that the concentration of estradiol may be as high as 120 to 140 pg/ml, compared with the value of approximately 10 to 20 pg/ml as seen in the cow at estrus.

Figure 9 depicts the changes in steroid hormone concentrations that occur during pregnancy in the mare. The values listed as E_1 include estrone as well as those estrogens peculiar to the mare, namely, equilin and

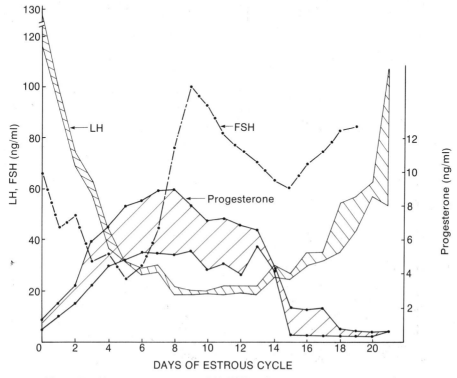

Figure 7. Nonpregnant mare — LH, FSH and progesterone concentrations.

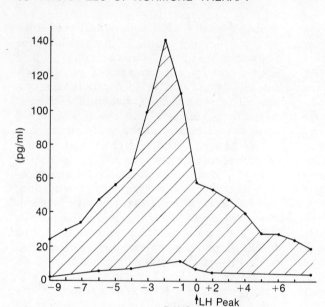

Figure 8. Nonpregnant mare — estradiol concentrations.

equilenin. The particular changes of consequence in the mare include the initial decline in progesterone that can be seen during the period from day 20 to 30, followed by a significant increase to the peak values at days 65 to 70. This sharp rise in progesterone is the result of progesterone secretion from the accessory corpora lutea that are formed in the ovary of the mare at this time. These elevated values are maintained until approximately day 130 to 140, after which the values decline quite rapidly, reaching rather insignificant levels by day 190 to 230. There is a subsequent rise in progesterone during the latter part of gestation, the significance of which is unknown. The concentrations of estradiol do show a rather steady rise through-out pregnancy until day 240, with subsequent

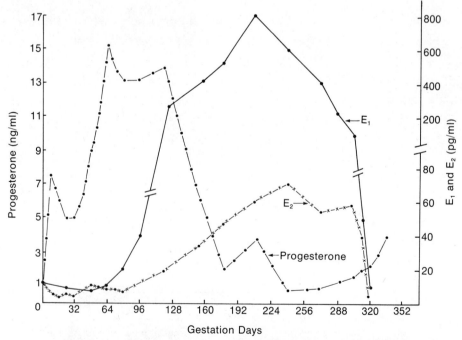

Figure 9. Pregnant mare — E_1, E_2 and progesterone concentrations.

gradual decline until day 300, after which the values decrease very rapidly.

Feline

Figure 10 presents data from a single report in the literature for the pregnant cat. Estrogen levels are high at the beginning of pregnancy, which would coincide with the time of estrus. These then decline and remain relatively constant during the major part of pregnancy, with a subsequent rise as parturition is approached and with a very steep rise occurring during the last week or so. There is then a beginning decline even before parturition occurs, so that the level returns to the same level seen during the midpart of pregnancy by the time that birth takes place. Progesterone, on the other hand, rises from a very low level at day 0 to a peak concentration on day 20 and then gradually declines, reaching basal levels once more at the time of parturition.

Ovine

Figure 11 presents the progesterone and LH values for the nonpregnant cyclic sheep. Progesterone levels rise rapidly to peak values of approximately 2 to 2.5 ng/ml, which are lower than values in the cow and are especially low when compared with values in the pig. The LH level peaks at the beginning of the estrous cycle on the day of estrus and then can be seen to increase once more at the end of the cycle as the next ovulation is occurring. FSH, prolactin and estrogen concentrations are reported in Figure 12, which shows the increased FSH level associated with estrus at day 0 and again on day 16. Estrogen levels are also elevated at the time of estrus (90 to 95 pg/ml) and show rather wide fluctuations during the midpart of the cycle, varying from 4 to 30 pg/ml during this time. There is a significant increase in prolactin that is associated with the time of estrus and is nearly superimposed on the LH spike (Fig. 11).

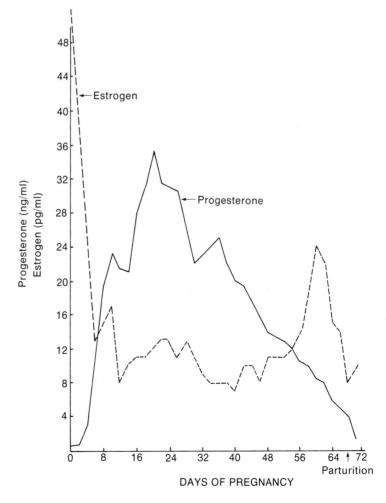

Figure 10. Pregnant cat — progesterone and estrogen concentrations.

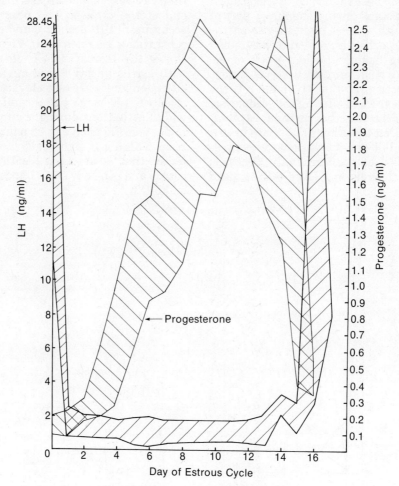

Figure 11. Nonpregnant sheep — LH and progesterone concentrations.

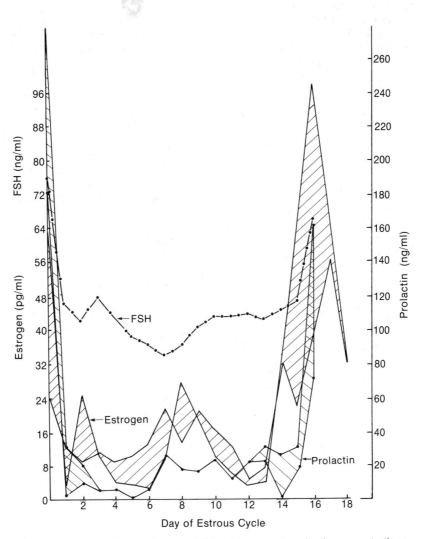

Figure 12. Nonpregnant sheep — FSH, estrogen and prolactin concentrations.

The estrogen and progesterone values for the pregnant sheep are shown in Figure 13. The gradual increase in progesterone throughout pregnancy is related to the increased capacity of the placenta in the pregnant sheep to produce progesterone and release it into the circulation. Thus, the progesterone curve is considerably different that that previously seen in the cow. Estrogen values during pregnancy are rather low and show very little change throughout the major part of gestation, with a sharp rise in estrogens occurring at the terminal end of pregnancy just prior to actual labor. The peak values occurring at this time do not differ greatly from the estrogen concentrations observed in the sheep at the time of estrus.

Porcine

Figure 14 depicts the progesterone, estrogen and LH curves for the nonpregnant pig. Estrogen levels peak at the time of estrus or just ahead of it and then subside to rather constant levels of approximately 20 pg/ml during midcycle. Progesterone values rise to maximal levels during the luteal phase of the cycle, with the maximum concentrations being in the vicinity of 30 ng/ml. The changes

in LH levels are similar to those in other species, with the spike of LH occurring at the time of estrus but lasting longer than we would expect to find it in the cow and with the next peak occurring at the subsequent estrous period. There seems to be a lack of fluctuation in LH during the midpart of the cycle, which is in contrast to cattle.

The progesterone and estrogen data are presented for the pregnant pig in Figure 15. Progesterone values average 12 to 14 ng/ml during the last 3 weeks of pregnancy, with a very abrupt decline occurring during the last 24 or 48 hours prior to parturition. Estrogen values remain relatively constant during much of pregnancy but do show a significant increase approaching the end of gestation, with particularly significant increases occurring during the last 2 to 3 weeks. This concentration usually peaks 1 to 2 days prior to the time of parturition and then begins to decline even before labor actually occurs.

PRINCIPLES OF HORMONE ACTION

Steroid Hormones

Since a given steroid hormone has the same structure regardless of the species,

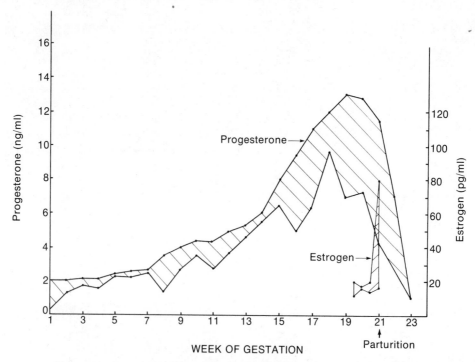

Figure 13. Pregnant sheep — progesterone and estrogen concentrations.

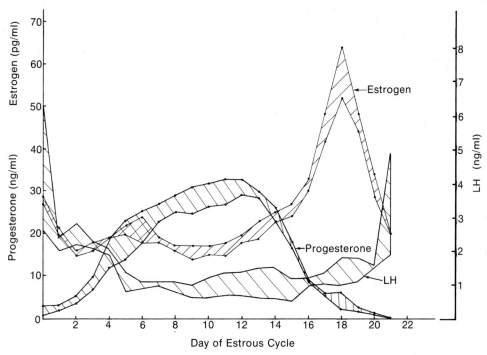

Figure 14. Nonpregnant pig — LH, estrogen and progesterone concentrations.

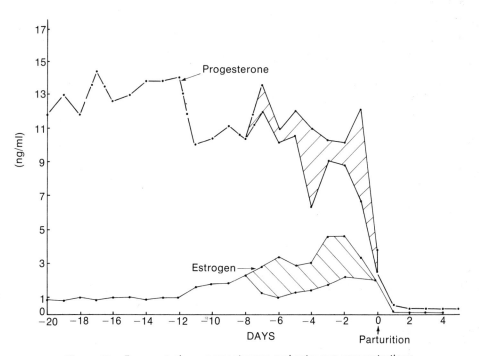

Figure 15. Pregnant pig — progesterone and estrogen concentrations.

there are no special precautions to be observed as to the source of material or the species to be treated. As indicated earlier, the half-life of these steroids may vary, depending on the individual animal or species. The rate of metabolic clearance also depends on the ability of the steroids to bind to proteins in the blood. Thus, natural glucocorticoids, e.g., hydrocortisone, can bind to a specific globulin such as corticoid-binding globulin and be rather slowly cleared. Other steroids, e.g., progesterone, may attach to serum proteins such as albumin and may be more rapidly cleared. Since these steroids can all be carried, to some extent, on the same proteins, the relative concentrations of other steroids may have a significant result on the clearance rate (half-life) of the steroid being used therapeutically.

In the following discussion, some indications for use, preparations available and side effects are presented for each group of steroid hormones. Names and addresses of companies supplying these preparations are listed in Appendix A. This is not an exhaustive listing, and the reader is encouraged to consult the other sections for more detailed information on each species.

Estrogenic Compounds

Indications for the use of estrogens are based on their biological activity. Briefly, estrogens are stimulatory to the uterus (myometrial tone, growth of uterine tissue and resistance to infectious agents), can cause regression of the corpus luteum in cattle, stimulate corpus luteum function in pigs, cause relaxation of the cervix, stimulate mammary gland development and are generally antagonistic to the effects of progesterone and androgens. Therefore, estrogens can be useful in the treatment of conditions such as metritis, pyometra, mummified fetus or elective abortion in cattle, alterations of corpus luteum (CL) lifespan and estrous cycle in cattle and prostatic hyperplasia in male dogs.

Preparations Available. Estrogens are available in repositol or shorter-acting preparations and as aqueous suspensions.

1. V-Estrovarin. Aqueous suspension containing 5.0 mg estrone (E_1) per ml.

2. Estradiol cypionate. Solution in oil containing either 2.0 or 4.0 mg estradiol cypionate/ml.

3. Estradiol valerate. 10, 20 or 40 mg/ml in oil.

4. Estradiol. 0.5 to 1.0 mg/ml as aqueous suspension or in oil.

Side Effects. Caution should be exercised concerning prolonged or excessive treatment since ovarian cystic follicles may occur, especially in cattle. Estrogen preparations may also result in decreased milk secretion or induction of abortion or be a cause of anemia in the dog.

Progestational Compounds

Progestogens have a calming or depressing effect on the myometrium and stimulate endometrial development. Their use may be indicated in cases of threatened abortion if due to inadequate progesterone levels. Oral forms have also had demonstrated effect on remission of ovarian follicular cysts.

Preparations Available. Progesterone is usually available as a repositol form for prolonged action or as a solution in oil for a shorter duration effect.

Side Effects. The major side effect is the predisposition to cystic hyperplasia and pyometra occurring in the bitch given long-term therapy.

Androgenic Compounds

Indications for androgens in veterinary medicine are rare. Although they may increase libido, their suppressive effects on gonadotropin secretion have generally given disappointing results when they were used to stimulate gametogenesis. At present, androgens are mainly of use for producing a satisfactory teaser animal by treating either a steer or a heifer with several repeated doses. In the female this will cause development of cystic ovarian follicles and nymphomania.

Preparations Available. Testosterone is available either as a solution or as a repositol treatment.

Side Effects. Use can result in suppression of spermatogenesis caused by negative feedback and suppression of gonadotropins from the pituitary gland. Inadvertent use in pregnant females may cause masculinization of the female fetuses.

Protein Hormones

When using protein hormones, the source of the preparation and the duration of the treatment must both be considered. Protein hormones may vary in their molecular composition or structure among species. If this difference is great enough, the protein may be unable to attach to the appropriate receptor site, or sites, and thus will be inactive. While this problem is not usually noted with gonadotropic hormones, it is of significance with other hormones, such as growth hormone.

Since the gonadotropic hormones are of large molecular size, they are antigenic and can stimulate the production of antibodies. Obviously this is only significant when a treatment is to be repeated several times. This is the basis for the poor response sometimes seen when cows are treated repeatedly for cystic follicles with an LH preparation or when pregnant mare serum gonadotropin (PMSG) is used repetitively for inducing ovulation.

Gonadotropins

Luteinizing Hormone (LH). These preparations are indicated for inducing ovulation of mature follicles or for treating cystic ovarian follicles. Although theoretically the use of LH and FSH together should result in stimulation of testicular function in the male, no significant evidence has yet been presented for such procedures.

Preparations Available. Preparations include:

1. Human chorionic gonadotropin (HCG). This material is prepared from the urine of pregnant women and is predominantly LH in biological activity. Molecular size is larger than that of pituitary LH, and the biological half-life is longer than that of natural LH.

2. Pituitary luteinizing hormone (PLH). This is produced from pituitary tissue of domestic animals.

Follicle-stimulating hormone (FSH). FSH is used for the stimulation of additional follicle growth in sows at weaning and to stimulate superovulation for embryo transfer. Little or no definitive data are available on the efficacy of such preparations in stimulating gametogenesis in the male.

Preparations Available. Preparations include:

1. Follicle-stimulating hormone-pituitary (FSH-P). This hormone is prepared by isolation from pituitary tissue of domestic animals.

2. Pregnant mare serum gonadotropin (PMSG). PMSG is isolated from serum of pregnant mares in the first half of pregnancy and has predominantly FSH-like action. This preparation will stimulate follicular activity in the female, although results are variable because of variation in potency of preparations and variability of individual responses.

Prolactin

This hormone might be useful in treating agalactia or hypogalactia but is not commercially available as a therapeutic agent. As an alternative, one can utilize phenothiazine-derivative tranquilizers, such as reserpine, which will stimulate release of endogenous prolactin. The efficacy of prolactin for stimulating lactation is questionable in cattle but may be beneficial in the sow.

Releasing Hormones

At this time not all of these compounds are commercially available. However, one substance in this group, gonadotropin-releasing hormone (GnRH) is available and offers promise in the treatment of follicular cysts or in treating other conditions in which LH-like hormones have been used. GnRH causes release of LH and FSH from the pituitary gland of the treated animal.

Since these releasing hormones have a very small molecular size (usually 10 amino acids or less) and have a similar structure in various species, there appears to be very little problem with antigen-antibody responses. Thus they maintain clinical efficacy even after repeated usage. It is expected that other releasing hormones will be available in the near future.

Prostaglandins (PG)

These substances are lipids produced from precursors such as arachidonic acid. Nearly all tissues in the body produce prostaglandins of one type or another. In the reproductive system, PGE_2 and $PGF_{2\alpha}$ are the primary substances of interest. Prostaglandins can cause regression of the cyclic CL in horses and cattle and result in synchronization of the next estrous period. They also cause contraction of smooth muscle, such as the myometrium in the uterus.

Preparations Available. At present two products are approved and available commercially for use in synchronizing estrus or inducing estrus in mares. These are Prostin $F_{2\alpha}$ and Synchroset. These products are useful only in mares with a functional corpus luteum.

Side Effects. These may include cramping of the intestinal musculature and sweating.

REFERENCES

1. Ash, R. W. and Heap, R. B.: Oestrogen, progesterone and corticosteroid concentrations in peripheral plasma of sows during pregnancy, parturition, lactation and after weaning. J. Endocrinol., 64:141, 1975.
2. Austad, R., Lunde, A. and Sjaastad, O.: Peripheral plasma levels of oestrodiol-17β and progesterone in the bitch during the oestrous cycle, in normal pregnancy and after dexamethasone treatment. J. Reprod. Fertil., 46:129, 1976.
3. Bassett, J. M., Oxborrow, T. J., Smith, I. D. and Thorburn, G. D.: The concentration of progesterone in the peripheral plasma of the pregnant ewe. J. Endocrinol., 45:449, 1969.
4. Bryant, G. D., Greenwood, F. C., Karr, G., Martinet, J. and Denamur, R.: Plasma prolactin in the oestrous cycle of the ewe: Effect of pituitary stalk section. J. Endocrinol., 51:405, 1971.
5. Chamley, W. A., Buckmaster, J. M., Cerini, M. E., Cummings, J. A., Goding, J. R., Obst, J. M., Williams, A. and Winfield, C.: Changes in the levels of progesterone, corticosteroids, estrone, estradiol 17-β, luteinizing hormone and prolactin in the peripheral plasma of the ewe during late pregnancy and at parturition. Biol. Reprod., 9:30, 1973.
6. Concannon, P. W., Hansel, W. and Visek, W. J.: The ovarian cycle of the bitch: Plasma estrogen, LH and progesterone. Biol. Reprod., 13:112, 1975.
7. Cunningham, H. F., Symons, A. M. and Saba, N.: Levels of progesterone, LH and FSH in the plasma of sheep during the oestrous cycle. J. Reprod. Fertil., 45:177, 1975.
8. Dobson, H., Midmer, S. E. and Fitzpatrick, R. J.: Relationship between progesterone concentrations in milk and plasma during the bovine oestrous cycle. Vet. Record, 96:222, 1975.
9. Evans, J. W., Faria, D. A., Hughes, J. P., Stabenfeldt, G. H. and Cupps, P. T.: Relationship between luteal function and metabolic clearance and production rates of progesterone in the mare. J. Reprod. Fertil., Suppl., 23:193, 1975.
10. Fathalla, M. A. R.: Utero-ovarian relationships in the cow with experimental cystic ovarian follicles. Ph.D. thesis, Ontario Veterinary College, University of Guelph, 1977.
11. Ganjam, V. K., Kenney, R. M. and Flickinger, G.: Effect of exogenous progesterone on its endogenous levels: Biological half-life of progesterone and lack of progesterone binding in mares. J. Reprod. Fertil., Suppl., 23:183, 1975.
12. Glencross, R. G., Munro, J. B., Senior, B. E. and Pope, G. S.: Concentrations of estradiol 17-β, oestrone and progesterone in jugular vein plasma of cows during the oestrous cycle and in early pregnancy. Acta Endocrinol. (Kbh), 73:374, 1973.
13. Hadley, J. C.: Total unconjugated oestrogen and progesterone concentrations in peripheral blood during pregnancy in the dog. J. Reprod. Fertil., 44:453, 1975.
14. Hansel, W. and Echternkamp, S. E.: Control of ovarian function in domestic animals. Am. Zoologist, 12:225, 1972.
15. Henricks, D. M., Guthrie, H. D. and Handlin, D. L.: Plasma estrogen, progesterone and luteinizing hormone levels during the estrous cycle in pigs. Biol. Reprod., 6:210, 1972.
16. Hoffmann, B. and Karg, H.: Endocrine balance of the cow at parturition. In Bosc, M. J., Palmer, R. and Sureau, C. (eds.): Avortement et Parturition Provoqués. Masson et Cie, Paris, 1974.
17. Hoffmann, B., Fortsch, J. E. and Karg, H.: Die Bestimmung von Glucocorticoidruckstanden mit einem biologischen Verfahren. 2. Mitteilung Untersuchungen beim Rind. Zbl. Vet. Med. A., 21:313, 1974.
18. Holtan, D. W., Nett, T. M. and Estergreen, V. L.: Plasma progestins in pregnant, postpartum and cycling mares. J. Anim. Sci., 40:351, 1975.
19. Kann, M. G.: Variations in plasma concentrations of LH and prolactin during the sheep oestrous cycle. C. R. Acad. Sci., 272:2934, 1971.
20. Karg, H., Hoffmann, B., Fortsch, J. E. and Hopwood, M. L.: Die Bestimmung von Glucocorticoidruckstanden mit einem biologischen Verfahren. 1. Mitteilung. Methodik, Untersuchungen beim Schwein. Z. Tierphysiol., 29:295, 1972.
21. McNatty, K. P., Allison, A. J. and Thurley, D. C.: Progesterone levels in peripheral plasma of Romney ewes during pregnancy. N. Z. J. Agr. Res., 15:831, 1972.
22. Mason, B. D., Krishnamurti, C. R. and Kitts, W. D.: Oestrone and oestradiol in jugular vein plasma during the oestrous cycle of the cow. J. Endocrinol., 55:141, 1972.
23. Molokwu, E. C. I. and Wagner, W. C.: Endocrine physiology of the puerperal sow. J. Anim. Sci., 26:1158, 1973.
24. Nett, T. M., Pickett, B., Siedel, G. and Voss, J.: Levels of luteinizing hormone and progesterone during the estrous cycle and early pregnancy in mares. Biol. Reprod., 14:412, 1976.
25. Noden, P. A., Oxender, W. D. and Hafs, H. D.: The cycle of oestrus, ovulation and plasma levels of hormones in the mare. J. Reprod. Fertil. Suppl., 23:189, 1975.
26. Pattison, M. L., Chen, C. L., Kelly, S. T. and Brandt, G. W.: Luteinizing hormone and estradiol in peripheral blood of mares during estrous cycle. Biol. Reprod., 11:245, 1974.
27. Scaramuzzi, R. J., Caldwell, B. V. and Moor, R. M.: Radioimmunoassay of LH and estrogen during the estrous cycle of the ewe. Biol. Reprod., 3:110, 1970.
28. Sharp, D. C. and Black, D. L.: Changes in peripheral plasma progesterone throughout the oestrous cycle of the pony mare. J. Reprod. Fertil., 33:535, 1973.
29. Shemesh, M., Lindner, H. R. and Ayalon, N.: Competitive protein-binding assay of progesterone in bovine jugular venous plasma during the oestrous cycle. J. Reprod. Fertil., 26:167, 1971.
30. Stabenfeldt, G. H.: Physiologic, pathologic and therapeutic roles of progestins in domestic animals. J.A.V.M.A., 164:311, 1974.
31. Stabenfeldt, G. H., Holt, J. A. and Ewing, L. L.:

Peripheral plasma progesterone levels during the ovine estrous cycle. Endocrinology, *85*:11, 1969.

32. Stabenfeldt, G. H., Hughes, J. D. and Evans, J. W.: Ovarian activity during the oestrous cycle of the mare. Endocrinology, *90*:1379, 1972.
33. Terqui, M., Dray, F. and Cotta, J.: Variations de la concentration de l'oestradiol 17-β dans le sang périphérique de la brebis au cours de cycle oestral. C. R. Acad. Sci., *227*:1795, 1973.
34. Thompson, F. N. and Wagner, W. C.: Plasma progesterone and oestrogens in sheep during late pregnancy: Contribution of the maternal adrenal and ovary. J. Reprod. Fertil., *41*:57, 1974.
35. Thompson, F. N. and Wagner, W. C.: Fetal-maternal corticosteroid relationships in sheep during late pregnancy. J. Reprod. Fertil., *41*:49, 1974.
36. Thorburn, G. D., Basset, J. M. and Smith, J. D.: Progesterone concentration in the peripheral plasma of sheep during the oestrous cycle. J. Endocrinol., *45*:459, 1969.
37. Verhage, H. G., Beamer, N. B. and Brenner, R. M.: Plasma levels of estradiol and progesterone in the cat during polyestrus, pregnancy and pseudopregnancy. Biol. Reprod., *14*:579, 1976.
38. Wetteman, R. P., Hafs, H. D., Edgerton, L. A. and Swanson, L. N.: Estradiol and progesterone in blood serum during the bovine estrous cycle. J. Anim. Sci., *34*:1020, 1972.

Endocrine Diagnosis in Reproductive Disorders

R. F. NACHREINER

Michigan State University, East Lansing, Michigan

The advent of the radioimmunoassay (RIA) has made it possible to quantitate microgram (μg, 10^{-6}gram), nanogram (ng, 10^{-9}gram) and picogram (pg, 10^{-12}gram) amounts of hormone per milliliter of blood. The sensitivity of the RIA procedure often requires as little as 10 microliters (μl) of serum. The RIA involves use of an antibody that is specific for the hormone to be measured. A radioactive isotope is attached to the specific hormone being measured and is allowed to bind to the antibody. As the concentrations of standards or unknowns increase in the medium, less radioactive hormone binds to the antibody. The amount of radiation that remains bound to the antibody can be used to calibrate a standard curve and to quantitate the amount of hormone in the unknowns. The procedure is precise enough to be able to go from day to day and week to week with reproducible results in laboratories that have validated assays and quality control regimens. The utilization of the RIA on a practical basis is available for (1) detection of luteal activity utilizing a progesterone assay of milk or serum, (2) detection of the presence of testicular interstitial cells in supposed castrates that are actually cryptorchids and (3) determination of low thyroid activity in some anestrous bitches or low fertility dogs.

MILK PROGESTERONE LEVELS

It is well documented that milk progesterone levels are closely correlated with plasma values in cows and mares. Absolute values are higher in milk than in serum. Recent data have shown that the progesterone tends to be associated with the milk fat; therefore, progesterone concentration will change from foremilk to strippings. It is important to standardize the procedure by using fat-free milk, composite milk samples, cream or fat. Since samples often need to be obtained at times other than at milking (e.g., insemination, therapy), the assays based upon milk fat appear to give the most precise results.

Use of Milk Progesterone Levels to Determine Early Pregnancy. These procedures are based on the presence of luteal function at the next expected estrus (day 20 after insemination, day 0) (Table 1).

When samples are obtained only at the time of anticipated estrus, the error in those declared not pregnant (low progesterone level) is low. However, the error in declaring cattle pregnant is high. Progesterone concentrations in samples from cattle that are not pregnant, although they have luteal tissue present, may have resulted from early

TABLE 1. *Use of Milk Progesterone to Determine Early Pregnancy**

	Pregnant (ng/ml)	Not Pregnant (ng/ml)	Unknown (ng/ml)
Milk	>11	<2	2–11
Fat	>120	<100	100–120

*Data from Hoffmann, B., Gunzler, O., Hamburger, R. and Schmidt, W.: Br. Vet. J., *132*:469, 1976.

embryonic death, abortion, elongated cycles, wrong sampling time and so forth. Increased accuracy can be obtained by obtaining a sample at the time of initial insemination (to assure the presence of estrus [low progesterone level]) and at the next anticipated estrus 20 days after insemination. Low progesterone concentrations on the initial sample and high progesterone levels on the 20-day sample are much more indicative of pregnancy.

Breeding during Luteal Phase. Management apparently continues to be a major factor leading to low fertility. Poor management is easily demonstrated when inseminations are being performed during the time when samples contain diestrous (luteal) levels of progesterone (milk > 2 ng/ml; milk fat > 30 ng/ml). It is highly unlikely that cattle would conceive at that time. In a study in Germany,[3] 13 per cent of the cows had nonestrous levels of progesterone at the time of insemination. When exposed to the hard data concerning problems in estrous detection, managers have improved their detection techniques.

Clinical Abnormalities. Ovarian abnormalities are often detected during routine rectal palpation. However, it is very difficult to determine whether the tissue is luteal or not. Apparently the luteal cyst can often be mistaken for a follicular cyst on rectal palpation. By obtaining a more accurate diagnosis, therapy would be more successful (Table 2).

DIAGNOSIS OF CRYPTORCHIDISM IN GELDINGS USING THE HCG RESPONSE TEST

Cox *et al.*[1] showed that administration of 12,000 IU of human chorionic gonadotropin (HCG) intravenously to intact stallions caused a rapid rise in testosterone concentrations within 15 minutes and that the levels were elevated above resting levels for 1 to 2 hours. In 35 "geldings" showing stallion behavior, the response to HCG caused by retained testicular tissue was similar to the stallion-type response. These cryptorchids, however, had less responsive gonad(s) than stallions did. Similar results were found in our laboratory using 10,000 IU of HCG intravenously (Table 3).

Resting levels do not appear to be significantly different from resting levels in castrates. However, the response to HCG is consistently at least two times the resting level in the cryptorchid, whereas the castrate does not show a significant response to HCG within 1 hour after HCG administration. However, one cryptorchid did not show a doubling of the resting level until 2 hours after HCG administration. Therefore, if convenient, a 2-hour sample should also be obtained. Geldings that continue to show stallion characteristics, although negative to HCG response at 30 and 60 minutes, should be rechecked to include the 2-hour post-HCG sample.

Ganjam *et al.*[2] reported on the use of total

TABLE 2. *Use of Progesterone Concentrations to Confirm Clinical Diagnosis**

	Clinical Diagnosis		
Laboratory Diagnosis	FOLLICULAR CYST (N = 86)	LUTEAL CYST (N = 50)	NO CLASSIFICATION (N = 50)
Follicular cyst	47	6	28
Luteal cyst	39	44	22

*Data from Hoffmann, B., Gunzler, O., Hamburger, R. and Schmidt, W.: Br. Vet. J., *132*:469, 1976.

TABLE 3. *Diagnosis of Cryptorchidism Using HCG Response Test*

HCG	Stallion	Complete Castrate	Castrate with Intact Epididymis	Cryptorchid
Pre-HCG	44 ± 20*	13 ± 5	12 ± 6	18 ± 9
30-min. post-HCG	143 ± 17	16 ± 5	11 ± 4	39 ± 13
60-min. post-HCG	191 ± 22	11 ± 7	11 ± 3	50 ± 18

*ng/100 ml, average ± standard error.

estrogens in diagnosing cryptorchid conditions in stallions. It appears that this is also a useful procedure. Total serum estrogens greater than 10 pg/ml are diagnostic for the presence of an abdominal testis.

HYPOTHYROIDISM LEADING TO REPRODUCTIVE DISORDERS

Common clinical features in hypothyroid humans include menorrhagia in the female and reduced libido and fertility in both sexes. A retrospective analysis of 4914 samples received from veterinarians between December, 1974, and October, 1976, showed 1867 samples in the hypothyroid range (based on low triiodothyronine [T_3] values). The normal range for thyroxine (T_4) and T_3 in our laboratory varies somewhat with season. Generally, it is 0.75 to 2.0 ng/ml for T_3 and 10 to 40 ng/ml for T_4. Only 37 samples were received primarily for detection of reproductive problems. Nineteen samples were received from bitches with irregular estrous cycles, and seven of these animals had low thyroid function. Eighteen male dogs with breeding problems were examined, and eight of these animals had low thyroid function. Practitioners reported that some of these dogs began cycling or had improved fertility after therapy was begun. However, an objective study was not performed. In a subsequent objective study of the effects of thyroidectomy on estrous cycles in 10 bitches, all cycled normally within 3 months of thyroidectomy. Serum hormone concentrations were indicative of classic primary hypothyroidism during this entire period. In a study of stallions at Cornell University,[4] thyroidectomy at 18 months of age decreased sexual desire and resulted in lethargy. However, semen characteristics, testicular histological findings and fertility were not affected. Apparently most animals can continue to reproduce, although hypothyroid. However, animals with abnormal reproductive function may have low thyroid function, and therapy may help these individuals.

SAMPLE HANDLING AND SHIPMENT

Procedures for handling and shipment of samples and hormone levels expected from different types of samples vary from laboratory to laboratory. It is imperative that practitioners utilizing an endocrine diagnostic service check with the laboratory to find out which type of sample to obtain and how these should be shipped. For instance, thyroid hormone concentrations are different in serum than in plasma. Also, refrigeration of samples for thyroid hormones is not necessary, but rapid deterioration of cortisol occurs if shipments are not kept cool. For progesterone analyses of milk, some laboratories use streptomycin as a preservative during shipment. As a rule, check with the laboratory prior to sample collection and shipment for specific instructions.

REFERENCES

1. Cox, J. E., Rowe, R. H., Smith, J. A. and Williams, J. H.: Testosterone in normal, cryptorchid, and castrated male horses. Equine Vet. J., *5*:85, 1973.
2. Ganjam, V. K. and Kenney, R. M.: Androgens and estrogens in normal and cryptorchid stallions. J. Reprod. Fertil. (Suppl.), *23*:67, 1975.
3. Hoffman, B., Gunzler, O., Hamburger, R. and Schmidt, W.: Milk progesterone as a parameter for fertility control in cattle. Br. Vet. J., *132*:469, 1976.
4. Lowe, J. E., Baldwin, B. H., Foote, R. H., Hillman, R. B. and Kallfelz, F. H.: Semen characteristics in thyroidectomized stallions. J. Reprod. Fertil. (Suppl.), *23*:81, 1975.

section **II**

CLINICAL PHARMACOLOGY

Consulting Editor
THOMAS E. POWERS

Clinical Pharmacology of Antibacterial Drugs and their Application in Treating Bovine Metritis

G. ZIV

Kimron Veterinary Institute, Bet-Dagan, Israel

INTRODUCTION

Diseases of the bovine reproductive organs are of great importance as causes of economic loss to the dairy cattle industry. The infectious microbial diseases that affect the fetus, such as brucellosis, vibriosis, trichomoniasis, leptospirosis and viral abortions, are usually controlled by diagnosis and herd preventive measures. The more common therapeutic problems encountered in the field are due to sporadic uterine infections,[39] which take the form of septic metritis, endometritis, pyometra and chronic metritis.

A discussion of chemotherapy of microbial infections of the uterus must begin with a consideration of etiological agents, as rational therapy depends on an accurate diagnosis. The fundamental principle in the treatment of any microbial infection is that therapy should be decided by isolation and determination of the causative organisms and *in vitro* testing of their susceptibility to antimicrobial agents.[47] Also of primary importance is knowing whether the pathogens that are isolated will be eliminated by concentrations of the antibacterial drug that can be safely achieved at the site of infection. In addition, in order to avoid drug residues in the organs of the cow, and in the milk, it is essential to understand the pharmacological principles that govern drug distribution and persistence after systemic (intravenous and intramuscular) and local (intrauterine) treatment. This discussion shall therefore deal with (1) the clinical significance and the types of organisms associated with infections of the reproductive organs of the dairy cow, (2) the antibiotic susceptibility patterns of these microorganisms, (3) time-concentration considerations of antibacterial agents in the body of the cow in general and in the uterus of the cow in particular after systemic and local treatment and (4) the potential public health consequences of antibiotic therapy in animals with bovine metritis.

ETIOLOGICAL CONSIDERATIONS

A number of studies have been conducted on the bacteriology of the bovine reproductive organs.[14, 34, 35] Results of several of these investigations suggest that 85 to 93 per cent of cows have uterine infections 2 weeks after parturition, but only 5 to 9 per cent are infected by 46 to 60 days postpartum.[10, 20] Some investigators claim that the uterus should be essentially sterile for optimal conception to occur.[17, 45] In studies in which bacteria isolated from the reproductive tract of dairy cows were related to the rate of fertility,[17, 45] it was shown that 38 per cent of the samples from the uterus of cows with a normal breeding history were sterile, compared with 5 per cent of similar samples from repeat breeder cows.[16] Other investigators contend that bacteria in the bovine genital tract have little or no effect on fertility.[11, 15] Some investigators have reported an improved conception rate following intrauterine administration of antibiotics or chemical solutions,[17, 39] but others report that postpartum antibiotic treatment of normally reproducing cows is of no benefit and may even be detrimental.[11, 39]

Host defenses are of great importance in determining the fate of damaged but viable bacteria and may at times outweigh the direct action of the chemotherapeutic agent.[39] Impaired defense mechanisms may be a major factor in the development of bovine uterine infections and in the failure of therapeutic agents to eliminate such infections.

Ovarian hormones affect uterine defense mechanisms.[18, 19] Under the influence of estrogens, the uterus possesses a high degree of bactericidal activity, which is less efficient when levels of progesterone are high.[39]

These defense mechanisms are inhibited by progesterone.[39] The healthy uterus of the postparturient dairy cow can control bacterial invaders rapidly by leukocytic infiltration, increased blood supply and relaxation of the cervix. The efficiency of these normal defenses are impaired by endocrine disturbances, age of the cow and defects in conformation of the reproductive organs. Therefore, predisposing factors may contribute to the likelihood of infection, the type of organisms causing infection and the failure of treatment when only antibacterial drugs are used for therapy.

The variety and prevalence of bacteria isolated from the bovine uterus after parturition were the subjects of several studies. The most frequent bacterial isolates included *Corynebacterium pyogenes*, coliforms, streptococci or combinations thereof.[45] The coliforms and streptococci, primarily normal digestive tract inhabitants, were probably nonpathogenic contaminants of the genital tract.[13, 45] *C. pyogenes* appeared to be the most harmful pathogen of the cow's reproductive tract. It was associated with the greatest gross changes,[39] formation of the pus in uterine discharges and reduced fertility.[45] Endometritis was diagnosed in 97.4 per cent of cows from which *C. pyogenes* had been isolated.[45]

ANTIBIOTIC SENSITIVITY PATTERNS

With very few exceptions, most data published concerning antimicrobial sensitivities of pathogenic micro-organisms of animal origin antedate the introduction and adoption of standardized testing methods in the course of routine laboratory diagnosis.[3] Therefore, a discussion of reports on the sensitivity of micro-organisms isolated from the genital tract of the cow is perhaps of limited value to clinicians. The resistance patterns of 237 bacterial isolates from the cervicovaginal mucus of cows to 14 antibiotics were determined by satisfactorily standardized procedures.[34] Antimicrobial drugs tested were: lincomycin (L), methicillin (Me), ampicillin (AM), chloramphenicol (C), erythromycin (E), gentamicin (GM), novobiocin (NB), penicillin (P), streptomycin (S), tetracycline (Te), bacitracin (B), kanamycin (K), colistin (CL) and a mixture of three sulfonamides, i.e., sulfamethazine, sulfadiazine

and sulfamerazine (SSS). The resistance pattern to these 14 antibacterial agents is given in Table 1.[34] It is worthwhile to discuss the resistance of each of the species tested to these drugs.

Resistance Patterns by Species

Micrococcus Species. Of the 24 isolates tested, 54.2 per cent were susceptible to lincomycin. Approximately 8 per cent of the isolates were resistant to ampicillin, whereas 34 per cent were susceptible to this drug. The majority of the isolates (72.2 per cent) were susceptible to erythromycin. Resistance to novobiocin was shown by 30 per cent of the isolates, whereas 70 per cent demonstrated an intermediate response and thus none were susceptible. Only 5 per cent of the isolates were resistant to penicillin, 79 per cent showed an intermediate response and 16 per cent were susceptible. Fifty-eight per cent of the isolates were susceptible to tetracycline, and the remaining 42 per cent were resistant to this drug.

Staphylococcus Species. Susceptibility to lincomycin and novobiocin was shown by 83.3 per cent of the 24 isolates of *S. epidermidis*. Resistance to penicillin was shown by 67 per cent of the isolates, whereas 33 per cent were of the intermediate type. The response to streptomycin was 75 per cent susceptible, 21 per cent resistant and 4 per cent intermediate. Resistance to triple sulfa was demonstrated by 13 per cent of the isolates, whereas 58 per cent were susceptible to tetracycline. Susceptibility to methicillin, chloramphenicol, erythromycin, gentamicin, bacitracin and kanamycin was demonstrated by all the isolates. The two *S. aureus* isolates were resistant to tetracycline and colistin, respectively; moderately susceptible to ampicillin, penicillin and streptomycin and susceptible to all other antibiotics used.

Streptococcus Species. Susceptibility to lincomycin was shown by 92 per cent of the 12 *S. bovis* isolates. Resistance to gentamicin was demonstrated by 83.3 per cent of isolates, and 16.7 per cent showed intermediate susceptibility. Susceptibility to novobiocin and tetracycline was shown by 92 per cent and 67 per cent of the isolates, respectively, but 33 per cent and 75 per cent were resistant to tetracycline and triple sulfa, respectively. In contrast to *S. bovis*

TABLE 1. Prevalence of Drug Resistance among 237 Bacteria Isolated from Bovine Cervicovaginal Mucus to 14 Antimicrobial Drugs (Bauer-Kirby Technique)*

Organism	No. of Isolates Tested	Antimicrobial Drug†													
		P	Me	AM	S	K	GM	NB	C	Te	L	E	B	CL	SSS
		PERCENTAGE OF RESISTANCE ISOLATES													
Micrococcus spp.	24	5	0	8	0	0	0	30	0	42	0	0	0	100	0
Staphylococcus epidermidis	24	67	0	54	21	0	0	0	0	41	0	0	0	100	13
Staphylococcus aureus	2	0	0	0	0	100	0	0	0	100	0	0	0	100	0
Streptococcus bovis	12	0	0	0	91	100	83	0	0	33	8	0	0	100	75
Streptococcus faecalis‡	19	100	100	0	100	100	100	15	0	47	94	0	0	100	100
Streptococcus acidominimus	12	0	0	0	16	92	0	0	0	0	0	0	0	100	100
Escherichia coli	40	100	100	9	3	0	0	100	0	80	100	100	100	100	2.5
Proteus spp.	5	60	100	0	60	0	0	20	0	100	100	100	100	100	60
Bacillus licheniformis	17	0	0	0	0	0	0	5	0	5	100	0	94	100	0
Bacillus firmus	12	0	8	0	41	0	0	33	0	8	83	0	100	100	0
Bacillus pumilus, Bacillus subtilis	20	0	0	0	0	0	0	0	0	0	100	0	100	100	0
Corynebacterium pyogenes	23	0	0	0	96	8	8	0	4	8	4	17	0	100	100
Kurthia spp.	13	0	0	0	0	0	0	0	0	0	0	0	0	100	77
Neisseria spp.	2	0	100	0	50	0	0	0	0	0	100	0	0	0	0
Branhamella spp.	5	0	100	0	40	0	0	0	0	0	100	0	0	0	0
Acinetobacter spp.	3	0	33	0	100	0	0	0	0	0	100	100	0	0	33

*Adapted from Panagala, V. S. and Barnum, D. A.: Can. Vet. J., 19:113, 1978.
†Key to drugs: Penicillin (P), methicillin (Me), ampicillin (AM), streptomycin (S), kanamycin (K), gentamicin (GM), novobiocin (NB), chloramphenicol (C), tetracycline (Te), lincomycin (L), erythromycin (E), bacitracin (B), colistin (CL) and mixture of sulfamethazine, sulfadiazine and sulfamerazine (SSS).
‡Includes Streptococcus faecium.

isolates, certain differences in response were shown by the 19 isolates representing *S. faecalis* and *S. faecium*. All isolates were susceptible to chloramphenicol, approximately 95 per cent were resistant to lincomycin and 47 per cent were resistant to tetracycline. The percentages of *S. faecalis* and *S. faecium* isolates susceptible to erythromycin and bacitracin were 95 and 63, respectively. The *S. acidominimus* isolates were susceptible to a majority of the antibiotics used. Resistance to triple sulfa and colistin was demonstrated by all isolates, whereas 92 per cent were resistant to kanamycin and 16.7 per cent to streptomycin. Susceptibility to gentamicin was shown by 92 per cent of the isolates, and 83 per cent showed intermediate susceptibility to streptomycin.

Escherichia, Proteus and Klebsiella Species. The 40 isolates of *E. coli* demonstrated a high degree of resistance to 50 per cent of the antibiotic agents used. Resistance was demonstrated to lincomycin, methicillin, novobiocin, erythromycin, penicillin, bacitracin and colistin by all isolates. All isolates were susceptible to chloramphenicol, gentamicin and kanamycin; approximately 90 per cent were susceptible to ampicillin and triple sulfa but 78 per cent were resistant to tetracycline. Resistance to streptomycin was shown by 3 per cent of the isolates, 4.2 per cent were moderately resistant and 58 per cent were susceptible. The response of the isolates representing the genus *Proteus* did not differ considerably from those produced by *E. coli*. The three isolates representing *Klebsiella* were resistant to lincomycin, methicillin, erythromycin, novobiocin, penicillin, tetracycline, bacitracin and colistin.

Bacillus Species. The 17 isolates of *B. licheniformis* were resistant to lincomycin and colistin. The resistance shown by the 12 *B. firmus* isolates was comparable to the resistance by *B. licheniformis*; all were resistant to bacitracin and colistin, and 83 per cent were also resistant to lincomycin. The *B. subtilis* and *B. pumilus* isolates were resistant to lincomycin, bacitracin and colistin.

Corynebacterium pyogenes and Kurthia Species. All 23 isolates of *C. pyogenes* were sensitive to penicillin, methicillin, ampicillin, novobiocin and bacitracin; all were resistant to colistin and triple sulfa and 97 per cent were resistant to streptomycin. The 13 isolates representing the genus *Kurthia* were resistant to colistin, and 77 per cent also demonstrated resistance to triple sulfa. All the *Kurthia* isolates were susceptible to the remaining 12 antibiotics used.

Neisseria, Branhamella, Acinetobacter and Pasteurella Species. The isolates representing these four genera occurred in very low numbers. The two *Neisseria* isolates were resistant to lincomycin and methicillin, and both isolates gave intermediate response to novobiocin and were susceptible to the remaining antibiotics. The genus *Pasteurella* was represented by a single isolate. Resistance was demonstrated to lincomycin and colistin, and intermediate resistance was shown to streptomycin, bacitracin and triple sulfa.

Resistance Patterns for All Isolates

In the total number of 237 isolates tested, approximately 66 per cent were resistant to one or more of the 14 antibacterial agents used. The range of resistance varied from 0.4 per cent for chloramphenicol to 95.8 per cent for colistin. An assessment of the extent of resistance to the 14 antibiotics used reveals a gradient of the following order: colistin 95.8 per cent, lincomycin 51.5 per cent, bacitracin 40.5 per cent, penicillin 34.6 per cent, triple sulfa 34.2 per cent, methicillin 32.1 per cent, streptomycin 31.2 per cent, tetracycline 28.7 per cent, novobiocin 24.9 per cent, erythromycin 23.2 per cent, kanamycin 18.6 per cent, gentamicin 13.1 per cent, ampicillin 8.0 per cent and chloramphenicol 0.4 per cent. The broadest spectrum of inhibitory activity was demonstrated by chloramphenicol, closely followed by gentamicin, kanamycin, ampicillin and erythromycin.

In addition, determinations were recently made[21] of the minimal inhibitory concentrations (MIC) of penicillin G, ampicillin, oxytetracycline, furazolidone and dihydrostreptomycin against several bacterial species isolated from the uterus of dairy cows. All the isolates tested were resistant to dihydrostreptomycin, and all but the streptococci were resistant to furazolidone. The minimal inhibitory concentrations of penicillin G and ampicillin were considerably lower than those of oxytetracycline (Table 2), but wide ranges in the MIC values were observed for each antibiotic tested.

TABLE 2. *Minimum Inhibitory Concentrations of Antibiotics for Bacteria Isolated from the Uterus of Dairy Cows**

Bacteria	No. of Isolates Tested	Antibiotic					
		Penicillin G		Ampicillin		Oxytetracycline	
		Mean	Range	Mean	Range	Mean	Range
		CONCENTRATION (μg/ml)†					
Corynebacterium	18	1.1‡	0.48–2.0	3.4	0.07–33.0	20.4	0.25–64.0
Pasteurella	9	0.78	0.19–3.0	0.14	0.04–0.62	25.7	0.46–140.0
Streptococcus	11	0.98	0.19–1.8	0.43	0.04–1.03	27.5	1.30–75.0
Escherichia coli	5	13.4§	4.30–30.0	7.95	1.03–33.0	75.5	6.0–150.0
Staphylococcus aureus	3	0.44	0.19–0.9	0.21	0.08–0.37	1.4	0.6–3.2

*Adapted from Kendrick, J. W.: Report to the California Milk Advisory Board, August, 1978.
†1 μg is approximately 15 International Units of penicillin G.
‡One value >1170 not included.
§One value >580 not included.

TIME-CONCENTRATION CONSIDERATIONS OF ANTIBIOTICS

Parenteral Administration

The parenteral administration of antibiotics does very little to enhance topical treatment of metritis[39] and is probably indicated only in cases in which there is septicemia or other extension of the infection.[39] Since antibacterial agents usually are not administered orally to ruminants for the treatment of local or generalized bacterial infections, this review will be limited to the intravenous (IV) and intramuscular (IM) routes only.

After an antibiotic is given IV or IM, it becomes mixed in the plasma where it is bound to proteins, adsorbed onto erythrocytes and distributed to various extravascular tissues to which it also may be bound (Fig. 1). The distribution results in an initial rapid fall in plasma concentration from the peak level, which occurs immediately after an IV infusion and 15 to 30 minutes after an IM injection for most antibiotics (Fig. 2). Subsequent decreases in serum levels are related to renal and biliary excretion and to a minor degree (for antibiotics) to biotransformation or metabolism. Extravascular tissue concentrations are dependent upon the concentration gradient from serum to tissue fluid, the degree of protein binding in serum and tissues, the diffusibility (which is determined by molecular size and pK' value) and the lipid solubility. Although there is a parallel decline of tissue and blood levels of antibiotics, these do not occur at the same time. There are areas of the body that avidly

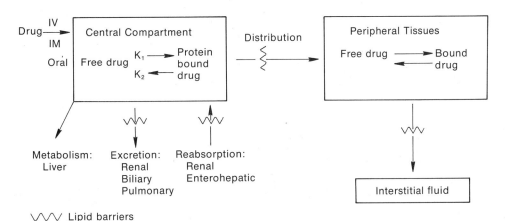

Figure 1. Drug distribution in the body.

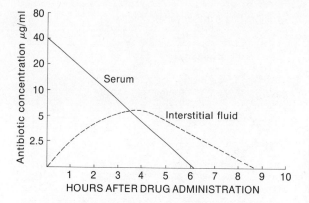

Figure 2. Simulated time-course of the serum and interstitial fluid concentration of an antibiotic after intravenous administration. Concentration is a logarithmic scale.

bind small fractions of a drug. Since the amount of drug bound is usually small, the rate of decline of drug concentration is not altered, but the locally bound drug may be important from a clinical pharmacological viewpoint.

A systematic search of the relevant veterinary literature has revealed only one publication dealing with the uptake of antibiotics by the endometrium of the cow after parenteral drug administration. A series of experiments was performed to determine the levels of sodium benzylpenicillin present in the endometrium of healthy, cycling cows

following the IM injection of a single dose of an aqueous solution at a rate of 22,000 IU/kg.[1] Tissue biopsy samples were obtained for a control before injection and at specific time intervals afterward. Blood samples were withdrawn from a vein immediately before taking the biopsy sample. Tissue biopsy samples were homogenized, and antibiotic concentration in serum and extracts of tissue homogenates were determined. The results are presented in Figure 3. The mean serum drug levels rose rapidly, reaching a peak of approximately 13.0 IU/ml at 15 minutes, whereas the mean peak levels in the

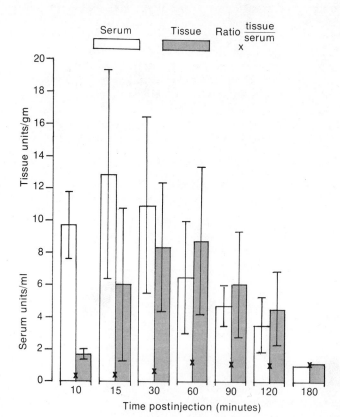

Figure 3. Serum and endometrial tissue concentrations of benzylpenicillin after intramuscular injection to cows at a dose level of 22,000 IU/kg. (From Ayliffe, T. R. and Noakes, D. E.: Vet. Rec., *102*:215, 1978.)

endometrium, 8.8 IU/gm, did not occur until 60 minutes after the injection but persisted at a higher level than the serum for a longer period of time. The ratios of mean tissue to mean serum levels are 0.18 at 10 minutes and 0.48, 0.76, 1.36, 1.29 and 1.30 at 15, 30, 60, 90 and 120 minutes, respectively. These results suggest that serum drug levels may be a poor indicator of the level of chemotherapeutic agent present within the tissues.

Most antibiotics currently used for the treatment of septic metritis follow the standard kinetics outlined. Thus, plotting the drug concentration in serum on a logarithmic scale versus time on a linear scale is linear after the period of absorption and distribution. The slope of the linear curve (β-phase) is a measure of the biological life of the antibiotic. The most commonly used measure is the time required for a 50 per cent decrease after absorption and distribution, which is referred to as the half-life of the drug. For example, in Figure 2 the half-life is 1 hour. The half-life of an antibiotic is extremely important in the determination of duration of pharmacological effect and in the adjustment of dosage programs. For most antibiotics the half-life of the agent is independent of the dose, concentration or route of administration. The half-lives of several antibiotics in adult ruminants are presented in Table 3.

Another pharmacological expression used with regard to antibiotics is the apparent volume of distribution. This refers to the relation between the amount of drug in the body and the plasma concentration. The apparent volume of distribution of a drug is usually expressed in liters/kg or as a percentage of body weight. Depending on the mathematical-kinetic model used to characterize distribution volume, antibiotics can be classified into at least three categories: (1) Those possessing distribution volumes equivalent to 30 per cent or less of body weight, including the aminoglycosides, the polymyxins and several penicillins (benzylpenicillin, carbenicillin) and cephalosporins (cephaloridine, cephacetrile); (2) antibiotics with distribution volumes in the range of 30 to 60 per cent of body weight, i.e., ampicillin, amoxicillin, cloxacillin, cephradine, lincomycin, clindamycin, novobiocin and rifamycin SV; and (3) antibiotics with large distribution volumes, i.e., the tetracyclines, macrolides and chloramphenicol. The apparent distribution volume of antibiotics in the latter class may be equal to or greater than

the total body volume and indicates that a proportionately larger amount of drug is present in the tissues.

In most instances, the clearance of antibiotics used in parenteral veterinary therapy is primarily dependent on the renal excretion of the agent. Because very few studies have been done concerning the effect of disease on renal clearance in cattle, the data achieved in normal animals must be used. Nonrenal clearance of antibiotics is principally by the liver and in the milk. There are exceptions for the latter in lactating farm animals. In the presence of combined im-

TABLE 3. *Half-Lives of Selected Antimicrobial Agents in Adult Ruminants*

Antibiotic	Half-Life (hours)
Penicillins:	
Benzylpenicillin	0.70
Phenoxymethylpenicillin	0.70
Ampicillin, amoxicillin, cloxacillin	1.25
Carbenicillin	0.55
Cephalosporins:	
Cephaloridine	0.60
Cephradine, cephapirin	0.80
Cephacetrile	1.20
Aminoglycosides:	
Streptomycin	2.4
Neomycin	3.2
Kanamycin	3.5
Aminosidine (paromomycin)	3.0
Gentamicin	2.0
Spectinomycin	1.2
Tetracyclines:	
Tetracycline	5.7
Oxytetracycline	4.1
Chlortetracycline	4.2
Doxycycline	9.0
Pyrrolidinomethyltetracycline	4.1
Tetracycline-L-methyl lysin	4.2
Minocycline	8.8
Macrolides:	
Erythromycin	2.0
Tylosin	1.8
Spiramycin	14.0
Polypeptides:	
Polymyxin B, colistin sulfate	5.0
Colistimethate	3.5
Others:	
Lincomycin, clindamycin	3.0
Novobiocin	3.2
Rifamycin SV	1.2
Rifampin	3.3
Chloramphenicol	3.5

pairment of renal and hepatic function, as may be the case in acute septicemia, the elimination via the milk may be significant for some antibiotics. For example, although 18 per cent of benzylpenicillin is metabolized, only 2 per cent of carbenicillin undergoes hydrolysis to penicilloic acid.[44] Thus, more of the carbenicillin accumulates in animals with hepatic failure. This difference in metabolism explains the difference in the range of serum levels and half-life of these two penicillins. In contrast, the difference in range of serum levels of tetracyclines is more closely related to serum binding, which will be discussed subsequently.

Tissue distribution of antibiotics can be considered as follows: Highly perfused lean tissues are the heart, lungs and hepatoportal system. Serum concentration reflects the level that an agent reaches in these areas. In contrast, poorly perfused lean tissues are muscle and skin, and poorly perfused fat tissues include adipose tissue and bone marrow. For practical purposes, bone, ligaments and cartilage have negligible perfusion.

One can only speculate on the degree of perfusion in the normal or infected postparturient uterus of the dairy cow. The involution of the maternal placenta and uterus, based on slaughter studies, appears to be as follows: Immediately after parturition the uterus is a large, flabby sac measuring nearly 1 meter long and weighing approximately 9 kg.[12] Early reduction in size results from peristaltic contractions at 3- or 4-minute intervals for 2 or 3 days.[46] The size decreases because of vasoconstriction and muscular contraction. Involution of the placenta occurs by several processes, i.e., disappearance of the caruncular stalk, dissolution of

the superficial layer of the caruncle and formation of uterine lochia. The maximum amount of uterine lochia, 1400 to 1600 ml, is present during the first 48 hours after parturition. This amount decreases to 500 ml by the eighth day postpartum. In infected uteri the process of placental disintegration may be hastened, although uterine involutional processes may be delayed. Because of these dynamic changes occurring in the reproductive tract of the postparturient dairy cow, it is likely that antibiotics administered parenterally can achieve satisfactory antibacterial concentrations at the site of infection. However, as data of this nature are completely unavailable, the rational use of antibiotics in the treatment of septic metritis must, at present, be based on the understanding of factors that influence serum and tissue levels of antibiotics. These factors are reviewed in the following section.

Protein Binding

The precise effect of protein binding of antibiotics is poorly understood.[40] Protein binding acts as a temporary means of storing the antibiotic agent and thereby prevents great fluctuations in the concentration of the free drug in body fluids. It should therefore be viewed as a dynamic process (Fig. 4). The affinity constants of an antibiotic for albumin will determine the degree of release of the agent. Only free antibiotic can exert its antibacterial action. Antibiotics must reach the bacterial receptor sites, all of which lie below the outer cell wall layers. If the antibiotic is bound to a large molecule such as albumin, the entry of the drug is prevented.

Antibiotics differ greatly in protein bind-

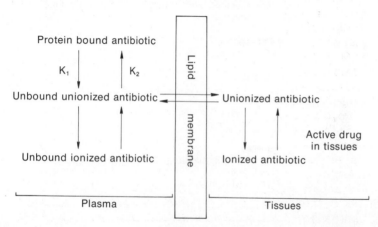

Figure 4. Antibiotic binding distribution.

ing from one class to another and also vary markedly within a class. Table 4 illustrates the protein-binding values given in the literature. For example, among the penicillins, ampicillin is 18 per cent bound, whereas cloxacillin is 71.3 to 78 per cent bound. Oxytetracycline is 21.2 to 22.4 per cent protein bound, whereas doxycycline is 84 to 90.2 per cent bound. Aminoglycosides and the macrolide antibiotics are bound to serum proteins to a very small degree, whereas novobiocin is more than 95 per cent bound. Great variation in these values has been reported, depending upon pH, protein concentration and the presence of other agents during determination. If other compounds are present in the serum that have receptor sites identical to that of the antibiotic, the relative amount of each compound that is bound will depend on the affinity constants of each substance. The amount of drug bound to serum protein may represent only a small fraction of the total amount of drug in the body. For example, if a drug is 50 per cent bound to albumin, only 10 per cent of the total drug in the body is bound. However, when 90 per cent serum protein binding is exceeded, 50 per cent of the total drug in the body is bound. If other sites also bind a drug, the free fraction is also greatly reduced. Thus, 42 per cent of a compound that was 50 per cent bound to serum protein and 50 per cent bound to another body compartment, such as muscle, would not be free to act. Data are not available on the extent of binding of antibiotics by the uterus and its lochial discharges.

The amount of free drug governs the level of drug in the tissues (Fig. 5), as the maximal concentration of free drug in tissue cannot exceed the level of free drug in serum. This is an important consideration since it might be expected that the leakage of serum into an area of the body would provide a higher concentration than would be expected based on diffusion of unbound drug. It is unlikely that inhibitory concentrations of antibiotic will be achieved in tissue if the concentration of free drug in serum is below inhibitory levels. It is extremely important to compare free drug rather than bound drug. For example, a drug that is 94 per cent protein bound has three times the active drug of a 98 per cent protein bound drug. Comparison is of 6 per cent free drug versus 2 per cent free drug. Keeping this in mind, when comparing a tetracycline such as oxytetracycline, which is 30 per cent protein

bound, with demethylchlortetracycline, which is 70 per cent protein bound, the difference is 70 per cent versus 30 per cent, or more than twice the free drug.

Protein binding is of great importance for drug distribution, since tissue barriers will exclude drug that is highly protein bound. For example, the passage of drugs into the cerebrospinal fluid (CSF) is low if the drugs are highly protein bound. However, some molecules do not enter the CSF even though protein binding is low. This indicates that other factors are equally important, such as the charge properties noted in Figure 4.

Protein binding will affect the duration of drug concentration in the blood and the rate of elimination of drugs from the body. Protein-bound antibiotics will not be removed by the glomeruli, since only unbound drugs are removed by glomerular filtration. However, renal clearance of many antibiotics is greatly influenced by tubular resorption and in the case of penicillins and cephalosporins by tubular excretion. This latter process is independent of protein binding, and even highly protein-bound drugs can be eliminated rapidly without eliminating a volume of plasma fluid that contains the drugs.

The factors mentioned thus far seem to indicate that high protein binding is a disadvantage. Nonetheless, maintenance of high serum levels for long periods is an important practical consideration for antibiotic therapy in a large animal practice. Even if the level of free drug needed to inhibit a pathogen is low, adequate levels in the interstitium may be present for a number of hours. From a public health viewpoint, however, it is reasonable to expect that the duration of antibiotic residues in the body is longer for drugs that are extensively protein bound to serum and tissue in comparison with antibiotics that possess minimal binding properties.

Tissue Distribution of Antibiotics

This subject has been extensively reviewed recently by Neu.[29] Studies of the distribution of antibiotics into tissue fluids were first performed in 1946, with the objective of measuring penicillin levels in wound exudates 8 hours after IM injection of small amounts of the drug. It was suggested at that time that the level of a drug in serum did not reflect levels in avascular sites.

Apparently, tissue levels of antibiotics, whether measured by implanted chambers

TABLE 4. *Binding of Antibiotics to Bovine and Ovine Sera as Determined by Equilibrium Dialysis and Ultrafiltration Methods**

Antibiotic	Type of Animal	No. of Animals	Concentration Tested (µg/ml)	Equilibrium Dialysis Method		Ultrafiltration Method	
				NO. OF ASSAYS	PERCENTAGE BOUND (MEAN ± SD)	NO. OF ASSAYS	PERCENTAGE BOUND (MEAN ± SD)
Penicillins:							
Penicillin G	Cows	4	2.0–4.0†	16	28.5 ± 3.8	32	32.6 ± 2.5
	Ewes	5	2.0–4.0	18	30.4 ± 2.5	30	36.8 ± 4.7
Phenoxymethylampicillin	Ewes	3	0.5–2.0	8	78.0 ± 7.6	15	81.0 ± 3.4
	Cows	2		6	18.0 ± 2.5	10	18.0 ± 2.0
	Ewes	4		10	13.8 ± 3.2	16	15.6 ± 3.8
Cloxacillin	Cows	4	10.0–20.0	12	71.3 ± 6.8	20	78.0 ± 5.4
	Ewes	4		12	72.6 ± 3.5	20	74.0 ± 4.0
Carbenicillin	Ewes	4	15.0–30.0	12	25.2 ± 3.8	10	34.2 ± 3.2
Cephalosporins:							
Cephaloridine	Ewes	4	1.5–3.0	12	0.0	12	6.2 ± 1.4
Cephalexin	Ewes	3	15.0–25.0	9	10.6 ± 1.2	9	12.6 ± 2.7
Tetracyclines:							
Tetracycline	Cows	4	2.5–5.0	12	31.6 ± 3.3	30	41.4 ± 2.1
	Ewes	6		16	27.5 ± 4.5	30	32.0 ± 4.0
Oxytetracycline	Cows	6	2.5–5.0	18	18.6 ± 2.2	30	22.4 ± 3.8
	Ewes	6		18	21.2 ± 3.2	30	24.6 ± 4.2
Chlortetracycline	Cows	6	1.0–4.0	18	46.8 ± 2.6	30	51.2 ± 5.4
	Ewes	6		18	45.6 ± 3.0	30	49.6 ± 3.8
Demethylchlortetracycline	Ewes	3	1.0–4.0	9	68.8 ± 2.6	12	70.2 ± 5.8
Methacycline	Ewes	3	2.0–4.0	8	79.2 ± 2.8	12	88.8 ± 3.5
Doxycyline	Ewes	4	0.5–1.5	12	84.0 ± 3.8	16	90.2 ± 2.4
Minocycline	Ewes	3	1.0–2.5	8	72.8 ± 2.0	12	80.2 ± 4.5
Aminoglycosides:							
Dihydrostreptomycin	Cows	4	2.5–5.0	16	8.0 ± 2.5	30	10.2 ± 2.0
	Ewes	6		24	11.6 ± 3.2	30	15.0 ± 3.8
Neomycin	Cows	2	5.0–10.0	6	44.8 ± 2.6	10	50.0 ± 3.4
	Ewes	4		8	49.4 ± 3.6	16	54.2 ± 4.4
Kanamycin	Ewes	3	2.5–5.0	12	0.0	12	4.0 ± 1.0
Paromomycin	Ewes	3	2.5–5.0	12	36.6 ± 2.8	12	38.0 ± 5.2
Spectinomycin	Cows	6	12.5–25.0	24	6.0 ± 2.0	24	8.4 ± 1.8

Drug	Animal	n	Range	n	Value	n	Value
Macrolides:							
Erythromycin	Cows	4	1.0–4.0	12	18.0 ± 1.6	18	20.4 ± 2.8
	Ewes	6		12	23.0 ± 3.4	18	24.8 ± 3.6
Oleandomycin	Ewes	3	5.0–7.5	6	20.0 ± 1.2	12	23.6 ± 3.4
Triacetyloleandomycin	Ewes	2	10.0	6	32.4 ± 1.4	8	34.6 ± 2.2
Spiramycin	Cows	6	2.5–5.0	18	37.6 ± 4.2	30	38.0 ± 3.8
	Ewes	6		18	29.8 ± 3.4	30	32.6 ± 4.6
Tylosin	Cows	2	2.5–5.0	6	33.5 ± 2.2	20	44.0 ± 2.0
	Ewes	6		18	38.0 ± 5.0	30	45.4 ± 3.8
Polypeptides:							
Polymyxin B	Cows	2	6.2–12.5	6	54.0 ± 3.0	8	74.6 ± 6.2
	Ewes	4		12	32.8 ± 4.4	12	42.2 ± 3.8
Colistin sulfate	Cows	2	6.2–12.5	6	56.0 ± 2.8	8	69.8 ± 5.6
	Ewes	4		12	60.4 ± 2.6	12	71.6 ± 4.2
Colistimethate	Ewes	4	6.2–12.5	12	34.0 ± 4.2	12	42.8 ± 3.8
Others:							
Lincomycin	Ewes	5	2.0–4.0	ND‡	—	15	34.2 ± 3.2
Clindamycin	Ewes	5	1.2–2.5	ND	—	15	46.0 ± 3.0
Chloramphenicol	Cows	4	20.0–40.0	16	36.6 ± 3.2	18	38.2 ± 2.6
	Ewes	4		8	32.2 ± 2.8	19	33.8 ± 1.8
Novobiocin	Ewes	3	2.5–5.0	12	96.4 ± 3.8	12	97.8 ± 2.0
Fusidic acid	Ewes	4	15.0–30.0	16	95.8 ± 3.8	24	98.0 ± 4.2
Vancomycin	Ewes	2	10.0–20.0	ND	—	8	54.8 ± 3.0
Ristocetin	Ewes	3	10.0–20.0	9	Undialyzable	ND	—
Rifamycin SV	Ewes	2	1.0–4.0	ND	—	4	72.6 ± 4.6
Rifampin	Ewes	2	0.1–0.4	ND	—	4	84.2 ± 5.6
Rifamide	Ewes	2	2.0–4.0	ND	—	4	70.2 ± 4.6

*From Ziv, G. and Sulman, E. G.: Antimicrob. Ag. Chemother., 2:206, 1972.
†International units.
‡Not done.

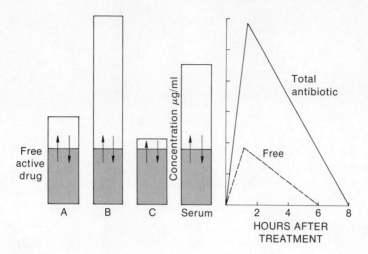

Figure 5. Distribution of drug in tissues as influenced by protein binding.

or abrasion techniques, are lower than serum levels and reflect the amount of free drug.[7, 8, 23, 24, 37] Larger doses of an agent will produce high serum levels that, in turn, will yield higher tissue levels, provided the administered dose formulation is quickly and almost completely absorbed after IM injection or the drug is administered IV. It is also clear that peak tissue levels are achieved approximately 1 to 2 hours after injection, and the tissue levels decline slowly over a number of hours. Data presented in Figure 3 for the relation between benzylpenicillin levels in bovine endometrial tissue and serum are in accord with the conclusions derived from experimental animal studies. There is a great need for similar data to be generated concerning the concentration of other antimicrobial agents in uterine tissue.

Data presented in Table 5 can be considered as an attempt to assess the duration of "effective" tissue antibiotic levels. The data were compiled from the relevant published information on serum antibiotic levels in ruminants following a single IM administration of several antibiotic formulations often used in large animal practice in various countries. Unbound drug levels in serum were taken to represent drug levels in tissue. It was considered that the percentage binding was not affected by serum drug concentrations, and no allowances were made for the possible synergistic effects of administration of combined antibiotics or the perfusion of tissue involved. For each antibiotic a range of minimal inhibitory concentration (MIC) values was selected on the basis of the approximate MIC expected using the more susceptible strains among some common

bacterial pathogens, excluding resistant variants.[2]

In spite of these arbitrary assumptions and uncertainties, the approximate duration of "effective" tissue drug levels may be considered as guidelines in the rational selection of antibiotics and antibiotic formulations for the parenteral treatment of postparturient septic bovine metritis (see Tables 1, 2 and 5). It appears that treatment with compounds containing chloramphenicol, ampicillin, gentamicin or kanamycin is most likely to be efficacious. Data presented in Table 5 also suggest that different formulations of ampicillin, chloramphenicol and oxytetracycline administered IM can result in significant differences in duration of free drug levels in serum. Thus, treatment with sodium ampicillin produced peak drug levels that were approximately two-fold higher than those seen after an almost equal dose of ampicillin trihydrate was injected. The latter formulation results in free drug concentration at the level of 2.0 μg/ml for 6 hours, as compared with 3 hours for the former compound. However, free serum drug concentrations at the level of 4.0 μg/ml could not be reached by the administration of ampicillin trihydrate at 12.5 mg/kg, whereas a 10 mg/kg-dose of ampicillin sodium maintained that level of free drug for 1.5 hours. An IV injection of chloramphenicol base at 50 mg/kg was able to maintain a free drug level of 8.0 μg/ml for 5 hours. However, after a similar dose of the same formulation was administered IM, peak total (bound and free) drug concentrations ranged between 3.8 and 5.6 μg/ml only. On the other hand, the IM injection of the water-soluble sodium

TABLE 5. *Peak Serum Antibiotic Concentrations and Duration of Free Drug Concentrations in Bovine Serum in Relation to Minimal Inhibitory Concentrations (MIC)**

Antimicrobial Agent	Route of Drug Administration	Dose	Peak Serum Concentration (μg or IU/ml)	MIC (μg or IU/ml)	Duration of Free-Drug Concentration in Serum for Given MIC Value (hours)	Reference
Benzylpenicillin sodium, aqueous solution	IM	6×10^6 IU/cow	1.0	0.05 0.10 0.50	6 4 1	41
"	IM	9×10^6 IU/cow	1.4	0.05 0.10 0.50	10 6 2	41
Benzylpenicillin procaine, aqueous suspension	IM	3×10^6 IU/cow	0.3	0.05 0.10 0.50	10 4 0	41
"	IM	6×10^6 IU/cow	0.5	0.05 0.10 0.50	24 12 0	41
"	IM	9×10^6 IU/cow	0.6	0.05 0.10 0.50	24 12 0	41
Benzylpenicillin benzathine, aqueous suspension	IM	9×10^6 IU/cow	0.03	0.05	0	41
Penethamate hydriodide (DAEEH) aqueous suspension	IM	3×10^6 IU/cow	0.4	0.05 0.10 0.50	8 4 0	41
"	IM	6×10^6 IU/cow	0.5	0.05 0.10 0.50	18 15 0	41
"	IM	9×10^6 IU/cow	1.6	0.05 0.10 0.50	30 24 10	41
Ampicillin/amoxicillin sodium, aqueous solution	IV	10 mg/kg	35.0	1.0 2.0 4.0 8.0	2.0 1.5 0.5 0.25	31

Table continued on following page.

TABLE 5. *Peak Serum Antibiotic Concentrations and Duration of Free Drug Concentrations in Bovine Serum in Relation to Minimal Inhibitory Concentrations (MIC)* (Continued)*

Antimicrobial Agent	Route of Drug Administration	Dose	Peak Serum Concentration (μg or IU/ml)	MIC (μg or IU/ml)	Duration of Free-Drug Concentration in Serum for Given MIC Value (hours)	Reference
Ampicillin/amoxicillin sodium, aqueous solution	IM	10 mg/kg	6.5	1.0 2.0 4.0 8.0	4.5 3.0 1.5 0	31
Ampicillin/amoxicillin trihydrate, aqueous suspension	IM	12.5 mg/kg	3.5	1.0 2.0 4.0	12.0 6.0 0	31
Cephacetrile sodium, aqueous solution	IV	8.5 mg/kg	50.0	2.0 4.0 8.0 16.0	1.5 1.0 0.75 0.5	51
"	IM	8.5 mg/kg	20.0	2.0 4.0 8.0 16.0	2.5 1.5 1.0 0.5	51
Dihydrostreptomycin, neomycin, kanamycin, aminosidine, gentamicin, aqueous solution	IV	20 mg/kg	150.0	0.5 1.0 2.0 4.0 8.0 16.0	12.0 8.0 3.0 2.0 1.0 0.5	55
"	IM	10 mg/kg	30.0	0.5 1.0 2.0 4.0 8.0 16.0	12.0 10.0 8.0 6.0 6.0 4.0	55
Oxytetracycline HCl, organic solvent	IV	20 mg/kg	22.0	0.5 1.0 2.0 4.0 8.0	8.0 4.5 2.5 1.5 0.5	56

Drug	Route	Dose				Ref.
"	IM	20 mg/kg	0.8–6.2†	0.5 1.0 2.0 4.0	4–12† 2–6† 1–4† 0	50
"	IM	10 mg/kg	0.8–5.2†	0.5 1.0 2.0	2–6† 0–4† 0–2†	50
"	IM	5 mg/kg	0.8–1.3†	0.5 1.0	0–6† 0	50
Erythromycin base, organic solvent and erythromycin lactobionate aqueous solution	IV	10 mg/kg	12.0	0.5 1.0 2.0 4.0 8.0	8.0 5.5 3.0 1.0 0.5	30, 50
Erythromycin base, organic solvent	IM	10 mg/kg	2.4	0.5 1.0 2.0 4.0	12.0 4.0 1.5 0	30
Erythromycin lactobionate, aqueous solution	IM	10 mg/kg	5.0	0.5 1.0 2.0 4.0	12.0 6.0 4.0 2.0	50
Tylosin base, organic solvent and tylosin tartrate, aqueous solution	IV	20 mg/kg	22.0	0.5 1.0 2.0 4.0 8.0	10.0 8.0 6.0 4.0 1.5	30, 54
Tylosin base, organic solvent	IM	20 mg/kg	2.5	0.5 1.0 2.0 4.0	12.0 9.0 1.5 0	30
Tylosin tartrate, aqueous solution	IM	20 mg/kg	5.6	0.5 1.0 2.0 4.0	12.0 8.0 4.0 2.5	30
Spiramycin base, organic solvent and spiramycin adipate aqueous solution	IV	20 mg/kg	16.0	1.0 2.0 4.0 8.0	36.0 12.0 2.0 1.0	30, 49

Table continued on following page.

TABLE 5. Peak Serum Antibiotic Concentrations and Duration of Free Drug Concentrations in Bovine Serum in Relation to Minimal Inhibitory Concentrations (MIC)* (Continued)

Antimicrobial Agent	Route of Drug Administration	Dose	Peak Serum Concentration (µg or IU/ml)	MIC (µg or IU/ml)	Duration of Free-Drug Concentration in Serum for Given MIC Value (hours)	Reference
Spiramycin base, organic solvent	IM	20 mg/kg	1.6	1.0 2.0	18.0 0	30
Spiramycin adipate, aqueous solution	IM	20 mg/kg	4.4	1.0 2.0 4.0 8.0	36.0 18.0 4.0 0	49
Lincomycin HCl and clindamycin phosphate, aqueous solution	IV	10 mg/kg	8.0	0.25 0.5 1.0 2.0 4.0	8.0 6.0 3.0 2.0 1.0	30
Lincomycin HCl and clindamycin HCl, aqueous solution	IM	20 mg/kg	12.0	0.25 0.5 1.0 2.0 4.0 8.0	12.0 10.0 8.0 6.0 4.0 1.5	30, 53
Chloramphenicol base, organic solvent	IV	20 mg/kg	30.0	2.0 4.0 8.0 16.0	12.0 8.0 5.0 2.0	36
Chloramphenicol base, organic solvent	IM	10 mg/kg	1.7	2.0	0	9, 43
"	IM	25 mg/kg	2.2	2.0	0	42
"	IM	50 mg/kg	3.8–5.6†	2.0 4.0	6–10† 0–6†	50, 57
Chloramphenicol sodium succinate, aqueous solution	IM	50 mg/kg	25.0	2.0 4.0 8.0 16.0	24.0 12.0 6.0 4.0	57

*Following single parenteral injection of antibiotics to adult ruminants.
†Dependent on the type of organic solvent and the number of injection sites.

succinate ester of chloramphenicol at 50 mg/kg resulted in free drug level of 8.0 μg/ml for 6 hours. It must be stressed, however, that some of the antibiotics most likely to be efficacious in treating bovine septic metritis are not licensed for use in food-producing animals in several countries.

Intrauterine Administration

Many antibacterial products have been infused into the uterus of cows for treatment of metritis or of failure to conceive after one or more matings (repeat breeders). This subject has been reviewed extensively recently[33, 45] and will not be included in the present article.

A wide range of antiseptics have been used locally to control the bacterial flora in the treatment of retained placenta and have also been used to control bacterial flora in the uterus following removal of the retained fetal membranes. These early drugs consisted of products such as charcoal, boric acid, acriflavine, bismuth subnitrite, silver oxide and various chlorine, iodine, iodoform and perborate preparations. The latter release much gas on contact with tissue debris and cause foaming similar to that resulting from the use of hydrogen peroxide.[39] One factor to consider when selecting products for uterine infusion is the product's effect on the uterus. It has been stated that products causing a severe inflammatory reaction in the uterus should be avoided.[39]

Because of their effect on tissue debris, a number of enzyme products containing urea, yeast, pepsin and papain have been advocated.[39] However, it is doubtful that these varied preparations greatly alter the course of the disease.[39]

Sulfanilamide, sulfathiazole, sulfamerazine and sulfamethazine have been used locally in the uterus by some practitioners, although others indicate that these drugs are rather insoluble, tend to settle in the apex of the horn and are of questionable value.[39] Various intrauterine combination products containing tetracycline, furazolidone, iodochlohydroxyquinoline, chloramphenicol, streptomycin, neomycin, polymyxin B, kanamycin and dapsone, with and without estrogens and corticosteroids, are commercially available to certain practitioners throughout the world, and variable claims are made regarding their clinical and bacteriological efficacy.

Penicillin, streptomycin and tyrothricin have been used extensively in the local treatment of retained placenta. Penicillin is usually quickly inactivated by penicillinase produced by the infective organisms in the uterus, and streptomycin and tyrothricin are rather irritating in large amounts. More recently, administration of 1 to 3 gm of the broad-spectrum antibiotics such as oxytetracycline, chlortetracycline, chloramphenicol and several nitrofurans has been recommended. For immediate response these are used as an infusion in 200 to 500 ml of saline or warm water. It has been claimed that boluses or powder produce a slightly slower response.[39] If the uterus is filled with a large amount of fetid fluid, this should be gently siphoned off before local antibiotic treatment.[39] In early cases, posterior pituitary extract (Pituitrin) and/or IM estrogens and the IV injection of calcium borogluconate seem to be of value in producing tonus in the atonic uterus.[39]

Several studies have shown that hormones, sulfonamides and antibiotics are rapidly absorbed from the uterus into the bloodstream.[4, 5, 22, 27] Because of the extensive increase in blood supply and enlarged surface area, it was thought that the early postpartum uterus would be an efficient organ for drug absorption.[38] With shedding of the placenta at birth, large areas of the endometrium are disturbed and/or removed, thus exposing extensive capillary beds. As the postpartum uterus involutes or returns to its normal nongravid state, it was expected that efficiency of absorption capability would be diminished, since the surface area is greatly reduced, the endometrium is reorganizing and the blood supply is greatly diminished. Contrary to these expectations, it was found that absorption efficiency of the uterus was poorest in the early postpartum period and increased with postpartum time.[38]

It appears from these investigations that the physiological state of the immediate postpartum uterus is not conducive to the absorption of certain antibacterial agents such as penicillin, dihydrostreptomycin and oxytetracycline as it is at later times in the involution period. However, absorption of sulfamethazine,[38] dapsone and chloramphenicol[50] is considerably quicker. It was

TABLE 6. *Amount and Duration of Antibiotics in Lumen of Uterus of Postparturient Dairy Cows**

Infusion in 30-ml Water	Hours after Treatment						
	6	12	18	24	30	36	42
	TOTAL AMOUNT IN UTERINE LUMEN (μg)						
Dihydrostrepto-mycin (1 gm)	1440	700	500	200	0	–	–
Crystalline peni-cillin G (1 million units)	2240	920	300	20	0	–	–
Procaine penicillin (1 million units)	2480	1525	620	370	48	0	–
Oxytetracycline (600 mg)	–	–	60,000	15,000	4000	1000	0

*Adapted from Kendrick, J. W.: Report to the California Milk Advisory Board, August, 1978.

postulated that the difference between absorption rates of sulfamethazine and absorption rates of penicillin, dihydrostreptomycin and oxytetracycline is due to the greater volume of sulfamethazine solution infused.[38] Since there is a large volume of mucinous material in the early postpartum uterus, a dilution factor or protein interaction with the drugs may be involved.[38] However, intrauterine treatment with a 3-gm bolus of dapsone or 2.5 gm of chloramphenicol dissolved in 20 ml of polyethylene glycol resulted in very quick absorption of these drugs from the uterus.[50]

Results of a single study[21] are available on the amount of penicillin, dihydrostreptomycin and oxytetracycline in the lumen of the uterus (Table 6) and the concentrations of these drugs in biopsy samples of the endometrium of cows treated between 21 and 35 days postpartum (Table 7). Penicillin is maintained at therapeutic levels in the lumen of the uterus for 24 hours and oxytetracycline for 36 hours. In the tissue of the uterus, penicillin is maintained at effective levels for 30 hours, whereas oxytetracycline could not be detected in the uterine tissue.[21]

Another potential factor influencing the rate of drug absorption may be the physiological state of the endometrium. Denudation and reorganization of the endometrium, as well as capillary constriction and recession, may play a role in the absorption process. A partially chelated preparation of oxytetracycline has been studied[28] and is reported to be very effective clinically, presumably because it is not readily absorbed from the uterine cavity. Data are limited concerning the comparative clinical and bacteriological

TABLE 7. *Amount of Duration of Penicillin in Biopsy Samples of Endometrium of Postparturient Dairy Cows**

Infusion in 30-ml Water	Hours after Treatment						
	6	12	18	24	30	36	42
	CONCENTRATION μg/gm OF ENDOMETRIAL TISSUE						
Crystalline penicillin (1 million units)	1000	652	480	300	200	–	
Procaine penicillin (1 million units)	900	649	500	320	250	33	

*Adapted from Kendrick, J. W.: Report to the California Milk Advisory Board, August, 1978.

efficacy of intrauterine antibacterial agents in the treatment of postparturient metritis and retained placenta.[38] One can only postulate, therefore, about the most desirable pharmacological properties of these drugs, particularly whether quick absorption from the uterus is advantageous as compared with slow absorption properties. Clearly, a broad spectrum of antibacterial activity, proper disintegration and dispersion inside the uterus and lack of irritation are essential prerequisites of any intrauterine product. It can also be argued that drugs that are slowly absorbed from the uterine cavity are more likely to result in the maintenance of therapeutic drug levels in the endometrial tissue over several days than are drugs that were shown to be quickly absorbed. On the other hand, if it is decided not to administer antibiotics parenterally along with intrauterine antibiotic treatment, drugs possessing quick absorption properties are more likely to penetrate the infected subendometrial tissues. However, for maintaining effective tissue drug levels, multiple treatments are probably indicated, using the quickly absorbed drugs.

PUBLIC HEALTH CONSIDERATIONS

Parenteral Administration

During the past few years several reports and reviews were published that dealt with the pharmacokinetic aspects of drug residues in food-producing animals.[6, 26, 31, 32] Although control mechanisms of governmental agencies and implementation of control procedures vary from one country to another, the concept of withdrawal times and limitations for use of drugs for animals, particularly antibiotic drugs, is well established. Public health considerations must weigh heavily in the selection of antibiotics for parenteral treatment of bacterial infections in dairy cows, and recommended guidelines should be consulted regarding dosage schedules, routes of drug administration and the pre-slaughter withholding periods.[25] These guidelines are suitable for the treatment of metritis in dairy cows.

It must be recognized, however, that during septic and toxemic infections in the cow, particularly in the immediate postpartum period, drug elimination and excretion mechanisms may not be functioning as effectively as in the subacutely infected or the normal cow.[31] In acutely infected, emergency-slaughtered cows, the majority of which had postparturient metritis and mastitis, drug residues at the intramuscular injection site, in the major excretory organs (liver and kidneys) and in the muscle persisted much longer than in normal animals similarly treated.[32]

Intrauterine Administration

Antibiotics absorbed into the general circulation have a potential for being excreted in the milk. A number of sulfonamides were shown to pass from the uterus into the blood and were present in the milk in measurable amounts.[27] Penicillin-dihydrostreptomycin (1 million units and 1 gm, respectively) or oxytetracycline (100 mg) was not detected in milk 12 hours or more after their infusion into the uterus of cycling cows.[22] Intrauterine infusions of sulfamethazine (66 mg/kg in a volume of approximately 150 ml), oxytetracycline (500 mg in a volume of 20 ml), penicillin G (1 million units) and dihydrostreptomycin (2.5 gm), both as 20-ml aqueous solutions, were detected in milk in only trace amounts, but sulfamethazine was present at high concentrations for 48 hours.[38] In a large field trial,[21] three types of uterine infusions were administered: (1) 625 mg of oxytetracycline and 25 ml of furacin with sufficient water to make 100 ml, (2) 1.7 million units of procaine penicillin and 1.3 gm of dihydrostreptomycin in 40 ml of water and (3) 1.8 million units of procaine penicillin and 2.25 mg of dihydrostreptomycin in 60 ml of water. Infusions were made 6 hours before milking time. Penicillin was the sole drug detected in the milk and at the first milking only. It was claimed that only crystalline penicillin and not procaine penicillin contributed to the appearance of the drug in the milk.[21] It appears therefore that the extent of antibiotic residues in the milk of cows following administration of accepted doses into the uterus is dependent on the degree of drug absorption from the uterine cavity, the ability of the drug to cross the blood-milk barrier and the sensitivity of assay methods. Data are not available on antibiotic residues in the carcass after intrauterine treatment, but it was shown that the recovery of penicillin, oxytetracycline and dihydrostreptomycin in the urine 24 hours after treatment accounted for 33, 26 and 63 per cent of the infused doses, respectively.[21] These findings suggest that antibiotic residues may be present in the body after intrauterine treatment for a considerably longer period than in the milk.

REFERENCES

1. Ayliffe, T. R. and Noakes, D. E.: Some preliminary studies on the uptake of sodium benzylpenicillin by the endometrium of the cow. Vet. Rec., *102*:215, 1978.
2. Barry, A. L.: The Antimicrobic Susceptibility Test: Principles and Practice. Philadelphia, Lea & Febiger, 1976.
3. Biberstein, E. L., Franti, C. E., Jange, S. S. and Ruby, A.: Antimicrobial sensitivity patterns in *Staphylococcus aureus* from animals. J.A.V.M.A., *164*:1183, 1974.
4. Bierschwal, C. H. and Uren, A. W.: The absorption of chlortetracycline (Aureomycin) by the bovine uterus. J.A.V.M.A., *129*:373, 1956.
5. Bierschwal, C. H., Dale, H. E., and Uren, A. W.: The absorption of sulfamethazine by the bovine uterus. J.A.V.M.A., *126*:398, 1955.
6. Bourne, W. A., Bevill, R. F., Sharma, R. M., Gural, R. P. and Dittert, L. W.: Distribution of sulfonamides in food producing animals: Pharmacokinetics of sulfamethazine in lambs. Am. J. Vet. Res., *38*:967, 1977.
7. Bryant, R. E. and Hammond, D.: Interaction of purulent material with antibiotics used to treat *Pseudomonas aeruginosa* infections. Antimicrob. Ag. Chemother., *6*:702, 1974.
8. Craig, W. A. and Kunin, C. M.: Dynamics of binding and release of the polymyxin antibiotics by tissues. J. Pharmacol. Exp. Ther., *184*:757, 1973.
9. DeCorte-Baeten, K. and Debackere, M.: Chloramphenicol plasma levels in horses, cattle and sheep after oral and intramuscular administration. Zbl. Vet. Med. (A), *22*:704, 1975.
10. Elliott, L., McMahon, K. J. and Gier, H. T.: Uterus of the cow after parturition: Bacterial content. Am. J. Vet. Res., *29*:77, 1968.
11. Gibbons, W. J., Attleberger, M. H. and Kiesel, G. K.: The bacteriology of the cervical mucus of cattle. Cornell Vet., *49*:255, 1959.
12. Gier, H. T. and Marion, T. B.,: Uterus of the cow after parturition: Involutional changes. Am. J. Vet. Res., *29*:83, 1968.
13. Griffin, J. F. T., Hartigan, P. J. and Nunn, W. R.: Non-specific uterine infection and bovine fertility. Theriogenology, *1*:91, 1974.
14. Griffin, J. F. T., Murphy, J. A. and Nunn, W. R.: Repetitive in vivo sampling of the bovine uterus under field conditions. Br. Vet. J., *130*:259, 1974.
15. Groden, A. P., Olds, D. and Mochow, C. R.: Causes of fertilization failure in repeat breeding cattle. J. Dairy Sci., *51*:778, 1968.
16. Gunter, J. T., Collins, W. J. and Owen, J.: A survey of the bacteria in the reproductive tract of dairy animals and their relationship to infertility. Am. J. Vet. Res., *16*:282, 1955.
17. Hardenbrook, A.: The diagnosis and treatment of non-specific infections of the bovine uterus and cervix. J.A.V.M.A., *132*:459, 1958.
18. Hawk, H. W., Turner, G. D. and Sykes, J. F.: The effect of ovarian hormones on the uterine defense mechanism during the early stages of induced infection. Am. J. Vet. Res., *21*:644, 1960.
19. Hawk, H. W., Brinsfield, T. H., Turner, G. D., Whitmore, G. W. and Norcross, M. A.: Effect of ovarian status on induced acute inflammatory responses in cattle uteri. Am. J. Vet. Res., *25*:362, 1964.
20. Johans, C. J., Clark, T. L. and Herrick, J. R.: Factors affecting calving interval. J.A.V.M.A., *151*:1692, 1967.
21. Kendrick, J. W.: Dairy cattle fertility: The cause, prevention and treatment of uterine disease. Report of the California Milk Advisory Board, August, 1978.
22. Kendrick, J. W. and Pier, A. C.: Antibiotic levels in milk following intrauterine infusion. Calif. Vet., *13*:27, 1960.
23. Kornguth, M. L., Monson, R. A. and Kunin, C. M.: Binding of antibiotics to soluble protein in the rat liver. J. Infect. Dis., *129*:552, 1974.
24. Kunin, C. M. and Finland, M.: Clinical pharmacology of the tetracycline antibiotics. Clin. Pharmacol. Ther., *2*:51, 1962.
25. Mercer, H. D.: Antimicrobial drugs in food producing animals: Control mechanisms of governmental agencies. Vet. Clin. North Am., *5*:3, 1975.
26. Mercer, H. D., Baggot, J. D. and Sams, R. A.: Application of pharmacokinetic methods to the drug residue profile. J. Toxicol. Environ. Hlth., *2*:787, 1977.
27. Miller, G. E. and Rouse, G.: Passage of drugs from the bovine uterus into blood, milk and urine. J. Dairy Sci., *53*:652, 1970.
28. Miller, G. E., Bergt, G. P., Rose, W. M., Brunson, D. B. and Messer, R. G.: Distribution of oxytetracycline in bovine plasma, milk, and urine following its intrauterine administration in two forms. J. Dairy Sci., *56*:659, 1973.
29. Neu, H. C.: Clinical pharmacokinetics in preventive antimicrobial therapy. South. Med. J., *70*(Suppl. 1):14, Oct., 1977.
30. Nouws, J. F. M.: Tissue distribution and residues of some antimicrobial drugs in normal and emergency-slaughtered ruminants. Thesis., Vet. Faculty, State Univ. of Utrecht, The Netherlands, 1978.
31. Nouws, J. F. M. and Ziv, G.: A kinetic study of beta-lactam antibiotic residues in normal dairy cows. Zbl. Vet. Med. (A), *25*:312, 1978.
32. Nouws, J. F. M. and Ziv, G.: Pre-slaughter withdrawal times for drugs in dairy cows. J. Vet. Pharmacol. Ther., *1*:47, 1978.
33. Oxender, W. D. and Seguin, B. E.: Bovine intrauterine therapy. J.A.V.M.A., *176*:217, 1976.
34. Panangala, V. S. and Barnum, D. A.: Antibiotic resistance patterns of organisms isolated from cervico-vaginal mucus of cows. Can. Vet. J., *19*:113, 1978.
35. Panangala, V. S., Fish, N. A. and Barnum, D. A.: Microflora of the cervico-vaginal mucus of repeat breeder cows. Can. Vet. J., *19*:83, 1978.

36. Pilloud, M.: Pharmacokinetics, plasma protein binding, and dosage of chloramphenicol in cattle and horses. Res. Vet. Sci., *15*:231, 1973.

37. Reynolds, A. V., Hamilton-Miller, J. M. T. and Brumfitt, W.: Diminished effect of gentamicin under anaerobic and hypercapnic conditions. Lancet, *I*:447, 1976.

38. Righter, H. F., Mercer, H. D., Kline, D. A. and Carter, G. G.: Absorption of antibacterial agents by the bovine involuting uterus. Can. Vet. J., *16*:10, 1975.

39. Roberts, S. J.: Veterinary Obstetrics and Genital Diseases. Ann Arbor, Mich., Edwards Bros., Inc., 1971, Ch. 13.

40. Rolinson, G. N. and Sutherland, R.: The binding of antibiotics to serum proteins. Br. J. Pharmacol., *25*:638, 1965.

41. Schipper, I. A., Filipovs, D., Ebeltoft, H. and Schermeister, L. J.: Blood serum concentrations of various benzylpenicillins after their intramuscular administration to cattle. J.A.V.M.A., *158*:494, 1971.

42. Sevcik, B., Dvorak, M. and Plisek, K.: The levels of chloramphenicol in blood serum of cows, dogs and poultry and in cow's milk after intramuscular application. Vet. Med. (Praha), *15*:83, 1970.

43. Sisodia, C. S., Gupta, V. S., Dunlop, R. H. and Radostits, O. M.: Chloramphenicol concentration in blood and milk of cows following parenteral administration. Can. Vet. J., *14*:217, 1973.

44. Standiford, H. C., Jordan, M. C.and Kirby, W. M. M.: Clinical pharmacology of carbenicillin compared with other penicillins. J. Infect. Dis., *122*:9, 1970.

45. Studer, E. and Morrow, D. A.: Postpartum evaluation of bovine reproductive potential: Comparison of findings from genital tract examination per rectum, uterine culture, and endometrial biopsy. J.A.V.M.A., *172*:489, 1978.

46. Venable, J. H. and McDonald, L. E.: Postparturient bovine uterine motility — normal and after experimentally produced retention of the fetal membranes. Am. J. Vet. Res., *19*:308, 1958.

47. Wilkowske, C. J. and Hermans, P. E.: Antimicrobial agents in the treatment of obstetrics and gynecologic infections. Med. Clin. North Am., *58*:711, 1974.

48. Zimelis, V. M. and Jackson, G. G.: Activity of aminoglycoside antibiotics against *Pseudomonas aeruginosa:* Specificity and site of calcium and magnesium antagonism. J. Infec. Dis., *127*:666, 1973.

49. Ziv, G.: Pharmacokinetic profile of spiramycin in dairy cows and ewes. Cahiers Med. Vet., *43*:377, 1974.

50. Ziv, G.: Unpublished data.

51. Ziv, G. and Nouws, J. F. M.: Clinical pharmacology of cephacetrile in ruminants. Zbl. Vet. Med. (B), *24*:798, 1977.

52. Ziv, G. and Sulman, F. G.: Binding of antibiotics to bovine and ovine serum. Antimicrob. Ag. Chemother., *2*:206, 1972.

53. Ziv, G. and Sulman, F. G.: Penetration of lincomycin and clindamycin into milk in ewes. Br. Vet. J., *129*:83, 1973.

54. Ziv, G. and Sulman, F. G.: Serum and milk concentrations of spectinomycin and tylosin in cows and ewes. Am. J. Vet. Res., *34*:329, 1973.

55. Ziv, G. and Sulman, F. G.: Distribution of aminoglycoside antibiotics in blood and milk. Res. Vet. Sci., *17*:68, 1974.

56. Ziv, G. and Sulman, F. G.: Analysis of pharmacokinetic properties of nine tetracycline analogues in dairy cows and ewes. Am. J. Vet. Res., *35*: 1197, 1974.

57. Ziv, G., Bogin, E. and Sulman, F. G.: Blood and milk levels of chloramphenicol in normal and mastitic cows and ewes after intramuscular administration of chloramphenicol base and chloramphenicol sodium succinate. Zbl. Vet. Med. (A), *20*:801, 1973.

58. Ziv, G., Gordin, S., Bechar, G. and Bernstein, S.: Binding of antibiotics to dry udder secretion and to udder tissue homogenates. Br. Vet. J., *132*:318, 1976.

Drug Therapy during Pregnancy and the Neonatal Period

LLOYD E. DAVIS

University of Illinois at Urbana-Champaign, Urbana, Illinois

HUBERT C. STANTON

Shell Development Company, Modesto, California

During the past 20 years, the number of active drugs available to the veterinarian has increased rapidly. Currently there are more than 7200 prescription drugs and drug combinations available. Seventy per cent of these were unknown or unavailable 15 years ago. The plight of the veterinarian is further increased by the fact that he is called upon to diagnose and treat ailments occurring in a variety of animal species in which drug disposition and dosage requirements differ. Additional considerations, important to the specialty of theriogenology, are the unique relationship of the mother to the fetus and the special characteristics of the newborn animal.

Growth and development characterize the perinatal period and have important implications for drug therapy in veterinary obstetrics and pediatrics. First, drugs or other foreign chemicals may be administered to or ingested by the dam during any stage of gestation and thereby influence the developing embryo or fetus. Second, drugs are frequently administered during parturition, so the offspring may be affected by the drugs given to the mother. Lastly, drugs may be given to the offspring during the neonatal period or may be secreted into the milk and ingested by the nursing animal.

The following discussion addresses itself to drug actions and adverse effects on the developing animal, pitfalls likely to be encountered in therapy during the perinatal period and pharmacological principles needed to use drugs rationally in the pregnant or neonatal patient.

PRENATAL CLINICAL PHARMACOLOGY

The developing offspring is an obligate parasite of the dam. As such, it is completely dependent on the physiological integrity of the mother for the maintenance of an appropriate internal environment. Exposure of the dam to foreign chemicals may affect development or function of the offspring during embryogenesis, fetal life or at the time of parturition.

Dysmorphogenesis

The action of a dysmorphogenic agent on the conceptus depends on the developmental stage of the embryo, the genetic susceptibility of the embryo and the physiological, nutritional and pathological status of the dam. The period during which chemical substances can affect development of the embryo or fetus is frequently quite short. Ontogenesis is a continuum of precisely orchestrated biochemical events that succeed one another at a rapid rate. Accordingly, each organ undergoes a "critical period" of differentiation at precise times following conception, and it is at these times that the conceptus is most vulnerable to environmental influences.[12, 15]

Gestation may be considered as consisting of four periods: blastogenesis, embryogenesis, metamorphosis and fetal growth. Following fertilization, the zygote undergoes cleavage as it passes from the oviduct into the uterus as a free blastocyst. The blastocyst implants or attaches to the endometrium and commences the process of embryogenesis. During this period the embryo undergoes very rapid and important transformations. These processes will be briefly illustrated using the pig as a model because the development of this species has been well characterized. Although other species undergo similar changes, the temporal relationships may be different. The comparative time intervals for the four major events for various species are tabulated in Table 1.

The primitive streak is completed and the notochord is forming by time of attachment (11 to 12 days). The primordial nervous system; sense organs; circulatory, excretory and digestive systems and limb buds are formed from the twelfth to the twentieth day. The period of metamorphosis (days 20 through 35) is marked by differentiation and organogenesis. The enamel organs are formed for subsequent tooth development, the nasal septum becomes complete, the chambers of the heart are separated, ossification of bone commences, skeletal muscle is formed, and the mammary gland primordia appear, as do the primordia of the endocrine glands. By the thirty-fifth day the facial clefts are closed and the palate is completed. The fetal period, extending from the end of metamorphosis to birth, is characterized by growth of the fetus. Most organs are differentiated prior to this time. During fetal life, the gut is withdrawn from the umbilical hernia (36 to 50 days), the external genitalia become differentiated (39 to 95 days) and histogenesis of the nervous system proceeds.

Teratogenic agents affect the conceptus in different ways, depending upon the stage of gestation. Exposure of the blastocyst to certain drugs prior to attachment may interfere with implantation and terminate pregnancy. Chemicals are most likely to induce morphological changes in the embryo during the midembryonic period when organogenesis is most active. There is increasing awareness that certain chemical substances, including methyl mercury, lead, nicotine and perhaps some pesticides, may induce more subtle physiological changes when administered to the dam in the latter period of pregnancy after the organs of the embryo are formed but during a critical period in the development of the organ function. The developing nervous system seems particularly susceptible to insult, and permanent but subtle changes in postnatal behavioral patterns may result. Impaired endocrine development may not be obvious until the animal approaches sexual maturity.

It is difficult to assess the importance of drugs and other chemical substances in producing embryonic death or anomalous development in domesticated animals because many other factors can influence development. These include genetic defects, radiation, infections, vitamin deficiencies and maternal endocrine disorders. An additional problem is that a number of plants ingested during grazing are capable of producing teratogenic effects in horses, cattle, sheep and swine. Little work has been done on evaluating the teratogenicity of drugs in any domesticated animal. Nearly all our knowledge has been derived from

TABLE 1. *Developmental Periods in Domesticated and Laboratory Animals**

Species	Initial Attachment or Implantation (days)	End of Embryonic Period (days)	End of Metamorphosis (days)	Birth (days)	Usual Number of Fetuses
Dog	14–21	20	30	63–68	2–12
Cat	13–17	18	22	64–66	4–6
Horse	25–70†	26	35	329–345	1
Ox	30–36	30	45	278–290	1
Sheep	17–20	21	32	147–155	1–2
Goat	10–15	21	32	147–152	1–2
Swine	20–24	20	35	112–116	8–12
Monkey	9–10	28	40	164	1
Man	7–8	36	60	267	1
Rabbit	7–8	10	14	32	1–12
Rat	4.5–6.5	12.5	16.5	22	8–12
Mouse	4.5	9	13.5	22	10–16

*The values given in the table provide a general indication of the length of the various periods. Except in the case of swine, primates and rodents, the precise intervals are not well defined.
†Values for the horse vary widely among different authors.

studies performed in chicks and laboratory rodents, and in most cases we do not know the relevance of this information as applied to other species. A number of drugs and other chemical categories that may have a high index of suspicion as potential teratogens based on studies conducted in laboratory animals are listed in Table 2. These drugs and chemical compounds should be employed with caution after breeding.

PLACENTAL TRANSFER OF DRUGS

During attachment of the blastocyst to the endometrium, the fetal membranes fuse with the uterine mucosa to form the placenta, which permits exchange between the fetal and maternal circulations. Placentation varies considerably among species, both in gross morphology and in the number of membranes separating maternal from fetal blood.[10] Drugs and other chemical substances must traverse these membranes to enter the fetal circulation. Therefore, it is important for the veterinarian to appreciate species differences as a basis for interpreting the experimental literature. The number of placental tissue layers separating the maternal and fetal circulations determines the histological classification of placental types (Table 3). It is erroneous, however, to assume that the complex placentae are less efficient or represent better

TABLE 2. *Substances Shown to be Embryotoxic in Laboratory Animals**

Class of Compound	Specific Examples	Class of Compund	Specific Examples
Hormones	Estrogens Progestogens Androgens Corticosteroids	Antimalarials	Quinine
		Insecticides	Aldrin Carbaryl Dieldrin
Vitamins	Vitamin A (excessive doses) Vitamin D (excessive doses)		Endrin Methylparathione
Central-acting drugs	Phenytoin Diazepam Thalidomide Glutethimide Meclizine	Herbicides	2,4-D Diquat Paraquat 2,4,5-T
	Trimethadione Amphetamines	Fungicides	Captan Difolatan Folpet
Antimetabolites	6-mercaptopurine Azaserine Nitrogen mustard Urethane Cyclophosphamide		Griseofulvin Methyl mercury Thiram
		Solvents	Dimethylsulfoxide Chloroform
Anti-inflammatory drugs	Salicylates Phenylbutazone	Metals	Arsenic Cadmium Chromium Copper Mercury Lithium Lead Selenium
Chemotherapeutic agents	Sulfadiazine Sulfamerazine Penicillin Tetracycline Streptomycin Actinomycin D		
Oral anticoagulants	Warfarin		
Oral hypoglycemics	Tolbutamide Carbutamide		

*Modified from Wilson, J. G.: Federation Proceedings, *36*:1698, 1977 and Cahen, R. L.: Clin. Pharmacol. Therap., *5*:480, 1964.

TABLE 3. *Placentation in Common Domesticated and Laboratory Animals**

Species	Morphological Type	Membranes
Ox	Epitheliochorial	Maternal: Endothelium Epithelium
Sheep	Epitheliochorial	
Goat	Epitheliochorial	Fetal: Chorion Endothelium
Horse	Epitheliochorial	
Swine	Epitheliochorial	
Dog	Endotheliochorial	Maternal: Endothelium Fetal: Chorion Endothelium
Cat	Endotheliochorial	
Rabbit	Hemoendothelial	Maternal: None Fetal: Endothelium
Rat	Hemoendothelial	
Mouse	Hemoendothelial	
Man	Hemochorial	Maternal: None Fetal: Chorion Endothelium
Monkey	Hemochorial	

*Modified from Hamilton, W. J., Boyd, J. D. and Mossman, H. W.: Human Embryology. 3rd Ed. Baltimore, Williams & Wilkins, 1962, pp. 459–467.

diffusion barriers to foreign chemicals than the simple one-membrane types. The physiological characteristics of each placenta must be determined from electron micrographs in conjunction with biochemical transport studies.[17]

Concepts of the placental "barrier" have been revised considerably as a result of research conducted over the past 20 years. Most drugs will readily diffuse across the placental membranes, as the molecular size of most drugs is relatively small and most are lipid-soluble. The concentration of a given drug in the fetal circulation and tissues will depend on many factors, including molecular size and lipid solubility of the drug, placental blood flow, extent of protein binding of the drug and disposition of the drug in the dam. The placenta may be freely permeable to a certain drug, yet the amount reaching the fetal circulation may be very low because the drug is extensively bound to albumin in the maternal circulation. Similarly, a drug may not attain significant concentrations in the fetus if it was rapidly metabolized or excreted by the mother. Conversely, a teratogenic metabolite of safe-parent drug may be formed by the mother and passed across the placenta to the fetus. Since drug metabolism pathways differ widely among species, it is conceivable that a teratogenic metabolite may be formed in one species but not in another.[11] As a general rule, the fetus has a very limited capacity for drug metabolism so that it may receive prolonged exposure to parent drugs or their metabolites passing the placenta.[9]

Because of the complex relationships between the drug, the dam and the fetus, one cannot obtain a clear understanding of placental permeability to a given substance by merely sampling blood from the mother and from the umbilical vein. A valid approach for quantifying placental transfer involves the maintenance of steady-state concentrations in maternal blood together with intermittent sampling of blood from the fetus.[1] It was learned from such investigations that constant maternal blood concentrations of some drugs may be hazardous to the fetus. For example, under such circumstances diazoxide produced destruction of pancreatic islet cells with resultant diabetes in fetal lambs,[4] chlorpromazine caused fetal tachycardia and degenerative changes in the fetal liver and phenylbutazone produced renal damage in the ovine fetus.[5] Fortunately, drug disposition in the mother is such that foreign chemicals are transformed or excreted before they can attain steady-state concentrations in the fetus.

An important clinical corollary of these experimental observations is the increased risk to the fetus of drugs administered to a pregnant female whose ability to eliminate these substances is compromised by disease. Drugs given to a mother suffering from renal insufficiency or hepatic disease may be eliminated from her body so slowly that steady-state concentrations of the drug are established. This would greatly increase the exposure of the fetus to the drug.

DEVELOPMENT OF DRUG RECEPTORS IN THE FETUS

When a drug enters the fetal circulation, several factors determine the pharmacological effects elicited in the organism: (1) the capacity to nonspecifically bind or metabolically inactivate the drug, (2) the ability to mobilize transmitter substances in the case of indirectly acting drugs or to convert inactive prodrugs to active species, (3) the kinetic characteristics and density of tissue drug receptors and (4) the capacity of the end organ to respond to stimuli to carry out its functions. There is some information about the first listed factor in a few species, but little can be said about the other factors at this time.

Both alpha and beta adrenergic receptors are present in the fetal lamb by the middle of gestation. Injection of isoproterenol, epinephrine, levarterenol or methoxamine into the fetal circulation will elicit characteristic cardiovascular effects. The sympatheticoadrenal system probably plays a major role in regulating the circulation of the fetus, but this has not been defined. It is known that norepinephrine causes constriction of the ductus arteriosus and ductus venosus.[3] Blockade of these receptors by various drugs will impair the ability of the fetus to respond to stress from hypoxia or hemorrhage.

The sympatheticoadrenal system of the newborn pig is, in many respects, immature. Although this neonate is capable of synthesizing and inactivating catecholamines, it may have difficulty in mobilizing stored transmitter from the adrenal gland in response to stress. There is also some emerging evidence that the newborn pig may not be fully capable of mobilizing or utilizing its energy reserves at birth because of low adrenergic metabolic receptor sensitivity.[15] Similar results have also been reported for rats and dogs.

Cholinergic receptors, acetylcholine and acetylcholinesterase are present in embryos at a very early stage that antedates the innervation of developing tissues. Skeletal muscle, smooth muscle and the heart of the fetus respond to the effects of cholinergic drugs and cholinesterase inhibitors. The cholinergic system is probably important in homeostasis of the fetus. Drugs that modify these functions may be deleterious to the fetus.

Adrenocorticotropic hormone (ACTH), vasopressin, renin and angiotensin II are all present in the fetus by the middle of gestation. Corticosteroid levels in plasma of fetal lambs are low but dramatically increase a few days before parturition.

Of particular interest is the observation that fetal tissues contain appreciable quantities of prostaglandins. Prostaglandin-E_1 (PGE_1) constricts the umbilical-placental blood vessels, dilates the pulmonary vasculature and maintains the patency of the ductus arteriosus. The administration of prostaglandin synthetase inhibitors (such as aspirin or indomethacin) may interfere with the regulation of these structures. Indomethacin has been successful in inducing closure of a patent ductus arteriosus in human infants several days postpartum.

The fetus is a complex system that is capable of regulating its functions by means of intrinsic autonomic and hormonal mechanisms. Because our knowledge of fetal physiology is rudimentary, we have little basis for predicting the pharmacological effects of various drugs on the fetus at this time.

EFFECTS ON FETUS OF DRUGS ADMINISTERED DURING PARTURITION

The veterinarian should consider possible effects on the fetus of drugs administered to the mother at the time of parturition. We are fortunate in that most deliveries are uneventful and do not require the use of drugs. Drugs may be employed during cesarean section, and an occasional pregnant animal may be receiving drug therapy for a chronic condition unrelated to the pregnancy.

Most general anesthetic agents will cross the placenta and depress the central nervous system of the newborn. The volatile inhalant anesthetics are subsequently eliminated unchanged from the lungs of the neonate and are the least troublesome in terms of prolonged depression. Intravenous anesthetic agents that require biotransformation (barbiturates) or renal excretion (ketamine) are likely to produce prolonged depression of the offspring following delivery and should be avoided. Ketamine has been shown to accumulate in the placenta and attains concentrations in the fetal plasma and brain similar to those in maternal plasma.

Opiates readily enter the fetus from the maternal circulation and produce respiratory depression in the newborn. Unlike the barbiturates, opiate depression is readily reversed by administering naloxone or nalorphine to the offspring following delivery. Meperidine has been found to inhibit constriction of the ductus arteriosus, whereas morphine had no effect. Such constriction was associated with the anticholinergic effects of meperidine. However, the clinical significance of this effect is unknown.

Autonomic drugs administered to the mother prior to or during parturition may affect various regulatory mechanisms of the fetus during delivery. Most adrenergic drugs are not transferred across the placenta, but their use as pressor agents in the mother may be harmful to the fetus be-

cause fetal asphyxia has been described as a result of severe vasoconstriction of placental vessels. Atropine and several adrenolytic agents (e.g., phenothiazines) readily enter the fetal circulation and may exert pharmacological effects in the neonate during and following parturition. Anticholinesterase agents (some organophosphorous compounds, neostigmine) cross the placenta and may produce myasthenia in the infant.

Tranquilizers will cross the placenta and produce undesirable effects in the newborn. Chlorpromazine has produced prolonged sedation and retinopathy. Diazepam, chlordiazepoxide and phenytoin readily cross into the fetus and produce neonatal depression.

Local anesthetics, if rapidly absorbed into the maternal circulation, will produce bradycardia, acidosis and central nervous system depression of the fetus. Thus, use of intravenous lidocaine for the management of cardiac arrhythmias in the mother during parturition would be a distinct hazard for the fetus.

Corticosteroids administered to the dam will enter the fetus and may suppress the hypothalamic-pituitary-adrenal axis. Salicylates produce bleeding tendencies in the newborn, with resultant hemorrhage following delivery.

Certain antibiotics should be avoided late in pregnancy because of potential harm to the fetus. Tetracyclines may produce abnormal dentition in the offspring. Furthermore, parenteral administration of tetracycline has been observed to cause fulminating hepatitis characterized by fatty metamorphosis in the dam. This condition is usually fatal. Streptomycin and gentamicin may produce deafness in the neonate, and nitrofurantoin can produce hemolysis in the newborn.

Digitoxin and digoxin cross the placenta. Concentrations of digitoxin in the heart of the fetus have been observed to be twice that found in the maternal heart. The neonate will slowly eliminate the glycoside from its body and should be closely monitored during the first week or two of life.

Oxytocin may be employed to correct uterine inertia. The extensive use of this hormone in veterinary obstetrics over a long period of time would indicate that it does not produce adverse effects on the newborn. However, oxytocin will cause constriction of the umbilical vessels, and this could compromise an already hypoxic fetus.

PEDIATRIC CLINICAL PHARMACOLOGY

The newborn animal differs from older individuals of the same species in a number of significant ways that increase the uncertainties associated with drug therapy. The neonatal period may be defined as extending from birth through 1 month of age, irrespective of species. In many respects this interval constitutes a transition from fetal life, during which the animal was protected chemically and physically, to an independent being requiring adaptation to its surroundings in order to survive. During this time there are a number of deficiencies present that may compromise the animal's ability to eliminate drugs from the body and that may alter the expected responses to the drug.

Functional Considerations

The problems most commonly encountered with drug therapy during the neonatal period are those of toxicity. Many of these adverse effects can be understood and therefore anticipated if the veterinarian is aware of how the neonate differs from a mature animal as a responding system.

The so-called blood-brain barrier that prevents the diffusion of many drugs and endogenous compounds into the brain of the adult is poorly developed in the fetus and in the newborn. It decreases in permeability throughout the neonatal period and is similar to that of the adult by 8 weeks of age. Thus, many substances that are normally excluded from the central nervous system will enter the brain of a very young animal. Bilirubin, penicillin, tetracyclines, sulfonamides and many other substances may thus produce neurotoxicity in the newborn, whereas these effects would be rare in an adult.

The respiratory enzymes of the brain are poorly differentiated at birth in some species. These enzymes include carbonic anhydrase, cytochrome oxidase, succinic dehydrogenase and adenosinetriphosphatase (ATPase). This deficit has a marked effect on the action of various convulsants and the ability of the neonate to withstand anoxia. The newborn is less susceptible to convulsants such as strychnine and is resistant to the effects of anoxia, carbon monoxide, cyanide and nitrobenzene. This ability to withstand hypoxia is associated with (1) the ability of the neonatal brain to undergo anaerobic metabolism, (2) the glycogen storage in the cardiac ventricles and (3) a lower rate of degradation of adenosine triphosphate (ATP).

Not all newborn animals are resistant to anoxia and this reflects the degree of maturity at birth. Thus, functionally mature neonates such as monkeys, guinea pigs, lambs, kids, calves, foals and piglets are quite sensitive to the effects of anoxia. Animals that are more immature at birth (puppies, kittens, rabbits, rats and mice) can withstand anoxia for periods up to 28 minutes.[8, 15] Opiates and barbiturates will greatly increase the duration of apnea in the asphyxiated neonate.

The cardiovascular system of a healthy animal is competent at birth and the reflexes are active. Following birth, respiratory efforts are initiated by clamping of the umbilical cord and exposure to cold. It is interesting that strong tactile stimuli will elicit gasping but will not cause sustained respiratory movements. Depressant drugs that block reflex activity may result in a failure to sustain respiration.

Newborn animals have a greater surface-to-body weight ratio than adults and hence have a greater physical problem maintaining their body temperature. Body temperature is maintained in homeothermic animals by balancing heat production and heat loss. In newborn animals the capacity to limit heat loss is small. Therefore, the capability of the newborn animal to increase heat production is of paramount importance for survival. The animal born into a cold environment responds by increasing its oxygen consumption, which results in an increase in heat production. The two principal mechanisms by which the increase in metabolic rate takes place are shivering and the lipolysis of brown adipose tissue. In animals species whose skeletal muscle is well developed at birth (foal, calf, kid, lamb, and piglet), shivering is the only means of increasing heat production. The piglet has no brown fat. Rats, kittens, rabbits and probably puppies are dependent on metabolism of their brown adipose tissue for thermogenesis. The heat production is caused by re-esterification of fatty acids or their oxidation. Thus, a supply of both oxygen and glucose is required. Furthermore, this metabolic response to cold is mediated by the sympathetic nerves.

It is therefore evident that any drug or other factor that will decrease the volume or distribution of the cardiac output or the availability of oxygen or glucose will also decrease the animal's capacity to maintain body temperature by (1) impairing the metabolism of brown fat or (2) depriving the muscles of energy required for shivering. Factors to be considered are hemorrhage, general anesthetics, asphyxia, inability to suckle and drugs with adrenergic blocking activity. Drugs that depress central nervous system or skeletal muscle function will depress or eliminate shivering. Examples of these agents are anesthetics, aminoglycoside antibiotics and muscle relaxants. It is not necessary to treat the newborn itself with these drugs, as the offspring may be affected by drugs that have crossed the placenta from a dam that was receiving medication immediately prior to parturition.

The newborn animal is more prone to develop methemoglobinemia and hemolysis because of at least three factors: (1) the fetal type of hemoglobin oxidizes more rapidly to methemoglobin, (2) the increased hemoglobin content of erythrocytes is associated with a decreased rate of reduction of hemoglobin and (3) there is a deficiency in methemoglobin reductase. The ultimate cause of the hypersensitivity of neonatal erythrocytes to oxidant drugs is unknown but may be related to hypoglycemia or to deficient enzyme systems in the erythrocyte. Drugs that may produce methemoglobinemia and/or hemolysis in the neonatal animal include sulfonamides, nitrofurans, methylene blue, ascorbic acid, acetylsalicylic acid, naphthalene derivatives, acetophenetidin, phenothiazines and antihistaminics.

Drug Disposition during the Neonatal Period

Most of the problems encountered with drug therapy during the neonatal period are associated with failure of the therapist to take into account the immaturity of systems responsible for the elimination of the drug. Other factors that may differ in the neonate are the absorption and distribution of drugs.

Absorption of Drugs

During the period immediately following birth, the permeability of the small intestine is much greater than it will be a few days later. Decrease in permeability is stimulated by the ingestion of colostrum, and the period of increased permeability to drugs corresponds to the time during which proteins can be absorbed intact from the gastrointestinal tract in those species that are immunologically naive. Blood levels of succinylsulfathiazole (an enteric sulfonamide) were studied following oral administration of the drug to newborn piglets and for several days following birth.[6] On the day of birth and the next day the drug was found in the blood in appreciable quantities. Thereafter it was undetectable, as was the case in adult animals. Thus, during the first 2 days of life, systemic effects might occur following oral administration of drugs that normally are not absorbed from the gut. Such drugs might include enteric sulfonamides, neomycin, streptomycin, carbenicillin and some nitrofurans.

Another factor to consider is drug absorption in young ruminants. During the neonatal period the rumen is neither developed nor functional. Consequently, in terms of drug absorption the immature ruminant functions more like a monogastric than a ruminant animal. Drugs will be more efficiently absorbed following oral administration than would be expected for a mature ruminant. Therefore, one must not take a usual oral dose of a drug suggested for a mature ox, sheep or goat and simply adjust it on the basis of weight for a calf, lamb or kid. It would be more reasonable to employ a dose equivalent to that recommended for a monogastric species.

Distribution of Drugs in the Body

The problem of increased blood-brain barrier permeability has already been discussed. Drugs that are normally excluded from the brain of older animals will permeate the brain of the neonate and should be used with care.

Body water is another feature of the very young animal that is important to drug distribution. At birth, water constitutes a higher percentage of the body weight than it does later in infancy. Furthermore, at this time the extracellular fluid volume is greater than the intracellular volume. This will affect the blood concentrations of drugs that are distributed in the extracellular space. For example, it was found that blood concentrations of salicylate (at a given dosage rate) were lowest in the newborn and increased throughout the first 4 to 6 weeks of life.[7] This corresponded to the relative decrease in extracellular fluid volume during the same period. Thus, if penicillin were administered at the rate of 10,000 units per pound to a 5-day-old foal, the plasma concentration would be expected to be less than for a yearling at the same dosage rate.

Biotransformation

Probably the greatest single factor altering pharmacokinetics during the neonatal period is the deficiency of enzymes responsible for the biotransformation of foreign chemicals. These enzymes convert lipid-soluble drugs to metabolites, which are more water-soluble and hence more easily excreted by the kidneys.

Enzymes that catalyze the oxidation and conjugation of drugs are associated with the smooth endoplasmic reticulum of hepatocytes. An enzyme, cytochrome P450, mediates the hydroxylation of many drugs. Drugs representing several pathways of metabolism were studied in homogenates of livers obtained from piglets from 2 weeks' prepartum through 6 weeks postpartum.[14] It was found that at birth these hepatic tissues were unable to metabolize most all of the drugs studied and were almost totally deficient in cytochrome P450. Drug-metabolizing enzymes developed rapidly and by 30 days of age the liver homog-enates metabolized drugs at about the same rate as adult tissue. Because of this phenomenon, the lethal dose of barbiturates is much lower in animals during the neonatal period, and neonates will sleep much longer than older animals even when given lower dosages.

Similar results were obtained when the duration of blood levels of salicylate was studied in foals, kids, piglets and puppies as a function of age.[7] Drug concentrations declined slowly in the blood of newborn animals, and elimination became more rapid at 1, 2 and 3 weeks of age. By 30 days of age the rates of elimination approximated those observed in adult animals of the same species. On the basis of these studies, one must modify dosage regimens during the first month of life, but thereafter the young animals may be treated by the same regimens employed in an adult of the same species.

Excretion

Renal function is deficient at birth and develops during the first 1 or 2 months of life. There appear to be species differences in the degree of maturity of the kidneys at birth. Equine and ruminant animals have considerable excretory competence at birth, whereas puppies and kittens are quite deficient in this function. Deficiencies in tubular secretory mechanism or glomerular filtration would decrease the rate of elimination of drugs from the body.

Drug Excretion into Maternal Milk

The excretion of drugs into maternal milk is important within the present context because of the potential effects on nursing offspring. Many substances are secreted or diffuse from the maternal blood into the milk of lactating animals. Concentrations of foreign chemical in milk can attain relatively high values shortly after administration to the dam. A number of drugs and pesticides that are readily excreted into the milk have been studied and are listed in Table 4. One can thus see the diversity of substances to which offspring might be exposed while nursing.

Rasmussen[13] in Denmark has conducted extensive investigations of mammary excretion and absorption of drugs. The princi-

TABLE 4. *Some Drugs and Pesticides Excreted into Maternal Milk**

Class	Compound Studied	Class	Compound Studied
Alkaloids	Atropine	Hormones	Stilbestrol
	Colchicine		Estradiol
	Ergot		Progesterone
	Morphine		
	Nicotine	Inorganic ions	Arsenic
	Pilocarpine		Bismuth
	Strychnine		Copper
	Theobromine		Iron
			Mercury
Anthelmintics	Hexachloroethane		Manganese
	Phenothiazine		Lead
	Tetrachloroethylene		Antimony
	Thiabendazole		Selenium
			Zinc
Cathartics	Aloe		Bromine
	Cascara sagrada		Iodine
	Danthron		
	Ricinoleic acid (castor oil)	Miscellaneous drugs	Aspirin
			Boric acid
Antibiotics	Cephaloridine		Ethanol
	Chloramphenicol		Ethyl ether
	Chlorotetracycline		Urea
	Cycloserine		Chloral hydrate
	Dihydrostreptomycin		Chloroform
	Erythromycin		Chlorpromazine
	Kanamycin		Caffeine
	Lincomycin		Methenamine
	Neomycin		Phenacetin
	Novobiocin		Phenylbutazone
	Oxacillin		Phenytoin
	Oxytetracycline		Warfarin
	Penicillin		
	Spiramycin	Chlorinated	Aldrin
	Streptomycin	hydrocarbon	Chlordane
	Tetracycline	insecticides	DDT
			Endrin
Antihistaminics	Antazoline		Dieldrin
	Diphenhydramine		Heptachlor
	Methapyrilene		Lindane
			Methoxychlor
Barbiturates	Barbital		Toxaphene
	Pentobarbital		
	Phenobarbital	Organophosphorous	Coumaphos
		insecticides	Diazinon
Chemotherapeutics	Dapsone		Malathion
	Isoniazid		Parathion
	Nitrofurans		Ronnel
	Pyrimethamine		Ruelene
	Sulfonamides		Trichlorfon
	Trimethoprim		
Diuretics	Bendroflumethiazide		
	Furosemide		

*Modified from Rasmussen, F.: Studies on the Mammary Excretion and Absorption of Drugs, Copenhagen, Carl Fr. Mortensen, 1966.

ples of drug diffusion from blood into milk or in the reverse direction are the same as for other biological membranes. Lipid-soluble molecules diffuse across the epithelial membranes of the alveoli and reach equilibrium ratios between milk and blood. These ratios are determined by pH of the milk, protein binding and sequestration in butterfat. Generally, basic substances attain higher milk:plasma ratios than do acidic compounds. This is discussed in detail in reviews by Baggot[2] and Rasmussen.[13]

Ingestion of milk containing drugs, plant alkaloids or pesticides by nursing offspring can represent a real threat to the neonate for the reasons just indicated. Antimicrobial drugs can disturb the flora of the gut of suckling animals. Intoxication of the infants can occur in the absence of symptomatology in the dam. A classic example of this is the presence of bleeding tendencies in piglets nursed by a sow that has ingested warfarin.

GUIDELINES FOR THERAPY IN OBSTETRICS AND PEDIATRICS

The disposition of drugs and other foreign chemicals between the mother and fetus is complex and not well understood. The neonatal animal is a special therapeutic problem because of immaturity of systems essential for drug elimination and increased susceptibility to drug intoxication. Because of the many uncertainties imposed by these considerations, it would seem prudent to adopt a very conservative approach to the pregnant or neonatal patient. Astute assessment of benefit/risk considerations is particularly important under these circumstances, and drug therapy should not be instituted for trivial reasons. If at all possible, *avoid drug therapy* in patients under 30 days of age.

In many cases there probably is very little that we can do to avoid possible teratogenic effects of drugs because the most susceptible period of the embryo occurs at a time when signs of pregnancy may not be obvious in the dam. The practitioner should avoid use of drugs that are potentially teratogenic in patients following breeding. This will minimize the possibility of drug-induced deformity or fetal wastage.

Likewise, parsimony in the selection of

drugs for management of a patient during parturition will lessen problems associated with the postnatal care of the offspring. Drugs employed at this time should not require biotransformation for their elimination from the body.

When drug therapy is essential to save the life of a neonatal patient, try to select a drug that doesn't require metabolism. For example, tetracycline would be preferred to chloramphenicol. Remember also that the newborn animal is probably immunodeficient and therefore bactericidal drugs would be indicated. Because of increased risks of drug therapy during the first 2 to 3 weeks of life, particular care should be taken to identify the etiological agent in order to maximize the benefit/risk ratio. When employing chemotherapy in the neonate, the dosage regimen should be modified by increasing the interval between doses rather than decreasing the size of the dose in order to compensate for the slower rates of elimination.

Drugs that are known oxidants should be avoided in patients late in pregnancy and in neonates, as such compounds may produce hemolysis and methemoglobinemia. These include substances such as nitrites, nitrofurans, sulfonamides, acetaminophen, acetophenetidin, methylene blue, phenothiazines and antihistaminics.

REFERENCES

1. Almond, C.H., Boulos, B.M., Davis, L.E. and Mackenzie, J.W.: New surgical technique for studying placental transfer of drugs *in vivo*. J. Surg. Res., *10*:7, 1970
2. Baggot J.D.: Principles of Drug Disposition in Domestic Animals. Philadelphia, W.B. Saunders Co., 1977.
3. Boreus, L.O. (ed.): Fetal Pharmacology. New York, Raven Press, 1973.
4. Boulos, B.M, Davis, L.E., Almond, C.H. and Jackson, R.L.: Placental transfer of diazoxide and its hazardous effect on the newborn. J. Clin. Pharmacol., *11*:206, 1971.
5. Boulos, B.M., Davis, L.E., Larks, S.D., Larks, G.G., Sirtori, C.R. and Almond, C.H.: Placental transfer of chlorpromazine, pentobarbital, and phenylbutazone with fetal electrocardiographic changes as determined by direct lead tracing. Arch. Int. Pharmacodyn. Ther., *194*:403, 1971.
6. Davis, L.E.: Unpublished observations.
7. Davis, L.E., Westfall, B.A. and Short, C.R.: Biotransformation and pharmacokinetics of salicylate in newborn animals. Am. J. Vet. Res., *34*:1105, 1973.
8. Dawes, G.S.: Foetal and Neonatal Physiology. Chicago, Yearbook Medical Publishers, 1968, pp. 141–159.

9. Gillette, J.R. and Stripp, B.: Pre and postnatal enzyme capacity for drug metabolite production. Federation Proceedings., *34*:172, 1975.
10. Hamilton, W.J., Boyd, J.D. and Mossman, H.W.: Human Embryology. 3rd Ed., Baltimore, Williams & Wilkins, Chapt. XVI, 1962.
11. Hucker, H.B.: Species differences in drug metabolism. Ann. Rev. Pharmacol. Toxicol., 10:99 1970.
12. Krêcêk, J.: The theory of critical developmental periods and postnatal development of endocrine functions. *In* Tobach, E. (ed.): Biopsychology of Development, New York, Academic Press, 1971, pp. 233–247.
13. Rasmussen, F.: Studies on the Mammary Excre-
tion and Absorption of Drugs. Copenhagen, Carl Fr. Mortensen, 1966.
14. Short, C.R. and Davis, L.E.: Post-natal development of drug-metabolizing enzyme activity in swine. J. Pharmacol. Exp. Ther., *174*:185, 1970.
15. Stanton, H.C.: Factors to consider when selecting animal models for postnatal teratology studies. J. Environ. Pathol. Toxicol. 1978, *2*:201, 1978.
16. Stanton, H.C. and Woo, S.K.: Development of adrenal medullary function in swine. Am. J. Physiol., *234*:E137, 1978.
17. Wynn, R.M.: Morphology of the placenta. *In* Assali, N.S. (ed.): Biology of Gestation. Vol. 1, New York, Academic Press, 1968, pp. 93–181.

Some Interactions, Incompatibilities and Adverse Effects of Antimicrobial Drugs

RAMESH C. GARG and THOMAS E. POWERS

Ohio State University, Columbus, Ohio

Antimicrobial drugs are very commonly used in veterinary practice. They are used systemically as well as locally for controlling a variety of infections. Intrauterine use of these drugs may be indicated when pathogens are harbored in the genital tract of female animals. In addition, antibiotics have been infused in the uterus of farm animals to improve their breeding efficiency.[10] In view of such a wide use of antibiotics in treating various gynecological infections in animals, it is important for the veterinarian to weigh carefully the beneficial versus the possible adverse effects, if any, of these drugs. Although antibiotics are a relatively safe class of drugs, the following points need to be considered carefully before and during therapy with these drugs:

1. Identification of the pathogen or pathogens present in the uterus and/or other parts of the genital tract.
2. Effects of various estrous cycle stages on the efficacy of antimicrobial drugs.
3. Disposition of drugs after parenteral and intrauterine administration.
4. Incompatibility of antibacterial agents with one another and/or with other chemicals.
5. Interactions of antimicrobials with other drugs that are simultaneously administered or present in the body of the animal.
6. Antagonism and synergism in antimicrobial therapy.
7. Adverse effects of antimicrobial drugs, if any.

The first three considerations are discussed in detail in separate articles of this section. The present discussion will be limited to the remaining items listed.

INCOMPATIBILITY OF ANTIMICROBIAL DRUGS WITH OTHER DRUGS AND SUBSTANCES

When antimicrobial drugs are intended for intrauterine or intramammary infusion, there is a tendency to use more than one antimicrobial agent. Sometimes these drugs are even mixed in one syringe and administered as a single medication. This is probably done in an attempt to broaden the antibacterial spectrum of the drug and to increase effectiveness of therapy. However, in most cases, a combination of antimicrobial drugs is no more effective than its single most effective component. The antimicrobial agents often combined include penicillin, tetracycline, streptomycin, nitrofurans and sulfonamides. Substances used to make the drug into a solution or suspension form suitable for infusion may be normal saline, distilled water, 5 per cent Ringer's solution, 5 per cent dextrose saline solution, lactated Ringer's solution, polyethylene glycol and others. Although these seem to be inert substances, it is known that in certain cases they may result in a physical or chemical change in an active member of the drug combination.

Incompatibility is associated with physical or chemical change in the drug or drugs, rendering them inactive. In some cases, visible signs appear such as precipitation, colloidal formation, color changes or gas formation.[14] But many reactions that take place during *in vitro* mixing of two or more drugs are invisible. For example, certain sulfonamides and penicillins are incompatible because the high pH of sulfonamides inactivates the penicillins, whereas carbenicillin inactivates gentamicin and methicillin inactivates kanamycin without any visible change. Some important examples of incompatibilities that can be expected with mixing of drugs are presented in Table 1. Detailed general information on this subject is available in the reference text by Martin.[9] Soluble salts of penicillin G are relatively stable at a slightly acidic pH range, but these become unstable in dextrose saline solution because of high pH or extremely low pH (3.5 to 5.5).

Occurrence of such chemical incompatibilities can be reduced to a great extent by not mixing them in the same syringe or bottle. The different chemicals should be administered separately, preferably at a suitably spaced time interval.

ANTIMICROBIAL DRUG INTERACTIONS

As with other drugs, the interaction between two or more antimicrobial drugs may occur anywhere from the time of their administration until they are eliminated from the body. These interactions are conveniently divided into two categories: (1) pharmacokinetic interactions, in which one drug alters the disposition of another by modifying its absorption, distribution, metabolism or excretion and (2) pharmacodynamic interactions, which occur at the site of action. As this subject has not been investigated as thoroughly in animals as in human beings, much of the information is based on data from human studies.

Drug interactions can be expected when two such drugs are present within one formulation or when they are administered as separate preparations simultaneously or at fixed time intervals. When infections such as severe endometritis, pyometra or mastitis are associated with systemic changes and septicemia, parenteral routes of therapy may be indicated, and all types of interactions as just discussed could be expected. Factors such as protein binding in serum, hepatic and renal function, urine pH and dosage and route of administration may contribute to the clinical outcome of drug interaction. The drug interactions can result in one or more of the following: (1) increase in therapeutic efficacy, (2) decrease in therapeutic response, (3) increase in toxic and adverse effects or (4) decrease in toxic and adverse effects.

In addition to drug-drug interactions, the antimicrobial agents may interact with the biological material such as mucus, mucopurulent exudate and other matter present at the site of infection, such as in pyometra. Presence of pus and necrotic tissue may inactivate some antibiotics. In recent studies[4] purulent material has been shown to inactivate the aminoglycoside antibiotics. This is probably due to binding of drug to the nucleic acid debris and to acid proteins. Antibacterial activity of several antibiotics after oral administration is decreased by simultaneous intake of milk and dairy products owing to chelation by bivalent ions such as calcium. Also, the udder tissue homogenates were shown to bind large proportions of the aminoglycosides and polymyxins.[17]

Binding of the antimicrobial agents at the tissue site may render them inactive for killing the pathogen present. The binding effect of membranes upon polymyxin antibiotics and on polyene antifungals renders these agents inactive for practical purposes.

Factors other than plasma protein or tissue binding of these drugs that may lead to decreased antimicrobial activity are the pH, presence of purulent exudate, intracellular location of the pathogen and decreased blood flow to the affected area of the body. The aminoglycoside antibiotics are less active in an acid environment; this group of drugs is many times more active at a pH of 8 than at an acid pH. Thus, although these essentially nonprotein-bound agents may diffuse well into the areas of blood clot and uterine lochia, the conditions present in the

TABLE 1. *Some Antimicrobial Drug Incompatibilities of Veterinary Significance*

Antimicrobial Drug	Incompatible With
Amphotericin B	0.9% NaCl solution, tetracycline HCl, potassium penicillin G, nitrofurantoin
Ampicillin sodium	Don't use additive with other drugs
Bacitracin	Polyethylene glycols (inactivate it)
Carbenicillin	Gentamicin, erythromycin
Cephalothin sodium	Calcium chloride, calcium gluconate, colistimethate sodium, erythromycin gluceptate and lactobionate, kanamycin sulfate, polymyxin B sulfate, sodium or potassium penicillin G, tetracycline, vitamin B complex with ascorbic acid
Chloramphenicol sodium succinate	Extremes of pH, erythromycin glucoheptonate and lactobionate, hydrocortisone sodium succinate, novobiocin sodium, polymyxin B sulfate, procaine HCl, 25% sodium sulfadiazone, tetracyclines, Vancomycin HCl, vitamin B complex preparations
Kanamycin sulfate	Cephalothin sodium, colistimethate sodium, dextrose, hydrocortisone sodium succinate, methicillin sodium, nitrofurantoin sodium, sulfisoxazole
Methicillin	Kanamycin, 0.9% NaCl solution, tetracyclines
Methicillin sodium	Acid media, hydrocortisone sodium succinate, kanamycin sulfate, oxytetracycline HCl, sodium bicarbonate, tetracycline HCl, vancomycin HCl
Nitrofurantoin sodium	Ammonium chloride, amphotericin B, dextrose in lactated Ringer's solution, dextrose solutions containing ascorbic acid and vitamin B complex, calcium chloride, Polymyxin B sulfate, streptomycin sulfate, vitamin B complex with vitamin C in dextrose solutions
Novobiocin sodium	ACTH, ammonium chloride, calcium gluconate, chloramphenicol sodium, dextrose solutions, erythromycin glucoheptonate, hydrocortisone sodium acetate, lactated Ringer's solution, procaine HCl, streptomycin sulfate, tetracycline HCl, vancomycin HCl, vitamin B complex with ascorbic acid
Penicillins	5% dextrose with bicarbonate, sulfonamides
Penicillin G (sodium or potassium salt) buffered	Acid and alkaline media, amphotericin B, ascorbic acid, tetracyclines, vancomycin HCl
Polymyxin B sulfate	Cephalothin sodium, chloramphenicol sodium succinate, nitrofurantoin sodium, chlortetracycline HCl, prednisolone sodium phosphate, tetracycline HCl
Streptomycin sulfate	Calcium gluconate, erythromycin glucoheptonate, nitrofurantoin sodium, novobiocin sodium, sulfadiazine sodium, sulfisoxazole diolamine
Tetracycline HCl	Amphotericin B, calcium salts, cephalothin sodium, chloramphenicol sodium succinate, erythromycin glucoheptonate, hydrocortisone, methicillin, nitrofurantoin sodium, novobiocin sodium, penicillin G, polymyxin B, sodium bicarbonate, 5% sodium chloride, sulfadiazine sodium, sulfisoxazole, vitamin B complex
Tylosin	Tetracycline, streptomycin, sulfonamides

TABLE 2. *Antimicrobial Drug Interactions*

Antimicrobial Drug	Interactant Drug	Results In
Aminoglycosides	Curariform agents, methoxyflurane Calcium salts	Increased neuromuscular blockade Decreased neuromuscular blockade
Amphotericin B	Corticosteroids Digitalis glycosides	Increased K^+ depletion Increased K^+ depletion, digitalis toxicity
Chloramphenicol	Barbiturates Tolbutamide Dicumarol Phenytoin	Increased sleeping time Increased hypoglycemia Increased blood clotting time Decreased metabolism of phenytoin
Colistin	Cephalothin	Increase in renal toxicity of colistin
Doxycycline	Barbiturates	Increased breakdown of doxycycline
Erythromycin	Clindamycin Lincomycin Penicillin	Possible antagonism Possible antagonism Possible antagonism
Gentamicin	Cephalothin	Increased incidence of gentamicin renal toxicity
Griseofulvin	Cephalosporins Phenobarbital	Increased nephrotoxicity Decreased absorption of griseofulvin and potentiation of barbiturate
Neomycin	Digitalis glycosides Penicillin V	Decreased absorption of digitalis Decreased absorption of penicillin V
Nitrofurantoin	Antacids	Decreased absorption of nitrofurantoin
Penicillin	Neomycin Erythromycin and tetracycline	Decreased absorption of penicillin Possible antagonism
Polymyxin	Succinyl choline Tubocurarine	Increased neuromuscular blockade Increased neuromuscular blockade
Sulfonamide	Ammonium chloride Methanamine Antacids	Increased crystalluria Increased crystalluria Decreased absorption of sulfonamides

Tetracyclines	Methoxyflurane
	
	Iron salts
	Calcium salts
		Renal damage and prolonged
		  anesthesia
		Decreased absorption of
		  tetracycline

Trimethoprim	Thiazides or furosemide	Increased incidence of thrombocytopenia

infected uterus may significantly reduce the effectiveness of these antibiotics in destroying the coccal and enteric organisms.

Chloramphenicol, after oral administration to the adult ruminant, is inactivated in the rumen.[7] Some interactions of veterinary significance are listed in Table 2.[3, 6, 16]

In addition to direct interactions, some antibiotics and other antimicrobial agents can alter the values of various laboratory tests generally used to evaluate the clinical condition of animals. Several observations of this type derived mainly from human studies[11] are listed in Table 3. Antibiotics that inhibit protein synthesis may cause impaired synthesis of endogenous proteins, e.g., tetracyclines may interfere with prothrombin production. For more information, the reader is referred to reference texts by Martin[9] and by Aronson *et al.*

TABLE 3. *Effect of Antimicrobial Drugs on Laboratory Tests**

Drug	Laboratory Tests†	
Ampicillin	Increased:	SGOT, leukocyte count
	Decreased:	None
Chloramphenicol	Increased:	Alkaline phosphatase, bilirubin, SGOT, SGPT
	Decreased:	Erythrocyte, leukocyte and thrombocyte counts; urobilinogen
Erythromycin	Increased:	Alkaline phosphatase, bilirubin, prothrombin time, SGOT, SGPT, leukocyte count
	Decreased:	None
Neomycin	Increased:	BUN, urine casts, urine protein
	Decreased:	Cholesterol
Penicillin	Increased:	Alkaline phosphatase, Coombs' test, urine glucose, urine protein
	Decreased:	Erythrocyte and leukocyte counts
Sulfonamides	Increased:	Amino acids, bilirubin, SGOT, leukocyte count, prothrombin time, urine crystals, brownish urine, urine glucose, urine protein, urine erythrocytes
	Decreased:	Protein-bound iodine, erythrocyte and thrombocyte counts
Tetracyclines	Increased:	BUN, phosphate, coagulation time, leukocyte count, prothrombin time, urine glucose, urine protein
	Decreased:	Calcium, potassium

*Adapted from Paul, J. W.: Proceedings 10th Annual Convention, American Association of Bovine Practitioners, 1977.

†Abbreviations: SGOT = serum glutamic-oxaloacetic transaminase, SGPT = serum glutamic-pyruvic transaminase, BUN = blood urea nitrogen.

SYNERGISM AND ANTAGONISM IN ANTIBACTERIAL DRUG COMBINATIONS

Synergism is defined as the supra-additive effect when two drugs are administered in combination. Jawetz[8] described in detail the mechanisms of synergism that are observed in antimicrobial drugs. The most clearly understood example is the synergism between sulfonamides and trimethoprim, a diaminopyrimidine compound (Fig. 1). Both of these compounds block sequentially at two different steps in the same metabolic pathway leading to the synthesis of folinic acid, which is needed by the bacteria for its growth and survival.

Sulfonamides, because of structural resemblance, competitively block the incorporation of para-aminobenzoic acid (PABA) in the folic acid molecule. Trimethoprim blocks the next step leading to the formation of folinic acid by inhibiting the folate reductase enzyme.[5] The synergism results in changing the bacteriostatic effect of these drugs to a bactericidal effect.

Synergistic response is also seen when two drugs with distinctly different modes of action are combined. Penicillins, which cause the disruption of the cell wall, increase the bactericidal rate when combined with antibiotics that act intracellularly, such as aminoglycosides. Drugs such as methicillin increase bactericidal activity when combined with penicillins by inactivating a beta lactamase enzyme produced by some organisms that is capable of inactivating penicillins.

Antagonism can be said to occur when the combined effect is less than that of the single most effective drug of the combination.

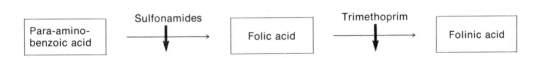

Figure 1. Synergism between sulfonamides and trimethoprim.

Chloramphenicol and tetracyclines are considered to antagonize penicillins and aminoglycosides. Other examples of antagonism include: (1) the simultaneous use of lincomycin and erythromycin results in decreased antibacterial activity and (2) local anesthetics (procaine and its derivatives) and para-aminobenzoic acid when given simultaneously with sulfonamides will result in inhibition of the activity of the sulfonamide. Synergism and/or antagonism of antimicrobial drug combinations is dependent on the species and strain of organisms as well as the concentration and specific drugs involved. Two drugs may be synergistic against one strain and antagonistic against another strain of organism.[12]

ADVERSE EFFECTS OF ANTIMICROBIAL DRUGS

Although antibiotics are considered relatively safe drugs, Stowe et al.,[15] based on reports from practicing veterinarians, have reported various adverse effects of antimicrobial drugs in animals. Polymyxins have been reported to be nephrotoxic after systemic administration. Oxytetracycline solutions given intrauterinely for control of uterine infection produced severe irritation of the endometrium. Uterine biopsies showed the presence of edema and superficial endometrial necrosis.[13] Tetracycline and aminoglycoside antibiotics can induce neuromuscular blocking effects. These cause inhibition of calcium and competitively block the skeletal muscle receptors.[1] Tetracyclines, by interacting with calcium, can also lead to hypotension and decreased cardiac output. The aminoglycosides can cause ototoxicity, nephrotoxicity and curariform types of neuromuscular paralysis. These toxicities may be enhanced when used in combination with other drugs such as (1) furosemide, which produces an increased incidence in nephrotoxicity, and (2) anesthetics and analgesics, which cause an increased incidence in neuromuscular paralysis.

CONCLUSION

To avoid most of the adverse antimicrobial drug reactions, it is suggested that selection of antibiotics be done with due consideration of the most probable etiological agent or agents. Personal formulary should be avoided, and a minimal number of drugs should be administered to the animal at one time.

It would appear that drug interactions and incompatibilities are very likely to occur when one practices polypharmacy. For this reason, it is proposed that, as far as possible, one should not mix two or more drug solutions unless their compatibility is known. Likewise, the administration of two or more drugs simultaneously to treat animals should be avoided except when required, and then one should use only those combinations in which an adverse drug interaction is not expected.

More knowledge regarding this area of clinical pharmacology is needed. The veterinarian should constantly be aware of the documented potential problems and very observant for possible new adverse responses.

REFERENCES

1. Adams, H. R.: Acute adverse effects of antibiotics. J.A.V.M.A., *166*:983, 1975.
2. Aronson, C. E., Powers, T. E., and Shiedy, S. F.: *In* The Complete Desk Reference of Veterinary Pharmaceuticals and Biologicals 78/79. Media, Pa., Harwell Publishing Co., 1978.
3. Braude, A. I.: Antimicrobial Drug Therapy. Vol. VIII, Philadelphia, W. B. Saunders Co., 1976, p. 139.
4. Bryant, R. E., and Hammond, D.: Interaction of purulent material with antibiotics used to treat *Pseudomonas aeruginosa* infections. Antimicrob. Agts. Chemother., 6:702, 1974.
5. Bushby, S.: Biochemical basis of chemotherapy and bacteriology concepts of trimethoprim-sulfonamide combinations. Proceedings of Symposium on Trimethoprim/Sulfonamide. Burroughs Wellcome Co., Research Triangle Park, N. C., 1978, pp. 4–15.
6. Davis, L. E.: Important interactions of antibiotic drugs. Clin. Pharm. Newsletter, *1*:1, 1975.
7. Davis, L. E., and Jenkin, W. L.: Some considerations regarding drug therapy in ruminant animals. Bovine Pract., 9:57, 1974.
8. Jawetz, E.: Actions of antimicrobial drugs in combinations. Vet. Clin. N. Am., 5:35, 1975.
9. Martin, E. W.: Hazards of Medication. Philadelphia, J. B. Lippincott Co., 1972.
10. Oxender, W. D., and Seguin, B. E.: Bovine intrauterine therapy. J.A.V.M.A., *168*:217, 1976.
11. Paul, J. W.: Clinical considerations regarding drug interactions in the bovine patient. Proceedings 10th Annual Convention, American Association of Bovine Practitioners, 1977, pp. 10–14.
12. Powers, T. E.: Pharmacological rationale for using trimethoprim-sulfonamide combinations. Proceedings of Symposium on Trimethoprim/Sulfonamide. Burroughs Wellcome Co., Research Triangle Park, N.C., pp. 50–54.

13. Seguin, B. E., Morrow, D. A., and Oxender, W. D.: Intrauterine therapy in the cow. J.A.V.M.A., *164*:609, 1974.
14. Stowe, C. M.: Indications, compatibilities and incompatibilities of antibiotics and sulfonamides. Proceedings, Drug Usage by Practitioners, Iowa State Univ., Ames, Iowa, 1976.
15. Stowe, C. M., Farnsworth, R., Hardy, R., Klausner, J., Larson, V. L. and Werdin, R. E.: Adverse drug reactions. *In* Kirk, R. W. (ed.): Current Veterinary Therapy VI, Small Animal Practice, Philadelphia, W. B. Saunders Co., 1977, pp. 153–160.
16. Teske, R. H., and Carter, G. G.: Effect of chloramphenicol on pentobarbital induced anesthesia in dogs. J.A.V.M.A., *159*:77, 1971.
17. Ziv, G., Gordin, S., Bechar, G., and Bernstein, S.: Binding of antibiotics to dry udder secretion and to udder tissue homogenates. Br. Vet. J. *132*:318, 1976.

Problems of Drug Residues in Animals

RICHARD TESKE

Food and Drug Administration, Beltsville, Maryland

INTRODUCTION

The use of drugs in food-producing animals therapeutically and in controlling diseases, as well as in increasing the efficiency of production and improving the quality of food products derived from animals, is considered essential in modern animal agriculture. In 1975 the animal health industry in the United States represented a sales volume at the manufacturer level in excess of 1 billion dollars. Feed additive products (other than nutritional feed additives) represent a sales volume in excess of 200 million dollars. This use is, of course, accompanied by the risk that residues (of parent compound and/or metabolic products thereof) may occur in edible products derived from animals.

REGULATION OF FOOD ADDITIVES

Responsibility for the regulation of new animal drugs and medicated feeds originated under the new drug provisions of the Federal Food, Drug and Cosmetic Act of 1938. At that time provisions of the Act enabled the Food and Drug Administration (FDA) to prevent the marketing of new animal drugs until their safety in the animal species for which they were recommended had been demonstrated. It was not until enactment of the Food Additives Amendment in 1958 that drug residues in food products derived from animals came under regulation. Under the Food Additives Amendment, animal drugs that cause residues in edible products are classified as food additives. Section 402 of the Act as amended provides that food products are considered to be adulterated if they contain residues of a new animal drug, or of a metabolite or degradation product thereof, which is unsafe as defined under Section 512. New Drugs are "unsafe" for a particular use unless there is, in effect, an approved New Animal Drug Application.

Approval of a New Animal Drug Application under Section 512 may include establishment of tolerances and/or withdrawal periods or other use restrictions required in order to assure that the proposed use of the drug will be safe with respect to residues in edible products. First of all the drug itself must be thoroughly characterized, as follows:

1. *Identification of the drug.* The sponsor must establish the identity of the drug, including common name; chemical name following nomenclature of chemical abstracts; other names in use, including trade names; empirical and structural (if known or proposed) formulas; and molecular weight.

2. *Definition and description of the drug.* The sponsor must provide a complete description of the drug, including a description of physical characteristics (physical state, color, odor, taste); a description of the manufacturing process, including a list of all substances used together with specifications; and the equations of all chemical reactions involved. Any production controls and stability data employed to assure a reproducible product and quality control measure-

ments should be described. The vehicle and any and all excipients and inert ingredients must also be listed and defined.

3. *Physical, chemical and/or biological properties.* The sponsor must provide data on the stability of the drug as well as appropriate information concerning other physical and chemical properties such as melting point, boiling point, solubility, specific gravity, refractive index, viscosity, optical rotation, pH, absorption spectra and fluorescence spectra. Also required is information on biological activity, including active sites on the molecule.

Requirements for Establishment of Drug Withdrawal Periods

The methods and procedures involved in establishment of a drug withdrawal period in food-producing animals are extensive and quite complex. A firm wishing to market a drug for use in food animals must prove that the drug and/or its metabolites will not cause harmful or potentially harmful residues or that any residues that do occur during treatment will be reduced to acceptable levels (as established by approval of a tolerance) or eliminated upon withdrawal of the drug. The primary questions that must be answered with respect to a given drug are:

1. What are the residues and in what amounts do they occur in edible products?

2. What is the tissue residue pattern during the depletion phase following drug withdrawal?

3. What potential adverse effects may be expected to occur as a result of exposure to these residues?

Metabolism in the Target Species

It is obvious that the answers to the first question can be obtained only by conducting careful and thorough metabolism studies in the animal species in which it is to be used. The objective of such studies is to describe the metabolism of the drug, to identify metabolites and biotransformation products and to determine the distribution of parent compound and metabolites in all edible products. Use of radiolabeled chemicals may be preferred for such studies in order to achieve adequate specificity and sensitivity. In using radiolabeled chemicals, care must be exercised in the choice of label position to insure that it is adequate to follow those

chemical moieties that are of toxicological interest and provide adequate specific activity to determine residue patterns at low levels. Thus, in labeling a compound such as sulfamethazine with ^{14}C, the most desirable location for the label would be in the benzene ring.

The purity and stability of the label are also of critical concern in such studies. For example, carbon 14 is often preferred as a label because of its stability, but limitations with respect to specific activity frequently restrict its use. With tritium, however, high levels of specific activity can be obtained, but unless the label is stable within the molecule, as it is for example with prednisolone 6,7^{3}H, exchange with water may occur. Purity of the labeled compound can pose similar problems in that contamination of the labeled compound with unreacted isotope can result in misleading or false information. For example, free ^{131}I that is present as a contaminant with a compound labeled with ^{131}I will be selectively taken up by the thyroid, leading to the conclusion that the thyroid contains residues of either the parent compound or a biotransformation product.

Application of Pharmacokinetics to the Drug Residue Problem

Development of drug residue data is one of the single most costly steps both in time and resources in drug development for food animals. Pharmacokinetic concepts could be utilized effectively both to extend and to improve the quality of data achieved in conventional drug residue protocols.[2]

First, what are some of the potential deficiencies that may result from relying on conventional methods alone? To begin with, conventional methods require extensive manpower and resource expenditures (residue extraction from tissue is a tedious and time-consuming procedure) and provide data applicable only to the particular dose, formulation, treatment regimen and test conditions used in the study. Within usual therapeutic dosage ranges, the depletion pattern for lower doses of a drug will comply with a withdrawal period established for a higher dose. However, the depletion pattern following higher doses will not necessarily comply with withdrawal periods established for lower doses. Furthermore, depletion patterns established for one route of administration or one drug formulation will not necessarily comply with withdrawal periods established for other routes of administration or other drug formulations. Also, there is frequently considerable animal-to-animal variation in residue tissue levels and excretion patterns. Conventional methods, however, often fail to allow for a critical evaluation of such variation. Furthermore, studies conducted by conventional methods generally add little to the data base concerning the behavior of a given drug in the system, that is, absorption and elimination rates and extent of distribution. In the absence of such information, the therapeutic regimens recommended for many veterinary drugs have been established on the basis of assumptions based on extrapolated data. For example, although much is known about the effects of sulfonamides in experimental animals and humans, relatively little is known about their effects in domestic animals. Of course, many sulfonamide drugs were introduced into veterinary therapeutics prior to 1958. At that time requirements for residue and safety data were minimal and generally inadequate by today's standards. Applications of sulfonamide drugs in veterinary medicine were generally based on information generated on laboratory animals and on accepted principles of sulfonamide activity rather than on controlled studies defining time-dose-effect relationships for commercial dosage forms in target species.

Finally, the drug withdrawal period that is based on data from conventional studies may be biased by the performance of animals in the experiment that are atypical with respect to their metabolic capacity for handling the drug. Clearly, there are a number of areas in which the data derived from conventional drug residue studies alone may be inadequate. Pharmacokinetic studies, when used as an adjunct to conventional studies, can provide additional data and also contribute significantly to the interpretation of conventional data.

Establishment of Tolerances

The degree of toxicity testing required, the residue compounds to be examined and the selection of animal species to be employed in the studies are determined by the data base available. If residues occur at levels above 0.1 parts per million (ppm) under conditions of proposed use, including the proposed withdrawal time, finite tolerances must be established. The following studies are required to provide a basis for establishment of finite tolerances.

1. A lifetime feeding study in a rodent species (usually the rat).
2. A three-generation reproduction study (may be conducted with the lifetime feeding study).
3. A feeding study in a nonrodent species (usually the dog), 6 months or longer in duration.
4. Teratological studies in two or more species.

Those compounds that are suspected carcinogens require a lifetime feeding study in a second rodent species (usually the mouse). A finite tolerance can be established only for those compounds that are negative with respect to carcinogenesis. The tolerance is determined by applying a safety factor (usually at least 1:100) to the "no-effect" level demonstrated in the most sensitive species tested. The "no-effect" level is defined as the highest dosage level tested that resulted in no deleterious biological effects.

Negligible Tolerance

Drugs that are used therapeutically (as opposed to chemicals such as growth promotants that are used on a continuous basis in large segments of the food animal population) or are used only in very young animals pose less potential for sustained exposure of humans to residues. Such drugs may qualify for establishment of a "negligible tolerance" based on 90-day toxicity studies conducted in one rodent and one nonrodent species. A "negligible tolerance" may not exceed 0.1 ppm in tissue or 0.01 ppm in milk and is determined by applying a safety factor of 2000 to the "no-effect" level demonstrated in the 90-day toxicity studies.

Carcinogens and the Delaney Clause

Section 409 of the Federal Food, Drug and Cosmetic Act establishes criteria and prescribes procedures for the approval of food additives that have been shown to be safe. The Delaney Clause of Section 409, enacted in 1958, flatly prohibits the approval of any additive that "is found to induce cancer when ingested by man or animal or if it is found, after tests which are appropriate for the evaluation of safety of food additives, to induce cancer in man or animal." Prior to 1962 the anticancer clause of Section 409 did not distinguish between compounds added directly to human food and compounds that might indirectly enter human food following administration, as feed additives or drugs, to food-producing animals. The act was interpreted as forbidding the FDA to approve the use of a carcinogenic animal drug whether or not such a compound might leave any residues in the edible tissues of the animal. In 1962, the United States Congress, as part of the Drug Amendments of 1962, modified Section 409, focusing on the likelihood that a compound would produce detectable residues. Section 409 was modified to provide that the proviso prohibiting approval of carcinogens shall not apply with respect to the use of a substance as an ingredient of feed for animals that are raised for food production if the Secretary of HEW finds that no residue of the additive will be found (by methods of examination prescribed or approved by the Secretary by regulations) in any edible portion of such animal after slaughter or in any food yielded by or derived from the living animal. Until March 23, 1977, the sensitivity of methods prescribed by the Secretary to demonstrate that edible products derived from animals treated with carcinogenic compounds will be free from residues was determined primarily by what could be achieved given the current "state-of-the-art" in analytical chemistry. Effective March 23, 1977, new regulations specifying the criteria and procedures to be used in evaluating assay methods for carcinogenic

residues in food-producing animals were promulgated. These procedures define the methods that are to be used in establishing "safe" levels of exposure. The methods involve estimation of theoretical upper limits of risk from a theoretical exposure based on extrapolation from a real dose-response curve in an appropriate laboratory animal species. Thus, the lower limit of sensitivity required for the assay method to assure that no residues occur in food products is determined.

These regulations were revoked by the commissions on May 26, 1978, because of administrative omissions in the record. The statement of revocation indicated the Agency's intent to repropose these regulations.

REFERENCES

1. Food and Drug Administration: Contracts 70-204 and 71-69, University of Illinois, Department of Veterinary Pharmacology, College of Veterinary Medicine, Urbana, Illinois, 1970–1974.
2. Mercer, H. D., Baggot, J. D. and Sams, R. A.: Application of pharmacokinetic methods to the drug residue profile. J. Toxicol. Environ. Health, 2:787, 1977.
3. Pilloud, M.: Pharmacokinetics, plasma protein binding and dosage of oxytetracycline in cattle and horses. Res. Vet. Sci., 15:224, 1973.
4. Ziv, G., Shani, J. and Sulman, F. G.: Pharmacokinetic evaluation of penicillin and cephalosporin derivatives in serum and milk of lactating cows and ewes. Am. J. Vet. Res., 34:1561, 1973.

EMBRYO TRANSFER

Consulting Editor

K. J. BETTERIDGE

Introduction to Embryo Transfer in Farm Animals

K. J. BETTERIDGE

Agriculture Canada, Animal Diseases Research Institute (Eastern), Ottawa, Ontario, Canada

Embryo transfer is the process by which embryos are collected from one female (the donor) before they have become attached to her uterus and are transferred to other females (recipients) to complete their gestation. The aim of this section is to describe embryo transfer sufficiently to provide veterinary practitioners, students or research workers with:

1. Familiarity with the advantages and disadvantages of the procedure that will help them to advise clients.

2. Information of use in deciding whether or not to become more involved with embryo transfer.

3. A preliminary manual of techniques for those who do become involved.

It should be understood at the outset that the provision of a proper embryo transfer service to clients is too demanding to be a part-time occupation. Thus the reader seeking information with which to advise clients can use this section as a basis for consultation with colleagues in embryo transfer organizations who might do the work. Those who elect to become involved in providing an embryo transfer service can use the procedures described as a base upon which to build their own modifications and improvements, but further involvement will require further reading. A review of the literature on which this section is based can be found in the three monographs listed at the end of this article.[5, 6, 7]

Embryo transfer in laboratory species will not be considered in this section, but the procedure has been reviewed by Chang and Pickworth.[1] Embryo collection and transfer in nonhuman primates has been described by Kraemer *et al.*,[3] Hurst *et al.*[2] and Marston *et al.*[4]

TERMINOLOGY

It may be helpful to recapitulate some embryological terms used in this section. An oocyte or *ovum* or *egg* is shed from the graafian follicle in the ovary. It and the spermatozoon that fertilizes it in the fallopian tube (or oviduct) are *gametes* that unite to form a *zygote* or fertilized ovum. Cleavage into *blastomeres* proceeds until these cells are too numerous to count, at which stage they form a ball called a *morula.* Further development leads to *blastulation,* or the formation of a cavity, the *blastocoele,* within the ball, which then becomes an early *blastocyst.* At one pole of the blastocyst is the *inner cell mass,* a clump of cells that will give rise to the embryo proper. The remaining wall of the blastocyst, the *trophoblast,* forms the embryonic membranes. With expansion, the blastocyst hatches from the *zona pellucida* and enlarges to a *blastodermic vesicle* on which the *embryonic disc* is visible as the development of the inner cell mass.

For simplicity, the term "embryo" will be used synonymously with the terms "fertilized egg," "fertilized ovum," "morula," "blastocyst" and "blastodermic vesicle" and to differentiate these from unfertilized eggs.

"Transfer" has been preferred to "transplantation" because the latter term can imply procedures used in organ transplantation.

HISTORY OF EMBRYO TRANSFER

Walter Heape performed the first embryo transfer (between rabbits) in 1890 at Cambridge University. It was 40 years before others began similar work, with sporadic attempts at perfecting transfer techniques in laboratory animals in the 1930's. The earliest attempts at transfers in farm animals were rewarding, success being achieved in sheep and goats as early as 1932.

The war years curtailed progress and it was not until the 1950's that further advances were made. The first successful transfers in pigs and cattle were reported in 1951 from the Soviet Union and the United States, respectively. In the following year, an indication of the potential of the technique was implicit in a report of successful long-distance transportation of rabbit embryos by air. The 1950's also saw the development, principally at Cambridge, of techniques in sheep that produced consistently satisfactory results, and by 1961 it was shown to be possible to transport sheep embryos successfully from Britain to South Africa, using a rabbit to incubate the embryos in her fallopian tube.

During the 1960's, some success with nonsurgical collection and transfer methods in cattle, sheep and goats was achieved. The value of the surgical technique as a research tool was firmly established by workers who used it in investigating the interrelationships of the embryo, uterus and ovary in early pregnancy in sheep and pigs. In 1969, the possibility of transporting pig embryos internationally in test tubes was demonstrated. In the same year, Rowson and his colleagues at Cambridge described surgical techniques in cattle that produced excellent pregnancy rates and were to be the tools of the trade during the boom of commercial interest in embryo transfer in cattle during the first half of the 1970's.

The commercial boom of the early 1970's was occasioned by the profitability of proliferating "exotic" (European) breeds of cattle that were being admitted in limited numbers through quarantine into North America and, via Great Britain, into New Zealand and thence to Australia. Directly and indirectly, the boom has had considerable impact on progress in developing transfer techniques and has made it possible to appraise the advantages and limitations of embryo transfer under more extensive conditions that were possible before. Exportation of bovine embryos of one breed, in recipients of another, was described in 1972. Four years later, commercial exportation of bovine embryos in test tubes began. Following the development of successful freezing techniques for mouse eggs, calves and lambs were also obtained from frozen embryos in 1973 and 1974. The first successful transfers of horse embryos were also reported in 1974 and the first international transportation of horse embryos (again using a rabbit as an incubator) in 1976. Also in 1976, nonsurgical collection and transfer techniques in cattle began to yield results similar to those achieved surgically, and, in the same year, the possibility of sexing bovine embryos before transfer was demonstrated. The first successful transfer of a nonhuman primate embryo was reported in 1975.

APPLICATIONS OF EMBRYO TRANSFER

Proliferating Desirable Genotypes

This, the most obvious direct application of embryo transfer to animal production, usually involves superovulating the donor female in order to increase the number of embryos available for transfer, especially in monotocous species. However, proliferation may also be accomplished by repeatedly collecting single embryos during successive cycles in untreated donors. Commercial embryo transfer companies depended on this application for rapid proliferation of "exotic" breeds of cattle, as previously mentioned. These beef breeds were in high demand because of their reputed performance and their market value. The latter was inflated by costs of importation coupled with a scarcity resulting from the limited numbers that could be brought in through the necessary quarantine stations. For a time, the market could bear the high costs of using embryo transfer to this end. Embryo transfer has also been used in several countries to proliferate particular breeds or strains of sheep. Australian workers, for example, used it to produce 277 lambs from 86 polled Merino ewes.

Genetic Improvement

The genetic gains that may be made by embryo transfer have often been exaggerated but have been reviewed in perspective by R. B. Land (in Monograph 1).[5] In developing countries, transfer techniques offer the possibility of immediate breed substitution by the use of indigenous females as recipients of imported embryos.

In cattle breed improvement programs in developed countries, embryo transfer could be used to increase the reproductive rate of females and thence the intensity of selection among them. It has been shown that the production of about six offspring per donor could double selection intensity and the rate of response to genetic selection for traits, such as growth, that can be measured in both sexes. This would be especially worthwhile in improving elite herds from which the gain could be spread over a large population by the use of artificial insemination (AI). Although intensity of selection for sex limited traits such as milk yield could also be increased by embryo transfer, it is generally concluded that the gains would be marginal and certainly less than could be achieved by optimizing selection schemes using conventional reproduction.

Progeny testing of donor females could be made feasible by the use of embryo transfer and could increase the accuracy of female selections, but, again, it is felt that this would add little to the easier progeny testing of males in large-scale breeding programs and, in any case, would be beset by the problem of unreliable yields of progeny from individual cows.

Selection for twinning should be possible using embryo transfer, but progress would be slow and subject to limitations to be discussed next. Selection for twinning may be merited in beef cattle but not in dairy herds, in which selection should continue to be concentrated on milk production.

Future technical developments should reduce costs but are unlikely to lead to big improvements in the *rate* of genetic gain. The availability of large numbers of embryos from elite cows would, however, increase the average genetic merit for the population over which it can be spread.

With improved preservation techniques, it should be possible to use frozen embryos for genetic controls because improved animals could be assessed by contemporary comparison with preserved representatives of the foundation stock. Freezing would also facilitate the establishment of gene banks, e. g., by preserving embryos of declining breeds.

Twinning in Cattle

Embryo transfer is being intensively evaluated as an alternative to genetic selection or gonadotropin treatment for increasing beef production by twinning. It has the considerable advantage of allowing the location of the embryos to be controlled. This is important because the capacity of a single uterine horn to support twin pregnancy is very limited, and embryos rarely migrate from one horn to the other in the cow's uterus. Thus, to achieve twin pregnancy reliably, it is preferable to place the two embryos in different horns. This is readily accomplished with transferred embryos but will occur only by chance (i.e., in 50 per cent of cases) in cattle that ovulate the two eggs themselves.

Nonsurgical techniques can now be used to induce twinning, either by transfer of two embryos to unmated recipients or by transfer of an additional embryo to mated recipients, taking care to introduce it into the horn contralateral to the recipients' own ovulation. Though may producers feel that twinning in cattle brings more problems than profit, Sreenan (in Monograph 1)[5] has pointed out that the problems (retained placenta, calf mortality, impaired production and reduced fertility in the dam) occur mainly in cows managed as though they were carrying singletons. If it is known which cows are carrying twins, it seems that proper management (particularly adequate nutrition) largely prevents the problems.

Freemartinism, which makes twinning a poor method of producing breeding stock or dairy cattle, is of little consequence to beef production. The technique of sexing embryos before transfer (see Section IV) makes it possible to avoid freemartinism, thus providing a further advantage of embryo transfer over alternative methods of inducing twinning. The desirability of inducing twinning by embryo transfer therefore depends principally on economics, discussed by Bowen later in this section.

Import and Export

As indicated in the historical context just discussed, the feasibility of moving livestock internationally as embryos is well established. Improving techniques for maintaining embryos in culture and for preserving them by freezing will certainly lead to an extension of this application, when the necessary expertise exists at the place of origin and at the destination.

The possibility of inadvertently transmitting disease along with the embryos raises important issues as far as animal health regulations are concerned. The likelihood of this occurring has not yet been properly evaluated, but it will certainly vary from disease to disease. Thus, on the one hand, mouse embryos can evidently be taken from a cytomegalovirus-infected uterus and develop normally in an *in vitro* culture system, probably being uninfected. On the other hand, some viruses have been shown both to penetrate the early embryo through the zona pellucida and to be introduced into the zygote via the spermatozoon in rabbits and mice.

Bacterium-like particles have also been found in early rat blastocysts. It is probable that a large proportion of such early infections are self-limiting as a result of embryonic death. Nevertheless, there is a danger that these embryos could survive, become tolerant of the infection and spread it to others after birth. Other viruses have been shown to be vertically transmitted in mice.

These facts have to be borne in mind by authorities faced with regulating a new form of international livestock trade. More work on the hazards of disease transmission is needed, but, in the interim, it would seem prudent to treat the importation of embryos with the same precautions that are required for "normal" animals from that particular country. Usually this would include health certification of sires, dams and perhaps their herds of origin, together with quarantine of recipients, if appropriate. Quarantined recipients would also serve as test animals for any transmissible disease associated with the embryos. Eventually, it may be possible to treat frozen embryos like frozen semen, holding them long enough before transfer to insure that their sires and dams were not incubating disease at the time of collection.

Disease Control

This application of embryo transfer might seem paradoxical, considering the preceding paragraphs. However, embryo transfer has proved a safe way of introducing new bloodlines into specific–pathogen-free pig herds, presumably because the specific pathogens in question are not carried by the embryos or the uterine flushes in which they are recovered. Similarly, it may prove possible to transfer "clean" embryos from infected dams of other species in order to rescue desirable genetic stock.

Treatment of Infertility

Embryo transfer as a new tool for obtaining offspring from certain infertile cows has been described by workers at Colorado State University (Monograph 1).[5] The infertility should be the result of disease, injury or aging and not of genetic origin. Success rates are lower than those obtained from healthy donors, and many of the infertile cows have to be treated and observed for extended periods to establish normal estrous cycle lengths before they are superovulated. These factors increase costs, and so this application is likely to remain limited to donors whose offspring can command a high price.

There is no technical reason why this application could not be useful in mares as well, but the attitudes of most of the authorities controlling horse breeding are likely to postpone its use for some time.

Research

Embryo transfer has already proved a powerful research tool. Improving techniques promise that its application in this less direct aspect of animal production will continue to expand. Obviously many of the applications already listed (e.g., genotype proliferation and movement of animals) can be of value in research, but embryo transfer also offers some unique possibilities to the investigator. So far, these have been exploited more in work with sheep and pigs than in the larger species because of expense and the fact that efficient techniques for cattle and horses have become available only recently.

Maternal and genetic influences on any particular characteristic can be differentiated by embryo transfer. In sheep, transfer of embryos of one breed into recipients of another has been used to show that birth weight depends largely on the genotype of the lamb but is also influenced by the breed of the recipient and by litter size. Similarly, fleece characteristics have been shown to be influenced by maternal environment during gestation. Finnish Landrace lambs absorb exceptional amounts of maternal immunoglobulins after birth, and transferring pure Finnish Landrace embryos to ewes of other breeds has demonstrated that this is due to qualities of the lamb and not of the mother.

It is often difficult to determine whether infertility is caused by fertilization failure, an adverse effect on the uterus or an adverse effect on the embryo. Collecting and evaluating ova and embryos from infertile ewes and, if necessary, transferring them to normal recipients has helped define the cause of infertility following such diverse influences as heat stress, age, poor nutrition, lactation and progestogen treatment. Similar use of the technique should be possible in investigating infertility caused by infectious disease.

Embryo transfer has already contributed a great deal to what we know about the establishment of pregnancy and its early maintenance, a time of considerable economic loss in animal breeding. Transfers of progressively older embryos has shown that an embryo needs to be present in the uterus by day 12 after estrus in sheep or by day 16 in cattle if it is to be able to prevent luteolysis and a return to estrus. The necessity of close synchrony between the developmental stages of embryos and uteri in all species has become obvious as a result of embryo transfer. The endocrinology of this interrelationship is still under investigation using the technique. Transfer experiments have contributed to the demonstration that the uterus brings about luteolysis through a local (not systemic) pathway in sheep. These studies played a part in developing the concept of a luteolytic role for prostaglandin-$F_{2\alpha}$ ($PGF_{2\alpha}$), a concept that has since had a major influence on animal production.

Our understanding of later events in pregnancy has also benefited from embryo transfer experiments. In pigs, both the minimum number of embryos necessary to maintain pregnancy (two to four) and the fact that the number of corpora lutea does not limit litter size have been determined in this way. In sheep, breeds that generally have only one or two lambs are capable of carrying additional offspring when receiving them by transfer, indicating that ovulation rates rather than uterine capacities make some breeds more prolific than others. Interbreed transfers in sheep have been used to show that gestation length is controlled by the fetus and not by the mother.

Specialized experimental animals can be produced by embryo manipulation and transfer. Chimeric sheep, of considerable immunological interest, have been born following injection of cells from one embryo into another before transfer. Dissimilar twins can be produced by embryo transfer, as previously described, and in cattle, most are chimeric as a result of fusion of placental blood vessels. They are therefore mutually tolerant of each other's tissues and of use in surgical and immunological studies. Combining twinning with sexing (see Section IV) offers the possibility of producing freemartins at will for the study of the pathogenesis of this condition. The ability to produce twins also makes it possible to study the management of twin-bearing cattle, an area of animal husbandry about which little is known.

GENERAL PROCEDURAL STEPS

Selection of the donor of embryos for transfer will, of course, depend on the application. So will the decision concerning whether or not she is to be superovulated or allowed to produce her normal complement of eggs. In either case, the donor needs to be inseminated (naturally or artificially) with chosen semen. Embryos then have to be collected surgically or nonsurgically in an appropriate flushing medium at an optimal time after insemination. Collected embryos have to be identified in the flushes, evaluated and maintained in a suitable medium pending transfer. At this point they may be subjected to manipulations, such as sexing, and may be cooled or frozen for longer periods of storage, in which case they will have to be warmed or thawed immediately before transfer.

Careful attention must be paid to the conditions under which embryos are handled. All glassware must be thoroughly washed, preferably using tissue culture detergents (e.g., 7X), with a final rinsing in double-glass-distilled water before sterilization by dry heat or autoclaving. Media may be either purchased or made from high-purity chemicals dissolved in glass-distilled water, preferably triple-distilled.

Recipients must have been in estrus at the same time as the donor, and it is therefore essential to know their reproductive histories and to have sufficient recipients for the number of embryos to be transferred. The maintenance of a large recipient herd constitutes the major expense of running an embryo transfer unit. Proper attention to its management and exclusion of disease are correspondingly important.

After transfer, recipients have to be observed for return to estrus and later subjected to a suitable pregnancy test.

For breed society registrations or international trade, it may be necessary to have progeny, sires, dams and recipients blood-typed (to establish parentage) and also certified free of specified diseases.

In the following articles, these steps will be considered, species by species, in the order in which they are encountered in practice.

REFERENCES

1. Chang, M. C. and Pickworth, S.: Egg transfer in the laboratory animal. *In* Hafez, E. S. E. and Blandau,

R. J. (eds): The Mammalian Oviduct: Comparative Biology and Methodology. Chicago, The University of Chicago Press, 1969.

2. Hurst, P. R., Jefferies, K., Eckstein, P. and Wheeler, A. G.: Recovery of uterine embryos in rhesus monkeys. Biol. Reprod., *15*:429, 1976.

3. Kraemer, D. C., Moore, G. T. and Kraemen, M. A.: Baboon infant produced by embryo transfer. Science (N.Y.), *192*:1246, 1976.

4. Marston, J. H., Penn, R. and Sivelle, P. C.: Successful autotransfer of tubal eggs in the rhesus monkey *(Macaca mulatta)*. J. Reprod. Fertil., *49*:175, 1977.

5. Monograph 1. Betteridge, K. J. (ed.): Embryo Transfer in Farm Animals — A Review of Techniques and Applications. Monograph No. 16, Agri-

culture Canada, Ottawa, 1977 (available from Information Division, Canada Department of Agriculture, Ottawa, K1A OC7, Canada).

6. Monograph 2. Rowson, L. E. A. (ed.): Egg Transfer in Cattle. Publication No. EUR 5491, Commission of the European Communities, Luxembourg, 1976 (available from Office for Official Publications of the European Communities, 5, rue du Commerce, B. P. 1003, Luxembourg).

7. Monograph 3. Society for the Study of Animal Breeding: Embryo Transfer — With Particular Reference to Cattle. British Veterinary Association. London (available from The British Veterinary Association, 7 Mansfield St., London WIM OAT, England).

Procedures and Results Obtainable in Cattle

K. J. BETTERIDGE

Agriculture Canada, Animal Diseases Research Institute (Eastern), Ottawa, Ontario, Canada

SELECTION OF DONORS

Except in experimental conditions, the choice of donor is likely to be dictated by the owner's requirements. However, it must be confirmed, both by clinical examination and by attention to their reproductive histories, that prospective donors (other than those being committed to transfer for treatment of infertility) are reproductively sound.

Surgical considerations are becoming very much less important as nonsurgical collection methods supervene. If surgery is contemplated, it must be remembered that midline incisions giving adequate exposure of the uterus are far easier in heifers than in cows with large udders. Lactating cows are poor candidates for surgical collection for additional reasons: they respond poorly to superovulation treatments (to be discussed), they may become ketotic when starved prior to surgery and their recovery from surgery may be prolonged and complicated by hypocalcemia for reasons that are not clear. In donors that have undergone surgery before, surgical difficulties may arise, both from adhesions and from the necessity of cutting through, or close to, an old incision.

Embryos can be satisfactorily collected

from donors at slaughter, if indicated, after excising the uterus and ovaries under aseptic conditions. There are encouraging signs that entire follicles, dissected from normal ovaries from the abattoir, may be cultured under special conditions and used to provide matured oocytes that can be fertilized when transferred to an estrous recipient. Rabbits and lambs have been obtained in this way, but it cannot yet be regarded as a practical source of embryos for cattle.

Calves can readily be superovulated and can provide reasonable yields of embryos following suitably modified methods of insemination. However, pregnancy rates following transfer of such embryos have been very disappointing, and so calves cannot be recommended as donors.

SUPEROVULATION AND INSEMINATION OF DONORS

Superovulation remains a weak link in the chain of events influencing the outcome of embryo transfer in cattle. Responses to all available gonadotropins are still notoriously variable, although they have become somewhat more consistent since the advent of prostaglandins (PG) for synchronization of the estrous cycle.

Treatments

The gonadotropin most often used to stimulate follicular growth in cattle is pregnant mare serum gonadotropin (PMSG). The usual dose is 2000 ± 500 IU given as an intramuscular (IM) injection in a small volume (2 to 5 ml) of physiological saline. Best results are obtained by giving PMSG on one day between days 9 and 12 of the estrous cycle (day 0 = first day of estrus). Luteolysis must then be induced by PG (25 to 30 mg $PGF_{2\alpha}$ or the manufacturer's recommended dose of an analog such as cloprostenol) injected IM 40 to 48 hours later. PG's are effective in lower doses by intrauterine infusion and at one time, when they were very expensive, were given by that route for economic reasons. Recent cost reductions make it unlikely that any resultant savings justify the inconvenience of intrauterine treatment. Estrus usually follows on the second (occasionally on the first or third) day after administration of PG.

If PG's are prohibited or are otherwise unavailable, PMSG treatment is timed to coincide either with natural luteolysis or with the withdrawal of a synchronizing progestational agent. During the natural cycle, PMSG is usually given on day 16, but then the interval to the onset of estrus can vary between 1 and 8 days. The most reliable progestational agents to use are progesterone itself or the synthetic steroid norethandrolone (SC 21009, Searle). Progesterone can be administered either intravaginally (in sponges or silicone rubber coils that contain 2 to 3 gm of the hormone and release it slowly) or as 17 to 30 daily IM injections of 40 mg in oil. Norethandrolone is implanted subcutaneously (SC) in the ear, as two implants, each containing 6 mg of the steroid. All these treatments should begin during the luteal phase of the cycle. The intravaginal and SC implants are left in for 8 to 10 days and are preceded by an injection of estrogen (e.g., 5 mg of estradiol valerate) or an estrogen-progestogen combination to lyse the corpus luteum (CL) present at the time of insertion. PMSG is injected either 2 days before withdrawal of the intravaginal or SC implants or on the day before the last progesterone injection. Estrus usually follows within 1 to 3 days of withdrawal or 2 to 4 days after the last progesterone injection. With these progestogens, estrus ensues earlier in animals treated with PMSG than in synchronized animals receiving no PMSG. Synchronization by progestogens is also less precise with use of PMSG than without it and may be less precise than that produced by PG.

As an alternative to PMSG, gonadotropins of pituitary origin may be used. These have much shorter half-lives in the circulation and therefore have to be given as a series of injections. Colorado workers, for example, have obtained good results with a preparation containing a mixture of follicle-stimulating hormone (FSH) and luteinizing hormone (LH) activities in the ratio of 5:1. This is given as 10 injections over 5 days, commencing between days 9 and 11 of the estrous cycle. The dose required is 5, 4, 3, 2 and 2 mg twice daily, with PG being given on the third day. Moore, in Australia, has found a horse anterior pituitary (HAP) preparation to be effective when given as three equal daily SC injections totaling 60 to 107 mg and beginning on the day before PG injection or on the day before the last injection of a synchronizing regimen of progesterone. Attempts to circumvent the repeated injections by using various vehicles to release the pituitary gonadotropins more slowly have not been very successful.

There is no evidence that any improvement in superovulation rates is obtained by using an ovulation-inducing hormone at the time of estrus after administration of PMSG or its equivalent. Human chorionic gonadotropin (HCG) or gonadotropin-releasing hormone (GnRH) have both been used for this purpose, probably unnecessarily.

More than two-thirds of donors treated with PMSG and PG, or by the alternative regimens just described, come into estrus. Some of the remainder ovulate silently. Some workers give an estrogen injection (e.g., 400 μg of estradiol) at the time when the induced estrus is anticipated on the grounds that it increases the incidence of overt estrus and thereby improves fertilization rates.

Insemination

Not surprisingly, excellent fertilization rates are given by natural service; more variable ones by AI. This probably reflects not only the quality of semen but also the accuracy of estrus detection. In most applications of embryo transfer, AI with selected semen (usually frozen) will be necessary, and it is usual to repeat inseminations at 12-hour intervals during and immediately after estrus. It is also usual to use at least twice the quantity of semen used on nonsuperovulated cows at each insemination. Recent studies have shown that a single insemination with fresh semen or two inseminations with frozen semen at 12-hour intervals can give satisfactory results, but much depends on the quality of the chosen semen.

Results of Superovulation

A major difficulty of discussing ovulation rates following superovulation is caused by the variation in response among donors on exactly the same treatments. Average ovulation rates can be misleading if they represent the mean of excessive and inadequate responses and may give little indication of the probability of obtaining an optimal response from any particular donor. A good working range of ovulation rates to aim for is 3 to 20 ovulations per donor. Anything less than 3 cannot be considered a superovulatory response, and rates much in excess of 20 are often accompanied by poorer fertilization rates and, perhaps, by lower embryo recovery rates, although the evidence for the latter point is equivocal. If the response rate is generally within this range, "excessive" responses will mostly be below 40 and can provide useful yields of embryos. If the working range is set higher by increasing the dose of gonadotropin, animals with responses above the upper limit of the range are more likely to be unusable because fertilization and recovery rates will fall, perhaps because grossly enlarged ovaries make it difficult for eggs to be picked up by the fimbriae and also lead to a highly abnormal endocrine environment. Some workers have also noticed a tendency for the pregnancy rate given by transferred embryos to decline as the dose of PMSG given to the donor increases.

Recent literature (Monograph 1) indicates that the general experience has been to obtain an average ovulation rate of 11 to 12 per responding donor. The proportion of animals failing to respond is poorly documented but ranges between 10 and 40 per cent for heifers and is higher for mature cows. Fertilization rates (of recovered eggs) average 75 per cent.

Sources of Variation in Response to Gonadotropins

Contrary to earlier indications, there is no evidence of a seasonal difference in responsiveness.

Breed differences are well established. British Friesians respond less well than either Charolais or Hereford × Angus; Angus less well than Herefords and Maine-Anjou significantly less well than Chianina, Limousin and Simmental. Again, however, the great variation within breeds must be remembered. Also, Shea *et al.* (Monographs 1 and 2) found that their Maine-Anjou donors gave rates of fertilization, embryo recovery and pregnancy in recipients at least equal to results given by the more responsive breeds. This illustrates the fact that the criterion of success in superovulation techniques must always be the yield of viable embryos, not merely the ovulation rate.

Nutritional effects on responsiveness are manifest only after radical changes such as starvation.

Different preparations of gonadotropins can vary a great deal in effectiveness. For PMSG, the evidence is that this results from variations in extraction and purification procedures and not from variations in ratios of FSH:LH activities. Variations of up to 350 per cent of labeled potency have been described in some FSH preparations.

Much more work is necessary to elucidate the causes of the enormous variation in responsiveness of individuals to gonadotropic stimulation. Only then might it be possible to tailor treatments to individual's requirements and to forecast responses accurately.

EMBRYO COLLECTION

Choosing the Time of Embryo Collection

Embryos usually pass from the oviducts into the uterus between days 3 and 5, but up to 10 per cent may remain in the oviduct until at least day 8 in superovulated heifers. In a series of 27 superovulated *cows*, however, all recovered eggs were found in the uterus at slaughter on days 7 to 12. The oviduct cannot be flushed nonsurgically and so surgical methods must be used up to day 5.

Rates of recovery of eggs and embryos at surgery or slaughter decline steadily between days 3 and 7 (e.g., from 78 per cent to 50 per cent in one series) and then remain relatively steady until at least day 12. After about day 10, recoveries tend to be more efficient at slaughter than at surgery, probably because of the surgical difficulties of inserting collection catheters low enough in the horns and body of the uterus to avoid missing some of the more widely distributed embryos.

The "quality" of recovered embryos, as judged by culture *in vitro,* has been shown by French workers to decline between days 5 and 9, the drop in survival rate being particularly sharp between days 6 and 7.

Embryos usually hatch from the zona pellucida between days 7 and 9 and are more difficult to recognize immediately after hatching.

Pregnancy rates given by transferred embryos increase between days 3 and 5 or 6 and then seem to remain approximately constant.

Consideration of these facts leads to the conclusion that the optimal time for surgical collection and immediate transfer is day 5 or 6. However, recent developments give overriding advantages to nonsurgical collection techniques a few days later (see following paragraphs). Consequently, exposure to the inherent risks of surgery has become much less warranted except for special purposes, e.g., in research or in obtaining embryos from donors that are infertile as a result of uterine pathology. The following description of surgical collection will, therefore, be brief.

Surgical Collection of Embryos

Facilities

Surgical facilities for embryo transfer, close to an animal holding area, should provide for "production-line" surgery. Three separate areas (one for induction of anesthesia and surgical preparation, one for surgery and one for recovery) are required, together with mobile tables allowing anesthetized cows to be moved from area to area. A laboratory, equipped with a stereomicroscope, incubator and the glassware necessary for handling embryos, should be adjacent to the surgery. An office and a room for preparing and sterilizing media and for cleaning, packing and autoclaving surgical instruments and drapes are also needed.

Methods

Midline surgery under general anesthesia is the method of choice. Donors should be deprived of food for 48 hours and of water for 24 hours. Anesthesia is induced by means of a concentrated solution of barbiturate (e.g., 25 per cent sodium thiopental at a dose of 10 mg/kg body weight) given intravenously (IV) and is maintained by standard closed-circuit gaseous anesthesia (halothane in oxygen ± nitrous oxide) or by an intravenous (IV) drip of an agent such as glycerol guaiacolate. A 15-cm midline incision is made immediately cranial to the udder, with full aseptic precautions. The uterus is gently drawn into the incision and anchored there to avoid repeated handling. Anchoring can be by means of umbilical tape passed through the mesometrium, ligated around the body of the uterus and tied to a stainless steel rod placed across the incision. Alternatively, a blunt instrument, such as a pair of needle holders, is pushed through the mesovarian ligament and rested across the incision to anchor one side of the tract at a time.

If embryos are to be collected from the oviduct, a cannula made of glass or polyethylene tubing (outside diameter [OD] 2 to 4 mm; inside diameter [ID] 1 to 3 mm), with a fire-polished, flared end, is passed through the fimbria and held in the ampulla between the finger and thumb or by vasectomy forceps. Its outer end is positioned over a round-bottomed collection dish. Flushing medium (20 to 50 ml) is introduced by syringe, and a blunted 18-gauge needle is introduced into the distal 5 to 10 cm of uterine horn, which is pinched off with the fingers below the point of penetration. (Blunted needles are better than sharp ones, which tend to leave the uterine lumen by penetrating the endometrium.) Avoiding excessive pressure, the medium is milked through the uterotubal junction until a steady flow is obtained out through the cannula into the dish. Some trauma around the ovary and fimbria is inevitable by this method and can lead to adhesions that impair fertility.

After day 5, nearly all embryos can be collected from the uterus. Medium is flushed into the horn, as just described, but as near its tip as possible, and is collected through a Foley catheter (size 16- or 18-French gauge) introduced into the base of the horn through a puncture made bluntly with closed hemostats. This avoids trauma to the oviduct. If necessary, a small volume (5 ml) of medium can be used to flush any residual embryos from the oviduct into the uterus before the main flush. For this purpose, a laboratory animal feeding needle (14 to 16 gauge with a ball on its tip) is suitably atraumatic to pass through the fimbria into the ampulla.

Throughout surgery, tissues are handled minimally and kept moistened with saline containing heparin (10 USP units/ml) in an effort to avoid fibrin formation and subsequent adhesions. Repair of the incision is by standard methods.

Results of Surgical Collection

The literature shows that recovery rates of eggs and embryos can be anticipated to amount to 50 to 70 per cent of ovulations. Combined with an average ovulation rate of 11 to 12, this means collecting about 6 to 8 embryos and unfertilized eggs per flushed donor. At a fertilization rate of 75 per cent, the average yield recorded is about 5 embryos per flushed donor (range 2 to 8).

The number of times that surgical recovery can be repeated on one donor is limited by adhesion formation and is variable but unlikely to exceed three times. After two collections it is usual to recommend that the donor be bred to carry her own calf.

Nonsurgical Collection of Embryos

Advantages and Disadvantages

The principal advantages of nonsurgical methods are that the elaborate facilities, costs, risks and postoperative adhesions associated with surgery are avoided. On-the-farm collections therefore become possible, lactating cows that are bad surgical subjects can be used and, most importantly, collections can be repeated many times from the same donor.

The disadvantages are: considerable manipulative skill is required (especially in heifers), sterility is more difficult to maintain, large volumes of flushing medium have to be used and searched for embryos, ovarian responses cannot be ascertained by inspection and embryos cannot be recovered from the oviducts.

Apparatus

The basic principle of approaches to nonsurgical collection has remained the same since the first attempts by Rowson and Dowling in the late 1940's. A catheter, fitted with an inflatable cuff, is introduced into the uterine horn. The cuff is inflated to seal off the horn, flushing medium is infused through the catheter into the lumen distal to the seal and then is collected through the same catheter. Most approaches have been through the cervix, but one method bypasses the cervix with a transvaginal incision.

Results were discouragingly variable and generally poor until 1972, when Sugie and his colleagues in Japan reported an average of 6.2 ova per recovery in 45 of 60 superovulated cows. Various modifications of their apparatus followed (e.g., Fig. 1A), and yields of eggs and embryos amounting to about 50 per cent of ovulations have been obtained with these. The difficulty of passing a catheter through the cervix in some animals, particularly heifers, has led to various methods aimed at improving results.

One approach devised by Testart and colleagues in France, (Fig. 1C) has been to bypass the cervix by making a dorsal incision in the vagina under epidural anesthesia. A special apparatus, constructed from a cuffed teat cannula held on a finger ring, is introduced by hand through the incision. Grasping the uterine horn directly, the cannula is pushed through its wall into the lumen. After inflating the cuff, the hand is withdrawn from the ring and the uterus is flushed with 20 to 50 ml of medium, using the freed hand to pinch off the uterotubal junction and to elevate it to help recovery. Recoveries of 40 to 50 per cent of eggs ovulated have been obtained with this apparatus.

A second approach has been that of Alexander in England, who designed a long, semi-rigid, detachable tip on a rigid catheter; a combination that facilitates negotiation of the cervix and the curve of the uterine horn without fear of penetrating its wall. The holes through which medium flows are closed during introduction (to avoid obstruction by mucus) and can then be opened from outside the cow. Excellent recoveries have been obtained with the apparatus but probably no better than those possible with the simpler, cheaper and more readily available catheters described in the following paragraph.

The third approach has been to revert to basic principles and the Rowson and Dowling type of catheter. Remarkable improvements in results have been independently achieved by many groups since 1975, all agreeing that success depends on dexterity, patience and practice. Two-way or three-way rubber urethral catheters of the Foley or Rusch type are a convenient, ready-made source of the apparatus and are obtainable in various sizes. One of the "ways" (channels) is used to inflate the cuff, so a two-way catheter is a single, cuffed tube while a three-way system has two channels for fluid

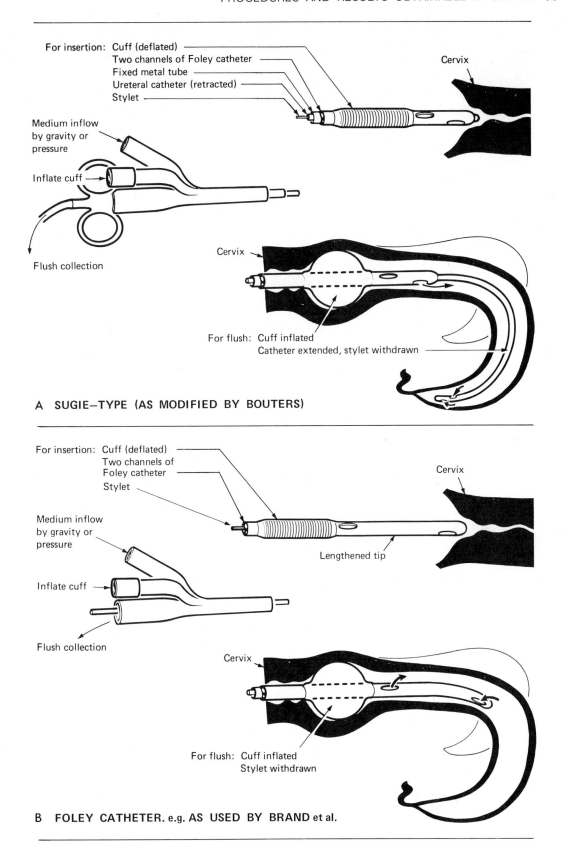

For insertion: Cuff (deflated)
Two channels of Foley catheter
Fixed metal tube
Ureteral catheter (retracted)
Stylet

Cervix

Medium inflow
by gravity or
pressure

Inflate cuff

Flush collection

Cervix

For flush: Cuff inflated
Catheter extended, stylet withdrawn

A SUGIE—TYPE (AS MODIFIED BY BOUTERS)

For insertion: Cuff (deflated)
Two channels of
Foley catheter
Stylet

Cervix

Medium inflow
by gravity or
pressure

Inflate cuff

Flush collection

Lengthened tip

Cervix

For flush: Cuff inflated
Stylet withdrawn

B FOLEY CATHETER. e.g. AS USED BY BRAND et al.

Figure 1. Three basic designs of apparatus for non-surgical collection of embryos from cattle. (From Monograph 1.)
Illustration continued on the following page.

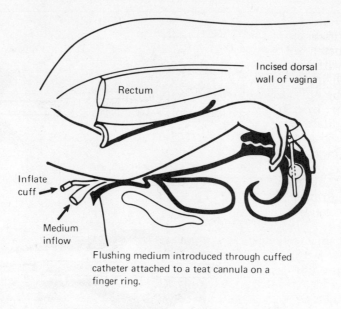

Flushing medium introduced through cuffed catheter attached to a teat cannula on a finger ring.

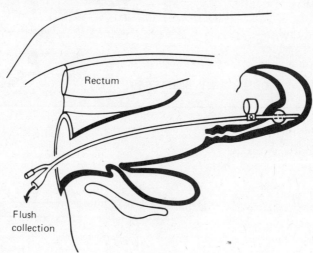

Uterine horn elevated and utero—tubal junction occluded with fingers during collection of flush.

C TRANSVAGINAL METHOD (TESTART AND GODARD—SIOUR, 1975)

Figure 1. *Continued*

and can be used for continuous irrigation (Fig. 1*B*). Sizes can be selected according to the size of donor but are usually between 3.6 and 6.0 mm OD. Collection procedures will be described for these specific types of catheter but generally apply to any transcervical method.

Procedure

The donor is restrained in a chute and given an epidural anesthetic (5 to 10 ml of 2 per cent lidocaine [Xylocaine]). Sedation is rarely necessary. The vulva and perineum are thoroughly cleaned and disinfected. The rubber catheter is slightly stretched over a metal stylet and clamped to it at its outer end. This prevents the tip of the stylet from emerging accidentally from the distal side opening of the catheter during insertion. A metal tip may be added to the standard catheter to guard against penetration of the rubber by the stylet. To prevent contamination of the catheter inside the vagina, it is introduced into the cervix via a 4-cm diameter vaginal speculum. After withdrawing the speculum, the catheter is manipulated through the cervix with the help of rectal palpation and guided into the base of one uterine horn until the cuff can be inflated with 7 to 20 ml of air. In small animals, it may be necessary to dilate the cervix with a tapered solid metal rod before the catheter can be introduced. In large, parous cows, vulsellum forceps may be needed on the cervix to pull the uterus into the pelvic cavity. With the stylet withdrawn, the person inserting the catheter retains control of the catheter and uterus *per rectum* while an assistant begins the flush.

Flushing with a two-way catheter is by a simple in-out flow. The uterine horn is distended with 50 to 75 ml of medium, introduced either by syringe or by gravity flow from a vessel held about 1 m above the inlet. The degree of distention can be felt *per rectum*, and volumes are adjusted to avoid possible rupture of the uterus. Medium is collected through siliconized tubing into sterile separation funnels at ground level. It flows by siphoning when the syringe or infusion tubing is disconnected from the catheter and replaced by the collection tubing. The flow can be helped by elevating and gently massaging the uterine horn. A Y-junction at the outer end of the catheter is useful for attaching infusion and collection tubes simultaneously, clamping off one with hemostats as appropriate. The flush is repeated about six times.

With a three-way catheter, infusion and collection tubes are connected to two channels of the catheter (Fig. 1*B*). Medium is run in by gravity, and uterine distention is brought about initially by occluding the outlet tubing. When the outlet is opened, the horn is flushed by a continuous flow (up to 500 ml) of medium, which is collected as in the two-way system. A syringe attached to a side arm off the inlet tubing has been found useful for creating turbulence within the uterus and for clearing blockages.

In the system illustrated in Fig. 1*A*, the ureteral catheter is advanced as far into the tip of the uterine horn as possible, after initially positioning the outer catheter as just described. The ureteral catheter has to be rigid enough to be advanced without kinking as its stylet is withdrawn, but not so rigid that it might perforate the uterine wall. As indicated (Fig. 1*A*), the principal flushing direction is from the base of the horn to the tip, but an additional reverse flush is felt to help recovery by creating local turbulence near the uterotubal junction. It is doubtful whether the complications justify use of this system, when the simpler methods produce equally good yields of embryos.

Temporary interruptions of flow can occur in any nonsurgical system as a result of plugging by mucus or improper positioning of the catheter in the uterine lumen. These have to be dealt with by rectal manipulation and a certain amount of hydrostatic ingenuity, but taps and valves that might trap or damage embryos should be avoided.

To flush the second uterine horn, it is usual to deflate and withdraw the first catheter and introduce a second one because the stylet cannot be reinserted safely. Repositioning of the original catheter into the second horn after deflation is possible if the stylet can be reinserted (e.g., in models with an added metal tip).

Results of Nonsurgical Collection

The number of embryos recovered as a proportion of the number of ovulations in superovulated donors can be assessed accurately only in experimental conditions when donors can be slaughtered afterwards to examine the ovaries. However, experienced workers estimate their recoveries to be between 50 and 70 per cent of palpated corpora lutea (CL), and this is corroborated by similar recovery rates achieved in nonsuperovulated cows. In other words, nonsurgical recoveries are now as efficient as surgical ones. Nonsurgical flushing has no adverse effect on fertility, but to guard against accidentally establishing a metritis, most workers use a bacteriocidal infusion through the catheter after flushing.

HANDLING AND SHORT-TERM STORAGE OF EMBRYOS

Media

Part of the reason for lack of success in early attempts at embryo transfer in cattle was probably due to the use of media containing bovine serum, which is toxic for embryos unless heat-inactivated at 56°C for 30 minutes. Tissue culture medium-199 (TCM-199) gave good results and was widely used when more extensive work first began. Recently, however, an enriched phosphate-

TABLE 1. *Enriched Phosphate-buffered Saline (Whittingham's PB1) Used as a Medium for Embryo Transfer in Cattle and Other Species*

Constituent	Formula Weight	Molarity in Final Solution	Weight (gm)	Volume Triple-distilled Water for Solution (ml)
*NaCl	58.44	136.89	8.00	
*KCl	74.56	2.68	0.20	
*Na$_2$HPO$_4$	141.96	8.09	1.15	
*KH$_2$PO$_4$	136.09	1.47	0.20	
Bovine serum albumin (Fraction V)			3.00	800 (Solution 1)
Glucose	180.16	5.56	1.00	
Na pyruvate	110.04	0.33	0.036	
Neomycin sulfate (or alternative antibiotic)			0.20	
*CaCl$_2$	110.99	0.90	0.10	100 (Solution 2)
*MgCl$_2$ • 6H$_2$O	203.31	0.49	0.10	100 (Solution 3)

Preparation 1. Make up solutions 1, 2 and 3 separately; cool to 4°C and then mix. This prevents precipitation.

2. Adjust pH to 7.1 to 7.2 with NaHCO$_3$ or HCl if necessary.

3. Confirm that osmolality is about 290 mOsm/kg (theoretically 310 mOsm/kg).

4. Sterilize by filtration through cellulose acetate (Millipore) filters, pore size 0.45 μ.

5. Store at −20°C for up to 3 months.

*These are the constituents of Dulbecco's phosphate-buffered saline.

buffered saline (PBS) (Table 1) has been shown to be superior to TCM-199 for culturing bovine embryos *in vitro* and has all but replaced it in transfer work.

Temperatures

Media should be warmed to body temperature before use, but there are no data to suggest whether flushes should be kept at 37°C, at room temperature of about 20°C, or at an intermediate temperature of 30°C. Each holding temperature has its advocates, and there is general agreement that sharp fluctuations in temperature should be avoided.

Handling

Embryos rapidly settle out of collection media. In surgical flushes they can therefore be found in the bottom of the round-bottomed collection dishes when examined under a stereomicroscope at magnifications of ×12 to ×50 with transmitted illumination. They can be aspirated into a siliconized, flame-polished Pasteur pipette of appropriate bore. Using this pipette, they are transferred to fresh medium in another dish to separate them from cellular debris. Blood in the flush can severely hamper locating embryos and should be diluted out to help the search. Elongated blastodermic vesicles found after day 13 are handled in wider-bore pipettes. Beyond day 14 (which would be for research purposes only), these vesicles are often long enough to become very tangled, and so flat-bottomed collection dishes should be used, giving them room to spread out.

The large volumes resulting from nonsurgical flushes are best collected into separating funnels because, after settling, the medium can be searched in small aliquots run off from the bottom and therefore likely to contain the embryos. Nonsurgical flushes tend to contain more mucus and cellular debris than those collected surgically, making location of embryos a little more difficult.

In Vitro Storage Time

For all practical purposes, embryos should be transferred as soon as possible after recovery. Pregnancy rates from transferred embryos tend to fall after more than 2 hours in TCM-199, but embryo survival in enriched PBS remains constant for at least 7.5 hours after collection.

Addition of about 20 per cent heat-inactivated fetal calf serum to the enriched PBS provides a medium in which bovine embryos at the morula stage can be cultured for at least 48 hours at 37°C with only an 8 to 15 per cent diminution in pregnancy rates after transfer. However, this is not advocated or necessary for routine work. The same medium allows blastocysts to be cooled to 0°C for up to 48 hours with almost 50 per cent survival, and, with further work, short-term storage will undoubtedly improve the possibilities of long-distance embryo transportation. Some precautions that are necessary in preparing media containing serum are described on page 81.

EVALUATION OF EMBRYOS

The only methods that have been used to evaluate the quality of bovine embryos after collection are morphological. Beyond the differentiation of unfertilized from fertilized ova, such methods therefore are subjective and depend very much on experience. In su-perovulated cattle, there is likely to be a considerable range of developmental stages on any given day of development. This variation, illustrated for the first 10 days in Figure 2, even occurs among embryos from the same donor. After about day 12, the blastodermic vesicle begins to expand longitudinally. Its growth is logarithmic, and very large differences in size are encountered. The appearance of healthy embryos at various developmental stages is shown in Figure 3.

Shea *et al.* (in Monograph 2) have studied how direct assessments of embryos relate to subsequent pregnancy in a large commercial unit. They scored embryos, usually collected on day 5, on a scale of one to five on the basis of compactness, symmetry and density of blastomeres. Although higher-scored embryos as a group generally produced greater success rates than lower-scored groups, this pattern was not invariable, especially when pregnancy rates were low. Shea and colleagues found the best predictor of an embryo's viability to be its stage of development; the less advanced the embryo on a given day, the less its chances of surviving. Retarded embryos also develop less well than more advanced ones in culture systems. Despite these broadly useful indications of an embryo's quality, the fact that some very poor-looking ones survive always makes it difficult to discard a potentially valuable embryo. This probably accounts, in part, for pregnancy rates in commercial

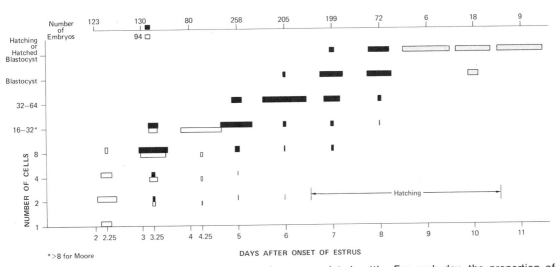

Figure 2. The cleavage and hatching of embryos in superovulated cattle. For each day, the proportion of recovered embryos in each developmental stage is represented by the length of the horizontal bar. (From Monograph 1.)

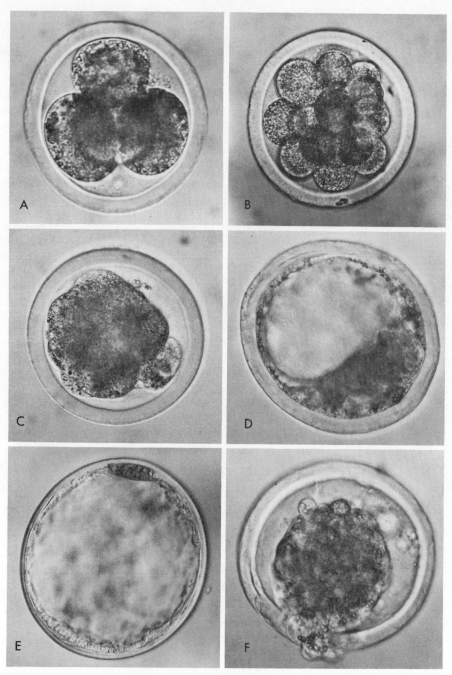

Figure 3. Cattle embryos at various transferable stages of development. *A,* 4-cell egg, day 3 (× 283). *B,* 16-cell egg, day 5 (× 290). *C,* Morula, day 6. Cells have compacted and have lost their visible individual outlines (× 270). *D,* Early blastocyst, day 7 (× 283). *E,* Blastocyst, fully expanded within the zona pellucida, day 10. Note the prominent inner cell mass (× 283). *F,* Hatching blastocyst, day 10. Note the cells extruding through the zona pellucida (× 283).

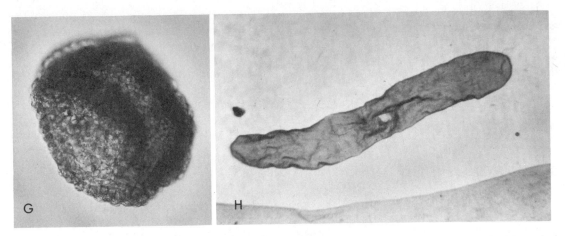

Figure 3. *Continued.* *G,* Hatched blastocyst, day 12, with typical wrinkled appearance ($\times$ 140). *H,* Elongating blastodermic vesicle, day 14, with a prominent embryonic disc. Part of a much larger embryo from the same donor can be seen at the bottom of the photograph ($\times$ 7.6). (From Monograph 1.)

units tending to be lower than in units devoted to more selective experimental use of embryo transfer.

Development in culture systems (*in vitro* or in the rabbit oviduct) is often used to assess embryo viability after experimental manipulations, such as cooling or freezing, because these are more convenient and economical than transfer. Ultimately, however, transfer has to be used to show that embryos judged viable in such systems can, in fact, produce calves.

Fixing and staining representative individuals from groups of embryos to assess them is, of course, only useful experimentally, but it is possible that some vital dyes could be used on living embryos without affecting them adversely. There is a need for more work on this and on other biochemical and biophysical parameters that might reflect viability by measuring the metabolism of bovine embryos.

SYNCHRONIZATION AND SELECTION OF RECIPIENTS

Transfers can be made reasonably successful only if the preceding estrus in the donor and recipient occurred within 2 days of each other. Experimentally it has been shown that results are (1) best when donors and recipients are exactly synchronous, (2) reasonable when they are out of phase by $\pm$ 1 day and (3) too poor to be usable when they differ by $\pm$ 2 days. Under large-scale commercial conditions, Shea *et al.* (in Monograph 2) obtained pregnancy rates of 62 per

cent in 1126 recipients that had been in estrus on the same day as the donors, 60 per cent in 334 recipients in estrus the day before the donors and 49 per cent in 556 recipients in estrus the day after the donors. Other commercial users claim that results obtained with recipients in estrus 1 day later than the donor are just as good as in exactly synchronous ones. This, they claim, has the important practical advantage of allowing an unused "+1" asynchronous animal to be used the next day as a synchronous "0" recipient for that day's donor.

Synchronization of donors and recipients, then, should be as precise as is practicable. This can be achieved in two ways: either by having a herd of recipients large enough so that there are sufficient animals in estrus naturally on any given day or by using synchronizing agents to induce estrus in groups of animals as they are needed. Both methods, but especially the first, require close attention to herd management and estrus detection and accurate recording systems.

Synchronization can be induced by the agents already discussed for donors, remembering that the same synchronization treatment induces estrus earlier in donors that have received gonadotropin than in recipients that have not. PG, for example, should be administered to recipients about 16 hours before giving it to the donor to induce estrus on the same day. Most workers who have compared pregnancy rates in artificially synchronized and naturally cycling recipients have found no difference between them.

Before admitting new animals to a recipient herd, they should be certified free of diseases that could ruin the operation of a unit, for example, tuberculosis, brucellosis, bluetongue, leptospirosis or anaplasmosis.

SURGICAL TRANSFER OF EMBRYOS

Surgical Methods

Most workers have used a midline approach to the recipient's uterus, just as described for surgical collection. A blunt probe (e.g., the reverse end of a suture needle or a blunted 16-gauge hypodermic needle) is used to perforate the uterine wall to admit the tip of the sterile Pasteur pipette containing the embryo. A syringe attached to the pipette is used to expel the embryo into the uterus in a minimal volume (0.2 ml) of medium. Positive pressure is maintained as the pipette is withdrawn to avoid reaspirating the embryo. Pipettes are examined under the stereomicroscope after use to confirm that embryos are not retained.

Others prefer a flank approach under paravertebral or local infiltration anesthesia with the recipient in the standing position. This may be slightly quicker and requires less elaborate facilities. However, exposure and maintaining proper asepsis is often more difficult, especially in range cattle. The embryo may be inserted by Pasteur pipette or via a 0.5 ml inseminating straw attached to a flexible polyethylene tube with a syringe fitted to its other end.

Closure following either approach is by routine surgical methods.

Site of Transfer

Single embryos should be transferred to the horn on the same side as the CL because survival rates are higher there than in the contralateral horn, though how much higher is disputed. Flank incisions are therefore made on the side where the CL has been palpated preoperatively. Young (day 5 to day 7) embryos should be inserted near the tip, rather than at the base, of the uterine horn, although evidence concerning whether or not this is critical is, again, controversial.

Twin embryos should be to transferred to separate horns (see page 71).

Results of Surgical Transfer

Transfers of twin embryos on days 4 to 7 have consistently resulted in pregnancy rates of 70 to 90 per cent and embryo survival rates of 40 to 60 per cent. Transfers of single embryos, however, at least under commercial circumstances when even "doubtful-looking" embryos must be used, can be expected to result in only 50 to 60 per cent of recipients becoming pregnant. So many factors can affect the outcome that it is usually difficult to define which particular ones are involved in making one group's results better than another's.

NONSURGICAL TRANSFER OF EMBRYOS

There have been reports of attempts at nonsurgical transfer through the cervix since 1949, but the first successful procedure was not until 1964. In the 1950's and early 1960's, it was believed that uterine infection and expulsion of the embryo into the vagina as a result of cervical stimulation were responsible for the lack of success. Inflation of the uterus with carbon dioxide decreased expulsion after transfer and improved results a little, but pregnancy rates remained low (less than 40 per cent pregnancies after twin transfers). Some success was also achieved with methods that bypassed the cervix, but the key to the more successful recent results appears to be the realization that transcervical transfers need to be delayed until after day 5 at the earliest and, preferably, until days 7 to 10. Brand and his colleagues at Utrecht have shown that spontaneous electrical activity in the myometrium declines between estrus and day 5, which may partially explain the physiological basis for better results obtained later in the luteal phase of the recipients. Provided that proper precautions are taken, infection is not a major cause of failure. This has been shown by performing bacteriological studies of transfer pipettes and by demonstrating that sham transfers do not affect pregnancy rates in bred heifers.

Three types of nonsurgical transfer apparatus have been used recently. The first comprises concentric metal cannulae through which a ureteral catheter is advanced well into the uterine horn to deposit the embryo. The second uses a transvaginal incision to bypass the cervix, and the third is a Cassou AI gun (or a modification of it), which, because of its simplicity and efficacy, seems likely to supersede the others.

In the concentric system, the outer metal tube acts as a vaginal speculum and is 30 cm long, 8 mm OD and 6 mm ID. The second tube is 35 cm long, 4 mm OD and 3 mm ID and the innermost tube is 51 cm long, 2.5 mm OD and 2 mm ID, just big enough for the ureteral catheter (70 cm long, No. 5- or 6-French gauge) to pass through it. Under epidural anesthesia and after thorough cleansing of the vulva and perineum, the vaginal speculum is introduced as far as the external os of the cervix with the aid of rectal manipulation. The second tube, with a paper cap taped to its distal end, is introduced through the first as far into the cervix as is possible without being traumatic (about 1 to 2 cm). The paper cap prevents mucus from entering the lumen or this tube and contaminating the third tube, which is inside it. The third tube can be extended through the paper, through the cranial portion of the cervix and 2 to 3 cm into the uterine horn ipsilateral to the CL. The ureteral catheter is passed into the third tube directly from its sterile pack and is advanced as far into the uterus as possible, while the horn is straightened *per rectum*. The embryo is flushed slowly through the ureteral catheter in about 1 ml of medium, followed by 0.5 ml of air from a Pasteur pipette. It is important to flush the catheter into a watch glass after withdrawal to check for possible retention of the embryo. Pregnancy rates of up to 43 per cent with single embryos have been obtained with apparatus of this type.

The transvaginal approach of Testart *et al.* is basically similar to their collection procedure. It has yielded embryo survival rates of 47 per cent when used on cows bred 5 to 10 days previously, establishing a twinning rate of 60 per cent.

The Cassou AI gun (Fig. 4) is being used increasingly for transfer, and modifications of the narrower gun designed originally for sheep AI are being made specifically for this purpose. The straw is first shortened by about 1.5 cm and is used to aspirate the embryo in a small volume of medium between air bubbles before being loaded into the gun. The gun is used just as for AI, except that it may be covered with a sterile paper tube that is not punctured until the cervix is reached. After day 7, it does not seem necessary to advance the gun far into the horn to expel the embryo. In unmated recipients, twin transfers have given pregnancy rates of up to 60 per cent with 45 per cent embryo survival. Very similar results have been obtained in previously mated recipients and, in a direct comparison, have been shown to almost match the results of surgical transfer.

MANAGEMENT OF PREGNANT RECIPIENTS

Timing of rectal examinations to diagnose pregnancy must depend on the relative importance of disposing of nonpregnant animals (which are expensive to maintain) and the possible risk of misdiagnosis at examinations made too early. The usual compromise is examination at 6 to 8 weeks.

Any undue stress, such as long-distance transportation, should be avoided during the first trimester of pregnancy.

A few workers have recorded a considerable incidence of abortions following transfer, but the significance of these is difficult to assess in the absence of control (normally established) pregnancies. Others have presented good evidence that fetal losses are not increased following transfers. For economic reasons, remarkably few experimental reports give calving rates (as opposed to pregnancy rates), but these should be forthcoming from commercial units.

A method for diagnosing twin pregnancy in cattle would help in the proper management of recipients carrying twins. Otherwise, recipients need be managed no differently from other pregnant heifers, unless they are carrying calves of a much larger breed. In this case elective cesarean sections may be called for, perhaps after initiating parturition by usual methods of induction with dexamethasone.

Blood typing requirements will be specified by the breed societies.

PERSONNEL REQUIREMENTS

These are discussed by Bowen later in this section.

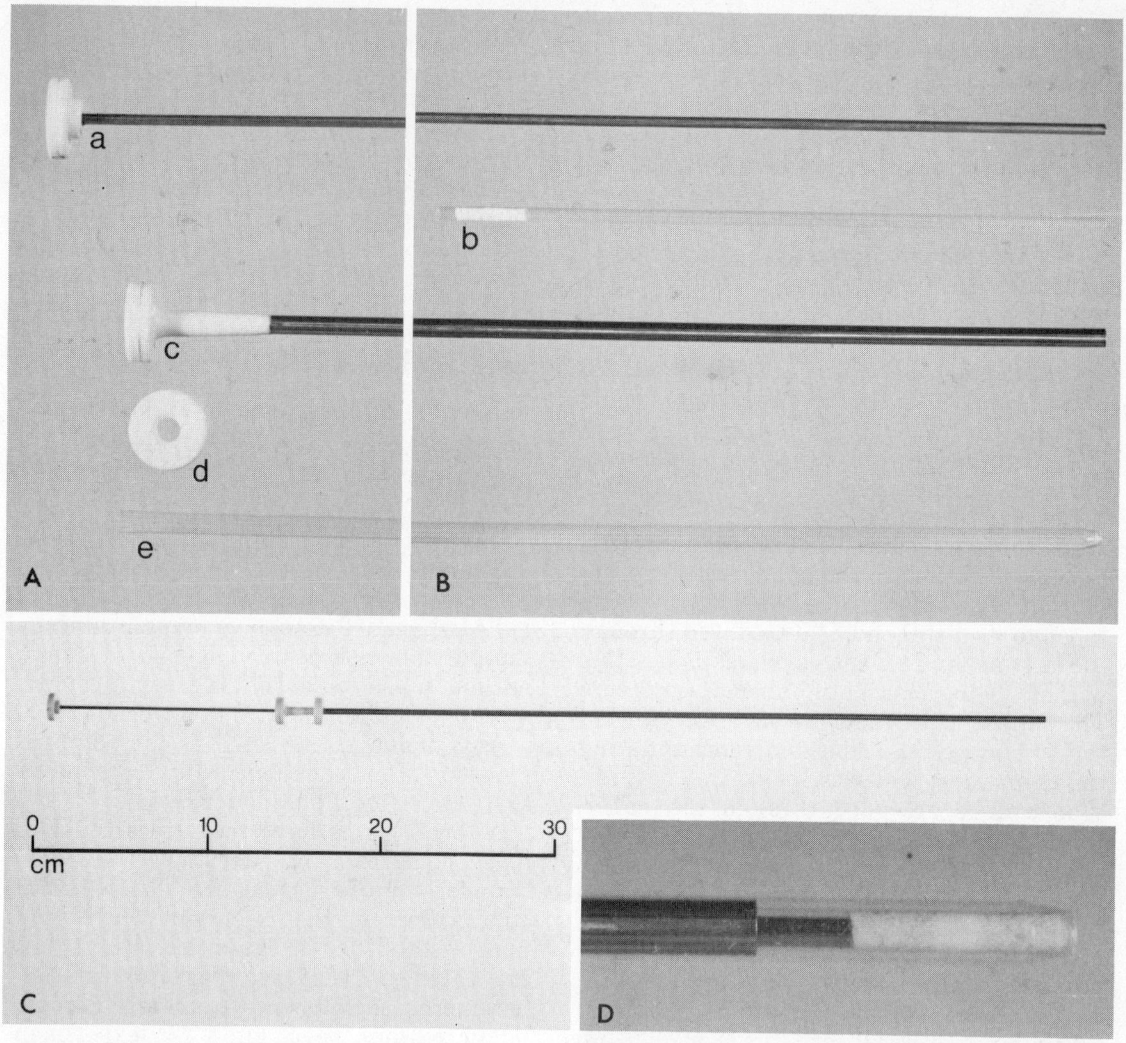

Figure 4. Cassou AI gun used for nonsurgical embryo transfer in cattle. *A* and *B,* The proximal and distal ends, respectively, of its component parts. These are: (*a*) a stainless steel plunger with a plastic hub, (*b*) a 0.5 ml plastic straw with a white plug of polyvinyl alcohol between two lengths of wick, (*c*) a stainless steel barrel with a plastic hub, (*d*) a plastic locking ring and (*e*) a clear plastic pipette with a tapered tip. The straw, after being filled with medium containing the embryo, fits into the distal end of the barrel. The clear plastic pipette holds it there by fitting over the barrel and being locked to the hub of the barrel by the ring. The plunger expels the contents of the straw by pushing the plug through to its distal end. *C,* The assembled gun with the plunger inserted as far as the proximal end of the straw, ready to expel its contents. *D,* The distal end of the gun after discharge. The plug can be seen pushed to the end of the straw that protrudes from the barrel inside the plastic pipette. In practice, the straw and pipette are usually shortened to achieve better rigidity and would extend only just beyond the metal barrel. (From Monograph 1.)

REFERENCES

1. Monograph 1. Betteridge, K. J. (ed.): Embryo Transfer in Farm Animals — A Review of Techniques and Applications. Monograph No. 16, Agriculture Canada, Ottawa, 1977 (available from Information Division, Canada Department of Agriculture, Ottawa, K1A OC7, Canada).

2. Monograph 2. Rowson, L. E. A. (ed.): Egg Transfer in Cattle. Publication No. EUR 5491, Commission of the European Communities, Luxembourg, 1976 (available from Office for Official Publications of the European Communities, 5, rue du Commerce, B. P. 1003, Luxembourg).

Procedures and Results Obtainable in Sheep and Goats

N. W. MOORE

University of Sydney Farms, Camden,
New South Wales, Australia

In general, similar procedures are involved in embryo transfer in sheep and goats, and any difference between the two species results from more frequent and extensive use of the technique in sheep.

SUPEROVULATION OF DONORS

During the breeding season, superovulation can be readily achieved by treatment with gonadotropins during the latter stage of the luteal and early part of the follicular phase of the estrous cycle. Pregnant mare serum gonadotropin (PMSG) and anterior pituitary extracts (e.g., horse anterior pituitary — HAP) are effective in both species, with PMSG having the advantages of availability and ease of administration. PMSG is given as a single subcutaneous (SC) or intramuscular (IM) injection on day 12 or 13 of the estrous cycle in the ewe, day 17 or 18 in the goat doe. HAP, presumably because of more rapid inactivation, needs to be given as three equal SC injections on consecutive days, commencing on day 12 in the ewe and day 17 in the doe. PMSG is commercially available in purified form; HAP is not, and must be prepared in the laboratory from slaughterhouse material. Procedures for the extraction of pituitaries are relatively simple and have been described previously.[1] The dose should be adjusted to the size and breed of the donor. In the Merino ewe weighing 40 to 50 kg, 1200 to 1300 IU of PMSG or 60 mg total dose of HAP should provide a mean of 10 to 12 ovulations. In the larger and more prolific Border Leicester weighing 70 to 80 kg, 1500 to 1700 IU of PMSG or 80 mg of HAP should give 12 to 15 ovulations. Similarly, in the doe, 1000 to 1100 IU of PMSG or 45 mg of HAP in the Angora of 25 to 30 kg should give 10 to 12 ovulations; and 1500 IU of PMSG or 60 mg of HAP in the larger and more prolific milch breeds should result in about 15 ovulations. As in other species,

there is substantial variation among individuals in their ovulatory response to standard doses of gonadotropin. In both species, an ovulating injection of luteinizing hormone (LH) or human chorionic gonadotropin (HCG) appears to have little or no beneficial effect on the ovulatory response to either PMSG or HAP.

The time of ovulation can be controlled, which is of value in predicting precise dates for transfer. Progesterone administered daily by IM injection (12 mg/day) or progestogen-impregnated intravaginal pessaries (e.g., Synchro-Mate, Searle) are generally effective. PMSG should be given, or HAP treatment commenced, on the day before the last progesterone injection or the day before removal of pessaries. Progestogen treatment should be continued for 2 to 3 days beyond the expected date of estrus. When the expected date of estrus is not known, the time over which daily progesterone injections are given, or pessaries are left inserted, should be at least 14 days in the ewe and 17 days in the doe. The majority of ewes and does will be in estrus 48 to 60 hours after the end of progesterone treatment, and there are indications that estrus following use of pessaries occurs some 12 hours earlier, at 36 to 48 hours after withdrawal. The ovulatory response in progestogen-treated animals is somewhat less variable than in normally cycling animals, presumably because of more precise control of the time elapsing between gonadotropin treatment and estrus.

In the ewe, and probably in the doe, similar progestogen and gonadotropin treatments are successful in inducing superovulation outside the normal breeding season. Ovulatory response to gonadotropins in the anestrous ewe appears to be comparable to that in the cyclic animal.

Recently, the prostaglandin (PG) analog cloprostenol (Estrumate, ICI), given as a single IM injection of 100 μg between days 4 and 13 has proved effective in synchronizing estrus in ewes treated with PMSG 24 to 72 hours previously. Virtually all animals come into estrus, 85 per cent of them within 36 hours of the administration of PG, and embryos recovered from them are normal.

PG is also luteolytic in goats but has not yet been used to any degree with gonadotropins to superovulate them at predetermined times.

Superovulation has been reported in 10- to 16-week-old prepuberal lambs given 750 to 1000 IU of PMSG after progesterone pretreatment (10 mg/day for 3 to 18 days). Surgical insemination (see following paragraphs) of the lambs resulted in a 77 per cent fertilization rate, and recovered embryos developed normally following transfer.[2] No information is available on the prepuberal doe.

In mature animals, age can influence ovarian response. In animals older than 6 or 7 years, ovulatory response is likely to be low, and it appears that higher doses of gonadotropin will not restore the response to that observed in younger females.

INSEMINATION OF DONORS

Natural Service and Artificial Insemination

If females are to be mated naturally, but not allowed continuous access to males, it is advisable to hand-mate at about 12 hour intervals until the ewe or doe will no longer accept the male. AI should be carried out twice, with 12 to 24 hours elapsing between inseminations, using at least 0.2 ml of semen containing at least 400×10^6 motile sperm at each insemination.

Surgical Insemination

In the ewe, failure of fertilization often occurs, particularly in animals showing a high ovulatory response to treatment. This appears to be due to faulty transport of spermatozoa through the cervix and can be overcome by surgical insemination directly into the uterine lumen. The uterus is exposed through a midventral incision under local anesthesia, e.g., 2 per cent lidocaine (Xylocaine), with the animals restrained in a special laparotomy cradle. Semen (0.01 to 0.02 ml) is injected by Pasteur pipette into each uterine horn 3 to 4 cm from the uterotubal junction. Barbiturates are not recommended for anesthesia because of their potential inhibitory effect on ovulation. The ovaries should not be exposed, and handling of the reproductive tract should be kept to a minimum, because rapid transport of ova within the tract can follow manipulation near the time of ovulation. Surgical insemination results in fertilization rates in excess of 90 per cent and should be adopted as routine practice when large numbers of embryos are required.

When precise control over the time of ovulation has been achieved, surgical insemination has further advantages. A proportion of superovulated ewes (approximately 10 to 15 per cent) usually fail to exhibit estrus and so would not be inseminated by natural service or by AI relying on estrus detection. Surgical insemination, however, can be successfully performed without reference to the time of estrus on the second day after discontinuing progestogen treatment in synchronized ewes, and so nonestrous ewes are not lost to this process. Ovulatory responses and fertilizability of ova shed by nonestrous ewes are similar to those of ewes that do exhibit estrus.

In the doe, fertilization failure following superovulation is not a severe problem, perhaps because the cervix is more patent in the doe than in the ewe and therefore offers less of a barrier to sperm transport.

EMBRYO COLLECTION

Choosing the Time of Embryo Collection

In the ewe, and probably in the doe, the survival and development of transferred embryos are dependent upon their age and are modified by the site to which they are transferred. Sheep embryos collected on day 3 or earlier (embryos of 8 cells or less) should be transferred to the oviducts, resulting in about 60 per cent developing into lambs. Those on day 4 or later (embryos of 16 to 20 cells or more) should be transferred to the uterus, with consequent survival rates of 70 to 75 per cent. Besides giving higher survival rates, transfers to the uterus are easier than those to the oviduct. Although survival rates are high, the collection and transfer of embryos beyond days 7 to 8 can cause major problems of identification and handling and generally should not be attempted. Thus, day-4 to day-6 collections and uterine transfers are optimal for most purposes.

Procedures

The procedures used for the collection of embryos from the ewe and doe are essentially similar to those described for cattle. Under general anesthesia, the reproductive tract is exposed by a midventral incision. General anesthesia is preferable to the local type because it precludes movement of the animal during the collection procedures. The cannulae used in the oviduct are about 2 mm outside diameter (OD) and are inserted 3 to 4 cm into the ampulla. In both species it is possible to express 5 to 10 ml of flushing media injected into the lumen of the uterine horn out through the oviduct. Precautions against adhesions are necessary, and standard surgical methods are used to close the incision.

Flushing is normally carried out 3 to 7 days after mating. After day 4 the majority of embryos of both species will have entered the uterus and, from then on, the uterine horns, as well as the oviducts, should be flushed.

These procedures should result in the recovery of approximately 80 per cent of embryos, regardless of the time after mating at which collection is attempted. Collections can be carried out beyond day 7 but, by then, many embryos will have developed into expanded blastocysts. These may collapse during collection, making them difficult to identify in the medium.

In both species, the number of embryos recovered rarely exceeds the number of corpora lutea (CL), indicating a low incidence of polyovular follicles. In the doe, however, CL are not as well defined as in the ewe, and some difficulty may be experienced in counting them, particularly after day 4.

Little is known of how many collections can be made from individual animals. The two main factors limiting repeated collections could be the development of refractoriness to gonadotropins and the presence of adhesions resulting from previous collections. If refractoriness does not develop (and there is limited evidence suggesting that this is the case) and if care is exercised in surgery, two or three effective collections from individual donors should be possible. Nonsurgical collection would limit adhesion problems, but there seems little hope of developing nonsurgical collection procedures in either the ewe or the doe.

HANDLING AND SHORT-TERM STORAGE OF EMBRYOS

Media

Various media have been used for the collection and storage of embryos prior to transfer. Homologous blood serum has been used successfully but has now been replaced by balanced salt solutions enriched with serum or serum albumins. Media should have a pH within the range 7.2 to 7.8 and an osmolality of about 300 mOsm. Dulbecco's phosphate-buffered saline (see Table 1, page 82) enriched with 15 to 20 per cent of serum from the species or 3 mg/ml of bovine serum albumin satisfies these requirements and is the most widely used medium for collection and storage of sheep and goat embryos. When serum is used, some precautions have to be exercised in its preparation. Serum is usually sterilized by passage through asbestos filters (e.g., Seitz filters), and it is advisable to discard the first 300 to 400 ml of filtrate because of the reported content of growth-inhibiting substances in the filters. Cellulose acetate filters (e.g., 0.45 μ Millipore filters) can be used, but, because of clogging, it is difficult to filter more than 40 to 50 ml of serum through individual filters. After filtering, serum can be stored frozen (-10 to $-20°C$) for use as required in the preparation of media. Antibiotics (100 IU of potassium penicillin and 50 IU of streptomycin sulfate/ml) are added to the medium, with a final filtering through cellulose acetate filters of about 0.3 μ pore size. Completed medium can be stored frozen for several months or refrigerated (5 to 8°C) for 3 to 4 days.

Handling

Embryos are handled as described for cattle and stored at 25 to 30°C prior to transfer.

In Vitro Storage Time

There is little information available concerning the effect of time elapsing between collection and transfer on the subsequent viability of sheep and goat embryos. Generally, media used for flushing and storage are similar to those that will support development during *in vitro* culture. Therefore, storage for several hours prior to transfer, if not associated with rapid changes in temperature, should have no marked effect upon subsequent viability.

The addition of about 20 per cent of blood serum from the appropriate species to enriched phosphate-buffered saline (PBS) provides a medium in which sheep or goat embryos can be cultured or cooled to 5 to 10°C. Cooling and warming rates of 0.5 to 1.0°C per minute have proved effective, but the duration of storage without marked loss if viability is restricted to 3 to 4 days. Even so, such short-term storage could be of practical use for transport of embryos and might allow transfer to less advanced recipients some days later.

EVALUATION OF EMBRYOS

The stage of development of embryos in relation to the time elapsing between mating and recovery (Table 1) and their general appearance are the major means of assessing viability. Occasionally, one or more relatively underdeveloped embryos are collected with others at the expected stage of development, e.g., 2-cell embryos with those of 8 cells or 8-cell embryos with blastocysts. Although little information is available about the capabilities of the underdeveloped embryos to fully develop to lambs or kids, studies of *in vitro* cultures would suggest that most of them are not viable. In the ewe, embryos with unequal-sized blastomeres or small anucleate particles are frequently encountered (Fig. 1), but the indications are that they are "atypical" rather than abnormal and are capable of full development to

normal lambs. Gross abnormalities of sheep embryos do occur, and many are the result of the involvement of more than one sperm in the fertilization process. However, it is doubtful if polyspermic ova progress beyond the pronuclear stage, in which case they would be indistinguishable from unfertilized ova and hence rejected for transfer. The incidence of atypical and abnormal embryos in the doe is not known. In neither species is there any evidence to suggest an effect of gonadotropin treatment on the incidence of abnormalities.

In the ewe, detailed information is available on the stage of development of embryos in relation to the time elapsing between the onset of estrus and collection (Table 1 and Fig. 1). In the goat, the limited data available suggest a similar rate of development but with embryos collected at equivalent stages being some 12 to 24 hours less advanced than sheep embryos. This is accounted for by later ovulation in goats. In both species ovulation occurs near the end of estrus, but the duration of estrus in the doe is usually at least 12 hours longer than in the ewe. In both species, embryos appearing to be at least 24 hours younger than expected are of suspect viability and probably unsuitable for transfer.

SYNCHRONIZATION AND SELECTION OF RECIPIENTS

Potential recipients should be capable of carrying and rearing young and preferably should be of a size similar to, or larger than, their respective donors. There appears to be no disadvantage in using recipients of breeds different from the donors.

TABLE 1. *Stage of Development of Sheep and Goat Embryos Collected at Various Times after Onset of Estrus*

Day of Collection*	Sheep	Goat
2	2–4 cells	1–2 cells
3	8 cells	4–8 cells
4	8–20 cells	8–20 cells
5	Early morulae (>20 cells)	20 cells–early morulae
6	Late morulae (cells condensed)–early blastocysts (limited expansion)	Morulae
7	Expanded and hatching blastocysts	Late morulae–expanding blastocysts
8	Hatched blastocysts	Hatching and hatched blastocysts

*Day of onset of estrus = day 0.

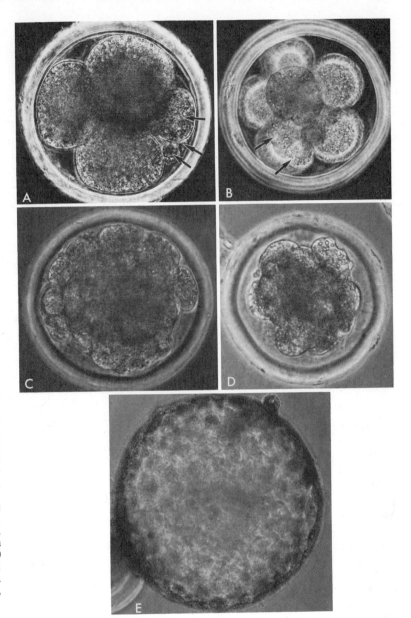

Figure 1. Sheep embryos at various transferable stages of development. *A,* 4-cell egg, day 2. Note the small particles (arrowed) making this an "atypical" rather than an abnormal embryo. *B,* 8-cell egg, day 3. This embryo is also atypical although at the expected stage of development. *C,* Early morula, day 5, containing more than 20 cells. *D,* Late morula, day 6, showing condensed inner cell mass. *E,* Expanded, hatched blastocyst, day 8. Note the loss of the zona pellucida. All photographs × 350 magnification. (Photographs *A* and *B* by kind permission of Dr. I. D. Killeen, from his Ph.D. thesis, University of Sydney, 1969).

The major factor affecting survival and development of transferred embryos is the degree of synchrony of estrus between donors and recipients. In the ewe, irrespective of age of embryos, greatest survival rates are achieved when the donor and recipients are less than 24 hours out of synchrony. Critical data are not available for the doe, but there are indications that the doe may tolerate as much as 36 hours' asynchrony.

About 10 potential recipients should be available for each donor. Synchronization treatment of recipients may be necessary when their numbers are limited or the transfer program is intense. Daily progesterone injections (12 mg/day for 16 to 18 days) or, more conveniently, intravaginal pessaries are effective for the control of estrus in cyclic females of both species, and the ability of treated recipients to support transferred embryos does not differ from that of naturally cycling females. Most ewes and does are in estrus 2 to 3 days after removal of pessaries or 3 to 5 days after the final progesterone injection. In order to synchronize estrus in donors and recipients, progestogen treatment of the recipients should be discontinued 1 day earlier than in their potential donors.

Apart from periods during which recipients are not showing full breeding activity, little or no advantage is to be gained from using gonadotropins together with progestogen treatment. Estrus and ovulation can be induced in anestrous ewes and does by relatively low doses of PMSG (400 to 700 IU) given on the day before, or day of, the conclusion of progestogen treatment. However, in practice it is probably not advisable to conduct transfer programs outside the normal breeding season. This is because there are suggestions, in both species, that survival rates of embryos in females following the induction of estrus, particularly of those in deep anestrus, may be reduced.

In sheep, the PG analog cloprostenol has been used (as in donors) to a limited extent to synchronize recipients, and acceptable pregnancy rates have been obtained.

When the time of estrus in donors and recipients is artificially controlled, transfer operations can be precisely programmed some time in advance.

TRANSFER OF EMBRYOS

Because of the tortuous nature of the cervix of both species, transfer is restricted to surgical procedures, such as those described for donors, carried out under general or local anesthesia. Local anesthesia has the advantages of low cost and rapidity, but necessitates proper restraint of animals in a laparotomy cradle. Transfer by minor surgery with laparoscopic techniques may be possible but has not yet been reported.

Transfer can be conveniently made by Pasteur pipette attached by flexible tubing to a 2-ml syringe. Each embryo is transferred by using approximately 0.01 ml of medium to the oviducts (up to and including day 3) or to the uterine horns 3 to 5 cm from the uterotubal junction (day 4 and later). A smooth-ended pipette inserted 2 to 3 cm into the oviduct via the fimbria should be used for tubal transfers, while a sharp-ended pipette stabbed through the uterine wall into the lumen is appropriate for uterine transfers.

The number of embryos transferred to individual recipients will depend upon their natural ability to support multiple pregnancies, and the potential of recipients to support multiple pregnancies should be taken into account before deciding on the number of recipients required for transfer programs. Little information is available on transuterine migration of embryos in the ewe and doe, but when two or more embryos are transferred, it is probably advisable to distribute them equally between the two oviducts or horns.

MANAGEMENT OF RECIPIENTS

No special attention other than that accorded to naturally pregnant females needs to be given to pregnant recipients.

During the breeding season, nonreturns to service can provide an early indication of pregnancy. Peripheral plasma progesterone levels on the eighteenth day after estrus in the ewe and on the twenty-second day in the doe should be more accurate for early pregnancy diagnosis. At later stages, x-ray examinations, rectal probes, ultrasonic apparatus, laparotomy or laparoscopy can be used to diagnose pregnancy, but such procedures can be costly and time-consuming and can suffer from varying degrees of inaccuracy.

PERSONNEL REQUIREMENTS

These are similar to those described in the following article on pigs.

REFERENCES

1. Moore, N. W. and Shelton, J. N.: Response of the ewe to a horse anterior pituitary extract. J. Reprod. Fertil., 7:79, 1964.
2. Trounson, A. O., Willadsen, S. M. and Moor, R. M.: Reproductive function in prepubertal lambs: ovulation, embryo development and ovarian steroidogenesis. J. Reprod. Fertil., *49*:65, 1977.

Procedures and Results Obtainable in Pigs

B. N. DAY

University of Missouri, Columbia, Missouri

SELECTION OF DONORS

The type of donor to be selected for embryo transfer will vary with the application of this procedure, as discussed in the introduction to this section. The sow should be reproductively sound and in good health for best results, especially as collection of embryos has to involve anesthesia and surgery. However, it should also be recognized that embryo transfer may provide a means of prolonging the reproductive life of superior sows that cannot reproduce for reasons other than a failure to produce normal eggs.

Both gilts and sows may be used as donors, but surgery is generally easier in gilts. When gilts are to be used, it is preferable that they be mature enough to have exhibited at least one normal estrous cycle. Gilts and sows with irregularities in the reproductive cycle should be recognized as poor risks for use in an embryo transfer program and should therefore be used only for special reasons.

Repeated embryo recovery is possible in pigs, but there is little information that can be used to predict the number of collections that might be expected from a gilt or sow. Adhesions around the reproductive tract have an adverse effect on egg transport and fertilization, as well as on manipulation of the reproductive tract at a subsequent recovery, and are the main problem hampering repeated operations. The use of surgical techniques that minimize adhesions is therefore particularly important when repeated collections are planned.

SUPEROVULATION AND INSEMINATION OF DONORS

Treatments

Superovulation can be induced in gilts by subcutaneous (SC) injection of 1500 IU of pregnant mare serum gonadotropin (PMSG) on day 15 or 16 of the estrous cycle. Lower doses of PMSG (1000 to 1200 IU) should be used in particular lines of gilts if the larger dose results in excessive ovarian stimulation. Estrus can be expected to be advanced by about 1 day as a result of the PMSG injection. Sows can be superovulated at weaning by an injection of 1200 IU of PMSG given SC on the morning of the day following removal of the pigs. Initially, for optimal results superovulated gilts and sows within a herd should be bred only when in estrus. Human chorionic gonadotropin (HCG) may then be introduced into the treatment schedule for more precise control of the time of ovulation, with the time of the HCG injection set to coincide with, or precede slightly, the expected onset of estrus. This will usually be 3.5 to 4 days after PMSG injection in gilts and 3 days following PMSG administration in sows. Ovulation can be expected to occur 40 to 42 hours after the injection of HCG.

Inexplicable variations in the ovulation rate occur in gilts and sows of similar age, breeding, management and reproductive stage that are given the same dose of PMSG. With the higher doses of PMSG, an average ovulation rate of between 20 and 30 may be expected, with a range as wide as 10 to 50. The standard deviation of ovulation rate is frequently increased three- to five-fold by superovulation. Use of a standard treatment regimen will help to minimize, but will not eliminate, the variation in response to PMSG.

Insemination

To help insure high fertilization rates in superovulated gilts and sows, matings or inseminations can be made every 12 hours during the first 2 days of estrus. The most important single insemination is at 24 hours following the onset of heat or the injection of HCG.

Standard artificial insemination (AI) procedures may be used for donor gilts. Using repeated inseminations of 100 ml of diluted, unstored semen containing at least 4 billion live sperm, conception rates and fertilization rates of recovered eggs in the 75 to 95 per cent range have been obtained in several studies.

EMBRYO COLLECTION

Choosing the Time of Embryo Collection

Embryo recovery can be timed either from the onset of estrus or from the injection of HCG in order to obtain the desired cleavage stage. More variation from predicted developmental stages should be expected when schedules are based on the onset of estrus. Embryos enter the uterus from the oviduct 66 to 90 hours after the onset of estrus or, on average, approximately 48 hours after ovulation.

To recover 4- to 8-cell embryos for transfer, the uterine horns of donors should be flushed approximately 90 to 96 hours following the onset of estrus or about 48 hours after ovulation. Both 2- and 4-cell eggs are present at 3 days following the onset of estrus, and a high proportion of the recovered embryos will be at the morula stage 5 days after the beginning of estrus.

Embryo transfer at the 4- to 8-cell stage is recommended primarily because embryos can be evaluated with less difficulty at this stage. Equally successful results have been obtained by the transfer of embryos of earlier cleavage stage to the oviducts of recipient gilts. However, reduced pregnancy rates have been observed following the transfer of blastocysts to synchronous recipients 6 days or more after the onset of estrus.

Surgical Collection of Embryos

Anesthesia is induced by an IV injection of 1.0 gm of sodium pentothal (or other effective agent) via an ear vein. A short length of tubing connecting the syringe to the needle is very helpful in preventing the needle from being dislodged by sudden movement of the pig during the infusion. The donor is then connected to a closed-circuit anesthetic unit by means of a mask, intranasal tubes or an endotracheal tube. Anesthesia may be maintained with halothane in nitrous oxide and oxygen, according to standard procedures. The ovaries and uterus are exposed by a midventral incision, using aseptic surgical procedures.

When embryos are to be recovered from the oviduct (Fig. 1), only a small portion of the reproductive tract need be exposed in order to insert a glass cannula with a flared end into the oviduct. The cannula is only inserted a short distance (2 to 3 cm) into the ampulla, particularly if very recent ovulations are evident, and is secured there with a ligature. Insertion of the cannula is usually easier if the infundibulum is not dislodged from the ovary. Eggs are flushed from the oviduct by injecting warmed (37°C) flushing medium (20 to 30 ml) into the isthmus of the oviduct through a 22-gauge needle at a point close to the uterotubal junction. The flushing medium is collected in a glass bowl and examined to determine if a second flush is needed. Alternatively, two flushings can be made routinely before examination. It is only in exceptional cases that missing eggs are recovered after a second flush.

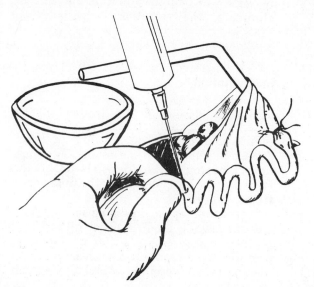

Figure 1. Recovery of embryos from the oviduct in a pig. For explanation, see text.

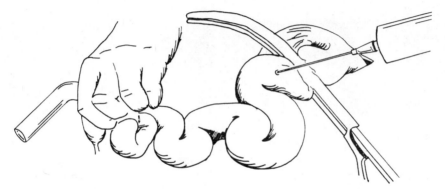

Figure 2. Recovery of embryos from the uterus in a pig. For explanation, see text.

To recover eggs from the uterus (Fig. 2), the uterine horn is occluded about 20 cm from the uterotubal junction with intestinal forceps. A blunted needle attached to a syringe is then inserted into the infundibular opening of the oviduct and 20 ml of medium is flushed through into the uterus. By gently stripping the fluid toward the intestinal forceps, embryos are removed from the area adjacent to the uterotubal junction and are kept away from that area by constricting the uterus with the thumb and forefinger. The end of a scalpel handle is used to make a longitudinal opening in the wall of the emptied part of the uterus about 5 cm from the uterotubal junction and a flared glass cannula (inside diameter 8 to 10 mm) with a curve of about 45° is inserted. The size of the cannula required will vary between gilts and sows, depending on the size of the reproductive tract. Pinching the uterine wall with the thumb and forefinger before penetration and then inserting the cannula immediately help to minimize contamination of the cannula with blood. The cannula may be held in place by an assistant or secured there with appropriate towel forceps. The medium in the uterus is then allowed to flow back toward the uterotubal junction and an additional 20 ml is infused into the uterus at a point adjacent to the intestinal forceps. As in other species, a blunt needle should be used for the uterine injection. The flushing medium is stripped toward the cannula, and the embryos are collected through it into a glass bowl for examination. After removal of the cannula, the uterine wall is sutured.

HANDLING AND SHORT-TERM STORAGE OF EMBRYOS

Media

Several media have been used successfully for embryo recovery and transfer in pigs, including TCM-199, Tyrode's and Brinster's solutions.

Handling

Examination of the flushings for embryos is made with a stereomicroscope and can be extremely difficult if collections are contaminated with cellular debris or blood. Bloody flushings should be diluted with fresh medium and then reduced in volume by aspirating off the top portion of fluid, which would not contain the embryos. Severe contamination usually results in failure to locate the embryos. Once found, embryos are transferred to a warmed glass bowl containing fresh medium, using methods already described for cattle. They should be stored at 35 to 37° C until transferred.

In Vitro Storage Time

The procedures involved permit transfer of recovered embryos to recipients within 1 hour or less following recovery. Embryos have been held successfully for longer periods without taking special precautions, but the practice is not to be encouraged un-

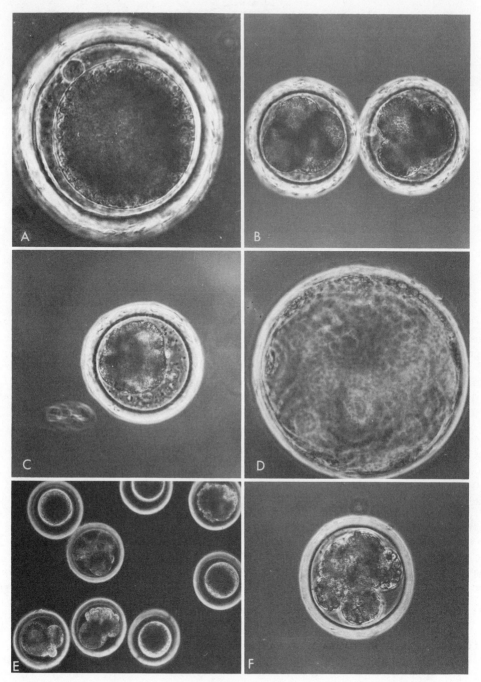

Figure 3. Pig embryos at transferable stages of development and degenerating pig eggs. *A,* An uncleaved pig egg recovered from the oviduct and probably fertilized. Note the prominent polar body and numerous spermatozoa in the zona pellucida ($\times$ 500 approx.). *B,* Two 4-celled pig eggs. Blastomeres are of equal size, dense, and well defined in comparison with the fragmenting egg shown in *F.* Spermatozoa are evident in the zona pellucida ($\times$ 300 approx.). *C,* A morula recovered from the uterus. Individual blastomeres are not obvious in the compact group of cells, and normal morulae may appear similar to unfertilized and fragmenting eggs. Spermatozoa are evident in the zona pellucida ($\times$ 300 approx.). *D,* An expanded blastocyst recovered from the uterus. The zona pellucida is still intact but thinner. The blastocoele is well developed ($\times$ 500 approx.). *E,* Uncleaved and fragmenting pig eggs at lower magnification. Note the absence of spermatozoa in zonae pellucidae and the lack of cellular organization in fragmenting eggs ($\times$ 175 approx.). *F,* A fragmenting pig egg. Compare the appearance and density of spermatozoa in the zona pellucida with *B* and *C.* The absence of well defined blastomeres indicates atypical cleavage ($\times$ 300 approx.).

less necessary for special reasons. For research purposes, pig embryos have been cultured for 24 hours at 37°C in a humidified atmosphere of 5 per cent CO_2 and 95 per cent air with no apparent decrease in embryo survival rates following transfer.

EVALUATION OF EMBRYOS

The 4- to 8-cell cleavage stage is the preferred time for evaluation of embryos in a transfer program. At the 4-cell stage in particular, there is usually little uncertainty regarding normal cleavage. Recovery at earlier stages may necessitate evaluation of 1-cell eggs, and at later cleavage stages it is more difficult to determine if blastomeres of unequal size are due to asynchrony in cleavage or to fragmentation. Also, individual blastomeres are less distinct, and normal morulae may appear similar to degenerating, unfertilized eggs (Fig. 3).

SYNCHRONIZATION AND SELECTION OF RECIPIENTS

Asynchrony in the occurrence of estrus or the injection of HCG in donor and recipient animals should be no more than 24 hours.

Gilts or sows may be used as recipient animals. Frequently, only gilts are used as recipients, and the time of ovulation is controlled. Prepuberal gilts aged 6 to 7 months may be injected with 750 IU of PMSG given SC followed 96 hours later by 500 IU of HCG administered IM. The time of the HCG injection is then considered to be "onset of estrus" for purposes of arranging synchrony with donors. Weaning may also be used to synchronize donor and recipient sows, or gilts and sows in a recipient herd that are synchronized with donors by chance may be used.

The effective synchronizing agent methallibure (Aimax, ICI) is no longer available. An alternative method, using gonadotropins and prostaglandins (PG), is under development and may be useful in transfer work. PG is luteolytic in pigs only between days 11 or 12 and 14 or 15, which is too short a period for practical use in synchronizing groups of normally cycling animals. To overcome this, PMSG and HCG are used to induce accessory corpora lutea (CL), which postpone estrus in all animals. Twelve days after giving HCG, PG can cause all the CL to regress, resulting in a high degree of synchronization and normal fertility.[1]

Recipient gilts should be examined during surgery to determine that CL of normal appearance are present. Considerable variation may be observed in the degree of luteal development present in donor and recipient gilts exhibiting estrus at the same time. Even so, substitution may sometimes be made for recipient animals that appear to differ extremely from the donor in their cyclic development, as indicated by ovarian examination.

TRANSFER OF EMBRYOS

Embryos are transferred to the recipient by use of a fire-polished Pasteur pipette through a puncture wound in the uterine wall about 10 to 15 cm from the uterotubal junction. The technique is as described for cattle (see page 86). All embryos can be transferred at one site, since spacing within the uterus will occur by intrauterine migration.

Alternative methods of uterine transfer have been used, including the insertion into the oviduct of a silicone rubber tube containing the embryos and medium. The tubing is attached to a syringe containing a larger volume of medium, and after the tubing is securely located within the oviduct, the medium containing the embryos is flushed into the uterine horns. A similar procedure that has been used successfully is to introduce the tubing into the uterine lumen through a small puncture wound made in the isthmus of the oviduct adjacent to the uterotubal junction.

Transfers of younger embryos to the oviduct are made by introducing the pipette into the lower ampulla. After expelling the embryos, the ampulla is constricted with the thumb and forefinger as the transfer pipette is withdrawn.

Effective nonsurgical transfer procedures have not been developed for swine, although it has been demonstrated that it is possible to obtain pregnancy by introducing the embryos through the cervix.

MANAGEMENT OF PREGNANT RECIPIENTS

Ultrasonic techniques are available to diagnose pregnancy at 30 to 60 days gestation in recipient animals not returning to estrus. Pregnant recipients are managed as for normal pregnancy.

PERSONNEL REQUIREMENTS

Transfers can be easily accomplished by a team consisting of a surgeon and two assistants whose responsibilities include preparing and anesthetizing animals for surgery, assisting with embryo recovery, evaluating

recovered embryos and transferring embryos to the recipients. The most intensive training required is in the evaluation of embryos.

REFERENCE

1. Guthrie, H. D. and Polge, C.: Control of oestrus and fertility in gilts with accessory corpora lutea by prostaglandin analogues, ICI 79,939 and ICI 80,996. J. Reprod. Fertil, *48*:427, 1976.

Procedures and Results Obtainable in Horses

K. J. BETTERIDGE

Agriculture Canada, Animal Diseases Research Institute (Eastern), Ottawa, Ontario, Canda

Relatively little work has been done on embryo transfer in horses for two main reasons. First, it has proved very difficult to superovulate mares; second, authorities who govern horse breeding have been notoriously reluctant to countenance "new" techniques such as artificial insemination (AI), let alone one that was first reported to be successful in 1974. Most of the developmental work reported has been by Oguri and Tsutsumi in Japan and Allen and coworkers at Cambridge, England. (see Allen's review in Monograph 1).

TREATMENT OF DONORS

Superovulation

The mare is very insensitive to gonadotropic stimulation. The only successes so far have been produced by use of crude or partially purified extracts of equine pituitary glands injected daily for 14 days during anestrus or for 6 days during the estrous cycle. Up to four ovulations per mare have been induced in this way, but transfer work to date has relied upon recovery of single, spontaneously produced embryos.

Induction of Single Ovulations

In the other farm animals, the timing of ovulation in relation to estrus is fixed closely enough to permit the use of estrus as a substitute for ovulation in dividing the follicular from the luteal phase of the estrous cycle. Such an approximation cannot be used in mares because of their long and variable periods of estrus. Human chorionic gonadotropin (HCG), 2000 to 3000 IU given IV or IM on about the third day of estrus, usually induces ovulation 24 to 72 hours later and helps a great deal in timing breeding and embryo collection arrangements. Its use with prostaglandins (PG) in synchronizing ovulation in donors and recipients will be described later.

Insemination

Standard natural breeding or AI procedures are used, either on alternate days during estrus, or when follicular rupture is anticipated from rectal palpation or at the time of HCG injection.

EMBRYO COLLECTION

Choosing the Time of Embryo Collection

Embryos enter the uterus 6 days after ovulation in the mare. Unfertilized eggs are retained in the oviduct for many months.

Transfers for most purposes are likely to be made 6 days or more after ovulation. This is because nonsurgical techniques for recovering and transferring uterine embryos are relatively easy and successful. Also, success rates seem to increase with time after ovulation, at least within the first 6 days. The upper age limit of embryos that can be transferred successfully is not known.

Surgical Collection of Embryos

These are likely to be limited to experimental use. Under general anesthesia induced with a barbiturate (e.g., methohexitone sodium, 5 mg/kg of body weight) and maintained with halothane in oxygen (with or without nitrous oxide), a 15- to 20-cm midline incision is extended caudally from just cranial to the umbilicus. Abdominal retractors and moist packs help in exposing the uterus, which is anchored to the retractors by umbilical tape ligated around the uterine body as far caudally as possible.

Uterine embryos can be recovered through a two-way Foley catheter inserted through a puncture in the base of the horn on the side of ovulation and are held in position with a ligature behind the fully inflated balloon. Medium (30 to 50 ml) is introduced and recovered through the same catheter. Alternatively, a glass or plastic cannula with a smooth, flared end can be substituted for the Foley catheter for collection. Medium is flushed toward it through a blunt 18-gauge needle introduced near the tip of the horn.

Embryos cannot be flushed back up the oviduct from the uterus because the uterotubal junction acts as a one-way valve. Therefore, within 6 days of ovulation, they have to be flushed from the oviduct into the uterus and collected through a cannula or Foley catheter inserted as just described, but nearer the tip of the uterine horn. A laboratory animal feeding needle or a blunt 18-gauge needle, passed into the ampulla through the fimbria and held there between the finger and thumb, is used for the flush. Exposure of the ovaries and oviducts for this purpose (and for confirming the site of ovulation) can be difficult in young mares. For research purposes, when it is essential to know that an embryo was, in fact, recovered from the oviduct, it is possible to flush in the reverse direction, using a fine cannula passed through the uterotubal junction exposed by a small uterine incision.

Surgical repair is by standard procedures, but postoperative antibiotic coverage is necessary in mares.

Nonsurgical Collection of Embryos

A large, easily dilatable cervix and straight, tubular uterine horns make the mare well suited to nonsurgical recovery techniques. Larger bore versions (10 mm outside diameter [OD]) of the cuffed tubes described for cattle can be introduced *per vaginum,* held in position *per rectum* and used for either in-out or continuous flow irrigation. The balloon cuff, inflated to a diameter of about 6 cm, can be used either in the cervix or in the base of each horn in turn. Volumes used for flushing have ranged between 100 and 1500 ml. Between 40 and 90 per cent of mares flushed later than 6 days after ovulation have yielded embryos. The fact that embryos have been recovered in up to five successive flushes from individual mares is particularly encouraging.

HANDLING, SHORT-TERM STORAGE AND EVALUATION OF EMBRYOS

Embryos are handled as in the other species.

Storage and evaluation have not been critically investigated in horses. Japanese workers have used physiological saline supplemented with either 2 per cent gelatin or mare's serum to recover embryos. Their successful transfers occurred when the medium was made up of equal parts of mare's serum and Ringer's solution containing penicillin. Cambridge workers used TCM-199 initially and then changed to enriched phosphate-buffered saline (PBS) (see Table 1, page 82), in parallel with their work with cattle.

Embryos recovered from the oviduct have first to be distinguished from old, retained, unfertilized eggs. It can also be difficult to determine whether early embryos are cleaving or fragmenting. Fortunately, an embryo recovered from the uterus is not likely to be developing abnormally and, as a blastocyst, has a very characteristic appearance. Unlike the other farm species, the equine embryo remains spherical in shape until it attaches to the uterine wall. Early

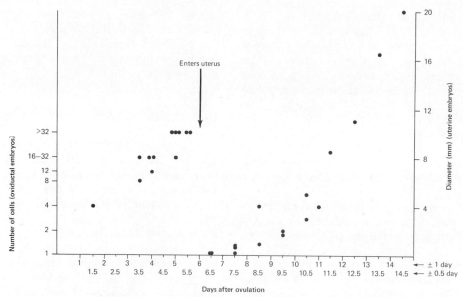

Figure 1. The cleavage and growth of embryos in pony mares. Each point represents a single embryo. (From Monograph 1.)

developmental stages are depicted in Figs. 1 and 2.

SYNCHRONIZATION OF RECIPIENTS

The degree of synchrony necessary for successful transfer in horses has not been determined but is assumed to be similar to that necessary in other farm animals. Insuring that donor and recipient ovulate within a 48 hour period has, until now, been difficult. Recently, however, a double prostaglandin (PG) treatment (based on analogous approaches to synchronizing random groups of cattle) has proved an effective means of synchronizing ovulation in groups of mares during the breeding season. All mares in the group are given a luteolytic dose of the PG analog fluprostenol (Equimate, ICI) on a given day designated as day zero. This will be luteolytic only in animals with a 4- to 13-day-old corpus luteum (CL). They will come into estrus 3 days later, while the others either progress into their luteal phase (if they had younger CL when treated) or return to estrus to their own accord (if they had more advanced CL when treated). HCG (2500 IU, IM) is given on day 6 to help synchronize ovulation in estrous animals, and about 75 per cent of mares ovulate 24 to 72 hours

later. On day 14, all mares have CL that are more than 4 days old, produced either spontaneously or in response to treatment. A second course of treatment (PG on day 14, HCG on day 20) therefore results in luteolysis in all mares, in synchronized onset of estrus in about 60 per cent and in synchronized ovulation in about 80 per cent of those treated.

TRANSFER OF EMBRYOS

Surgical Methods

These are exactly the same as those used in the other species but are unlikely to be utilized very widely in view of the success with nonsurgical techniques. Deposition in the oviduct has been used for embryos collected 1 or 2 days after ovulation. All embryos at later stages have been transferred to the uterus. At Cambridge only one transfer in eight was successful between 1 and 3 days after ovulation compared with six in eight between days 4 and 6.

Nonsurgical Methods

Simply depositing the embryo into the body of the uterus by means of a cattle insemination pipette through the cervix has

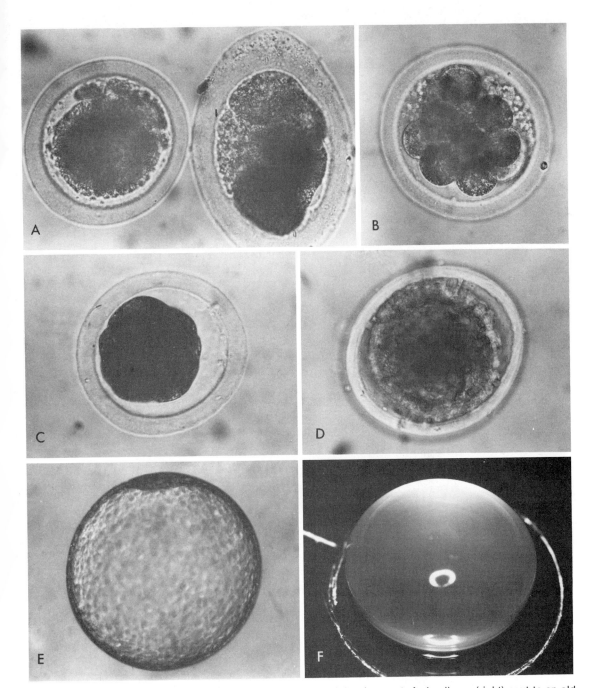

Figure 2. Horse embryos at various transferable (?) stages of development. *A*, 4-cell egg (right) next to an old, unfertilized egg flushed from the oviduct of the same mare 1½ days ± ½ day after ovulation (× 284). *B*, 12-cell egg from the oviduct 4 days ± 1 day after ovulation (× 288). *C*, Morula from the oviduct 5 days ± 1 day after ovulation (× 288). *D*, Early blastocyst from the uterus 6½ days ± ½ day after ovulation (× 275). *E*, Expanded blastocyst from the uterus 7½ days ± ½ day after ovulation (× 86). *F*, Expanded blastocyst from uterus 12½ days ± ½ day after ovulation (× 3.4). (From Monograph 1.)

led to success in eight of eleven (72 per cent) attempts (see Allen in Monograph 1). No special effort need be made to place the embryo ipsilateral to the CL, probably because transuterine migration of the embryo often occurs in the mare under normal circumstances. There is little doubt that the efficiency of nonsurgical techniques in the mare could make embryo transfer a relatively easy tool to use in reproductive work in horses, especially if the two impediments mentioned at the beginning of this article can be overcome.

REFERENCE

1. Monograph 1. Betteridge, K. J. (ed.): Embryo Transfer in Farm Animals — A Review of Techniques and Applications. Monograph No. 16, Agriculture Canada, Ottawa, 1977 (available from Information Division, Canada Department of Agriculture, Ottawa, K1A OC7, Canada).

Long-Term Storage of Frozen Embryos

N. W. MOORE

University of Sydney Farms, Camden, New South Wales, Australia

INTRODUCTION

The effective storage of embryos would have numerous applications. Synchronization of recipients with donors would not be necessary, and embryos could be held and transferred as suitable recipients became available. Storage would provide a method of cheap and rapid transport of animals, and potentially valuable animals (including rare breeds and species) could be retained for future use. Further, while embryos are stored prior to use, their parents or sibs or both, could be tested for disease and for production characteristics.

Short-term storage for the various species has been described earlier in this section and is already being used for the transport of embryos at temperatures of about 5 to 10°C.

Successful frozen storage of mammalian embryos was first achieved in the mouse, then in sheep, cattle and goats, but not in pigs because of an inability to cool pig embryos below 15°C without loss of viability. Although relatively few embryos of farm animals have been frozen with subsequent normal development after thawing, most of the factors likely to affect viability have been identified.

Cryoprotective Agents

Enriched phosphate buffers similar to those used for liquid storage have been used for frozen storage, but cryoprotectants need to be added before freezing and removed after thawing. Two cryoprotectants have been used: dimethylsulfoxide (DMSO) at concentrations of about 1.5 M, and glycerol at 1.0 M. They serve to prevent intracellular development of ice crystals that would damage cells. DMSO has been successfully used with sheep and cattle embryos and glycerol with cattle and goat embryos, but in none of the species have strict comparisons been made between the protective capacities of the two cryoprotectants.

Optimal Developmental Stages of Embryos for Freezing

To date, appreciable survival rates have been achieved only with late morulae and early blastocysts collected 6 to 8 days after mating. Earlier and later stage embryos appear to be more susceptible to the freezing or thawing procedures or both, presently in use.

Freezing and Thawing Rates

Survival has been achieved with cooling rates of between 0.1 and 0.3°C/minute and warming rates of 1 to 12°C/minute. It is likely that very slow cooling is required to dehydrate embryos and hence minimize damage from intracellular ice formation before the whole embryo becomes frozen. During the cooling procedures, the induction of ice crystallization in the freezing medium at temperatures of about −3 to −7°C is necessary to achieve survival. In the three species in which success has been achieved, there are indications of differences in cooling and warming rate requirements. With cattle morulae and early blastocysts, cooling rates of about 0.15°C/minute have been successful when DMSO has been used as a cryoprotectant. When glycerol has been used, survival has been achieved with a cooling rate of 0.3°C/minute. Sheep embryos at a similar stage of development have survived cooling at 0.3°C/minute in media containing DMSO, while, in the goat, glycerol and a cooling rate of 0.2°C/minute have been used successfully. However, far too few embryos have been used in the limited number of studies reported to make firm recommendations.

In general, embryos are cooled at slow rates to approximately −60°C and then more rapidly (about 1°C/minute) to about −100°C before transferring them directly into liquid N_2 for storage.

Limited survival of sheep embryos has been obtained following rapid thawing by placing the embryos directly into warm water, but until thawing rates are more fully investigated, slow thawing procedures would seem to be more appropriate.

FREEZING AND THAWING PROCEDURES

Small glass tubes containing 2 to 3 ml of storage medium are generally used, but for ease of identification and safety, the use of ampules and straws similar to those used for storage of semen should be investigated.

Addition of Cryoprotectant

DMSO or glycerol should be added at about 30°C to allow rapid penetration. DMSO is added by moving the embryos through dishes containing increasing concentrations of DMSO in the medium (0.25, 0.50, 0.75, 1.00, 1.25 and 1.50 M) and leaving the embryos to equilibrate in each dish for 4 to 5 minutes before transfer into the next higher concentration. Glycerol has been added by the slow addition (over 15 to 20 minutes) of medium containing twice the required concentration of glycerol (2.0 M) to embryos held in a similar volume of medium devoid of glycerol. Although different procedures have been used for the addition of the two cryoprotectants, no reasons have been

given for this, nor have strict comparisons been made between procedures.

Cooling

Several cooling procedures have been described. The procedure adopted must depend upon the facilities available and the ability to follow predetermined cooling requirements.

The cooling tubes can be held in racks over liquid N_2 and raised or lowered as required. They can be held in ethanol (constantly stirred) and cooled by the addition of solid CO_2 to an outer jacket or directly to the ethanol, or they can be held in an ethanol bath over liquid N_2. Partial or complete automation of freezing procedures may be possible, but it is essential that there be little or no lag between an adjustment and the consequent temperature change within the cooling tubes. Commercially available freezing units for embryos are an expensive but more convenient means of achieving these temperature changes (see Appendix A).

Crystallization in the freezing tubes at −3 to −7°C is initiated by seeding with small crystals of frozen medium or by application of forceps cooled in liquid N_2 to the outside of the vial. Cooling should continue during the seeding process. To achieve the faster cooling rates below −60°C, the tubes held in racks or in ethanol over liquid N_2 can simply be lowered; those held in ethanol and cooled by solid CO_2 will have to be transferred to vessels containing liquid N_2. In commercial freezing units, cooling rates are controlled automatically.

Storage

Once in liquid N_2, no special precautions other than those used for storage of semen need be taken. However, it will be necessary to develop effective and universal methods of identifying embryos according to their source, breeding, and time of freezing.

The effect, if any, of the duration of storage in liquid N_2 on subsequent viability of embryos is not known, but apparently normal young have developed from embryos stored for 12 months and more. It might be reasonable to assume, by analogy with other cellular material that has been stored frozen, that there will be little loss of viability during extended periods of storage.

Thawing

In general, thawing procedures have been less controlled than those of freezing. Thawing rates of about 10 to 12°C/minute can be achieved by holding the freezing tubes at room temperature in test tubes previously cooled in liquid N_2, while rates of 2 to 4°C/minute can be obtained by transferring the freezing tubes to an ethanol bath previously cooled to about -100°C by immersion in liquid N_2. More precise and controlled rates of warming can be achieved by transferring the tubes to racks or ethanol baths held over liquid N_2.

Once the tubes have reached -5 to 0°C, they are allowed to warm to 30°C at 0.5 to 1.0°C/minute. The cryoprotectant should be removed by the reverse of the procedures used for its addition. Potentially viable embryos should regain their pre-storage integrity within approximately 2 to 3 hours of thawing. The proportion of embryos regaining their integrity that subsequently develop to normal young following transfer to recipients appears to be similar to that of unstored embryos.

Results

Results from studies on frozen storage of embryos of farm animals have been extremely variable, and far too few embryos have been frozen to provide meaningful indications of expected rates of success. When optimum procedures have been used, it would seem that less than 50 per cent of embryos survive freezing and thawing. It is imperative that survival rates be increased before the practical implications of frozen storage can be fully exploited. Improvements will result only from concentrated experimentation using large numbers of embryos. A major factor presently limiting experimentation is our inability, particularly with cattle, to harvest large numbers of embryos reliably from individual animals.

Possible Future Developments

K. J. BETTERIDGE

Agriculture Canada, Animal Diseases Research Institute (Eastern), Ottawa, Ontario, Canada

SEXING OF EMBRYOS

This is already possible in more advanced cattle and sheep embryos, as described and discussed in Section IV. It is possible that analogous techniques will be applied to other species and, using microsurgical techniques, to younger embryos.

PRODUCTION OF IDENTICAL TWINS

Identical twins are ideal for making comparisons between animals in many research applications. To produce them at will would be valuable. It is possible to separate individual blastomeres at the 2- to 4-cell stage and have them develop into separate individual blastocysts. At least two lambs have been born following such a procedure. However, there are too many problems involved with technique to regard it as a potential method of producing identical twins in the immediate future. Work with mice suggests that the later in development the separation is made, the less likely it is that a single blastomere will give rise to an embryo. The possibility of "cloning" (producing large numbers of identical offspring from one divided embryo) therefore seems very remote.

In studies involving the examination of large numbers of expanded blastodermic vesicles, occasional ones with twin embryonic discs have been observed. Whether these produce identical twins has not been determined, and, in any case, to select twins in this way would hardly be practicable.

There are encouraging preliminary reports from West Germany indicating that identical twin cattle may result from the microsurgical bisection of a morula or blastocyst within its zona pellucida.

PHENOCOPYING

In amphibia, it has been shown that substitution of a somatic cell nucleus for the nucleus of a developing egg results in an embryo with a genotype identical to the donor of the somatic cell nucleus. Nuclear transplantation is made easier in amphibia by large cell sizes, but, recently, limited success has also been achieved in rabbits. Nuclei of embryonic rabbit cells have been introduced into unfertilized rabbit eggs by both microinjection and virus-induced fusion and have undergone some development. An ability to produce "carbon copies" of individual animals in this way would have enormous implications but is not likely to become a reality for many years yet.

PRODUCTION OF HOMOZYGOTES

In mice, it is possible to remove one pronucleus microsurgically from one-celled, fertilized eggs. The remaining pronucleus can be induced to form a diploid nucleus by incubation in medium containing cytochalasin B. Only females will continue to develop because YY cells lack essential genes carried on the X chromosome. Transfer of the resulting blastocysts has produced litters of homozygous female mice, making this a powerful genetic tool in highly inbred laboratory strains, but analogous applications in less inbred domestic species may be limited by adverse effects of some recessive genes in homozygotes.

The Economics of Embryo Transfer

J. M. BOWEN

Texas A&M University
College Station, Texas

INTRODUCTION

The economic value of embryo transfer will depend on the balance between its costs and the benefits to be gained from the applications described in the introduction to this section. Obviously the contribution that embryo transfer can make is affected by many factors other than strictly financial ones. Nevertheless, in a free market, potential advantages of embryo transfer can only be assessed in a balanced way when all of its costs are known.

In order to reach any conclusions about the costs and returns of embryo transfer, a model unit must be envisaged, and to it must be applied reasonable (if hypothetical) production figures that would be achievable with the staff described and given reasonable success rates in superovulation and conception. Costs and results might differ considerably among embryo transfer units. The figures used in the following model can, therefore, only be applied to a particular organization after suitable modification.

Calculations have been based on an interest rate of 7.5 per cent on capital, realizing that this is subject to wide variation. Annual costs have been divided by the numbers of pregnancies that can be anticipated (from assumptions to be described), thus showing the cost of each calf obtained by embryo transfer. Cost estimates for the model have been calculated for both the United Kingdom and North America for comparative purposes. Methods of raising and utilizing capital will not be considered.

The economics of embryo transfer are changing rapidly, parallel to developing techniques. In view of this, the cost of setting up a traditional (or what might now be considered a historical) cattle transfer unit, based wholly on surgical methods, will be considered. Afterwards, the cost estimates will be modified in light of progress in embryo transfer techniques.

PROJECTED ANIMAL NUMBERS, OPERATING SCHEDULE AND SUCCESS RATES

A surgical unit necessitates superovulating donors and maintaining large numbers of recipients to keep it in full activity. The following scale of operation will be assumed:

Donor cows operated upon each month	24
Recipients needed in heat on any one day	15–20
Recipients per donor	6–7
Pregnancy rate per donor	3.5
Resultant annual total of pregnant recipients	1008

Up to 20 potential recipients should be in heat on any one day in case a particular donor yields that many embryos. Theoretically, this number of recipients could be provided by a herd of 420 animals; in practice the number needs to be closer to 500.

The average number of cattle used per operation is about six or seven, or 170 per month, all of which must be replaced as the month goes on. In view of this, it is necessary to have on hand some 600 recipients. If this recipient pool is to be operated as a closed herd, all animals must be certified free of disease before entering the premises. Therefore, an additional 170 animals each month will be in quarantine, awaiting entry into the herd. In addition, there will be recipients awaiting pregnancy diagnosis 2 months after surgery and pregnant recipients awaiting shipment to their owners. At the assumed production rate, these represent 340 and 84 animals respectively. Each month, 86 nonpregnant recipients will be either readmitted to the recipient herd or sold as empty heifers and replaced. Thus, the cattle on hand at any one time comprise:

Recipient pool	600
Replacements in quarantine	170
Recipients awaiting pregnancy check	340
Pregnant recipients awaiting shipment	84
Total	1194

Allowing for donors, this means holding about 1200 cattle. The costs of such an enterprise can be divided into capital expenditures and running expenses.

CAPITAL COSTS

Land. First, a farm unit must be purchased or leased. In an extensive system of management, the farm needs to be at least 200 acres (or on poorer soils 800 to 1000 acres) in order to accommodate the animals adequately. The alternative is to manage the cattle intensively, preferably in a feedlot. This requires more capital at first but is considerably more convenient for checking heat and for handling cattle. The cost of acquiring land can be estimated as shown in Table 1.

Buildings and Equipment. The capital costs of these are estimated in Table 2.

Donor Costs. These will usually be bought by the client rather than by the embryo transfer company. Their cost will be subject to wide fluctuations, but estimates of £1,000 or $4,000 each are considered for illustrative purposes. Using these figures, the capital cost of 50 donors is £50,000 or $200,000, with the respective interest costs being £3.72 or $14.88 per pregnancy.

Depreciation of donors must also be taken into account because experience has shown that it is unlikely, as a general rule, that a donor can be used successfully more than three times. There is also a cumulative traumatic effect of repeated surgeries, and it can be calculated that the depreciation is 50 per cent after one operation, 80 per cent after two operations and, after three operations, the animal's value can be written off completely. Depreciation of the donors can therefore be calculated as shown in Table 3.

RUNNING COSTS

Recipient Costs. In view of the high turnover of animals and in order to simplify calculations, all the recipient costs will be considered as a running expense, using North American prices as an example.

From earlier projections of animal numbers and their rate of use and success

TABLE 1. *Estimating Costs of Acquiring Land*

	United Kingdom (Pounds)			North America (Dollars)		
	CAPITAL COSTS	INTEREST COSTS	INTEREST COSTS PER PREGNANCY	CAPITAL COSTS	INTEREST COSTS	INTEREST COSTS PER PREGNANCY
200 acres	100,000	7,500	7.44	100,000	7,500	7.44
800 acres	–	–	–	32,000	2,400	2.38
Feedlot	–	–	–	50,000	3,750	3.72

TABLE 2. *Estimating Costs of Buildings and Equipment*

	United Kingdom (Pounds)	North America (Dollars)
Building	30,000	30,000
Chute	300	900
Operating table	100	450
Anesthetic machines (2)	2,000	4,000
Sterilizer	1,000	3,000
Instruments	500	1,500
Microscopes	2,000	6,000
Glassware	200	600
Miscellaneous	1,000	1,000
Initial expenses	1,000	3,000
	38,100	50,450
Depreciation per annum (33.3%)	12,700	16,816
Interest on capital	2,858	3,784
	15,558	20,600
Depreciation and interest costs/pregnancy	15.43	20.44

TABLE 3. *Calculating Depreciation Costs of Donors*

	United Kingdom (Pounds)			North America (Dollars)		
	VALUE	DEPRECIATION	COST/ PREGNANCY	VALUE	DEPRECIATION	COST/ PREGNANCY
Original	1,000	0	–	4,000	0	–
After 1 operation (3.5 calves)	500	500	142.86	2,000	2,000	571.43
After 2 operations (7 calves)	200	800	114.28	800	3,200	457.14
After 3 operations (10.5 calves)	0	1,000	95.24	0	4,000	380.95

rate, the investment in recipients at $300 each can be calculated as follows:

	Dollars
Cost of original 600	180,000
Annual cost of replacements (170/month × 12 = 2040)	612,000
Recipients awaiting pregnancy diagnosis for 2 months (340)	102,000
Pregnant recipients awaiting shipment (84)	25,200
	919,200
Less sale of empty recipients (86/month × 12 = 1032 at $150 each)	154,800
Total capital cost of recipients	764,400
Capital cost of recipients/pregnancy	758.33

It was shown previously that, at any one time, there will be 1194 recipients on hand, representing an investment of $358,200. The interest charges on this amount to $26,865 or $26.65 per pregnancy.

British cattle prices are fluctuating widely but, for discussion, will be taken as amounting to a capital cost of £470 per pregnancy with a consequent interest cost of £20 per pregnancy.

Wages. These costs are among those that reflect how busy the embryo transfer unit is. Since many costs in the running of a center are fixed, all personnel should be kept as fully employed as possible to at least reduce their cost on a per pregnancy basis. Costs may be estimated as shown in Table 4.

Feeding Costs. These expenses may be estimated as £2.00 or $1.35 per head per day. The capital cost of feed on hand will also be subject to interest charges. Thus, the cost of feeding 1194 recipients is shown in Table 5.

Drugs, Materials and Miscellaneous. Annual costs to maintain the production rate projected are shown in Table 6.

Preparation Costs. The expenses of preparing the building, instruments, glassware and animals for surgical transfers throughout the year are shown in Table 7.

Transport Costs. Each operating day, it can be anticipated that moving 15 heifers a distance of 30 miles will be necessary. Allowing £0.50 or $1.00 per mile and 2 hours of a worker's time, this amounts to £25 or $54 per day for 288 operating days per year. Additional costs will be incurred on a less regular basis, making transportation expenses as shown in Table 8.

SUMMARY OF CAPITAL AND RUNNING COSTS

From the preceding figures, the costs per pregnancy are tabulated in the first two columns of Table 9. Commercially, these costs will have to be augmented by a profit of 33.3 per cent, making the sale price of each pregnant recipient £1,931.75 or $2,134.85.

If the donors are owned by the center, interest charges and depreciation (e.g., for two operations) will increase the cost of each pregnancy to £1,566.81 or $2,073.14. The sale prices under these circumstances would therefore be £2,089.08 or $2,764.19.

SAVINGS EFFECTED WITH PROSTAGLANDINS

The use of prostaglandins (PG) allows the embryo transfer unit to reduce dramatically the number of animals on hand at any one time by synchronizing a certain number of recipients to supplement those exhibiting estrus naturally. Whether PG results in a fall in the pregnancy rate in sychronized re-

TABLE 4.   *Estimating Annual Costs of Personnel*

Personnel	United Kingdom (Pounds)	United States (Dollars)
Head veterinarian	10,000	30,000
Assistant veterinarian	5,000	20,000
Embryologist	3,000	20,000
Head stockman or cowboy	3,000	12,000
Farm hands or cowboys (4)	7,400	42,000
Secretarial staff (2)	3,000	20,000
	31,400	144,000
Cost of wages/pregnancy	31.15	142.86

TABLE 5. *Estimating Costs of Feeding Recipients*

	United Kingdom (Pounds)		North America (Dollars)	
	COST	COST PER PREGNANCY	COST	COST PER PREGNANCY
Annual cost	871,620	864.70	588,343	583.67
Interest charges on 3 months' feedstuffs on hand	16,343	16.21	11,031	10.94

TABLE 6. *Estimating Annual Costs of Drugs, Materials and Miscellaneous Requirements*

	United Kingdom (Pounds)	North America (Dollars)
Phosphate-buffered saline	50	100
PMSG	1,600	2,420
Halothane (Fluothane)	4,320	14,170
Suture materials	1,000	2,880
Miscellaneous	2,000	5,000
Total	8,970	24,570
Total annual cost/pregnancy	8.90	24.38

TABLE 7. *Estimating Annual Costs of Preparation*

	United Kingdom (Pounds)	North America (Dollars)
Washing and sterilizing	500	500
Cleaning staff	2,400	12,000
Heating	1,800	1,200
Electricity	1,200	1,200
	5,900	14,900
Total annual cost/pregnancy	5.85	14.78

TABLE 8. *Estimating Costs of Transportation*

	United Kingdom (Pounds)	North America (Dollars)
15 heifers each operating day	7,200	15,552
Other transportation	2,000	10,000
Total	9,200	25,552
Total annual transportation cost/pregnancy	9.13	25.35

TABLE 9. *Comparison of the Costs per Pregnancy in Various Forms of Embryo Transfer Units*

Expenditure	Surgical Unit		Prostaglandin Unit	Feedlot Liaison	Veterinary Practice (Nonsurgical Collection)
	POUNDS	DOLLARS	DOLLARS	DOLLARS	DOLLARS
Land, interest on capital	7.44	7.44	7.44	3.72	–
Buildings and equipment— depreciation and interest on capital	15.43	20.44	20.44	20.44	–
Recipients—capital cost	470.00	758.33	669.04	453.57	634.52
Recipients—interest charges	20.00	26.65	19.96	9.46	17.60
Wages	31.15	142.86	142.86	157.74	71.43*
Feeding—annual cost	864.70	583.67	437.02	207.27	385.20
Feeding—interest charges on feedstuffs on hand	16.21	10.94	8.19	3.89	7.22
Drugs, materials, etc.	8.90	24.38	24.38	24.38	11.90
Preparation	5.85	14.78	14.78	14.78	–
Transport	9.13	25.35	25.35	50.70	14.28
Prostaglandin costs	–	–	10.00	–	15.71
Total cost of each pregnancy	1,448.81	1,614.84	1,379.46	945.95	1,157.86
Savings effected	–	–	235.38	668.89	456.98

*Fee paid/pregnancy.

cipients is disputed. In any case, it could be argued that some fall is more than justified by the savings incurred. The herd of potential recipients cannot be reduced to less than 300 to 350 animals if it is to provide 170 cows a month, and so the costs would be as follows:

Recipient Costs. The capital cost of 300 recipients is $90,000, half that previously tabulated. The rate of use and replacement remains the same, so the capital cost of recipients per pregnancy with the reduced herd becomes $669.04.

The number of cattle on hand at any one time in the smaller herd will be 894, some 300 fewer than before, representing an investment of $268,200. The interest is therefore reduced to $20,115 or $19.96 per pregnancy.

Feeding Costs. The annual cost of feeding the smaller herd is reduced to 894 × 1.35 × 365 = $440,519 or $437.02 per pregnancy. Similarly, the amount of feed on hand for 3 months is reduced, and so interest charges on it fall to $8,259 or $8.19 per pregnancy.

Prostaglandin Costs. If seven animals are treated for each operating day at $5 per dose, the annual cost is 7 × 5 × 288 = $10,080 or $10 per pregnancy.

Summary of Savings. Other costs remain as before, so the savings effected can be seen in the third column of Table 9.

SAVINGS EFFECTED BY USING FEEDLOT HEIFERS

One of the simplest and most effective means of cutting recipient costs is to build the embryo transfer unit in conjunction with an existing feedlot. Then it is only necessary to employ someone to check the heifers for estrus in the feedlot and to remove them as required 2 days before surgery. Compensation to the feedlot operator would vary between $50 and $150 for each animal operated upon, and the nonpregnant animals would be returned to the feedlot to be fattened and slaughtered as before. If the embryo transfer unit is responsible for feeding the animals postoperatively up to the time of pregnancy diagnosis, the following calculations can be made:

Recipient Costs. The 1032 recipients that do not become pregnant each year will cost 1032 × 150 = $154,800 in compensation. The 1008 pregnant heifers will be purchased for $302,400, making a total of $457,200 or $453.57 per pregnancy.

Annual interest charges will be reduced because, at any one time, the unit will hold only 340 animals awaiting diagnosis and 84 pregnant animals awaiting shipment home. These 424 animals represent an investment of $127,200, with interest charges of $9,540 or $9.46 per pregnancy.

Wages. An extra person in the feedlot would cost $15,000 annually or $14.88 per pregnancy.

Feeding Costs. The annual cost of feeding 424 animals is 424 × 1.35 × 365 = $208,926 or $207.27 per pregnancy. Three months' food supply represents an investment of $52,231, with interest charges of $3,917 or $3.89 per pregnancy.

Transport Costs. If these double (which is unlikely), they would add $25 to the cost of each pregnancy.

Summary of Savings. Other costs, again, remain as before, and so the savings are shown in the fourth column of Table 9.

COSTS OF NONSURGICAL EMBRYO TRANSFER

The preceding costs could be supported only by an "artificial" market, as was discussed in the introduction to this section. Since the end of the "boom," there has been a renewed effort to reduce costs by using nonsurgical methods, especially in dairy cows.

A small nonsurgical unit, focusing its attention on the recovery of single embryos, could be set up alongside a veterinarian's clinic. Processing perhaps two donors a week would be possible with a smaller staff and would blend in very well with a large animal practice. Dairy animals could be presented on the day of nonsurgical collection and returned home immediately afterwards. Such a unit would not need more than 30 to 50 recipients on hand and could adjust its work timetable to suit local conditions. Alternatively, it would be feasible to run a small unit that visited farms to collect the embryos, transferring them to the farmers' own recipients. If the farmers had sufficient replacement heifers to be used as recipients, PMSG could be used for superovulating the donor. Such intraherd transfers could dramatically reduce the main cost of embryo transfer — that of feeding and maintaining recipients. However, a unit attached to a veterinary clinic doing two collections a week from superovulated donors for 9 months of the year (i.e., 72 collections per year, producing 252 pregnancies) would remain costly because of the need to maintain recipients. This can be seen in the following cost accounting:

Recipient Costs. The original 50 would cost $15,000. A total of 504 recipients would be used for transfers from 72 collections and

would cost $151,200 to replace. The 252 nonpregnant recipients would realize $37,800 when sold. At any one time, with the unit holding a 2-month output of recipients awaiting diagnosis (84 animals) and a 1-month output of pregnant recipients (21 animals), this brings the total capital cost to $159,900 or $634.52 per pregnancy. Interest charges on the 197 animals on hand amount to $4,433 per year or $17.60 per pregnancy.

Wages. These would mostly be absorbed by the veterinary practice, with the substitution of a veterinarian's fee of $250 per collection or $17.43 per pregnancy.

Feeding Costs. To feed 197 animals for 1 year would cost 197 × 365 × 1.35 = $97,072 or $385.20 per pregnancy. Holding feedstuffs for 3 months involves capital of $24,268, with annual interest charges of $1,820 or $7.22 per pregnancy.

Drugs, Materials and Miscellaneous Costs. Excluding PG, these are estimated at about $40 per collection or $3,000 annually ($11.90 per pregnancy).

Transport Costs. These would be similar to those incurred in the surgical system, approximately $50 per collection day or $14.28 per pregnancy.

Prostaglandin Costs. At $5 per dose, and allowing for the treatment of one donor and 10 recipients per collection, this amounts to 72 × 11 × 5 = $3,960 or $15.71 per pregnancy.

Summary of Nonsurgical Costs in a Veterinary Practice. The annual cost of producing 252 pregnancies (3.5 per collection) is shown in the last column of Table 9.

Larger units would need not only more recipients but also facilities for housing and milking donors, making costs even closer to those of a surgical unit.

COSTS OF EMBRYO FREEZING COMBINED WITH NONSURGICAL TECHNIQUES

Embryo freezing will no doubt go a long way toward changing and improving the concept of embryo transfer and greatly facilitating the global transport of cattle, while at the same time reducing the risks that have always been associated with cattle movements. Contributing to this expectation is the fact that the additional expense of the freezing equipment and laboratory facilities, compared with the major cost of the recipient herd, is minimal. Reduced shipping charges should, therefore, more than compensate for freezing costs.

Projected Animal Numbers, Operating Schedule and Recovery Rates. In an embryo freezing unit, superovulation would greatly increase the number of embryos available for freezing at little cost increase to the unit. Since the day-7 embryo is suitable for freezing, the following approximate schedule would allow the collection of multiple embryos resulting from superovulation in successive estrous cycles:

Day 0	Inseminate at natural estrus
Day 7	Collect single embryo
Days 8 and 10	Administer PMSG and PG
Days 12 and 13	Inseminate at induced estrus
Day 20	Collect multiple embryos
Day 32	Inseminate at natural estrus and repeat the timetable

About seven embryos should be the average nonsurgical yield, thus this timetable would theoretically provide eight embryos or, with repetition, 17 embryos within 2 to 3 months. Such a schedule should be well-suited to the high-producing dairy cow. Possible drawbacks to such a system would be refractoriness to repeated PMSG treatments (which is unproved) and longer cycles following superovulation (which could be abbreviated with use of PG). With this system, it is projected that 20 donors at any one time would be sufficient for one superovulated donor per day, 288 days per year, yielding 2000 embryos. The nonsuperovulated donors would be in addition to these, but their yield is included in the 2000 embryos for purposes of discussion. Over the year, 118 donors would be needed to provide this number of embryos at the rate or production just projected.

Freezing eliminates the need for having synchronous recipients on collection days, so a herd of 80 recipients at any one time would be adequate.

Land. The smallest acreage projected for the original surgical transfer unit would be adequate, at a projected cost of $60,000 with interest charges of $4,500.

Buildings and Equipment. Milking fa-

cilities will have to be provided, so the cost of buildings would remain at $30,000. Commercially available freezing units are included because of their convenience. Temperature measuring equipment is added for controlling other types of freezing system and for developmental work. In summary:

Buildings	30,000
Microscopes	6,000
Freezer	3,000
Pyrometer and attachments	5,000
Pyrograph	3,000
Glassware, etc.	1,000
Liquid nitrogen containers	4,500
Total	52,500
Depreciation per annum	17,500
Interest on capital	3,938
Total depreciation and interest costs	$21,438

Wages. The payroll for a veterinarian, embryologist, cryobiologist, two dairymen, two farm hands and a secretary would total $100,000 annually.

Feeding Costs. Feedstuffs for the 20 donors will cost $9,855; the 3-month supply on hand will incur interest charges of $185 per annum.

Drugs, Preparation and Collection Materials Costs. These are estimated as:

Liquid nitrogen (6300 liters)	1,890
PMSG and PG ($12.50 per treatment)	3,600
Catheters, etc.	3,000
Media	1,500
Straws and /or ampules	1,000
Miscellaneous supplies	1,000
Heating and sterilizing	1,000
Total	$12,990

Transport Costs. At $25 per working day this will be $7,200.

Summary of Collection and Freezing Costs. These are as follows:

Land—interest on capital	4,500
Buildings and equipment—depreciation and interest on capital	21,438
Wages	100,000
Feeding—annual cost	9,855
Feeding—interest on feedstuffs on hand	185
Drugs, materials, etc. and preparation	12,990
Transport	7,200
Total	$156,168
Total cost per embryo for 2000 embryos collected	$78.09

Costs of Transferring and Transporting Frozen Embryos. As has been discussed earlier in this section, it is really too early to know what pregnancy rates to expect with large-scale application of the technique. For illustrative purposes, a pregnancy rate of 33 per cent for all frozen embryos will be assumed, i.e., 666 per year or 2.3 per collection or 5.6 per donor. The collection cost for each pregnancy is thus 156,168 ÷ 666 = $234, but transfer costs must be added to this.

Assuming that 60 per cent of all embryos frozen will be transferred, 2000 embryos will require 1200 recipients. If the place of transfer is local and similar to the collection center, its capital and running costs can be taken to be the same as the collection center, with additional feeding costs of $30,000 to cope with 80 recipients at any one time. Transfer costs are therefore 186,168 ÷ 666 = $280 per pregnancy. Thus, the total cost of obtaining a calf from a frozen embryo would be $514 plus the cost of a recipient, or $814 based on previously assumed prices.

Transport costs must be added if the frozen embryos are to be exported. For export from Canada to the Middle East, for example, 2000 ampules would require three liquid nitrogen containers costing about $800 each to dispatch by air freight. The additional expense of 2400 ÷ 666 = $3.60 per pregnancy is insignificant.

In comparison, Auld Croft Farms (personal communication) have stated that to move 490 pregnant recipients by air from North America to the Middle East would cost $435,000. Unfortunately, it can reasonably be assumed that 10 to 15 per cent of these recipients will abort as a result of the journey, leaving about 417 pregnant animals that cost $1,043 each to transport. When the cost of the transfer is added to this, the advantage of shipping frozen embryos is obvious.

bryo transfer to increase beef production by low-cost twinning. They concluded that an embryo transfer unit, working with nonsurgical recovery and transfer methods, could have operating costs as low as £68 per calf. Even at this price they felt that it would be uneconomical for commercial beef production. Their hypothetical scheme entails the recovery of 4500 eggs per annum from two donors per day and transfer into synchronized recipients by a team of only three people, which would be no mean feat. As cited, their cost estimates do not take into account some real expenses that would arise with the service they envisage. In treating the National herd as a single herd, they appear to have oversimplified the situation, making it analogous to an intraherd transfer scheme in which both the donor and recipient costs could be discounted. In addition, they anticipate obtaining a 60 per cent conception rate for nonsurgical transfers, which may be optimistic.

The present analysis of costs has, necessarily, been made on hypothetical model systems, but it is hoped that this will provide the reader with an indication of expenses that will be incurred and economies that might be effected.

The high costs of embryo transfer are likely to restrict its use to specialized purposes over the foreseeable future. There is no shortage of such purposes in research, and the savings that could be brought about by transporting frozen embryos have been demonstrated. With the demise of the surgical embryo transfer unit, it remains to be seen in what applications the more flexible nonsurgical techniques will be economically feasible.

A broader difficulty facing the agricultural economist is knowing how to justify this tool of increased productivity in a world that appears to have an overabundance of meat and milk.

DISCUSSION

According to Cox,[1] Wilmut and Hume have considered the prospects of using em-

REFERENCE

1. Cox, S.: Costs limit scope for ova transplants. Farmers Weekly, *85*(22):85, 1976.

section IV

CYTOGENETICS

Consulting Editor

W. C. D. HARE

Cytogenetics*

W. C. D. HARE

Animal Pathology Division, Health of Animals Branch, Agriculture Canada, Animal Diseases Research Institute, Ottawa, Ontario, Canada

INTRODUCTION

Cytogenetics, or cellular genetics, started as a branch of genetics toward the end of the nineteenth century with studies into the cytological basis of Mendel's laws of inheritance. For the first half of the twentieth century most cytogenetic studies were done on plants, invertebrates or lower vertebrates. Mammalian cytogenetics, of which both human and veterinary cytogenetics are a part, has developed mainly within the last 20 years.

Cytogenetics is the field of study concerned with (1) the structure and properties of chromosomes, (2) chromosomal behavior during somatic cell division (mitosis) in growth and development and germ cell division (meiosis) in reproduction (Figs. 1, 2, 3, 4), (3) chromosomal influence on the phenotype and (4) the factors that cause chromosomal changes. Veterinary cytogenetics is the application of cytogenetic studies to clinical problems affecting domesticated animals.

The intent of this chapter is to show how cytogenetic studies can be a useful diagnostic tool in animal reproduction and how they can be, and have been, used to understand the pathogenesis of some types of infertility, embryonic and fetal death, abnormal sexual and somatic development and hybrid sterility. The application of cytogenetic studies to prenatal sex determination and detection of chromosomal abnormalities is also considered. Finally, the techniques used to prepare material for cytogenetic studies and the methods used in analysis are described, and suggestions are made for the selection, handling and submission of tissues for cytogenetic studies.

A glossary of terms is provided at the end of this article. The system of nomenclature used to describe the chromosomal complement and any abnormalities is explained briefly here.

In describing a complement, the number of chromosomes is given first, followed by a comma and the sex chromosome constitution, e.g., a bull: 60,XY. The autosomes are specified only when there is an abnormality present. When whole chromosomes are added or missing, plus (+) or minus (−) signs are placed before the chromosome designation, e.g., a cow with trisomy 18: 61,XX,+18. When parts of a chromosome are added to or deleted from, + or − signs are placed after the chromosome designation. The short arms are designated p, the long arms q. If there is any doubt about the identification of a particular chromosome, a question mark (?) is put before it. Therefore a cow with a deletion of the long arm of what is thought to be chromosome 13 would read 60,XX,?13q−. When two or more different cell populations are present, they are listed in numerical or alphabetical order, e.g., sex chromosome chimerism in a freemartin: 60,XX/60,XY. There are a number of nomenclature symbols that are used to indicate structural changes. Some of these are: translocation, t (rob, tan and rcp are optional alternatives to "t" for Robertsonian, tandem fusion and reciprocal translocations, respectively); inversion, inv; insertion, ins; dicentric, dic (resulting from a translocation, tdic); centromere, cen; and duplication, dup. These are written in lower case immediately before the chromosome designation. If more than one chromosome is involved, a semicolon (;) is used to separate the designations, e.g., a bull heterozygous for a centric fusion between autosomes 1 and 29: 59,XY,t(1q;29q) or 59,XY,rob(1q;29q).

INFERTILITY AND STERILITY

When infertility is indicated by a reduction in the expected litter size in multiparous species and by increased early returns to service in primiparous species, fertilization failure or early embryonic death due to chromosomal abnormalities should be considered as a possible cause.

Male and female animals heterozygous

*Dr. W. C. D. Hare thanks Drs. A. H. Corner, M. D. Eaglesome, Wendy E. Hare, R. A. McFeely and D. Mitchell and Mrs. E. L. Singh for reading the manuscript and making constructive suggestions and Mrs Singh for help in preparing the karyotypes.

Metaphase Chromosomes

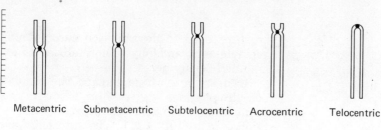

Metacentric   Submetacentric   Subtelocentric   Acrocentric   Telocentric

Figure 1. The morphological classification of mitotic metaphase chromosomes based on centromeric position.

for a genetically balanced autosomal abnormality are usually phenotypically normal. However they can produce unbalanced products of meiosis (Figs. 5, 6) that, if they are capable of maturation and fertilization, will give rise to genetically imbalanced embryos that may die *in utero* or be congenitally malformed.

Not all animals heterozygous for balanced autosomal abnormalities are infertile. In the male, if the unbalanced products of meiosis fail to mature or if they mature but are incapable of fertilization, lowering of fertility will not be noted because there will be an adequate number of balanced spermatozoa available to take their place. However, in the female, since there are fewer ova maturing at any one time, a failure to mature or be fertilized could result in lowered fertility. Therefore, the effect of each type of genetically balanced autosomal abnormality has to be evaluated independently. Male and female animals homozygous for a genetically balanced autosomal abnormality will produce only balanced meiotic products and will be fertile. Reports of chromosomal findings in cases of infertility and sterility, as just defined, are summarized in Table 1.

Diagnosis

Chromosomal analysis of blood leukocytes will readily determine the presence of autosomal abnormalities resulting in numerical or gross structural changes, but the effect of these abnormalities on fertility has to be determined either by chromosomal studies on cells in meiosis or by studies of litter size or nonreturns to service in a statistically significant number of animals with appropriate controls. It must be borne in mind, however, that genetically balanced autosomal changes that do not result in numerical or gross structural alterations can also produce unbalanced gametes. These may be detected in chromosomes during mitosis by using banding techniques or may be determined more readily in chromosomes during meiosis.

EMBRYONIC AND FETAL MORTALITY

Embryonic and fetal death accounts for a substantial loss in animal production. Various etiological factors can be involved, and, as a result, estimates of the percentage loss that occurs differ considerably. In the mare, dog and cat, the loss probably averages 10 to 15 per cent and in the cow, ewe, doe and sow approximately 20 to 30 per cent. Studies done on man and in the pig suggest that in all species a proportion of the loss is probably due to chromosomal abnormalities.

In man, it is estimated that 15 to 20 per cent of all conceptions fail and that 20 to 25 per cent of spontaneous abortions have chromosomal abnormalities. The vast majority (95 to 96 per cent) of these are numerical changes, such as monosomy, polysomy, polyploidy (simple and in mosaic or chimeric form) and mixoploidy, and only 4 to 5 per cent are structural.

In the pig, nine (10 per cent) of eighty-eight 10-day-old blastocysts showed chromosomal abnormalities. Another 2.3 per cent were degenerating, and the possibility that this was due to chromosomal defects could not be excluded. Among the nine, eight had numerical and one had structural abnormalities: four triploidy, three tetraploidy, one diploidy/triploidy and one deletion. In a similar study of seventy-six 25-day-old embryos, eight (10.5 per cent) were dead and one (1.3 per cent) had a chromosomal abnormality.

Monosomies and polysomies are probably due to nondisjunction during meiosis or the

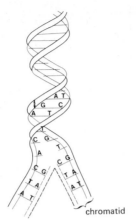

DNA replication
Figure 2.

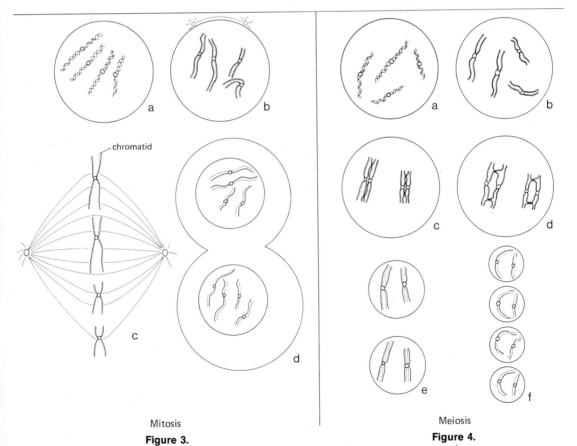

Mitosis

Figure 3.

Meiosis

Figure 4.

Figure 2.   The double helical structure of a molecule of deoxyribonucleic acid (DNA) in the process of replication. Adenine (A), thymine (T), guanine (G) and cytosine (C).

Figure 3.   Some of the stages of mitosis: *a,* prophase; *b,* late prophase; *c,* metaphase and *d,* telophase.

Figure 4.   Some of the stages of meiosis: *a,* zygotene; *b,* pachygene; *c,* diplotene; *d,* diakinesis; *e,* telophase I and *f, telophase II.*

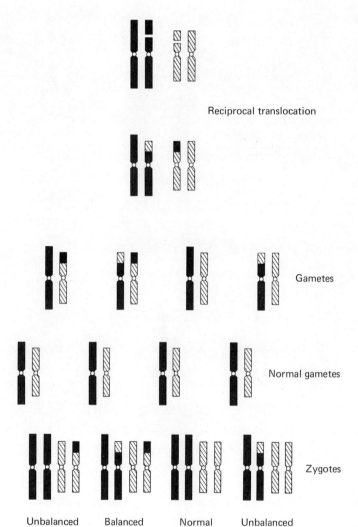

Reciprocal translocation

Gametes

Normal gametes

Zygotes

Unbalanced   Balanced   Normal   Unbalanced

Figure 5. Diagram of the possible segregation patterns for the gametes of a reciprocal translocation heterozygote during meiosis and the types of zygote they can form with normal gametes.

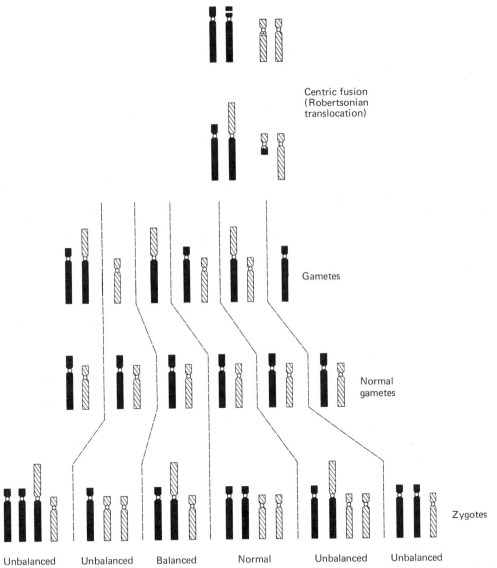

Centric fusion
(Robertsonian
translocation)

Gametes

Normal
gametes

Zygotes

Unbalanced   Unbalanced   Balanced   Normal   Unbalanced   Unbalanced

Figure 6. Diagram of the possible segregation patterns for the gametes of a centric fusion heterozygote during meiosis and the types of zygote they can form with normal gametes.

TABLE 1. *Chromosomal Findings in Infertility and Sterility*

Species	Sex	Chromosomal Complement	Remarks
Horse	M	–	None reported
	F	63,Xp−q−	Irregular estrus and follicular regression
Cattle	M and F	59,XY,t(1q;29q)	Reduced fertility
	M and F	59,XY,t(2q;4q) 59,XY,t(14q;20q) 59,XY,t(27q;29q) 59,XY,t(1q;25q) 59,XY,t?(7—11q;20—25q)	Number of affected animals too small to determine effect on fertility
	F	59,XX, dic(6;16)	
	M	60,XY/59,XY,t(14q;20q)	Reduced fertility
	M and F	59,XY with autosomal tandem fusion	Reduced fertility
	M	60,XY with autosomal pericentric inversion	Infertile
	M	60,XY with increased frequency of autosomal chromatid gaps and breaks	Reduced fertility
	M	60,XY/60,XX in hemopoietic tissues	Bulls twin to freemartins with nonspecific reduced fertility or sterility
	F	59,XX,t(1q;29q) and an X-autosome translocation	Repeated returns to service and one stillborn calf
Sheep	M and F	Two different centric fusions and one dicentric fusion (Robertsonian translocations)	Fertility of heterozygous rams unaffected; fertility of heterozygous ewes may be affected
Goat	M and F	Centric fusions	Evidence regarding effect on fertility inconclusive for bucks; embryonic mortality in does heterozygous for one centric fusion reported as higher
Pig	M	38,XY/38,XY,t(6q+;15q−)	100 per cent embryonic mortality
	M	37,XY,−18/38,XY/39,XY+18 37,XY,−18/38,XY	50 per cent reduction in litter size production
	M	38,XY,t(1p−;6q+) 38,XY,t(13q−;14q+)	Heterozygotes had reduced fertility
	M	38,XY,t(11p+;15q−)	Father and son with reduced fertility
	F	38,XX+cen 38,XX/38,XX+cen	Reduced first litter size
Dog	M and F	Several centric fusions reported	No information of the effect on the fertility of the heterozygotes
Cat	M and F	–	None reported

Meiotic Non-disjunction

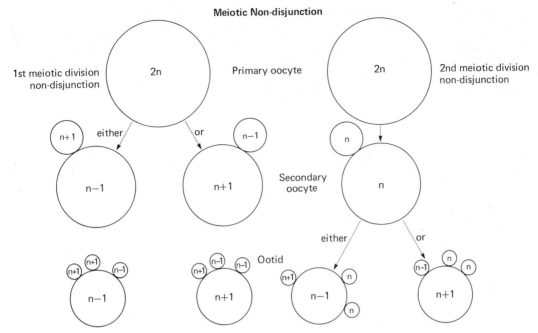

Figure 7. The mechanism of nondisjunction, which occurs during the first or second meiotic division and results in either monosomy or trisomy.

early cleavage stages (Figs. 7, 8). Triploidy can be caused by two sperm entering (polyspermy) and fertilizing (polyandry) one egg or by suppression of the second polar body and one sperm fertilizing a diploid egg (polygyny) (Fig. 9). The incidence of both polyandry and polygyny is known to be increased by aging of the gametes. This is more likely to happen in animals that ovulate spontaneously, e.g., mare, cow, ewe, goat, sow and dog, than in animals in which ovulation is induced, e.g., the cat, and especially when artificial insemination is used rather than natural service. In man, in whom the likelihood of coitus is not limited by estrus, the possibilities for aging of the gametes are considerable. Tetraploidy probably occurs because of suppression of the first cleavage division of a diploid zygote; the chromosomes duplicate and divide, but the cell does not. It has been shown that tetraploidy of fertilized ova can be induced by heat treatment, and one can speculate that an elevated body temperature due to fever or environmental circumstances might do the same. Tetra-

Mitotic Non-disjunction

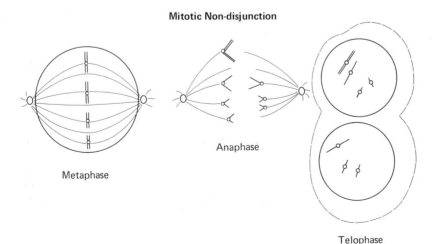

Figure 8. The mechanism of mitotic nondisjunction leading to either monosomy or trisomy.

Triploidy

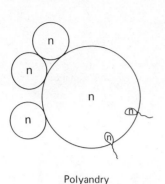

Polyandry

Polygyny

Figure 9. Triploidy resulting from polyandry or polygyny.

ploidy can also occur because of fusion of diploid zygotes or fertilization of a haploid ovum by three spermatozoa.

Mixoploids arise from a mitotic error during an early cleavage division of the zygote. Chimeras, which resemble developmental mixoploids, are formed by the fusion of two zygotes. Diploid/triploid chimeras can be formed by the fusion of a diploid zygote with a triploid zygote or by the second polar body failing to extrude and subsequently fusing with one of the blastomeres from the first cleavage division.

Structural rearrangements (Fig. 10) may be due to random or nonrandom spontaneous breakage and reunion, and the genotype may play a role in these, but it is also well known that other factors such as certain viruses, drugs, chemicals and radiation cause chromosomal damage. Certain viruses are known to be associated with early embryonic death, but it has not been shown, as yet, that these deaths are also associated with chromosomal abnormalities.

Animals heterozygous for a balanced translocation are potential candidates for producing genetically imbalanced gametes that, in turn, can form unbalanced zygotes that will die. Examples of this have been described under the heading of infertility and sterility.

The pathogenesis of early embryonic death is likely due to the fact that the genetic imbalance created by the chromosomal abnormality is such that embryogenesis is arrested either immediately or in its early stages. The types of chromosomal abnormalities associated with fetal death more closely resemble those observed in congenital malformations. Based on the observation that embryonic cell lines with chromosomal abnormalities grow more slowly than diploid embryonic cell lines, the lethal effect may be due to (1) placental development taking place more slowly than fetal development with the resultant death of the fetus or (2) a decreased cell growth rate leading to asynchronous development with disturbances in the embryonic induction mechanisms leading to reduced size and cell numbers in various organs.

Diagnosis

A diagnosis of embryonic or fetal death due to chromosomal abnormalities depends on the ability to demonstrate the presence of abnormalities that are inconsistent with life in the embryonic or fetal material.

Embryonic material has to be obtained by experimentation. Chromosome preparations are made by a direct method or following cell culture. Fetal material can be used for chromosomal analysis provided that it is sterile. Cells from some tissues, such as bone marrow, can be processed directly. Cells from other tissues, including blood, have to be cultured.

CONGENITAL ABNORMALITIES

Testicular Hypoplasia

A bilateral reduction in the size of scrotal testes without any other apparent phenotypic abnormality is sometimes associated with chromosomal aberrations. The small size of the testes is usually detected at puberty when the glands fail to enlarge. The most common association is with an aneuploid sex chromosome complement (e.g., 2n+1,XXY) or variants with an aneuploid sex chromosome complement (e.g., 2n,XY/2n+1,XXY). In man, such sex chromosome aneuploids are associated with Klinefelter's syndrome, for which consistent features are gynecomastia, small testes with aspermatogenesis and hyalinized seminiferous tubules but intact Leydig cells, as well as elevated levels of urinary gonadotropins. In animals, hyalinization does not seem to be a regular feature, but the seminiferous tubules are reduced in number and typically are lined by Sertoli cells with little or no germinal epithelium. Interstitial tissue appears to be increased, and Leydig cells are intact but may be hyperplastic and clumped. Hormone assays have usually not been done. Less marked

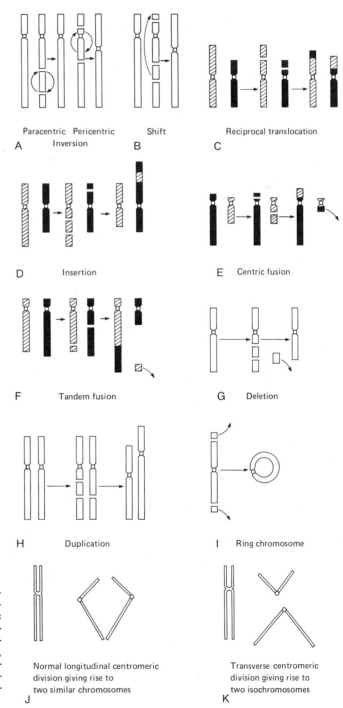

Figure 10. Diagrams to illustrate how various structural chromosomal rearrangements occur: *A,* paracentric and pericentric inversion; *B,* shift; *C,* reciprocal translocation; *D,* insertion; *E,* centric fusion; *F,* tandem fusion; *G,* deletion; *H,* duplication; *I,* ring chromosome and *J,* normal centromeric division versus a transverse centromeric division that gives rise to isochromosomes.

bilateral testicular hypoplasia, in which germinal epithelium is present but spermatogenesis is incomplete, has been seen in association with autosomal aberrations, "sticky" chromosomes, multipolar nuclear spindles in spermatocytes and a lack of homology between maternal and paternal chromosomes that occurs in some interspecific hybrids, e.g., mule.

Chromosomal abnormalities that have been reported in association with bilateral testicular hypoplasia are summarized in Table 2.

Gonadal Dysgenesis

This designation includes phenotypic female animals with a history of anestrus and the following features: normal vulva and vagina, underdeveloped uterus, absent or small inactive gonads that have no follicular development and are unresponsive to hormones, absence of or poorly developed secondary sexual characteristics due to a lack of estrogens and elevated levels of urinary gonadotropins. Chromosomal studies have shown that a number of these animals have aneuploid or unexpected sex chromosomal complements. In man, phenotypic females with ovarian dysgenesis and sex chromosomal abnormalities have been divided into three groups based on their clinical features and the histology of their gonads: (1) those with ovarian dysgenesis, short stature, webbed neck and other somatic anomalies (Turner's syndrome); (2) those with ovarian dysgenesis, short stature and few or no other somatic anomalies and (3) those with ovarian dysgenesis, normal or increased stature and no other somatic anomalies. The latter form of dysgenesis is usually referred to as pure gonadal dysgenesis. The most common sex chromosomal abnormality in groups 1 and 2 is 45,X, but 45,X mosaicism with structurally normal sex chromosomes, 45,X/46,XX; 45,X/46,XY, also occurs fairly frequently. In group 3 the majority of patients have normal sex chromosomal complements 46,XX and 45,XY, but a few have 45,X; 45,X/46,XY or 45,X/46,XX complements. Occasionally cases of gonadal dysgenesis are accompanied by clitoral enlargement.

The chromosomal complements reported in association with gonadal dysgenesis in domestic animals are summarized in Table 3.

Ovarian Hypoplasia

Under this designation will be considered animals that are phenotypic females with a history of occasional or very irregular estrus. The external and internal genitalia are normal female but may be underdeveloped. The ovaries are small, smooth and usually without palpable follicles. On histological examination the ovaries show a reduced number of follicles, very few of which are normal and most of which are degenerating or degenerated. The chromosomal findings are summarized in Table 4.

Diagnosis of Congenital Abnormalities

Cytogenetic studies can be of value in clarifying the cause of some cases of testicular hypoplasia, gonadal dysgenesis and ovarian hypoplasia. A venous blood sample and a piece of fascia, skin or mucous membrane should be submitted for cell culture and chromosomal analysis together with a full history, clinical findings and, whenever possible, all or part of the gonads for microscopic examination. Chromosomal analyses may also be of value in differentiating between gonadal dysgenesis and testicular feminization because the genetic sex of the latter is always male.

INTERSEXES

Traditionally the term "intersex" has been used almost synonymously with the term "hermaphrodite" to describe animals whose genital organs have some of the characteristics of both male and female, but in this article the term "intersex" will be expanded to include "sex reversed" animals, i.e., animals whose chromosomal or nuclear sex is the opposite of their gonadal sex.

Sex chromosomal aberrations are found quite frequently in intersexes because an abnormality of the sex chromosomes can be expected to affect the differentiation of the gonad, which, in turn, will affect the development of the Wolffian and Müllerian duct systems, the urogenital sinus and the primordia of the external genitalia. Maleness has to be induced in the bipotential undifferentiated reproductive system. Induction

TABLE 2. *Chromosomal Aberrations in Testicular Hypoplasia*

Species	Chromosomal Complement	Remarks
Stallion	–	None reported
Bull	60,XX/60,XY 61,XXY 60,XY/61,XXY 60,XX/60,XY/61,XXY	Reported in association with marked bilateral hypoplasia
	59,X/60,XY/61,XXY	Associated with but apparently not a direct cause of hypoplasia in related bulls
	"Sticky" chromosomes, multipolar nuclear spindles	Observed in association with less severe hypoplasia characterized by thin, watery ejaculate
Ram	59,XXY	Seen in some cases of marked bilateral hypoplasia
	Centric fusions	"Hourglass" testes with spermatocyte arrest and cryptorchidism seen in association with translocations, but cause and effect relationship not demonstrated
Buck	60,XX	Marked bilateral hypoplasia seen in extreme masculinized form of intersex condition in polled goats
	62,XXXY/63,XXXXY	Reported in association with hypoplastic scrotal testes, well-developed teats and milk secretion
Boar	–	None reported
Dog	79,XXY	Bilateral hypoplasia
Tom	38,XX/38XY 39,XXY 38,XY/39,XXY 38,XY/39,XYY 38,XX/57,XXY 38,XX/57,XYY 38,XY/57,XXY 38,XX/38,XY/39,XXY 38,XY/39,XXY/40,XXYY 38,XX/38,XY/39,XXY/40,XXYY	Reportedly associated with bilateral hypoplasia in sterile tortoise-shell or calico (T-C) cats. Orange and black coat colors require the presence of two X chromosomes.
	38,XY (presumed 38,XY/38/XY chimera) 39,XX/38,XY 38,XY/57,XXY	Some T-C male cats are fertile presumably because of a predominating influence of the XY cells

TABLE 3. *Chromosomal Findings in Gonadal Dysgenesis*

Species	Chromosomal Complement	Remarks
Mare	63,X 63,X/64,XX 63,X/64,XY	Anestrus; small, flacid uterus and cervix; gonads unresponsive to hormones
	64,XY	Similar findings to above, but no histologic examination of gonads; therefore possible testicular feminization
Cow	60,XX	Vulva, vagina, poorly developed udder and teats; anestrus; gonads unresponsive to hormones
Sow	37,X	Anestrus, infantile genitalia, short bowlegs
Queen	37,X	One case, lived only 3 days; therefore speculative as to future gonadal development
Ewe	–	No reports
Doe	–	No reports
Bitch	–	No reports

TABLE 4. *Chromosomal Findings in Ovarian Hypoplasia*

Species	Chromosomal Complement	Remarks
Mare	65,XXX	Irregular estrous cycles, no conceptions, normal external genitalia, underdeveloped uterus, small ovaries
Cow	60,XY	Anestrus, normal external genitalia, underdeveloped udder and teats, small uterus, inactive ovaries with degenerate follicles
	61,XXX	Small but normal body conformation, only one recorded estrus at 18 months, underdeveloped uterus, both ovaries small and spindle-shaped—one with one follicle and one corpus luteum, the other with only ovarian stroma
		61,XXX also found in heifer that was fertile
	High frequency of chromatid gaps, breaks and deletions in long arm of one X chromosome	Sterile
Ewe	–	No reports
Doe	–	No reports
Sow	–	No reports
Bitch	–	No reports
Queen	–	No reports

is caused by secretions from the fetal testes, and there are many stages of development during which the masculinization process can go wrong and cause intersexuality. Femaleness, on the other hand, is basic, and a female reproductive tract will develop in spite of differential or functional failure of the fetal ovaries.

The external appearance of the intersex animal can range from that of a normal female to that of a normal male. Virilization of the female urogenital sinus and primordia of the external genitalia can cause an enlargement of the clitoris, an increase in the anogenital distance and a failure of the cranial one-third of the vagina to develop. Incomplete masculinization of the male can result in lack of scrotal development; subcutaneous, inguinal or abdominal testes; small penis and prepuce and hypospadias. Internally the findings depend upon the type of gonadal tissue present and its effect on the duct systems: these can range from a virtually complete Müllerian duct system to a virtually complete Wolffian duct system.

Hermaphrodites are classed as "true," "male pseudo-" or "female pseudo-" according to the type of gonadal tissue present.

True hermaphrodites have both ovarian and testicular tissue and account for many of the intersex cases. This is to be expected since the presence of both types of tissue can be looked upon as incomplete masculinization of the gonads at the time of their differentiation. The chromosomal complements 2n,XX; 2,XX/2n,XY and 2n,XX/2n,XY/2n+1,XXY have been found in association with true hermaphroditism.

Male pseudohermaphrodites have only testicular gonadal tissue. They account for the majority of intersex cases because they result from the incomplete inhibition of the Müllerian duct system or the incomplete masculinization of the Wolffian duct system, the urogenital sinus or the external genitalia by fetal testicular secretions. The chromosomal complements 2n,XX; 2n,XY; 2n−1,X/2n,XY; 2n,XX/2n,XY; 2n,XY/2n+1,XXY, 2n−1,X/2n,XX/2n+1,XXY; 2nXX/2n,XY/2n+1,XXY and 2n+2,XXXY have been observed in association with male pseudohermaphroditism.

A type of male pseudohermaphroditism known as testicular feminization is not caused by a lack of fetal testicular secretions but by a reduction or lack of sensitivity to the secretions by receptor organs in the Wolffian duct system, urogenital sinus and primordia of the external genitalia. The external appearance is that of a normal female, and the chromosomal complement is 2n,XY. Testicular feminization is an inherited defect that is consistent with either an autosomal dominant sex-limited mutation or an X-linked recessive mutation. Cases have been reported in horses, cattle, sheep and pigs.

The well-known freemartin syndrome, which occurs quite frequently in cattle and occasionally in sheep, goats and pigs, represents anatomically either true hermaphroditism or male pseudohermaphroditism, depending on the extent to which the female gonad has been masculinized by a factor from the male twin. The extent to which the rest of the genital system is masculinized depends on the secretions from the freemartin's own gonads, but invariably the caudal two-thirds of the vagina are present. Freemartinism occurs only with vascular exchange between fetuses of unlike sex. Consequently red and white blood cell chimerism is a feature, and 2n,XX/2n,XY chromosomes are found in hemopoietic cells, but only 2n,XX chromosomes are found in cells of different embryonic origin, with the exception of germ cells in which the presence of 2n,XY cells has been observed in the gonad. However, it should be noted that blood cell chimerism can occur without freemartinism in a small percentage of heterosexual twins in cattle and invariably occurs in heterosexual twins in horses.

Female pseudohermaphrodites have only ovarian tissue and are rarely encountered because they occur only with masculinization of the genital system due to exogenous androgens or with excessive endogenous androgen production, e.g., congenital adrenal hyperplasia.

Occurrence in Specific Species

The chromosomal findings reported for true hermaphrodites and male pseudohermaphrodites, exclusive of testicular feminization and freemartinism cases, are summarized in Tables 5 and 6.

A number of cases have been described in which the genetic sex was the opposite of the gonadal sex. The vast majority of these "sex reversals" have been male pseudohermaphrodites with a 2n,XX chromoso-

TABLE 5.   *Chromosomal Findings in True Hermaphroditism*

Species	Chromosomal Complement	Remarks
Horse	64,XX	Only one or two degenerate follicles in testicular gonads
	64,XX/64,XY	One testis, one ovotestis
Cattle	60,XX/60,XY 60,XX/90,XXY	Cryptorchids with no female external genitalia, but ovary, ovotestis, uterus, cervix, cranial vagina and seminal vesicles
Sheep	–	No reports
Goat	60,XX/60,XY	Male type horns, female type beard, small udder and vagina, enlarged clitoris
	60,XX	Polled with female external genitalia, enlarged clitoris, lactating mammary glands; these represent the extreme female form of intersexuality associated with the homozygous polled condition in female goats, most of which are male pseudohermaphrodites
Pig	38,XX 38,XX/38,XY 38,XX/39,XXY 37,X/38,XX/38,XY	Many not recognized in life because external genitalia are female and ovaries often functional; clitoris usually enlarged and sometimes penile
Dog	78,XX 78,XX/79,XXY	True hermaphrodites account for 25 per cent of intersexes; female external genitalia, enlarged clitoris often with an "os"
Cat	38,XX/57,XXY	Single case, type of gonadal tissue not reported, therefore either true hermaphrodite or male pseudohermaphrodite.
	38,XX/38,XY	Single case with one ovary and one testis

mal complement in several tissues. In goats, the autosomal dominant gene for polledness is also responsible for intersexuality when the gene is homozygous in genetic females. It appears to act like a Y chromosome by activating the gene on the X chromosome that causes medullary stimulation and testicular tissue development in the indifferent gonad. Sex reversal associated with male pseudohermaphroditism is also a common occurrence in pigs: it is probably caused by a pleiotropic autosomal recessive gene expressing itself variably with regard to intersexuality in the homozygous female by modifying the action of the X chromosome to form testicular tissue in the undifferentiated gonad. Several cases of sex reversal in male pseudohermaphrodite cocker spaniel dogs have also been reported. In three cases, the dogs were related in a manner consistent with

an autosomal recessive gene expressing itself in the homozygous female in a manner similar to that described for the goat and pig. In the horse, too, several male pseudohermaphrodites have been found to be genetic females.

Two heifers with ovarian hypoplasia and twin heifers with nonpalpable gonads but with cyclic patterns of estrogen and progesterone levels in the blood (indicative of some ovarian activity) have been described as being 60,XY.

Chromosomal findings have been reported in a few cases of female pseudohermaphroditism.

Cattle

One female pseudohermaphrodite has been reported. Clinically there was no vulva or penis, but a subcutaneous urethra

TABLE 6. *Chromosomal Findings in Male Pseudohermaphroditism Exclusive of Freemartinism and Testicular Feminization*

Species	Chromosomal Complement	Remarks
Horse	64,XX 64,XY/65,XXY [63,X]/64,XX/64,XY/[65,XXY]* 64,XX/[64,XY]/[65,XXY] [63,X]/64,XX/65,XXY 66,XXXY	Cryptorchidism and marked stallion behavior with either an enlarged clitoris in a reduced vulva with an increased anogenital distance or a reduced penis in the perineal region
Cattle	60,XY 60,XX/60,XY 60,XX/60,X?inv(Xp—q+)	Cryptorchidism with either a small vulva and enlarged clitoris or perineal hypospadias
Sheep	54,XX/54,XY	Possible freemartin since chromosomal studies restricted to blood leukocytes
	54,XX	Apparent sex reversal
Goat	60,XX	Autosomal gene for polledness is responsible for intersexuality in homozygous genetic females and infertility in homozygous genetic males; gene is of variable penetrance and expression with regard to degree of intersexuality, so phenotype varies from almost normal male to almost normal female
	62,XXXY/63,XXXXY	Hypoplastic scrotal testes, well-developed teats, milk secretion; no information on other genitalia, therefore unconfirmed as male pseudohermaphrodites
Pig	38,XX	Sex reversal similar to that seen in polled goats; probably caused by a pleiotropic autosomal recessive gene expressing itself with regard to inter-sexuality in the homozygous female
	39,XXY 38,XX/38,XY	Variable masculinization of the female genital tract
Dog	78,XY 78,XX	All sex reversed (78,XX) cases have been in cocker spaniels, three of which were related in a manner consistent with an autosomal recessive gene expressing itself in the homozygous female
Cat	38,XX/57,XXY	See Table 5.

*Brackets indicate uncertainty as to whether or not these cells represented cell populations.

extended down the perineal region and opened a few centimeters cranial to the abdominal teats. Autopsy revealed ovaries without signs of cyclic activity, oviducts, uterus, cervix and cranial vagina. Chromosomal studies showed 60,XX/90,XXY cell populations in the musculature, kidney and right gonad.

Pig

A single female pseudohermaphrodite has been reported. It had a 38,XX chromosomal complement.

Dog

Only two cases of female pseudohermaphroditism that could not be explained by exogenous factors have been described. The external genitalia were of a male type, but the penis was small and no "os" was evident. A vestigial scrotum was present, but no testes could be palpated. Internally the genitalia consisted of ovaries, oviducts, uterus and cranial vagina. The urethra passed through the caudal part of the vagina where it was enveloped by the prostate. The adrenal glands were normal on histological examination. One animal had 78,XX chromosomes; the other was sex chromatin-positive. There are a number of cases with anatomical changes similar to those just described and with a 78,XX chromosomal complement in which it is known that the bitch received androgens or progestins during gestation.

Diagnosis

Chromosomal analysis can be an aid in the differential diagnosis of certain conditions. It may be important to differentiate between testicular feminization and gonadal dysgenesis because the former is known to be hereditary whereas the latter is not.

Animals with testicular feminization and gonadal dysgenesis usually have a similar history of anestrus, poorly developed udder and teats and a normal-appearing vulva with no enlargement of the clitoris. In testicular feminization, the vagina usually ends blindly, the Müllerian duct derivatives are absent or rudimentary, the gonadal tissue is testicular, the urinary 17-ketosteroid levels are elevated and levels of gonadotropins are normal to slightly elevated. In gonadal dysgenesis, the Müllerian duct derivatives are present but infantile, the gonadal tissue is undifferentiated ovarian stroma, the urinary 17-ketosteroid levels are low and gonadotropin levels are elevated. A differential diagnosis can be made based on a microscopic examination of the gonadal tissue and determination of the hormone levels, but when this is impractical, chromosomal analysis of peripheral blood leukocytes may provide the answer. In testicular feminization the chromosomal complement is invariably 2n,XY, whereas in gonadal dysgenesis the following complements have been recorded: 2n−1,X; 2n,XX and 2n−1,X/2n,XX. However cattle with ovarian hypoplasia have been 2n,XY.

It is not unusual to have to determine whether or not a heifer is a freemartin, especially in those cases in which the virilization is not well marked. Chromosomal analyses performed on peripheral blood leukocytes and fibroblasts will enable the determination to be made. Sex chromosome chimerism in the blood leukocytes, but not in the fibroblasts, is a sound indication of freemartinism, whereas sex chromosome chimerism in both blood leukocytes and fibroblasts will determine that freemartinism is not present.

Chromosomal analyses can also be of value in differentiating the 2n,XX male pseudohermaphrodites from those with a Y chromosome in their complement. Since the former condition is hereditary, sex chromosome determination could aid in elimination of the problem. A number of cells from a variety of tissues have to be analyzed to be as certain as possible that a Y chromosome is not present.

Whenever tissues are submitted for chromosomal analysis, they should be accompanied by a full description of the genitalia and whenever possible by the entire gonads for microscopic examination.

OTHER CONGENITAL ABNORMALITIES

Some chromosomal changes are consistent with life, but they affect the normal development of the individual and cause congenital malformations. On the other hand, it should not be assumed that the presence of a chromosomal abnormality and a congenital anomaly means that the abnormality caused the anomaly. Such a relationship has to be shown by breeding experiments, if these are possible, or by the accumulation of data showing that the chromosomal abnormality is consistently associated with the congenital anomaly.

Chromosomal abnormalities are associated with a number of congenital anomalies in man, and several well-known syndromes are recognized as being caused by particular chromosomal changes, e.g., Down's syndrome or mongolism with trisomy G21 and the cri du chat syndrome with a deletion in the short arm of chromosome B5.

In domestic animals, chromosomal abnormalities have been observed in association with a number of congenital anomalies, and these are summarized in Table 7, but there are few examples in which a cause-and-effect relationship has been shown to exist.

Diagnosis

Tissues from congenitally malformed animals should be submitted for chromosomal analysis whenever possible. Only thus can the role of chromosomal abnormalities in causing congenital abnormalities in domestic animals become known, and it is conceivable that at some time in the future this knowledge can be used in prenatal screening for chromosomal abnormalities, either during embryo transfer or by culturing cells obtained by amniocentesis.

PRENATAL CYTOGENETIC STUDIES

Prenatal cytogenetic studies have been done on amniotic fluid cell cultures obtained by transabdominal amniocentesis for a number of years in human medicine. These studies are indicated in high risk groups such as mothers over 35 years of age, for whom the chance of having a child with one of the trisomy syndromes is increased, and mothers who are carriers of X-linked recessive disorders, in which case it may be desirable to therapeutically abort male fetuses.

In veterinary medicine, amniocentesis for cytogenetic purposes is practical only in large animals, although it has been done in a bitch at 40 days of pregnancy. Based on the present lack of knowledge of the frequency of chromosomal abnormalities in aborted fetuses during the latter two-thirds of pregnancy and in liveborn animals with congenital anomalies, the only justification for doing cytogenetic studies on fetal fluid cells would seem to be the economic advantages to be derived from early sex determination. In cattle, fetal sex determination should be made before 120 days of gestation to allow time for the fetus to be aborted safely if it is of unwanted sex.

Cattle

Sex determination by sex chromatin analysis in fetal fluid cells is not practical in cattle because of the coarse granular appearance of the nuclear chromatin. Therefore such determination has to be made by the sex chromosmal analysis of cultured fetal fluid cells.

Two approaches to obtaining fetal fluids have been described, a transvaginal approach through the dorsal fornix in cows and a trans-sacrosciatic approach in heifers. The first 1 to 2 ml of aspirated fetal fluids should be discarded as a precaution against maternal cell contamination, and several cultures should be set up from each sample to increase the opportunities for clones of fetal cells to become established should maternal cells be present. Blood-stained samples should be viewed with extreme caution and, if possible, discarded and the sample retaken. Also, when male cells are not observed during chromosomal analysis, numerous cells from each culture and from several passages should be studied to minimize the possibility of misinterpreting maternal cells for female fetal cells. Some workers claim that sufficient cell growth for chromosomal analysis is regularly obtained in 4 to 7 days, whereas the experience gained from other cattle studies and many human studies indicates that a more realistic expectation is 14 to 18 days. With experience and care, the culture success can be expected to be about 90 per cent and the accuracy in fetal sex determination about 95 per cent.

The sex of bovine embryos can also be determined by chromsomal analysis at the time of their transfer from donor to recipient. Using strict aseptic procedures, a small fragment of trophoblast is removed from the blastocyst without damaging the inner cell mass. The cells of the fragment are then processed to display the chromosomes. Approximately 66 per cent of day-12, 65 per cent of day-13, 63 per cent of day-14 and 55 per cent of day-15 biopsied embryos have

TABLE 7. *Chromosomal Aberrations Associated with Other Congenital Anomalies*

Species	Congenital Anomaly	Chromosomal Complement	Remarks
Horse	–	–	None reported
Cattle	Lethal extreme brachygnathia with other anomalies	61,XX or 61,XY+?(13—24) 60,XX or XY/61,XX or XY,+?(13—24) 60,XY/61,XY,+?(1—6) 61,XY,+?	Several cases* Single case* Single case*
	Ventricular septal defect, patent foramen ovale, umbilical hernia	61,XX,+?(13—18)	Single case*
	Dwarfism characterized by short legs, epiphyseal nonunion, delayed puberty, plus abnormalities of the optic papilla	61,XX or XY,+?23	Several cases*
	Acardiac monster Anidian monster	Monosomy for chromosome number one	Single case each
	Polymelia and other abnormalities	60,XX,?8—	Single case
	Multiple abnormalities of central nervous system	59,XX,tan(1q;7q) Increased polyploidy	Single case Several cases
	Hereditary exfoliative dermatosis	Negative heteropyknotic segment in long arm of one X chromosome	Several cases
	Cryptorchidism with shortening of penis	60,XY/62,XX	Single case
	Cryptorchidism with shortening and retroflexion of the penis	60,XY(blood) 60,XX/61,XX,+cen (other tissues)	Single case, possible twin to a bull
	Muscle hyperplasia	Increased polyploidy	Several cases
Sheep	Short upper jaws	54,XX or XY/54,XX or XY,?13—	Several cases
Goat	–	–	No reports
Pig	Polymelia and other anomalies, meningocele, double muscle atresia ani, cryptorchidism		Negative or inconclusive
Dog	Hydrocephalus, hypospadias, lack of scrotal development	117,XXY/156,XXYY	Stillborn
	Hydrocephalus	78,XY/156,XXYY	Littermate to above died shortly after birth
	Tetralogy of Fallot, patent foramen ovale, cleft palate Ventricular septal defect	77,XY,rob?(2q;10q) 79,XY,+cen	Two cases in survey of 15 dogs with congenital cardiac defects
Dog	Bone chondroplasia	77,XX,rob?(1q;19q)	Single case*†
	Ectopic ureter	77,XX,rob?(1q;19q)	Single case*†, its dam, anatomically normal, also had the chromosome translocation
Cat	Macerated fetal runt	39,XY,+11	Single case

*Chromosomes not banded, therefore impossible to be sure which autosomes involved.
†Both cases in miniature poodles, possible existence of a Robertsonian translocation in the breed.

been sexed successfully. Indications are that embryos less than 0.9 mm in length do not provide good material for successful biopsy and chromosomal analysis using present techniques. Embryo survival rates following the transfer of biopsied embryos have been 34.5 per cent for day-14 and day-15 embryos and 18.1 per cent for day-13 embryos. However, the numbers involved are small, and the transfers have been made under different conditions and without proper controls, so valid conclusions cannot be drawn. Recently, 60 per cent of day-6 and day-7 embryos have been sexed successfully and given a pregnancy rate of 71 per cent following transfer. The sexing of bovine embryos has an obvious potential, with the ultimate objective of combining sexing with freezing and a satisfactory pregnancy rate following transfer.

Sexing embryos during transfer has also been done in sheep. It also holds possibilities for other species, but the task is more difficult because the sex chromosomes are not as readily distinguished from the autosomes as they are in cattle.

HYBRIDS

Interspecific hybridization rarely occurs under natural conditions and usually takes place in captivity or as a result of experimentation. Hybridization may result in hybrid inviability with the embryo or fetus dying *in utero*. This applies especially to males. Hybrids of both sexes tend to show reduced fertility, but complete sterility occurs more frequently in males than in females.

From a cytogenetic standpoint it is apparent that minor differences in parental sets of chromosomes can be overcome so that the hybrids are fertile or have only reduced fertility, while major differences in parental sets lead to a breakdown in gametogenesis due to failures in synapsis of the first meiotic division and sterility. On the other hand, apparent morphological similarity of parental sets does not guarantee hybrid fertility for reasons that are not well understood.

Horse

Hybrids resulting from crossing the domestic horse (*Equus caballus*) with Przewalski's horse (*E. przewalski*), the donkey (*E. asinus*) and the Grévy zebra (*E. grevyi*) are considered.

The *E. przewalski* × *E. caballus* hybrid is fertile. Indications are that the chromosomal complement of *E. caballus*, 2n = 64 with 26 atelocentric and 36 acrocentric autosomes (Fig. 11), was derived from a centric fusion rearrangement of two pairs of acrocentric autosomes in *E. przewalski*, 2n = 66 with 24 atelocentric and 40 acrocentric autosomes. As a result, there is chromosome homology. The hybrid has a diploid number of 2n = 65 and is equivalent to a heterozygote for a centric fusion. It is fertile presumably because any imbalanced gametes that are formed fail to mature.

However, the *E. caballus* × *E. asinus* hybrids, the mule and the hinny, are sterile. The chromosomal complement of *E. asinus*, 2n = 62, has 48 atelocentric and 12 acrocentric autosomes, which is considerably different from that of *E. caballus*. Consequently, the chromosomal complements of the mule and the hinny have many unevenly matched pairs, leading to incomplete homologous pairing during meiosis and a block in spermatogenesis and oogenesis. Surprisingly, spermatozoa are occasionally found in the male mule and hinny, and a few oocytes manage to survive in the female mule and hinny, leading to follicular development and estrus at irregular intervals.

Cattle

The hybrids considered are those resulting from crossing domestic cattle (*Bos taurus*) with Zebu cattle (*B. indicus*), the American bison (*Bison bison*) and the European bison (*Bison bonasus*).

The *B. taurus* × *B. indicus* hybrid is fertile. Both *B. taurus* and *B. indicus* have a chromosome number of 2n = 60 with 29 acrocentric autosomes (Fig. 12). The X chromosomes are similar, but the *B. taurus* Y is a small submetacentric chromosome and the *B. indicus* Y is a small acrocentric chromosome, approximately the same size as the submetacentric Y. The difference could be the result of a pericentric inversion.

The *B. taurus* × *Bison bison* female hybrid is fertile, but the male is sterile. Females also predominate in the F$_1$ progeny. Both *Bison bison* and *B. taurus* have a chromosome number of 2n = 60. The only apparent difference in banded chromosomes is in the Y chromosome, which is acrocentric in *Bison bison* because of a short arm deletion. Cattalos are the progeny of crosses in which both parents are part bison and part cattle.

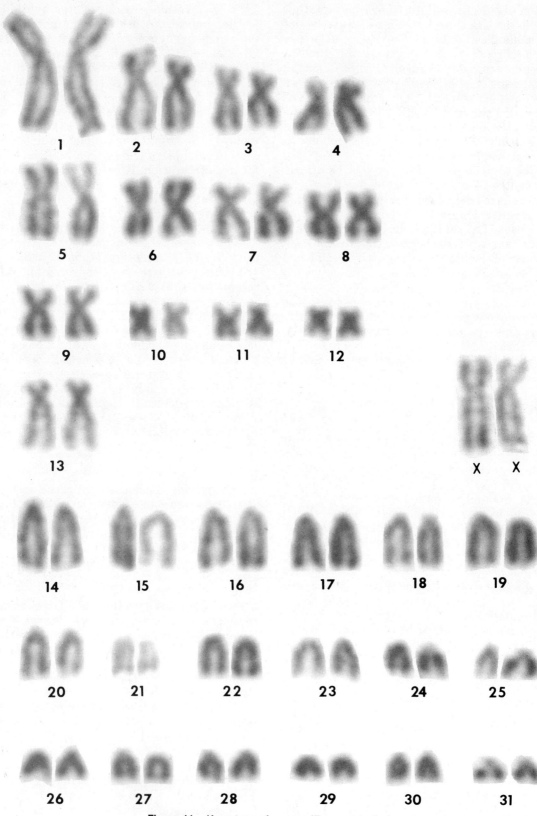

Figure 11. Karyotype of a mare (*Equus caballus*).

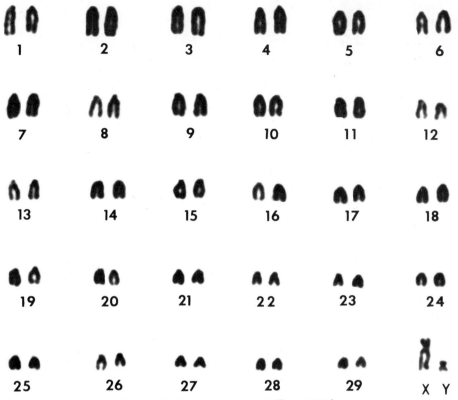

Figure 12. Karyotype of a bull (*Bos taurus*).

When the percentage of bison or cattle blood in the cattalo is below 14 per cent, the male is frequently fertile. Studies indicate that the male infertility is not due to a lack of homologous pairing during meiosis but rather to a gamete maturation problem. Active meiosis and spermatogenesis have been observed with a total absence of spermatozoa in the epididymis and in ejaculates. The reciprocal cross, bison bull and domestic cow, results in hydramnios with a high fetal mortality and risk to the dam.

The chromosome complements of domestic cattle and the European bison appear to be identical, as are several blood group factors. The *B. taurus* × *Bison bonasus* and *Bison bonasus* × *B. taurus* female hybrids are fertile, but the males are sterile, both in the F_1 generation and the first backcross generation.

Sheep

Hybrids resulting from crossing sheep (*Ovis aries*) with goats (*Capra hircus*) are considered.

A number of attempts have been made to cross sheep with goats. Conception readily occurs when does are inseminated with ram semen, but the fetus usually dies about the end of the sixth week of pregnancy. Death has been attributed to maternal antibodies crossing the placenta and hemolyzing the fetal red blood cells. However, there are a few reports of liveborn hybrids. Their chromosomal complement is 2n = 57 with 3 metacentric and 52 acrocentric autosomes. The female hybrid is fertile, but spermatozoa from the male are incapable of fertilization. With G-banding it can be seen that there is considerable banding homology between the sheep chromosomal complement 2n = 54, with 6 metacentric and 48 acrocentric chromosomes, and the goat chromosomal complement 2n = 60, with 60 acrocentrics. The three metacentric pairs of sheep chromosomes appear to have been formed by centric fusions of the goat chromosomes 1;3, 2;8 and 5;11, respectively (Figs. 13, 14).

Ewes inseminated with buck semen generally fail to conceive, although a few fertilized eggs have been observed.

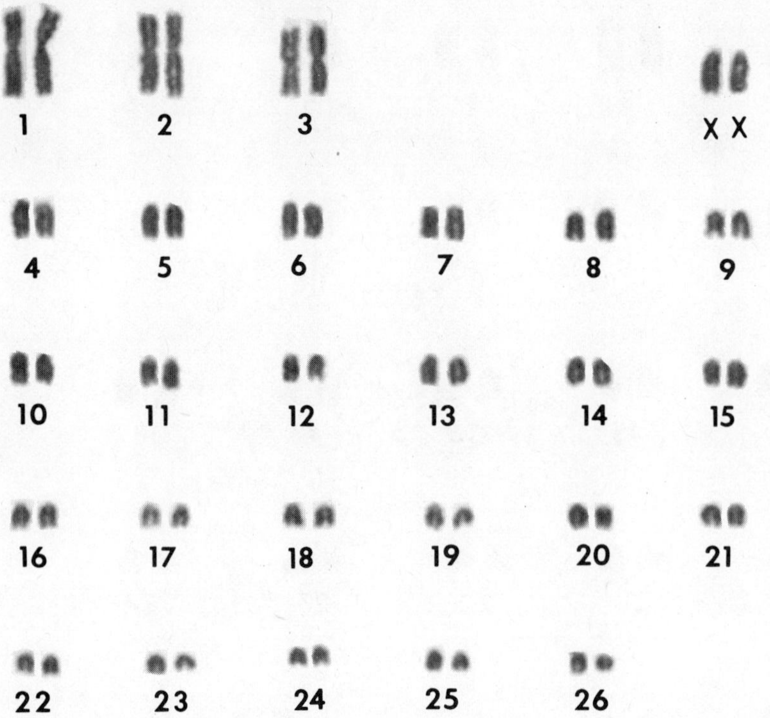

Figure 13. Karyotype of a ewe (*Ovis aries*).

Pig

Hybrids produced by crossing the domestic pig (*Sus scrofa*) with the European wild pig are fertile. Chromosomal studies show that the European wild pig has a chromosomal complement of 2n = 36, with 26 atelocentric and 8 acrocentric autosomes, as opposed to the domestic pig with a chromosome number of 2n = 38, with 24 atelocentric and 12 acrocentric autosomes (Fig. 15). The wild pigs are homozygous for a centric fusion (15q;17q) in the domestic pig karyotype. The hybrids have 37 chromosomes, 25 atelocentric and 10 acrocentric autosomes, and are heterozygous for the centric fusion.

Dog

The chromosomal complement of the domestic dog (*Canis familiaris*), 2n = 78 with 76 acrocentric autosomes, a large submetacentric X chromosome and a small submetacentric Y chromosome (Fig. 16), appears morphologically identical in unbanded chromosomes with the karyotypes of the Asiatic jackal (*C. aureus*), the wolf (*C. lupus*), the dingo (*C. dingo*), the red wolf (*C. niger*), the African hunting dog (*Lycaon pictus*) and the coyote (*C. latrans*).

Reciprocal crosses with fertile hybrids are possible between *C. familiaris* and *C.* *aureus, C. dingo, C. lupus* and *C. niger*. The cross between a male dog and a female coyote yields fertile female hybrids, but the fertility of the male hybrids is in some doubt. The reciprocal cross has been reported to give fertile hybrids.

Cat

Hybrids resulting from crossing the domestic cat (*Felis catus*) with the leopard (*F. bengalensis*), the jungle cat (*F. chaus*), the steppe cat (*F. libyca candata*), the bobcat (*F. lynx rufa*) and the European wild cat (*F. silvestris*) have been reported. Female hybrids from the male jungle cat × female domestic cat and male steppe cat × female domestic cat were fertile, but the fertility of the male hybrids was not recorded. The fertility of the hybrids resulting from the male bobcat and male European wildcat crossed with female domestic cats is not recorded. The domestic cat has a chromosomal complement 2n = 38 with 32 atelocentric autosomes and 4 acrocentric autosomes (Fig. 17). All cats studied from the Northern hemisphere have 38 chromosomes, while many from the Southern hemisphere have 2n = 36. There is considerable similarity suggestive of homology among the *Felidae* karyotypes, and the differences that exist

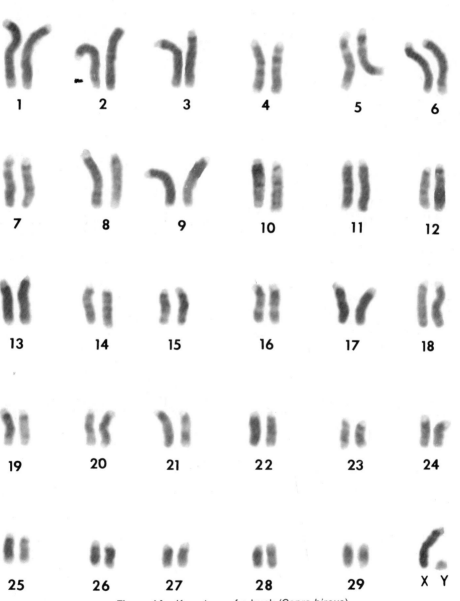

Figure 14. Karyotype of a buck (*Capra hircus*).

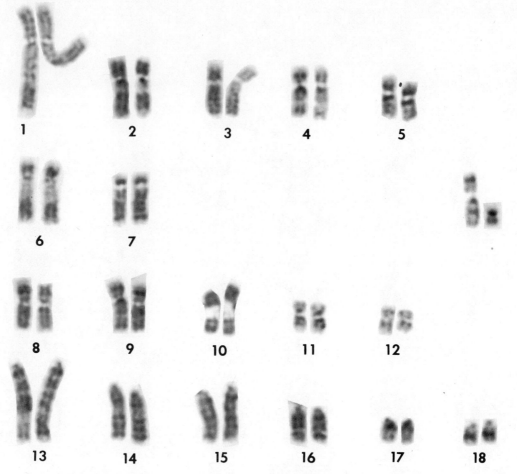

Figure 15. Karyotype of a boar (*Sus scrofa*) with G-banded chromosomes.

are probably the result of pericentric inversions, centric fusions, reciprocal translocations and deletions. For example, there are reports of hybrids resulting from the cross between *F. lynx rufa*, 2n = 38 with 32 atelocentric and 4 acrocentric autosomes, and the ocelot (*F. pardalis*), 2n = 36 with 34 atelocentric autosomes.

TECHNIQUES

The most frequently used source of dividing cells for routine chromosomal analysis is peripheral blood mononuclear leukocytes cultured for 72 hours at 37°C. Standard tissue culture procedures are used, but the actual method varies from one laboratory to another and from one species to another. Therefore it is sound policy to consult a laboratory with personnel experienced in culturing leukocytes from domestic animals. Tissue culture kits for processing human

peripheral blood are available commercially (see Appendix *B* for names and addresses of suppliers), and they have been used successfully with domestic animal bloods.

The principles involved in culturing peripheral blood leukocytes and in the preparation of chromosomes are the same regardless of laboratory or species. Blood is collected in sterile tubes containing 10 to 20 IU/ml of sodium heparin in aqueous solution. Either whole blood or mononuclear leukocytes separated from red blood cells are put into tissue culture medium that is supplemented with serum and antibiotics. A mitogen such as phytohemagglutinin (PHA), pokeweed (PWM) or concanavalin A is added to stimulate the lymphocytes to undergo division. The cultures are incubated at 37°C, and the maximum response is usually obtained at about 66 to 72 hours. Colchicine, colcemid (a derivative of colchicine) or a similar drug is then added for one to a few hours of further incubation prior to harvesting the cells. Colcemid prevents the formation of the cell spindle and halts cell division in metaphase, which is the stage at which the chromosomes are most readily visible. Colcemid also causes contraction and separation of the chromatids, so that too concentrated a solution or too long an exposure time can cause poor chromosome preparations. Following their exposure to colcemid, the cells are suspended in a hypotonic solution, which has the effect of swelling the cells by osmosis and dispersing the chromosomes. It may also cause some shortening of the chromatids. After the hypotonic treatment, the cells are fixed in acetic alcohol and then the chromosomes are flattened on a microscope slide by allowing a drop of the alcoholic cell suspension to fall onto a wet slide, whereupon the drop spreads out and the cells are flattened.

Chromosomes can also be obtained for analysis by a direct method from tissues in which the cells are actively dividing, such as bone marrow and other hemopoietic tissues. The biopsied material is transferred to tissue culture medium that is supplemented with serum and colcemid and incubated at 37°C for one to a few hours. Thereafter the cells are handled as described for the preparation of chromosomes from blood leukocyte cultures.

Meiotic preparations from testicular tissue are obtained by squeezing the cells out of the seminiferous tubules that are in a hypotonic solution. The cells are later fixed in acetic alcohol, and the slides are made as before.

Chromosome preparations from other tissues are obtained by growing the cells in long-term culture. Tissues used frequently

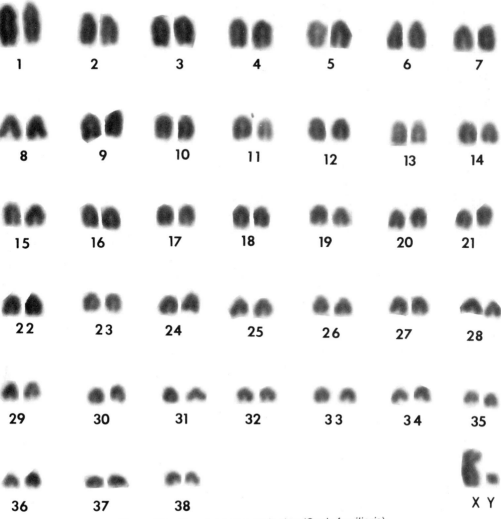

Figure 16. Karyotype of a male dog (*Canis familiaris*).

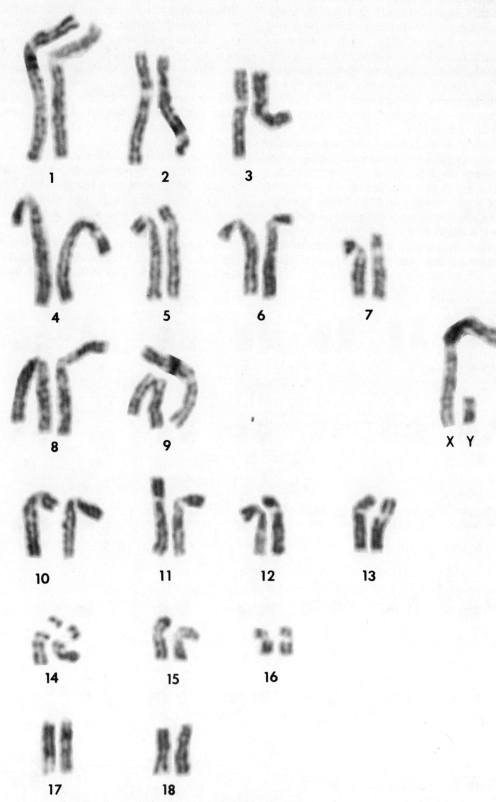

Figure 17. Karyotype of a male cat (*Felis catus*) with G-banded chromosomes.

because they are readily accessible in the live animal are skin, mucous membrane (buccal, vaginal) and fascia. Only about 2 mm³ of tissue is required, but it has to be biopsied under strict aseptic conditions. Other tissues obtained at surgery or autopsy can also be used if they are sterile. Cultures can be initiated from cell suspensions obtained by disaggregating the tissue cells with the enzyme trypsin. This method is useful only when there is a relatively large volume of tissue. Otherwise the tissue is cut up into very small pieces that either are sandwiched between coverslips in a tissue culture tube or flask or are allowed to adhere to the surface of the tissue culture flask before the tissue culture medium is added. The cells usually grow out in a few days and cover the surface of the vessel in 2 to 3 weeks. They are then subcultured by trypsinizing them off the glass, resuspending them in tissue culture medium and reseeding them into two or three flasks. A mitotic peak usually occurs 15 to 24 hours after reseeding, at which time colcemid is added for one to a few hours. The cells are then trypsinized off the surface of the flask and handled for chromosome preparation as described before.

Chromosomes can be stained with any DNA stain. However, it is now standard practice to "band" the chromosomes because the differential banding patterns facilitate the detection of structural chromosomal rearrangements. Several types of banding patterns can be produced, and it may be necessary to use more than one to obtain the information required for analysis. The commonly used patterns are as follows:

1. Q-bands are produced by staining with the fluorescent dyes quinacrine mustard or quinacrine hydrochloride (Fig. 18). Quinacrine binds to DNA by intercalation, and it is thought that pale or negative fluorescence is associated with decreased or inhibited binding due to nonhistone protein-DNA interactions.

2. G-bands are produced by staining with Giemsa after treating the chromosomes with any one of a number of techniques that denature proteins (Figs. 15, 17, 19, 20, 21). It has been suggested that light staining areas occur when the treatment has denatured the nonhistone proteins so that they more effectively cover the DNA and prevent the binding of dye.

3. R-bands are the reverse of G-bands and are produced by staining with Giemsa or acridine orange after treating the fixed chromosomes in different ways (Fig. 22). The mechanism of staining with Giemsa is thought to be the same as in G-banding, except that the denaturation of the nonhistone proteins is altered by the different pH, temperature and salt concentrations used in R-banding.

4. C-bands are produced by treating the fixed chromosomes to extract DNA, followed by staining with Giemsa (Figs. 23, 24). C-bands appear when constitutive (centromeric) heterochromatin is stained because of nonhistone protein-DNA interactions protecting the DNA from extraction and enhancing its staining reaction.

After staining, the preparations are cleared in xylene, and the slides are mounted with a coverglass and synthetic balsam. The chromosomes are analyzed by using a microscope with good objectives, preferably flatfield. Detailed studies are made at magnifications of 1000 to 1250 ×.

Sex chromatin studies in the live animal are possible in the dog and cat by using oral epithelial cells and in all species by using polymorphonuclear leukocytes.

Buccal smears are made by pooling several scrapings on a precleaned microscope slide and spreading them quickly in a thin layer over a large area. The cells are fixed for at least 15 minutes in 95 per cent ethanol or equal parts of 95 per cent ethanol and ether and then are air dried before hydrolyzing in 5N HCl at 22°C for 20 minutes. The slide is then passed through several changes of distilled water to get rid of the acid, and the cells are stained for 5 minutes in 1 per cent cresylecht violet. The cells are then differentiated in two changes of 95 per cent ethanol for 5 minutes and in absolute alcohol until the microscopic cell structure is well defined. The preparation is cleared in xylene, and the slide is mounted with a coverglass and balsam. The slides are examined under oil immersion. The presence of the characteristic chromatin mass, the Barr body, adjacent to the nuclear membrane indicates a chromatin-positive cell.

Accessory nuclear lobules or drumsticks are visible in routine blood films stained with Wright's stain. They appear as deep staining masses about 1.5 μ in diameter attached by a fine filament to a nuclear lobe.

Text continued on page 152.

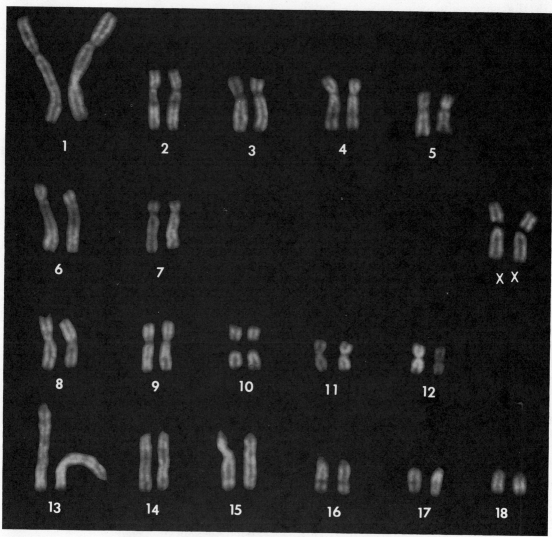

Figure 18. Karyotype of a sow with Q-banded chromosomes.

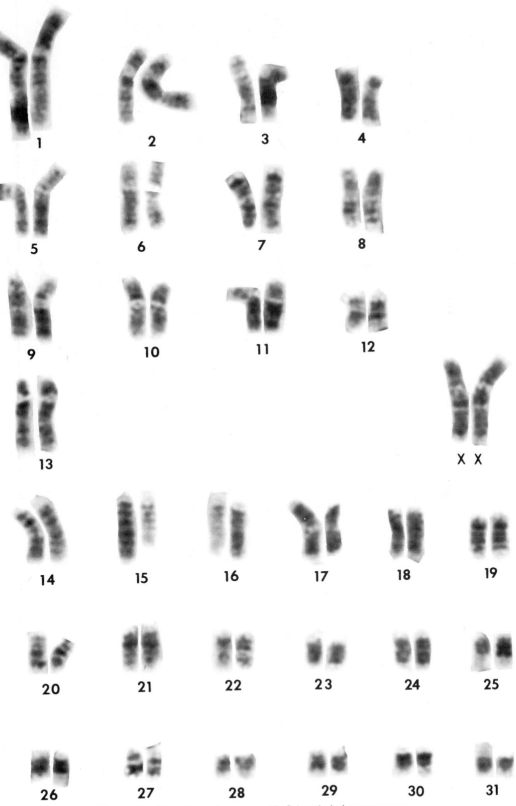

Figure 19. Karyotype of a mare with G-banded chromosomes.

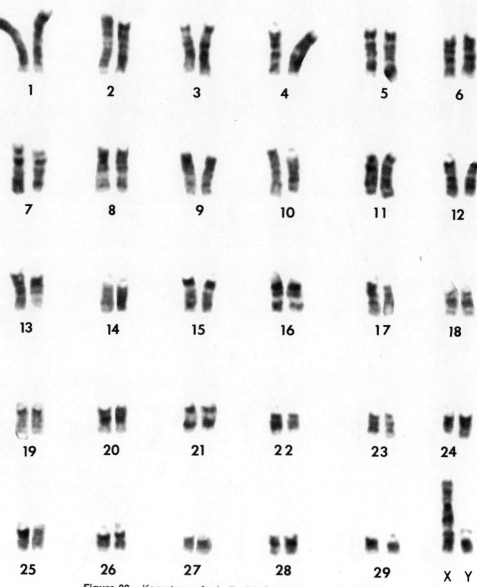

Figure 20. Karyotype of a bull with G-banded chromosomes.

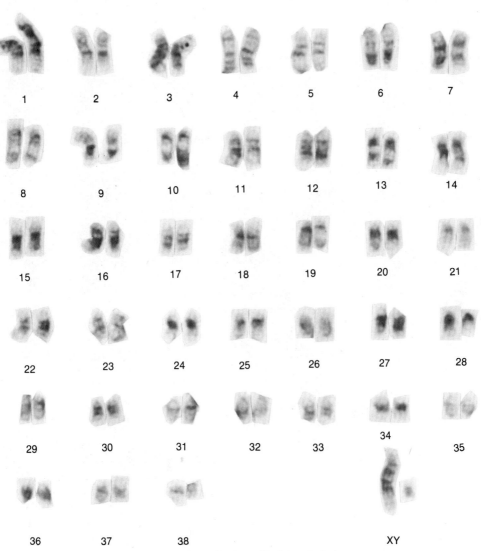

Figure 21. Karyotype of a male dog with G-banded chromosomes.

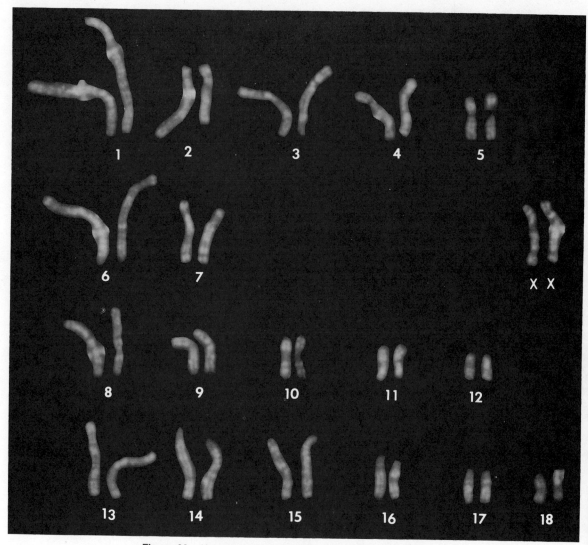

Figure 22. Karyotype of a sow with R-banded chromosomes.

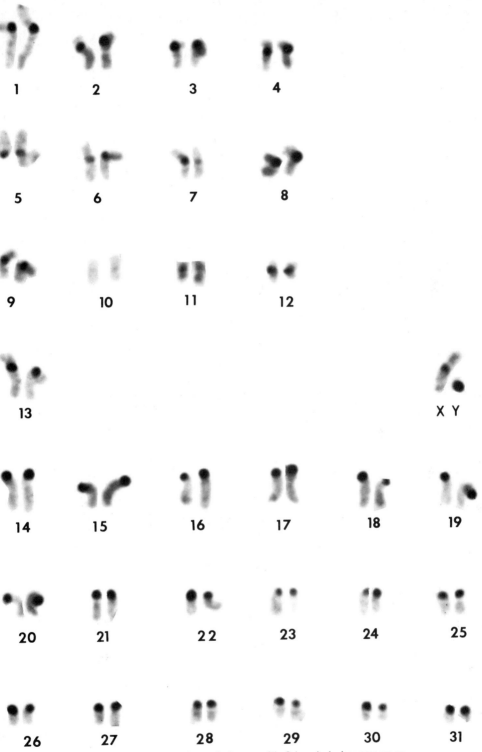

Figure 23. Karyotype of a male horse with C-banded chromosomes.

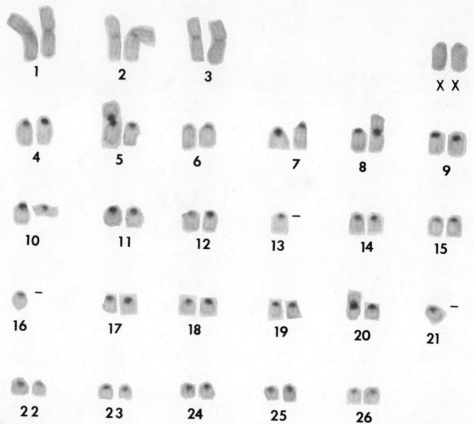

Figure 24. Karyotype of a cell line from a female lamb with C-banded chromosomes. Note the comparatively small amount of centromeric heterochromatin in chromosome pairs 1, 2, 3 and the sex chromosomes XX and the translocations: tdic(5;16); rob(8q;13q) and rob(20q;21q).

SUBMISSION OF SAMPLES

The cytogenetics laboratory must be contacted and arrangements made prior to submitting samples for analysis.

Venous blood can be sent by mail, air freight, parcel post, and so forth provided it is packaged to prevent freezing in winter or overheating in summer. Ideally it should be kept at 4°C and received in the laboratory within 48 hours of being drawn. The blood can be drawn into sterile 15-ml vacutainer tubes to which 150 IU of sterile sodium heparin in aqueous solution has been added. It is important to note that a sodium heparin solution with phenol as a preservative should not be used. It is also important that the skin over the vein should be thoroughly cleaned and sterilized before taking the blood.

Tissues for culture and cytogenetic studies must be obtained by sterile technique. A piece measuring 2 mm³ is adequate. It should be placed in a sterile 15-ml culture tube with a leakproof screw cap, e.g., a sterile 2-dr specimen vial with leakproof screw cap or an equivalent container filled to the top with tissue culture medium supplemented with 10 per cent serum and antibiotics (final concentration 100 IU of penicillin and 100 mg of streptomycin per ml.)

Tissues for histology should be cut into thin slices and fixed in 10 per cent buffered formalin or Bouin's solution and shipped in a leakproof container.

GLOSSARY OF TERMS

Acentric fragment: a chromosome segment without a centromere.

Acrocentric chromosome: a chromosome with its centromere located very close to the end of the chromosome (Fig. 1).

Aneuploid (aneuploidy): cells or individuals with one or two chromosomes more or less than the species number.

Atelocentric chromosome: a chromosome

with its centromere not at the end of the chromosome. In this article the term is used to describe all but acrocentric and telocentric chromosomes.

Autosome: any chromosome with the exception of the sex chromosomes.

Balanced chromosomal rearrangement: a structural chromosomal change in which there is no apparent loss or gain of genetic material.

Barr body: see sex chromatin.

Centric fusion: a translocation involving two acrocentric chromosomes that takes place when breaks occur close to the centromere in the long arm of one and the short arm of the other, followed by an exchange and reunion to form an atelocentric chromosome and a very small metacentric chromosome or a centric fragment (Figs. 6, 10*E*, 24).

Centromere: the region of each chromosome with which the spindle fibers become associated during mitosis and meiosis. It is seen as a constriction in metaphase chromosomes (Fig. 1).

Chimera (chimerism): an individual having two or more populations of cells derived from two or more zygotes.

Chromatid: one of the two visible longitudinal strands seen forming the arms of chromosomes during mitosis and meiosis (Figs. 2, 3, 4).

Chromatid break: a discontinuity with misalignment in one of the chromatids.

Chromatid gap: a discontinuity without misalignment in one of the chromatids.

Chromosome: a structure in the nucleus of the cell that consists of DNA, histone proteins, nonhistone proteins, and some RNA. The DNA consists of functional units called genes that are linearly arranged. Chromosomes are normally paired, one derived from each parent.

Chromosome band: a part of a chromosome that is clearly distinguished from adjacent parts by a lighter or darker staining intensity (Figs. 15, 18, 20, 24).

Chromosome break: a discontinuity with misalignment involving both chromatids.

Chromosome gap: a discontinuity without misalignment involving both chromatids.

Deletion: the loss of a segment of a chromosome. Deletion can be terminal if the segment is lost from the end of the arm or interstitial if it is lost from another part of the arm (Fig. 10*G*).

Dicentric chromosome: a chromosome with two centromeres (Fig. 24).

Diploid (diploidy): a cell or individual having twice the normal haploid (gametic) number of chromosomes for the species. The chromosomes are in pairs, one member of each pair derived from the mother and one from the father. The symbol is 2n. The diploid numbers for the various domestic species are: horse–64, cattle–60, sheep–54, goat–60, pig–38, dog–78, and cat–38.

DNA: deoxyribonucleic acid, which is a polymer of deoxyribonucleotides constituting the primary genetic material. It is present in chromosomes as two long linear molecules (strands) arranged in the form of a double helix (Fig. 2).

DNA replication: the process by which prior to cell division, the DNA strands separate and a new complementary strand is made for each other so that there are two pairs of strands, one the mirror image of the other. Each pair forms a chromatid (Fig. 2).

Duplication: the insertion of a deleted fragment into an homologous chromosome (Fig. 10*H*).

Endoreduplication: DNA replication without nuclear division.

Euploid (euploidy): a cell or individual with the haploid number of chromosomes or whole multiples of haploid number.

Haploid (haploidy): a cell having the gametic number of chromosomes for the species. The symbol is n.

Heteroploid (heteroploidy): a cell or individual with any chromosome number other than the diploid number.

Idiogram: a diagrammatic representation of a karyotype.

Insertion: a segment from one chromosome that is inserted into a nonhomologous chromosome (Fig. 10*D*).

Isochromosome: a chromosome with equal and genetically identical arms. It is formed when the centromere divides transversely rather than along the long axis of the chromosome during cell division (Fig. 10 *J*, *K*).

Inversion: reversal of a chromosome segment and the gene sequence contained therein following chromosome breakage and reunion. This is known as paracentric inversion if the centromere is not in the segment and pericentric inversion if it is (Fig. 10 *A*).

Karyotype: the systematic arrangement of metaphase chromosomes from a single cell in homologous pairs following photography (Figs. 11 to 24).

Meiosis: the two successive cellular divisions that result in a primary spermatocyte or oocyte giving rise to a spermatid or ootid.

Division I is reductional, division II equational (Fig. 4).

Metacentric chromosome: a chromosome in which the two arms are equal in length (Fig. 1).

Metaphase: the stage in meiosis and mitosis at which the chromosomes are arranged along the equator of the cell attached by their centromere to the spindle. At this stage the chromatids are shorter, uncoiled and lie parallel to each other (Fig. 3).

Mitosis: cellular division as it occurs in somatic cells, whereby each daughter cell has the same chromosomal complement and therefore genetic material as the parental cell (Fig. 3).

Mixoploid (mixoploidy): in the strict sense an individual or a population of cells containing cells that differ in their chromosome number. In this article the term is used synonymously with "mosaic."

Monosomy: loss of one chromosome from a pair. The cell or individual is monosomic for that particular chromosome. Monosomy occurs as a result of nondisjunction (Figs. 7, 8).

Mosaic (mosaicism): an individual or tissue with populations of cells differing in chromosome number and/or structure that are derived from a single zygote (compare with chimera).

Nondisjunction: the irregular distribution of sister chromatids during mitosis or of homologous chromosomes during meiosis that results in aneuploid cells, i.e., one daughter cell becomes trisomic and the other daughter cell monosomic for a particular chromosome (Figs. 7, 8).

Nuclear drumstick: see sex chromatin.

Polyandry: fertilization of an ovum by more than one sperm (Fig. 9).

Polygyny: the union of one sperm with two or more female pronuclei within the ovum (Fig. 9).

Polyploid (polyploidy): a cell or individual having more than two complete sets of chromosomes.

Polysomy: a gain of one or more chromosomes in a pair, e.g., trisomy.

Polyspermy: the entry of more than one sperm into an ovum (Fig. 9).

Reciprocal translocation: an exchange of segments between two chromosomes. These may or may not produce changes in the size and shape of the chromsomes involved (Figs. 5, 10C).

Ring chromosome: structure formed as a result of breaks in both arms of a chromosome and union of the proximal ends (Fig. 10I).

Robertsonian translocation: see centric fusion.

Sex chromatin: a small condensed mass of chromatin that stains heterochromatically in interphase nuclei, sometimes referred to as the "Barr body" or "drumstick." It represents the inactivated X chromosome. The Barr body is seen adjacent to the nuclear membrane in a proportion of female cells. The number of Barr bodies per nucleus is one less than the number of X chromosomes. The nuclear drumstick is seen in a proportion of female polymorphonuclear leukocytes as a small appendage attached to a nuclear lobe by a fine neck.

Sex chromosomes: the pair of chromosomes involved in sex determination. In most mammals the female sex chromosomes XX form a homologous pair (Fig. 11) but the male sex chromosomes XY do not (Fig. 12).

Shift: the movement of a segment of a chromosome to another part of the same chromosome (Fig. 10B).

Submetacentric chromosome: a chromosome in which one arm is only one-half to one-third as long as the other arm (Fig. 1).

Subtelocentric chromosome: a chromosome in which one arm is only one-third to one-seventh as long as the other arm (Fig. 1).

Tandem fusion: a translocation in which there is a break near the centromere in the arm of one chromosome and a break near the end of the arm of another chromosome followed by a transfer of the arm and subsequent reunion of the broken ends (Fig. 10F).

Telocentric chromosome: a chromosome in which the centromere is at the end of the chromosome (Fig. 1).

Tetraploid (tetraploidy): a cell or individual having four complete sets of chromosomes in the nucleus.

Triploid (triploidy): a cell or individual having three complete sets of chromosomes in the nucleus (Fig. 9).

Trisomy: a gain of one chromosome in a pair. The cell or individual is trisomic for that particular chromosome. Trisomy occurs as a result of nondisjunction (Figs. 7, 8).

Unbalanced chromosomal rearrangement: a structural chromosomal change in which there is loss or gain of genetic material, e.g., deletions, duplications, isochromosomes (Fig. 10G, H, J, K).

X-chromosome inactivation: the compensatory mechanism whereby the products of X-linked genes are made equal in the XX and XY sex chromosome complements. In all mammals except marsupials, inactivation of the maternally or paternally derived X chromosome is random. Normally, even when there are more than two X chromosomes, only one X is active.

Zygote: the diploid cell formed by the fusion of a male and a female haploid gamete.

REFERENCES

1. Basrur, P. K.: Innovations in cytogenetics and their applications to domestic animals. 1st World Congress on Genetics Applied to Livestock Production, Madrid, 1974.
2. Bishop, M. W. A.: Genetically determined abnormalities of the reproductive system. J. Reprod. Fertil. (Suppl.), *15*:51, 1972.
3. Benirschke, K.: Comparative Mammalian Cytogenetics. New York, Springer-Verlag New York, Inc., 1969.
4. Bruère, A. N.: The discovery and biological consequences of some important chromosome anomalies in populations of domestic animals. 1st World Congress on Genetics Applied to Livestock Production, Madrid, 1974.
5. Eaglesome, M. D., and Mitchell, D.: Collection and cytogenetics of fetal fluids from heifers during the third month of pregnancy. I Collection. Theriogenology, 7:196, 1977.
6. Fechheimer, N. S.: Causal basis of chromosome abnormalities. J. Reprod. Fertil. (Suppl.), *15*:79, 1972.
7. Gluhovschi, M., Bistriceanu, M. and Palicica, R.: Les troubles de la reproduction chez les animaux domestiques, dus à des modifications du genome. Cah. Méd. Vét., *44*:155, 1975.
8. Gray, A. P.: Mammalian hybrids. 2nd Ed. Slough, England, Commonwealth Agricultural Bureaux, 1972.
9. Gustavsson, I.: Chromosomal errors in the reproduction of the domestic pig. *In* Boué, A. and Thibault, C. (Eds.): Les Accidents Chromosomiques de la Reproduction. Paris, Inserm, 1973.
10. Hamerton, J. L.: Human Cytogenetics. Vols. I and II. New York and London, Academic Press, 1971.
11. Hare, W. C. D., Mitchell, D., Betteridge, K. J., Eaglesome, M. D., and Randall, G. C. B.: Sexing two-week old bovine embryos by chromosomal analysis prior to surgical transfer: Preliminary methods and results. Theriogenology, *5*:243, 1976.
12. Makino, S.: Human Chromosomes. Amsterdam, Oxford North Holland Publishing Co., 1975.
13. McFeely, R. A. and Kanagawa, H.: Intersexuality. *In* Hafez, E. S. E. (Ed.): Reproduction in Farm Animals. 3rd ed. Philadelphia, Lea and Febiger, 1974.
14. Marcum, J. B.: The freemartin syndrome. Anim. Breed. Abst., *42*:227, 1974.
15. Moore, K. L.: The Sex Chromatin. Philadelphia, W. B. Saunders Co., 1966.
16. Moustafa, L. A., Hahn, J., and Roselius, R.: Versuche zur Geschlechtsbestimmung an Tag 6 und 7 alten Rinderembryonen. Tierärztl. Wschr., *91*: 236, 1978.
17. Ricke, G. W.: Numerical aberrations of gonosomes and reproductive failure in cattle. *In* Boué, A. and Thibault, C. (Eds.): Les Accidents Chromosomiques de la Reproduction. Paris, Inserm, 1973.
18. Rieck, G. W.: Chromosomenanomalien und ihre pathologischen Folgeerscheinungen bei den Haustieren. 1st World Congress on Genetics Applied to Livestock Production, Madrid, 1974.
19. Rieger, R., Michaelis, A., and Green, M. M.: A Glossary of Genetics and Cytogenetics. 3rd Ed. New York, Springer-Verlag New York Inc., 1968.
20. Singh, E. L. and Hare, W. C. D.: Collection and cytogenetics of fetal fluids from heifers during the third month of pregnancy. II Cytogenetic studies. Theriogenology, 7:203, 1977.

section **V**

BOVINE

Consulting Editor
DAVID A. MORROW

Physical Examination of the Bovine Female Reproductive System

INGEMAR SETTERGREN

Royal Veterinary College, Uppsala, Sweden

The fertility and infertility examinations in the bovine female require a thorough, methodical approach. It is suggested that the following method of examination be utilized:

HISTORY

The history is an important part of the examination, as reliable and detailed information facilitates and forms the basis of the diagnosis. Some of the more important parts of the history include:

Age. It is necessary to know the age of the animal in order to be able to evaluate the findings of the examination. The size of the nonpregnant sexual organs depends to a large extent on the animal's age. For example, the normal size of the uterus of an old cow would definitely be abnormal in a heifer. The ovaries also increase in size with age. The uterine horns in a heifer are normally symmetrical, but after one or more calvings the horns are usually of different sizes.

In some chronic herd infections such as vibriosis, the cows may have an almost normal fertility, whereas the heifers show a marked repeat breeding.

Parturition. The calving date should always be recorded whenever possible. The events surrounding the time of parturition are important for the fertility during the subsequent breeding period. The gestation length should correspond to what is normal in the breed. An abortion is always a serious abnormality, but a moderate shortening of the gestation length is also an important symptom if it occurs in several animals in a herd.

A difficult calving can influence fertility. Any help during parturition from the owner or from a veterinarian should be recorded. Retained placenta causes an ingrowth of bacteria into the uterus and also lengthens the puerperium. Many such cases in a herd indicate some type of general disturbance. Twin pregnancy in cows usually causes retained placenta.

Puerperium. The time from parturition until the uterus has returned to its normal nonpregnant size is about 3 weeks in the cow. The normal discharge during the puerperium, the lochia, is brownish to red in color and decreases markedly after about 10 days. If the discharge continues for some time and becomes pus-like, metritis should be suspected.

Heat Periods and Services. The date of the first heat after parturition and all service dates should be recorded. Normally most cows will show heat 30 to 40 days after calving, but usually an ovulation without outer signs of heat will have occurred prior to that. In the individual cows the interval between services should be noted. Service intervals of 28 to 32 days or 45 to 50 days indicate embryonic deaths. Many cases of prolonged service intervals in a herd may be due to a specific infection, e.g., vibriosis. Increased repeat breeding with normal service intervals can be caused by infertile semen or poor heat detection. It must be remembered that some cows will exhibit estrus during the first part of pregnancy. The service dates can be used to establish the fertility of individual bulls. When several bulls are used in a herd or if there has been a change of bulls, it is important to estimate the fertility of the individual bulls.

General Diseases. Not only diseases of the genital tract but also general diseases will influence fertility. For instance, parturient paresis and ketosis will lengthen the time from parturition to the first ovulation. Diseases causing loss of body weight may be the reason for anestrus and prolonged calving intervals.

Nutrition and Management. Whenever there are infertility problems in an entire herd, the feeding practices and the management should be checked. Poor quality silage and hay, flooded pastures and infected drinking water may cause herd infertility.

Heat detection may be the single most important management factor. For instance, if artificial insemination (AI) is used and the heat periods are constantly reported too late, this may simulate an infertility problem in the herd.

Milk Production and Growth of Calves. The milk production of dairy cattle and the calf crop and growth of the calves of beef cattle should also be recorded in the history.

GENERAL CLINICAL EXAMINATION

It is not necessary to perform a general health examination in otherwise healthy cows examined for infertility. On the other hand, outbreaks of infectious diseases such as viral diarrhea and infectious bovine rhinotracheitis (IBR) might cause abortions and infertility in a herd, which necessitates further investigations. The occurrence of coital infections such as vibriosis and trichomoniasis, as well as of brucellosis, in the herd during the preceding year should, of course, be recorded.

SPECIAL CLINICAL EXAMINATIONS

Visual Inspection

Inspection is a very important step in the examination of the sexual health of an animal, and any veterinarian working in the field of animal reproduction should train himself to observe the relevant symptoms.

Initially the general conformation of an animal may tell something about the condition of the sexual organs. In some cases of cystic ovarian degeneration, the cow has a masculine appearance accompanied by a deep voice. Heifers that do not produce estrogens from the gonads, e.g., in cases of freemartinism or total ovarian hypoplasia, have a steer-like appearance with a narrow pelvis and long legs.

During late pregnancy the pelvic ligaments become relaxed and the vulva edematous, especially about the time of parturition. At the end of the puerperium, about 3 weeks after calving, the ligaments and the vulva should return to normal conditions. If the pelvic ligaments do not return to normal within a month of calving or if they become relaxed after having been normal for some time, an endocrinological disturbance, usually caused by cystic ovaries, should be suspected.

Different types of discharge from the vulva can be observed. During proestrus there is normally a small amount of a clear, watery discharge that dries and forms whitish crusts on the tail and around the ischial tuberosities. At the time of standing heat, the mucus has increased very much in volume and viscosity and forms clear strings that may hang all the way from the vulva to the floor. A postestrous bleeding is frequently observed in cattle 36 to 48 hours after the end of heat.

Pathological conditions may cause different types of discharge from the vulva. In cases of metritis, there is a constant or intermittent flow of pus from the vulva. In animals with cystic ovaries, one may often observe a mucous discharge, which is not as clear as that during heat but is more opalescent.

The size of the udder and the teats will sometimes help to diagnose reproductive abnormalities. A small, empty udder in a cow served 7 to 9 months ago indicates that she is not pregnant. A freemartin or a heifer with total ovarian hypoplasia has much smaller teats than the normal heifers of comparable age.

Rectal Examination

Proper protective clothing should be used, consisting of rubber boots and a rubber or plastic apron. For all detailed palpation of the genital organs, rubber sleeves and gloves should also be worn. Plastic sleeves can be used for single inseminations and treatments, but these are not suitable for diagnostic work and may also damage the rectal mucosa.

Record keeping is a very important part of the examination. Small tape recorders are now available that can be carried on a string around the neck, and the results of each examination can be dictated into the recorder.

Before inserting the hand in the rectum, the glove should be well lubricated. Fecal material is removed with the hand still in the rectum, otherwise air will be sucked in and the rectum will become quite distended. If the rectum becomes filled with air, the hand is moved back and forth several times, at the same time pressing the rectal wall dorsally against the sacrum.

The examination of the genital tract must be done systematically to insure that all parts are examined properly. The following procedure is recommended:

Procedure

After the fecal material has been removed from the rectum, the cervix is located. This is a firm cylindrical structure situated medially in the pelvic cavity. The length and diameter of the cervix in a nonpregnant cow are 8 to 12 cm by 4 to 6 cm, respectively, and in heifers 6 to 8 cm by 3 to 4 cm, respectively. The caudal end of the cervix is located with the thumb, and the external os is examined to establish whether it is opened or closed and if there is a prolapse of a cervical ring.

The next step is to retract the cervix as much as possible and grasp the area between the uterine horns with two fingers to get hold of the intercornual ligament. There are two portions of this ligament; a dorsal one, which is thin, and a ventral one, which is thicker and stronger. The ventral portion is used for retraction and rolling up of the uterus, but it may be necessary to pull the upper portion carefully to be able to reach the ventral segment. Rolling up of the uterine horns should always be done in nonpregnant animals and in animals during early pregnancy to enable palpation of the total length of the uterine horns. If it is not possible to reach the intercornual ligament directly, one of the broad ligaments can be used for retraction of the uterus, and the hand is moved medially via the adjacent uterine horn and the ventral portion of the intercornual ligament grasped.

After rolling up the uterus, both horns are examined from the base to the tip. Utilizing the tip of the uterine horn, it is now easy to examine the lower part of the oviduct. Usually 5 to 10 cm can be evaluated. The uterus is examined for size and symmetry of the horns, consistency and thickness of the wall and for possible content.

The next step is to examine the ovaries, which are found lateral and caudal to the tip of the horns. The ovaries are rounded or cylindrical structures measuring 2 to 5 cm in length along the attached border, 1.5 to 4 cm in height from the attached to the free border and 1.5 to 3 cm thick from the anterior to the posterior side. The normal structures that are found in the ovaries are follicles and corpora lutea. The smallest palpable follicles are 5 to 6 mm in diameter, and the largest normal follicles are about 20 mm in diameter. Normal follicles are rounded, smooth structures with good tension. Fluctuation can be felt by palpation.

Atretic follicles and follicles close to the time of ovulation are soft and flattened. After ovulation the collapsed follicle is smaller than the preovulatory follicle. It is often called the corpus hemorrhagicum, but the bovine collapsed follicle contains very little blood compared with other species that have a real corpus hemorrhagicum. The corpus luteum develops from this structure and reaches a maximum size of 20 to 30 mm during midcycle (Fig. 1). The consistency of the corpus luteum is liver-like until regression starts at about day 17 of the cycle, when it becomes rather firm. The corpus luteum of pregnancy is rounded and embedded in the ovary; it feels more edematous than the cyclic corpus luteum, especially at 3 to 5 months of pregnancy.

When the ovaries are examined, the ovarian bursa should be checked. This is done by retracting the ovary and placing the thumb in front of it to prevent it from slipping forward. Three fingers are then slid forward, while pressing against the floor of the pelvis. The fingers are then spread, and the open end of the ovarian bursa is now felt. If the bursa is open normally, it feels like a thin string on the dorsal side of the fingers.

Changes in the Sexual Organs during the Normal Estrous Cycle

The practicing veterinarian must be able to estimate the approximate stage of the estrous cycle of a cow or a heifer after rectal examination. A short description is given in the following paragraphs, and the stages are illustrated in Figures 1 and 2.

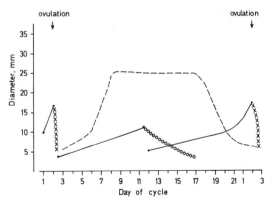

Figure 1. The largest follicle and the corpus luteum during the sexual cycle in cattle: ——————, normal follicle; ...., atretic follicle; xxxxxxxxxxxxx, ovulated follicle and ----------------------, corpus luteum.

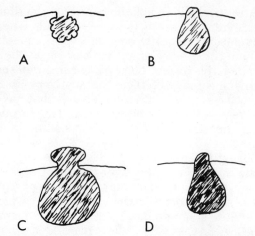

Figure 2. Shape and relative size of the corpus luteum during the sexual cycle in cattle. (*A*) Day 2 to 3 of the cycle, (*B*) day 6 to 7 of the cycle, (*C*) day 10 to 16 of the cycle and (*D*) day 18 to 19 of the cycle.

Proestrus. During proestrus, there is an increased tonus of the uterus and the horns become coiled. A relatively large follicle with tense consistency can be palpated in one of the ovaries. The corpus luteum is small, firm and often triangular in shape. A clear, watery discharge from the vulva can often be observed.

Estrus. At estrus, the follicle increases rapidly in size and becomes soft prior to ovulation. The uterus is contracted and firm with an uneven surface caused by contractions of the circular muscle layer. Clear mucus with high viscosity is discharged from the vulva.

Postestrus. During postestrus, the follicle has ovulated and the new corpus luteum is forming. It is small and difficult to palpate for the first days after ovulation. Sometimes the corpus luteum feels like clotted blood at palpation. Immediately after ovulation, the uterus is still contracted and has a more even structure than before. It is also common to find the cervix in an almost vertical position at this time. Later, the uterus becomes flabby. A bloody mucous discharge is observed in many cows, especially during winter months.

Days 6 to 11 of the Cycle. The corpus luteum is usually palpable now and increases in size up to day 8 to 10. At the same time it attains its liver-like consistency and rounded shape (Fig. 2). All follicles from the preceding cycle greater than 5 mm in diameter have undergone atresia, and a new group of follicles begins to grow from the third or fourth day of the cycle. The largest follicle is indicated in Figure 1 and continues to grow to day 11. At this time it becomes atretic, after which it is soft and flattened on palpation.

Days 12 to 19 of the Cycle. A new group of follicles has started to grow. The largest one can always be palpated and will be ovulated at the next estrus (Fig. 1). The corpus luteum retains its size up to day 16 or 17 and often has a crown (Fig. 2*C*). When the corpus luteum is reduced in size, the process usually begins in the peripheral part, whereby it becomes triangular and at the same time firmer than before (Fig. 2*D*).

Palpable Abnormalities of the Genital Organs

Ovarian Hypoplasia. In total hypoplasia the ovaries are very small and spindle-shaped and have no normal structures (Fig. 3). The uterus is anatomically normal but very small. In unilateral or bilateral partial hypoplasia, one or both ovaries are smaller than normal, but there may be some remnants of functional structures. The uterus is of normal size.

Freemartinism. The entire genital tract is malformed, but there is a great variation in the abnormalities found. The gonads may vary from ovary-like structures to structures resembling testicles with epididymides. The gonads are very small and often are difficult to palpate. The tubular part of the genital tract is always extensively malformed. In most cases the cervix and corpus and the caudal part of the horns are missing. There are always seminal vesicles present.

Ovarian Atrophy. This condition is found in high-producing dairy cows during winter and spring or in herds in which deficiencies in nutrition occur. Both ovaries are

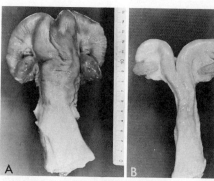

Figure 3. Sexual organs of a normal heifer (*A*) and of a heifer with bilateral total ovarian hypoplasia (*B*).

small and equal in size and have a smooth surface and firm consistency.

Cysts of the Ovaries. Two types of cysts, follicular and luteal, develop from unruptured follicles. Follicular cysts occur in one or both ovaries. They are often multiple, thin-walled and have a relatively large diameter, measuring 3 to 7 cm. The cysts are rare in heifers and first-calvers, increase up to the fifth lactation and then remain at the same level.

Luteal cysts are smaller in size than follicular cysts, measuring 2.5 to 4 cm in diameter. They are thick-walled, and usually only one or two cysts are present at a time. It is generally possible to differentiate between the two types, but sometimes partly luteinized transitional types occur, which makes the diagnosis difficult.

Cystic Corpora Lutea. These are formed from ovulated follicles that do not become solid but retain a fluid-like cavity in the center. They are difficult to diagnose clinically unless the cysts are large and thin-walled. Cystic corpora lutea do not alter the estrous cycle and are not found in pregnant animals.

Tumors. Various tumors are sometimes found in the ovaries. Most common is the granulosa cell tumor, which is found in cattle of all ages. It is usually large, relatively firm and nodular. The theca cell tumor is less common, rather soft in consistency and fast growing.

Segmental Aplasia of the Paramesonephric Duct. The best known type of segmental aplasia is the so-called white heifer disease, which received its name from the relatively high frequency in white Shorthorn heifers. It may, however, occur in any breed. The aplasia can occur anywhere along the duct system but is most common in the cervical area. The remaining parts of the uterine horn often become filled with secretions, which may simulate pregnancy.

There are also other types of segmental aplasia. An abnormality that is found in all breeds is uterus unicornis, in which one uterine horn is completely missing. These animals may very well become pregnant.

Occasionally, part of one or both oviducts is missing. If a small part is missing, hydrosalpinx results.

Inflammatory Changes of the Uterus. The most common inflammatory change is chronic endometritis, of which different degrees can be distinguished.

In first degree endometritis, the uterus is thick-walled and flabby but without palpable content. A continuous vaginal discharge is not present, but at the time of estrus the mucus is mixed with pus.

Second degree endometritis is characterized by an obvious enlargement of the uterus, comparable to a 5 to 6 weeks pregnancy. Discharge of a purulent exudate occurs at all stages of the cycle.

Third degree endometritis is primarily called pyometra. The uterus is more or less distended by a purulent exudate and compares in size to 2 to 4 months pregnancy. However, the uterine wall is thicker than in pregnancy, and there is no fetal bump. Usually both horns are involved, but involvement is not necessarily symmetrical. The purulent discharge is not continuous but can be heavy at times. The best chance of observing the exudate is when the cow is lying down.

Hydro- and Mucometra. In this condition the uterine wall is very thin and is filled with a fluid that varies from watery to mucous-like. The amounts of fluid may vary from very small volumes to several liters. Hydro- or mucometra is usually caused by long-lasting ovarian cysts. In extreme cases the thin wall makes it impossible to palpate the uterus.

Abnormalities of the Cervix. Most common is a lack of fusion of the two paramesonephric ducts, which causes different types of duplications. Such duplications occur in all breeds with differing frequencies. The most common type is a duplication of the external os, which can be diagnosed if the recommended examination procedure is followed. The duplication can include the entire cervix and also the corpus uteri and the vagina. It seems, however, that the external os of the cervix is always engaged, which makes it easier to diagnose the condition clinically.

Sometimes one or two of the cervical rings may be missing, and the cervix then feels very short. An S-shaped cervix has been found in several breeds, which makes artificial insemination impossible or very difficult.

Vaginal Examination

Vaginal examination is often neglected, but it is a useful aid, not only in order to confirm malformation of the vagina and the cervix or to collect material for microbiological investigation but also to help in heat detection. The best instrument to use is a glass speculum measuring 45 to 50 cm in length with a built-in source of light or a flashlight for illumination.

In cases of suspected segmental aplasia involving the vagina and the cervix or duplication of the cervix, vaginal examination will help to confirm the findings at palpation. For animals with vaginitis or endometritis, vaginal examination will reveal the degree of inflammation and the amount and type of exudate.

In herds with problems of heat detection, vaginal examination is very useful in order to establish the stage of the estrous cycle. During proestrus the mucosa in the anterior vagina and around the external os is pink in color, moist and shows some mucous secretion. During standing heat the mucosa becomes redder, the external os is relaxed and a stream of clear mucus can be seen coming from the cervix. The mucus often collects in a pool in the anterior part of the vagina. During postestrus the hyperemia of the vagina disappears and the color becomes pale. The amount of mucus decreases and is often mixed with blood. During the luteal phase, the vaginal mucosa is pale and is covered with tenacious mucus that is grayish or opalescent in color.

SAMPLING OF SPECIMENS FOR LABORATORY EXAMINATION

Sometimes it is necessary to collect material for further microbiological, serological or histological investigations. The mucous agglutination test is used for the diagnosis of vibriosis and trichomoniasis. For this purpose a sterile gauze tampon is placed in the anterior part of the vagina for at least 20 minutes. Heifers that have been served 6 weeks or more prior to the examination should preferably be selected for the test. The tampons are sent to a laboratory for testing of the presence of antibodies in the vaginal mucus.

REFERENCES

1. Bane, A. and Rajakoski, E. The bovine estrous cycle. Cornell Vet., *51*:77, 1961.
2. Zemjanis, R.: Diagnostic and Therapeutic Techniques in Animal Reproduction. 2nd Ed. Baltimore, The Williams and Wilkins Co, 1970.

Initiation of Puberty and Postpartum Estrus in Beef Cattle

C. C. KALTENBACH
University of Wyoming, Laramie, Wyoming

INTRODUCTION

Puberty and postpartum anestrus are two of the most important factors affecting reproductive efficiency in beef cattle. The hormones that control the onset of puberty and initiate postpartum estrus have similar secretory patterns prior to and during both of these important physiological events. Because of the similarity from both a physiological and economic standpoint, it seems appropriate to discuss these events simultaneously.

FACTORS INFLUENCING PUBERTY

Puberty is generally defined as the condition of first being or the period of first becoming capable of reproducing sexually. In heifers, puberty is reached at the time of first ovulation. This initial ovulation often occurs without being accompanied by estrus; therefore, puberty should be considered as the time when first estrus and ovulation occur simultaneously. Puberty in heifers is controlled or influenced by both genetic and environmental factors.

The genetic influence on age at puberty is exerted by both breed of sire and breed of dam. There is also a heterosis (hybrid vigor) effect on age at puberty in addition to that exerted by increases in average daily gain. In general, large breeds are

TABLE 1. *Influence of Level of Feed on Age and Weight at Puberty in Straightbred and Crossbred Hereford and Angus Heifers**

Variable	Straightbred	Crossbred
Age at puberty (days)		
High nutrition	381	381
Low nutrition	572	424
Weight at puberty (lb)		
High nutrition	658	726
Low nutrition	590	559

*Adapted from Wiltbank, J. N., Kasson, C. W. and Ingalls, J. E.: J. Anim. Sci., 29:602, 1969.

older and heavier at puberty than are smaller breeds.

The environmental factors affecting puberty are exerted primarily by growth rate, which has a definite influence on age at puberty. A significant relationship between the level of feed (i.e., growth rate) and the age at puberty has been established in several studies; however, the magnitude of response to different rates of gain prior to puberty is influenced by breed (Table 1).

High ambient temperatures have been shown to increase age at puberty slightly in European cattle and markedly in Zebu cattle. Disease may also delay puberty, although this effect is exerted mainly by its influence on growth rate. Another major factor determining the age at first estrus appears to be the season of the year in which the animal is born. Calves born during increasing day length (spring) reach puberty up to 2 months earlier than those born during decreasing day length. The manner in which season of birth affects age at puberty is unknown.

FACTORS INFLUENCING ONSET OF POSTPARTUM ESTRUS

The onset of the first postpartum estrus is influenced by several factors, including level of nutrition before and after calving, body condition at calving, lactation, dystocia, breed and age of the cow. The level of nutrition both before and after calving has a dramatic effect on the length of the interval between calving and the first postpartum estrus. In one recent study it was shown that for each 10-day interval occurring 60 to 90 days postpartum, the likeli-

hood of estrus was significantly increased as body condition at calving improved from thin to moderate to good, emphasizing the importance of precalving nutrition.[6] The limiting nutrients in a beef cattle enterprise are generally energy and phosphorus. Phosphorus is particularly important in areas that are deficient in this mineral when high calcium feeds such as legumes are fed. Protein deficiencies can also affect the postpartum interval, especially in first-calf heifers.

Lactation exerts a dramatic effect on the postpartum interval. Removal of the mammary gland prior to parturition shortens the postpartum interval dramatically.[5] Nonsuckled and suckled cows in this study had intervals of 25 and 61 days, respectively, compared with 14 days for those in which the mammary gland was removed. The frequency of milking or suckling is also related to the length of the anestrous period. Cows milked twice each day have shorter intervals than cows nursing one calf, which, in turn, have intervals similar in duration to cows milked four times daily. Cows nursing two or more calves have longer intervals than cows nursing single calves.

Other factors include dystocia, age and breed effects. Dystocia not only delays return to estrus but also lowers conception rates. First-calf heifers invariably have longer postpartum intervals than do multiparous cow. The most dramatic breed effects have been observed between *Bos taurus and Bos indicus* breeds, with the latter having extended postpartum intervals.

HORMONE PROFILES

The endocrine events associated with puberty and postpartum anestrus have been examined in several laboratories. Unfortunately, in most of these studies, blood samples were not taken at sufficiently frequent intervals to assess important but transient changes that occur in secretory patterns of the hormones regulating these physiological events. Two recently completed studies, one in heifers[1] and the other in postpartum cows,[3] have attempted to overcome these deficiencies. In both of these studies blood samples were taken every 6 hours daily and at 15- or 20-minute intervals for 4 hours once each week. Samples were collected from the period of approximately 50 days before until 10 days after first estrus in the heifers and from parturition until estrus in the cows.

Quantification of luteinizing hormone (LH), follicle-stimulating hormone (FSH), gonadotropin-releasing hormone (Gn-RH), prolactin, progesterone and estradiol-17β in the heifers revealed significant changes only in LH and progesterone levels. Although peripheral levels of LH fluctuated markedly during the prepuberal period, this hormone was characterized by two distinct peaks. An initial peak occurred 9 to 11 days prior to the second or "pubertal" peak, which resulted in ovulation and initiation of normal cyclic ovarian activity. There were also two distinct transitory elevations in peripheral levels of progesterone lasting from 2 to 5 days. The first elevation returned to baseline immediately prior to the "priming" peak of LH, whereas the second elevation preceded the "pubertal" peak of LH. Distinct changes in the secretory pattern of LH occurred coincident with the second elevation in progesterone. Although LH continued to be secreted in frequent bursts, the magnitude of these bursts was reduced. This was interpreted as establishment of phasic LH release characteristic of the normal cyclic cow.

Blood samples obtained in the cow study were quantified for LH, prolactin, progesterone, cortisol, estradiol-17β and estrone. Prolactin was of particular interest, as this hormone appears to have antigonadotropic effects that precipitate the well-characterized amenorrhea-galactorrhea syndrome in women. Lactation and suckling stimulate prolactin release, and since there is evidence suggesting that high levels of prolactin may delay postpartum estrus in ewes, it was theorized that a similar effect might occur in cattle. The secretory patterns of prolactin that were observed in the cow study could best be described as variable. Onset of postpartum estrus could not be related to frequency, magnitude or duration of secretory peaks or to mean levels of prolactin.

It is thus difficult to ascribe any particular role to prolactin regarding the onset of postpartum estrus. A similar conclusion was reached for cortisol and estradiol-17β, as there were no appreciable changes in either of these steroids during the postpartum interval.

On the other hand, based on observations in heifers, secretion of LH appears to be very important. Peripheral levels of LH following parturition were initially very low. This pattern was followed by a period of intense secretory activity that lasted 2 to 3 weeks. There was an abrupt decrease in the frequency and magnitude of the secretory peaks characteristic of this period approximately 6 days prior to estrus and ovulation. The decrease in LH secretory activity immediately preceded a transitory elevation in progesterone that lasted only 4 days.

Interestingly, the onset of LH intense secretory activity in these cows appears to be triggered by estrone. A significant elevation in estrone beginning 13 ± 1 days after parturition was observed in all six cows in this study. This peak of estrone, lasting only 1 or 2 days, was immediately followed by an increase in LH secretory activity in four of the six cows whose postpartum intervals were less than 50 days. The two additional cows whose postpartum intervals were 68 and 70 days, respectively, did not respond to the increase in estrone. These cows, however, continued to have peaks of estrone at 7- to 9-day intervals. LH was triggered by the second estrone peak in one cow and by the third peak in the remaining cow.

A theory regarding the endocrine events associated with the first postpartum estrus can thus be developed. Ovarian follicular activity, which begins within approximately 10 days following parturition and continues throughout the postpartum period, probably contributes a peak of estrone with each wave of follicular development. The peak of estrone, in turn, alters the function of the hypothalamus, leading to increased LH secretory activity. LH secreted in this manner sensitizes the ovary for a period of 2 to 3 weeks, resulting in a short-lived elevation of peripheral progesterone levels. The progesterone again alters hypothalamic function, possibly leading to an increase in secretion of FSH, which results in a final burst in follicular growth, culminating in ovulation. This ovulation is usually accompanied by estrus, although a relatively high incidence of silent ovulations has been reported in several studies. The great variation observed in the length of the postpartum interval among animals may be explained by failure of the hypothalamus to "read" the initial surge in estrone. In fact, several surges of estrone

TABLE 2. *Occurrence of Estrus and Pregnancy in Prepubertal Heifers Treated with Syncro-Mate B**

	Treatment	
Variable	CONTROL	SYNCRO-MATE B†
No. heifers	14	16
No. in estrus		
0–4 days	0	15
0–21 days	0	16
No. pregnant		
0–4 days	0	8
0–21 days	0	12

*Adapted from Gonzalez-Padilla, E., Ruiz, D., LeFever, D., Denham, A. and Wiltbank, J. N.: J. Anim. Sci., 40:1110, 1975.
†Implant containing 6 mg of Norgestomet for 9 days and injection of 5 mg of estradiol valerate and 3 mg of Norgestomet on day of implantation.

may be required in some animals. Sensitivity of the hypothalamus in this regard could easily be affected by the level of nutrition, suckling stimulus and other environmental factors.

HORMONAL INDUCTION OF ESTRUS

Numerous hormonal treatments have been tested for their ability to induce puberty and postpartum estrus. These treatments usually consist of a progestogen used in combination with estrogen, pregnant mare serum gonadotropin (PMSG), or estrogen and PMSG.

Successful induction of puberty was obtained in early trials when PMSG was given at the end of a progestogen regimen that was administered either by injection or by feeding. These early treatments have mostly been replaced by hormonal treat-

ments designed for estrous synchronization. Of these, the most widely used appears to be the Syncro-Mate B system (Table 2). Within limits, this treatment alone appears to be quite effective. An additional injection of estradiol at the end of this progestogen regimen had no beneficial effect in terms of estrous response but did reduce conception rates at the induced estrus. Results similar to those shown in Table 2 have also been obtained when PMSG was given at the end of the Synchro-Mate B regimen.[4] Failure of the PMSG to exert an obvious additive effect coupled with the relative unavailability of this hormone and the probability of obtaining superovulation, which may be detrimental to fertility, makes this a questionable practice.

The necessity for including estrogen at the beginning of the progestogen treatment has been tested only on a limited scale. Evidence in one study[3] indicated that estrogen may not be needed for effective induction of pubertal estrus. Estrogen is needed, however, to initiate regression of corpora lutea in cycling animals. Since most treated groups will probably contain a few animals that have already reached puberty, it seems advisable to routinely include the estrogen injection at the beginning of the progestogen treatment.

The response obtained following use of Syncro-Mate B and similar treatments is definitely influenced by age and weight of the heifers at the time of treatment (Tables 3 and 4).

A good response can be expected in prepubertal heifers that have reached an optimum age but lack the requisite weight and in heifers that are sufficiently heavy but are too young. Heifers that are both young and light will not respond as favorably.

The Syncro-Mate B treatment also ap-

TABLE 3. *Effect of Age on Estrus and Pregnancy in Brangus Heifers**

	Yearlings		2-Year-Olds	
Variable	CONTROL	TREATED	CONTROL	TREATED
No. heifers	28	24	20	19
In heat 0–25 days (%)	28	71	40	100
Pregnant 0–25 days (%)	3	42	15	63

*Adapted from Gonzales-Padilla, E., Ruiz, D., LeFever, D., Denham, A., and Wiltbank, J. N.: J. Anim. Sci., 40:1110, 1975.

TABLE 4. *Effect of Body Weight on Estrus and Pregnancy**

Weight (lb)	No. Heifers	In Heat (%) 0–25 DAYS	Pregnant (%) 0–25 DAYS
400–485			
Control	15	20	0
Treated†	11	64	54
486–574			
Control	28	14	3
Treated	29	75	57
575–660			
Control	26	38	15
Treated	22	100	56
661–750			
Control	16	50	30
Treated	13	100	54

*Adapted from Gonzalez-Padilla, E., Ruiz, D., LeFever, D., Denham, A. and Wiltbank, J. N.: J. Anim. Sci., *40*:1110, 1975.

†As described in Table 2.

pears to be an effective inducer of estrus and ovulation in the postpartum cow. The data in Table 5 were obtained from lactating beef cows whose postpartum interval averaged 70 days at the end of the treatment period.

These data provide an example of what might be expected in a group of lactating cows that were thin at calving. The 35 per cent incidence of estrus by 94 days in the control cows is unacceptable.

As with all induction treatments, the ultimate response is dependent upon lactation status, level of nutrition and the interval between calving and initiation of treatment. A further improvement in response to the progestogen treatment might be obtained by temporarily weaning the calves for 48 hours following implant removal (see following article).

In some instances the addition of PMSG

TABLE 5. *Effect of Syncro-Mate B Treatment on Postpartum Estrus*

Treatment	No. Cows	Percent Showing Estrus
Syncro-Mate B	143	65*
Control	72	35†

*Days 1–4 post-treatment
†Days 1–24.

(500 to 750 IU) on the last day of progestogen treatment may also increase the percentage of cows showing estrus. However, lack of standardization and availability and the potential for superovulation probably preclude the routine use of this hormone.

Several studies have now been conducted to determine if CB-154 (2-Br-α-ergocryptine), an ergot derivative that inhibits prolactin secretion, will shorten the postpartum anestrous interval. Results to date have been disappointing, regardless of whether the CB-154 was administered alone or in combination with a progestogen treatment. These results, combined with previous data that failed to establish a relationship between blood levels of prolactin and duration of the postpartum interval, indicate that prolactin plays only a minor role, if any, in determining the duration of anestrus in the postpartum cow.

Although the data presented in this article were derived primarily with the use of Norgestomet, there is no reason to believe that this particular compound is any worse or any better than other progestogens, synthetic or natural. It is obvious, however, that some form of progestogen is required for effective induction of estrus in both prepubertal heifers and postpartum cows.

REFERENCES

1. Gonzalez-Padilla, E., Wiltbank, J. N. and Niswender, G. D.: Puberty in beef heifers. I. The interrelationship between pituitary, hypothalamic and ovarian hormones. J. Anim. Sci., *40*:1091, 1975.
2. Gonzalez-Padilla, E., Ruiz, R., LeFever, D., Denham, A. and Wiltbank, J. N.: Puberty in beef heifers. III. Induction of fertile estrus. J. Anim. Sci., *40*:1110, 1975.
3. Humphrey, W. D., Kaltenbach, C. C., Dunn, T. G. and Niswender, G. D.: Characterization of hormonal patterns in the beef cow during postpartum anestrus. (Submitted for publication).
4. Mauleon, P.: Recent research related to the physiology of puberty. *In* The Early Calving of Heifers and Its Impact on Beef Production. Commission of European Communities, 1975, p. 37.
5. Short, R. E., Bellows, R. A., Moody, E. L. and Howland, B. E.: Effects of mastectomy on bovine postpartum reproduction. J. Anim. Sci., *34*:70, 1972.
6. Whitman, R. W., Remmenga, E. E. and Wiltbank, J. N.: Weight change, condition and beef cow reproduction. J. Anim. Sci., *41*:387, 1975 (Abstr.).
7. Wiltbank, J. N., Kasson, C. W. and Ingalls, J. E.: Puberty in crossbred and straightbred beef heifers on two levels of feed. J. Anim. Sci., *29*:602, 1969.

Control of Estrus in Cattle

C. C. KALTENBACH

University of Wyoming, Laramie, Wyoming

INTRODUCTION

Methods for controlling the estrous cycle in cattle were first initiated in the 1940's by a research team at the University of Wisconsin. Many of the problems confronting early workers in the field are still with us today; however, significant advances have been made. It is the purpose of this article to discuss various methods that have been developed, as well as some of the problems associated with estrous cycle control.

BENEFITS

Facilitation of artificial insemination (AI) is usually given as justification for development and use of estrous synchronization techniques. The benefits of AI are well known, and this in itself may be sufficient justification. Another, perhaps equally important, reason for wanting to use estrous synchronization lies in the area of herd management, particularly as it applies to beef herds.

Total pounds of calf weaned per cow exposed is the ultimate measure of success in a cow-calf enterprise. Weaning weight, which is the product of calf age and average daily gain, can be increased most rapidly by increasing the average age of all calves at weaning (Table 1). This is most easily accomplished by utilizing a short breeding season and by increasing the proportion of cows conceiving during the early part of the breeding season.

The advantage of heavy weaning weights is also evident when the calves are 18 months of age (Table 2). In this instance, steer calves were divided into weight classes by 50-pound increments based on their weaning weights. These data indicate that the calves that are heaviest at weaning are also the heaviest at 18 months of age. Similarly, the light calves at weaning are still light at 18 months of age. Therefore, heavy weaning weights are advantageous regardless of whether calves are sold at weaning or at 18 months of age. Similar data are available for heifer calves, which is particularly advantageous with regard to age at puberty.

Therefore, estrous synchronization, in combination with a short breeding season, can increase calf weight at weaning and 18 months of age and increase the proportion of female offspring that reach puberty prior to onset of the breeding season. In addition, a short breeding season increases the average period of time between calving and the beginning of the subsequent breeding season. This increase in time is beneficial in the annual struggle with the postpartum anestrous cow.

METHODS

Prostaglandins

Physiological Responses

Prostaglandins are extremely potent "hormone-like" substances that occur naturally in a wide variety of tissues and body fluids. Chemically, prostaglandins have been identified as C_{20} unsaturated fatty acids, with a cyclopentane ring at C8–C12.

Prostaglandins have a wide range of physiological activities. The most important property, to those interested in animal reproduction, is the ability of prostaglandin-$F_{2\alpha}$ ($PGF_{2\alpha}$) to cause functional and morphological regression of the corpus luteum (CL). The luteolytic properties of $PGF_{2\alpha}$ were first demonstrated by Pharris and Wyngarden in the pseudopregnant rat. A similar action of this compound was soon demonstrated in numerous other species, including the sheep, horse and cow.

TABLE 1. *Effect of Age on Weaning Weight of Beef Calves**

Calving Period	Number	Weaning Weight (lb)	Age (days)	Average Daily Gain (lb)
1st	10,157	404	212	1.58
2nd	6,881	371	190	1.57
3rd	3,470	328	164	1.56

*From C. O. Schoonover, University of Wyoming (unpublished data).

TABLE 2. *Effect of Weaning Weight on Subsequent 18-Month Weight of Steer Calves*

Weight Class (lb)	Number	Weaning Weight		18-Month Weight	
		GROUP MEAN (lb)	DEVIATION FROM OVERALL MEAN (lb)	GROUP MEAN (lb)	DEVIATION FROM OVERALL MEAN (lb)
< 300	38	262	−82	589	−100
301–350	32	330	−14	660	−29
351–400	29	318	+34	740	+51
401–450	19	418	+74	778	+89
> 451	10	466	+122	842	+153
Total/average	128	344		689	

The dose of $PGF_{2\alpha}$ required for luteolysis in the cow is dependent on the site of deposition. Partial luteolysis is obtained with only 300 μg if the compound is administered directly into the corpus luteum. Intrauterine administration of 5 mg of $PGF_{2\alpha}$ produces a consistent luteolytic response, whereas 30 mg is generally considered to be a minimally effective subcutaneous or intramuscular dose.

The sequence of changes in progesterone, estrogen and luteinizing hormone (LH) levels that culminates in ovulation after $PGF_{2\alpha}$ administration is similar to those observed following normal CL regression in untreated cows. Transitory increases in prolactin, growth hormone and glucocorticoid concentrations have also been observed following $PGF_{2\alpha}$ administration. Luteolytic doses of $PGF_{2\alpha}$ given intramuscularly cause no major changes in blood pressure, heart rate or body temperature.

Synchronization of Ovulation

Discovery of the luteolytic properties of specific prostaglandins was rapidly followed by experiments designed to determine if these compounds could be used effectively to synchronize estrus in cattle. Several synthetic analogs of $PGF_{2\alpha}$ have also been produced. The most notable of these appears to be cloprostenol (Estrumate). This analog and a THAM salt preparation of the parent compound, $PGF_{2\alpha}$, have been used widely in estrous synchronization trials.

Intrauterine administration was employed in several early studies; however, the readily apparent disadvantages of this procedure coupled with an increase in availability of these compounds has led to general acceptance of the intramuscular route.

Although both $PGF_{2\alpha}$ – THAM salt and cloprostenol are effective luteolytic agents, neither compound will prevent formation of the corpus luteum and both are therefore ineffective during the first 5 days of the estrous cycle. They are effective only in cows having a functional corpus luteum, which also rules out their use in postpartum anestrous cows and prepubertal heifers.

Problems associated with detection of estrus are the greatest deterrent to use of AI, particularly in beef cattle, and the greatest stimulus for development of effective estrous synchronization procedures. Detection of estrus following synchronization presents a similar problem. This has led to general agreement among investigators that a system involving fixed-time insemination following treatment will be the most acceptable method.

Since prostaglandins are not effective if administered before day 5 or beyond day 18 of the cycle, up to 30 per cent of cyclic cattle may fail to be synchronized by a single injection. Furthermore, in some trials, synchrony following a single injection has not been precise. This has led to the use of two injections of prostaglandin administered at a 10- to 12-day interval. Theoretically, all animals should have a functional corpus luteum (days 5 to 18 of the cycle) when the second injection of prostaglandin is administered. In practice this appears to be the case, and precision of synchrony tends to be improved following the second injection.

In addition to precision of synchrony, the period of time relative to treatment during which the peak of estrous activity occurs is also important, particularly if one wishes to use fixed-time inseminations. The time at which the peak of activity occurs has been observed to shift by as much as 24 hours. There is no obvious reason as to why this occurs; however, such a shift may explain the variable results obtained following either single or double inseminations at a fixed time. Single insemination times at either 72 or 80 hours have been compared in most instances with a double insemination at 70 and 88 hours or 72 and 96 hours following prostaglandin administration. In some studies higher fertility has been obtained with a single insemination, whereas in other trials conception rates have been higher following two inseminations. The variation in results is probably due to both precision of synchrony and peak of estrous activity.

In addition to the double injection procedure followed by fixed-time insemination, numerous other systems have been tested. These include: (1) synchronization with two injections of prostaglandin and insemination after detection of estrus, (2) insemination after detection of estrus for 5 days followed by one injection of prostaglandin and insemination after estrous detection for the next 5 days and (3) examination of the ovaries by rectal palpation and treatment of only those cows that have corpora lutea. One or two injections of prostaglandin can be used in this system, and insemination can be at a fixed time (single or double) or following detection of estrus.

Progestogens

Methods of Administration

In contrast to prostaglandins, progestogens block ovulation and suppress estrus. Administration of exogenous progestogens for a period of time sufficient to allow natural regression of the CL in all treated cows, followed by removal of the exogenous source, will synchronize estrus in the entire herd.

In early studies progesterone was administered by daily subcutaneous or intramuscular injections. This tedious process was soon replaced by oral administration of synthetic progestogens added to feed. Problems associated with uniform intake led to the development of subcutaneous implants and intravaginal devices.

The most widely used implant is one made of Hydron, a synthetic polymer. Each implant contains 6 mg of Norgestomet (SC-21009), a potent synthetic progestogen. Insertion of the implant is normally accompanied by an intramuscular injection containing 3 mg of the Norgestomet and 5 or 6 mg of estradiol valerate. This treatment bears the trade name Syncro-Mate B. The implant is small enough to pass through a 9-gauge thin-wall needle, and it is usually placed subcutaneously on the back of the ear. To prevent infection, it is recommended that the ear either be scrubbed with an antiseptic soap solution or clipped and sprayed with an appropriate antiseptic. The entire process can be accomplished at the rate of one animal per minute. The animals must be restrained in a squeeze chute equipped with a head catch. Additional head restraint is usually unnecessary. The retention rate of properly inserted implants exceeds 99 per cent. The implants can be removed from animals at the rate of three per minute.

Intravaginal administration of progestogen was initially accomplished with sponge pessaries similar to those developed for use in sheep. Difficulties associated with retention of the sponge led to development of stainless steel spirals (3.2 cm × 30.5 cm) coated with silicone rubber. This progesterone releasing–intravaginal device (PRID) was developed by Abbott Laboratories, and it contains natural progesterone as opposed to a synthetic progestogen. The large surface area of the PRID allows sufficient absorption to maintain blood levels of progesterone that will inhibit estrus. The PRIDs, which are coiled to a diameter of 5.0 cm, are inserted with the aid of a speculum, and they are easily removed by pulling on a previously attached nylon cord that remains outside the vagina. Initial problems with retention appear to be solved, and losses are generally less than 5 per cent.

Duration of Treatment

In early studies, progestogens were usually administered for at least 18 days. This is a sufficient period of time for the corpora lutea of all treated animals in a herd to regress naturally. Although administration of progestogen for this period of time normally resulted in precise synchrony following cessation of treatment, a significant reduction in fertility was commonly observed. Failure of sperm transport, a common cause of subfertility in progestogen-synchronized sheep, does not appear to be a significant factor in cattle. There is evidence that the cleavage rate of fertilized ova is slower than normal in cattle that have received progestogen in excess of 14 days.

The duration of progestogen administration is thus an important factor in post-treatment fertility. Wiltbank and his co-workers demonstrated that the duration of progestogen administration could be reduced from 18 days to 9 days if an injection of estrogen, which induces regression of the corpora lutea, is given on day 1 of treatment. Although estrogen is an effective luteolytic agent, it will not effectively block formation of new corpora lutea. A large dose of progesterone given in combination with estrogen will inhibit corpus luteum formation. The combined injection of Norgestomet and estrogen was thus incorporated in the Syncro-Mate B treatment to achieve satisfactory synchronization in cattle treated during the early days of the estrous cycle.

Initial work with the PRID also incorporated an injectable consisting of a combination of 5 mg of estradiol valerate benzoate and 50 mg of progesterone. In recent experiments the progesterone injection has been eliminated, and the estrogen is administered with a gelatin capsule attached to the PRID. Extension of the treatment period from 9 to 12 days, in the absence of the progesterone injection, provides sufficient precision in the estrous response. Further extension of the treatment to 14 days with elimination of both estrogen and progesterone at the beginning of therapy is currently being tested; however, insufficient data are available to determine if this is a feasible treatment.

Insemination Times

Insemination approximately 12 hours after onset of the synchronized estrus has generally resulted in conception rates comparable to nonsynchronized control animals. Difficulties associated with estrous detection have stimulated efforts to estab-

lish appropriate hours for fixed-time inseminations.

Insemination at estrus has been compared with insemination at 56 or 56 hours and 74 hours following removal of PRIDs. Conception rates following the single insemination at 56 hours have been comparable to those obtained with the double insemination, and in most instances they have exceeded those obtained following insemination at estrus in dairy cows and heifers. Insufficient data are available to determine if a single timed insemination following this treatment is adequate in lactating beef cows.

Only very limited data are available concerning conception rates with a double insemination following removal of implants containing Norgestomet. A single insemination at 48-hours postimplant removal in heifers has provided acceptable conception rates in some trials. Similar, but limited, data have been obtained in lactating beef cows inseminated at 54 hours after implant removal.

A promising new technique, referred to as SHANG, is currently being tested in lactating beef cows. This procedure involves isolation of all calves at implant removal. Calves are returned to their dams following a single timed insemination at 48 hours. In preliminary trials, calf removal increased the percentage of cows showing estrus, provided better synchrony of estrus and increased conception rates (Table 3). Calf health does not appear to be impaired if feed and water are provided during the 48-hour period.

Unfortunately, the rather dramatic increase in conception rates observed in the

TABLE 3. *Pregnancy Rates in Lactating Beef Cows Following Syncro-Mate B**

Treatment	Number	Per Cent Pregnant		
		2 DAYS	5 DAYS	25 DAYS
Control	624	–	8	42
SMB-Estrus†	683	–	30	49
SMB-Time‡	654	41	41	56

*Summary of eight herds in 1976. (Data courtesy G. D. Searle & Co.)

†Single insemination following detection of estrus.

‡Single insemination 48 to 54 hours after implant removal. Calves separated from cows between implant removal and insemination.

TABLE 4. *Pregnancy Rates in Syncro-Mate B–Treated Lactating Cows with and without Calf Removal or GnRH*

Item	Treatment			
	CONTROL	CALF REMOVAL*	GnRH†	INSEMINATION AT ESTRUS
Number of cows treated	128	128	120	117
Per cent inseminated	49	100	100	54
Per cent pregnant‡				
First service	38	30	28	32
First 20 days of breeding	38	49	52	53

*Single insemination 48 to 54 hours after implant removal and separation of calves.

†GnRH (125 μg) administered 36 hours after implant removal. Single insemination 12 hours after GnRH administration.

‡Pregnancy rates based on cows treated.

early trials has not always been duplicated in subsequent studies (Table 4). Additional information is required to determine if specific factors such as nutritional status, postpartum interval, breed and period of calf removal affect the response obtained with the SHANG treatment.

Control of Ovulation

Synthesis and release of LH are controlled by a hypothalamic peptide. Isolation and identification of this hypothalamic-releasing factor led to synthesis of gonadotropin-releasing hormone (GnRH), which has been used in combination with both prostaglandins and progestogens for precise control of ovulation.

A single intramuscular dose (100 to 125 μg) of GnRH given 30 to 40 hours after removal of implants or PRIDs initiates LH release, which is followed by ovulation approximately 32 hours later. A similar response is obtained in prostaglandin-treated cattle if GnRH is given 60 hours after prostaglandin administration (Fig. 1).

The precise release of LH allows a single insemination approximately 12 to 18 hours after GnRH administration. In most studies, conception rates following use of GnRH are comparable, and often exceed, those obtained when single inseminations are performed, either at estrus or at a fixed time. More data are needed to determine if GnRH administration provides sufficient benefit, compared with fixed-time insemination, to justify the additional expense. Approval for use by regulatory agencies may also be a determining factor.

Selection of Appropriate Treatment

At this point in time it is impossible to recommend any single treatment or procedure as the one of choice. In fact, it is doubtful if any single procedure will ever fit all occasions.

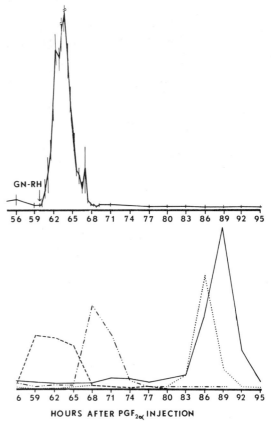

Figure 1. Peripheral levels of LH following administration of $PGF_{2\alpha}$. Heifers in bottom panel (n = 4) received $PGF_{2\alpha}$ only, whereas heifers in top panel (n = 4) received an additional injection of GnRH.

Choice of drug will depend primarily on the percentage of cattle that are cycling prior to treatment. Herds in which a large proportion of the animals are either anestrous or prepubertal will not respond sufficiently to treatment with prostaglandins. In contrast, because of relatively short withdrawal times and simplicity of administration, prostaglandins may be the treatment of choice in dairy herds and beef herds composed mainly of pubertal heifers and nonlactating cows.

Numerous factors, including available personnel, handling facilities, proximity of holding pastures, relative costs and personal preference will all have to be considered in the selection of appropriate insemination procedures. Detection of estrus is particularly difficult following synchronization of large numbers of cattle, and a certain percentage of animals in heat will invariably be missed. Fixed-time inseminations are therefore appealing; however,

selection of either single or double inseminations and whether to use GnRH (if available) or SHANG in lactating beef cows will be necessary.

Nutritional status and herd health will also dictate if any synchronization procedure is appropriate. Good herd management is a prerequisite for all of the estrous synchronization procedures currently being tested. None of these procedures will ever be a remedy for poor management practices.

REFERENCES

1. Gordon, I.: Controlled breeding in cattle. Part 1. Hormones in the regulation of reproduction, oestrus control, and set-time artificial insemination. Anim. Breed. Abs., *44*:265, 1976.
2. Manns, J. G. and Hafs, H. D.: Controlled breeding in cattle: A review. Can. J. Anim. Sci., *56*:121, 1976.

Testosterone Treatment of Cows for Detection of Estrus

JACK H. BRITT

North Carolina State University, Raleigh, North Carolina

From observations of behavior in ovariectomized ewes given estrogens or androgens, Signoret[4] concluded that sexual activty was enhanced after treatments with testosterone. Similar conclusions were made after he gave androgens to cows.[5] Thus, a potentially practical application of these observations resulted after it was found that androgen-treated cows were effective in detecting estrus in their herdmates.[5]

The author and associates[1, 2, 3] have conducted a series of experiments to determine methods for inducing increased mounting (sexual) activity in cows by treatments with testosterone or testosterone derivatives and to determine whether these cows are useful as aids in detection of estrus in herds of beef or dairy cattle.

SELECTION OF ANIMALS FOR TREATMENT

The principal advantages of utilizing a cow rather than a bull or steer for detection of estrus include: (1) safety, (2) the ready availability of physically sound cull cows in most herds, (3) the avoidance of having to castrate or surgically alter detector animal, (4) the relatively rapid rate at which a normal cow can be "transformed" into a detector animal and (5) the reduced risk of venereal disease transmission. Cows or mature heifers may be utilized, but cows are preferred because they have had more sexual activity (estrous cycles, pregnancy, and so forth) and usually have established their position in the social order of the herd, although this may change after treatment. The animal selected for treatment should be medium in size in relation to herdmates, physically sound (especially the feet and legs), nonlactating and open. In dairy herds, an animal of choice would be a first or second lactation cow destined to be culled for low milk production or chronic mastitis. Freemartins and cows with ovarian follicular cysts may be potentially useful detector animals, but such animals have not been studied after androgen treatment. In beef herds, a cow can be chosen between the calving and breeding periods, based on her performance; cows that lose their calf soon after calving are good candidates for treatment. The animal chosen should be gentle enough to handle regularly.

TREATMENT REGIMENS

Procedures for treatment have been divided arbitrarily into an induction phase and a maintenance phase. The induction phase is designed to initiate increased mounting behavior and sexual activity, and the maintenance phase is designed to perpetuate this behavior.

We have adminstered treatments via intramuscular (IM) and subcutaneous (SC) injections and by intravaginal implants or pessaries (Fig. 1). All methods have proved to be effective in inducing mounting behavior as long as blood levels of testosterone remain above about 3 ng/ml during the first 3 weeks of treatment. The preferred route of treatment is injection because intravaginal implants or pessaries are not retained well after mounting activity begins. Ear implants containing testosterone are not effective since they do not sufficiently elevate blood testosterone levels.

In our initial studies we administered testosterone propionate in oil (IM) to mature Angus-Holstein cows at the rate of 200 mg on alternate days for 3 weeks. This dose was approximately 0.4 mg/kg at each injection. In subsequent studies we have observed that larger doses can be given at less frequent intervals without altering the end result. For example, 500 to 600 mg of testosterone propionate in oil (IM) once weekly for 3 weeks has been effective, as has a single treatment with 2 gm of testosterone enanthate in oil given in three or four injection sites. The choice of products used should be based on their release rate and carrier. Testosterone derivatives are released slower than crystalline testosterone when administered in an oil base. The release rate after an IM injection is more rapid than after a subcutaneous dosage. Products administered in alcohol carriers (depot products) crystallize after injection, and the injected product is delivered as if from an implant.

Basically, the dosage can be evaluated for its effectiveness by observing behavior in treated animals. Within 10 days after initiation of treatments, animals receiving an effective dose should show increased sexual activity, such as attempts to mount other animals, as well as some signs of heat, including clear mucous discharge from the vulva. If these signs do not appear by 2 weeks, the treatment dose is probably not sufficiently large to be effective.

Once increased mounting activity has been elicited in the detector cow or heifer by an induction regimen, this activity can be maintained with less frequent treatments of long-lasting androgens. We have utilized testosterone enanthante (SC) in oil at the rate of 500 mg (1 mg/kg) every 2 weeks to maintain increased mounting behavior.[2]

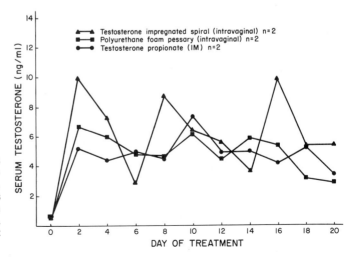

Figure 1. Serum testosterone levels after administration of testosterone impregnated intravaginal Silastic spirals, testosterone impregnated foam pessaries or testosterone propionate (200 mg, IM on alternate days). (From Kiser, T. E., Britt, J. H. and Ritchie, H. D.: J. Anim. Sci., *44*: 1030, 1977.)

TABLE 1. *Percentage of Cows Detected in Estrus and Conception Rates for Cows Observed by Three Estrous Detection Procedures*

Method of Estrous Detection	Total No. Cows	Inseminated Cows		Conception Rate (%)
		NO.	%	
Herdsman	31	21	67	62
Surgically altered bull	30	21	70	62
Testosterone-treated cow	29	24	84	67

Similar doses of other long-lasting testosterone derivatives should be equally effective in maintaining the desired behavior in treated animals. Since minimum effective doses required to maintain mounting behavior have not been determined, the dose should be based primarily on the behavior response of the treated animal and should be given only "to effect."

MANAGING THE DETECTOR ANIMAL

The correct ratio of detector animals to breeding females depends on several factors, including the duration of daily exposure periods, animal density, percentage of herd pregnant and amount of "rest period" given to detector animals. In one study,[2] we continually exposed each testosterone-treated cow (Angus-Holstein crossbred fitted with a halter-mounted marking device) to 29 females of breeding age during an artificial insemination (AI) period of 54 days. Similar sized groups of breeding-age cows either were exposed to a surgically altered bull (vasectomy and penile fixation) or were observed 1 hour twice daily by herdsmen (Table 1). Eighty-four per cent of the cows

TABLE 2. *Detection Method for Cows Detected in Estrus during a 33-Day AI Period**

Method	No. Cows Detected	Percentage of Total
Standing only	57	27.6
Marked only	41	19.8
Standing and marked	93	44.9
Other	16	7.7
Total	207	100.0

*Ratio of detector cows to breeding-age females = 1:60.

exposed to the testosterone-treated cow were inseminated during the AI period, compared with 70 per cent and 67 per cent for those exposed to a bull or observed by a herdsman, respectively. Conception rates did not differ among the three groups. It was noted that all cows marked by the testosterone-treated cow or surgically altered bull were also observed in standing heat by the herdsman — probably because the detector animal directed the herdsman's attention to those cows in heat.

In another study,[2] the ratio of testosterone-treated detector animals to breeding-age females was 1:60 during a 33-day AI period. Under these circumstances, not all cows in heat were marked by the detector animals fitted with halter-mounted marking devices (Table 2). Overall, 44.9 per cent of the cows detected in heat were both marked and observed in standing heat, whereas 27.6 per cent were observed standing only and 19.8 per cent were observed with marks only. The remaining 7.7 per cent were detected in heat by other signs, including mucous discharge from the vulva, ruffled hair on the rump and mud streaks on the flank. Nevertheless, we concluded that the testosterone-treated cows were effective aids in estrous detection since 20 per cent of the cows bred during the AI period were detected solely on the basis of ink marks applied by the detector animals.

The accuracy of estrous detection by testosterone-treated detector animals was determined by exposing two treated cows to a herd of crossbred beef cattle composed of 26 pregnant and 62 nonpregnant females. During a 20-day period, 74 per cent of the nonpregnant females were marked by the detector cows, whereas not one of the pregnant animals was marked (Table 3). Blood samples collected from 18 of the animals marked were assayed for serum progesterone concentration in order to verify that the cows were in estrus at the time they

Reproductive Status	Total No. Cows	Marked Cows	
		NO.	%
Nonpregnant	62	46	74
Pregnant	26	0	0

were marked. Results from the progesterone determinations indicated that all animals were marked during estrus.

REGULATIONS AFFECTING USE OF TESTOSTERONE IN COWS

The United States Food and Drug Administration has not specifically approved the use of testosterone or testosterone derivatives for the purpose of inducing mounting behavior in cows for detection of estrus. Regulations governing the use of testosterone or testosterone derivatives in cattle should be observed.

RECOMMENDATIONS OR GUIDELINES

1. Choose physically sound, nonlactating animals for treatment. Heifers should have reached sexual maturity before treatment.

2. Treatment dosages should be based partially on behavioral response of treated animals. Higher doses given initially should increase male-like behavior in animals, and lower dosages should be used to maintain this behavior.

3. If the detector-animal-to-breeding-animal ratio is high (for example, 1:50), rotation of detector animals may provide the best performance. A detector animal could be rested for 1 week and then rotated with another detector animal on alternate weeks.

4. Detector animals should not be penned with bulls, either alone or with the breeding group.

5. Halter-mounted marking devices should be checked frequently for an adequate supply of ink. Ink usage increases during periods of increased estrous activity and during periods when the ambient temperature increases.

REFERENCES

1. Kiser, T. E., Britt, J. H. and Ritchie, H. D.: Testosterone induction of mounting behavior in cows for use in estrous detection. Research Report 288, Report of Beef Cattle–Forage Research 1975, Michigan Agricultural Experiment Station, East Lansing, Mich., 1975, pp. 19–30.
2. Kiser, T. E., Britt, J. H. and Ritchie, H. D.: Testosterone treatment of cows for use in detection of estrus. J. Anim. Sci., *44*:1030, 1977.
3. Kiser, T. E., Britt, J. H., Welch, R. A. and Ritchie, H. D.: Estrous detection with testosterone treated cows. J. Anim. Sci. (abstract), *41*:362, 1975.
4. Signoret, J. P.: Effet de la nature de l'hormone-oestrogene ou audrogene-et du rythne d'injections sur l'apparition d'elements de comportment sexuel male ou femelle chex la brebis ovariectomisee. Proc. VIIth Intern. Cong. Anim. Reprod. & A. I. *1*:401, 1972.
5. Signoret, J. P.: Nouvelle methode de detection de l'estrus chez les bovins. Annal. Zootech., *24*:125, 1975.

Altering Estrous Cycles in Cows by Intrauterine Infusion

BRAD SEGUIN

University of Minnesota, St. Paul, Minnesota

MECHANISM OF ACTION

Intrauterine (IU) infusion has been used for several decades in attempts to stimulate estrous activity in cows as well as mares. In the past 10 to 20 years much has been learned about the physiological relationship between the uterus and ovaries in cattle. The uterus controls the duration of corpus luteum (CL) function by producing a luteolytic factor (possibly prostaglandin-$F_{2\alpha}$) near the end of diestrus. With demise of the CL the sequential events of proestrus occur, leading to another estrus and ovulation. With greater knowledge of this utero-ovarian relationship has come a greater understanding of how IU infusion in cows is able to result in altered estrous cycles. When true anestrus with ovarian atrophy exists, IU infusion is not likely to initiate estrous activity. Estrus will follow IU infusion of certain preparations, however, in cases of unobserved estrus. Several investigations have shown that estrus will occur 6 to 10 days after IU infusion (especially when irritating substances are used) if a CL is present at the time of infusion. The likely mechanism of action is that endometrial irritation caused by the infused preparation stimulates production and release of the uterine luteolytic factor to cause CL regression and, thus, the onset of estrus.

An irritation mechanism for this response, as opposed to a distention mechanism, is indicated in the cow by several investigations. Very small volumes (<1.0 ml) of irritating substances such as alcohol and iodine solutions are capable of altering estrous cycles when infused IU. In contrast, large volumes of nonirritating preparations such as physiological saline (250 ml) infused IU do not cause altered cycles. Also, insemination of cows with semen (approximately 1.0 ml) containing excessive debris and pathogenic bacteria can cause alteration of estrous cycles by inducing endometritis. Estrous cycles in mares can be altered by IU infusion of saline, uterine biopsy or perhaps merely by cervical manipulation. A difference in uterine sensitivity to stimulation between the bovine and equine species may therefore exist.

In cattle, IU infusion of a dilute iodine solution (DIS, 5 ml of Lugol's solution in 250 ml of physiological saline) on day 4 of the estrous cycle (estrus = day 0) results in a shortened cycle of 10 to 11 days (Table 1). The same treatment on day 15 of the cycle results in a slight extension of the cycle to about 25 days. Normal cycle lengths occur, however, if infusion of DIS occurs at estrus or on day 10 to 11. Serum progesterone profiles in these treatment groups (Fig. 1) indicate that these cycle alterations are true indications of ovarian (CL) function following the treatments. Endometrial biopsies indicate that infusion of DIS at all stages of the cycle causes necrosis of the endometrium. The responses following infusion on day 4, 10 or 15 may appear somewhat confusing, i.e., shortened, unaltered and lengthened cycles after infusion on day 4, 10 and 15, respectively. However, the interval from infusion to estrus in each case is fairly uniform, 7 to 10 days.

TABLE 1. *Effect of Dilute Iodine Solution (DIS)* Infusion on Length of Estrous Cycle in Cows*

Treatment	No.	Cycle Length		Interval from DIS to Estrus
		INFUSION	SUBSEQUENT	
DIS-estrus	5	22.4	20.6	22.4
DIS-day 4	8	10.6†	22.4	6.6
DIS-day 15	9	25.1†	22.9	10.1
Control	9	21.3	21.6	–

*DIS was 5 ml of Lugol's solution in 250 ml of physiological saline.
†Significantly (p < 0.05) different than controls.

Subsequent research in Sweden indicates that endometrial irritation causes alteration in prostaglandin-$F_{2\alpha}$ patterns during the estrous cycle. After infusion of DIS of day 4, prostaglandin appears to be released about day 6 to 7, or approximately 10 days earlier than usual. Infusion of DIS on day 15 results in a delayed release of prostaglandin.

Preparations that are known to cause endometrial irritation and the previously described alterations in estrous cycles include iodine preparations such as the DIS just referred to and antibiotic preparations in alcohol or propylene glycol bases, such as oxytetracycline in propylene glycol preparations (Liquamycin Injectable). IU infusion of a 0.2 per cent nitrofurazone preparation on day 3 of the cycle in seven cows resulted in cycles of 7, 11, 12, 16, 17, 21 and 21 days duration. Cycle length may have been more consistently reduced if this preparation had been infused on day 4 or 5. Infusion of this preparation on day 1 or 2 of the cycle did not affect cycle length. Pro-

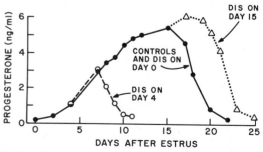

Figure 1. Serum progesterone concentrations in cows given intrauterine infusion of dilute iodine solution (DIS) on days 0, 4 or 15 of the estrous cycle.

ducts that have been tested on day 4 and found not to cause cycle alteration include physiological saline solution, a nitrofurazone-estradiol in peanut oil preparation (Utonex) and aqueous penicillin (procaine penicillin G, UPS in aqueous solution).

CLINICAL APPLICATION OF ESTROUS CYCLE ALTERATION BY INFUSION

Japanese investigators studied the possibility of using IU infusion of an iodine solution for synchronizing estrus in cows with breeding difficulties, such as unobserved estrus. Of 282 cows treated during the luteal phase of the cycle, 198 (70 per cent) were observed in estrus 6 to 11 days after treatment. Cows observed in estrus were inseminated, and 52 per cent conceived on first service. Thus, it appears that the endometrium was able to recover from the iodine irritation in time to allow fertilization and embryo development.

Induction of luteolysis is an effective method of causing early termination of an unwanted pregnancy, for example, in cases of mismating. IU infusion of DIS or some other irritating substance on or after day 4 following breeding will stimulate luteolysis followed by estrus, thus disrupting a possible pregnancy.

IU infusion of irritating substances such as iodine solutions might also have application in treating the relatively rare persistent CL condition in cattle. In cows, persistent CLs probably occur only when some form of uterine pathology inhibits the uterine luteolytic factor, for example, in cases of pyometra. Since these applications (synchronization of estrus, early disruption of a possible pregnancy and pyometra therapy) utilize uterine irritation to induce the uterine luteolytic factor, administration of prostaglandin-$F_{2\alpha}$ or its analogs (potent luteolysins) would provide a more direct and probably more consistent method of inducing CL regression. Presently, prostaglandin-$F_{2\alpha}$ and its analogs are not commercially available in the United States for use in cattle. These prostaglandin products are available for use in cattle in some other countries, however.

Another potential application of these irritating preparations might be as a method for inducing a chemical endometrial curettage in cases of chronic endometritis. Controlled evaluation of such procedures are not available, however. Infusion of iodine solutions has been used by veterinarians for treating cases of metritis in cattle for years, even preceding the use of antibiotics for this purpose. Few controlled comparative evaluations of the efficacy of iodine solutions for this purpose are available.

The postbreeding infusion is another situation in which irritation induced by IU infusion might be of concern. Since such infusions usually occur within 24 to 36 hours of estrus, which is during the period before the CL has developed, stimulation of the luteolytic factor appears to be a minor consideration. The irritation itself may however affect the uterine environment for the developing embryo. Endometrial epithelium is capable of rapid regeneration, which may allow normal embryonic development and implantation. Evaluation of the effects on fertility of irritating preparations used as postbreeding infusions is an area that requires further investigation.

SUMMARY

Estrous cycles and CL function in cows can be altered by IU infusion of irritating substances. The likely mechanism of action is that endometrial irritation induced by the infused preparation stimulates the uterine luteolytic factor to cause CL regression and thus the onset of estrus. IU infusion of irritating substances may have application when luteolysis is desired, i.e., for synchronizing estrus in cases of unobserved estrus, for disrupting an unwanted pregnancy and for treating cows with pyometra. Implications of endometrial irritation in cases of chronic endometritis or following postbreeding infusion are mainly unknown. Compounds that cause endometrial irritation when infused IU in cows (such as iodine or alcohol-based solutions) are likely to result in alteration of estrous cycles and CL function. Estrus is likely to occur 6 to 10 days after infusion of such products if a CL is present at the time of infusion. Nonirritating aqueous or oil-based preparations are not likely to cause estrous cycle alteration when infused IU in cows.

REFERENCES

1. Ginther, O. J.: Utero-ovarian relationships in cattle: Physiologic aspects. J.A.V.M.A., *153*:1656, 1968.
2. Ginther, O. J.: Utero-ovarian relationships in cattle: Applied veterinary aspects. J.A.V.M.A., *153*:1665, 1968.
3. Ginther, O. J. and Meckley, P. E.: Effect of intrauterine infusion on length of diestrus in cows and mares. Vet. Med./Sm. Anim. Clin., *67*:751, 1972.
4. Nakahara, T., Domeki, I. and Yamauchi, M.: Synchronization of estrous cycles in cows by intrauterine injection with iodine solution. Nat. Inst. Anim. Hlth. Quart., *11*:219, 1971.
5. Seguin, B. E., Morrow, D. A. and Louis, T. M.: Luteolysis, luteostasis and the effect of prostaglandin $F_{2\alpha}$ in cows after endometrial irritation. Am. J. Vet. Res., *35*:57, 1974.

Etiology of Retained Bovine Placenta

EBERHARD GRUNERT

Clinic of Obstetrics and Gynecology of Cattle, Hanover, Germany

DEFINITION

In cattle the fetal membranes are expelled physiologically within a period of 12 hours after delivery of the fetus. Retention of the entire afterbirth or of parts of the fetal membranes for longer periods must be considered to be pathological. Partial retention is observed particularly on the placentomes in the ovarian end (apical section) of the pregnant horn. It is, however, not always possible to establish a sharp time limit between the end of the physiological and the beginning of the pathological state in every case of retained bovine afterbirth. In most cases placental retention should be considered as a clinical symptom of a more generalized disease, e.g., infections, metabolic diseases, nutritional deficiencies, allergies or other disorders and seldom as a disease of its own. Therefore, in determining the etiology of retained placenta, one should think of both direct and indirect causes.

OCCURRENCE AND INCIDENCE

Retention of the fetal membranes is observed more frequently in the bovine than in other species. Dairy cattle are affected more commonly than are beef cattle. In brucella-free areas, the frequency of retained placenta after apparently normal parturition is reported to be between 3 and 12 per cent, with an average of 7 per cent. The incidence of retained afterbirth in cattle following abnormal deliveries (i.e., twin parturition, cesarean section, fetotomy, other serious dystocias, abortion and premature calving) and in herds infected with brucellosis is high, ranging between 30 and 50 per cent or even more. The same is true for other infections that may cause abortion or premature parturition, e.g., *Campylobacter fetus*, *Listeria* and IBR/IPV. An enzootic outbreak of retained placenta in herds that are free of the common enzootic infections causing abortion is observed when calf diarrhea or acute mastitis, or both, are common and when management problems or nutritional deficiencies, or both, can be found. Cows that have had a previous retained afterbirth have an increased chance of the placenta being retained after subsequent calvings.

ETIOLOGY

In the majority of cases, placental retention in cattle is caused by a disturbance of the loosening mechanism in the placentomes. Some of the processes that lead to retained placenta should have taken place in the placentomes days or weeks or even months before parturition or premature delivery, e.g., in instances of metabolic and deficiency diseases.

The Loosening Process in Placentomes

An undisturbed loosening mechanism is essential for timely, spontaneous expulsion of the afterbirth. This mechanism is already apparent during the last months of pregnancy when preparatory changes take place in the placental epithelium and connective tissues. The maternal and fetal connective tissues in the placentomes become progressively collagenized up to the time of parturition. The maternal epithelial lining of the crypts nearest the caruncular stalk is flattened. In addition, many binuclear giant cells appear, whose resorptive and phagocytic activities are manifested by the development of polynuclear giant cells shortly before the detachment process. With the onset of parturition and following hormonally induced imbibition, the tissues of the placentomes become loose — a process that appears to be essential for the undisturbed expulsion of the fetal membranes.

During the stage of dilation and particularly during the contractions of the uterus, there is a constantly changing uterine pressure that leads to alternating anemic and hyperemic conditions and temporary changes in the surface area of the fetal chorionic villi. As a result, the attachment of the chorionic epithelium in the maternal crypts becomes impaired. During the expulsion period, the first signs of the mechanical processes of detachment become evident in the vicinity of the caruncular stalk. These processes are probably facilitated by the fact that the caruncles are pressed against the fetus following uterine contractions. A placentome that is not pathologically altered will therefore expand peripherally as a result of this flattening. This change in shape is apparently possible only if the hormonally induced relaxation of the maternal connective tissue allows the sideward expansion of the caruncular stalk, which was more compact before parturition (Fig. 1). An essential factor after expulsion of the fetus and rupture of the umbilical cord is the anemia of the fetal villi, which results from lack of blood circulation into the fetal capillaries. By shrinking of the blood vessels, the surface area of the chorionic epithelium also becomes greatly reduced. The postpartum uterine contractions complete the process of detachment of the membranes. The reduction in size of the uterus leads to a decrease in size of the caruncle stalk (Fig. 2). These purely mechanical processes of detachment of the fetal membranes should not be underestimated.

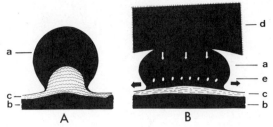

Figure 1. Change in shape of a caruncle. (*A*) Before parturition and (*B*) during the expulsion period: (*a*) area of villi and crypts, (*b*) myometrium, (*c*) connective tissue of the caruncular stalk in connection with the subepithelial connective tissue of the uterine wall, (*d*) fetal membranes and fetus and (*e*) loosening processes in the area of the stalk. (Schematic drawing after Schulz, L. Cl. and Merkt, H.: Vet. Med., *11*:712, 1956.)

Disturbance of the Loosening Process in Placentomes

A disturbance of the detachment mechanism in the placentome can be infectious or noninfectious, direct or indirect. Among the direct causes of retained placenta are:

Immature Placentomes. This important cause of retention of fetal membranes occurs mostly in noninfectious abortions or premature parturition, i.e., in instances of a shortened gestation period. The average duration of pregnancy could depend on the breed and might be influenced by specific bulls. The frequency of placental retention is dependent upon the duration of pregnancy up to the time of expulsion of the fetus (Fig. 3). The incidence has been found to be nearly 15 per cent in cows that abort

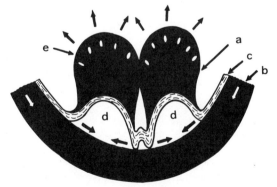

Figure 2. Change in shape of a caruncle during the postpartum uterine contractions: (*a*) area of villi and crypts, (*b*) myometrium (in stage of intensive contractions), (*c*) connective tissue (see Figure 1), (*d*) formation of cavities during uterine contractions and (*e*) loosening processes in the periphery of the caruncle. (Schematic drawing after Schulz, L. Cl. and Merkt, H. Vet. Med., *11*:712, 1956.)

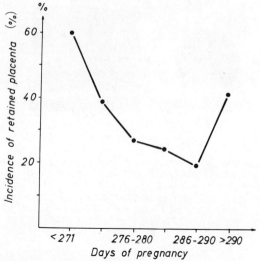

Figure 3. Relationship between the duration of pregnancy and the occurrence of retained placenta in German black pied cattle.

between day 121 and day 150 of pregnancy, whereas it rises to 50 per cent or more in those animals that abort between day 240 and day 265 of the gestation period. The afterbirth falls away normally as long as abortion occurs before day 120 of gestation.

Changes that are normally induced by estrogens, such as the imbibition of the maternal connective tissue and swelling of the connective tissue fibers, as well as the

absorption of water by the cells, are found to be absent in immature placentomes removed immediately after parturition and examined histologically. The histological study reveals deficient hormonal preparation of the maternal placental connective tissue. The collagen fibers of the caruncles are wavey and clearly contoured, particularly in the caruncular stalk. They become swollen, acquire indistinct contours and become nearly linear after hormonal sensitization. These caruncles, which are not prepared for detachment, do not seem to permit mechanical loosening in the area of the stalk during the expulsion period. Maturity occurs approximately 2 to 5 days before the end of breed-dependent average gestation length. Therefore, the earlier that premature parturition occurs, the higher the percentage of retained placenta. The transformation of placental connective tissue is thought to be an important prerequisite for uncomplicated delivery of fetal membranes. In addition, the nearly complete disappearance of the maternal crypt epithelium is decisive for the correct timing of the expulsion of the placenta (Figs. 4, 5, 6). The number of epithelial cells in cases of retained placenta after premature parturition corresponds approximately to the number of epithelial cells during the eighth month of gestation (Fig. 7).

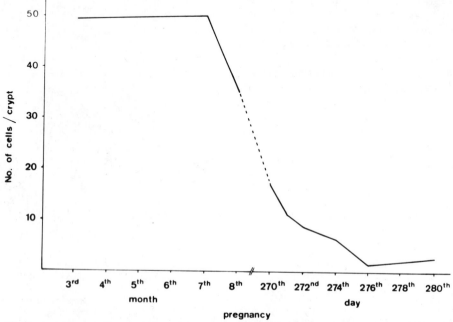

Figure 4. Number of epithelial cells per crypt of the maternal placenta during pregnancy.

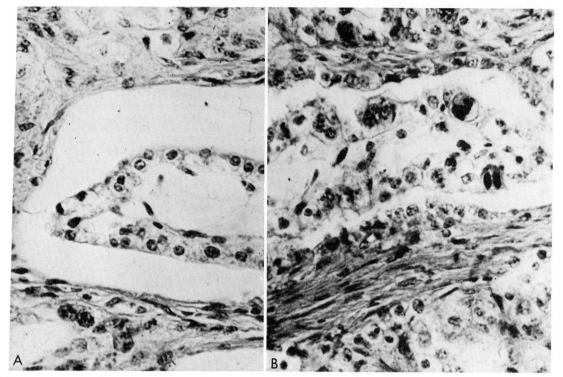

Figure 5. Parts of placentomes near caruncular stalk. *(A)* Mature placentome (disappearance of the maternal crypt epithelium), and *(B)* immature placentome (complete epithelial layer in the maternal crypt).

Edema of the Chorionic Villi. Often one finds severe, noninflammatory edema of the fetal cotyledons. This can be seen in placentomes recovered shortly after calving, especially in cows following cesarean section or in animals that have had a longstanding uterine torsion. In these cases the edema extends to the ends of the chorionic villi, and the fetal membranes therefore remain firmly attached to the surface of these placentomes.

Necrotic Areas between the Chorionic Villi and the Cryptal Walls. The presence of small areas of necrotic epithelium between the chorionic villi and the cryptal walls is observed in animals with retained placenta. These alterations presumably occur antepartum and are often the main symptom of a more generalized disease. The observation of blood extravasations preceding the necrosis in a firmly attached placenta indicates the presence of a weak hemorrhagic diathesis. Thus, necrosis might be an effect of an allergic reaction.

Advanced Involution of the Placentomes. An additional cause of retained fetal membranes is an already advanced involution of the placentomes. In these cases placentomes recovered shortly after delivery show proliferative processes in the

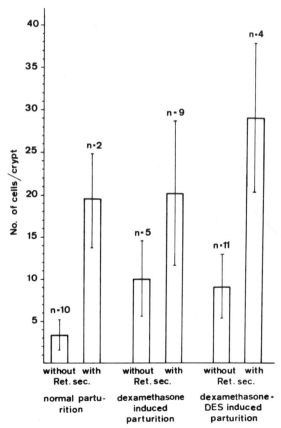

Figure 6. Number of epithelial cells per crypt of the maternal placenta after spontaneous and dexamethasone-induced parturition.

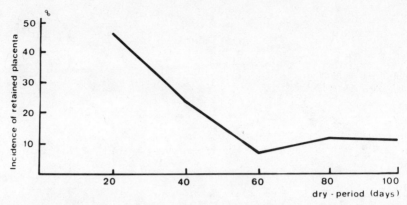

Figure 7. Relationship between the duration of the dry period and the occurrence of retained placenta in cattle. (According to Kudlac, E.: Tierzüchter, 25:15, 1973.)

maternal connective tissue when examined histologically. Because the maternal septal tissue becomes thicker, fetal villi can be trapped within it, thus complicating the process of detachment.

Hyperemia of the Placentomes. Hyperemia of the placentomes is seldom considered to be the cause of placental retention. This could occur before parturition or perhaps could even be caused by the too rapid closure of the umbilical blood vessels. The surface area of the fetal capillaries increases as a result of their congestion with blood. The villi may therefore remain incarcerated in the crypts.

Placentitis and Cotyledonitis. In placentitis and cotyledonitis the degree of the inflammatory reaction may vary from slight alterations to severe necrosis. The lesions may be localized in the cervical or apical part of the pregnant horn or may be diffuse. The nongravid horn is not always involved, and the degree of placentitis in this horn is usually not as severe as in the gravid horn. Affected cotyledons or portions of them are necrotic and of a yellow-gray color. In mold infections the placentomes are greatly enlarged and necrotic, have swollen margins and are firmly incarcerated. The inflammation may involve only the villi, small, localized portions of the cotyledon or all of the placentome. The edematous placental stroma contains increased numbers of leukocytes.

Germs are transmitted to the placenta during gestation from primary foci that may be localized in various parts of the body of an infected animal. For example, pyogenic bacteria such as *Corynebacterium pyogenes*, coliform bacteria, cocci and other organisms come from diseased udders or infected claws or from wounds or peritonitis. Infections of the placenta may also originate from disorders of the gastrointestinal tract, such as diarrhea caused by bacteria, molds and other organisms, particularly when spoiled food is fed or the diet has been changed suddenly. If the placentitis develops before parturition, the fetal membranes are edematous, necrotic or leathery and sometimes hemorrhagic.

Uterine Atony Associated with Normal Detachment of the Fetal Membranes

Uterine atony without any form of disturbance of the detachment process is considered to be the cause of 1 to 2 per cent of all cases of retained placenta. The fetal membranes are either already detached and cannot be expelled because of the absence of uterine contractions, or the mechanical process of detachment is hindered by the insufficiency of the uterine contractions and muscle tone. In this case it is possible to remove the cotyledons from the caruncles without causing any harm by pulling slightly on the fetal membranes.

Mechanical Prevention of Placental Expulsion

This occurs in very isolated instances, at most constituting 0.5 per cent of all cases of placental retention. The fully or nearly detached cotyledon becomes trapped in a

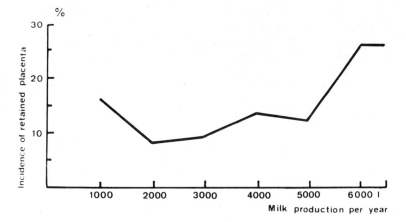

Figure 8. Relationship between milk yield and the occurrence of retained placenta in cattle. (According to Kudlac, E.: Tierzüchter, *25*:15, 1973.)

rapidly closing passage of the nonpregnant or invaginated uterine horn, or in a double cervical canal or behind a fleshy band in the vagina. Such complications are usually caused by very large cotyledons. Occasionally the retention occurs because membranous parts of the placenta wrap around the caruncles. Very seldom retention may also occur after cesarean section, when parts of the membranes become sutured within the hysterorrhaphy wound.

Indirect Causes of Retained Placenta

The indirect causes of retained placenta that can lead to the changes just described in the placentomes are illustrated in Figure 8 and are summarized in Table 1.

THERAPY OF RETAINED PLACENTA

On day 1 postpartum one can start a 5-minute trial to loosen the placenta manually. Regardless of the outcome, 40 gm of a sulfonamide or 2 to 4 gm or 2 to 4 million IU of an antibiotic is deposited in the uterus. This treatment should be repeated on days 3, 6 and 9 postpartum (pp) when necessary, in addition to manual trials of loosening the afterbirth.

On day 10 to 12, the retained placenta can be withdrawn in most cases, following which an antibiotic should be instilled into the uterus.

Iodine or antibiotic treatment is recommended, when necessary, 6 weeks pp.

If prednisolone is injected (day 1 pp — 100 mg; days 3 and 5 — 50 mg; day 7 — 25 mg) in addition to local antibiotic treatment, putrescence, caruncular necrosis and

TABLE 1. *Indirect Causes of Retained Placenta in Cattle*

A. *Intensive stress (especially in older animals) and nutritional factors.* Management problems, short dry period in dairy cattle (less than 5 weeks), transport stress, change of locality in advanced pregnancy, high milk production, deficiency of vitamins and minerals (carotene, vitamin A, iodine selenium and vitamin E), imbalances in calcium and phosphorus metabolism effects of imbalanced feeding.

B. *Duration of pregnancy and its influencing factors.* Shortened gestation period (parturition occurs more than 5 days before the end of breed-dependent average gestation length) caused by stress from vaccination or other manipulations, panic and so forth or by hormonal induction of premature birth; infections that may cause abortion or premature parturition (particularly brucellosis); toxic causes (some chemicals and drugs, e.g., heavy metals, chlorinated naphthalenes); allergies and anaphylactic reactions (warble fly allergy, *Brucella* antigens); urticaria from different sources (e.g., green or rotten potatoes); hormonal disturbances (estrogen or progesterone deficiency); prolonged gestation (exceeding 290 to 295 days) caused by aplasia or severe hypoplasia of the adrenal gland or of the pituitary gland; vitamin A deficiency; hereditary factors.

C. *Miscellaneous causes.* Excessive distention of the uterus (multiple births, hydrallantois and hydramnios, fetal giants and fetal double monsters); trauma of the uterus with secondary infection during dystocia; uterine inertia (hereditary, nutritional, circulatory, hormonal); hereditary factors (higher incidence of retained placenta in daughters of dams that have shown retained placenta); sex of fetus (higher incidence following birth of male calves); rate of daylight change; seasonal influences; stillbirth; cesarean section.

accumulation of lochia in the uterus can be diminished or excluded.

On day 7 to 8 diethylstilbestrol (50 mg) can be injected to widen the cervical canal, which will make the removal of the afterbirth on or about day 10 much easier.

PROPHYLAXIS

Prophylaxis includes versatile, biological-rich, limited nutrition for pregnant animals; sufficiently large animal boxes; daily outlet (also during wintertime); avoidance of transport; sufficiently extended dry period (6 to 8 weeks); avoidance of bacterial infections and parturition hygiene. In addition, one injection of 2 million IU of vitamin A should be given intramuscularly 4 to 8 weeks antepartum.

REFERENCES

1. Cohen, P.: Een statistisch onderzoek omtrent Retentio Secundinarum en enige andere, met de voortplanting samenhangende, processen bij het rund. Thesis. Utrecht, 1956.
2. Jubb, K. V. F. and Kennedy, P. C.: Pathology of Domestic Animals. New York and London, Academic Press, 1970.
3. Julien, W. E., Conrad, H. R., Jones, J. E. and Moxon, A. L.: Selenium and vitamin E and incidence of retained placenta in parturient dairy cows. J. Dairy Sci., *59*:1954, 1976.
4. Kudlac, E.: Ursachen, Vorbeuge und Behandlung der Nachgeburtsverhaltung beim Rind. Tierzüchter, *25*:15, 1973.
5. Roberts, S. J.: Veterinary Obstetrics and Genital Diseases. 2nd Ed. Ann Arbor, Mich., Edwards Brothers, Inc., 1971.
6. Schulz, L. Cl. and Merkt H.: Morphologische Befunde an extirpierten Plazentomen, zugleich ein Beitrag zur Ätiologie der Retentio secundinarum beim Rind. Vet. Med., *11*:712, 1956.

Therapy for Retained Placenta

ALLEN G. SQUIRE

Chino Valley Veterinary Group, Ontario, California

Treatment for the retention of the fetal membranes, as much as any other condition in food animal practice, causes the veterinarian to become an educator and public relations expert in addition to his primary duty as a practitioner. Methods of treatment now practiced include most that have ever been described, and all have some merit, depending on the veterinarian and the client involved. The basic goals of any therapeutic regimen should be the return of the cow to reproductive usefulness as soon as possible and the prevention of secondary complications that can lead to economic losses from lowered milk production and delayed conception.

MANUAL REMOVAL

Although practiced by many veterinarians upon client demand, manual removal, the venerated tradition of "cleaning" by physically separating the caruncle and fetal cotyledon, is slowly beginning to fall by the wayside with the advent of new research, more enlightened practitioners, and the education of dairymen. The basic technique is graphically described by Roberts[2] and will not be covered here except to mention that an increase in complications is associated with this practice. Metritis, septicemia, toxemia, uterine abscesses, perimetritis and other attendant complications such as delayed involution and conception have been described by several workers as occurring in a greater percentage of cows from which the placenta has been manually removed than in cows from which the placenta is allowed to separate naturally.

In the opinion of this author and of many others, the only time that manual removal should be practiced is when the attending veterinarian fortuitously finds the entire placenta free and only hindered in its expulsion by a partially closed cervix. In this case the placenta can be gently "teased" through the cervix, with care being taken not to traumatize the cervix or vagina during the procedure. Roberts states that the veterinarian should ". . . have the courage of his convictions in these cases" and only attempt removal in cases in which the placenta has a few loose attachments.[2]

CONSERVATIVE TREATMENT

Two major obstacles to conservative treatment are client acceptance and a lack of a unified opinion about the most advantageous therapeutic regimen. The problem of client acceptance of new, less radical methods of treatment can best be handled by client education concerning the disadvantages of manual removal of the placenta. The obstacle of lack of a unified opinion regarding treatment, though seemingly insignificant, has been magnified by endless clinical reports and testimonials concerning the efficacy of an ever-growing list of hormones and antimicrobial agents.

Hormones, especially oxytoxic drugs and estrogens, have often been included in retained placenta therapy, either solely or in conjunction with antimicrobial agents. When associated with uterine atony due to hypocalcemia, placental retention has been shown to respond to oxytocin, often given in conjunction with therapeutic doses of calcium borogluconate. The uterine tone is increased, and expulsion of the fetal membranes is thus facilitated. Oxytocin used for this purpose is administered at a rate of 30 to 50 units subcutaneously or intramuscularly at intervals of 2 hours for as many as four repeated doses. Oxytocin is of little benefit after 24 to 48 hours postpartum. Ergonovine at a dosage of 1 to 5 mg, has been used for a more lasting oxytocic effect and appears to be much more beneficial than oxytocin in cases of diseased or atonic myometrial tissue. Estrogens are a logical choice for use because of their ability to increase uterine tone, myometrial activity and uterine circulation, thereby making the uterus more resistant to infection. Estradiol in doses of 1 to 4 mg has been used as often as three to four times with no untoward effects; however, excessive doses could cause reduced subsequent fertility.

An extensive list of antiseptics and antibiotics has been used in the therapy of placental retention, both by intrauterine and parenteral routes. Both routes have local and systemic effects, making it necessary to observe milk withdrawal times for antibiotic residues. Among the most prominent drugs used have been sulfonamides, iodines, penicillin and tetracyclines. Several sulfonamides have been used both systemically and locally, and in Hammermann's study[1] these preparations were shown to result in higher subsequent fertility than manual removal in conjunction with various intrauterine treatments. Lugol's iodine, given as 500 ml of a 2 to 4 per cent solution for intrauterine infusion every 2 to 3 days until the placenta drops, has been shown to be an effective antimicrobial agent. Among the most conservative methods of treatment described is the use of penicillin parenterally; however, local effect is questionable because of the penicillinase production of the uterine organisms.

Recently, use of the broad-spectrum tetracycline family of antibiotics has been shown to decrease the incidence of metritis and also to allow subsequent fertility of treated cows with retained placentae to approximate that of herdmates not having placental retention. In agreement with previous studies by Beattie and Leaming, Gould *et al.*, Easterbrooks and Plastridge and Banerjee, it was demonstrated that cows with placental retention at 24 hours postpartum treated every other day by placing gelatin capsules containing 2 to 3 gm of tetracycline hydrochloride in the uterus had a fertility rate equal to that of their herdmates not having a placental retention. An equal group of cows having no treatment had a lowered fertility rate, as measured by services per conception, open interval and percentage of first service conception.

STUDY OF EFFECTS OF THERAPY ON FERTILITY

In a recent study by Squire[3] of five California dairies, 179 cows with placental retention from among 1663 calvings (11 per cent incidence) were randomly placed into three treatment groups: a tetracycline bolus group; a group that received a vaginal examination only, with no attempt at removal of the fetal membranes, and a control group (Table 1). Only data from the 129 cows that conceived were included in the calculations of services per conception and open intervals. The group receiving intrauterine boluses every other day until one treatment after the placenta was expelled (49 cows) averaged 1.8 services per conception and 46 per cent first service conception rate, with an average of 93 days open. The vaginal examination group (40 cows) averaged 2.3 services per conception, 33 per cent first service conceptions and a 113-day open in-

TABLE 1. *Effects of Placental Retention and Therapy on Fertility in California Dairy Cows*

Group	Number	Services per Conception*	First Service Conception Rate (%)	Open Interval (days)
Tetracycline†	49	1.8	46	93
Vaginal examination	40	2.3	33	113
Controls	40	2.2	39	111
Herdmates‡	1396	1.9	50	100

*Only data from cows conceiving were included in days open and services per conception calculations.
†2.5 gm in gelatin capsules every other day until one treatment after placenta was expelled.
‡Cows calving at the same time as those with retained fetal membranes.

terval. The control group (40 cows) averaged 2.2 services per conception, 39 per cent first services and a 111-day open interval. This is in comparison to an average of 1.9 services per conception, 50 per cent first service conception rate and 100-day average open interval of the 1396 herdmates that conceived.

Although 50 of the 179 cows studied were not confirmed pregnant, 35 of these cows were culled for reasons other than fertility. The 15 cows not conceiving represent an infertility rate similar to that of the herdmates (8 per cent of the cows in the study versus 6 per cent of the 1484 herdmates). The overall cull rate of the cows in the study (infertility plus all other reasons) was 27 per cent (50 of 179 cows), which is quite consistent with Southern California dairy cull rates and managerial practices.

In summary, this study appears to indicate that the combination of intrauterine boluses and close observation as a routine postpartum treatment for placental retention can result in ensuing fertility rates approximating those of herdmates not retaining fetal membranes. More research is needed to compare the efficacy data of the other substances that are currently commonly used for treatment.

ADMINISTRATION TECHNIQUE

Ease of administration as well as cleanliness must be considered in all methods of treatment of placental retention. The author prefers the method of tying the cow's tail over the back to the opposite front leg. The vulvar area is then prepared with a suitable antiseptic scrub, and the boluses or capsules are introduced into the cervix and into the uterine horns with a clean plastic sleeve. The need for extra administration equipment such as tubes, pumps and bottles is eliminated, and the possibility of contamination is greatly reduced by this method.

COMPLICATIONS

The most common early complication of retained placenta is metritis, as evidenced by elevated temperature, depression, excessive fetid uterine discharge and general signs of toxemia. The animal should be treated symptomatically as needed with parenteral antibiotics and sulfonamides, intravenous fluids and dextrose solutions and gentle intrauterine treatment, preferably with an antiseptic or antimicrobial solution. In cases in which an excessive amount of foul-smelling uterine fluid is present, use of a soft plastic stomach tube and gravity suction techniques, followed by administration of ergonovine at a dosage of 5 to 10 mg, will assist in evacuation of the uterus. Tetracycline boluses or capsules, although of a slower onset than solutions, quite often aid in controlling the infection within a short time. Most other complications are a result of metritis and will be greatly reduced in incidence and severity by this early and thorough therapy.

Although rare in most localities, tetanus can result from uterine invasion by *Clostridium tetani*, usually during calving in a contaminated area. In endemic areas, including much of Europe and parts of the Southwestern United States, tetanus antitoxin at a dose of 1500 to 3000 units is advisable as a preventive measure for cows with retained placenta.

Delayed involution and pyometra are frequent sequelae to retained placenta, especially in herds in which placental retention goes untreated or unnoticed. Routine veterinary examination of the genital tract at 25 to 30 days postpartum will reveal those animals with abnormal uterine findings, and proper therapy can be promptly instituted.

RECOMMENDATIONS

In conclusion, the author's recommendations for treating placental retention in dairy cattle will follow those just outlined. Two or 3 gm of a broad-spectrum antibiotic bolus, preferably tetracycline, should be placed in the uterus at least every other day until the placenta has fallen away and any metritis subsides. A placenta that adheres firmly should not be manually removed, nor should manual removal be attempted in animals with severe metritis. In the case of septicemia, prompt systemic therapy is necessary with penicillin, tetracyclines or sulfonamides. Uterine lavage with a tetracycline solution is very beneficial but must be performed gently to avoid damaging or further irritating the uterus. Routine examination of these cows 25 to 30 days postpartum is essential and can increase subsequent fertility by early detection of uterine abnormalities followed by prompt treatment.

REFERENCES

1. Hammermann, J.: Treatment of retained placenta with special reference to the fertility of the cow. Proceedings 9th Nordic Veterinary Congress, Copenhagen, 1962, II 534.
2. Roberts, S. J.: Veterinary Obstetrics and Genital Diseases. 2nd Ed. Ann Arbor, Mich., Edwards Brothers, Inc., 1971.
3. Squire, A. G.: Retained placenta: A comparison of tetracycline treatment and no treatment on subsequent fertility of the cow. Unpublished, 1980.

Treatment of Bovine Pyometra with Prostaglandins

BORJE K. GUSTAFSSON
University of Illinois, Urbana, Illinois

The classic bovine pyometra, also called true pyometra, is an infectious uterine disorder characterized by the accumulation of purulent exudate in the uterus, persistence of the corpus luteum (CL) and anestrus. The retention of the CL is most probably due to a reduction or inhibition of the synthesis or release of the uterine luteolytic factor, prostaglandin-$F_{2\alpha}$ ($PGF_{2\alpha}$), caused by pathological changes in the endometrium. According to recent investigations, pyometrial fluid appears to contain relatively large quantities of $PGF_{2\alpha}$. Therefore, an alternative explanation for the retained CL might be a faulty transfer of $PGF_{2\alpha}$ to the ovary. The diagnosis of pyometra is often erroneously used for cows having chronic endometritis with a slightly or moderately enlarged uterus caused by a thickening of the uterine wall. These animals, which often have a mucopurulent discharge from the vulva, demonstrate a form of purulent endometritis with little, if any, accumulation of fluid in uterus. Such cows are usually cycling, although the cycle length may be irregular.

OCCURRENCE

Bovine pyometra occurs most commonly during the early postpartum period (15 to 60 days postpartum), often following peripartal disturbances such as dystocia, retained placenta or acute puerperal metritis. True pyometra can also occur at various intervals after breeding. These cases are often associated with embryonic death, which may result from an infection introduced at breeding or one already present in uterus at breeding. Inseminations erroneously performed during the luteal phase of the cycle can also result in pyometra. If a pregnant cow is inseminated or treated by intrauterine infusion, abortion is the likely result and is often followed by pyometra.

ETIOLOGY AND PATHOGENESIS

Postpartum pyometra is a consequence of puerperal infections. In countries in which brucellosis (*Brucella abortus*) exists, this microorganism must always be suspected to be the primary cause of infection, but other microorganisms can be secondary invaders. In brucellosis-free countries a variety of infectious microorganisms can be responsible for the postpartum infections. These include hemolytic streptococci, hemolytic staphylococci, coliforms, *Corynebacterium pyogenes* and *Pseudomonas aeruginosa*. There may occasionally be animals infected with clostridia or different types of fungi. *Corynebacterium pyogenes* is probably the most common cause of bovine pyometra and can be the cause of pyometra in several cows within a herd.

Postbreeding pyometra, which is much more uncommon, is usually caused by the same microorganisms as postpartum pyometra. It should be remembered that in countries in which trichomoniasis occurs postbreeding pyometra is a common result of *Trichomonas fetus* infection.

True pyometra seldom shows spontaneous recovery unless the cyclic activity starts and can continue for months without any change in the condition.

CLINICAL SIGNS AND DIAGNOSIS

There are usually no general signs of illness, even in cows with a considerably enlarged uterus. The retention of the CL causes anestrus. In most cases of postpartum pyometra a purulent discharge is observed, particularly when the cow lies down. The discharge is usually thick, mucoid and creamy. The color is yellow, white, grayish-white, greenish-gray or reddish-brown. In other cows the cervix is closed and there is no discharge of pus from the vulva. In cases of embryonic death, the discharge may contain remnants of fetal membranes and tissue debris.

Rectal examination reveals a distended and fluctuating uterus. The size can correspond to that of pregnancy from about 6 weeks to approximately 5 months. The uterine wall is usually thickened, compared with the pregnant condition. It is, however, more atonic than in a normal pregnancy. The consistency of the uterine content is usually thicker than that of a normal pregnancy. Both horns may be equally enlarged, but asymmetrical enlargement of one horn is more common. A CL can be palpated in one of the ovaries. In the majority of cases, vaginal examination reveals a slightly enlarged and somewhat open external os of the cervix and a mucopurulent discharge around the os and in the anterior vagina. Other cows have a completely sealed, very tight cervix, like that of pregnancy. In postbreeding pyometra it is sometimes possible to palpate fetal parts and parts of the fetal membranes.

DIFFERENTIAL DIAGNOSIS

Palpation findings may simulate a normal pregnancy. However, the uterine wall usually feels thicker, and the uterine content is also thicker than in pregnancy. The fetal membrane slip, cotyledons and fremitus in the uterine artery that are characteristic of pregnancy are lacking in cases of pyometra.

Mucometra or hydrometra is another condition characterized by accumulation of fluid in the uterus. Except for cases in connection with obstruction or segmental aplasia of the tubular tract, this condition occurs most frequently in chronic cases of ovarian cysts. Usually the uterine wall is remarkably thin (atrophied), especially in cows with mucometra in connection with cystic ovaries. In the latter case the status of the ovaries will make the differential diagnosis easier. It should be noted that a pyometra may occasionally exist even if no CL can be palpated. Furthermore, it is not uncommon to find that the CL is smaller than at midcycle.

TREATMENT

Treatment with Conventional Methods

In the past, several different methods have been used to treat pyometra. Local treatment of the uterus (infusions) with different antiseptic solutions, together with draining the pus from the uterus, was for a long time the only treatment available. The prognosis with these forms of treatment was usually poor. German literature reports a clinical recovery percentage of 20 to 30 per cent. The conception rate was less.

Better results were obtained with parenteral administration of various estrogens — a common current method. Estrogens may have a luteolytic effect, resulting in estrus with strong uterine contractions. However, the effect is not consistent, especially when small doses of estrogen are administered. It depends also on the type of estrogen used (which limits the general value of the treatment) as certain estrogens, for example diethylstilbestrol, are not approved for veterinary use in all countries.

Besides the variable effect, the estrogens have other great disadvantages. The main risk involved is that the infection can spread to the oviducts, ovaries and ovarian bursa and cause sterility because of adhesions and inflammation. It has been reported that this risk may be greater with long-acting estrogens.

Doses of estrogens reported to have effect are, for example, 20 to 100 mg of diethylstilbestrol intramuscularly (IM) and 5 to 15 mg of estradiol benzoate or estradiol cypionate IM. It appears that repeated injections give the best results, but it also increases the risks of side effects considerably (see previous discussion). After the uterus has emptied about 1 week after the estrogen treatment, it is common to infuse the organ with disinfectant solutions, such as Lugol's solution, or with antibiotics to speed up the recovery. Sometimes the estrogens have been combined with an IM injection of oxytocin. The clinical recovery rate with estrogens seems to be about 50 per cent. In general it appears best to wait at least two to three estrous periods after evacuation of the uterus before breeding the cow. Fifty to 60 per cent of the clinically recovered cows can then be expected to become pregnant.

The most effective of the conventional methods to empty the uterus in cases of classic pyometra is enucleation of the corpus luteum. This has also been used extensively in the past. However, there are side effects with this treatment that have limited its use considerably. Hemorrhage and adhesions are well-known disadvantages of the CL-enucleation. Therefore, this treatment is considered to be contraindicated except as a last attempt after other methods have failed.

Treatment with Prostaglandins

Prostaglandins are unsaturated fatty acids that are synthesized by several different tissues in the body. As far as reproduction is concerned, the most interesting production site is the uterus. Prostaglandin-$F_{2\alpha}$ ($PGF_{2\alpha}$) is most probably the uterine luteolysin in cattle. Parenterally administered $PGF_{2\alpha}$ causes luteolysis and estrus within 2 to 3 days. The practical application of $PGF_{2\alpha}$ in veterinary medicine is to a great extent based on its luteolytic action. A prerequisite for the use of $PGF_{2\alpha}$ in cattle is therefore that a functional CL be present. Other effects, such as a direct stimulation of the myometrium, do occur but are not likely to be important in cases of pyometra, although they might contribute by increasing the uterine tone and relaxing the cervix. Further investigations are necessary, however, to evaluate the potential direct effects on the myometrium and cervix.

Besides the natural $PGF_{2\alpha}$, structurally related substances have been synthesized. In general, these synthetic analogs to $PGF_{2\alpha}$ have a strong luteolytic effect. Both $PGF_{2\alpha}$ and its synthetic analogs are being marketed in several countries. It should, however, be pointed out that the public health authorities in most countries are still awaiting the results of studies on the residue concentration of prostaglandins or its metabolites in milk and meat before approving the preparations for routine use. Other countries have already approved the use of $PGF_{2\alpha}$ or its analogs in animals.

The first reports of the use of prostaglandins for treatment of pyometra came in 1974, when it was reported that IM and intravenous (IV) $PGF_{2\alpha}$ was very effective in causing luteolysis and in evacuating the uterus in cattle with pyometra. Later reports have confirmed this effect. Uterine evacuation starts as early as about 24 hours after the injection, and cows frequently come in heat 3 to 4 days after injection. They apparently ovulate at this estrus. At present it seems that doses between 12.5 and 30 mg of $PGF_{2\alpha}$ THAM-salt IM should be used. It is probable that a dose of 25 mg or more will give the most constant effect, but there are indications that lower doses might be as effective. Much lower doses could probably be used if the intrauterine route proves to be as effective in cases of pyometra as it is during normal diestrus. It appears that one treatment is enough to establish normal cyclicity if the condition has not lasted too long. Some cows may need several treatments at intervals of 10 to 14 days. Even if the condition is detected fairly early, it may sometimes be advantageous in hastening recovery to induce estrus several times within a short period of time. This could shorten the time from treatment to conception. As far as is known today, it seems that the best time to breed the cows would be at the first or second estrus after the induced one, depending on whether the discharge is normal or not. That could mean about 7 weeks from treatment to breeding. Two or three $PGF_{2\alpha}$ treatments at an interval of about 10 days would probably shorten this period.

Synthetic analogs of $PGF_{2\alpha}$ have been used with good results for treatment of pyometra. The standard luteolytic dose for cattle of the products currently used (cloprostenol) is 500 μg (0.5 mg) IM. The CL responds with luteolysis in the same way as with natural $PGF_{2\alpha}$. A single treatment seems to be enough in most cases to establish normal cyclicity. Estrus occurs approximately one cycle length after the induced ovulation. The second estrus has been reported to result in secretion of normal cervical mucus. As regards repeated treatments, the same applies to the analogs as to the natural $PGF_{2\alpha}$ (see previous discussion).

Whether supportive treatment with antibiotics administered systemically or locally should be used after the evacuation of uterus remains to be investigated. In the studies reported here, no supportive antibiotic therapy has been given.

The treatment of bovine pyometra with prostaglandins is a fairly new method. Therefore, it is too early to draw definite conclusions concerning the results. There is no doubt, however, that the effect as far as evacuation of the uterus is concerned is excellent (> 90 per cent) provided a functional CL is present. In most cases normal cyclicity resumes after the treatment. Furthermore, the nontraumatic nature of the prostaglandin treatment has great advantages compared with the manual enucleation of the CL.

Pregnancy results obtained so far seem to be rather good and promising for the future use of $PGF_{2\alpha}$ or its analogs as a therapeutic agent for pyometra. In one study 65 per cent of 20 cows inseminated after such treatment became pregnant, and an average number of 2.2 inseminations per pregnancy were required. The best results were obtained with inseminations during the second or third heat after treatment. In another study, 5 of 12 cows bred at the first heat after the injection (the induced heat) became pregnant. In general, breeding at the induced heat is not recommended. In any case it would probably be better to wait at least another 10 to 14 days, at which time a second prostaglandin injection can be given (see previous discussion).

Further studies are desired to clarify the relationship between the size of the dose given and the clinical response, the clinical effect of intrauterine administration of the prostaglandins and the potential effect of a combination treatment (for example, prostaglandin/oxytocin, prostaglandin/estrogens) and to evaluate the recovery rate and conception results under different conditions. It might very well be possible to increase the efficacy of the treatment. One question of interest in this context is the potential use of prostaglandins in cases of chronic endometritis with no apparent accumulation of fluid in the uterus and with normal estrous cycles. It is well known that the spontaneous recovery in many such cases is good after the cow has gone through several cycles. Endogenous estrogens produced near the time of estrus apparently enhance recovery. It could therefore be useful to increase the number of estrous periods within a short period of time with prostaglandins. Under favorable conditions it would be possible to bring the cow into heat every tenth day instead of the normal 21-day interval. That could speed up the recovery and reduce the time from calving to breeding in cases of moderate or mild chronic endometritis, which usually require a long time from calving to breeding.

REFERENCES

1. Arthur, G. H.: Veterinary Reproduction and Obstetrics. Baltimore, The Williams & Wilkins Co., 1975.
2. Bäckström, G., Edqvist, L. E. and Gustafsson, B.: Prostaglandin $F_{2\alpha}$ ($PGF_{2\alpha}$) as a therapeutic agent for pyometra in cows. Proceedings 12th Nordic Veterinary Congress, R *41*:277, 1974.
3. Cooper, M. J., Hammond, D., Harker, D. B. and Jackson, P. S.: The use of ICI 80,996 (cloprostenol) in the treatment of various forms of infertility in cattle. Proceedings 8th International Congress on Animal Reproduction. Communication Abstracts p. 58, 1976.
4. Cooper, M. J. and Furr, B. J. A.: The role of prostaglandins in animal breeding. Vet. Rec., *94*:161, 1974.

5. Gustafsson, B., Bäckström, G. and Edqvist, L. E.: Treatment of bovine pyometra with prostaglandin $F_{2\alpha}$: An evaluation of a field study. Theriogenology, 6:45, 1976.
6. Heap, R. B. and Poyser, N. L.: Prostaglandins in pyometrial fluid from the cow, bitch and ferret. Br. J. Pharmac., 55:515, 1975.
7. Roberts, S. J.: Veterinary Obstetrics and Genital Diseases. 2nd Ed. Ann Arbor, Mich., Edwards Brothers, Inc., 1971.

Anestrus in Cattle

R. ZEMJANIS
University of Minnesota, St. Paul, Minnesota

Because of its high incidence and the resulting loss, anestrus is the most costly infertility problem in cattle. It is well documented in dairy cattle by the use of detailed reproductive records. However, anestrus also exists in beef cattle.

It has been customary to think of postpartum anestrus whenever anestrus is discussed. Actually, postpartum anestrus represents a relatively small percentage of the total cases of anestrus. The following classification has been proposed:[11]

1. *Preservice anestrus*. In this category belong all animals that have not been observed in heat at the time of planned breeding. In addition to postpartum cows, this group also includes heifers.

2. *Postservice anestrus*. This category represents an absence of observed heat in serviced animals that have failed to conceive. Included are two groups of animals: (a) cows and heifers returning to heat 36 or more days following service and (b) animals that are found to be nonpregnant upon pregnancy examination.

The incidence of both categories has been estimated for dairy cattle populations. The author has recorded a 12.6 per cent incidence of preservice anestrus and 30.8 per cent incidence of postservice anestrus in herds with average fertility.[11] In problem herds the incidence is much higher. These data are consistent with other reports. In general, they represent herds with better than average production and management.

Anestrus leads to delay in conception and, in dairy cattle, to a loss of production that can be expressed in production days lost. The exact number of production days lost has not been estimated for the herds providing the incidence data. It is, however, safe to assume that a minimum of 30 days is lost for each case of preservice anestrus. The actual figures are certainly much higher.

The minimum time lost because of postservice anestrus could be arbitrarily set as 42 days, corresponding to two estrous cycles. Actually the loss is much higher. For instance, pregnancy examination conducted at 45 days following service permits a loss of at least three estrous cycles, equivalent to approximately 63 days in the nonpregnant animal.

Considering that practically every third animal experiences postservice anestrus resulting in extension of the calving interval by almost 2 months, the economic impact of this disorder is obvious.

CLINICAL APPROACH TO ANESTRUS

Anestrus is a symptom or sign observed as a problem by personnel in charge of breeding in a herd. To accept this as a diagnosis constitutes a professional error.

Each case of anestrus must be considered as one of the two following possibilities: (1) signs of estrus are not exhibited or (2) signs of estrus are exhibited but are not observed. It is obvious that rational management of anestrus is impossible unless which of these categories exists is determined. This may be difficult, but thorough clinical examination combined with tactful but detailed evaluation of observation and breeding practices will provide answers in most cases.

The clinical examination involves systematic exploration of the uterus, ovaries and other parts of the reproductive organs for signs that indicate that the cyclic function of the ovaries is *not* occurring.

Conditions associated with absence of cycling are listed in Table 1.

Cows with true, or organic, anestrus are relatively easy to manage. They are easily diagnosed, and in many cases there are

TABLE 1. *Causes of Arrested Ovarian Function*

---

1. Normal pregnancy
2. Abnormal causes:
   Luteal cysts
   Follicular cysts (certain cases)
   Bilateral atrophy of ovaries
   Freemartinism
   White heifer disease (certain cases)
   Pyometra
   Fetal mummification and maceration

---

proven methods of therapy. Unfortunately, true, or organic, anestrus accounts for only 10.5 per cent of all cases of anestrus.

The remainder of the anestrous cows possess a normal genital tract and have ovaries carrying the various functional structures that are associated with normal cycling. They present a real dilemma to the attending veterinarian. Since cyclic changes occur, are all these cases caused by failure to observe estrus? Two conditions associated with cyclic structures in the ovaries must be considered before discussing the problems of heat observation. One is the so-called retained corpus luteum, and the other is silent estrus. Both are widely used as diagnoses and also as excuses. In order to diagnose "retained corpus luteum" and to differentiate it from the functional yellow body, the structure of approximately the same size and consistency must be found in the same area of the same ovary on at least two subsequent examinations spaced 10 to 14 days apart. Experience in this clinic involving a considerable number of animals and examinations indicates that the retained corpus luteum is indeed very rare. This has been confirmed by other workers.

"Silent estrus," or quiet ovulations, is physiological during the immediate postparturient period in both dairy and beef cattle. Its significance as the cause of anestrus at the time of planned breeding is highly questionable. A study by Cornell workers[6] indicated that the incidence of "silent heat" is negligible by the end of the fourth month after parturition. There is also evidence that the incidence of silent estrus can be reduced to a minimum by increasing the number of heat observation periods from one to several a day.

What are the problems leading to failure to observe estrus in cycling cows? Since management practices are involved, specific errors and deficiences in heat observation may be difficult to single out. All possibilities must be considered and explored.

First, great variation exists among animals in both intensity and length of estrus. Continuous observation has shown that estrus is not suddenly turned on, nor does it cease in similar manner following a plateau of strong excitement that reaches a peak, as indicated by displayed receptivity.[7, 8] There are waves of estrual excitement interspersed with periods of quiescence. The intensity of estrus and the expression of heat signs are also influenced by the time of day, environment, pecking order and other factors — all affecting the ease of observation. Estrous signs are most intense before 6:00 AM and after 6:00 PM.

Detecting weak estrus requires the complete attention of the best observers. Even good observers will fail to notice signs of estrus if observation is done when the animals are relatively quiescent during a normal estrus. It is equally obvious that even normal signs of estrus will remain unnoticed if animals are observed only briefly or at the wrong time or are not observed at all.

Clinical experience strongly suggests that inadequate observation (for example, during the weekend) is the most important single cause of anestrus in cycling animals. Many "anestrous" animals, when examined on Mondays, have been found to exhibit uterine and ovarian changes indicating recent estrus and ovulation. Likewise, genital examination has frequently revealed estrus in animals presented as being anestrous.

Common errors and deficiencies of heat observation practices are listed in Table 2.

Tact, patience and understanding of all these possibilities are required during evaluation of observation practices. Information regarding general management practices on the farm is extremely valuable in many cases.

TABLE 2. *Common Errors and Deficiencies of Heat Observation Practices*

---

1. Inadequate time for observation:
   a. Only one daily observation period
   b. Observation period too short
   c. Other responsibilities during observation period
2. Ignorance
3. Negligence
4. Combination of the above

CLINICAL MANAGEMENT OF ANESTRUS

It should be obvious that the success of any measures will greatly depend on the accuracy of the etiological diagnosis, that is, whether pathological findings or deficient observation is involved.

The Noncycling Animal

In general, anestrous animals demonstrating clinical evidence that the cyclic function of the ovaries is either arrested or absent are easy to manage. Clear-cut diagnoses provide a basis for rational prognostic and therapeutic considerations.

Thus, there is no treatment for freemartinism, white heifer disease, bilateral hypoplasia of the ovaries and other types of congenital abnormalities. Most cases of pyometra can be successfully treated. Likewise, there is proven therapy for cystic ovaries, both of the follicular and luteal type.

Ovarian atrophy in heifers is the result of nutritional deficiencies, principally energy or protein, or both. Minerals such as phosphorus and some trace elements have been incriminated. Ovarian atrophy is also observed in young cows during the peak period of their lactation. Both correction of ration and mineral supplementation are effective, although recovery may take 2 to 3 weeks. In cases of atrophy, hormone therapy has been ineffective and, on occasion, even harmful.

The Cycling Animal

Observed estrus allowing properly timed service is the ultimate goal of any clinical measures. Any and all of these measures should lead to increased observation efficiency. A multidirectional approach is needed because of the complexity of the problem. This is outlined in Table 3 and is explained in detail as follows.

Intensification or Induction of Estrus

This step involves hormone therapy, either by application or by induced withdrawal. Several hormones have been tried, often without clear-cut clinical indications, particularly when cycling animals are treated.

TABLE 3. *Clinical Measures to Improve Detection of Estrus*

1. Intensification or induction of estrus
2. Improving observation
   a. Improve observer
   b. Adequate observation
   c. Facilitate observation
   d. Anticipate next estrus
3. Prevention of anestrus

Hormone Therapy

ESTROGENS. Follicular extracts, diethylstilbestrol and natural estrogens have been used and recommended. Close scrutiny of reported results demonstrates that although estrogens are capable of inducing psychological signs in many animals, the induced estrus is seldom accompanied by ovulation, unless the hormone is administered coincidentally during proestrus. Timing and dosages for utilization of the luteolytic effect have so far not been worked out. Estrogen therapy has been observed to induce cystic degeneration of ovaries.

FOLLICLE-STIMULATING HORMONE. Theoretically, follicle-stimulating hormones (FSH) should induce and support follicular growth leading to estrus. In the form of pregnant mare serum gonadotropin (PMSG), FSH has been used by several workers and also in this clinic. PMSG has been administered in single or repeated doses, ranging from 600 to 1000 IU. Purified follicular stimulating hormone (PFSH) (Armour) has been given in 50-mg amounts. The effectiveness of FSH therapy appears to be highly questionable.

THYROID. The role of the thyroid gland in female reproduction is still controversial. Early work indicated that thyroidectomy in cows resulted in anestrus. This led to the recommendation that the hormone be used for treatment of anestrus. The suggested dosages have ranged from 2 to 5 grains daily, administered orally. Results obtained in this clinic are discouraging.

A summary of results of hormone therapy obtained in this clinic is given in Table 4. All cases in which estrus or service was recorded within 23 days following treatment were considered as successfully treated. The table includes data on conception rates from the first three services following treatment. The results are not encouraging. Comparable

TABLE 4. *Effect of Hormone Therapy for Induction of Estrus*

| | | | Per Cent 1st Service Conception | |
| | | | COWS IN ESTRUS | |
Hormone	Cows Treated	Per Cent Estrous within 23 Days	WITHIN 23 DAYS	ALL TREATED
Estrogen	83	73.5	47.5	25.3
FSH	74	58.1	46.5	48.5
Thyroid	86	61.7	45.3	27.9

evaluation of results obtained by other workers reveals a similar lack of success.

Luteolytic Therapy. Considerable time, effort and money have been devoted to attempts to develop methods of estrous synchronization. An important incentive for these attempts, however, has been the general recognition of the difficulties of heat detection in both dairy and beef cattle. Enucleation of the corpus luteum, administration and withdrawal of progestins and utilization of the luteolytic activity of prostaglandins have all been used for synchronization as well as for induction of estrus.

ENUCLEATION. Manual removal of the corpus luteum is one of the oldest approaches used in endocrinological research and therapy. It is a relatively safe procedure if it can be performed with minimum effort, as trauma to the ovaries and local hemorrhage are unavoidable if force is applied. Most reports reviewed indicate that enucleated animals are in heat between 2 and 8 days following treatment, with the majority being observed in heat between 3 and 5 days. Results from this clinic and from selected references are given in Table 5.

The data indicate that enucleation of the corpus luteum is a reliable method of inducing physiological estrus. Excellent results have been obtained in this clinic by servicing enucleated animals on day 4 following treatment, even in the absence of observed estrus. Animals are rebred on the fifth day if they show signs of estrus on this day.

PROGESTINS. The same compounds and treatment regimens that have been tried in synchronization studies have also been used in attempts to induce estrus. However, it is beyond the scope of this presentation to review all of them. The relatively wide spread of first estrus following withdrawal reduces the value of this method for induction of estrus and ovulation at predetermined times. The low fertility of services on the first withdrawal estrus is also disadvantageous.

PROSTAGLANDINS. Prostaglandins, primarily PGF_2, are luteolytic in most animal species, including the bovine species. Several trials have demonstrated that extremely precise synchronization can be obtained by administration of PGF_2 during the luteal phase from day 5 to 15 of the estrous cycle or twice at 10-day intervals. Predictability of the induced estrus has stimulated studies of fertility of services at a predetermined time. The conception rates obtained have been reasonably good.[2]

If prostaglandins pass the scrutiny of the Food and Drug Administration and if their use can be made practically and economically feasible, they could truly be a "wonder drug," removing most, if not all, of the woes and worries about detection of estrus and timing of service.

INFUSION OF THE UTERUS. Infusion of large volumes of substances into the uterus is a widely accepted method of inducing estrus in mares. The effect of such a treatment in cows is not established. Timing of the infusion and selection of the substance, which is placed into the uterus, influence the results obtained. Early observations in this clinic of the effect of postservice infusions in repeat breeders clearly indicated that a certain number of cows infused before day 5 of

TABLE 5. *Effect of Enucleation of Corpus Luteum*

Cows Treated	Per Cent Estrous within 23 Days	First Service Conception Rate	Authors
51	70.0	50.0	Wright[9]
155	64.9	52.1	Gibbons[1]
2746	62.5	49.7	Teige et al.[5]
212	79.6	69.1	Zemjanis et al.[13]

the estrous cycle had another estrous period within a week after infusion.[10] Subsequent research demonstrated that the effect of altering the cycle length was due to the irritating properties of iodine, nitrofurazone or oxytetracycline solutions.[4] Japanese workers concluded that 20 to 40 ml of Lugol's solution was ineffective if infused on days 1, 13 and 19 of the estrous cycle. Shortened cycles were observed in animals treated between the second and fourth day of the cycle. Infusions during luteal phase resulted in estrus 8 to 11 days later.[3] In view of the greater effectiveness of infusions during metestrus, it appears that other mechanisms of action are involved in addition to luteolysis.

Although there is no doubt that uterine infusions alter the estrous cycle in cattle, there is no specific treatment that can currently be recommended.

Improving Observation

It is obvious that effective observation of estrus is essential for success in any type of treatment or management of anestrus. Even the most reliable therapy will be ineffective if observation fails.

Improving the Observer. There is great difference in the efficiency with which different individuals observe for estrus. Knowledge of all signs of estrus, as well as the circumstances in which they will be displayed and therefore best observed, is essential. Thus, for example, the herdsman should know that he should look for the restless animal in a resting herd. He should also know that animals tend to display estrus when moved around in the yard or holding area.

Another factor is the effect of the weekend, which constitutes greater than one-fourth of the week. Animals are more or less intentionally neglected by substitutes and even by regular farm help. Providing a bonus or any kind of reward for each animal serviced during weekends has resulted in many more services during this time period.

Adequate Observation. The duration of the observation period should allow ample time for observation of all animals in the herd. Half an hour is a must, particularly if the observer has to cover several areas and also attempts to move animals. The person in charge of observing estrus should be freed of any other responsibilities. There should be at least two, and preferably more, observation periods scheduled daily. Controlled experiments have amply demonstrated the need for several daily observation periods. A recent study in Australia comparing continuous with twice-a-day observation revealed that the latter practice resulted in failure to observe heat in 46 per cent of cows.[7, 8] It also led to recording mistaken estrus in 12 per cent of cases. Inseminations following incorrectly observed estrus are not only infertile but may also result in uterine infections if insemination is done during the luteal phase.

Facilitating Observation. Managerial practices facilitating observation include use of heat detecting devices and teaser bulls. Heat-detecting devices (see Appendix B) generally consist of a plastic capsule of two compartments that must be carefully attached to the skin of the rump to prevent premature loss of the device. Pressure applied by the mounting animal breaks the partition between the two compartments, allowing the contents to mix. This results in a red coloring. Patience may be needed to obtain maximum benefit from the device. Australian workers concluded that the device increases the efficiency of estrous detection considerably.[7, 8]

Teasers equipped with proper marking devices (see Appendix B) aid considerably in facilitating observation. Because of the danger of transmission of venereal diseases, bulls that are only vasectomized should not be used. Surgical deviation of the penis or locking of the penis in the sheath produces reliable teasers. Both aggressiveness, which increases with age, and decline of libido limit the use of teasers to no more than a season. Ovariectomized cows primed with androgens or nymphomaniac animals are equally effective and less dangerous than teaser bulls.

Anticipation of Next Estrus. Detection of estrus in an individual anestrous animal is considerably more effective if the time when the animal must be closely observed can be narrowed from the entire estrous cycle to a few or single days.

Prediction of next estrus on the basis of uterine and ovarian findings is a veterinary service that has been greatly effective in this clinic. It has been well received by clients, who demand it as routine service, and it compares favorably with any other known method of improving estrous detection (Table 6).

The technique has been described elsewhere. Prediction is more accurate when animals are examined at the time when changes are most dramatic, such as proestrus, estrus and metestrus.

Intelligent use of individual records and heat expectancy charts is essential for top reproductive efficiency. Observed estrus that is too early for breeding and service dates should be recorded on heat expectancy charts. Expected estrus is then calculated on the basis of these entries and heat prediction information, and the number or the name of the involved animal is entered in the space provided for the predicted day or days.

Prevention of Anestrus

Even if a foolproof method of inducing physiological estrus were available for treatment of anestrous animals, the time lost cannot be regained. This loss can, however, be considerably reduced by preventive measures. In fact, this is the area in which veterinary preventive programs are most beneficial to the clients. Because there are two categories of animals involved, the preventive approach to preservice anestrus and postservice anestrus must be different.

Preservice anestrus can be virtually eliminated. An alert client keeping and consulting reproductive records can identify all females that have not been observed in heat by 1 month before planned breeding. These animals are then reported to the attending veterinarian for examination and, if needed, treatment without time loss. An outline illustrating the preventive approach to preservice anestrus is given in Table 7.

TABLE 7. *Measures toward Prevention of Preservice Anestrus*

1. Establishing individual reproductive records.
2. Educating clients in keeping these records. Calving, heat and service dates should be entered.
3. Educating the client to consult the records and to "read the signs of danger." Absence of recorded estrus at the end of 60 days of postparturient period is a good example of a danger sign.
4. Examination of all animals that had not been observed in heat.
5. Treatment of curable abnormalities causing anestrus.
6. Prediction of next heat.
7. Improvement of observation practices.

different problem. In contrast to preservice anestrus, a failure to observe estrus in serviced animals is not considered a danger sign. On the contrary, it is generally accepted as an indication of conception and as such is used worldwide to determine nonreturn rates. The high incidence of postservice anestrus points out the fallacy of such an assumption. The clients are helpless in these cases, as they are entirely dependent upon veterinarians as far as detection of postservice anestrus is concerned. Early pregnancy diagnosis is the key to prevention of postservice anestrus.

Ideally, all serviced animals failing to conceive should be detected before the first estrus after service. At present, there are no practical methods permitting definite diagnosis at that time. Rectal palpation and the determination of milk progesterone levels between 19 and 23 days do, however, provide information suggesting pregnancy or indicating return to estrus. Follow-up examinations in this clinic indicate that the information obtained from these examinations is accurate in all cases in which findings suggest return to estrus. In cases in which ovarian and uterine changes are comparable with pregnancy, pregnancy is confirmed in 85 to 90 per cent of animals.

A definite diagnosis is possible before the next estrus, that is, the second expected estrus following service. The techniques of examination at 19 to 23 days and early pregnancy diagnoses have been described elsewhere.[12]

TABLE 6. *Effect of Heat Prediction on Detection of Estrus*

		Per Cent 1st Service Conception	
Cows Treated	Per Cent Estrous within 23 Days	COWS IN ESTRUS WITHIN 23 DAYS	OF ALL TREATED
522	78.5	69.1	55.7

REFERENCES

1. Gibbons, W. J.: Reproductive problems in cattle. Vet. Med., *49*:323, 1954.
2. Lauderdale, J. W., Seguin, B. E., Stellflug, J. N., Chenault, J. R., Thatcher, W. W., Vincent, C. K. and Loyancano, A. F.: Fertility of cattle following PGF$_{2\alpha}$ injection. J. Anim. Sci., *30*:392, 1974.
3. Nakahara, T., Domeki, I. and Yamauchi, M.: Effects of intrauterine infection of iodine solution on the estrous cycle of the cow. N.I. Anim. Health Quart., *11*:211, 1971.
4. Seguin, B. E., Morrow, D. A. and Oxender, W. D.: Intrauterine therapy in the cow. J.A.V.M.A., *164*:609, 1974.
5. Teige, J. and Jakobsen, K. R.: Investigation on the effect of enucleation of corpus luteum in dairy cattle. Proceedings. III International Congress Animal Reproduction, 1956.
6. Trimberger, G. W. and Fincher, M. G.: Regularity of estrus, ovarian function and conception rates in dairy cattle. Cornell University Agric. Exper. Sta. Bull., 1956, p. 911.
7. Williamson, N. B., Morris, R. S., Blood, D. C. and Cannon, C. M.: A study of oestrous behavior and oestrus detection methods in a large commercial dairy herd. 1. The relative efficiency of methods of oestrus detection. Vet. Rec., *91*:50, 1972.
8. Williamson, N. B., Morris, R. S., Blood, D. C., Cannon C. M. and Wright, P. J.: A Study of oestrous behaviors and oestrus detection methods in a large commercial dairy herd. Oestrous signs and behavior patterns. Vet. Rec., *91*:58, 1972.
9. Wright, J. G.: Observations on the clinical aspects of reproductive disorders in cattle. Vet. Rec., *57*:313, 1945.
10. Zemjanis, R.: Repeat-breeder syndrome. N.Y. State Veterinary Medical Association Annual Conference, Ithaca, N.Y., 1958.
11. Zemjanis, R.: Incidence of anestrus in dairy cattle. J.A.V.M.A., *139*:1023, 1961.
12. Zemjanis, R.: Diagnostic and Therapeutic Techniques in Animal Reproduction. 2nd Ed. Baltimore, The Williams & Wilkins Co., 1970.
13. Zemjanis, R., Fahning, M. L. and Schultz, R. H.: Anestrus, the practitioner's dilemma. Vet. Scope, *XIVI*:14, 1969.

Ovarian Cysts in Dairy Cows

BRAD SEGUIN

University of Minnesota, St. Paul, Minnesota

Ovarian cysts are a common, clinically recognized endocrine cause of infertility in dairy cows. Surveys indicate that 5 to 10 per cent of dairy cows are affected during the postpartum and breeding periods. Ovarian cysts, ovarian cystic degeneration or dysfunction, cystic ovaries and "cystic" cows are general terms used to describe the condition; follicular cysts and luteal cysts are specific forms of the condition. The disorder is characterized by persistence (usually $\geq$ 10 days) of an ovarian follicular structure, or structures, that is usually larger than the normal mature follicle ($\geq$ 2.5 cm in diameter) in the absence of a corpus luteum (CL). The presence of a cystic-type structure in conjunction with a mature CL is usually a nonpathological situation. Abnormal estrous behavior, varying from lack of estrus (anestrus) to abnormally frequent estrus or estrus-like activity (nymphomania) to masculinization (virilism), is associated with the condition. Palpable uterine changes ranging from edema shortly after the onset of the cystic condition to marked lack of uterine tonus as the condition becomes chronic are frequently detected. Shortening of the uterine horns and occasionally an accumulation of uterine secretions (mucometra) may also be noted.

TYPES OF OVARIAN CYSTS

Three types of ovarian cysts (follicular and luteal cysts and cystic corpora lutea) are frequently described, only two of which (follicular and luteal cysts) are generally considered to be pathological (Fig. 1). Follicular and luteal cysts develop from follicles that fail to ovulate and may continue to enlarge after the anticipated ovulation. Follicular cysts have a thin wall, are fluctuant on palpation and are more likely to rupture during rectal manipulation; whereas luteal cysts have a layer of luteal tissue in the cyst wall, making them more resilient on palpation. Follicular cysts are probably more likely to appear as multiple cysts than are luteal cysts. Both types of cysts may share a common etiology (deficiency of luteinizing hormone [LH] secretion at estrus), with follicular cysts possibly resulting from a greater relative LH deficiency than that causing luteal cysts. Clinically, follicular and luteal cysts are rarely differentiated and are usually treated similarly.

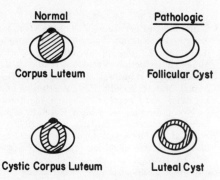

Figure 1. Types of bovine ovarian cysts. The cross-hatched areas represent luteal tissue, and the blackened areas represent ovulation papillae.

Cystic CLs form after ovulation, when for unknown reasons a fluid-filled cavity forms within the developing luteal tissue. An ovulatory papilla or crown marking the ovulation site is frequently detectable by palpation and is useful clinically to differentiate cystic CLs from follicular and luteal cysts. The presence of a cystic CL is usually considered a nonpathological condition, since it has been shown that luteal tissue from cystic CLs is fully capable of producing progesterone, and some researchers have stated that cystic CLs do not adversely affect estrous cycle length or pregnancy.

ABNORMAL ESTROUS BEHAVIOR

The degree of the various types of abnormal estrous behavior reported in affected cows has varied greatly. The general trend seems to be for more cows with cysts to be anestrous in recent years, as opposed to exhibiting nymphomania. This observation probably reflects the increased palpation and evaluation of cows during the early postpartum period as part of reproductive herd health programs. As a consequence, earlier and thus more effective treatment has probably resulted. When postpartum examinations are not routinely done, "cystic" cows showing frequent, irregular signs of estrus are more likely to attract the attention of dairymen and veterinarians than are anestrous "cystic" cows.

Recently, methods have been developed that enable researchers to measure hormone concentrations in small quantities of blood. Consequently, several investigations of the endocrine status (progesterone, LH and es-

trogens) of cows with cysts have been reported. Summation of these reports indicates that the progesterone level is frequently low (especially with follicular cysts), the LH level is normal to slightly elevated and estrogen concentrations are variable (normal to slightly elevated, but not markedly elevated) in cows with ovarian cysts. Slight elevations in the LH level probably reflect lack of negative progesterone feedback on the hypothalamic-pituitary axis. Levels of androgens (i.e., testosterone and androstenedione) in cows with cysts were very low (probably normal) in one survey. These endocrine findings seem true regardless of the type of behavior exhibited. At this time no clear endocrine difference has been reported for "cystic" cows that are anestrous versus those exhibiting nymphomania or virilism.

ETIOLOGY OF THE CYSTIC CONDITION

The etiology of follicular and luteal cysts has not been conclusively determined. A commonly accepted hypothesis is that cysts result from a deficiency in the preovulatory LH surge near the onset of estrus, and, as a result, ovulation does not occur. The therapeutic efficacy of LH, the histological evidence of increased "hormone" granules and the endocrine evidence of increased concentrations of gonadotropins in the anterior pituitaries of affected cows support this hypothesis.

Many factors have been observed to be positively correlated with the incidence of ovarian cysts, although mechanisms by which these factors exert an influence on incidence rates are not established. The condition is more common in mature cows (after the second lactation), more common in the early postpartum period (and therefore at times of high rates of milk production and heavy grain intake) and more common in the fall and winter months. In one study, cows with follicular cysts produced significantly more milk than herdmates during lactations in which they were cystic, but their milk production was not different from herdmates during precystic lactations. Thus, it appeared that circumstances associated with the cystic condition may have been responsible for increased production. In another study, ovarian cysts were more common in cows that had complications near calving.

An hereditary influence has been demonstrated. In a study of lifetime reproductive records of 144 dams and their 245 daughters in a large purebred Holstein herd, 43 dams had ovarian cysts and 26.8 per cent of their 82 daughters had been affected. The remaining 101 dams had no history of ovarian cysts, and only 9.2 per cent of their 163 daughters developed ovarian cysts. In Sweden, the incidence of ovarian cysts decreased from 10.8 per cent in 1954 to 5.1 per cent in 1964 to 3.3 per cent in 1974 after adoption of a policy whereby bulls used as artificial insemination (AI) studs were culled if their daughters had a greater than average incidence of ovarian cysts. Also, bull calves were not considered for AI use if a tendency toward ovarian cysts was evident in their pedigree.

Iatrogenic induction of cysts by clinical use of estrogens is frequently cited. Researchers have found that when estrogens are given to cows during late diestrus and early proestrus a high percentage of animals develop ovarian cysts. Injection of estrogens at other stages of the estrous cycle did not result in the development of ovarian cysts. The relationship between the clinical use of estrogen-type drugs such as diethylstilbestrol (DES) for a variety of postpartum reproductive conditions and the incidence of ovarian cysts in dairy cows has been surveyed. The incidence of ovarian cysts did not differ between a group of 323 cows given DES and 447 herdmates not given DES (7.7 per cent and 7.3 per cent, respectively). It was concluded that the risk of inducing ovarian cysts by estrogen therapy should not deter its clinical use (especially early in the postpartum period).

Ingestion of feedstuffs containing estrogen-like substances is sometimes suspected when a herd has a high percentage of cows with ovarian cysts. Although some legume forages such as alfalfa and some clovers contain estrogenic activity, analysis of such feeds from herds with a high incidence of ovarian cysts has not demonstrated these forages to be the source of the problem.

TREATMENT PROCEDURES

Therapy for ovarian cysts is aimed at stimulating or simulating development of a functional CL.

Manual Rupture of Cysts. The earliest form of therapy was manual rupture of the cyst via rectal manipulation. A relatively low recovery rate (37 per cent) has been reported for cows treated in this manner, although many practitioners and other researchers have reported higher success rates. Reviewing several previous studies, Schjerven reported that 63 per cent of 829 cows with cysts treated by manual rupture became pregnant.[6a]

Possible complications from manual rupture of cysts include hemorrhage and adhesions. Realistically, such complications are probably much less likely after rupture of cysts, at least follicular cysts, than with enucleation of CLs.

Very large (4 to 6 cm in diameter) follicular cysts are frequently detected at 20 to 40 days postpartum, and it may prove difficult not to rupture these cysts in the course of examination. In such cases, manual rupture of early, thin-walled follicular cysts seems to have few, if any, disadvantages and may shorten recovery time and allow the cow to begin cycling normally by the time of desired breeding. However, controlled experiments comparing manual rupture of early follicular cysts versus no treatment or other treatments are not available. It should be recognized that the spontaneous recovery rate of ovarian cysts is greatest (up to 40 to 50 per cent) during this early postpartum period. In one trial in which cows with ovarian cysts were not treated but were palpated every week, 30 per cent recovered spontaneously within 30 days of first diagnosis, an additional 39 per cent recovered in 30 to 300 days and 31 per cent failed to recover by 300 days postpartum. Some cows that appear to respond positively to manual rupture may be among those destined to recover on their own. Manual rupture of cysts, especially thick-walled luteal cysts, should not be performed when excessive force is required.

Administration of Luteinizing Hormone. Administration of LH, as human chorionic gonadotropin (HCG) or a pituitary extract (PLH), has been commonly used to treat cows with ovarian cysts since the mid-1940's. HCG is a protein hormone (molecular weight of 30,000) rich in LH activity and is present in urine from pregnant women. Pituitary LH extracts, usually from sheep or swine, contain follicle-stimulating hormone (FSH) and other pituitary protein hormones as well as LH. Both HCG and PLH preparations have antigenic properties. The clinical ramifications of this antigenicity, although long suspected following repeated treatments, have not been clarified. The desired consequence of HCG or PLH therapy is stimulation of development of luteal tissue (luteinization), either within the cystic structure, or structures, or in other follicles that may be present at the time of treatment. The ability of HCG to cause luteinization, as evidenced by increases in serum progesterone levels in cows treated for ovarian cysts, has been demonstrated (Fig. 2). Luteinization of cysts usually occurs without ovulation, whereas luteinization of other noncystic ovarian follicles present at the time of treatment may occur with or without ovulation. Thus, a normal CL may be detected from 7 to 14 days after treatment in some cows. Absence of a distinct CL at these times should not be judged as evidence of treatment failure, as a cyst can luteinize without marked changes in palpable characteristics. This observation, plus the fact that many cows will not show a normal estrus until about 20 days (Fig. 3) after treatment, has led to the recommendation that cows not be retreated for cysts before 3 to 4 weeks unless signs of nymphomania persist.

Fertility after successful treatment, i.e., if the estrus is normal, does not appear to be reduced. Some early authors have recommended that breeding be delayed for one or two estrous cycles after treatment of cows with cysts to avoid an increased rate of twinning. More recent investigations have not confirmed this observation. To minimize chances of recurrence of cysts, it seems best

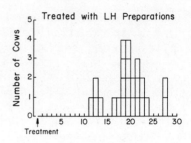

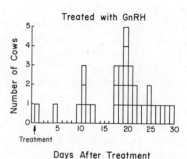

Days After Treatment

Figure 3. Distribution of estrus in cows with ovarian cysts after treatment with luteinizing hormone (LH) preparations of gonadotropin-releasing hormone (GnRH).

to start breeding cows at the first apparently normal estrus after treatment. Dosages of 5000 units intravenously (IV) and 10,000 units intramuscularly (IM) of HCG or PLH appear to be relatively equivalent, as indicated by clinical response, and somewhat superior to lower doses given by these respective routes. Recovery rates vary according to the endpoint used. A high percentage (probably ≥ 90 per cent) of treated cows develop luteal tissue after treatment. A portion of these (55 per cent in one study [Table 1]) will be observed in estrus within 30 days of treatment, and probably 55 to 60 per cent of those bred will conceive at the first service. Thus, in one study (Table 1) 30 per cent (100 × 0.55 × 0.55 = 30) of cows treated for cysts with LH preparations conceived within 1 month of treatment. A larger proportion of those treated (possibly 80 to 90 per cent) will eventually conceive if given enough time.

Administration of Progesterone and Progestins. Progesterone and progestins have been used to treat cows with ovarian cysts. The intention here is to mimic CL production of progesterone, prevent estrous behavior and cause the pituitary to store LH for later release. After 14 to 21 days of progesterone influence, it is hoped that estrus with ovulation will occur in 3 to 5 days. In

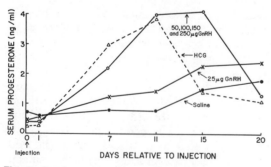

Figure 2. Average serum progesterone concentrations in cows with ovarian follicular cysts after intramuscular injection of 0 (saline), 25, 50, 100, 150 or 250 μg of gonadotropin-releasing hormone (GnRH) or 10,000 units of human chorionic gonadotropin (HCG), five cows per treatment (n = 35).

one study, 100 cows with cysts that exhibited nymphomaniac behavior were given a single IM injection of a long-acting form of progesterone (1 mg per pound of body weight). In most cases, signs of nymphomania ceased in 36 to 72 hours. A tendency for uterine infections to occur was noted following administration of progesterone. In another study, cows with follicular cysts were given daily subcutaneous injections of 50 or 100 mg of progesterone in oil per day for 14 days. Regardless of the dosage used, about 60 per cent of the 40 cows in each group began normal estrous cycles within a few days of the last injection, and about 50 per cent of those treated conceived at an average of 45 days after treatment. Of 30 untreated control cows (with cystic ovaries), only four began normal cycles and conceived. Orally active progestins such as melengestrol acetate (MGA), medroxyprogesterone acetate (MAP) and others are capable of inhibiting estrus in normal cows and, based on experience from a limited number of individual cases, may be equally as effective as injected progesterone for treating cows with cysts. Controlled clinical trials using oral progestins to treat cows with ovarian cysts have not been reported. At the present time in the United States, orally active progestins are not commercially available for the purpose of estrous synchronization or treatment of ovarian cysts in cattle.

Combinations of the aforementioned treatments, i.e., HCG and progesterone plus manual rupture, are commonly used in many European and Scandinavian countries. In a Norwegian study, HCG (1500 to 3000 units) plus progesterone (125 to 250 mg) was given IV, together with rupture of the cysts, and 83 per cent of 70 cows treated with this regimen recovered.

Administration of Gonadotropin-Releasing Hormone. In the last 5 years, researchers have isolated the hypothalamic factor (hormone) that controls release of LH by the pituitary. This hormone called gonadotropin-releasing hormone, or GnRH, is a decapeptide (10 amino acids, molecular weight of 1182). GnRH can be synthesized and has similar LH-releasing activity as the purified hypothalamic extract. One of the first potential veterinary applications of GnRH investigated was its use as a treatment for ovarian cysts in cattle. Several researchers have now shown that single IM injections of GnRH are capable of consistent-

TABLE 1. *Reproductive Performance of Cows with Ovarian Cysts after Treatment with LH Preparations or GnRH**

Treatment	No. of Cows	No. Detected in Estrus by 30 Days	Average Days to First Estrus[†]	First Service Fertility Rate[†] (No. Pregnant/ No. Bred)
LH	49	27 (55%)	19.8	11/20 (55%)
GnRH	57	38 (67%)	19.1	19/32 (60%)

*From Seguin, B. E.: Ph.D. Thesis, Michigan State University, 1975.

†For cows detected in estrus within 30 days of treatment.

ly causing elevated serum LH levels in cows with ovarian cysts, with subsequent formation of luteal tissue in a high proportion of those treated. The LH release occurring after administration of GnRH is of relatively short duration (2 to 4 hours) and is similar to the preovulatory LH surge that occurs near the onset of estrus in cattle. GnRH effectively stimulates luteal tissue formation, either by causing luteinization (without ovulation) of the cyst or by luteinizing or ovulating other follicles present at the time of treatment. The luteal tissue that is produced functions similarly to a normal CL, as indicated by serum progesterone levels (see Figure 2).

Most clinical trials in the United States have used a dosage of 100 μg in a single IM injection, whereas some European researchers have used dosages 10 to 15 times greater (1.0 to 1.5 mg). Parameters of clinical response reported have included nearly all (approximately 100 per cent) of treated cows releasing LH in response to GnRH, most (90 to 95 per cent) developing active luteal tissue, 75 to 85 per cent of treated cows responding positively (occurrence of estrus or palpable indication of change), 67 per cent of treated cows exhibiting a normal estrus within 30 days of treatment (usually at about 20 days after treatment) and normal rates of fertility at the first estrus after treatment (59 per cent of cows in one study). Thus, as with HCG treatment, reports on therapeutic effectiveness of GnRH can vary depending on the parameter reported. In one study (see Table 1), 67 per cent of cows with follicular cysts treated with GnRH were observed in estrus within 30 days of treatment, and the first service conception rate during that period was 60 per cent. Thus, approximately 40 per cent of cows treated with GnRH in this study conceived within 1 month of treatment ($100 \times 0.67 \times 0.60 = 40$). As more time and services are allowed, higher percentages of treated cows will have conceived. Therefore, GnRH and HCG, in dosages of 100 μg and 10,000 units, respectively, given IM, appear to be relatively equivalent in their therapeutic efficacy based on both endocrine and clinical parameters.

Based on relatively limited evaluation, the effect of GnRH in treating cows for ovarian cysts does not appear to be affected by previous unsuccessful treatment with HCG or other LH preparations. The reverse of this, i.e., use of HCG after unsuccessful use of GnRH, is also not well studied. GnRH may have advantages over HCG and other LH preparations in that GnRH is probably less antigenic (lower molecular weight of 1182 and faster clearance rate) and can be produced synthetically. GnRH is also less disruptive to normal CL function if a misdiagnosis is made and a cow with a normal CL is treated. In this situation, the LH preparations (HCG) can cause extended CL function and delay the next estrus by 5 to 10 days.

GENERAL CONSIDERATIONS AND SUMMARY

Early detection and treatment of ovarian cysts appear to give the best assurance of recovery. This implies the need for an awareness by dairymen of cows not detected to be cycling, i.e., those cows exhibiting abnormal estrous behavior. It also supports the need for evaluation of the postpartum reproductive status of cows, i.e., a reproductive herd health program. It should be remembered that in areas where these programs are employed and all cows are checked during the postpartum period, the apparent incidence of cysts in the herd will probably rise, owing to better surveillance. The cause of ovarian cysts is not established. Although early treatment appears warranted, some clinicians prefer not to use hormonal therapy during the very early postpartum period, relying on spontaneous recovery or manual rupture early and use hormonal therapy later, near breeding time, when needed. Breeding at the first estrus after treatment appears warranted in order to minimize the

economic loss, minimize chances of redevelopment of cysts and make use of pregnancy to prevent recurrences. It should be remembered that cows can have a cyst, or cysts, on one ovary and cycle normally or conceive and maintain a pregnancy from other portions of ovarian tissue. It is not uncommon to find the cyst still detectable, along with a new CL, 30 days after treatment. These cows should be considered as recovered and should not be retreated.

Currently in the United States, the most common treatment for ovarian cysts is probably administration of LH, either as human chorionic gonadotropin (HCG) or as pituitary LH extract. Manual rupture of cysts, especially the follicular type during the early postpartum period, is also very common. The treatment prognosis with LH preparations is that about two-thirds of treated cows have a normal estrus within 30 days of treatment and have normal fertility at that estrus. Many cows responding to treatment will be in estrus about 20 days after treatment. GnRH, which appears to be equally as effective as the LH preparations, shows promise as an alternative method of therapy for cows with this condition.

REFERENCES

1. Brodie, B., Hatch, R. D., Thurmon, J. C. and Erwin, B. G.: Estrogen therapy and follicular cysts in cows. Mod. Vet. Prac., Oct., 1970, pp. 54–55.
2. Garverick, H. A., Kesler, D. J., Cantley, T. C., Elmore, R. G., Youngquist, R. S. and Bierschwal, C. J.: Hormone response of dairy cows with ovarian cysts after treatment with HCG or GnRH. Theriogenology 6:413, 1976.
3. Johnson, A. D. and Ulberg, L. C.: Influence of exogenous progesterone on follicular cysts in dairy cattle. J. Dairy Sci., 50:758, 1967.
4. Jubb, K. V. and McEntee, K.: Observations on the bovine pituitary gland. I. and II. Corn. Vet., 45:570, 1955.
5. Morrow, D. A., Roberts, S. J., McEntee, K. and Gray, H. G.: Postpartum ovarian activity and uterine involution in dairy cattle. J.A.V.M.A., 149:1596, 1966.
6. Roberts, S. J.: Veterinary Obstetrics and Genital Diseases. 2nd Ed. Ann Arbor, Mich., Edwards Brothers, Inc., 1971, pp. 421–433.
6a. Schjerven, L.: A clinical study on cystic ovarian disease in dairy cattle. Ph.D. Dissertation, College of Veterinary Medicine, Oslo, Norway, 1971.
7. Seguin, B. E., Convey, E. M. and Oxender, W. D.: Effect of gonadotropin-releasing hormone and human chorionic gonadotropin on cows with ovarian follicular cysts. Am. J. Vet. Res., 37:153, 1976.
8. Whitmore, H. L., Tyler, W. J. and Casida, L. E.: Incidence of cystic ovaries in Holstein-Friesian cows. J.A.V.M.A., 165:693, 1974.

"Repeat-Breeding" or Conception Failure in Cattle

R. ZEMJANIS

University of Minnesota, St. Paul, Minnesota

Theoretically, any unsuccessful service constitutes a reproductive problem. However, not all unsuccessful services are reported. Individual failures to conceive seldom cause concern. Failures from two services are considered to be more serious, particularly so if several animals are involved, and no progressive cattle breeder ignores animals failing to conceive from three services. For practical purposes, conception failure in cattle can be considered as synonymous with "repeat-breeding", which has been defined as failure to conceive from three or more regularly spaced services in the absence of detectable abnormalities.

The incidence of conception failure varies between herds and within herds from year to year. Table 1 summarizes the incidence in four large populations of cattle. Hewett's[5] and the author's[16] data indicate an increasing incidence with increasing age, size of herd and production.

Economically, repeat-breeding is one of the most important reproductive problems. Every case is associated with extension of the calving interval by at least three estrous cycles, or approximately 2 months.

Etiologically and pathogenetically, conception failures are complex. Although it is the female that fails to conceive, the causative factor may be found in the male, or the failure may also be caused by inadequate management. In general, causes of individual failures are confined to the female, whereas group or herd failures point toward a common cause, such as infertility of the bull or inadequacy of management. Therefore, the role of female, male and management factors must be determined in all attempts to arrive at an etiological diagnosis.

Pathogenetically, conception failure or repeat-breeding is the result of either fertilization failure or early embryonic death. In cattle, the latter must occur before the sixteenth or seventeenth day after service in order to allow regular return to estrus.

The following discussion is restricted to female factors.

DISORDERS IN THE FEMALE CAUSING CONCEPTION FAILURE

The etiology of conception failure in the female is complex. Physiological events leading to conception are numerous, involving many systems and organs. Their function is governed by the neuroendocrine system, which is responsible for the proper sequence and synchrony of the numerous events and functions. Errors or failures are possible in such a complex system, and any of the many functions and events may be affected. Each single failure is capable of causing conception failure. Etiological diagnosis requires that all possible causes are considered. In spite of the considerable advances gained in reproductive physiology during the recent decades, there are many events that are not fully understood. The abnormal events and functions are even less well understood. In addition, simple and practical diagnostic methods are lacking, even for the better understood malfunctions and disorders. The following discussion must be read with this in mind.

Disorders of the Ovary

Defective Oogenesis

Theoretically, defective eggs can be expected to cause conception failure; however, meaningful experimental evidence linking defective eggs with conception failure is difficult to obtain for obvious reasons. There is, however, circumstantial evidence that some fertilization failures and early embryonic deaths may be caused by defective oogenesis.

TABLE 1. *Incidence of "Repeat-Breeding"*

Total Cattle	"Repeat-Breeders" (%)	Reference
5744	10.2	Hewett[5]
5858	15.1	Zemjanis[16]
5844	11.6	Boyd and Reed[2]
4811	5.0	Francos[4]

The etiology is unknown, although genetic factors appear to account for certain cases. The clinical diagnosis of disorders of oogenesis is impossible, and there is no treatment available.

Degeneration of Ovulated Normal Eggs

Aging of eggs, accompanied by degenerative changes, may take place because of delayed ovulation or late service. Unless the aging process is advanced, the fertilizability of the egg is not impaired. However, conceptuses resulting from fertilization of aged eggs seldom survive, and the early embryonic death rate is high. This phenomenon has been effectively demonstrated in experimental animals. However, observations in cattle are lacking. Lowered fertility has been associated with high ambient temperatures. A recent study indicated that the critical period when damage was inflicted occurred during the first 6 days following service. The role of febrile diseases on fertilization has not been investigated.

Disorders of Ovulation

Anovulation, one of the two disorders of ovulation, results in fertilization failure and, therefore, could theoretically cause conception failure. The significance of anovulation in the etiology of conception failure is, however, not clear.

Delayed ovulation also presents a controversial problem. A high incidence of delayed ovulation, exceeding 18 per cent, has been reported by South African workers.[15] Observations in the author's clinic revealed a much lower incidence, as less than 2 per cent of delayed ovulations were detected in several hundred repeat-breeder cattle. Differences in breeds of cattle and in their environment may explain the diverging observations.

Clinical diagnosis of ovulation failures requires that the same follicle be detected in the same ovary upon at least two subsequent examinations, one at the peak of estrus and another between 24 and 36 hours later. Absence of the previously identified follicle and replacement of the same by a soft depression with a crater in its central portion indicate that ovulation had occurred normally. Palpation of the ovaries between 36 and 72 hours following services may result in diagnostic errors. The opening of the follicular wall created by ovulation occasionally closes, and blood and proliferating luteal tissue fill the follicular cavity. The soft dome thus raised may be mistaken for a follicle. Diagnoses of ovulation failure made on the basis of one single observation are highly questionable.

The etiology of ovulatory failures has not been established, but they appear to be caused by the same endocrine malfunction that results in the development of follicular cysts. It is plausible that luteinizing hormone (LH) therapy commonly used for treatment of cystic follicles would be effective in cases of ovulation failure. However, by the time a diagnosis of ovulation failure can be made, the entrapped egg is aged, if not dead. Therefore, prophylactic rather than curative therapy is justified to assure that ovulation will occur at the next estrus. The prophylactic therapy must be given early in the next heat period. Intravenous administration of 1000 to 2500 IV of human chorionic gonadotropin (HCG) or of a comparable dose of other LH-acting hormone preparations has been effective in author's clinic.

Inflammation of the Ovary (Oophoritis, Ovaritis)

Severe bilateral inflammation of the ovaries causes sterility by interfering with both oogenesis and ovulation. In unilateral cases and when only a part of the gonad is involved, the prognosis is guarded but by no means hopeless. Whenever the mesosalpinx or salpinx is involved in the inflammatory process, the situation is more serious.

The incidence of ovaritis is generally low.[18] Trauma caused by unduly rough manipulations during palpation, and particularly by indiscriminate attempts to enucleate yellow bodies or to manually rupture cystic ovaries, is the most common cause of oophoritis. However, general fibrosis has been found in animals that have never before been palpated, suggesting other causes such as ascending or systemic infection. Acute inflammation is clinically characterized by swelling of the affected gonad and increased sensitivity to touch. Fresh adhesions may or may not be palpated. Increased consistency, often accompanied by well-organized adhesions to surrounding structures, is characteristic of chronic cases of ovarian inflammation. Adhesions, on occasion, are so extensive that they form a fibrous mass in which the ovary cannot be identified. Since there is no therapy, the prognosis is generally guarded to poor, depending on the extent and degree of the inflammation.

Disorders of the Oviducts

The oviducts are responsible for collection of the ovulated eggs and their transport to the site of fertilization. They are also involved in sperm cell transport and capacitation. Once conception occurs, the zygote depends upon the oviduct for its survival and timely descent to the uterus. To fulfill their function, oviducts must be anatomically normal and must have normal hormonal support. Obstruction and interference with normal peristaltic and segmental motility and secretion cause conception failures. The clinically detectable anatomical abnormalities include hydrosalpinx, perisalpingitis (or ovarian bursitis) and salpingitis.

Hydrosalpinx

Hydrosalpinx is defined as distention of the oviduct by an accumulation of fluid entrapped in the obstructed oviduct. The entire salpinx or segments of different length and number may be involved. To distinguish pyosalpinx from other types of hydrosalpinx is clinically impossible. The general incidence of hydrosalpinx is low. The author and co-workers found hydrosalpinx in less than 1 per cent of genital organs examined clinically.[18] Postmortem examination has revealed a slightly higher incidence.

The history of cases observed by the author tends to incriminate trauma and ascending infection as major causes of hydrosalpinx. It is prudent to assume that microorganisms invading the uterus also find their way into the oviducts and contribute to the etiology of hydrosalpinx. Hydrosalpinx, along with perisalpingitis, is a prominent sign of "Epivag" observed in South Africa (to be discussed later in article). In many cases lesions are bilateral, and the affected animals are rendered sterile.[9]

Clinical diagnosis of the more severe cases of hydrosalpinx does not present any difficulties. The small cyst-like expansions of the oviduct are easily overlooked unless both oviducts are explored carefully in their entire length. The small parasalpingeal cysts in the mesosalpinx should not be confused with those involving the oviduct itself.

The prognosis in bilateral cases is obviously poor and is guarded when the lesion is unilateral. There is no therapy for hydrosalpinx. Oviductal or tubal obstructions exist without clinically evident hydrosalpinx. This has led to attempts to adapt some of the tubal patency tests used by gynecologists for diagnosis in cattle. So far, their practical value is negligible.

Perisalpingitis (Ovarian Bursitis)

This lesion results from adhesion formation between the mesosalpinx and mesovarium, often including the fimbriae and ovary. Adhesions located at the opening of the ovarian bursa cause marked narrowing of this structure. Perisalpingitis affects fertility mainly by interfering with tubal motility. In normal cattle the reported incidence of perisalpingitis is low.[18] It is considerably higher among cattle of low fertility.

Trauma and ascending infection are common causes of perisalpingitis. Localized blood and exudate from inflamed oviducts organize and form adhesions.

Clinically, perisalpingitis is diagnosed by careful exploration of the mesosalpinx and mesovarium, which form the bursa. The technique involves first grasping the ovary without disturbing its site and then sliding all four fingers into the bursa along the ventral aspect of the mesovarium. Any adhesions present between it and the mesosalpinx are encountered directly. The entrance to the bursa is then explored by a slight turn of the hand and simultaneous spreading of all four fingers.[17] When the size of the opening is normal, the fingers can be spread apart without much interference. In severe cases only two or three fingers can be inserted into the opening. The extent and degree of adhesion formation are noted during the process of exploration.

The prognosis depends upon the severity of the lesion and also upon whether only one or both oviducts are affected. In the author's experience occasional animals have conceived in spite of the presence of bilateral, relatively severe perisalpingitis.

There is no treatment for this disease.

Salpingitis

Salpingitis can be defined as inflammation of the oviduct without obstruction and resulting hydrosalpinx. Many cases of salpingitis are not associated with clinically detectable changes. There are very few reports concerning the incidence of salpingitis, and this can be explained by the difficulties of diagnosis. Upon postmortem examination of their experimental "repeat-breeder" cows, Tanabe and Casida[13] found oviduct problems in 10 per cent of the cows examined. It is apparent that microorganisms infecting the uterus also gain entrance into the oviducts.

Clinical diagnosis is possible only in cases in which the oviducts are enlarged, i.e., pachysalpingitis. It should, however, be attempted in all cases of conception failure. Direct palpation of the oviducts is possible, although it is difficult to follow the course of the oviduct *in situ*. The oviduct can be more conveniently explored by the method described for examination of the ovarian bursa.

The prognosis is guarded in all cases, as there is no specific treatment.

Functional Disorders of the Oviducts

It is generally known that both the rate and composition of oviduct secretions are dependent upon the levels of estrogens and progestins. Likewise, it has been established that these hormones control the motility of the oviducts. Low doses of estrogens slow down the rate of the descent of the zygote, whereas larger doses are known to flush the zygote prematurely into the uterus and even as far as into the vagina. Progestins, in general, hasten the descent.

Theoretically, it is possible that endocrine imbalance of both hormones is responsible for infertility by their effects on oviducts.

In spite of recent advances made in the methodology of hormone assays, the finer details of the changing hormone levels required for proper function of the oviducts have as yet not been elucidated.

Disorders of the Uterus

A normal uterine environment is required for survival and transport of sperm cells and for maintenance of pregnancy. Thus, anatomical and functional disorders of the uterus may cause conception failure by interfering with fertilization or by causing early embryonic death.

Metritis and Endometritis

The role of inflammation of the uterus in the etiology of infertility has been a controversial subject for a long time. It has been questioned by many practicing veterinarians who failed to obtain results from intra-uterine therapy. Roberts believes that by the time of the third and fourth services uterine infections are eliminated by self-healing and, therefore, have little significance as causes of "repeat-breeding."[11]

Yet there are a considerable number of repeat-breeding animals with clinically evident uterine infection. Histopathological examination of biopsy and postmortem materials has revealed a greater incidence of inflammatory changes in infertile than in fertile animals. Likewise, the effect of specific infections such as brucellosis, campylobacteriosis, (vibriosis) tuberculosis and trichomoniasis is generally known and established. Therefore, metritis as a cause of conception failure cannot be ignored.

Etiology. The incidence of metritis as a cause of conception failure is rather difficult to establish. Most of the available data originate from histopathological studies that found the disorder in 30 to 70 per cent of cases. A host of microbial agents have been incriminated as etiological agents. In addition to *Brucella abortus, Mycobacterium tuberculosis* and *Campylobacter fetus* var. *venerealis,* a great number of miscellaneous microorganisms such as *Corynebacterium pyogenes, Escherichia coli* and *Pseudomonas aeruginosa,* as well as staphylococci and streptococci, have been isolated from the uterus. The role of leptospiras as a cause of endometritis needs clarification, since *Leptospira hardjo* infection has been reported in herds with low fertility. Endometritis is also found initially following introduction of *Trichomonas fetus* organisms into the genital tract of the cow. Mycoplasmal organisms have been isolated from the bovine uterus, although the significance of the infection as a cause of infertility has not been definitely established.

Several viruses are known to cause endometritis. Thus, Kendrick and McEntee induced severe endometritis in 11 of 12 heifers by inseminating them with semen containing infectious bovine rhinotracheitis (IBR) virus.[6] Similarly, bovine viral diarrhea-mucosal disease (BVD-MD) virus, when added to semen, caused mild metritis in inseminated animals.[1] An IBR-like virus has been reported to cause infertility in cattle in Africa.[9] This disease, originally named "Epivag" (to be discussed later), is accompanied by endometritis, which is one of the major lesions. It can be expected that better diagnostic methods and more persistent search will result in the discovery of additional viruses.

Transmission is strictly venereal in cases of campylobacteriosis (vibriosis) and trichomoniasis. Although other means of transmission may be more common for most of the other infections, many of them are semen-borne. Semen-borne infections are particularly dangerous if animals are not in estrus when inseminated and if the resistance of the uterus is lowered.

Corynebacterium pyogenes, as well as many of the other miscellaneous bacteria, gain their entrance during the puerperium, particularly in confined cattle. Under certain conditions, *C. pyogenes* may develop into a herd infection.

Diagnosis. The clinical diagnosis of metritis is difficult, as overt clinical signs are often not apparent. Palpation findings are generally negative. Exceptions are those cattle in which a small amount of fluid can be detected in one or both horns. The author has found scanty amounts of purulent material *in uteri* from slaughtered animals that appeared normal upon antemortem palpation. Therefore, until hysteroscopic methods are developed, observed purulent discharge from the external os of the cervix remains the only practical, undisputable evidence of endometritis. Consequently, vaginal examination should be conducted in all cases of conception failure. Uterine biopsies have limited application in the field.

A history of dystocia, retained placenta or purulent discharge during the immediate postpartum period, as well as observations by persons who inseminate animals, lends support to the diagnosis. It must be noted, though, that observation of pus-like material in the form of a small bleb on the withdrawn insemination pipette is misleading in many cases. So also is the appearance of a whitish vulvar discharge from animals within 12 to 24 hours following natural mating.

Because of the complex etiology, a single general approach to the search for the etiological agent cannot be recommended. Selection of an approach must be guided by the history, clinical findings and epidemiological observations. Serological tests in one form or another are available for the diagnosis of brucellosis, leptospirosis and some of the viral infections. The presence of microbes, detected either directly or by culture, must be demonstrated in cervicovaginal samples collected at estrus (campylobacteriosis) or during diestrus (trichomoniasis) from recently exposed animals or in pyometra exudate when trichomoniasis is suspected. Miscellaneous organisms are detected by microbiological examination of cervicouterine samples aspirated as aseptically as possible into insemination pipettes conveniently sealed by heating and compressing their ends. Swabs obtained from the anterior vagina and the external os provide less reliable materials. In individual cases of conception failure, etiological diagnosis is seldom attempted. Epidemiological investigation must be conducted whenever group or herd infertility is encountered.

Prognosis. The prognosis in cases of metritis depends upon the specific infectious agent involved and the severity, as well as the duration, of the inflammatory process. Complete functional recovery of the endometrium is unlikely in cases of long duration.

Therapy. The value of intrauterine therapy for treatment of conception failure is as controversial as the role of infection in the etiology of the problem. There are as many reports recording success as failures. Although it is clearly indicated in cases of uterine infection, intrauterine medication cannot be effective when conception failure has other causes. Furthermore, it must be understood that success in the treatment of uterine infection can be expected only if and when: (1) the causative agent is susceptible to the drug used, (2) the drug is used in effective concentration and (3) the entire endometrium and the rest of the internal tubular tract are exposed to the drug.

In practice, the drug must often be selected without the benefit of an etiological diagnosis and sensitivity test results. Selection must be arbitrary, and most workers use either broad-spectrum drugs or combinations for broadest possible coverage. Currently the problem of selection is compounded by regulations concerning drug residues, applicable also to uterine administration. Scrutiny of the scanty available literature[10] reveals that of the commonly used intrauterine drugs only sulfa drugs and nitrofurans appear in milk in appreciable levels for more than 24 hours after administration. No residues or barely detectable traces are found in the milk 24 hours after administration of penicillin, streptomycin, oxytetracycline and tetracycline. Nevertheless, with proper precautions, antibacterial drugs are used to save lives or to restore mammary function. There is no good reason why intrauterine therapy should be avoided when indicated.

Because of the etiological complexity of uterine infections, it is impossible to offer specific recommendations in regard to the choice of drugs. The author follows simple rules of thumb: (1) Lugol's solution is the first choice in cases without a clear-cut diagnosis of uterine infection, (2) when the etiological agent and its sensitivity are known, the choice is obvious — use the most effective drug and (3) in cases of uterine infection without an etiological diagnosis, the first choice is penicillin combined with chloramphenicol or neomycin and, second, oxytetracycline, tetracycline and chloramphenicol singly. A recent report of the comparative *in vitro* effectivity of intrauterine drugs commonly used against mixed microflora obtained from cervicovaginal swabs ranks penicillin in combination with broad-spectrum drugs as most effective, tetracyclines and chloramphenicol as weak seconds and nitrofurans and penicillin-streptomycin combinations as least effective.[8]

There are no experimental data available to indicate effective intrauterine concentration. In the absence of such evidence, the author has used one-tenth of the recommended systemic daily dose of a drug as the basis for estimation of concentration. In general, a factor of one is applicable, i.e., 1 million IU of penicillin, 1 gm of streptomycin, chloramphenicol or oxytetracycline used separately.

Exposure of the entire surface to the antimicrobial drug is achieved by first filling both horns with the solution or suspension and then depositing it in the remainder of the tubular tract. As a rule, 20 ml and 40 ml are adequate for treatment of heifers and adult cows, respectively.

The time of the intrauterine treatment, in the author's experience, depends upon the recent reproductive history of the "repeat-breeder" animal. Animals found to be non-pregnant upon routine pregnancy examination and those that had not been serviced when last in heat should be treated without delay, disregarding the stage of the estrous cycle. Close observation is recommended for repeat-breeder animals serviced at last estrus. Those returning in heat are rebred, and examination and treatment are scheduled for the day after service. Such an approach has several advantages. Loss of an additional 3 weeks is avoided by utilizing the estrous period for service. In addition, timing of service and ovulation can be checked. Intrauterine infusion of a great variety of drugs on days 1 to 2 after service has not interfered with conception, in the author's experience. Conception rates of treated animals have exceeded those of untreated controls.[16] Postservice infusion has been associated with shortened estrous cycles.[12, 16] This effect, in animals treated by the author, has not been limited to irritant agents such as Lugol's solution and oxytetracycline.

Repeat treatments following culture and sensitivity tests are required in stubborn cases of infection. In the author's opinion the disadvantages of indwelling catheters outweigh the advantages.

Inadequate Endocrine Support to the Uterus

Theoretically, endocrine imbalance can act by both pathogenetic mechanisms. It may interfere with sperm transport, survival and capacitation and thereby cause fertilization failure. On the other hand, conception failure may reflect early (before day 16) embryonic death caused by inadequacy of the uterine environment. Detailed and continuous monitoring of hormone levels during estrus, mating and ovulation to substantiate the former possibility has not been reported. A study of progesterone replacement by Cates[3] demonstrated that reduction of the daily progesterone dose from 100 to 75 mg resulted in embryonic resorptions observed on day 35 of pregnancy. Progesterone levels during the luteal phase following service tend to be lower in repeat-breeder animals than in those conceiving. Whether this reflects the cause or consequence of conception failure remains to be determined.

Several workers, including the author, have administered supplemental progesterone to repeat-breeding animals.[16] The results have been inconclusive. Our present knowledge does not indicate progesterone therapy for conception failure.

Parametritis, Perimetritis and Uterine Abscess

These conditions, as such, do not cause conception failure unless the inflammatory process involves the ovaries, oviducts and ovarian bursae or an abscess drains into the uterus. The incidence of these diseases is low, and their significance on the fertility of the affected cattle is minimal.

Tumors of the Uterus

Uterine tumors are extremely rare in cattle. The principal tumors are malignant lymphoma, leiomyoma and carcinoma. As causes of conception failure, uterine tumors have little, if any, significance.

White Heifer Disease

This inherited, congenital segmental aplasia of the tubular genital tract is seldom encountered in repeat-breeder animals.

Disorders of the Cervix

Diseases of the cervix theoretically may cause infertility by obstructing passage of sperm, by creating a spermicidal environment or by causing failure of the cervix to seal the external orifice of the uterine cavity.

Double Cervix and Double External Os

These two types of maldevelopment do not interfere with the success of natural mating. The double external os may create mechanical difficulties when insemination pipettes are introduced. The orifices lead to a single interior cervix and do not interfere with sperm transport to both horns.

The incidence of these abnormalities is low. In one survey conducted by the author and co-workers, only two cases were observed in 20,913 genital tracts examined.[18] Diagnosis is made by rectal palpation, with vaginal examination providing supporting evidence.

Segmental Aplasia of the Cervix

This form of white heifer disease leads to sterility, but the complaint is practically never of conception failure.

Cervicitis

The role of cervicitis in the etiology of conception failure is not clear. It can be speculated that acute cervicitis at the time of natural mating or artificial insemination could interfere with conception. Clinical diagnosis of acute endocervicitis is practically impossible. The significance of the detectable anatomical deformities of chronic cervicitis is difficult to evaluate. In many instances, marked deformities are found in pregnant animals. Distortion of the form, size and consistency of the cervix in chronic cervicitis is rarely associated with hydrometra. This indicates that the cervical canal is very seldom, if ever, obstructed. On the other hand, infectious endocervicitis occurring along with infectious metritis cannot be ignored. The etiology of infectious cervicitis is similar to that of metritis and has been discussed previously.

Diagnosis of cervicitis is readily made by rectal palpation in all cases associated with detectable distortion of form, size and consistency of the organ. Stenosis without marked changes in the general appearance of the cervix can seldom be diagnosed clinically. Vaginoscopy is required for diagnosis of the purulent or mucopurulent endocervicitis that accompanies metritis.

As pointed out previously, care must be taken in assessing the role of diagnosed cervicitis in cases of conception failure. There is no treatment that will correct the markedly distorted cervix or eliminate the scar tissue. Intrauterine therapy for metritis can also be expected to act upon concurrent cervicitis.

Paracervical and Pericervical Abscesses

Unless they drain into the cervical canal, uterus or vagina, these abscesses have no effect on fertility of the involved animal. Their general incidence is rare.

There is no direct treatment for these abscesses. Systemic therapy with anti-infective drugs may be indicated.

Disorders of the Vagina and Vulva

The author is in full agreement with the opinion expressed by Roberts,[11] who stated that localized disorders of the posterior tubular genital tract have little and transient, if any, effect on the fertility of the affected animals. There are obvious exceptions, such as the total aplasia of the vagina in freemartins and the partial segmental aplasia in certain types of white heifer disease. Severe traumatic or infectious vestibulovaginitis is also an exception. The author has observed copious purulent discharge from animals with normally progressing pregnancies.

Vestibulovaginitis Concurrent with Cervicitis and Metritis

All ascending infections gain entrance to the uterus through the vestibulum and vagina. Therefore, most specific and nonspecific infections causing metritis also affect the vestibulum and vagina. In fact, the vagina is the first structure to be exposed to all venereally transmitted diseases affecting conception rate.

The incidence of this type of vestibulovaginitis is not known. It can be assumed that it approximates that of the specific and nonspecific infections affecting the uterus. Diagnosis can be made only on the basis of vaginal examination. The vaginal mucosa is hyperemic, but its integrity is not disturbed. Mucopurulent or purulent exudate is found primarily on the floor of the anterior vagina. Occasionally, pus flakes cover the floor of the vestibulum and contaminate the ventral commissure of the vulva. Since the etiology of this type of vaginitis is similar to that of metritis, the prognostic and therapeutic approach is generally the same as that discussed previously in the section on metritis.

Infectious Pustular Vulvovaginitis (IPV)

This disease was known to exist for several decades before Kendrick and co-workers described the epidemiology in 1958 and demonstrated that it was caused by a viral agent.[7] Although dramatic in its course, IPV is not associated with infertility or abortions.

Diagnosis of the disease is made on the basis of the typical clinical signs.

The prognosis is good, and the course of the disease is approximately 3 to 4 weeks. Local antibodies are formed. The effectivity of IBR vaccines for the control of IPV has not been tested clinically.

"Epivag" (Bovine Venereal Epididymitis and Vaginitis)

In the female this disease is characterized by severe vulvar discharge of mucopurulent

or purulent exudate and by stubborn infertility that is apparently caused by infection of the entire tubular tract. The disease has been reported only in South, East and Central Africa.

The etiological agent is a virus[9] that appears to be related to the IBR virus. Transmission, in contrast to IPV, is strictly venereal. Yellow, copious vulvar discharge often resulting in a smeared tail and thighs is the first sign observed. Inspection of the vestibulum and vaginoscopic examination reveal hyperemic mucosa and yellow flakes of exudate, but the typical pathological changes characteristic of IPV are absent. Rectal palpation during the initial stage gives negative results. Later, hydrosalpinx and perisalpingitis appear in a higher number of affected animals. Diagnosis is based on clinical signs and confirmed in the laboratory.

The prognosis is guarded to poor. As many as 25 per cent of the animals remain sterile as a result of bilateral oviduct lesions. There are no therapeutic or immunizing agents available for treatment or control of this disease.

Granular Vaginitis

Granular vaginitis, or granular venereal disease, has appeared in reports from all cattle-raising countries. Laymen and veterinarians have diagnosed the presence of this disease by spreading to vulvar lips and observing the granular-appearing lymph follicles on the floor of the vestibulum. Literally thousands of cows and heifers have been treated with powders, suppositories and various solutions, all recommended as specific treatment of granular vaginitis.

Critical evaluation has cast serious doubts as to the existence of granular vaginitis as a disease entity. Trautman found no correlation between the incidence of granular vaginitis and conception rate in 4,916 artificially inseminated cows.[14] The author made similar observations while investigating 23 herds allegedly affected by this disease.

Miscellaneous Infections

In recent years reports have appeared concerning isolation of several viruses and *Mycoplasma* variants. The pathogenicity of these organisms, however, has not been established; therefore, their role as causes of infertility for the present time remains obscure.

REFERENCES

1. Archbald, L. F., Gibson, C. D., Schultz, R. H., Fahning, M. L. and Zemjanis, R.: The effects of intrauterine infusion of BVD-MD virus on the oviducts and uterus of nonpregnant cows. Am. J. Vet. Res., *34*:1133, 1973.
2. Boyd, H. and Reed, C. B.: Investigations into the incidence and causes of infertility in dairy cattle — fertility variations. Br. Vet. J., *117*:18, 1961.
3. Cates, W. F.: Minimum daily exogenous progesterone requirement for implantation in the bovine species. Ph.D. thesis, University of Minnesota, 1963.
4. Francos, G.: Observations of reproductive disorders in dairy herds in Israel. Deutsche Tierarztl. Wochenschrift, *81*:135, 1974.
5. Hewett, C. D.: A survey of the incidence of the repeat-breeder cow in Sweden with reference to herd, size, season, age, milk yield. Br. Vet. J., *124*:342, 1968.
6. Kendrick, J. W. and McEntee, J. H.: The effect of artificial insemination with semen contaminated with IBR-IPV virus. Cornell Vet., *57*:1, 1967.
7. Kendrick, J. W., Gillespie, J. H. and McEntee, K.: Infectious pustular vulvovaginitis of cattle. Cornell Vet., *48*:458, 1958.
8. Koleff, W. K.: Comparative investigation of the effect of various antibiotics for therapy of endometritis in the cow. Tierarztl. and Umschau, *28*:80, 1973.
9. Mare, J. and Van Rensburg, S. J.: The isolation of viruses associated with infertility in cattle — a preliminary report. S. Afr. J. Vet. Med., *32*:201, 1961.
10. Righter, H. F., Mercer, H. D., Kline, D. A. and Carter, G. G.: Absorption of antibacterial agents by the bovine involuting uterus. Can. Vet. J., *16*:10, 1975.
11. Roberts, S. J.: Veterinary Obstetrics and Genital Diseases. 2nd Ed. Ann Arbor, Mich., Edward Bros. Inc., 1971.
12. Seguin, B. E., Morrow, D. A. and Oxender, W. D.: Intrauterine therapy in the cow. J.A.V.M.A., *164*:609, 1974.
13. Tanabe, T. Y. and Casida, L. E.: The nature of reproductive failure in cows of low fertility. J. Dairy Sci. *32*:237, 1949.
14. Trautman, E. C.: Granular vaginitis as a cause of infertility in dairy cattle. J.A.V.M.A., *124*:184, 1954.
15. Van Rensburg, S. W. J.: Ovulatory failure in bovines. Onderst. J. Vet. Res., *29*:55, 1962.
16. Zemjanis, R.: The problem of repeat breeding. New England Veterinary Medicine Association Annual Conference, 1963.
17. Zemjanis, R.: Diagnostic and Therapeutic Techniques in Animal Reproduction. 2nd Ed. Baltimore, The Williams & Wilkins Co., 1970.
18. Zemjanis, R., Larson, L. L. and Bhalla, R. P. S.: Clinical incidence of genital abnormalities in the cow. J.A.V.M.A., *139*:1015, 1961.

Abortion

R. B. MILLER

University of Guelph,
Guelph, Ontario, Canada

INTRODUCTION

The terms used in this discussion will coincide with those recommended by the Committee on Bovine Nomenclature.[4] Reproductive dysgenesis is an all-encompassing term used to describe all categories of reproductive failure regardless of cause and regardless of when these losses occur in the gestational period. Losses occurring from conception until embryonic differentiation is complete (approximately 45 days) are termed embryonic mortality. Those losses occurring during the fetal period, that is from differentiation until parturition, are divided into abortions and premature deliveries. An abortion is the explusion before full term of a conceptus incapable of independent life, whereas a premature delivery is the expulsion before full term of a fetus capable of independent life.

MAGNITUDE OF REPRODUCTIVE DYSGENESIS

David *et al.*[2] have reported that when using healthy cows and fertile bulls approximately 63 calves may be expected from 100 first inseminations. The early losses termed embryonic mortality are manifested as repeat breeders, and no physical evidence of the lost embryo may be present. The incidence of fetal abortions and premature deliveries born dead is reported to be between 7 and 12 per cent of cows identified as pregnant between 30 and 50 days after breeding.

CATEGORIES OF REPRODUCTIVE DYSGENESIS

The causes of abortion may be divided into several categories. These include genetic, thermal, nutritional, toxic substances and infectious causes.

Genetic Causes. Genetic factors include abnormalities of the chromosomes or genes that result in defects in the embryo or fetus. The proportion of reproductive dysgenesis attributed to genetic factors is very large and may constitute from one-third to two-thirds of the losses occurring after fertilization. These losses tend to occur early in gestation in humans, most taking place within the first month. The greater proportion of the losses that are due to genetic causes go unrecognized except for known hereditary conditions in which the fetus displays recognizable gross abnormalities.

Thermal Causes. Thermal causes of abortion are usually associated with a rise in temperature, rather than a fall. Pregnant cows exposed to high environmental temperatures have an increased body temperature and respiration and heart rates compared with nonpregnant cows. The greatest effects of heat stress on the reproductive system are associated with decreased fertility near the time of breeding. Heat stress, however, also delays puberty, causes anestrus and depresses estrous activity. There is some evidence to suggest that abortions may occur with sudden rises in temperature, although this manifestation is probably rare.

Nutritional Causes. Nutritional factors are more commonly associated with infertility than with abortion. The premating weight of heifers has a strong influence on pregnancy rate. Subsequent reproductive performance, however, tends to be little affected by the weight of the animal. Moustgaard[8] states that:

If during pregnancy malnutrition happens to coincide with the first third of gestation, i.e. during the sensitive periods of organogenesis, development of malformations and even fetal death may be the sequelae. In the fetal stage (2nd and 3rd trimesters) such deficiency may result in functional disturbances manifest mainly in such organ systems as have several sensitive periods. In extreme deficiency death may ensue or nonviable offspring may be born.

Roberts[9] reports that acute, severe starvation may result in abortion and that this acts as a protective mechanism to preserve the maternal animal's own body reserves. In the author's experience, emaciated animals may abort; however, following the abortion the animal remains recumbent, retains the fetal membranes and dies in a few days.

Abortion or premature delivery in these cases does not preserve the life of the animal but heralds the terminal event. Parturition induction at an earlier stage would be indicated.

The stage at which the deficiency develops and the acuteness and severity of the deficiency all determine the manifestations observed.

Vitamin A deficiency may result in abortion usually late in gestation. Stillbirth and the birth of weak, blind or otherwise malformed calves also occur.[8] The condition may be diagnosed by observing squamous metaplasia of the epithelium lining the parotid salivary duct on histological examination.

Iodine deficiency may result in the delivery of hairless, weak, stillborn or goitrous calves. Circumstantial evidence suggests that the ingestion of large amounts of goitrogenic plants (Brassicacae) may produce a similar result.[8]

Hastings in Faulkner[3] reports a condition manifested by the birth of dead, weak or premature calves and a high incidence of retained placenta that appeared to respond to vitamin E and selenium injections.

Lesions in the myocardium and skeletal muscle consistent with those observed in vitamin E and selenium deficiency are occasionally reported in aborted bovine fetuses. The significance of this lesion as a cause of abortion has not been documented experimentally in cattle.

Toxic Causes. Toxic substances or plants are frequently suspected of causing abortion but are usually difficult to document. Nitrates may fall into this category.[3] The effects of the consumption of pine needles, plants causing locoism and warfarin should also be considered.

The ingestion of pine needles *(Pinus ponderosa)* and subsequent abortion has been reported throughout western Canada and the United States. Sudden weather changes causing cattle to seek shelter, scarcity of feed, logging operations and sudden access to pine needles have all been reported as reasons for the consumption of the needles. The abortion rate may be very low or greater than 50 per cent. Abortions usually occur in the last trimester and may take place within 48 hours after ingestion of the plant. Experiments in mice show that fungi convert some constituents of pine needles into compounds that are toxic to fetal development. More recent work suggests that a heat-stable toxin in pine needle fiber may be the more important factor. The placenta is invariably retained, and there is frequently much hemorrhage. The diagnosis, until the toxin has been clearly identified, will be presumptive and associated with animals consuming pine needles.

Locoism is described as the disease produced by toxic varieties of plants in the genera *Oxytropis* or *Astragalus* belonging to the family Leguminosae. The effects of lathyrogens may be closely related.[14] Poisoning by locoweeds occurs in United States and Canada and is particularly prevalent when pastures are poor or during winter grazing. Locoweeds may be available and green in winter when other plants are dormant. After ingestion of the toxic plant, abortion or fetal abnormalities may occur, depending on the stage of gestation and the amount of plant being eaten. The incubation period for abortion is probably very long; however, evidence in sheep suggests that it is related to dose. The toxic effect may be exerted through the placental and fetal vascular systems. Luteal cells in the ovary, however, are extremely vacuolated, and this may interfere with progesterone production, thus disrupting the pregnancy. In sheep, in which most of the experimental work has been done, the abortion rate may approach 45 per cent, again depending on the time and level of feeding.[5]

The diagnosis is based on the presence of abortions and malformations consisting of lateral rotations of forelimbs, flexures of the carpal joints, contracted tendons, anterior flexure and hypermobility of the hock joints.[5] In malformed sheep there is cytoplasmic vacuolation in neurons, convoluted renal tubules, lymph node macrophages, splenic macrophages, pancreatic acinar cells and thyroid epithelium. Cytoplasmic vacuolation occurs in the corpus luteum, luteal cells and chorionic epithelium of pregnant sheep. It would appear that lesions may be reversible, and therefore losses can be reduced if animals are removed from pastures containing the toxic plants soon enough.

The ingestion of warfarin will produce abortion in cattle and is thought by some to be teratogenic for human infants. It is probably uncommonly seen as an abortifacient, occurring only following accidental ingestion after contamination of food by rat bait. The pathogenesis of the abortion and the usual trimester in which abortion occurs have not been investigated. A related compound, coumarin, occurring naturally on some moldy sweet clover has been associated with neonatal death.

Infectious Causes. The final category of losses due to abortion is that attributed to infectious agents. The proportion of abortions diagnosed as infectious is expanding as more and more agents are demonstrated in fetuses. By far the greatest proportion of the causes that are diagnosed fall into this category, but the size of the category in relation to other causes is not known as only about one out of four abortions is diagnosed.

Isolation of infectious agents or the demonstration of specific fetal antibody in an abortus does not mean that this agent has caused the abortion. Many agents pass through the fetal placental unit and do not appear to disturb the pregnancy. The duration of fetal illness from infection to the time of abortion frequently determines what will be found in the fetus. An organism that rapidly produces fetal death may be readily cultured from appropriate specimens. On the other hand, some organisms produce a prolonged fetal illness, and at the time the fetus is examined the organism cannot be cultured. Instead, fetal antibodies to the agent reveal that it has been present. As just mentioned, many agents may stimulate fetal antibody production by midgestation and not be involved in abortion. It is therefore necessary to correlate antibody levels to specific lesions and history.

INVESTIGATION OF REPRODUCTIVE DYSGENESIS

When faced with a single abortion on a farm, a complete investigation of the herd may not be warranted. Some laboratories prefer not to examine specimens from herds in which only one abortion has occurred but would rather wait until there is a second abortion. This is an attempt to reduce the large numbers of abortions handled by these laboratories and allows more time to concentrate on cases more likely to reflect a herd problem.

If it is decided to investigate the cause after the first abortion, the fetus plus the placenta should always be submitted. Including the placenta greatly increases the opportunity of reaching a diagnosis. If the cow does not discharge the membranes, asep-

Text continued on page 222.

TABLE 1. *Etiological Agents Associated with Abortion in Cattle*

Agent and Common Names	Prevalence	Source of Agent	Incubation to Abortion	Probable Pathogenesis	Usual History
BACTERIAL:					
Brucella abortus Brucellosis Bang's disease	All countries in which cattle are raised	Aborted fetus, uterine discharge, placenta, infected premises, milk	2 weeks to 5 months or longer	Organisms enter through mucous membranes, e.g. alimentary tract, go to lymph nodes, udder and uterus; grow well in placenta, causing placentitis	Abortion, birth of weak or dead calves, retained placenta, infertility
Campylobacter fetus var. venerealis Vibriosis Bovine genital vibriosis	Throughout the world	Infected crypts of the penis and fornix of the prepuce; infected bulls to heifers approximately 100%; infected cows to susceptible bulls considerably lower; bull to bull unlikely	3–8 months	Organism produces endometritis and septicemia	Infertility and failure of conception
Campylobacter fetus intestinalis	Widely distributed	Possibly intestine	Not established	Ingested and may cause a bacteremia from intestine to liver with subsequent infection of uterus and placentome	Rarely infertility, sporadic abortion
Corynebacterium pyogenes	Worldwide	Common on many of the mucous membranes of normal cattle		Probably usually hematogenous to caruncle, adjacent endometrium and placenta	Usually no signs before or after infection, occasionally preceded by systemic illness and/or followed by endometritis
Leptospira pomona canicola icterohaemorrhagiae grippotyphosa hardjo Leptospirosis	Most areas of the world, related to geographical areas	Infected cows, wildlife, swine, etc., contamination of water or feed by urine	2–5 weeks after initial infection	Penetration of abraded skin and mucous membranes	Icterus, anemia, fever may accompany or precede the abortion, may be no observed premonitary signs

Abortion Rate	Stage of Gestation in Which Abortion Occurs	Diagnostic Method Preferred: Microbiology (1) Serology (2) Lesions (3)	Duration of Carrier State	Recurrence of Abortion	Prevention and Control	Samples To Be Submitted
80% of un-vaccinated cows infected in first or second trimester will abort	6–9 months	(1) Isolation of organism from uterine fluids, milk, placenta, fetal lung, fetal stomach contents (2) tube agglutination titer of 1:100 or greater is evidence of infection and presumptive evidence of abortion	Spread by milk for prolonged periods, possibly for life	High rate of infertility, majority abort only once	Vaccination of females at 3–10 months with Strain 19 vaccine, remove infected animals, depopulate	Fetus and placenta, paired serum samples
Usually less than 10%	6–8 months	(1) Culture from fetus, placenta or abomasal contents; dark field examina-tion of abomasal contents (2) obtain vaginal mucus anti-bodies on a herd basis or for culture	May survive on cervix for a full gestation	Uncommon, convalescent cows resistant to reinfection	Vaccination, artificial insemination with anti-biotic-treated semen	Placenta and fetus for culture, vaginal mucus on herd basis
Sporadic	4–9 months	(1) Culture placenta, abomasal contents	Survives in gut for extended period	Not established	Sporadic, usually not necessary	Placenta and fetus for culture
Sporadic or multiple, up to 64%	Usually in the last trimester	(1) Culture from the placenta, as organism may not be in fetal tissues	Unknown	May be sterile, recurrence unknown	No vaccines used	Placenta and fetus
5–40%	Usually in the last trimester	(1) Culture urine from cow commonly up to 10 days, may be necessary for 3 months, also culture milk (2) microscopic agglutination test on serum in herd, acute and convalescent samples	Shed in urine for 2–3 months, also in milk	Immune to serotype causing the abortion but susceptible to the other types, infertility common after abortion	Isolate affected animals, bacterins available	Paired serum samples, placenta and fetus, fresh urine

Table continued on following page

TABLE 1. *Etiological Agents Associated with Abortion in Cattle* (Continued)

Agent and Common Names	Prevalence	Source of Agent	Incubation to Abortion	Probable Pathogenesis	Usual History
Listeria *monocytogenes* Listeriosis	Widespread throughout the world	Wide host range in animals, birds and fish; organism resistant to adverse environmental conditions; propagates in high pH silage; survives in dried feces for 2 years	May be very long, as appears to be stress related	Penetrates intact mucous membranes of respiratory or alimentary tract, latent infection established and stress results in placentitis and fetal septicemia	Pyrexia, depression and retained placenta may occur in the dam
FUNGAL:					
Aspergillus sp. 60–80% Mucorales 10–15%	Worldwide	Ubiquitous in nature, wet hay or straw	35 days after intravenous inoculation of spores, probably weeks or months after natural infection	Molds taken into lungs or mouth and then invade through lesions traveling to the placenta hematogenously	Tends to be seasonal in Northern Hemisphere; peak incidence in January, February or March when cattle confined; usually no prodomal signs
PROTOZOAN:					
Trichomonas foetus Trichomoniasis *Tritrichomonas foetus*	Worldwide	Infected bulls at breeding only, artificial insemination transmission from infected bulls is 1%	From breeding any time up to 7 months	Inflammation of vagina, cervix and endometrium produces a hostile intrauterine environment	Natural breeding and infertility most common with pyometra and abortion, abortions may be most common in older cows with partial immunity
VIRAL:					
Blue tongue	Widespread but not worldwide	Cullicoides from infected sheep or cattle, also by infected semen	Variable, may be very long	Viremia and infection of fetus	Signs in cow mild

Abortion Rate	Stage of Gestation in Which Abortion Occurs	Diagnostic Method Preferred: Microbiology (1) Serology (2) Lesions (3)	Duration of Carrier State	Recurrence of Abortion	Prevention and Control	Samples To Be Submitted
Sporadic or multiple, up to 50%	Most in latter portions of last trimester	(1) Isolation from fetus or placenta	May be in feces and milk, healthy carrier may be important reservoir	May recur in same animal and on same farm from year to year	No commercial bacterin, isolate known infected animals	Placenta and fetus for culture and histological studies
Sporadic to 5–10% of herd	May be 4 months' gestation to term	(3) Mycotic elements in typical placental, skin or lung lesions (1) Yeast and molds may be present in abomasal contents and not be the cause of abortion, care must be taken in interpretation	Probably not a factor	Recovery in severe cases may be slow and prolonged and permanent sterility may follow	Keep off moldy feed, at least temporarily	Placenta and fetus for culture and histological study
Very low	Usually in first half of gestation but may be up to 7 months	(1) Must find the organism in pyometra discharge, placental fluids or stomach contents	Males remain carriers for a long period, cows may retain the organism for 150 days	As animals lose immunity, may become reinfected	Artificial insemination from non-infected bulls	Uterine sample, placenta and fetus
Probably low, not established	Variable	(1) Virus isolation from fetus or from blood of dam	Calves infected *in utero* may be permanently infected	Unlikely	None	Blood samples from dam for culture, paired serum samples, fetus for culture

Table continued on following page

TABLE 1. *Etiological Agents Associated with Abortion in Cattle* (Continued)

Agent and Common Names	Prevalence	Source of Agent	Incubation to Abortion	Probable Pathogenesis	Usual History
Bovine viral diarrhea BVD-MDC BVD	Widespread throughout the world	Infected cattle housed or pastured together	4 days to 3 months after an outbreak	Viremia crossing the placenta as early as 58th day and up to 120 days	Febrile disease in herd prior to abortion and calves born with with brain damage
Infectious bovine rhinotracheitis red nose IBR IBR-IPV	Widespread throughout the world	Infected cows, any animal with a positive titer may be carrying the virus	2 weeks to 4 months	Virus carried in blood leukocytes localized in placental vessels, on entering fetus, kills fetus in 24 hours	Commonly follows respiratory conjunctival form of the disease, may be no signs in the cow, introduction of infected animals
Parainfluenza-3 virus infection PI-3	Agent widespread but significance in abortion not established	Probably respiratory tract	*In utero* inoculation required at 46–56 days	Viremia in the dam with establishment of infection in the fetus	Not established
CHLAMYDIAL:					
Chlamydia psittaci	Germany, United States, Italy, France, Yugoslavia, Israel, Spain	Not established but probably an infected or aborting animal	Experimental subcutaneous or intramuscular injection 40–126 days after inoculation	Parenteral or aerosol inoculation causes chlamydemia and organism localized in placenta	No illness in cows
UNKNOWN:					
Epizootic bovine abortion EBA	Probably localized to one area in California	Unknown	Not established	Not established	Occurs in cows pastured on native vegetation in foothills and mountains of California

Abortion Rate	Stage of Gestation in Which Abortion Occurs	Diagnostic Method Preferred: Microbiology (1) Serology (2) Lesions (3)	Duration of Carrier State	Recurrence of Abortion	Prevention and Control	Samples To Be Submitted
Usually very low	Usually early, but may be up to 4 months	(2) Febrile disease in cows with a two- to four-fold titer rise (3) serum neutralizing antibody in calves with brain abnormalities	May be up to 56 days in respiratory tract or urine for 2 days, could be transmitted in semen	Unlikely, as immune	Vaccination, after 8 months of age; don't vaccinate pregnant cows	Placenta and entire fetus, acute and convalescent sera from cow, sera from colostral-free calves with congenital abnormalities
5–60%	4 months to term	(1) Fluorescent antibody test on fetal kidney (3) lesions in the fetal liver and adrenal gland may be diagnostic (2) four-fold rise in titer from abortion to 2 weeks	Probably for life of animal	Unlikely	Vaccinate heifers at 6–8 months of age	Placenta and fetus, paired serum samples from cow
Probably low	Variable	(2) Paired serum samples in dam, serum antibody or virus in the fetus with typical lesions	Unknown	Unlikely, as low titer prevents infection	Vaccination	Paired serum samples, placenta and fetus
Probably <3%	7–9 months usually, but as early as 4 months	(2) Paired serum samples at abortion and 2 weeks later; fetus has antibody levels (1) culture as many tissues as possible, as have high failure rate	Not known	Probably not but may cause infertility	Vaccine not known but if exposed tetracyclines may be effective orally	Paired serum samples, culture fetus and placenta, fetal sera
Up to 75%	Last trimester	(3) Lesions consistent with the condition in a localized area (2) elevated fetal immunoglobulin-G	Not established	Seldom abort more than once	No vaccination	Complete history, placenta and fetus

tic removal of at least one cotyledon and its submission to the laboratory may help to reveal the agent. The inflammation associated with it may be the only evidence of the cause of abortion.

Along with the fetus and placenta, submission of amniotic fluid or, if not available, a vaginal or uterine swab is frequently helpful. Fresh urine samples are of value in some cases. A serum sample taken from the cow at the time of abortion and another taken 3 weeks later may also suggest the cause of abortion; however, the abortion may not occur until the convalescent stage of the disease. Caution is needed in interpretation of results from serum specimens as the association of high immunoglobulin levels with abortion may only be circumstantial. Along with these specimens, submit a complete history of the herd, the affected cow, the environment and the nutrition.

When faced with more than one abortion in a herd, go through the same procedures as just suggested but with the addition that consideration should be given to collecting serum samples from the remainder of a representative portion of the herd. Only a few of the recognized causes of abortion are associated with "abortion storms" or herd infertility. Occasionally these causes can be diagnosed readily, sometimes by a single placenta or fetus, e.g., brucellosis, vibriosis or infectious bovine rhinotracheitis. Sometimes, however, the diagnosis is much more elusive and requires patience and close cooperation between the livestock manger, clinician and laboratory to correlate data in order to uncover even circumstantial evidence pointing to a diagnosis, e.g., leptospirosis or bovine viral diarrhea.

The most commonly recognized causes of abortion are listed in Table 1, with some of the associated findings, submissions required for a diagnosis and other pertinent information. Details of the most commonly recognized conditions are discussed elsewhere in this book.

REFERENCES

1. Bruner, D. W. and Gillespie, J. H.: Hagan's Infectious Diseases of Domestic Animals. 6th Ed. Ithaca, N. Y., Cornell University Press, 1973.
2. David, J. S. E., Bishop, M. W. H. and Cembrowicz, H. J.: Reproductive expectancy and infertility in cattle. Vet. Rec., *89*:181, 1971.
3. Faulkner, L. C. (ed.): Abortion Diseases of Livestock. Springfield, Ill., Charles C Thomas, Publisher, 1968.
4. Hubbert, W. T. (chairman): Recommendations for standardizing bovine reproductive terms. Cornell Vet., *62*:216, 1971.
5. James, L. G., Shupe, J. L., Binns, W. and Keeler, R. F.: Abortive and teratogenic effects of locoweed on sheep and cattle. Am. J. Vet. Res., *28*:1379, 1967.
6. Jubb, K. V. F. and Kennedy, P. C.: The female genital system. *In* Pathology of Domestic Animals. 2nd Ed. Vol. I, New York, Academic Press, 1970, pp. 487–585.
7. Kirkbride, C. A. (ed.): Laboratory diagnosis of bovine abortion. Madison, Wisc., Am. Ass. Vet. Lab. Diagnosticians. 1975.
8. Moustgaard, J.: Nutritive influences upon reproduction. *In* Cole, H. H. and Cupps, P. T. (eds.): Reproduction in Domestic Animals. 2nd Ed. New York, Academic Press, 1969, pp. 489–516.
9. Roberts, S. J.: Veterinary Obstetrics and Genital Disease. 2nd Ed. Ann Arbor, Mich., Edward Bros. Inc., 1971.
10. Storz, J.: Chlamydia and Chlamydia-Induced Diseases. Springfield, Ill.: Charles C Thomas, Publisher, 1971.

Uterine Cultures and Histological Evaluation as Complements to Routine Postpartum Examinations

ERICH STUDER

Carnation Research Farm,
Carnation, Washington

DAVID A. MORROW

Michigan State University,
East Lansing, Michigan

INDICATIONS

Bacteriological cultures and histological examination of the uterus are diagnostic aids that supplement the routine postpartum examination by palpation *per rectum* and visual inspection of the posterior genital tract *via speculum*.

Culture and histological examinations are certainly important for the diagnosis of specific genital tract infections but are also prognostically helpful in treating individual valuable animals with breeding difficulties. Although references indicate that endometritis may be detected by gross examination of the genital tract,[7, 12, 15] it is generally agreed that the diagnosis of endometritis solely on the basis of rectal palpation is not always reliable.[7, 10, 12, 15] One researcher concluded that after 25 to 30 days postpartum only gross abnormalities could be detected by rectal palpation. Subtle involutionary changes and chronic endometritis cannot be detected by palpation.[10]

CULTURING TECHNIQUE

With cow restrained in stocks or a chute and the tail secured, the perineal area is washed with a disinfectant soap and water. The vulva is disinfected with 80 per cent isopropyl alcohol and finally with povidone-iodine solution (Betadine Solution). With an assistant parting the vulvar lips, a guarded culture instrument (see Appendix B for name and address of manufacturer) is advanced into the body of the uterus by cervical manipulation via the rectum, similar to introduction of an insemination pipette. The sterile swab is then pushed out of its protective sheath and moved about slightly. After the swab is retracted back into its sheath, the culture instrument is removed from the vagina while the vulvar lips are parted again. In some first-calf heifers the entire culture set cannot be passed through the cervix. In these animals the culture swab is advanced out of its sheath in the cervix and manipulated through the cervix into the uterine lumen. Culture media such as blood agar, veal infusion broth and fluid thioglycollate (see Appendix B for names and addresses of manufacturers) are inoculated following removal of the protective sheath cap. The culture swab is first streaked on blood agar for primary isolation, then dipped in veal infusion broth and finally dropped into fluid thioglycollate.

BACTERIAL IDENTIFICATION

Bacterial growth on blood agar from initial streaks is considered especially significant. The importance of growth on solid media only after subculturing from incubated broth is dependent on the specific organisms isolated. Identification of bacteria is achieved by standard bacteriological procedures. Veal infusion broth is used to grow the more fastidious aerobic or facultatively anaerobic organisms, whereas fluid thioglycollate affords growth of facultative anaerobes and strict anaerobes. For isolation of specific genital tract pathogens, special media must be used—CTA or Thiogel media (Appendix B) for *Campylobacter fetus* and Trichosel (Appendix B) for *Trichomonas fetus*. When the samples are to be forwarded to a laboratory and specific media are not available, a transport medium (Appendix B) should be inoculated.

HISTOLOGICAL TECHNIQUE

Following the culturing procedure, uterine samples can be obtained with a Universal Biopsy Instrument set (Appendix B). By cervical manipulation via the

223

TABLE 1. *Comparison of Gross Genital Tract Rating with Microscopic Inflammatory Rating in Postpartum Cows*

Factors Evaluated	Numbers	Correlation	Significance
Gross right horn versus inflammatory rating	104	0.27	<0.01
Gross left horn versus inflammatory rating	103	0.32	<0.01
Purulent exudate versus inflammatory rating, right horn	104	0.36	<0.01
Purulent exudate versus inflammatory rating, left horn	103	0.42	<0.01

rectum the instrument can be passed into the body of the uterus or into each uterine horn separately. The tip is opened, and by manual assistance via the rectum, the uterine wall in the intercornual area is pressed into the jaws of the biopsy device. The bit of endometrium clipped off when the jaws are closed will usually be several millimeters in all dimensions. The specimen is then immediately placed into Bouin's fixative solution. Bouin's solution is preferred because it results in fewer shrinkage artifacts compared with a softer fixative such as formalin.

HISTOLOGICAL EVALUATION

The evaluation must be performed by a trained individual. The importance of inflammatory cells within the section must be related to the estrous cycle stage at the time of sampling. Studies in normal reproducing cows showed that a varied number of neutrophils were present during the relatively short time preceding and following estrus. At other times these cells were practically nonexistent. However, the author concluded that neutrophils located in and beneath the surface epithelium, around glandular ducts and scattered in the superficial stroma may be physiologically normal even in high numbers.[13] Skjerven also reported that neutrophil infiltra-

tion during the luteal phase of the cycle should be considered pathological. A varying number of eosinophils in the stroma, irrespective of the stage of the cycle, may also be considered physiological, although there were never large numbers of these cells found during the luteal phase of the cycle. Lymphocytes appeared only in small numbers during all stages of the cycle. A more general occurrence of these cells, and especially the presence of multiple lymphatic follicles, was considered pathological and less favorable from a prognostic point of view.[13]

The presence of circumscribed accumulations of inflammatory cells in the stratum proprium and around glands and blood vessels, as revealed by uterine histopathological examinations, reduced the incidence of pregnancy in repeat breeder cows.[1, 2] Another study reported a significant relationship between encapsulated glands and breeding difficulties.[11] In a recent investigation[14] gross evaluation of the postpartum genital tract by palpation *per rectum,* vaginal speculum examination and visual inspection of vaginal discharges was significantly correlated to biopsy ratings (P<0.01) (Table 1). The gross purulent exudate rating was also directly correlated to bacterial isolation (r = 0.44, P<0.01). As the number of different organisms that were isolated increased, so did the purulent exudate rating (P<0.01). Of 113 isola-

TABLE 2. *Relationship between Specific Bacteria and Genital Tract Condition**

Numbers	Bacteria	Vagina	Cervix	Right Horn	Left Horn	Purulent Exudate	Total Grade
18	*Corynebacterium pyogenes*	0.28‡	1.39	0.83	0.50	1.00†	4.00†
41	Coliforms	0.07	1.07	0.66	0.37	0.54‡	2.80
24	Streptococci	0.08	1.17	0.58	0.29	0.29	2.42
30	Negatives	0.03	0.97	0.53	0.27	0.067	1.87

*Rating: 0–3 range.
†Sig. difference from negative (P<0.01).
‡Sig. difference from negative (P<0.05).

TABLE 3. *Comparison of Uterine Inflammatory Rating with Bacterial Isolation in Postpartum Cows*

Factors Evaluated	Numbers	Correlation	Significance
Right horn—inflammatory rating versus bacterial isolation	104	0.19	<0.05
Left horn—inflammatory rating versus bacterial isolation	103	0.03	<0.01
Combined right horn and left horn—inflammatory rating versus bacterial isolation	101	0.27	<0.01

tions, 83 were *Corynebacterium pyogenes,* coliforms, streptococci or combinations thereof. The coliforms and some streptococci are normal digestive tract inhabitants and may also be nonpathogenic contaminants of the genital tract.[4, 5, 8] Although many of the cows in these studies had multiple infections, *Corynebacterium pyogenes* was associated with the greatest gross changes (Table 2). This organism was especially associated with animals having increased purulent exudate compared with animals that were bacteriologically negative (P<0.01). Isolation of bacteria was also correlated with biopsy inflammatory scores (Table 3).

Similar to the gross rating, the highest inflammatory value was associated with *Corynebacterium pyogenes* (P<0.01) (Table 4). The severity of endometrial inflammation correlated well with the corresponding gross uterine evaluation (right horn, r = 0.27, P<0.01) (left horn, r = 0.32, P<0.01). The presence of polymorphonuclear cells was considered to be pathological, which was in agreement with previous studies.[11, 13] Also, the occurrence of multiple lymphocytic inflammatory follicles and diffuse mononuclear cells and the existence of periglandular fibrosis must be considered abnormal. Cystic glands with shallow epithelium are most indicative of hormonal imbalance.[3, 9]

Since the endometrial biopsy section rep-resents a small portion of the entire endometrium, its legitimate usefulness might be questioned. A study on slaughterhouse material revealed a good correlation between sections from the two horns and the body of the uterus, with the last pregnant horn having the most severe inflammatory change.[1] Since both the right and left uterine horns were biopsied in the recent investigation, the two sides could be independently compared with other factors and compared with each other. The inflammatory rating of the two horns was in close agreement (P<0.01), indicating that one sample from the body of the uterus reflects the entire endometrium. Both gross genital tract rating and microscopic inflammatory rating were higher for the right horn than for the left horn. This is likely due to the 61/39 right-horn-to-left-horn pregnancy rate in the herd.

RECOMMENDATIONS

Although routine culture and biopsy of the bovine uterus are impractical, these diagnostic procedures should be used under specific circumstances:

1. Diagnosis of specific herd fertility problems such as repeat breeding.

2. Evaluation of the endometrium of a valuable repeat breeder animal. Periglandular fibrosis, obliteration of glands and

TABLE 4. *Relationship between Specific Bacteria and Histological Rating in Postpartum Cows*

Bacteria	Right Horn			Left Horn		
	NO	%	RATING	NO.	%	RATING
Corynebacterium pyogenes	18	22.0	2.17*	17	20.7	2.12*
Coliforms	41	50.0	1.63	41	50.0	1.78†
Streptococci	23	28.1	1.61	24	29.3	1.58
Negatives	29	35.4	1.48	29	35.4	1.31

*Sig. difference from negatives (P<0.01).
†Sig. difference from negatives (P<0.05).

cystic alterations of glands are poor prognostic signs.

3. Use as a research tool for finding answers to fertility problems.

REFERENCES

1. Brus, D. H. J.: Biopsia Uteri of Cows. Rep. 2nd Int. Congr. Physiol. Anim. Reprod., 2, Copenhagen, 1952, p. 175.
2. Brus, D. H. J.: Biopsia Uteri. Haar betekenis bij de studie naar de oorzaken der steriliteit van het rund. Thesis, Rijksuniversiteit, Utrecht, Netherlands, 1954, p. 191.
3. Dawson, F. L. M.: The microbial content and morphological character of the normal bovine uterus and oviduct. J. Agric. Sci., 40:150, 1950.
4. Griffin, J. F. T., Hartigan, P. J. and Nunn, W. R.: Non-specific uterine infection and bovine fertility. Theriogenology, 1:91, 1974.
5. Griffin, J. F. T., Hartigan, P. J. and Nunn, W. R.: Non-specific uterine infection and bovine fertility. Theriogenology, 1:107, 1974.
6. Griffin, J. F. T., Murphy, J. A., Nunn, W. R. and Hartigan, P. J.: Repetitive in vivo sampling of the bovine uterus under field conditions. Br. Vet. J., 130:259, 1974.
7. Hardenbrook, H., Jr.: The diagnosis and treatment of nonspecific infections of the bovine uterus and cervix. J.A.V.M.A., 132:459, 1958.
8. Hartigan, P. J., Murphy, J. A., Nunn, W. R. and Griffin, J. F. T.: An investigation into the causes of reproduction failure in dairy cows. Irish Vet. J., 26:225, 1972.
9. Mochow, R. and Olds, D.: Effect of age and number of calvings on histological characteristics of the bovine uterus. J. Dairy Sci., 49:642, 1966.
10. Morrow, D. A., Roberts, S. J., McEntee, K. and Gray, H. G.: Postpartum ovarian activity and uterine involution in dairy cattle. J.A.V.M.A., 149:1596, 1966.
11. Moss, S., Sykes, J. F. and Wrenn, T. R.: Some abnormalities of the bovine endometrium. J. Anim. Sci., 15:631, 1956.
12. Roberts, S. J.: Veterinary Obstetrics and Genital Diseases. 2nd Ed. Ann Arbor, Mich., Edward Brothers, Inc., 1971, pp. 368–369.
13. Skjervcn, O.: Endometrial biopsy studies in reproductively normal cattle — Clinical, histochemical and histological observations during the estrous cycle. Acta Endocrinol. (Suppl.), 22:26, 1956.
14. Studer, E. and Morrow, D. A.: Relationship of bovine postpartum genital tract examination per rectum to endometrial biopsy and uterine culture results. J.A.V.M.A., 172:489, 1978.
15. Zemjanis, R. M.: Diagnostic and Therapeutic Technique in Animal Reproduction. 2nd Ed. Baltimore, The Williams and Wilkins Co., 1970.

Application of Embryo Transfer to Infertile Cows

R. A. BOWEN and PETER ELSDEN

Colorado State University, Fort Collins, Colorado

Bovine embryo transfer has become an established technique for potentiating a cow's reproductive performance. A majority of the research and commercial effort applied to embryo transfer has utilized normally cycling, fertile donors, but recent work has demonstrated the value of using embryo transfer techniques in the clinical management of infertile cows. Etiological factors involved in bovine infertility are numerous, and embryo transfer obviously cannot be expected to be applicable to all cases. Older cows that have become infertile as a result of chronic genital tract infections, trauma or senescent changes represent the type of infertility cases for which embryo transfer techniques can become valuable tools in diagnosis, prognosis and oftentimes therapy.

When a cow is presented for diagnosis and treatment of infertility, the first step is to determine whether she is indeed infertile. It is not too unusual to find that an "infertile" cow is pregnant! Basic management deficiencies such as poor nutrition or breeding with poor quality semen should be eliminated as a cause of the infertility. If the history of the cow and a thorough physical examination indicate that the animal is cycling normally and has been given an adequate opportunity to become pregnant, she can be assumed to be infertile, and embryo transfer can be considered. In some cases, therapy for a specific condition (such as metritis) is necessary before embryo transfer can be utilized.

Donors for embryo recovery should be checked for estrous behavior twice daily; it is best to observe at least two normal estrous cycles prior to superovulation. Several superovulation schemes are available. The superovulation treatment usually consists of injecting either pregnant mare serum gonadotropin (PMSG) or follicle-stimulating hormone (FSH), beginning 4 to 5 days prior to the expected onset of estrus. PMSG is given in a single dose, whereas FSH must be injected twice daily because of its short half-life. Prostaglandin-$F_{2\alpha}$ (PGF$_{2\alpha}$ can be used to control the estrous cycle during superovulation. Dosages for all of these hormones vary, depending on factors such as route of administration and frequency of injection. Cow weight does not seem to be an important variable, and dosages are generally not adjusted for differences in size. There are several different schedules of dosages for each hormone that produce similar results, and the following dosage information should serve as a general, but by no means absolute, guide for bovine superovulation:

1. PMSG — one intramuscular injection of 2000 IU.

2. FSH — a 4:1 mixture of FSH and luteinizing hormone is injected twice daily; on the first day 5 mg (based on FSH) is given b.i.d., the second day 4 mg b.i.d., the third day 3 mg b.i.d. and thereafter 2 mg b.i.d. until estrus.

3. PGF$_{2\alpha}$ — two intramuscular injections 4 to 8 hours apart of 20 and 10 mg of PGF$_{2\alpha}$ (free acid) beginning 2 days prior to the desired onset of estrus.

A typical schedule involving the use of prostaglandin treatment would be to inject 2000 IU of PMSG on day 10 of the cycle; subsequently, 48 and 56 hours after administration of PMSG, 20 mg and 10 mg of PGF$_{2\alpha}$ are injected intramuscularly. A majority of cows are in estrus 2 days following prostaglandin treatment. The response of the cow to superovulation treatment should be monitored by rectal palpation during the superovulation period. If no or very few follicles are detected at estrus, the cow should not be bred, and superovulation should be attempted during another cycle, perhaps with a different treatment.

The superovulated cow should be bred at least twice at half-day intervals following the onset of estrus. The rationale behind this type of breeding schedule is that the superovulated cow probably ovulates over a relatively extended period of time. Many embryo transfer centers use two or three standard insemination doses at each breeding. In problem cows an extended breeding period may be even more important. If the bull to be used is not highly fertile, fresh semen should be utilized when possible.

Embryo transfer has often been a useful aid in diagnosing, giving a reliable prognosis and in many cases obtaining additional progeny from cows with the following types of infertility:

Periovarian Adhesions. Adhesions involving the ovary and oviduct may induce infertility by interfering with transport of the ovulated egg into the oviduct. Such adhesions may be caused by ascending uterine infections, peritonitis or previous surgery. Surgical embryo recovery and cesarean section, especially if not done carefully, often induce adhesions of this type. Adhesions vary greatly in extent and can be either obvious or difficult to determine by rectal palpation. The laparotomy used for embryo recovery is an excellent means of diagnosing this problem and determining the extent of the adhesions. Superovulation increases the number of ovulations and thus the chance of an egg or eggs reaching the oviduct in a cow with periovarian adhesions. Embryos can therefore be recovered from many cows previously considered infertile. If adhesions are extensive and no embryos are recovered, slaughter is recommended.

Oviductal Obstructions. Obstruction of the oviducts is a relatively common cause of infertility in cows and heifers. This can range from a loose plug of cellular debris to total unilateral or bilateral obliteration of the oviductal lumen. Except in animals that develop a pronounced hydrosalpinx, such obstructions are impossible to detect by rectal palpation and are often diagnosed only after attempts to flush the oviducts for embryo recovery. Embryos are only rarely recovered from the side of an oviductal obstruction, but a precise diagnosis and prognosis are obtained. Obstructions due to plugs of debris can usually be flushed out, and this therapy often restores fertility or makes subsequent successful embryo recoveries possible. Resection of unilateral obstructions or ovariectomy on the affected side are other possibilities for therapy.

Idiopathic Infertility. Despite extensive research devoted to defining causes of bovine infertility, a specific etiology cannot be demonstrated in a majority of cases typified by the "repeat breeder" syndrome. Such cases must currently be classified as idiopathic. A subset of idiopathic infertility can be loosely ascribed to senescence. The age at

TABLE 1. *Summary of Results of Embryo Transfer in 25 Infertility Cases*

Diagnosis	No. Cows	No. Surgeries	Total Corpora Lutea (range)	Total Eggs (range)	Transferred Eggs (range)	Total Pregnancies (range)
Periovarian adhesions	6	7	50 (0–18)	22 (0–9)	18 (0–8)	8 (0–4)
Chronic metritis	3	3	25 (0–23)	24 (0–22)	14 (0–14)	7 (0–7)
Oviductal obstruction	6	8	75 (1–20)	27 (0–8)	10 (0–4)	4 (0–2)
"Senescence"	4	7	105 (6–29)	51 (1–21)	12 (0–7)	5 (0–3)
Idiopathic	6	9	61 (1–20)	33 (0–9)	21 (0–6)	13 (0–4)
Total	25	34	316	157	75	37

which a cow can be classified as senescent is debatable, but many old cows do seem to become infertile before they lose the ability to produce mature ova and ovulate. Idiopathic infertility in heifers is at the other end of the spectrum.

Embryo transfer has been used to obtain calves from heifers and cows with idiopathic infertility. In most of these cases, fertilized ova have been recovered from animals displaying normal estrous cycle lengths. This suggests that early embryonic death is often responsible for the infertility and that embryo transfer can rescue some embryos before their environment becomes lethal. The use of embryo transfer in mature, infertile cows of proven genetic superiority is the most rewarding application of the technique. Embryo transfer from heifers with idiopathic infertility is of questionable value, because of the possibility of propagating hereditable defects.

A summary of results following surgical embryo recovery and transfer in 25 infertility cases is given in Table 1. The category of transferred eggs includes quite a few that were retarded or in some way abnormal but for which it was believed that a pregnancy was at least possible. The low recovery rate (157 eggs from 317 corpora lutea) suggests that in many of these infertility cases the ovulated egg never reaches the oviduct and uterus. Perhaps the major point of this table is that although pregnancies can be ob-

tained from a population of cows with a certain type of infertility, it is not possible to give a reliable prediction for a single cow (that is, no pregnancies were obtained from many of these cows).

Nonsurgical embryo recovery methods are now available. These methods eliminate the formation of adhesions, which was the major disadvantage of embryo transfer. The success of nonsurgical methods should induce more owners of truly superior cows to consider embryo transfer. Embryos can be recovered nonsurgically from many infertile cows. In cows with lesions such as fimbrial adhesions or oviductal obstructions, fewer embryos than would be expected following ovarian palpation will be recovered or embryos may be recovered from only one uterine horn. The recovery of embryos from cows with idiopathic infertility may often be normal. Surgical embryo recovery techniques will, however, remain a valuable tool in diagnosis, prognosis and therapy of many cases of bovine infertility.

REFERENCES

1. Drost, M., Anderson, G. B., Cupps, P. T., Horton, M. B., Warner, B. V. and Wright, R. W.: A field study on embryo transfer in cattle. J.A.V.M.A., *166*:1176, 1975.
2. Newcombe, R.: Fundamental aspects of ovum transfer in cattle. Vet. Rec., *99*:40, 1975.

Pregnancy Diagnosis in the Cow

LESLIE BALL

Colorado State University,
Fort Collins, Colorado

GENERAL DISCUSSION

Pregnancy status can be determined in the cow by rectal palpation and by progesterone assay of either milk or blood serum. Progesterone assays are about 90 per cent accurate. Blood or milk is obtained 21 to 26 days postbreeding and sent to an endocrine laboratory for determination of progesterone levels. Plasma levels lower than 2 ng per ml are considered diagnostic for open cows. *Per-rectal* palpation for a corpus luteum is also about 90 per cent accurate during the period from 21 to 24 days postbreeding. The corpus luteum will be regressed if pregnancy has not occurred.

Per-rectal palpation of the uterus and its contents is the method of choice for pregnancy diagnosis and for estimation of duration of pregnancy in the cow. The most important factors involved in uterine palpation are proper anatomical orientation and a thorough, methodical approach. Most mistakes result from failure to adhere to these two principles. Both uterine horns should be palpated full length before a cow is declared either open or pregnant. To accomplish this, the rectum should be emptied and the uterus retracted if possible, especially in the cow that otherwise is difficult to palpate. It is important to not forcefully manipulate against peristaltic waves or in a rectum ballooned with air, as this usually results in both trauma and an inadequate examination. The ballooned rectum can usually be emptied by reaching forward and gently grasping the first peristaltic ring with a finger, then pulling slowly backward. Gentle stimulation of the rectal wall with the finger tips may also stimulate a peristaltic wave that will deflate the rectum.

RETRACTION OF THE UTERUS

The landmarks of greatest value in the rectal examination are the cervix, the shaft of the ilium and the pelvic brim. Retraction of the open or early gravid uterus into the pelvic inlet is essential for quick, accurate examination. Retraction can usually be accomplished in open cows and those pregnant less than 90 days. Beyond 90 days, the procedure becomes more difficult or impossible. By this time, however, placentomes and sometimes fetal parts and membranes can usually be palpated without retraction. Methods for retraction vary. The following procedures are suggested as guides; however, each person should develop effective techniques of his own. The essential principle is to achieve complete retraction without lodging the uterus beneath the broad ligament, where it is difficult or impossible to palpate properly.

We will assume left-handed palpation for purposes of description. The cervix is a firm, cylindrical structure about 8 cm in length. It is usually located on the midline near the pelvic brim. If not, it is over the brim or entirely within the pelvis. The pelvic inlet is swept with the edge of the opened palpation hand. Finger tips should not be used, as they may damage the rectal mucosa. If the cervix is not encountered at the pelvic brim, the procedure is repeated at various depths until it is located. The cranial end of the cervix is located, and the cervix is pulled caudally by exerting leverage against it (Fig. 1). In the process, the cranial end of the cervix is elevated against the side of the pelvis so that the tract is in a reversed S configuration (Fig. 1). The thumb is inserted under the upper curve of the S, and the fingers are then extended around the left horn of the uterus (Fig. 2). From this location the left horn can be palpated full length, or the fingers can be placed under the ventral intercornual ligament of the uterus and the horns tilted back for easy access. Alternatively, the thumb can be inserted between the horns to maintain retraction and the second horn palpated as was the first (Fig. 3).

When retraction by this technique is difficult or impossible, another technique is sometimes successful in some pregnant cows. The hand is inserted into the rectum and down over the brim of the pelvis, where the uterus is cupped in an angle formed by the arm and hand. The uterus

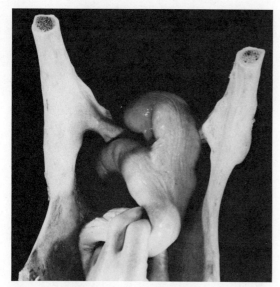

Figure 1. Retraction of the uterus, phase 1. The cranial end of the cervix is located, and the cervix is pulled caudally by applying traction against it. The tract is in a reversed S configuration when the manipulation is completed.

can then be retracted gently up and over the brim of the pelvis. There the fetus can be carefully palpated if accurate assessment of duration of pregnancy is required. The larger, fluctuant horn is worked gently between the fingers and doubled thumb until the fetus or amnion is located (Fig. 4).

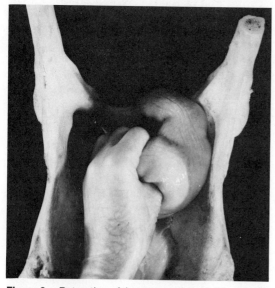

Figure 2. Retraction of the uterus, phase 2. The thumb is inserted under the upper curve of the S and the fingers are then extended around the left horn of the uterus by left-handed palpators.

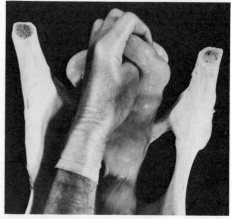

Figure 3. Retraction of the uterus, phase 3. The thumb is inserted between the horns to maintain retraction, and the second horn is palpated full length.

PREGNANCY DETERMINATION

The uterine horns should be palpated their entire length for consistency. If the horns are empty, they will have a meat-like consistency; if pregnancy exists, fluids will be present in one or both horns. These fluids result in a characteristic fluctuance of one or both uterine horns. A common mistake is that of attempting to slip fetal membranes without first detecting fluctuance. A false slip of the broad ligament or other structure is sometimes obtained, and an open cow is diagnosed as being pregnant.

There are four criteria that can be used to positively diagnose pregnancy: (1) palpation of the amniotic vesicle, (2) slip of

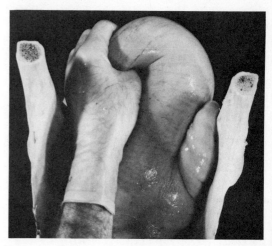

Figure 4. Palpation for the fetus or amnion. The larger fluctuant horn is worked gently between the fingers and doubled thumb until the fetus or amnion is located.

fetal membranes, (3) palpation of the fetus and (4) palpation of placentomes. For a gestation that is advanced beyond 5 or 6 months, the size and fremitus of middle uterine arteries also give positive evidence of pregnancy.

Palpation of the Amniotic Vesicle

Palpation of the amniotic vesicle is possible from about day 30 to day 65 of gestation. Before 30 days it is too small, and after 65 days it becomes too large and soft to palpate. The amniotic vesicle can usually be located in the pregnant horn in the vicinity of greatest fluid enlargement and thinnest uterine wall. It can be trapped in the palm of the hand or between the fingers and the thumb by working gently up or down the horn (Figs. 5 and 6).

Palpation of the amnion should not be used routinely to determine pregnancy because there is danger of rupture of either the amniotic vesicle or the fetal heart sac, resulting in abortion. Gentle palpation of the amnion is justified when it is necessary to predict duration of gestation. The approximate length of the vesicle can be measured by finger-widths (Table 1) to estimate duration of gestation accurately.

Slip of Fetal Membranes

There are no normal uterine-fetal membrane attachments in the interplacentomal

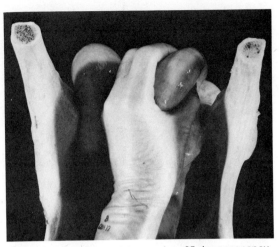

Figure 6. Palpation of the amnion, 65-day pregnancy. The amnion is trapped in the palm of the hand, and its size is estimated by finger-width comparison.

areas, and in these locations the chorioallantoic membranes can be "slipped." A portion of the fluid-filled part of the uterine wall (in early pregnancy, the entire cross section of the horn) is grasped gently and is then allowed to slip between the thumb and forefinger. The chorioallantois and then the uterine wall slip between the thumb and forefinger in turn, giving a characteristic sensation if the cow is pregnant. The sensation is similar to that of slipping a thin, taut string crossways between the fingers. As pregnancy advances, the membranes progressively fill both uterine horns, and the gravid horn becomes quite turgid. At 10 weeks it is often easier to detect pregnancy by slip of membranes in the nongravid horn, as it is less tense and smaller than the gravid one. With extensive experience in the use of membrane slip and palpation of the amnion, it is possible to diagnose pregnancy as early as 30 to 35 days postbreeding.

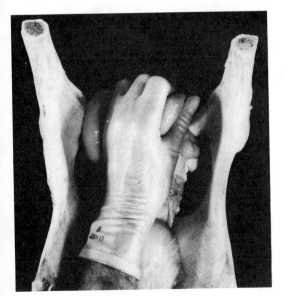

Figure 5. Palpation of the amnion, 50-day pregnancy. The amnion can be trapped in the palm of the hand or between the fingers and the thumb by working gently up or down the pregnant horn of the uterus.

TABLE 1. *Estimation of Duration of Pregnancy Using Amnion*

Duration (days)	Metric (cm)	Width (fingers or hand)*
35	≃ 0.7	½ finger
42	≃ 1.5	1 finger
48	≃ 3.5	2 fingers
53	≃ 5.5	3 fingers
58	≃ 7.5	4 fingers
62	≃ 9.0	Hand less thumb
65	≃ 10.5	Hand and thumb

*Figures for average sized hand.

TABLE 2. *Estimation of Duration of Pregnancy by Fetal Crown-to-Nose Measurement*

Duration (days)	Metric (cm)	Size (fingers or hand)*
68–70	≈ 1.5	1 finger width (tip)
80	≈ 3.5	2 fingers width (tip)
90	≈ 5.5	3 fingers width (tip)
100	≈ 7.5	4 fingers width (tip)
110	≈ 9.0	Hand less thumb
120	≈ 10.5	Hand and thumb (5 fingers)

*Figures for average sized hand.

Palpation of Placentomes

Small placentomes can be palpated at 70 to 75 days. They become a more important diagnostic criterion as gestation advances because their increased size and the increased flaccidity of the uterus make them easier to palpate. They are not as good a criterion for estimating duration of gestation as measurement of fetal head size (see Table 3). There is a tendency to underestimate duration of gestation by palpation of placentomes. A frequent error by persons who fail to orient themselves is mistaking placentomes for ovaries or vice versa.

Palpation of the Fetus

The fetus cannot be palpated until the amnion becomes flaccid enough to allow this manipulation. This usually occurs at about 65 to 70 days. From this point on, palpation of the fetus is valuable for both positive diagnosis and timing of duration of gestation. Digital measurement of the fetal head size (crown-nose length) is especially valuable in this respect (Table 2). To accomplish this, the horn containing the most fluid is gently searched by manipulating it between the fingers and folded thumb until the head is encountered (see Figure 4). The head is then measured as

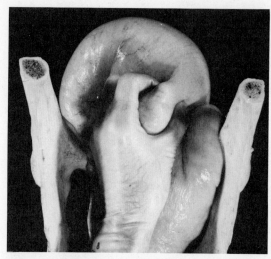

Figure 7. Palpation of the fetal head. After the head is located by manipulating the uterus between the fingers and folded thumb, it is measured as accurately as possible by finger-width comparison.

accurately as possible by finger-width comparison (Fig. 7, Table 3). This manipulation is safe when gently applied. Of 285 cows in which amnions (1/3) and fetal heads (2/3) were palpated, only one had aborted when the cows were repalpated 45 days later (Table 3). In many cows the fetus is out of reach between 5 and 7 months of gestation.

ESTIMATION OF DURATION OF GESTATION BY OTHER CRITERIA

Use of amnion and fetal head size for estimation of duration of gestation has been discussed. Palpation of some structures allows more accurate timing of stage of gestation than others (Table 4). In general, as gestation advances, estimation of duration becomes less precise because of physiological variation and difficulty in palpation of structures that allow more precise timing.

TABLE 3. *Accuracy of Pregnancy Diagnosis by Palpation of Amnion and Fetal Head*

Trial	No.	Duration of Pregnancy (days)	Method		Accuracy	
			AMNION	FETAL HEAD	AVE. MISS	RANGE
1	207	36–77	≈ 2/3	≈ 1/3	3.2	0–12
2	115	73–109	—	All	3.5	0–15
3	285	40–79	≈ 1/3	≈ 2/3	2.3	0–12

TABLE 4. *Estimation of Duration of Pregnancy in 175 Cows Bred 110 to 160 Days Prior to Palpation*

Structures Palpated	No.	Ave. Miss	Range
Head	85	5.3	0–12
Placentomes	18	7.8	0–18
MUA* and placentomes	13	9.2	1–30
Fetus-placentomes	31	7.8	1–25
Legs and MUA	11	7.2	0–12
Feet and legs	17	7.1	0–18

*MUA = middle uterine artery.

Palpation of the Middle Uterine Artery

Enlargement of the middle uterine artery can be palpated on the gravid side as early as 85 to 90 days of gestation. This artery is freely movable and lies in the area of the shaft of the ilium. Care should be taken to distinguish it from the external iliac artery that is attached to the ilium. The middle uterine artery progressively enlarges after the cow becomes pregnant (Table 5). Fremitus, the buzzing sensation resulting from turbulence produced by hypertrophy and rapid coursing of blood through the artery, can be palpated as early as 90 to 120 days after conception. The artery is held loosely between the fingers; too much digital pressure may produce a false fremitus. The artery is about the size of the small finger on the average hand by 6 months, the size of the middle finger by 7 months and thumb size by 8 to 8 1/2 months.

Size of the Uterus

Uterine size can be used to estimate the duration of gestation when the uterus can be retracted. The author has little confidence in this criterion, however. There is often considerable variation between the size of the uterus in two cows bred on the same day. Greater accuracy can be achieved by using amnion and fetal head measurements, since these structures are also palpable if the uterus is retractable.

Size of the Fetus

The crown-rump length of the fetus is related linearly with the age of the fetus.

When fetal length can be estimated accurately, duration of gestation can be calculated. The formula $\sqrt{L} \times 2$ (when L stands for length in inches) will give the approximate duration of pregnancy in months. It is, however, usually more difficult to estimate the total length of the fetus accurately than it is to measure the fetal head size.

Summary

The periods when cattlemen require accurately timed pregnancy diagnosis usually fall between 35 and 120 days. During these periods, quite precise estimations of duration of gestation can be made by measurement of the amnion and later the fetal head. Size of placentomes and estimations of fetal length can also be of some value during these times. During early pregnancy, determination of the size of the pregnant horn can be of value, although this is not as precise as the other methods. During later stages of pregnancy, determination of the size of the middle uterine arteries and of fetal parts such as the feet are of value; however, as the length of gestation increases, accuracy in timing decreases.

SOURCES OF ERROR IN PREGNANCY DIAGNOSIS

There are several sources of error in pregnancy diagnosis. The urinary bladder can be mistaken for the pregnant horn. However, the bladder is round (not tubular), has no cervix attached and has no bifurcation. The uterus is usually below and to the right of the urinary bladder. The rumen may likewise be mistaken for fetal parts. However, the rumen is doughy and is not attached to the cervix.

Several diseases of the uterus resemble pregnancy. Some of these are pyometra, hydrometra and various neoplastic growths and other pathological conditions of the uterus. When a fetus becomes mummified, it forms a hard mass in the uterus, but there are no fluids or membranes. Placentomes are also absent, and there is little or no enlargement of the middle uterine arteries. Adherence to the rules for positive diagnosis of pregnancy should avoid mistaking these conditions for pregnancy.

TABLE 5. *Changes during Gestation in the Cow*

Stage	Uterus	Fetus	Placentomes	Middle Uterine Arteries
30 days	Slight fluctuation, membranes can first be slipped	Cannot be palpated, owing to turgid amnion		No change
40 days	Pregnant horn 4–6 cm			Increased pulse
60 days	Pregnant horn 6–9 cm			Increased pulse
75 days	Starts over brim, pregnant horn 9–13 cm, begin boxing-glove stage	Ballot fetus	May be palpable, about 1 cm in diameter	
3 months	Pregnant horn 12–16 cm, may still be retractable	Fetus palpable, ≈ 13-cm long	2-cm diameter	Artery pencil size, fremitus in some cases
3½ months	Pregnant horn 14–20 cm, uterus less turgid, retraction difficult	Fetus palpable, ≈ 20-cm long		"
4 months	Not retractable	≈ 25-cm long, may be out of reach		Size of pencil, fremitus present, artery on nongravid side enlarged ≈ 1-cm diameter, fremitus distinct, tortuous, may find fremitus on nongravid side
5 months	On abdominal floor	May be out of reach		
6 months		Usually out of reach	Quite variable,	≈ 1.3-cm diameter, very distinct fremitus nongravid side ≈ 1-cm diameter
7 months		May be palpable	6 cm upward	"
8 months		Readily palpable, hoof well formed and reflexes good, incisors erupted in later stages	"	Distinct fremitus on nongravid side — ≈ 2-cm diameter

TABLE 6. *Effect of Palpation on Apparent Fetal Loss*

Apparent Loss	Fluctuance Only	Fluctuance plus Amnion	Fluctuance plus Membrane Slip	Totals
By Method[1]—No., Loss (%)	289 11 (3.8)[a]	333 20 (6.0)[ab]	307 28 (9.1)[b]	929 59 (6.4)
By Palpator[2]				
Palpator A Loss (%)	122 2 (1.6)	106 4 (3.8)	107 8 (7.5)	335 14 (4.2)[a]
Palpator B Loss (%)	75 4 (5.3)	91 5 (5.5)	99 8 (8.1)	265 17 (6.4)[ab]
Palpator C Loss (%)	79 5 (6.3)	126 11 (8.7)	87 11 (12.6)	292 27 (9.2)[b]
By Time of Palpation[3]				
35–51 days Loss (%)	140 6 (4.3)	206 16 (7.8)	136 19 (14.0)	482 41 (8.5)[a]
52–70 days Loss (%)	136 5 (3.7)	117 2 (1.7)	157 8 (5.1)	410 15 (3.7)[b]
Time of Abortion[4]				
Cows calving after palpation X̄ days to abort	265 51.8	305 50.0[a]	266 53.3[c]	836 51.6
Cows not calving after palpation X̄ days to abort	11 50.2	18 45.9[b]	27 49.2[d]	56 48.3

[1]Within row, values with different superscripts are different, $P < 0.025$.
[2]Within column, values with different superscripts are different, $P < 0.025$.
[3]Within column, values with different superscripts are different, $P < 0.05$.
[4]Within columns, values with different superscripts are different: a, b $P < 0.05$; c, d $P < 0.01$.

ABORTION INDUCED BY PALPATION

Palpation should be as gentle as possible. Previous work has indicated no difference in fetal attrition following palpation of the amnion compared with fetal membrane slip.[2] However, there was a slightly better survival associated with amnion palpation. In work being carried out at Colorado State University, we have found a similar trend.[1] However, palpation for fluctuance alone in cows in which a breeding date was recorded resulted in less fetal attrition than either amnion or fetal membrane palpation. It appears that the trauma induced by palpation of the amnion and especially of the fetal membranes may be a significant iatrogenic cause of fetal attrition. Rates of iatrogenic fetal attrition are relatively low for all methods. However, these manipulations should be carried out both gently, and efficiently. The effect of palpation on apparent fetal loss is presented in Table 6.

REFERENCES

1. Abbitt, B., Ball, L., Kitts, G. P., Sitzman, C., Wilgenburg, B., Raim, L. W. and Seidel, G. E., Jr.: Effect of three methods of palpation for pregnancy diagnosis per rectum on embryonic and fetal attrition in cows. J.A.V.M.A., *173*:973, 1978.
2. Callaghan, C. J.: Clinical observations on normal and abnormal reproduction in the dairy cow. Southwest. Vet., *XXII*:193, 1969.
3. Roberts, S. J.: Veterinary Obstetrics and Genital Diseases (Theriogenology). Ann Arbor, Mich., Edwards Brothers, Inc., 1971.
4. Zemjanis, R.: Diagnostic and Therapeutic Techniques in Animal Reproduction. Baltimore, The Williams and Wilkins Co., 1970.

Parturition Induction in Cattle

WILLIAM C. WAGNER
University of Illinois, Urbana, Illinois

GENERAL COMMENTS

In using glucocorticoids for induction of parturition in cattle, the same considerations should be kept in mind as always apply when administering these potent medications. Utilization of highly potent glucocorticoids may result in alterations of the leukocyte patterns, with an increase in circulating neutrophils and a decrease in the circulating lymphocytes that may persist for 1 to 3 days after a single injection. In addition, the animal usually will experience an elevated glucose level as a result of the gluconeogenic activity of the preparation used, as well as altered immunological responses.

Of particular concern in using these agents is the potential for retention of the fetal membranes following this premature parturition and the possibility of sequelae such as metritis that may occur. For this reason the glucocorticoid preparations most frequently used for induction of parturition in cattle carry a label warning specifically stating that the use of this preparation in late pregnancy is contraindicated. Because of this, the veterinarian should be careful to explain the possible effects and sequelae of such treatment to the owner prior to administration. Should undesirable side effects occur, the practitioner is considered to be the sole legally liable individual, since the drug company has already stated its position by giving this contraindication warning.

INDICATIONS

The timing of administration of these materials for parturition induction should be such that the calf will have a normal or near normal opportunity for survival. This generally means that one should time the administration of the drug so that the calf is born no more than 14 days prior to the expected date of parturition. A rule of thumb that has proved useful in field trials is to inject animals that are within 7 to 14 days of calving and then repeat this treatment in the next group 1 week later and so on until all of the animals have been treated. In this way animals are grouped for parturition, but the possibility of any significant number of animals calving more than approximately 12 days prematurely is eliminated. The other reason for timing the treatment at this stage is due to the changing sensitivity of the animal's system to glucocorticoids, i.e., treatment earlier in pregnancy might require a somewhat higher dosage to accomplish the same objective. Treatment with glucocorticoids requires the presence of a live fetus and a functional placenta. Thus it will not be of value in cases of mummified fetus.

THERAPEUTIC AGENTS AND EXPECTED RESULTS

Glucocorticoids

There are several types of glucocorticoid preparations that are available on the market that can be utilized for early induction of parturition in cattle. Most of the experience within the United States has been with the so-called short-acting preparations such as dexamethasone (Azium) or flumethasone (Flucort, Methagon). However in other areas, e.g., Europe, New Zealand and Australia, somewhat longer-acting preparations have been utilized that in general are of the dexamethasone trimethylacetate form or similar types of preparations. These are discussed separately as follows:

Short-acting Glucocorticoids

Dosage and Route of Administration. The dosage for dexamethasone is a minimum of 20 mg given as a single intramuscular injection. In some studies a dosage of 30 mg given as a single injection has yielded a higher rate of efficacy and may be preferable if one is handling large numbers of animals, in which case repeat treatments are less desirable. The dosage for flumethasone, either the Flucort or Methagon preparation, would be approximately 7.5 mg per animal, given as a single intramuscular injection.

Response. The response to these glucocorticoids usually is quite prompt. One can observe changes in the reproductive tract, including pelvic ligament relaxation, dilation of the vaginal canal and relaxation of the cervix, occurring rapidly within the 24 to 48 hours following injection. Usually parturition occurs in less than 70 hours after treatment, with the average interval being approximately 40 to 48 hours postinjection. Labor is usually uneventful, and expulsion of the fetus occurs quite readily. Calving difficulty scores that have been recorded during induced parturition in cattle have not indicated a significant increase or decrease in the scores, although there is frequently a higher incidence of minor aid or assistance given. We believe this reflects the fact that there is someone present observing the parturition and therefore is likely to give aid, even in situations in which it is not an absolute necessity.

Long-acting Glucocorticoids

Dosage and Route of Administration. These materials are given by intramuscular injection, usually in the amount of 20 mg of the dexamethasone preparation.

Response. Parturition will occur between 5 and 10 days following the injection, with the shorter interval occurring in those animals that are treated nearer to the expected date of parturition. Again, the usual signs of impending parturition can be observed, including pelvic relaxation, dilation of the birth canal and so forth.

Sequelae and Aftercare

Neonatal Survival. There is no indication of decreased survival rates in the calves resulting from induced parturition. Although there is some disagreement, it appears that induced parturition calves are able to attain normal levels of gamma globulin. Since there is a likelihood of large numbers of newborn calves being present within a small, confined area, it is possible for epidemics of diarrhea or pneumonia to occur. This does not indicate increased susceptibility but rather increased ease of transmission because of the concentration of a susceptible population. Usually if animals begin showing signs of diarrhea or pneumonia, rapid movement and dispersal of calves and dams over a larger area on pasture will result in prompt diminution of the problem and normal survival rates. The growth rate of the calves also seems to be normal, as demonstrated in those studies in which growth rates have been computed.

Placental Retention. There is a rather high rate of placental retention in most animals undergoing induced parturition, especially with the short-acting glucocorticoids. The retention of the fetal membrane seems to be the result of premature parturition rather than the induction procedure *per se* and may be alleviated by treatment with high doses of estrogenic hormones. The induction of parturition with long-acting glucocorticoids does not seem to result in the previously mentioned high incidence of placental retention, and this may be related to the increased period of time during which estrogen secretion can increase, resulting in normal or near normal estrogen levels at the time of onset of labor. As demonstrated by Grunert, it would appear that this final increase in estrogen is important in altering the attachment of the placenta in the cow and rendering it more easily expelled during the normal parturition (see reference below).

Fertility. Fertility following induced parturition appears to be unaffected. In the study reported by Wagner et al.[5] the conception rate in induced animals was identical with the conception rate observed in the same herd prior to and following the year during which parturition induction was performed. Furthermore, the fertility of induced animals does not seem to be altered by the retention of the placenta when compared with induced animals in which the placenta is expelled at the normal time. Studies on uterine histology have indicated a slight delay in uterine repair in the early postpartum period, but later on (40 to 50 days postpartum) the uterine repair seems to have occurred normally, and one cannot distinguish between induced and normal parturition animals.

Milk Secretion. The mammary glands seem to become well developed during this rapid induction process and will demonstrate filling with milk at the time of labor. The actual secretion of milk may not be as plentiful at the very onset, but there is no indication that total milk production is decreased when the entire lactation period is compared between natural and induced parturition cattle.

Prostaglandins

Although not yet cleared for clinical use, prostaglandins, especially those such as prostaglandin-$F_{2\alpha}$ ($PFG_{2\alpha}$), can be used for parturition induction in cattle. The dosage required for parturition induction is similar to that required for destruction of the corpus luteum in the cyclic bovine female. Thus a single injection of 20 mg of active $PGF_{2\alpha}$ should be sufficient to initiate parturition. The response is quite similar to that observed when using short-acting glucocorticoids, with parturition occurring at approximately 40 to 48 hours and with a significant incidence of placental retention occurring. Thus, for induction of parturition in normal animals there does not appear to be any significant advantage in using prostaglandins as compared with use of the short-acting glucocorticoids.

Other potential uses for prostaglandins that should be mentioned include their application in cases of fetal mummification. The glucocorticoids apparently require a viable fetus and placenta in order to exert their effect, whereas prostaglandins do not have this requirement in the cow. Therefore, one can initiate expulsion of a dead fetus or a mummified fetus with prostaglandins in the cow, whereas treatment of these cases with glucocorticoid preparations has been shown to be ineffective.

REFERENCES

1. Bailey, L. F., McLennan, M. W., McLean, D. M., Hartford, P. R. and Munro, G. L.: The use of dexamethasone trimethylacetate to advance parturition in dairy cows. Austral. Vet. J., *49*:567, 1973.
2. Carroll, E. J.: Induction of parturition in farm animals. J. Anim. Sci. (Suppl. I), *38*:1, 1974.
3. Kordts, E. and Jöchle, W.: Induced parturition in daily cattle: A comparison of a corticoid (flumethasone) and a prostaglandin ($PGF_{2\alpha}$) in different age groups. Theriogenology, *3*:171, 1975.
4. Muller, L. D., Beardsley, G L., Ellis, R. P., Reed, D. E. and Owens, M. J.: Calf response to the initiation of parturition in dairy cows with dexamethasone or dexamethasone with estradiol benzoate. J. Anim. Sci., *41*:1711, 1975.
5. Wagner, W. C., Willham, R. L. and Evans, L. E.: Controlled parturition in cattle. J. Anim. Sci., *38*:485, 1974.

Elective Termination of Unwanted and Pathological Gestation

LESLIE BALL

Colorado State University,
Fort Collins, Colorado

ARIE BRAND

State University of Utrecht,
Utrecht, The Netherlands

From time to time the veterinarian is requested to terminate gestation in cows. This can be accomplished by several different methods that are time dependent. For example, during the period from conception to about 5 months, the maintenance of pregnancy is dependent on progesterone produced by the corpus luteum. Either inhibition of production of progesterone by drug-induced luteolysis or by manual expression of the corpus luteum during this period produces abortion.

During the period from about 5 to 8 months, abortion is more difficult to induce. Extragonadal sources may supply progesterone during this period and help maintain pregnancy; thus, methods that cause luteolysis no longer work well. Neither is the fetoplacental unit mature enough yet to respond consistently to treatments that induce premature parturition. However, methods that activate mechanisms involved at normal parturition can be utilized after about 8 months of gestation. An advanced degree of placental maturation appears to be necessary; therefore, these methods are most effective only during the last month of normal gestation. Glucocorticoids and prostaglandins have been used to induce abortion during this period of gestation. They are also effective in some cases of pathological prolonged gestation in which the fetus is alive and the fetoplacental unit is viable.

A third mechanism for producing abortion is initiated by destruction of the fetus, which then becomes a foreign body to be expelled from the uterus. Mechanical methods that kill the fetus can be applied only during times when the uterus is easily retracted and while the fetus is relatively small. Consequently, they are limited to the second and third months of gestation.

The rapidity of action of different treatments is noteworthy. Following administration of prostaglandins or manual removal of the corpus luteum, abortion usually occurs on approximately the fifth day but may be delayed until the tenth day or longer after treatment with estrogens. In contrast, when the amnion is ruptured or the fetus is decapitated, abortion may take several weeks to occur. The typical differences in progesterone levels and times of abortion following treatment with estradiol valerate and prostaglandin-$F_{2\alpha}$ ($PGF_{2\alpha}$) are illustrated in Figure 1. Prostaglandin-$F_{2\alpha}$ causes a more rapid decline in blood progesterone levels and earlier abortion. It is likely that the mechanisms of induction of luteolysis are different in the two drugs; perhaps the estrogens must stimulate production or release of endogenous prostaglandins before luteolysis occurs.

In cattle, the indications for elective interruption of gestation can be classified into three categories: (1) mismating; (2) pathological gestation such as hydrops of fetal membranes, mummification or maceration of the fetus or prolonged pathological gestation and (3) induced parturition as a managment tool. The first two indications will be the subject of this article.

MISMATING

Interruption of pregnancy is desirable when an animal has been either mismated

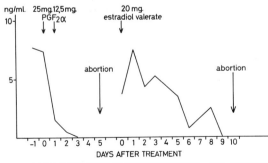

BLOOD PROGESTERONE AFTER ADMINISTRATION OF PGF₂α AND ESTRADIOL VALERATE IN TWO ANIMALS PREGNANT FOR 4,5 AND 5 MONTHS RESPECTIVELY

Figure 1. Differences in progesterone levels and times of abortion following treatment with estradiol valerate and $PGF_{2\alpha}$.

to an unwanted male or mated prematurely so that dystocia is likely to occur at the end of a gestation of normal length. The treatment chosen will be affected by duration of gestation, date planned for breeding or rebreeding, acceptable fertility, health risk, post-treatment performance and success rate. Treatments are primarily presented relative to duration of gestation, but the other factors will also be discussed.

Early Treatment after an Observed Breeding

Some mismated cows fail to conceive and may come into estrus if given sufficient time. Such expectant treatment can be used only if estrous detection is adequate and sufficient time is available between the time of mismating and the time desired for rebreeding because the cow must still be aborted if she happens to be pregnant. This approach has the advantage of not influencing the reproductive system by unnecessary treatments. Its major disadvantage is loss of time if the cow is pregnant.

If a cow fails to come into heat following a breeding, she can be treated either immediately or after a later examination for pregnancy. A mismated cow or heifer that should be bred soon to another sire requires a different approach to save time. The method selected should bring her into a fertile estrus as soon as possible.

Development of the conceptus can usually be halted by infusion of the uterus if the time of mismating is known. Irritant drugs such as 20 to 50 ml of 1 to 2 per cent Lugol's solution or 500 mg of tetracycline in 30 to 50 ml of saline have been used successfully. The infusion should be done on or soon after day 4 postestrus. Earlier infusion is less likely to destroy the conceptus because it may not yet be in the uterus. Uterine infusion with irritant drugs at appropriate times may also cause luteolysis, terminating gestation. Infusion should probably not be used after day 11 because the estrous cycle may be lengthened in open cows, resulting in further loss of time.

Thirty mg of $PGF_{2\alpha}$ given intramuscularly or 5 mg by intrauterine infusion after the fifth day postmating will cause regression of the corpus luteum and interrupt pregnancy. Infusion in the uterine horn ipsilateral to the corpus luteum is most effective.

Treatment with estrogens within 1 or 2 days after the mismating will usually prevent further gestation by interfering with ova transport and alteration of the uterine biochemical environment. Four to 8 mg of estradiol valerate or 40 to 80 mg of diethylstilbestrol is given intramuscularly. The effects of $PGF_{2\alpha}$ and estradiol valerate administration on serum progesterone levels are illustrated in Figure 1. The reduction in serum progesterone is associated with regression of the corpus luteum with both drugs.

Oxytocin, 100 to 200 mg/day, given from days 2 through 7, also causes regression of the corpus luteum, but this treatment is inconvenient and impractical. Manual enucleation of the corpus luteum will also terminate pregnancy but may be associated with ovarian adhesions, excessive maternal bleeding and even death. For these reasons it should not be used.

Injection of prostaglandins or infusion of the uterus with irritant drugs is probably the best method to stimulate early return to a fertile estrus after mismating. Estrogen treatments are associated with slower return to fertile estrus and may also cause development of cystic follicles. Uterine infusion is fairly effective and inexpensive but requires more time and skill than injection with hormones. Thus, drug effectiveness and technical competence, as well as economics, must be considered by the veterinarian when selecting a treatment.

With any of these methods, the cow should be re-examined 35 to 50 days after the mismating to make certain that abortion has occurred.

Treatment between 1 and 5 Months

Induction of abortion in cattle pregnant for 1 to 5 months is requested for different reasons. The treatment method may vary, depending on whether the cow is to be used as a breeding or a feeder (slaughter) animal. Fertility is not important in feeder heifers, allowing a wider latitude in selection of treatment.

The date of mismating may be unknown in some cows. In others, the cattleman fails to call a veterinarian when the mismating is observed. For prognostic reasons, the duration of gestation should be estimated as

accurately as possible when it is unknown because the success of treatment is decreased in some cows pregnant more than 5 months. Retained placenta, dystocia and metritis are also more likely to occur if abortion is induced as gestation advances. Thus, it is important to induce abortion as soon as possible in mismated breeding cows to obtain highest fertility following treatment.

Induced Abortion in the Breeding Cow

Prostaglandins are effective abortifacients in breeder cattle during the first 4 months of pregnancy. Single intramuscular dosages of 45 mg of $PGF_{2\alpha}$ are usually effective. Split intramuscular dosages of 25 mg the first day and 15 mg the second are more effective.

Prostaglandins are probably the drugs of choice for producing abortion in breeding cows during the first 4 months of gestation. The fetus is expelled at an earlier time and in a better state of preservation than with estrogens. There also seem to be fewer complications caused by metritis and retained placenta, and the postabortion health of the dam is thus improved.

Manual rupture of the amniotic sac (amnion) or manipulative decapitation, or both, can be used to terminate pregnancy effectively in cows between their thirtieth and ninetieth days of gestation. Abortion usually occurs between the fourteenth and thirty-fifth days after either of these manipulations. In contrast, enucleation of the corpus luteum results in rapid abortion and return to estrus. This difference in response is probably related to progesterone production, which is terminated abruptly by enucleation of the corpus luteum. A functional corpus luteum is probably maintained for a period of time after either fetal decapitation or rupture of the amnion. Fetal membranes may also continue to grow for a short time after rupture of the amnion.

Abortion rates approaching 100 per cent have been obtained after rupture of the amnion between days 30 and 65. Location of the amnion by an unskilled person is often a more difficult task than its rupture once it is found. Failure to abort probably results most often from failure to find and rupture the vesicle properly.

The uterus is first retracted and then searched carefully by palpating the fluc-

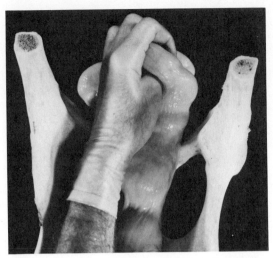

Figure 2. The amnion is located by palpating the fluctuant part of the pregnant horn between the cupped fingers and folded thumb.

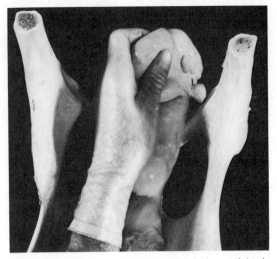

Figure 3. When located, the amniotic vesicle is trapped between the fingers and thumb and squeezed until it is felt to rupture. The fetus is then traumatized between the fingers and thumb.

tuant part of the pregnant horn between the cupped fingers and thumb (Fig. 2). The amnion is usually located in the part of the uterus containing the most fluid. When located, the amniotic sac is squeezed until it is felt to rupture (Fig. 3); then the fetus is traumatized between the fingers and thumb to insure fetal death and abortion.

Manipulative decapitation terminated pregnancy successfully in 100 per cent of 47 heifers pregnant 65 to 90 days. After 90 days, this method becomes more and more complicated because the fetus is often difficult to locate and position properly and the

fetal skeleton becomes more resistant to trauma.

The decapitation manipulation is illustrated in Figures 4, 5 and 6. By palpation of the pregnant horn between the dorsal surface of the flexed thumb and the fingers (Fig. 4), the fetal head and neck are located (Fig. 5). The neck is positioned between the forefinger and thumb, and the fetal head is separated from its body by pressure (Fig. 6). Abortion usually occurs within 2 to 4 weeks (Fig. 7).

The use of decapitation to terminate pregnancy in mismated cows is sometimes

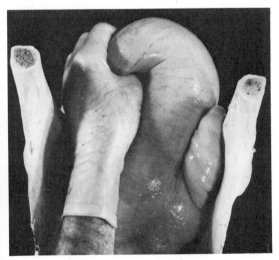

Figure 4. Location of the fetal head, phase 1. The pregnant horn is palpated between the flexed thumb and fingers until the fetal head is located.

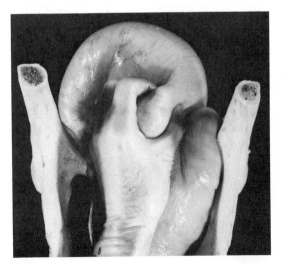

Figure 5. The fetal head and neck are located and secured between the fingers and thumb.

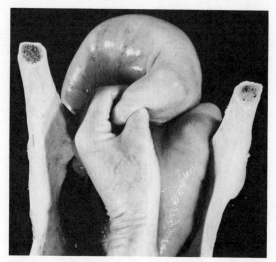

Figure 6. The fetal head is separated from the body by squeezing the neck between the fingers and folded thumb.

complicated by subsequent mummification, whereas rupture of the amnion is not. Mummification is rarely seen in beef heifers, but two of four Holstein dairy heifers pregnant about 100 days developed mummification following fetal decapitation (Ball, unpublished data).

The corpus luteum can be located by *per-rectal* palpation and enucleated into the abdominal cavity in cows less than 6 months pregnant. Abortion usually occurs about 5 days later. This method has several disadvantages, as indicated earlier. Bleeding becomes more copious as gestation progresses, and the corpus luteum is more difficult to express than at earlier

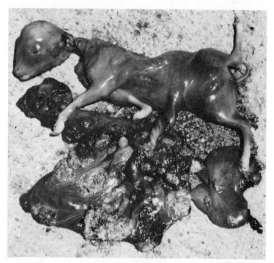

Figure 7. Abortion usually occurs within 2 to 4 weeks. The fetus and membranes may be somewhat autolyzed when the abortion occurs.

times. Fatal hemorrhage is more likely to occur in cows that have corpora lutea expressed late in gestation. For these reasons, as well as for those listed earlier, this method cannot be recommended as a routine manipulation, since better methods are now available.

Many cows pregnant 1 to 5 months will abort following a single intramuscular injection of 20 mg of estradiol benzoate, estradiol valerate or cyclopentylpropionate, and most will abort if the treatment is repeated in 4 days. Repository diethylstilbestrol in intramuscular dosages of 100 to 175 mg will also usually cause abortion. The smaller dosages are given to heifers pregnant 90 days or less; successively larger dosages are given as gestation and cow size increase. Treatment with diethylstilbestrol can often be repeated with successful results in cattle that fail to abort following the first injection.

There are significant disadvantages to the use of estrogens as abortifacients in breeding cows. Abortion is usually slow to occur, and the fetus is often aborted in a decomposed condition. Fetal membranes are more likely to be retained at later stages of gestation, and metritis occurs more often than with abortion induced with prostaglandins.

Induced Abortion in the Feeder Heifer

It is sometimes desirable to terminate gestation in feeder heifers. Nonpregnant (open) feeder heifers usually command a higher price at the time that they are purchased for the feedlot than heifers that cannot be guaranteed open. In addition, pregnant heifers that calve toward the end of a feeding period may be excessively fat, increasing the likelihood of death of both the calf and heifer. Postpartum uterine infections that decrease efficiency of postabortion gain are also commonly observed. Finally, pregnancy in feeder heifers may decrease efficiency of marketable gain, and dressing percentage is lower than in open heifers.

An ideal treatment for aborting feedlot heifers should be effective over a wide range of fetal ages, require a single, time-efficient application and be economical to use. The methods used to produce abortion in breeding cattle work as well in feedlot heifers, but each fails to meet at least one criterion for an ideal treatment at this time.

Prostaglandins appear to be potentially the most satisfactory drugs for this purpose, but current costs and restrictions by some governmental agencies will limit their use until these aspects change. Prostaglandins should then find wide acceptance as abortifacients in feedlot heifers.

Repository diethylstilbestrol has been widely used in the past for aborting feedlot heifers, but governmental restraints now prevent this usage in some countries. The esters of estradiol are fairly effective in causing regression of the corpus luteum and inducing abortion, but the dose levels required are high and they are not as effective in single dose treatments as repository diethylstilbestrol or prostaglandins. The major disadvantages of estrogenic hormones for inducing abortion in feedlot cattle are increased postpartum metritis and, possibly, decreased economic efficiency in treated cattle.

Pregnancy examination coupled with fetal decapitation or manual rupture of the amnion, when possible, is indicated prior to administration of any of the abortifacient drugs to feedlot heifers. Drug costs are reduced, and the feeder heifer is not subjected to potentially disruptive drugs if this procedure is followed. The disadvantages of manual methods are restriction of usage over a limited range of fetal ages and the requirement of special palpation skill.

Induced Abortion in Late Gestation

Almost any potent estrogen will cause abortion in late gestation if given persistently enough in large enough quantities. Daily dosages of 10 to 20 mg of esters of estradiol or 50 to 150 mg of diethylstilbestrol are usually effective after a period of time. Estrogens that must be given repeatedly are not practical for inducing abortion in feedlot heifers more than 5 months into gestation. Massive or repeated doses of glucocorticoids have also been used but are expensive and not too dependable in producing parturition until the last few weeks of gestation.

Since complications of metritis and retained placenta are common sequelae to abortions induced in late gestation with estrogens, the prognosis for fertility is decreased in breeding cattle and the perfor- mance of feeder heifers is sometimes reduced. These aspects should be considered before abortion is induced in either feeding or breeding cattle after 6 months of gestation.

Alternatives to induced abortion are either careful observation as calving time approaches followed by cesarean section if necessary or induced parturition 2 to 3 weeks before term. Dystocia may not be decreased by induced parturition near term, but the need for cesarean section is more often eliminated.

INDUCED ABORTION IN PATHOLOGICAL GESTATION

Pathological gestation must often be terminated. Examples of conditions that sometimes require termination are hydrops amnion and allantois, mummified or macerated fetus and some cases of prolonged pathological gestation of either genetic or nongenetic (teratogenic) origin.

Hydrops of the Fetal Membranes

Hydrops allantois is characterized by rapid enlargement of the abdomen, usually in late gestation. On *per-rectal* palpation, the uterus is swollen and turgid, and the fetus and placentomes are difficult or impossible to palpate. The uterus fills the abdomen, and its bifurcation is usually easy to palpate because of uterine swelling. If hydrops allantois is allowed to continue to develop, the prepubic tendon may rupture. Few cows survive when the disease has progressed to this point.

In contrast, hydrops amnion is characterized by slowly developing enlargement of the abdomen and a flaccid uterus in which the fetus and placentomes are usually easy to palpate *per rectum.*

Salvage slaughter should be considered in all cases of hydrops allantois because it is often complicated by dystocia, retained fetal membranes, severe metritis and shock at the time of either induced or natural parturition. Dehydration is also a fairly constant complication, requiring heroic fluid therapy in many cases. If the cow survives, lactation is usually depressed, and the prognosis for fertility is unfavorable.

Induction of Abortion by Drainage of Chorioallantoic Fluids

Puncture of the chorioallantoic membranes through the cervix induces drainage but also introduces bacteria into the uterus. Metritis and fetal maceration often develop; therefore, this method should not be used. A surgical approach is less likely to introduce bacteria into the uterus. A site is prepared for aseptic surgery in the right lower flank. A sterile trocar and cannula are inserted about 10 to 15 cm above the lower margin of the right flank fold through the abdominal wall into the chorionic sac, and the fluid is drained at a rate not exceeding 1 liter per minute. Care should be taken to insert the trocar into a location unoccupied by the fetus. In rare instances, cows recover following initial drainage of 15 to 20 liters of fluid; thus, this method may be tried in early cases. Removal of 30 to 50 liters of fluid usually induces abortion in 24 to 72 hours; if not, treatment may be repeated in 2 days.

Induction of Abortion by Use of Drugs

Parturition in cases of hydrops of fetal membranes can often be induced with the glucocorticoids dexamethasone (20 to 40 mg) and flumethasone (10 to 20 mg) in single or repeated intramuscular treatments. Lower dosages will often induce abortion, but success rates increase with the dosages just recommended. The veterinarian should be aware that these dosages are above those recommended by the manufacturers for routine treatments, and these drugs are not approved for this purpose in some countries. Prostaglandins are also usually effective; $PGF_{2\alpha}$ is given in intramuscular dosages of 30 to 45 mg. The dosages should be at the higher levels recommended for all of these drugs if gestation is less than 8½ months at the time of treatment. If the cow is refractory to the first treatment, the injection should be repeated at the higher levels after 48 hours. Estrogens have also been used to induce parturition in cases of dropsy of the fetal membranes but are not as satisfactory as glucocorticoids or $PGF_{2\alpha}$.

Clinical Aspects

The abdominal press may sometimes be absent with hydrops, possibly owing to the large atonic uterus that may be unable to push the fetus into the birth canal and stimulate the abdominal press. Maternal debility and sometimes failure of the cervix or birth canal, or both, to dilate may also be factors associated with depressed labor. In any event, the fetus may be difficult to reach in the standing cow when attempts are made to assist delivery. Success can usually be attained if the cow is induced to lie down.

The final delivery may be by either forced extraction or fetotomy. Assisted delivery should always be practiced as early as possible to decrease the likelihood of fatal complications following treatment. Cesarean section is usually contraindicated. The prognosis for cesarean section is unfavorable because the uterus is atonic and friable and fetal membranes are almost always retained. Metritis is also commonly observed, and the cow usually dies.

Fetal ascites, anasarca or maceration is frequently observed with hydrops allantois. These conditions seem to occur more often with single than with twin fetuses and may complicate delivery.

Prognosis

The prognosis for treatment of hydrops allantois by the surgical method is guarded but may be more favorable than with drug-induced abortion, according to data from the obstetrical clinic at Utrecht, the Netherlands.[7] Of 12 cows recently treated by the surgical method, eight recovered (breeding data were not available), two were salvaged by slaughter and two died. Parturition was successfully induced in all 12 cows; several required a second application of the treatment. Attempts were also made to induce parturition in five cows with dexamethasone and three with prostaglandins. Induction was successful in three of the five given dexamethasone and in all three given prostaglandins. One cow given dexamethasone died with a macerated fetus without going into labor, and another required the aseptic surgical technique described on this page to induce parturition after induction by dexamethasone was unsuccessful.

Three of six cows in which drug induction was successful died postpartum, and a fourth had to be slaughtered. Hypovolemic shock was the cause of death in two cows in which parturition was induced with PGF$_{2\alpha}$.

Fetal Mummification and Maceration

Fetal mummification or maceration should be suspected when the cow's abdomen does not enlarge at term or when she does not deliver a calf at the expected time after being diagnosed pregnant; anestrus is also present. The owner may request veterinary examination because premonitory signs of parturition do not develop as the cow approaches term. In fact, the mummified or macerated fetus is often carried beyond term.

The diagnosis is verified by rectal palpation. A firm mass may be felt in the uterus, but fluctuation and fremitus of the middle uterine arteries are absent. Neither placentomes nor fetal membranes can be palpated, but the head and sunken orbits of a fetal mummy can often be felt if the entire uterus can be retracted far enough. Retraction may be hindered because weight of the fetal mummy or macerated fetus often carries the uterus beyond reach, making differential diagnosis difficult.

Cervical forceps may be used to assist in the retraction procedure. The forceps is passed through the vagina to the cervix in closed position. One of the jaws is inserted into the external cervical os, the other into the fornix of the vagina and the forceps closed securely. Gentle traction on the handles assisted by *per-rectal* traction against the cervix will usually retract the uterus into position for palpation. A macerated fetus can present difficulties in differential diagnosis. Crepitation is usually present with a macerated fetus and is produced when the bones of the fetus rub or knock against each other on palpation. Examination of the cervix through a vaginal speculum is also helpful at times. A purulent discharge may be observed when a macerated fetus is present; this discharge may also soil the perineum and tail of the cow.

Fetal mummification has been treated with both estrogens and prostaglandins. Fifty mg of diethylstilbestrol or 5 to 10 mg of estradiol in a single dose will often cause expulsion of a mummified fetus. Repeated daily dosages of 50 mg of diethylstilbestrol will almost always result in expulsion, but overall dosages may be excessive by this method, ranging up to 800 mg in some instances. Expulsion of the mummy can be expected between the second and fourth day following a single injection in about 80 per cent of cows. Repository diethylstilbestrol in dosages of 100 to 150 mg has also been used.

Prostaglandin-F$_{2\alpha}$ has also been fairly effective in promoting expulsion of mummified fetuses. It has been given as an intrauterine treatment, 10.5 to 45 mg infused into the horn ipsilateral to the corpus luteum, or as an intramuscular injection of 25 to 35 mg. Expulsion of the mummy usually occurs in 3 to 4 days when this treatment is effective.

Whether estrogens or PGF$_{2\alpha}$ is used, expulsion of the mummy may not be complete. It is sometimes retained in the cervix, requiring manual or instrumental removal. Gentle manual dilation and teasing of the fetus through the cervix may be successful. Manipulation with a cervical forceps or obstetrical tongs will also sometimes allow delivery under these conditions.

Treatment of the cow with a chronic macerated fetus is seldom indicated. Damage to the endometrium is severe, and the cow seldom recovers enough to become pregnant again if the macerated fetus is expelled. In addition, treatment for removal of the contents is often not successful; therefore, salvage slaughter is usually indicated.

Dairymen sometimes insist on treatment of valuable cows. Large doses of diethylstilbestrol are sometimes effective in causing expulsion of the macerated fetus. Vandeplassche and coworkers[8] used 120 to 1400 mg of diethylstilbestrol divided into four to six doses given at 2-day intervals in five cows and obtained expulsion of the macerated fetus in two of them. Prostaglandins might also be used for this purpose, but it is unlikely that success would be much better. The structureless nature of the macerated fetus prevents its expulsion in most cows, even though the corpus luteum is regressed by the treatment.

Prolonged Pathological Gestation

Prolonged pathological gestation can be suspected when the cow fails to develop premonitory signs of parturition toward the end of a normal gestation period. There is little softening of the sacrosciatic ligaments, and the udder remains flaccid. The abdomen may continue to enlarge if a fetal giant is the cause of the prolonged gestation.

Prolonged gestation may result if either the fetal pituitary or the adrenal glands are hypoplastic. The bovine fetus may not become excessively large when the pituitary gland is hypoplastic, probably owing to lack of growth hormone, but continues to grow if the adrenal glands are hypoplastic.

These conditions can be either hereditary or congenital; many of the latter may be associated with ingestion of poisons that affect pituitary growth at critical periods during gestation. An example is the ingestion by sheep of *Veratrum californicum* on the fourteenth day of gestation. The fetus develops cyclopia and other head defects associated with prolonged gestation caused by faulty pituitary function. The fetal hypothalamic-pituitary-adrenal axis does not function properly in initiation of parturition; thus, gestation is prolonged. If prolonged gestation with fetal overgrowth is allowed to progress too long, it becomes impossible for the dam to deliver the fetus *per vaginam* and cesarean section is required. However, if parturition is induced by treatment of the cow with corticosteroids before 290 days of gestation, the fetus can often be extracted *per vaginam*. Dexamethasone (20 mg) or flumethasone (10 mg) will usually induce parturition. These dosages exceed the maximum levels recommended by manufacturers of these drugs.

PROLONGED NORMAL GESTATION

A major problem encountered by the veterinarian when prolonged gestation is suspected is reliability of breeding dates. A livestock owner may erroneously believe that a cow has a prolonged gestation if he fails to record a rebreeding date and then forgets that the cow was rebred. If a breeding date has been misrecorded by 21 days, induction of parturition at 290 days of gestation based on the recorded date will still result in a viable calf. However, if parturition is induced too soon in such a cow, the likelihood of neonatal death loss is increased.

When prolonged normal or pathological gestation is suspected, a careful *per-rectal* palpation should be performed. Fetal size and location, size of middle uterine arteries and placentomes and enlargement and softening of the cervix should be determined. Cows that have normal, slightly extended gestation periods have the usual external premonitory signs of parturition; those with pathological prolonged gestation do not. Parturition should be induced as soon as possible if the cow is in prolonged gestation, provided she is less than 300 days pregnant. If gestation is much extended, cesarean section should be performed without delay.

Normal gestation can be prolonged up to 2 weeks. Calves born from such gestations are likely to be larger than average and more often require cesarean section. Induction of parturition will usually reduce the percentage of cows requiring cesarean section and thus may be indicated if the owner is certain of the breeding date. Induction of normal parturition has been discussed in the preceding article.

REFERENCES

1. Ball, L. and Carroll, E. J.: Induction of fetal death in cattle by manual rupture of the amniotic vesicle. J.A.V.M.A., *142*:373, 1963.
2. Brand, A., de Bois, C. H. W. and Vandehende, R.: Indicaties voor prostaglandinen op het gebied van de voortplanting van landbouwhuisdieren. Tijdschr. Diergeneesk (Neth. J. Vet. Sci.), *100*:191, 1975.
3. Carroll, E. J.: Induction of parturition in farm animals. J. Anim. Sci. (Suppl. 1), *38*:1, 1974.
4. Dawson, F. L. M.: Methods for early termination of pregnancy in the cow. Vet. Rec., *94*:542, 1974.
5. Grunert, Von, E., Andresen, P. and Ahlers, D.: Moglichkeiten der konzeptionsverhutung der abortauslosung oder der vorzeiteigen gebutseinleitung beim rind. Dtsch. Teiraztl. Wschr., *81*:549, 1974.
6. Roberts, S. J.: Veterinary Obstetrics and Genital Diseases (Theriogenology). 2nd Ed. Ann Arbor, Mich., Edwards Brothers, Inc., 1971.
7. Schuijt, G.: Unpublished data on response of cows with hydrops allantois to different methods of induction of parturition.
8. Vandeplassche, M., Bouters, R., Spincemaille, J. and Bonte, P.: Induction of parturition in cases of pathological gestation in cattle. Theriogenology, *1*:115, 1974.
9. Wagner, W. C., Thompson, F. N., Evans, L. E. and Molokwu, B. C. I.: Hormonal mechanisms controlling parturition. J. Anim. Sci. (Suppl 1), *38*:39, 1974.

Delivery by Forced Extraction and Other Aspects of Bovine Obstetrics

GERRIT SCHUIJT

State University of Utrecht, Utrecht,
The Netherlands

LESLIE BALL

Colorado State University,
Fort Collins, Colorado

MECHANICAL ASPECTS OF NORMAL PARTURITION

Stages of Labor

Normal parturition (labor) is a continuous process but is often divided into three stages for purposes of description. These stages are arbitrary but fairly well defined and are classified as: stage 1, cervical dilation; stage 2, fetal expulsion and stage 3, expulsion of fetal membranes. They usually follow one another in the sequence given, but sometimes (when dystocia is present) fetal membranes are expelled or at least freed from their maternal attachments before a dead fetus is delivered. Dystocia occurs when any stage is slow to develop or fails to progress normally.

Stage 1: Cervical Dilation

Stage 1 begins when longitudinal and circular muscle fibers of the uterus start to contract and ends when the cervix is dilated and fetal parts enter the birth canal. Visible signs of labor are scanty or absent during stage 1. The pastured cow will usually seek an isolated place, and vaginal discharges increase with liquefaction and expulsion of the cervical plug. Occasionally, signs of colic are evident, especially in heifers. Restlessness and a tendency to lie down and get up frequently are also often observed. The duration of stage 1 is 2 to 6 hours and is sometimes longer in heifers.

Stage 2: Fetal Expulsion

Second-stage labor begins when fetal parts enter the birth canal and stimulate the abdominal press. The chorioallantoic sac is usually ruptured early in second-stage labor, and the unbroken amniotic sac is often forced through the vulva after the cow has been in labor for a short time. *Delivery should be completed within 2 hours after the amniotic sac appears at the vulva.* The feet of the fetus are forced through the amniotic sac, either just before or after it comes to the vulva.

During stage 1, uterine contractions first occur about every 15 minutes, but by the beginning of the second stage they occur about every 3 to 5 minutes. When point pressure is applied to the birth canal by fetal parts, the uterine contractions are accompanied by the abdominal press. The press is exerted more frequently as labor progresses, until it occurs every 1 1/2 to 2 1/2 minutes. A series of frequent presses followed by a short period of rest is characteristic of this stage of labor. The greatest frequency and force occur when the fetal head is being forced through the vulva.

Following delivery of the head, a short period of rest may ensue. Strong expulsive efforts are required again to force the thorax through the birth canal. Delivery of the hips and legs is usually uneventful, occurring soon after the chest passes through the vulva. Sometimes the cow will stop straining for a short time following delivery of the thorax, allowing the rear legs to rest in the birth canal. The umbilicus may remain intact throughout most of the delivery process, supplying some oxygen to the fetus. In some forced deliveries, traction can be relaxed when the thorax is delivered, and the calf can be stimulated to breathe while it is still receiving some support from placental circulation.

Guidelines for Intervention in Parturition. The bovine fetus will often live *in utero* for 8 to 10 hours after second-stage labor begins but is usually expelled within 4 hours. When progress of labor is interrupted or tedious, intervention may be necessary. An examination should be made and needed assistance given in accordance with the following specific conditions: First, if the cow has been in first-stage labor longer than 6 hours and does not begin to press, she should be examined. The signs of first-stage labor should be described carefully to clients so they recognize such signs when labor begins. Second, if the cow has been in second-stage labor for 2 or 3 hours and progress is very slow or absent, she should be examined. The birth canal of heifers is slower to dilate than that of cows, and parturition also progresses more slowly. Heifers should therefore be allowed a little more time than cows before intervention is practiced. Third, if the amniotic sac ("water" or "foot" sac) is observed hanging from the vulva or separating its lips and delivery is not completed in 2 hours, the cow should be examined.

These specific guidelines for intervention in protracted labor will be adequate in most instances. However, the cattleman should realize that interruption of normal progress of labor at any stage or time is pathological. When it happens, the cow should be examined as soon as possible.

Stage 3: Expulsion of Fetal Membranes

Fetal membranes are usually expelled within 8 hours following delivery of the fetus. If they are retained, treatment of the uterus with broad-spectrum antibiotics is indicated, but manual removal should not be practiced.

Observation and Handling

It is important for cattlemen to have a dystocia watch during calving time so that signs of labor can be observed and early intervention practiced, if necessary. The calving watch should allow observation of every expectant dam at intervals no greater than 3 hours; otherwise, time in second-stage labor cannot be defined accurately enough to prevent calf losses from intervention occurring too late.

Observation of cattle should be accomplished quietly. Range cattle should not be moved away from pastures to strange maternity facilities unless dystocia develops. When a parturient cow is removed from pasture to a maternity facility, labor often stops for a period of time. The occurrence of dystocia is increased by stabling range cattle before labor begins. In an experiment in which half the range cattle were allowed to calve without interference while the other half were taken to strange maternity facilities and disturbed by frequent periods of observation beginning several days before parturition was expected, the rate of dystocia was doubled in the latter group.

MATERNITY FACILITIES

The facilities required for controlling parturient cows vary, depending on the temperament of the cows indigenous to the area or ranch. In European countries and in some dairies in other countries, milk cows are gentled and taught to lead from birth. They can usually be led into a stable or pen and tied in a place providing adequate room to carry out obstetrical procedures. In contrast, most beef cows resist restraint violently; thus, maternity facilities must be designed to maintain control without causing excitement and excessive activity from attempts to escape.

Maternity Room

Most cattlemen provide some type of maternity facility. Many are relatively simple; others are very elaborate. Large beef cow operations, in which much of the initial intervention is practiced by laymen, require efficient systems. A maternity room should meet at least the following standards: It should be at least 18 feet (5.5 meters) square to allow adequate room to work behind the restrained cow. It should be well lighted, warm, easy to clean and sanitize and should have a sturdy stanchion head gate with straight, upright neckpieces for choke-free restraint of the cow in either standing or recumbent positions. The head gate should have sturdy hinged wings extending out from each side to help restrain the cow. (Fig. 1). These wings can be swung toward each other, forming an alleyway to the head gate. A head gate of this type can be mounted in an alleyway under a shed, as well as in a maternity room. In addition, a method to restrain lateral movement of cows during cesarean section or fetotomy is desirable. Sanitary facilities for storage of obstetrical equipment should be provided in convenient places.

A similar maternity room is desirable for dairy farms but is less essential if the cat-

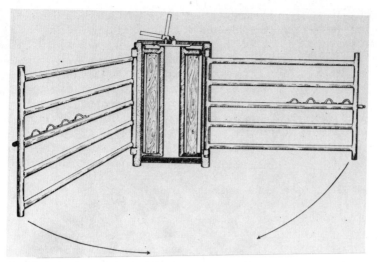

Figure 1. Hinged head gate for obstetrical manipulations. The movable wings can be swung away from the cow once her head is secured or when she goes down during obstetrical manipulations.

tle are gentle. A stable or pen that is clean and provides adequate room may be sufficient.

Sanitation of Calving Facilities

The calving facility and equipment should be kept clean to prevent transfer of infections from one cow to another. Concrete floors are easy to keep clean and disinfected, but the likelihood of damage to cows attempting to rise or move about on the slick floor surface is increased. Fresh straw should be placed in the room before each maternity case to assure good footing and provide a soft bed. Dirt floors provide more satisfactory footing but are much less sanitary. If used, they should be deeply bedded with clean, fresh straw before each use, and straw should not be allowed to remain on the floor between obstetrical cases. Disposable plastic sheeting may be laid over the straw behind the cow if she is down in a wet or muddy area away from the maternity room.

LUBRICATION

The amniotic fluid has good lubricating properties but is exhausted after prolonged labor. The need for obstetrical manipulation is usually associated with a need for additional lubrication.

Obstetrical Soaps and Mineral Oil. Obstetrical soaps are often used as lubricants but have two disadvantages. They are short-lived, requiring frequent reapplication, and they tend to remove the natural lubricants from the birth canal because of their cleansing capability. Shortly after their application, the birth canal is in worse condition than before. Mineral oil has good lubricating qualities but has caused oil granulomas in the endometrium. Decreased fertility might be expected following its use.

Expanding Lubricants. Expanding polymers derived from cellulose, e.g., carboxymethylcellulose, overcome some of the problems associated with soap and mineral oil. Their major disadvantage is that they require frequent reapplication. They are fairly tenacious and have good lubricating qualities but are soluble enough that they do not persist in the uterus and cause damage during the postparturient period. They can be compounded in thin solutions and pumped into the uterus if desired or used in thicker solutions to lubricate the obstetrician's hands and arms. The expanders are available in bulk form from various drug supply and chemical houses, and proprietary forms are available from most veterinary supply houses. A thick solution of carboxymethylcellulose is prepared by mixing 1 part by volume of the dry powder with about 25 parts of water. Four ml of glacial acetic acid is added per liter as a preservative. A thinner solution may be required for application with a pump.

Petroleum Jelly–Based Lubricant. A heavier petroleum jelly–based compound can be used for lubrication for fetotomies, birth canal dilation and difficult extractions. It is compounded by adding 1 part by volume of finely ground boric acid to 10 parts of white petroleum jelly (Vaseline). Addition of the boric acid is made easier by melting the petroleum jelly. The boric acid is omitted if the lubricant is to be used in mares.

The compound can be applied to the hands and arms of the obstetrician and to the vagina and internal fetal parts of the cow. It tends not to adhere to wet membranes and skin but gives excellent lubricating qualities when applied to the dry arm. It also provides protection to the examiner's skin in the presence of an infected uterus, allowing bare-armed manipulation with a greater degree of safety.

Application of Lubricant. The lubricating medium should be used liberally at the first sign of drying of the fetus and birth canal. Pumping of lubricant around the fetus with a stomach pump equipped with a rubber intranasal tube assures more even and thorough application of liquid lubricants. This procedure may also expand the uterus away from the fetus when it is very dry and tight, allowing easier fetal manipulation or placement of fetotomy wire. Pumping the lubricant around the fetus is more time consuming than hand application and is not required in most instances if the dystocia has not been prolonged.

INITIAL EXAMINATION

Anamnesis

The initial examination should include a history and thorough examination of the reproductive tract and fetus. Parity, duration of labor and previous attempts to assist delivery should be determined. Duration of gestation and pertinent observations on the course of gestation and labor should also be discussed with the client.

Sanitation during Obstetrical Manipulation

Many cows become infertile following obstetrical procedures, probably because of the introduction of bacteria into the uterus by unsanitary obstetrical techniques. The tail of the cow should be tied (over the back to the opposite front leg) to her neck and the perineal region cleaned carefully with a disinfectant soap and water before the examination. In many instances, the period of initial examination is the only time that the uterus is invaded, and plastic gloves can be worn to decrease contamination and protect the obstetrician from infectious diseases. However, they are not useful for extensive manipulations because they tear easily.

When extensive manipulations become necessary, it is impossible to keep from contaminating the uterus. However, contamination can be held to a minimum by keeping the arms clean and the surroundings sanitary. The cow should be prevented, if possible, from defecating over the arms of the obstetrician and the legs of the calf during obstetrical manipulations.

The Examination

After lubricating the arms, the birth canal should be examined for dilation and size of the pelvic opening, with special attention being given to cervical dilation and strictures in the vestibular region. In addition, a thorough search should be made for prior damage to the uterus and birth canal, especially in cows in prolonged labor or those in which lay assistance has been attempted.

Vital Signs

The obstetrician must decide during the initial examination which obstetrical procedure to utilize. This decision will be influenced by the vital status of the fetus. The live fetus should usually be delivered by mutation and forced extraction or by cesarean section; the dead fetus by mutation and forced extraction or by fetotomy. A flow diagram of parturition is presented in Figure 2.

The fetus may be examined for reflexes when vital status is in doubt. The feet may be pinched to produce a withdrawal reflex, the eyes palpated for a blink reflex and the mouth and tongue palpated or pinched to elicit suckling or tongue withdrawal reflexes. The anal sphincter may be felt to contract if a finger is placed in the rectum.

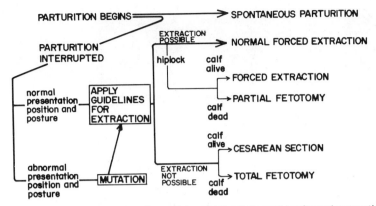

Figure 2. Flow pattern for parturition. When the calf cannot be delivered by forced extraction, the live calf is delivered by cesarean section and the dead one by fetotomy.

In the absence of these reflexes, one should palpate the thorax for a heartbeat or the umbilicus for a pulse before making a final decision on the vital status of the fetus.

Guidelines

Guidelines are necessary to allow the obstetrician to decide quickly during the initial examination which method to use for delivery of the fetus. The guidelines and techniques discussed hereafter are those utilized at the obstetrics clinic at the University of Utrecht, the Netherlands.

Guideline for Attempted Mutation. Abnormalities in presentation, position and posture should be diagnosed and corrected before traction is applied if the fetus is alive. When the fetus is dead and reposition is difficult or dangerous, partial fetotomy should be performed. Attempts to perform difficult mutations are tiring to the obstetrician and may endanger the life of the dam and fetus if they become too extended. If the obstetrician works at a mutation for a maximum of 1/2 hour without making progress, cesarean section or fetotomy is indicated. This decision can usually be made in much less time by the experienced person.

Guidelines for Extraction of Oversized Fetus in Anterior Presentation. The most common cause of dystocia is an oversized fetus. Dystocia due to fetal oversize is commonly mishandled by application of excessive traction or by application of traction before the birth canal is properly dilated. Consequently, many cows are badly damaged and many calves are killed. Common types of maternal damage are vulvar, vaginal and cervical tears, he-

matoma, postparturient vaginal necrosis and calving paralysis due to damage to femoral and obturator nerves. Most of this type of damage is preventable if guidelines are followed that dictate the use of proper obstetrical techniques.

To determine whether or not the fetus in anterior presentation can be delivered *per vaginam*, the cow is cast in right lateral recumbency. Chains are looped around the pasterns, with the pull coming off the dorsal (anterior) surface (Fig. 3). Traction is not applied to the head. Unilateral traction is then applied by one person to the bottom forelimb until the shoulder of the fetus is brought past the pelvic inlet. The shoulder can usually be felt to pass the ilium; if not, one can assume it has passed when the fetlock joint is extended about 10 cm outside the vulva. In large breeds, the joint may be extracted 15 cm or more before the shoulder has passed the ilium. Unilateral traction, full force, is then applied to the top forelimb by a second person. Extraction is nearly always possible if the second shoulder also passes the ilium into the birth canal; if not, a cesarean section or fetotomy should be started immediately. Similar diagnostic steps may be used in the standing cow with one exception, i.e., the weight of the fetus that is nearly oversized may prevent its shoulders from coming through the pelvic inlet. In this case, the cow should be cast on her side and the testing procedure repeated before resorting to cesarean section.

Guidelines for Extraction of Oversized Fetus in Posterior Presentation. The fetus in posterior presentation presents a more difficult problem because the umbilicus is impacted on the pelvic

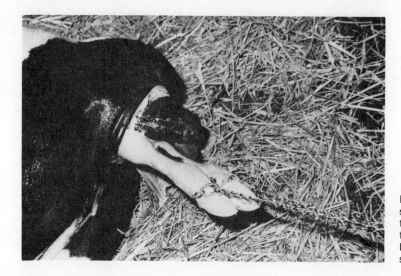

Figure 3. Attachment of chains should be around the pasterns, with the pull coming off the dorsum of the foot. The chain eyelets should be bent slightly to conform to the shape of the foot.

brim or ruptured while the head and thorax are still inside the dam. The diagnosis should be made in the recumbent cow.

The hips of the fetus are widest between its greater trochanters (see Figure 9). The maternal pelvic inlet has a wider dorso-pubic than bis-iliac diameter (Fig. 4). The guidelines for extraction in posterior presentation take these factors into consideration. The fetus is first rotated 90° into the dorso-ilial position so its greatest hip diameter corresponds to the greatest diameter of the maternal pelvis (see Figure 10). Extraction is usually possible when two people, pulling simultaneously in a caudal, slightly dorsal direction on the rotated fetus, are able to extract it far enough that its hocks are presented at the vulvar area.

However, cesarean section should be utilized if there is any doubt, because a difficult extraction usually kills the fetus. Excessive traction on the fetus in posterior presentation has been associated with joint and back lesions, diaphragmatic hernia, broken ribs, pulmonary bleeding, liver rupture and other damage to the fetus.[6]

Many persons believe that heifers tolerate relatively harder traction than cows because their bony pelvis has greater capacity to expand. This may be true, but maternal damage is seen more often in heifers than in cows because attempts have been made to extract oversized calves when cesarean section or fetotomy should have been used.

MANUAL DILATION OF BIRTH CANAL

When the fetus is to be delivered by traction, the state of dilation of the birth canal should be evaluated, and it should be dilated manually if necessary. The hands and arms of the obstetrician and the birth canal are kept well lubricated with the petroleum jelly–based lubricant previously discussed. The hands are clasped together by interlocking the fingers; then the arms are inserted into the vulva and vagina like a wedge, rotating as they are worked in and out. The clasped hands can also be inserted with the arms parallel; then the birth canal is expanded by pushing the elbows outward, bringing a persistent force against the nondilated parts (Fig. 5). Up to

MATERNAL PELVIC INLET

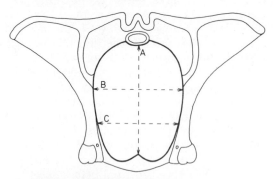

A. SACRO-PUBIC DIAMETER
B. DORSAL TRANS-ILIAL DIAMETER
C. VENTRAL TRANS-ILIAL DIAMETER

Figure 4. Maternal pelvic inlet. The sacro-pubic and oblique diameters are greater than the dorsal trans-ilial diameter, which in turn is greater than the ventral trans-ilial diameter.

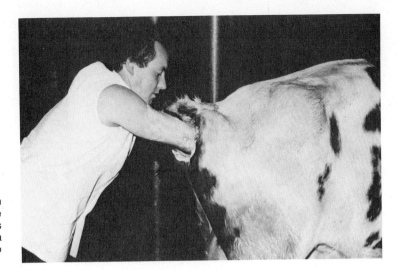

Figure 5. Dilation of the birth canal. The well-lubricated arms are inserted into the vagina, the fingers locked and the arms used as a wedge to apply dilation pressure to the birth canal.

20 minutes of manual dilation may be required. Extraction should not be attempted until dilation is adequate.

The two points of greatest resistance to delivery occur when the head passes through the vestibule and vulva and again when the thorax is delivered. There is little danger to the fetus in anterior presentation during this phase of extraction because its umbilicus is still attached and functional. This is important because slow extraction during this phase is essential to prevent damage to the birth canal if it is not sufficiently dilated. The obstetrician should make certain that the vestibule is dilating properly as the head and thorax pass through it. If not, moderate traction force is maintained on the legs of the fetus while the hand is worked around the head or thorax in the constricted area, lifting

and stretching it away from the fetus until it can pass safely.

The fetus in posterior presentation should also be extracted slowly until the hips are at the vulva to make certain that the birth canal is sufficiently dilated. If not, dilation is completed by manual methods.

FORCED EXTRACTION OF FETUS

Forced Extraction in Anterior Presentation

When forced extraction is chosen, the cow should not be given an epidural anesthetic unless absolutely necessary so that she is able to assist in the delivery. Obstetrical chains are placed around the pas-

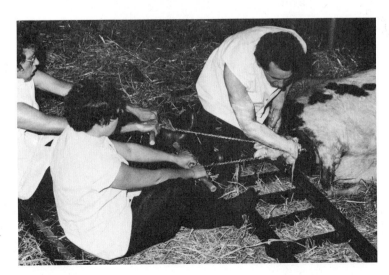

Figure 6. Foot purchase can be obtained by pulling against a ladder or plank placed against the cow, parallel with her rear legs.

PHASE I.   EXTRACTION OF A CALF IN ANTERIOR
            PRESENTATION, COW IN RIGHT RECUMBENCY.

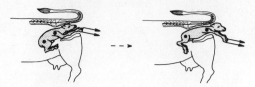

THE DIRECTION OF TRACTION IS SLIGHTLY VENTRAL
UNTIL THE SCAPULO-HUMORAL JOINTS HAVE
PASSED THE PELVIC INLET AND THE HEAD IS
OUTSIDE THE VULVA.

Figure 7. Extraction of the calf in anterior presentation. Phase 1.

TRANSVERSE SECTION THROUGH PELVIC
REGION OF CALF

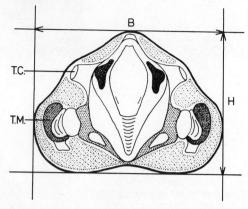

THE WIDTH, B, IS GREATER THAN THE HEIGHT, H.

T.C.-TUBER COXAE OF ILIUM
T.M.-TROCHANTER MAJOR OF FEMUR

Figure 9. Transverse section through pelvic region of the calf.

terns, with their eyelets on the dorsal surface of the forefeet (see Figure 3). The eyelets of the chains should be bent slightly so they conform to the curvature of the feet. Only one assistant is assigned to apply traction to each of the forelimbs, and head traction is not used because of the increased likelihood of damage to the fetus.

The cow should be cast on her right side before hard traction is applied. A ladder or plank placed against her buttocks parallel to her rear legs provides a foot brace for the traction assistants (Fig. 6). The obstetrician manipulates the fetus and controls the application of traction, which should be in a caudal and slightly ventral direction (Fig. 7). For easiest and safest delivery of the calf, hard traction should be applied only when the cow presses.

Rotation of the Fetus

A rotating force is applied by the obstetrician to the fetus when its head, neck and forelegs are through the vulva. This produces the dorso-ilial or dorso-sacral-ilial position *before* the hips of the fetus engage

the maternal pelvic inlet. Rotation allows the fetal hips to come through the maternal pelvic inlet at its wider diameter and helps to prevent fetal hiplock (Fig. 8, 9 and 10).

To obtain rotation, the obstetrician takes a position on the ventral side of the fetus and directs the traction assistants to pull when the cow presses. Traction on the upper leg of the fetus should be more dorsal, relative to the longitudinal axis of the calf, than traction on the bottom leg. The traction assistants should exchange chain handles following the casting procedure to adjust the traction on the individual fore-

PHASE 2. COW IN RIGHT RECUMBENCY.

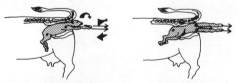

THE DIRECTION OF TRACTION IS STRAIGHT BACK-WARD. AS SOON AS THE HEAD IS OUTSIDE THE VULVA, TRACTION ASSISTANTS EXCHANGE CHAINS (TO FACILITATE ROTATION) AND THE CALF IS ROTATED ABOUT 90° WHILE THE THORAX IS EXTRACTED. USUALLY THE CALF WILL BE DELIVERED AT THIS TIME.

Figure 8. Extraction of the calf in anterior presentation. Phase 2.

FETAL EXTRACTION IN ANTERIOR PRESENTATION

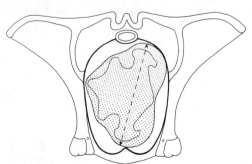

CALF ROTATED ABOUT 90° TO POSITION ITS HIPS TO COME THROUGH THE WIDEST DIAMETER OF THE MATERNAL PELVIC INLET.

Figure 10. Rotation of the fetus allows its hips to be extracted through the pelvic inlet at its greatest diameter.

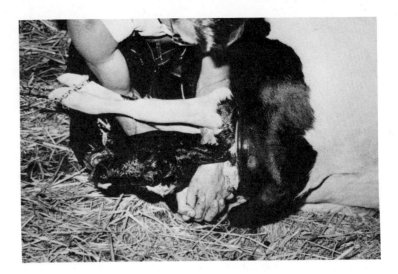

Figure 11. Rotation is begun before the fetal hips are engaged at the pelvic inlet.

legs in the proper direction. The slight crossing of direction of traction on the forelegs obtained by exchanging chain handles makes rotation of the fetus by the obstetrician easier. The obstetrician passes the hand and arm nearest to the cow either beneath or between the forelegs and then to the upper side of the fetal neck. The other hand and arm are passed beneath the fetal legs and neck, and the hands are clasped near the base of the neck (Fig. 11). The legs can then be used to lever the calf into the dorso-ilial position as it is extracted (Fig. 12).

Hiplock

When hiplock occurs in spite of these techniques, traction should be discontinued while the nostrils of the calf are cleared of mucus and membranes and the calf is induced to breathe. Breathing can usually be stimulated by tickling the nostrils or pouring cold water over the head of the fetus. There are two reasons why it is important not to apply traction except when the cow presses. First, continuous traction is generally unproductive and prevents the calf from breathing enough to stay alive. Second, the act of pressing pulls the maternal pelvic inlet more nearly perpendicular to her spinal column. This has the practical effect of making the pelvic inlet functionally (not literally) larger and allows easier delivery of the calf (Fig. 13).

The direction of traction should be adjusted so that the pull is caudal and somewhat dorsal; this direction of pull is more perpendicular to the pelvic inlet (Fig. 14). Rotation is maintained, preferably at the

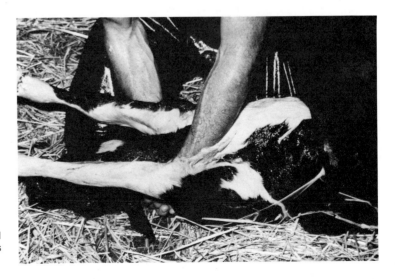

Figure 12. Rotation is completed when calf is turned on its long axis 60 to 90°.

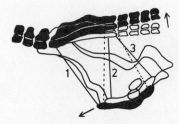

■ Pelvic position during abdominal press and expulsion

☐ Normal pelvic position

1 Sacro–pubic pelvic inlet diameter does not enlarge

2 Vertical pelvic diameter is almost as large as sacro-
   pubic pelvic inlet diameter during the abdominal press

3 The height of the pelvic outlet remains about the same
   during the abdominal press as during resting periods

Figure 13. When a cow presses, the pubis is pulled forward, enlarging the vertical pelvic diameter. The pelvic inlet and outlet diameters remain relatively unchanged.

dorso-ilial position. Palpation along the back of the calf is required to insure that its pelvis is rotated as far as is necessary. If not, repulsion against the fetal pelvis or torso sometimes displaces the locked pelvis far enough to make rotation easier. As many as three traction assistants may be required to deliver the hiplocked fetus, but traction is applied only when the cow presses.

Forced Extraction in Posterior Presentation

Forced extraction of the fetus in posterior presentation is done in reverse order to anterior presentation. The cow is cast in lateral recumbency. Everything should be ready before the final extraction is begun. Handles should be attached to chains close

PHASE 3. HIPLOCK

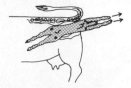

WHEN HIPLOCK OCCURS, THE DIRECTION OF TRACTION SHOULD BE CAUDAL AND SLIGHTLY DORSAL. THE CALF IS KEPT ROTATED ABOUT 90° AND TRACTION WITH UP TO 3 MEN IS APPLIED ONLY DURING PERIODS OF ABDOMINAL PRESS AS LONG AS THE CALF IS ALIVE.

Figure 14. Extraction of the hiplocked fetus in anterior presentation.

PHASE I. EXTRACTION OF A CALF IN POSTERIOR PRESENTATION

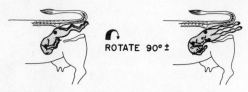

ROTATE 90°±

COW CAN BE IN EITHER RIGHT OR LEFT LATERAL RECUMBENCY. HIND QUARTERS ARE ROTATED 90°± BY CROSSING ITS LEGS AND APPLYING A ROTATIONAL FORCE WITHOUT TRACTION.

Figure 15. Extraction of the calf in posterior presentation. Phase 1. The calf is rotated 90° to take advantage of the greatest maternal pelvic diameter.

to the traction points so that they need not be repositioned when the fetus is half out of the cow. The birth canal should be adequately dilated. During the preliminary examination, the calf will have been rotated to the dorso-ilial position (Fig. 15) and its hips brought through the pelvic inlet by applying traction in a caudal, slightly dorsal direction (Fig. 16). When dilation is adequate and the hips have passed the pelvic inlet, the rear quarters are then rotated back to the dorso-sacral position by application of caudal, slightly ventral traction (Fig. 17). Excessive traction may damage the hip or stifle joints of the calf during early phases of delivery.

Once its hips are through the vestibule, the fetus should be extracted as quickly as possible to prevent asphyxiation. However, traction should be applied only when the cow is pressing to prevent damage to or fracture of the fetal spine at the lumbosacral junction.

There are likely to be more complications during forced extraction in posterior than in anterior presentation. Cranial parts of the fetus are still in the uterus

PHASE 2. EXTRACTION

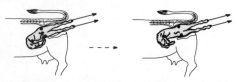

THE DIRECTION OF TRACTION IS CAUDAL AND SLIGHTLY DORSAL. WHEN THE HIPS PASS THE PELVIC INLET, THE CALF IS ROTATED BACK INTO DORSO-SACRAL POSITION.

Figure 16. Extraction of the calf in posterior presentation. Phase 2. If the fetal hips come into the birth canal when simultaneous traction is applied by two men, the fetus can usually be delivered.

PHASE 3. EXTRACTION

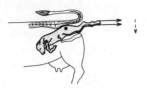

DIRECTION OF TRACTION IS FIRST CAUDAL THEN CAUDAL AND SLIGHTLY VENTRAL AFTER THE STIFLE JOINT PASSES THE VULVAR LIPS. ALTHOUGH PHASE 3 MAY NOT LAST TOO LONG, FORCED TRACTION IS APPLIED ONLY DURING THE ABDOMINAL PRESS.

Figure 17. After the fetal hips clear the pelvic inlet, the fetus is rotated to the dorso-sacral position by applying caudal, slightly ventral traction to the rear legs.

and birth canal when the fetal oxygen supply is lost because of rupture or impaction of the umbilicus; therefore, asphyxiation occurs more often. Mechanical damage to the fetus is also more likely to occur; probably because fetal body conformation and traction are less compatible with safe delivery than with a fetus in anterior presentation.[6]

The fetus in posterior presentation is sometimes not pushed far enough into the birth canal to dilate the cervix, vagina and vulva properly. Consequently, forced delivery should not be attempted until these parts are properly dilated (see Figure 5). Otherwise, the calf may be extracted so far that its umbilicus is stretched, broken or impacted on the pelvis, but completion of delivery is inhibited by lack of dilation.

USE OF FETAL EXTRACTOR

Use of the fetal extractor is discouraged. Many cattle are lost because of misuse of this device. Operators need to appreciate that excessive force can be applied with fetal extractors, resulting in laceration of the birth canal, maternal paralysis and damage to the fetus. Other disadvantages are limitation of traction to caudal and caudal-ventral directions and difficulty of rotation of the fetus when necessary. In spite of these disadvantages, the use of the fetal extractor is sometimes necessary when traction assistants are not available; however, no more force should be applied with them than could be applied by three strong people.

REFERENCES

1. Arthur, G. H.: Veterinary Reproduction and Obstetrics. Baltimore, The Williams and Wilkins Co., 1975.
2. Baier, W. and Schaetz, F.: Tieràrztliche Geburtskunde. Stuttgart, Ferdinand Enke Verlag, 1958.
3. Richter, J. and Gòetze, R.: Tiergeburtshilfe. Berlin, Paul Parey, 1960.
4. Roberts, S. J.: Veterinary Obstetrics and Genital Disease (Theriogenology). 2nd Ed. Ann Arbor, Mich., Edwards Brothers, Inc. 1971.
5. Rüsse, M.: Der Geburtsablauf beim Rind. Arch. exp. Veterinärmed. Bd *lg*; 1965, pp. 763 and 963.
6. Schuijt, G.: Assisted delivery of the calf by manual or mechanical traction. Netherlands J. Vet. Sci., *102*:677, 1977.

Surgical Procedures of the Reproductive System of the Cow

ROBERT S. HUDSON

Auburn University, Auburn, Alabama

The knowledgeable veterinarian approaches surgical intervention involving the reproductive system of the cow with caution, always considering whether the condition at hand materially detracts from the potential performance of the patient, whether the condition merits a reasonably good prognosis and whether the anticipated expense is justified. Keeping these factors in mind and considering the actual and potential values of the animal, the operator decides whether to recommend temporary or minimal repair to facilitate salvage or permanent and perhaps extensive repair to restore useful reproductive function. Although it is folly to instigate a complicated, and therefore expensive, procedure for an animal of marginal worth, the valuable animal and its owner deserve the benefit of the best the profession can offer.

Many of the indications for elective surgery arise from injuries sustained during assisted parturition. Far fewer injuries occur when birth is unassisted, indicating the need for prudence and patience in all obstetrical manipulations.

One should remember that injuries associated with dystocia frequently are multiple, and thorough examination is required to avoid overlooking one or more serious conditions while concentrating on a more obvious defect. Heroic restoration is a failure if the animal ceases to perform economically. The purpose of this portion of the text is to present some of the currently useful techniques for protection from injury and for restoration to reproductive health and function.

EPISIOTOMY

Surgical incision of the vulva is indicated during an obstetrical procedure when the vulva interferes appreciably with mutation or delivery of the fetus. Specific indications include marginal fetal oversize or insufficient dilation of the vulva due to hypoplasia or juvenility. Induration of the vulva or vestibule caused by previous trauma may also preclude sufficient dilation. The premise is that surgical incision is preferable to bursting or laceration. Considering the advantages of avoiding serious and costly injury to the perineum of the parturient heifer or cow, episiotomy is a simple and rewarding procedure, when indicated.

An episiotomy may be elected when the fetal head or, rarely, the gluteal prominence is presented at the vulva, and it appears likely that further traction will result in tearing of the vulva. It is usually difficult to assess the need for episiotomy prior to actual presentation of the fetal part. In the presence of a decomposing fetus, partial fetotomy is preferable to episiotomy because of the difficulty in securing first intention healing in the presence of gross contamination.

Surgical Technique. Choice of the mode of anesthesia presents a unique situation. Epidural anesthesia may be sluggish in onset, particularly if the patient is recumbent. Additionally, the effect of epidural anesthesia may adversely inhibit the desired abdominal pressing of the animal once delivery is resumed. Provided the limiting fetal part, for example the calvarium, is stretching the vulva and is serving as a template for incision, local infiltration of an anesthetic agent is probably ineffective and superfluous. Careful observation has revealed no evidence of reaction to pain from incision of the grossly stretched tissues. The stretching may provide insensitivity to pain. Following delivery, anesthesia may be required in order to suture the incision.

Since the objective of episiotomy is to avoid vulvar tearing, which tends to begin at the dorsal commissure and to extend dorsally into the anus and rectum, the incision is begun at a point along the free edge of the stretched vulva 3 to 5 cm from the dorsal commissure, using a scalpel or a sharp, straight scissors. Incising entirely through the vulvar lip, the incision is continued in a dorsolateral direction, the length of the incision depending on the need for enlargement of the orifice. A 7-cm incision is usually sufficient to allow delivery of the fetus without tearing of the vulva.

Following delivery, the incision is cleansed of foreign material such as fetal fluid and is sutured with a modified vertical mattress suture pattern, the deep thrusts of the pattern passing through skin, fibrous tissue and vestibular submucosa and the superficial thrusts passing through skin alone. If the patient is to receive little or no postoperative attention, absorbable suture material such as No. 1 chromic gut is used. Otherwise, nonabsorbable suture is preferred. Careful cosmetic closure is indicated to reduce the probability of excessive fibrosis and disruption of the symmetry of the vulvar cleft, which could predispose to pneumovagina. Aftercare includes the initial application of a topical antibiotic powder and examination of the patient by the veterinarian prior to the next breeding season.

PERINEAL LACERATIONS

Lacerations of the perineum have been classified according to location and degree of tissue disruption. First-degree lacerations are superficial wounds of the mucosa of the vagina or vestibule. Second-degree lacerations involve the entire wall of the vagina or vulva, or both. Third-degree defects result from laceration of the vagina and rectum as well as the anus, perineal body and vulva.

Torn or lacerated mucosa without further complications seldom requires specific treatment, and rapid healing is expected. Disruption of mucosa alone is unlikely to result in stenosis. If, however, the laceration is complicated by deep bruising of perivaginal or perivulvar tissues, severe necrosis often follows, with ascending infections of the genital or urinary tract and sometimes stenosis of the vagina. These sequelae can be avoided at times by vigorous attention to hygiene and by administration of systemic and topical antibacterial therapy.

Second-degree lacerations involving the entire vaginal wall frequently accompany forced delivery in undersized or overfat beef heifers but also may result from any obstetrical delivery when impatience or excitement guides the operator. Often the immediate effect is protrusion of perivaginal fat through the laceration. This protruding fat should be removed. Failure to do so may allow a pedunculated mass of fat to persist as the laceration heals, causing tenesmus and perhaps being mistaken for a neoplasm. The laceration, however recent, should not be sutured. Occasionally, severely bruised perivaginal fat becomes necrotic and fibrotic, causing persistent vaginal irritation, which in turn encourages tenesmus and vaginal prolapse. When irregular fibrotic masses are palpated in the perivaginal area, suggesting the condition just described, surgical removal is indicated. Under epidural anesthesia the vagina is manually prolapsed, the vaginal wall is incised and the mass is removed by blunt dissection. The incision is sutured with No. 1 absorbable suture material, using a horizontal interrupted mattress pattern.

Occluding Adhesions of the Vagina

Severe trauma deep in the vaginal vault sometimes includes circumferential tearing of the vaginal wall. Unattended healing may lead to extensive adhesion formation, which occludes a portion of the lumen.

Diagnosis. If the adhesions form following calving injury, fluid accumulates proximal to the occlusion, eventually causing a feeling of fullness for the cow. This may result in tenesmus, which is often the first sign of the problem. Upon manual examination of the vagina, the occlusion is readily evident. In most instances the adhered tissues are relatively weak and can be separated with moderate manual force, thus releasing the trapped fluid. The ease of separation and the ragged adhesions, together with a history of calving, should help differentiate the condition from congenital segmental aplasia.

Rarely, the laceration is located in the fornix of the vagina. The occlusion then forms just caudal to the external os of the cervix, effectively sealing the cervix. The anterior end of the vagina appears as a smooth blind pouch.

Prognosis. If the occlusion has caused excessive fluid accumulation in the uterus with accompanying endometrial atrophy or obstructive bilateral salpingitis, the prognosis is poor. Adhesions in the midportion of the vagina without serious lesions anterior to that point are amenable to correction. The primary problem is preventing recurrence of the adhesions. The following technique for maintaining re-established patency has proved to be of value in some cases.

Surgical Technique. Following epidural anesthesia and preparation of the perineum and accessible portion of the vagina, it is well initially to attempt manual separation of the adhered surfaces, especially if the injury is recent and the adhesions are still formative. It may be necessary to force closed forceps centrally through the area of adhesion, opening the forceps to tear open the occlusion. Any irregular pockets that have formed are flattened by incision of the mucous membrane. It is better to avoid excision of large areas of mucous membrane. Suturing is quite difficult and is not necessary.

Various pessaries have been designed for maintaining patency and preventing reformation of the adhesions. None of these has worked as well for the author as does an inflatable rubber beach ball, 25 cm long when deflated, that has a grommet on the end opposite the inflation tube. Following medication of the vagina with a lanolin-base antibiotic ointment, the grommet of the beach ball is drawn snugly against the cervix by a suture through the edge of the external cervical os, using 0.6 mm nonabsorbable suture material (Vetafil).[1] Once in place, the beach ball is inflated minimally, just enough to smooth the surface of the ball but not enough to cause severe pressure on the dilated vagina or to stimulate tenesmus when anesthesia wears off or to interfere with urination. Retention of the ball is insured by closing the vulva with interrupted vertical mattress tape sutures at the perineal hairline. The inflation tube should be easily accessible for the convalescent period.

Aftercare consists of daily cleansing of the

perineum, deflation of the beach ball, infusion of the vagina with an oil-base antibiotic medication and reinflation of the ball. The vulvar sutures and the ball can be removed in 7 to 10 days. The daily topical medication should be continued until healing is near completion.

Incompetence of the Constrictor Vestibuli Muscle

A properly functioning constrictor vestibuli muscle is a primary barrier to ascending contamination of the vagina. Located at the junction of the vestibule and vagina, the muscle, if undamaged, forms a constriction that is evident by its resistance when a cylindrical speculum is passed into the vagina.

Extensive lacerations in the area of this muscle or severe repeated stretching of the muscle at parturition may disrupt its function, predisposing to pneumovagina, chronic vaginitis and infertility. The condition often becomes apparent when there is additional dysfunction, such as malocclusion of the vulvar cleft caused by vulvar laceration, excessive episiotomy scars or innate conformational defects.

Surgical Technique. The veterinarian who is concerned with the effects of pneumovagina must decide whether to disregard the incompetent constrictor vestibuli muscle and depend on episioplasty alone. This is the preferred approach when pneumovagina is not severe enough to cause persistent ballooning and dilation of the vaginal vault and when there is no concomitant surgical problem of the anterior vagina or cervix. Conversely, when pneumovagina is severe in spite of a properly aligned vulvar cleft, a rapidly performed alleviating technique involves placement of a deep circumferential suture (Buhner suture) to create the competence originally provided by the constrictor vestibuli muscle.

Episioplasty consists of some form of the classic Caslick's operation in which approximately the dorsal two-thirds to three-fourths of the edges of the vulvar lips are trimmed, thus denuding a 0.5-cm strip. After this, the edges are brought together by using 0.6-mm nonabsorbable sutures in an interrupted vertical mattress pattern. Alternatively, when the vulva is small but incompetent, excessive tissue removal may be avoided by incising the mucocutaneous junctions in the prescribed areas, rather than trimming.

Formerly it was thought that partial closure of the vulvar cleft would necessitate artificial insemination. However, experience has demonstrated that natural service is quite possible.

Third-Degree Perineal Lacerations

Rectovaginal or rectovulvar lacerations usually occur when traction is applied to a fetus by an overzealous, excited or impatient operator. Most often the operator fails to allow sufficient time for dilation of the soft tissues of the birth canal once delivery is begun. Predisposition to injury may include a hypoplastic or stenotic vulva or an oversized fetus. It is extremely rare for a cow to sustain third-degree lacerations when calving is unassisted.

Most lacerations commence as the head of the fetus in the anterior longitudinal presentation approaches the vulvar cleft. The incidence of third-degree laceration with posterior presentation is low. The tearing begins at the dorsal commissure of the vulva and extends dorsally and cranially for a variable distance, dividing the anus, anal sphincter and rectum as well as the perineal body, vestibule and vagina. The divided tissues are severely bruised and devitalized. The immediate result will be a variable amount of tissue loss.

Management of Third-Degree Lacerations. When the operator, whether layman or veterinarian, discovers the extent of injury, there is an inclination to make immediate repair. However, the devitalized nature of the tissues at this time does not allow for optimum healing. In fact, immediate repair, which is often unsuccessful, may cause added loss of tissue, making subsequent repair more difficult. It is better to postpone surgical correction for 4 to 6 weeks, allowing for resolution of tissue damage.

Rectovaginal defects in cattle are not always a cause of infertility. In fact it sometimes is difficult to render an accurate prognosis. It is likely that the affected commercial cow that is in a herd with a limited breeding season will fail to conceive on schedule, with or without surgical repair. When breeding schedules are nonexistent, a cow of marginal value may be kept in the herd for a time without repair in hopes that she will eventually conceive against the odds. Valuable purebred animals should be restored surgically.

Once satisfactory resolution of inflammation is obtained, the cow is ready for surgery. There is little need for extensive preoperative preparation. Fasting to reduce fecal volume is contraindicated. Feces that is neither firm nor diarrheic is desirable to obviate immediate postoperative irritation. One last thorough examination of the entire reproductive tract is in order.

The patient is confined in a chute or stanchion in the standing position. If there is a calf at the side, it should be in full view of the dam. Epidural anesthetic (2 per cent procaine with ephedrine) in volume just sufficient for anesthesia of the perineum is administered, being careful to avoid anesthesia of the pelvic limbs. The tail is tied to one side by a neckrope. The perineal region and vaginal vault are cleansed by repeated flushing with a mild organic iodine surgical detergent (Betadine Scrub). Care must be taken to avoid excessive infusion of the detergent or rinse water into the rectum, as this may reflux during the procedure.

There is no need for the special longhandled instruments employed in similar procedures in the mare. The usual assortment of instruments used in routine general surgery is sufficient.

At the operator's option a tampon of 5-cm stockinette (Tomac tubular stockinette) stuffed loosely with cotton and tied with a 25-cm length of umbilical tape may be placed in the rectum cranial to the rectovaginal defect. The loose end of the tape is secured to one side of the perineal region outside the operative area, to be used after surgery for removing the tampon.

The operative area is exposed by placing tension sutures in the perineal skin near the mucocutaneous margin on each side of the disrupted dorsal commissure of the vulva and at the lacerated edges of the anus. These four sutures are anchored laterally near the tubera ischii to hold open the common cavity of the defect. The cranial limit of the defect is thus revealed as a "shelf" separating the rectal and vaginal lumina, caudal to which is the common cavity created by the laceration. The healed junctions of bright red rectal mucosa and pale vaginal and vestibular mucosa form a seam on each side of the common cavity extending to the perineal skin (Fig. 1). The free edge of the shelf is incised to a depth of 3 cm and extended laterally and

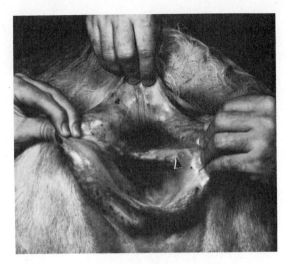

Figure 1. Third degree perineal laceration in a cow. Note common opening of rectum and vagina. Arrow marks healed junction of rectal and vaginal mucosae.

caudally on each side, following the lines of junction of the rectal and vaginal (or vestibular) mucosae (Fig. 2). The horizontal dissection is intended to provide flaps of tissue sufficient to allow reconstruction of the rectal floor and vaginal roof. Occasionally, especially following previously unsuccessful attempts at repair, excessive fibrous scar tissue may lie along the lines of dissection. The fibrous tissue is carefully removed with minimal excision of normal tissue in order to

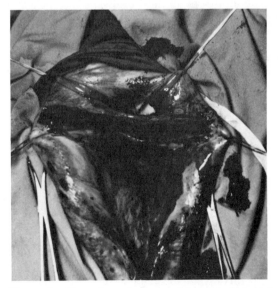

Figure 2. Dissection along margins of rectum and vagina forming flaps for reconstruction of rectal floor and vaginal roof. (From Hudson, R. S.: The Bovine Practitioner, 7:34, 1972.)

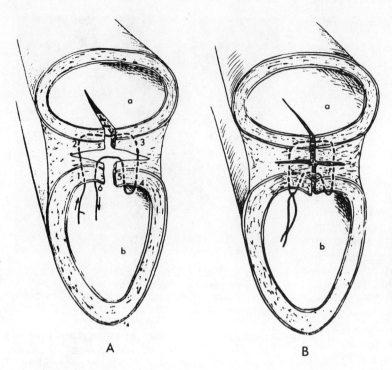

A   B

Figure 3. A, Pattern for closure of perineal laceration. (1) Deep thrust through left vaginal flap, (2) thrust through left perirectal tissue and rectal submucosa, (3) thrust through right rectal submucosa and perirectal tissue, (4) deep thrust through right vaginal flap into vaginal lumen, (5) superficial thrust through right vaginal flap and (6) superficial thrust from deep side of left vaginal flap to vaginal lumen. B, Closure of perineal laceration. Suture must not penetrate rectal mucosa. (From Hudson, R. S.: The Bovine Practitioner, 7:34, 1972.)

preserve as much tissue as possible to bridge the defect.

Synthetic nonabsorbable 0.6-mm suture (Vetafil) and a No. 2 or 3 half-circle cutting edge needle (fistula needle) are used in the modified vertical mattress suture pattern after the method of Goetze as described by Rosenberger (Fig. 3). A surgeon's knot is tied snugly by hand. Following each tie the defect is inspected carefully for proper alignment and apposition, as there is no opportunity for placement of sutures as an afterthought once the suture line is completed. The two tag ends of each suture are left long (8 cm) and are tied together at their ends to aid in identification of each surgical knot during removal. Both natural and synthetic absorbable suture materials have proved to be inferior to nonabsorbable sutures for this procedure, and the added effort of nonabsorbable suture removal is considered worthwhile.

It is important that the suture pattern effects abutment closure of the edges of the rectal mucosa. The suture must not penetrate the rectal mucosa. While the edges of vestibular mucosa are everted, excessive flap formation is of no value and tends to exert undue tension on the suture line.

The first one or two sutures are placed in the shelf cranial to its free edge in order to establish the pattern of tissue relationship prior to suturing the actual defect. It is thought that the cranial limit of the defect is most vulnerable to dehiscence. Sutures are placed at 1-cm intervals until the rectum and vestibule are reconstructed, with the perineal body in between, to within 1 cm of the perineal skin. Vertical dissection is then made, beginning at the anus and extending ventrally to the point of the original dorsal commissure of the vulva, or, if there is an indication of malocclusion of the vulvar lips, the dissection is extended farther, along the edges of the labia. The closure of the horizontal dissection is completed, after which the vertical perineal incision is closed with interrupted vertical mattress sutures of 0.4-mm nonabsorbable material (Fig. 4).

Aftercare consists of the initial application of an antibacterial powder, furazolidone (Topazone), to the perineal suture line and administration of systemic antibiotics for 5 days. Little advantage is gained by curious exploration of the horizontal closure during healing. Sutures are removed with long scissors in 10 to 14 days, following digital palpation of the individual knots in the vestibular mucosa. The cow may be serviced naturally at any time after the thirtieth postoperative day. Manual rectal examination of the internal genitalia or artificial insemination should be postponed until the fortieth day. There is no evidence of an increased inci-

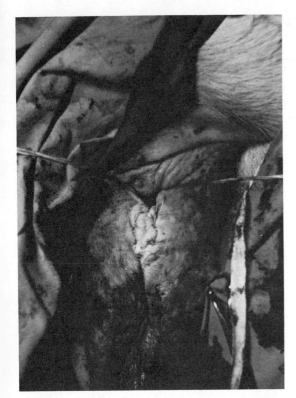

Figure 4. Closed perineal skin; vertical mattress sutures. Temporary guy sutures are holding anus open for visualization.

dence of dystocia following or related to the restoration.

Rectovaginal fistulae in the cow apparently are rare. The mode of perineal laceration in the cow, i.e., from the vulva cranially, does not provide for fistula formation. The fistulae in cows that have been encountered by the author have resulted from partial failure of repair of complete perineal disruption. The method of repair of fistulae has been surgical conversion to a complete disruption and repair as just described.

UROVAGINA

General Considerations. Pooling of urine in the anterior portion of the vagina is a rare but extremely serious cause of infertility. The condition is instigated by either congenital or acquired cranioventral tipping of the pelvis, so that the external urinary meatus is higher than the anterior pelvic floor, thus directing the urine flow inward. The collection of increasing volumes of urine in the anterior part of the vaginal vault in-

duces sacculation and eventual drooping of the dilated vaginal vault into the abdominal cavity. Hence, a vicious circle is formed, which is aggravated by pneumovagina. The external cervical os is bathed in urine that may permeate the cervical canal and fill the uterus. As much as 3.5 liters of urine has been formed in the vaginal pool in some patients.

In order to avoid procreation of heritable conformational defects, the veterinarian should try to determine whether the abnormal pelvic structure is due to heritable influence or trauma. In many instances there will be a history of trauma, such as sacroiliac luxation acquired during extreme traction in delivering a fetus, and occasionally after violent struggling by an animal that has been cast. The condition will be evident by noticeable protrusion of the tubera sacrale above the spinal column. The tipped pelvis gives the appearance of a "weak loin" (Fig. 5).

Correction of urovagina is quite successful. However, if the condition has persisted for a prolonged period, the prognosis for restoration of fertility is guarded. Fortunately the surgical procedure is relatively simple and inexpensive, justifying an attempt at complete restoration.

Surgical Technique. A transverse dam composed of a fold of vaginal mucosa is established cranial to the external urinary meatus in order to prevent cranial flow of urine (Fig. 6). Surgery is done under low epidural anesthesia with the cow in the standing position. Urine and debris are scooped from the vagina by hand. The perin-

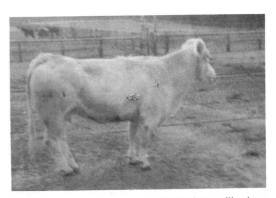

Figure 5. Charolais cow with bilateral sacroiliac luxation; injury sustained during forced fetal extraction. Acquired conformation predisposes to pooling of urine in anterior vagina. Note tipping of pelvis. (From Hudson, R. S.: The Bovine Practitioner, 7:34, 1972.)

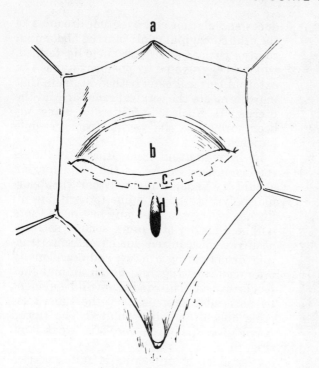

Figure 6. Surgical management of urine pooling in anterior vagina. Posterior view of open vulva showing technique of construction of transverse fold of vaginal floor: (a) dorsal commissure, (b) vaginal lumen, (c) transverse fold of vagina constructed by placement of continuous mattress sutures through base of fold and (d) suburethral diverticulum. (From Hudson, R. S.: The Bovine Practitioner, 7:34, 1972.)

eal region and vaginal vault are thoroughly and repeatedly flushed with an organic iodine surgical detergent. In order to deflate the greatly enlarged vagina, the cranial limit of the vagina is depressed, grasped with one hand and retracted, thus forcing out the air. Deflation is transitory, but it is helpful in elevating a transverse fold of mucosa on the vaginal floor. The fold should include the ventral 120° of the circumference of the vagina and is fixed in position by using a 12-cm half-curved, cutting-edge needle and 0.6-mm nonabsorbable suture material (Vetafil) in a continuous horizontal mattress pattern through the base of the fold. Approximately 8 cm of vaginal floor should be elevated to form the fold. The suturing is laborious, and provided the vagina is large enough, the use of both hands is helpful. Alternatively, vulsellum forceps may be helpful in maintaining the fold during establishment of the suture pattern. As the pattern is carried across the midline, the urethra must be avoided. The continuous suture is drawn taut, thus forming a semilunar dam about 5 cm high. The intent is to cause adhesion of the base of the fold for permanent structural change. Fortunately, the free edge of the dam tends to lean cranially, a safety factor for both cow and bull during coitus, should natural service be used. The suture is removed in 30 days. The

vagina is infused daily with a bland oil-base antibiotic medication.

If concomitant perineal injury causes pneumovagina, repair is required using the applicable techniques previously described. In the absence of primary pneumovagina, when only the dam is employed, the pooling of urine should cease immediately. This may be checked by manual rectal examination. The vagina, relieved of the continuing insult, should return to normal condition and tone.

PROLAPSE OF THE VAGINA

General Considerations. Protrusion of all or part of the everted vagina through the vulva is a common condition in certain pluriparous cows, especially those of the Hereford, Santa Gertrudis and Holstein breeds. Predisposing factors include vaginal injury at previous parturition; obesity, with a heavy deposition of perivaginal fat; extended intake of large volumes of low quality roughage; severe cold weather and poor conformation, including an excessively large and flaccid vulva. Studies have confirmed the influence of heredity on vaginal prolapse in some instances, particularly in certain bloodlines of Hereford cattle. Although this is cause for concern, it would be injudicious to diagnose every case of vaginal prolapse as being hereditary.

It is interesting to note that the common denominator in virtually every instance of vaginal prolapse is incompetence of the constrictor vestibuli and constrictor vulvae muscles. Thus, the varied causes of this incompetence represent the immediate predisposition.

Typically, vaginal prolapse is a condition of advanced gestation, occurring a few days to 2 or 3 months prior to parturition. This period coincides with increasing intraabdominal volume and pressure and with gradual slackening of the pelvic ligaments. Perhaps an excessive amount of estrogenic substances in the diet may stimulate vaginal prolapse.

Walker[10a] has classified vaginal prolapse based on progression, severity and prognosis.

FIRST-DEGREE PROLAPSE. The floor of the vagina protrudes intermittently through the gaping vulvar cleft, usually only when the cow is lying down. This stage may go unnoticed. The vagina becomes irritated by exposure to sun, wind, dust, cold temperature and fecal contamination. If parturition is not imminent, the continued vaginal irritation may produce tenesmus, which leads to the next stage.

SECOND-DEGREE PROLAPSE. The floor of the vagina is in continuous prolapse. If neglected, the bladder may be reverted into the prolapsus, kinking the urethra and interfering with urination. Exposure to external irritants is protracted. The problem is obvious even to the casual observer.

THIRD-DEGREE PROLAPSE. The cervix and almost the entire vagina are prolapsed. This may happen without progression through the first and second stages and is dependent on flaccidity of the vagina and lack of support of the perivaginal tissue. Third-degree prolapse is common in Santa Gertrudis cows with chronic cervical enlargement. If the cervical seal is materially disturbed, there is danger of imminent septic abortion. Regardless of the method of repair, the cow should be kept under close observation. Repeated attempts to detect viability of the fetus may aggravate the irritated vagina, but may be worthwhile. Signs of toxemia indicate fetal death.

FOURTH-DEGREE PROLAPSE. The prolapse is of prolonged duration. Deep necrosis has ensued, and there are adhesions between perivaginal tissue and adjacent organs, especially the bladder. Peritonitis is present or imminent. The prognosis for the dam is poor.

Frequently, unattended prolapse is complicated by prolapse of the rectum. Some authors favor amputation of the prolapsed rectum in these cases. This author chooses to dispense with amputation if at all possible, depending instead on replacement and purse-string suture.

Replacement of Vaginal Prolapse. Using epidural anesthesia the cleansed vagina is firmly but gently returned to its natural position with the hands. The fingers are kept together, or the fists are used in order to prevent bruising with the fingertips. The use of probangs is discouraged. Prolapse of long duration with severe edema may require patient and extended effort. Repeated covering of the exposed mucosa with a hygroscopic material such as sulfa urea powder is helpful.

Selection of Method of Retention. There are virtually dozens of ways of retaining the replaced vaginal prolapsus. This depends upon (1) the ingenuity of practitioners in a vexing situation and (2) the continued pursuit of the comprehensive "perfect" method. Vaginal prolapse characteristically appears during late gestation but sometimes occurs or recurs in the nongravid cow. Selection of a method of retention is somewhat dependent on the nearness to parturition and the frequency of observation that the convalescent patient will receive.

LACING OF THE VULVA. This technique is preferred by some operators when parturition or abortion is expected in a few days. Paired loops of doubled wide umbilical tape are placed in the thick skin at the hairline on each side of the vulva, and the loops are laced with 1-inch gauze. The advantages are simplicity and the intentional breaking of the lacing if the animal calves unattended. The disadvantages are that the retention is temporary and may have to be replaced, the lacing tends to collect feces and the irritation may induce resumption of tenesmus and prolapse.

HALSTED PATTERN. A series of umbilical tape sutures using the Halsted pattern is placed just dorsal to the dorsal commissure and along the vulvar cleft (Fig. 7). The sutures enter and exit through the thick skin at the hairline lateral to each vulvar lip. The

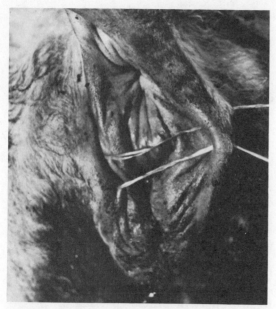

Figure 7. Halsted pattern for closure of vulva. Note sutures placed laterally at hairline.

area remains relatively free of gross fecal contamination. Sutures can be expected to last 3 weeks.

MODIFIED QUILL TECHNIQUE. Widely placed mattress sutures encircle vertically placed "quills" of rubber tubing or rope (Fig. 8). This is one of the most secure external fixation patterns.

BUHNER METHOD. This deeply placed circumferential suture has gained popularity with those who have used it. The objective is to insert a loop of tape that in effect simulates the action of the constrictor vestibuli muscle. Thus it can be used for correction of mild pneumovagina as well as retention of the replaced vagina. The technique is not to be confused with superficial purse-string sutures. The special equipment needed are a Buhner needle with the eye in the point and Buhner suture tape (tubular woven flattened nonabsorbable synthetic material).

After onset of epidural anesthesia, the perineal region is scrubbed and disinfected. A horizontal skin incision approximately 1 cm long is made midway between the anus and the dorsal commissure of the vulva. Another horizontal incision approximately 1.5 cm long is made at the same level as the ventral commissure of the vulva (cranial to the normally projecting ventral commissure).

The Buhner needle is introduced through the lower incision with the curvature directed in a lateral-medial direction (Fig. 9). With one hand in the vagina for guidance, the needle is embedded in the deep subcutaneous tissue, forced as far cranially as possi-

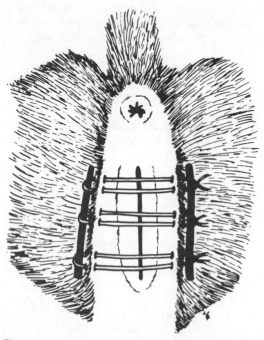

Figure 8. Modified quill pattern for closure of vulva. Rubber tubing is incorporated in suture line.

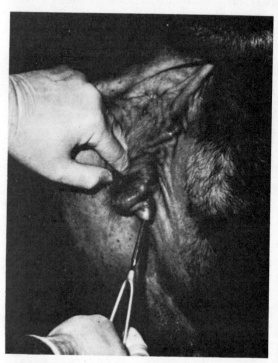

Figure 9. Buhner suture technique. Needle is directed through incision at ventral commissure of vulva and is forced as deeply cranially as possible before exiting through incision dorsal to dorsal commissure.

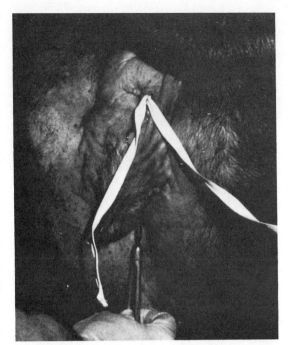

Figure 10. Buhner suture technique. Buhner suture material is threaded through exposed eye of needle. Note depth of tissue traversed.

ble and forced dorsally through the dorsal incision until the needle eye is well exposed.

A piece of antibiotic-soaked Buhner suture tape approximately 40 cm long is threaded through the needle (Fig. 10). While holding one end of the tape, the needle is withdrawn ventrally and the tape is removed from the eye of the needle. The needle without tape is introduced into the ventral incision and is forced dorsally on the opposite side, again emerging from the dorsal incision. The tape is again threaded into the eye of the needle, and the needle is withdrawn ventrally through the ventral incision (Fig. 11).

Tension is applied to each end of the tape, thus forcing the dorsal loop beneath the skin of the upper incision. The suture is tightened to permit entry of two or three fingers into the vulva, and a square knot or bow knot is used to maintain closure (Fig. 12). The constriction thus formed is circular (Fig. 13). When the square knot is used, it will actually be below the skin. The incisions may or may not be closed with simple interrupted sutures, depending on the individual surgeon's preference.

If the cow is close to calving (within 30 days), the bow knot is preferably used. Prior to calving this technique has disadvantages because extremely close observation of the patient and removal of the tape are necessary just prior to or at the time of parturition. The knot can be untied and gentle digital dilatation of the vulva will reduce tension.

For postpartum prolapses the square knot

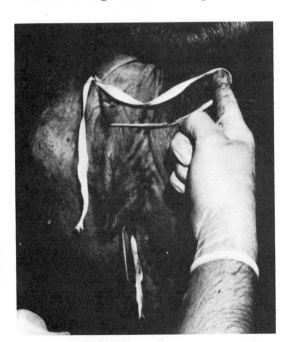

Figure 11. Buhner suture technique. Second limb of suture is carried around left side of vulva.

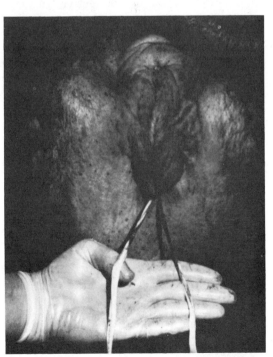

Figure 12. Buhner technique. The suture is pulled taut and tied at the ventral incision.

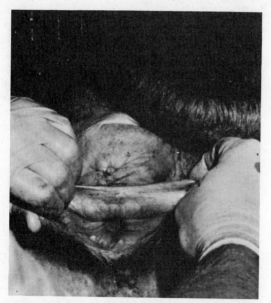

Figure 13. Completed effect of Buhner suture. Constriction resembles that of constrictor vestibuli muscle.

is used and is embedded under the skin. After a few days, the knot is not discernible except by close observation. If the cow is left in the breeding herd, normal copulation may occur and no hindrance to artificial insemination has been noticed. Often after the tape has been retained for 2 months or more, a moderate deposit of connective tissue is stimulated by the buried tape. The connective tissue band that is formed may be strong enough to prevent future prolapse, even after removal of the suture tape and infrequently it may be strong enough to cause dystocia. In such cases, episiotomy may be required.

CERVICOPEXY. Winkler[11] has described a technique in which the external os of the cervix is sutured to the prepubic tendon with a large U-shaped needle and nonabsorbable suture. This technique has not received the popularity that it deserves primarily because of initial discouragement of some of those who are trying it for the first time. One of the primary advantages is that postanesthesia tenesmus is minimal.

CESAREAN SECTION

Contrary to the tone of some authors of texts on obstetrics of 30 years ago, laparohysterotomy or cesarean section now enjoys a widely respected position among veteri-

narians as a means of fetal delivery. The procedure is employed frequently as the initial choice in handling critical bovine dystocia. Additionally, the experienced bovine practitioner takes satisfaction from the knowledge that the operation provides, in most cases, a satisfactory ultimate means of delivery of an otherwise inaccessible fetus.

Cesarean section, when truly indicated, generally meets acceptance by cattlemen as well. Since the operation frequently commands the highest fee among obstetrical procedures, the owner of a patient appreciates consideration of alternatives and even initial attempts at conventional delivery. However, the confident obstetrician wastes little time in deciding when cesarean section is indicated, thus avoiding further deterioration of the condition of dam and fetus.

Indications. Ideally, cesarean section is indicated when a live fetus cannot be delivered otherwise, when the dam presents a good surgical risk and when environmental factors are favorable for a major surgical procedure. Realistically, many cases in which the operation is indicated are less than ideal and require complexities of judgment. Cesarean delivery of a dead calf unduly upsets the cost:benefit ratio if a less costly alternative procedure (e.g., fetotomy at the hands of a skilled operator) would serve as well. This is particularly true with large dairy cows; less so with small beef heifers. Commonly in bovine practice, the patient is presented as a poor surgical risk because of general debilitation or prolonged neglected dystocia, but cesarean section may still be the most appropriate indication. Perhaps the most important disadvantage to such a situation is that the novice owner may unfairly condemn the procedure if an unfavorable termination ensues. Surgical invasion of the abdomen at low ambient temperature or when a brisk wind is stirring heavily contaminated air compounds surgical risk.

Fetal oversize is recorded as one of the most common indications for cesarean section. Among the causes are relative immaturity of the dam, genetic mismatching and prolonged gestation. The novice may presume that a fetus is too large for conventional delivery when the overall physical size or pelvic diameters of the dam are categorically small. This may not be the case; many very young heifers produce extremely small calves. In order to determine accurately whether a calf can be delivered by traction, the operator may attempt to draw the appropriate fetal parts, usually the head and extended forelimbs, into the pelvic canal. That is, the critical measurement of fetus versus maternal pelvis can be made by trying to deliver the calf. Good judgment dictates that this effort be done as quickly and gently as possible to avoid undue trauma to dam or fetus, should the final indication be cesarean section.

If the fetal head and extended forelimbs can be brought into the pelvic canal, delivery by traction is probable. One notable exception to this test is fetal muscular hypertrophy, "double muscling," in which the fetal hips and buttocks have the greatest transverse diameters of all fetal parts. This partial oversize allows the anterior parts of the fetus to be delivered with impunity, but then the extremely large hindquarters become impacted in the birth canal. Continued traction usually results in permanent unilateral femoral paralysis of the calf and may induce calving paralysis in the dam. Unfortunately the condition is difficult to anticipate prior to the operator's irreversible commitment to delivery by traction. When the condition is perceived as a herd problem, the veterinarian and owner or herdsman may instigate elective cesarean sections, or perhaps pelvic symphysiotomy.

A grossly putrescent and emphysematous fetus may be an indication for cesarean section, particularly if the uterine and cervical musculature are contracted, so that mutation is not accomplished safely. Again, this is a matter of good judgment. If the fetus can be removed readily by other than cesarean section, one avoids the high risk of peritonitis.

Cesarean section is clearly indicated when the uterus is ruptured, in order to avoid further trauma to the uterus, major uterine vessels and small intestines. Prolonged instances of torsion of the uterus, seen particularly in beef herds under careless surveillance, present a probable indication for cesarean section. While detorsion may be quite possible, the accompanying edema of the torsion area renders the tissue very friable and subject to rupture on delivery by traction.

Advanced hydrallantois suggests immediate cesarean section in the author's experience. While a more conservative means of inducing labor, such as use of estrogens and oxytocin, is a subjective alternative, the patient is usually physically weakened, owing to the reduced feed intake into the crowded rumen and the heavy weight of excessive intrauterine fluid. Every effort should be made to relieve the cow of the burden before involuntary recumbency, an extremely poor prognostic sign, develops.

The experienced obstetrician will encounter numerous other valid indications for cesarean section.

Choice of Surgical Approach. Certainly experience and personal preference influence each operator's selection of surgical approach. Key considerations include availability of restraint devices, operator control of the actions of the patient and accessibility to the gravid uterus. Some operators feel that the alert, even frenzied, beef heifer is an ideal candidate for the standing position, left flank approach in a squeeze chute; whereas a phlegmatic or exhausted cow might elect to lie down. The large, mature beef or dairy cow may also be more amenable to a standing position.

The flank approach may be used for animals in lateral recumbency. A distinct advantage of the left flank approach is that the rumen helps to hold the small intestine in place. In addition, should the animal develop rumen tympany during the operation, the opened left flank reduces respiratory embarrassment, and the rumen is readily accessible for deflation.

Ventral approaches include longitudinal midline and paramedian incisions, the latter being located either medial or lateral to the course of the left or right subcutaneous abdominal vein. The midline site is less vascular and probably can be incised and sutured more rapidly than paramedian locations. Unless there is a specific contraindication, left paramedian incisions are preferable to those on the right, in that during preparation and in the final stages of the operation the animal can rest in right lateral recumbency. The flank and ventral midline approaches will be described in detail.

Preoperative Considerations. Once a decision is made to perform cesarean section, the physical condition of the patient should be assessed. Although the procedure may be an emergency, haste should not preclude supplying any necessary antishock therapy, which can be continued during and after the surgery as needed.

Anesthesia. Usually epidural anesthesia and regional or local anesthesia are sufficient for most patients. General anesthesia and deep sedation are to be avoided when the fetus is alive. Xylazine is used extensively by some veterinarians but has the reported disadvantage of adversely increasing myometrial tone.

Flank Operation — Standing Animal. The patient selected for this approach should be of temperament and physical condition that indicate that the animal will remain standing during the procedure. Fractious animals should be confined in a clean squeeze chute with only a moderate amount of "squeeze," thus discouraging the animal's resting on the sides of the chute. Excessive restraint encourages the animal to lie down. All personnel should be warned to stay away from the patient's head to avoid causing the animal to charge and perhaps fall.

Epidural injection of 5 to 10 ml of 2 per cent procaine hydrochloride will reduce abdominal straining, defecation and tail movement and preserve the standing position. Next, the left paralumbar fossa and adjacent areas are clipped and scrubbed. Linear infiltration of the dorsal and cranial boundaries of the operative field with 2 per cent procaine hydrochloride provides satisfactory anesthesia. Paravertebral thoracolumbar block is an alternative.

If the animal is unruly, only the side bar of the chute should be draped. With tractable patients the operative field is covered with a waterproof absorbent shroud with a 30- to 40-cm incision opening.

Beginning at a point approximately 10 cm ventral to the lumbar transverse processes, all layers of the abdominal wall are incised along a 25- to 40-cm vertical line. Small heifers may require an oblique incision along the direction of the fibers of the external oblique muscle to gain adequate length of incision above the chute side.

Usually the pelvic limbs of the fetus are in the cranial portion of the gravid uterine horn, i.e., anterior fetal presentation. Grasping one or both pelvic extremities through the uterine wall, the appropriate portion of the uterus is rotated up and out through the incision. Avoiding placentomes and selecting the least vascular area of the exposed portion of the uterus, a longitudinal incision is made over the line from fetal foot to hock. A fetus with large buttocks may require a somewhat longer incision. Certainly the incision should be of sufficient length to prevent tearing of the uterus as the fetus is

removed. The fetal membranes are incised or torn and the fetus is withdrawn, preferably by an assistant, so that the operator can control the uterus and avoid intraperitoneal or intraincisional spillage of fetal fluid. As the fetus is removed, the umbilical cord is stretched and allowed to break 10 cm or so from the umbilicus, holding the cord at its abdominal end. The operator assures that a living calf receives adequate neonatal care.

If the fetus is alive, the placenta should be left undisturbed except for trimming frayed edges that could interfere with suturing the uterine incision. The serosal surface of the uterus is cleansed of blood clots and fibrin accumulation by rinsing with physiological saline and by rubbing with a gauze sponge. The operator may elect to place a broad-spectrum antibiotic in the uterus, particularly if the uterus is obviously septic.

A variety of inverting suture patterns are suitable for closing the uterine incision. Continuous patterns are preferable to interrupted sutures in their speed of application and exactness of closure. De Bois described a recurrent suture pattern that is successful. The incision may be closed with a Cushing suture, using No. 1 chromic gut. A contracting uterus requires one suture row; a debilitated organ requires two rows. Oxytocin (40 IU) may be given after suturing to hasten uterine contraction.

The abdominal incision is closed by simple continuous suture of the peritoneum and transverse abdominal muscle combined, using No. 1 chromic gut; by simple continuous or interrupted sutures of No. 2 or 3 chromic gut in the internal oblique muscle and the external oblique muscle and fascia, and by a continuous interlocking pattern in the skin, using nonabsorbable suture material. The procedure as described is suitable for the recumbent flank approach as well.

The weakened animal with advanced hydrallantois but with ability to stand should be operated with all haste in the standing position. Once an animal in this state becomes recumbent, the prognosis is poor. One may consider the right flank approach if the uterus distends the upper portion of that side. The unusually voluminous uterus may resist exteriorization. However, the fetus is usually small in such cases and can be removed intra-abdominally through a small uterine incision. As much fetal fluid as possible is left in the uterus, which is carefully sutured. One should anticipate spontaneous dilation of the cervix with gradual escape of the fluid within 24 hours. The patient should be observed and treated with intravenous fluids as needed.

Ventral Midline Approach. The young beef heifer is particularly suited to the ventral midline approach. This site is also useful when the operator encounters a large, greatly distended, septic uterus.

Low epidural anesthesia aids in preventing abdominal straining during the procedure. The patient is cast and restrained at an angle between right lateral recumbency and dorsal recumbency by tying the head and forelimbs anteriorly and the left hindlimb posteriorly. The right hindlimb is secured dorsally.

The ventral surface of the abdomen is clipped or shaved and scrubbed from the udder to a transverse line 12 cm anterior to the umbilicus. The midline is infiltrated with 2 per cent procaine hydrochloride from a point 7 cm anterior to the umbilicus to the base of the udder. A waterproof, absorbent shroud of sufficient size to cover the abdomen, udder and hindlimbs is put in place.

The skin incision is begun 5 to 7 cm anterior to the umbilicus and is carried posteriorly as needed. Following incision of the subcutaneous fascia, the abdominal tunic and peritoneum are incised longitudinally.

Upon opening the abdominal cavity, the free edge of the greater omentum is identified internal and posterior to the posterior commissure of the abdominal incision. This free edge is drawn anteriorly, thus exposing the uterus. The gravid horn is exteriorized by grasping a fetal part, usually one or both pelvic limbs.

Incision of the uterus, removal of the fetus and suturing of the uterine incision are much the same as in the flank approach. Following return of the uterus to the abdominal cavity, the greater omentum is drawn posteriorly over the exposed viscera.

The peritoneum and abdominal tunic together are closed, using a continuous overlapping mattress pattern with 0.6 mm or larger nonabsorbable synthetic suture. Care should be taken not to damage the suture material, which reduces its tensile strength. The closure is completed by applying a simple continuous pattern of the same suture material to the free overlapping edge and the underlying tunic. The skin and fascia are sutured with a continuous interlocking pattern, again using nonabsorbable 0.6 mm synthetic suture.

Aftercare. The dam is encouraged to rise as soon as possible. If the fetus is alive, it is often wise to milk some colostrum from the dam and give it to the calf via stomach tube with the idea that the intervention of the obstetrical procedure may delay natural acceptance of the calf by the dam.

Uncomplicated cases indicate a good prognosis. If the uterus is particularly debilitated and septic, one should anticipate possible severe septicemia for up to 1 week postdelivery.

REFERENCES

1. De Bois, C. H. W.: Oral presentation. Annual Conference, Society for Theriogenology, University of Missouri, October, 1973.
2. Bierschwal, C. J. and De Bois, C. H. W.: The Buhner method for control of chronic vaginal prolapse in the cow. Vet. Med. Small Anim. Clin., *66*:230, 1971.
3. Buhner, E.: Simple surgical treatment of uterine and vaginal prolapse. Tieraerztl. Umsch., *13*:183, 1958 (in German).
4. Friermuth, G. J.: Episiotomy in veterinary obstetrics. J.A.V.M.A., *113*:(Sept.)23, 1948.
5. Habel, R. E.: The topographic anatomy of the muscles, nerves and arteries of the bovine female perineum. Am. J. Anat., *19*:79, 1966.
6. Hudson, R. S.: Repair of perineal lacerations in the cow. Bovine Practit., 7:34, 1972.
7. Roberts, S. J.: Veterinary Obstetrics and Genital Diseases (Theriogenology). 2nd Ed. Published by author. Distributed by Edwards Bros., Ann Arbor, Mich., 1971.
8. Rosenberger, G.: Krankheiten des Rindes. Berlin, Paul Parey, 1970 (in German).
9. Sloss, V. and Dufty, J. H.: Elective cesarean operation in Hereford cattle. Austral. Vet. J., *53*:420, 1977.
10. Vandeplassche, M.: Embryotomy and Cesarotomy. *In* Oehme, F. W. and Prier, J. E. (eds): Textbook of Large Animal Surgery. Baltimore, The Williams & Wilkins Co., 1974.
10a. Walker, D. F.: Personal communication.
11. Winkler, J. K.: Repair of bovine vaginal prolapse by cervical fixation. J.A.V.M.A., *149*:768, 1966.
12. Woodward, R. R. and Queensberry, J. R.: A study of vaginal and uterine prolapse in Hereford cattle. J. Anim. Sci., *15*:119, 1956.

Periparturient Care of the Dam

MAARTEN DROST
University of Florida, Gainesville, Florida

PREPARTUM CARE

Prepartum care offers the opportunity to medically evaluate, supervise and maintain the optimal physical condition of the pregnant cow or heifer to insure delivery of a healthy calf. Although such care should start at the time of sire selection and breeding and should be followed by a balanced nutritional program and adequate exercise, particularly in heifers, it frequently is not provided until term approaches.

Emphasis should be placed on the following goals:

1. Client education.
   a. Nutrition.
   b. Immunization.
   c. Management.
2. Provision of a maternity area.
3. Supervision at calving time.

Maternity Area

The ideal calving area is a level pasture area, free from brush and bodies of water and near enough to the house to allow frequent observation and supervision of parturition. A spacious, dry, well-bedded boxstall is an acceptable alternative during periods of inclement weather or in total confinement operations.

Regular exercise should be provided.

The animal should be moved into the maternity area several days to 1 week prior to the anticipated time of calving. The hindquarters should be cleaned at this time to minimize contamination of the birth canal during parturition.

Signs of Impending Parturition

Accelerated mammary development is one of the earliest signs of impending parturition. Incipient enlargement occurs in heifers during the fourth month of gestation. In cows, enlargement of the udder may not become apparent until 2 to 3 weeks before parturition. Just prior to parturition, the udder secretion changes from a sticky serum discharge to colostrum, a thick, yellowish, opaque secretion.

Detection of changes in the sacrosciatic ligaments by simultaneous external and rectal palpation is an accurate method of determining the onset of parturition in most cattle. Slight relaxation first becomes evident a few days before term, when it is possible to displace the posterior border of the ligament up to 2.5 cm by using moderate pressure. A slight dropping of the muscles over this region and a slightly raised tailhead become apparent in a few animals at this time. The onset of progressive relaxation of the ligaments coincides with the onset of cervical softening and dilation.

Complete relaxation of the caudal border of the pelvic ligaments is generally followed by parturition within 12 hours.

Signs of discomfort and restlessness do not usually appear until the cervix has dilated sufficiently to admit a hand. Slight dorsal arching of the back is apparent at this time, but definite straining does not commence until the chorioallantois nears the vulva. Hydrostatic pressure by the fetal fluids contained within the intact membranes assists in complete effacement of the cervix. Stretching of the vagina reflexly evokes contractions of the abdominal muscles, and during one of these contractions the chorioallantois ruptures. Following rupture of this membrane, there is a temporary weakening or cessation of the abdominal press, which resumes as the amnion nears the vulva. The average interval between rupture of the chorioallantois and the amnion is about 1 hour.

Once the amniotic sac bursts, regular intermittent straining begins after a brief rest period. As labor progresses, there is a gradual increase in the frequency and duration of the abdominal contractions, and straining sometimes becomes nearly continuous during the last few minutes of parturition. The greatest delay in expulsion of the calf occurs when the head reaches the vulva. At this stage little outward progression takes place during each series of contractions, and the calf frequently recedes into the vagina between bouts. This feature is most obvious in heifers, in which stretching of the vulva

272

takes more time. Once the head of the calf has passed through the vulva, the rest of the body follows rapidly.

If no progress is made for 2 hours after the appearance of the amnion, assistance should be given.

Following delivery, the first attention should be directed toward the initiation of respiration in the calf (see following article).

IMMEDIATE POSTPARTUM CARE OF THE DAM

After the delivery of each calf the uterus must be checked for the presence of another fetus. At the same time the birth canal is examined for trauma. Next the udder is examined for the presence of colostrum and the possibility of blind quarters or mastitis.

If dystocia occurred, 50 units of oxytocin is administered parenterally to the dam to expel air, fetal fluids and blood from the uterus and to lessen the likelihood of uterine prolapse and retained placenta. The cow is made to stand, again to reduce the possibility of uterine prolapse, particularly after a forced extraction, and to assess the extent of possible nerve damage during delivery.

Intrauterine antibiotic therapy (2 gm of oxytetracycline) is given at this time if hygienic conditions are suboptimal or if prolonged assistance was required. It is important that the medication be placed between the endometrium and the fetal membranes and not merely dropped into the lumen of the uterus. Routine intrauterine antibiotic treatment of all cows in a herd after unassisted term delivery is not recommended. In the event of trauma to the birth canal, broad-spectrum systemic antibiotics are administered as well.

Trauma to the Birth Canal

Trauma to the soft tissues of the genital tract or to the bony pelvis may lead to fatal hemorrhage or infection or to disability due to fractures, dislocations or paralysis.

Minor lacerations and contusions are common, particularly to the vulva and cervix after forced extraction and fetotomy. Mild lacerations need not be sutured. However, they frequently become infected, especially if the tissues are traumatized and devital-

ized or if retention of the fetal membranes occurs. Infected lacerations result in swelling, pain and persistent straining. Treatment consists of use of parenteral broad-spectrum antibiotics and epidural anesthesia, which gives temporary relief from straining. In beef cattle with chronic tenesmus, 5 to 10 ml of ethyl alcohol may be injected epidurally; 4 ml is injected initially followed by 1-ml increments at 10-minute intervals just until the straining is abolished. Return of sensation to the tail will be delayed for several weeks after this treatment.

Lacerations of the vagina generally occur at the vestibulovaginal junction, particularly in fat heifers. A large fetus may be preceded by a cuff of perivaginal fat that ruptures during forced extraction when it is halted by the constriction of the vestibulovaginal junction just anterior to the urethral diverticulum. Perivaginal fat is extruded through the laceration in the vaginal mucosa. This fat should be trimmed out with scissors, and the procedure will be accompanied by very little bleeding. The defect occurs most frequently in the lateral wall of the vagina and may be repaired or left to heal without suturing. Systemic antibiotics are given.

Hemorrhage from the birth canal may be due to a torn caruncle or caruncular stalk or to the attempted premature removal of the fetal membranes. Occasionally, the intercornual septum is exceptionally long and extends almost to the internal os of the cervix. This predisposes it to rupture and to subsequent bleeding. To repair tears in the uterus that are located not too close to the cervix, the uterus may be made to prolapse by injecting 10 ml of epinephrine solution (1:1000 USP) intravenously and inverting the gravid horn. A handful of caruncles is grasped as close to the tip of the previously gravid horn as possible and gradually pulled into the birth canal where the presence of the mass elicits straining. This leads to complete prolapse of the uterus as the horn is steadily pulled posteriorly. Epinephrine renders the uterus completely flaccid. The procedure must not be preceded by the administration of either oxytocin or epidural anesthesia.

Administration of 50 units of oxytocin aids in control of hemorrhage by contracting the uterus and its vessels.

Lacerations of the cervix produce particularly serious and persistent hemorrhage.

Such trauma occurs when the cervix is incompletely dilated and the calf is forcibly extracted. Attempts at control are difficult but may be made by withdrawal of the cervix to the vulva, using cervical forceps under epidural anesthesia.

If bleeding occurs from a large vessel through a laceration in the vaginal wall, the vessel should be clamped by forceps. The handle of the instrument is sutured to the dorsal commissure of the vulva and left in place for 1 week.

With severe intrauterine hemorrhage the clot is left undisturbed for 24 hours, at which time it may be broken down and removed manually. This is followed by intrauterine antibiotic treatment. Blood transfusions are given as dictated by the hematocrit value and the condition of the patient. Most fatal hemorrhages occur intraperitoneally because of rupture of the large vessels in the blood ligament. This occurs most frequently with torsion or prolapse of the uterus. When such hemorrhage is suspected, the only hope of saving the animal is prompt laparotomy and ligation of the vessel.

REFERENCE

1. Dufty, J. H.: Determination of the onset of parturition in Hereford cattle. Austr. Vet. J., 47:77, 1971.

Perinatal Care of the Calf

MAARTEN DROST

University of Florida, Gainesville, Florida

At the time of parturition the fetus undergoes dramatic physiological changes after its relatively passive intrauterine existence. From its temperature-controlled, protected aquatic environment it is forced through a narrow birth canal into hostile surroundings. To insure uninterrupted oxygenation it must suddenly initiate respiration. Profound circulatory and digestive changes occur, and the neonate must respond to innumerable antigenic challenges.

When called upon to assist in the delivery of a calf, it is the task of the veterinarian to minimize adverse influences threatening the calf and to enhance its defenses.

ESTABLISHMENT OF RESPIRATION

Delayed passage through the birth canal in the face of a faltering placenta compromises oxygenation of the calf. Although the animal is able to breathe as soon as the nose passes the labia, expansion of the chest is restricted by the narrow birth canal. This situation is seriously aggravated when continuous forced traction is applied. As soon as the head passes the lips of the vulva, extraction should be interrupted, the nostrils cleared of mucus and cold water applied to the head.

Again, when the calf is completely delivered, primary attention is directed toward establishing respiration. Mucus and fetal fluids should be expressed from the nose and mouth by external pressure of the thumbs along the bridge of the nose and the flat fingers in the intermandibular space, sliding from the level of the eyes toward the muzzle. If the calf fails to start breathing on its own, it may be suspended by the hindlegs with the head off the ground. Next, excessive mucus and amniotic fluid are expressed from the airways by applying slow, bilateral pressure with the hands along the chest from the costal arches to the neck. This is done once and firmly. The airways are most effectively cleared by suction.

Respiration is stimulated by many factors, but only ventilation of the lungs, cooling and certain drugs allow us to render help immediately. The best stimulus for respiration is ventilation of the lungs. Cooling is a very important respiratory stimulus that can be achieved by simply pouring cold water over the head of the calf. Brisk rubbing of the skin or tickling of the nasal mucosa with a piece of straw also has a favorable effect. The phrenic nerve can be stimulated with a sharp tap on the thorax slightly dorsocaudal to where the heartbeat can be felt.

Several drugs are available to stimulate

respiration (doxapram hydrochloride, nikethamide, pentylenetetrazol). Administration of these products generally leads to the calf's taking several deep breaths. As every inspiration is a stimulus for the next one, these agents may have a favorable effect. It should be remembered that these respiratory stimulants are generally short acting, with a transient effect of 5 to 10 minutes.

The objection to use of all of these measures with the truly asphyctic calf is that application of artificial respiration is postponed too long. Progressive asphyxia may lead to cerebral damage, which further reduces the success of our attempts at resuscitation.

Forced Ventilation

Forced ventilation has the inherent danger of causing pneumothorax when the force with which the air is introduced into the lungs is too great. The resistance of the lungs, which have been atelectatic until now, is much greater than that of the abomasum, with the result that most of the air ends up in the stomach. Endotracheal intubation obviates this problem, but placement of the tube requires a certain amount of dexterity. The use of oxygen-rich air mixtures can frequently support our treatment but cannot take its place.

Artificial Respiration

The calf is placed in lateral recumbency, and the mouth and nostrils are cleared of mucus. An assistant holds the mouth open and extends the tongue of the calf to allow air to pass freely. While kneeling at the backside of the calf, the veterinarian uses one hand to grasp the humerus of the top leg, and the other hand is pushed a little way underneath the last rib. Next, the chest wall is elevated by lifting the front leg and the costal arch until the calf is almost lifted off the ground. This expands the chest. During a short pause the lungs are given the opportunity to expand. The latter expansion is slow because the lungs are still atelectatic. Next the thoracic walls are firmly compressed with flat hands. These movements are repeated approximately once every 5 seconds, whereby the major effort is aimed at the inspiration.

As a rule, no expiratory sound will be heard until after several resuscitory movements. Initially, very little air will be aspirated as the lungs begin to expand. This treatment may be maintained for 15 minutes while other methods to stimulate respiration are employed, e.g., cold water or drugs. When spontaneous respiratory movements occur after a few minutes, they are immediately supported, after which the rhythm of the artificial respiration is resumed.

The major advantage of this prompt intervention is that the lungs are immediately supplied with oxygen. In addition, the heart is massaged, and a pumping action is exerted on the large vessels of the heart, stimulating circulation.

After the frequency and depth of spontaneous respiration have reached an adequate level, the calf is briskly rubbed dry. The calf is then placed on its chest with the front legs extended and spread out and the hindlegs in a dog-sitting position extended alongside the body. This facilitates expansion of the chest. A handful of straw may be placed bilaterally in the axillae to keep a weak calf from falling over.

ASSESSMENT OF VIABILITY

Neonatal asphyxia is the result of inadequate gaseous exchange between the maternal and fetal circulation during parturition, i.e., caused by placental detachment. Oxygen uptake and carbon dioxide release are insufficient and lead to a respiratory acidosis. Gradually a metabolic acidosis also develops, as a result of the accumulation of acid products of metabolism originating from anaerobic fat conversion. A serious acidosis leads to central depression and constriction of arterioles, which in turn lead to a sharp decrease in the pulmonary circulation.

Depending on the degree of the hypoxia immediately after parturition, *dyspnea* is present, whereby the rate of respiration is very slow or absent; *muscle tone* is flaccid; reflexes are diminished or absent and the pulse may be less than 100 beats per minute. The prognosis becomes worse with the progressive absence of reflexes from the hindleg pedal reflex, to the front leg pedal reflex, to the swallowing reflex to the corneal reflex.

An edematous head and cyanotic swollen tongue may be due to wedging of the head in the birth canal, hence of a local nature. Treatment must be aimed at establishing ventilation, correcting the acidosis and improving the circulation.

A strict respiratory acidosis rapidly improves with proper ventilation. Metabolic acidosis may be corrected by slow intravenous injection of 4 to 5 gm of sodium bicarbonate solution in 50 ml of sterile water or 5 per cent dextrose solution.

AFTERCARE

Once respiration has been established, the umbilical stump is disinfected and dried by submersion in a clean cup of tincture of iodine. The calf is examined for the presence of cleft palate, contracted tendons or other congenital defects.

The newborn calf should be housed in a draft-free environment with an optimal temperature of 15°C and humidity of 70 per cent. It is important that the calf receive 2 liters (5 per cent of body weight) of its dam's colostrum immediately after birth.

Health Management of the Periparturient Cow and Calf in Large Herds

PAUL E. BLACKMER

Chino Valley Veterinary Group, Ontario, California

INTRODUCTION

Many veterinarians involved in dairy practice are familiar with the seemingly irrepressible economic-based trend of dairymen toward larger herd sizes, more intensive confinement and increased labor efficiency. Most typically, such operations have expanded or modified existing facilities piecemeal as cow numbers increased. In some instances, completely new operations have been built from the ground up. Unfortunately, in both cases the situation too frequently is one of a dairyman experienced in running smaller, less concentrated herds designing facilities for larger herds with more animal concentration and with which he has had little direct experience. Such situations predictably result in new herd health problems that the owner did not anticipate. The health of the periparturient cow and of the neonatal calf is most often the first aspect of herd health that is jeopardized when such ill-conceived animal concentration occurs.

It is the purpose of this article to call attention to specialized herd health practices developed at large dairies (having more than 1000 cows) that have been successful in maintaining herd health despite increased concentration of large herds.

The large dairies from which the data for this article were obtained are located in the semi-arid southwestern region of the United States. Perhaps nowhere else has the trend toward dairy cattle concentration been more dramatic or successful. Although this information is directly applicable to their style of dairying and climate, most of the practices to be described also apply and can be profitably adapted to smaller dairies in other areas. Because of their relatively unique style of dairying, as compared with the more traditional dairy farm areas of the northern and eastern United States, a brief description of the southwestern area's husbandry practices is in order to establish proper perspective.

Dairy cattle in this area are managed in what are called dry lot dairies. Herds in excess of 1000 milking cows are common, although not yet considered average. The cows typically are confined in outdoor dirt-based corrals with shades, which, if present, provide the only protection from a mild climate. The cow concentration in corrals averages one cow per 600 square feet of corral space, with 100-cow corrals being the most common size for the larger dairies. Locking stanchions usually make up the entire front or manger perimeter of the corral with the head openings spaced every 2 1/2 feet apart. The area directly behind the stanchions is the only cemented portion of the corral. The practice of pasturing milking cows is essentially nonexistent on dry lot dairies, although a small percentage of these dairies do keep some of their dry cows on small, irrigated pasture maintained in conjunction with waste water management. Most commonly, milk cows are kept in the corrals closest to the milking barns, and dry cows are farthest from the barn.

DRY COW MANAGEMENT

The management of the dry cow has considerable impact on the health of the periparturient cow and calf and is an integral part of the herd health management program.

Ideally, the dry cow program starts 1 to 2 weeks prior to actually drying off the cows. Late-lactation cows in advanced gestation are selected for drying off, based on breeding and production records. These records, plus the physical appearance of the cow, should be reviewed for each animal individually to determine if the cow should be culled or dried. Cows with a partially ruptured median suspensory ligament or a pendulous udder will be prone to udder and teat injury at freshening and even without injury represent a special labor problem to milk. Cows with locomotor problems likewise should be scrutinized to determine if drying or culling would be most profitable. Cows with chronic unresponsive mastitis should be culled rather than dried in most instances.

Once the decision to dry a cow is made, she should be moved to a drying-off string. Such a string accumulates cows for 1 to 2 weeks in preparation for weekly or biweekly drying off. The nutrition for this string should be roughages only. Concentrates should not be fed. The objective of moving the late-lactation cow to this string is to alter her social and nutritional status such that milk production decreases and drying off is more easily accomplished. Cows needing foot trimming should be taken care of before leaving this string. Also, each cow's pregnancy status should be reconfirmed by rectal palpation or "bumping."

Dry cow therapy is recommended for every quarter on every cow immediately after the last milking. It is advisable that a management person be present on days when cows are dried. At the time of treatment the date should be clearly marked on the cow's hip both for later reference in the dry corral and to signify that she has been dry-cow treated.

The practice of marking dates or symbols on cows in different colors using livestock marking crayons or aerosol spray paint is an extremely useful management aid in large herds. It is not, however, a substitute for individual cow record cards.

The subject of dry cow vaccinations should be mentioned, in that owners of many herds vaccinate cows at the time they are dried. The merit of cow vaccination at this period of gestation is that the antibody titers for the antigens used should be very high in the cow's colostrum at freshening. It is felt that such vaccinations can be very beneficial to the control of selected neonatal calf diseases. In the author's experience, dry cow vaccination for various *Salmonella* organisms has been useful in the control of calfhood salmonellosis.

Recent work has shown beneficial results in the control of retained placentae and postpartum metabolic disease by the injection of selenium and vitamin E preparations in dry cows. Such approaches to the health management of the periparturient cow and calf should not be overlooked. However, local conditions vary such that treatments that are beneficial in one area or management system may not be justifiable elsewhere.

The selective grouping of dry cows on large dairies is practical, economical and commendable from a herd health viewpoint. Four separate cow groups should be maintained: (1) cows just dried; (2) lean, dry cows; (3) fat, dry cows, and (4) cows that are 3 weeks or less away from calving.

The flow of dry cows after the last milking should begin at the corral for recently dried cows. The cows going into this corral should still have the date that they were dried clearly marked on them. This will enable one to make a more educated appraisal at a glance of whether a cow's udder is involuting properly or if a problem situation is arising. Enlarged, noninvoluting quarters should be examined to determine if additional treatment is necessary. Culturing for bacteria and mycoplasmal organisms may be indicated. Deficiencies in the drying-off policy should be suspected if more than a few cows appear as problem cows this soon after drying. The practice of teat-dipping all cows in this string at least once daily is recommended.

The diet for cows in this corral again should be roughage only. Combinations of legume hay, corn silage and/or nonlegume hay should be fed to approximate the National Research Council (NRC) requirements of net energy, crude protein, calcium, phosphorus and vitamin A for dry cows. Excessive amounts of calcium and protein are to be avoided because these have been incriminated as causes of milk fever and downer cow syndrome, respectively. In practice, feeding two to three parts of oat hay to one part of alfalfa hay often approximates the needs of this group of dry cows. Trace-mineralized, free-choice salt should be available.

After 2 weeks in the recently dried corral, most cows' udders have involuted, signifying that they are ready to be moved to either the fat dry cow corral or the lean dry cow corral. Booster vaccinations should be given at this time if dry cow vaccinations are practiced.

The only difference in nutrition for these two groups is that grain can be fed to the lean group, if necessary, in addition to the roughage diet just described, which is fed to all groups of dry cows. Three to 5 pounds of a dairy concentrate per head per day is recommended for dry cows in the lean group. The segregation used at this time, based on the cow's condition at the end of lactation, should be recorded so that a more enlightened use of production feeding during the subsequent lactation can be made to prevent excessively fat cows.

Approximately 2 to 3 weeks prior to calving, as their udders start to make up, the dry cows should be moved to a close-up corral. The nutrition of this corral should consist of roughage, using the same guidelines as for other dry cows, plus milk cow concentrate at a rate of one-quarter to one-third the amount fed to the fresh cow string. A high-phosphorus mineral supplement may be necessary in addition to free-choice, trace-mineralized salt. Grain feeding is increased at this time to gradually develop a rumen flora that will be compatible with the higher concentrate-to-roughage ratio that will be fed postfreshening.

CALVING AREA MANAGEMENT

The calving area is the bridge between the close-up dry cow corral and the milk cow strings. Ideally, it should be located directly adjacent to the close-up dry cow corral and be one of the most intensively managed areas of the dairy. It should be designed for year-round calving, with sanitation in mind, and should have facilities for proper handling and restraint of periparturient cows and neonatal calves. In a large herd such an area should be divided into four subgroups: (1) the close-up area, (2) the maternity area, (3) the fresh cow area and (4) the calf-holding area (Fig. 1).

Close-up Area

Close-up dry cows should enter this area from the close-up dry cow corral when it is apparent that they are within several days of calving. In practice, twice weekly segregation from the close-up dry cow corral is necessary to accomplish this most efficiently. The rationale for this grouping is to have a small group of cows in a small area that can be closely observed and easily moved to the maternity area within hours of parturition.

This close-up pen should be dirt-based as much as possible for the comfort and safety of the cow. The population density in this pen should be about one-half that of the milk cow corrals; otherwise, the manure build-up can become incompatible with keeping cows clean. This area should be free of holes, which may result in heavily pregnant cows being trapped in lateral recumbency and becoming bloated. The pen should be sloped enough to allow for good drainage during rainy periods. There should be a roof over the end of the pen away from the drainage, so that a dry place is always available for cows to lie down. This roof should also serve as a shade in hot weather.

The individual cow records should be reviewed as cows approach the calving area. Notations on the record from previous years can alert the calving area attendant of the possibility of milk fever occurring in certain cows based on prior calvings. Also, checking production data at this time should serve to call attention to which cows are the most valuable and thus deserve special considerations. Cows that are already leaking substantial amounts of colostrum should be recorded as such, both on the record and on the cow herself. Calves from these cows should be considered as candidates for bottle feeding of colostrum from other cows. The cows should be teat-dipped daily prior to calving

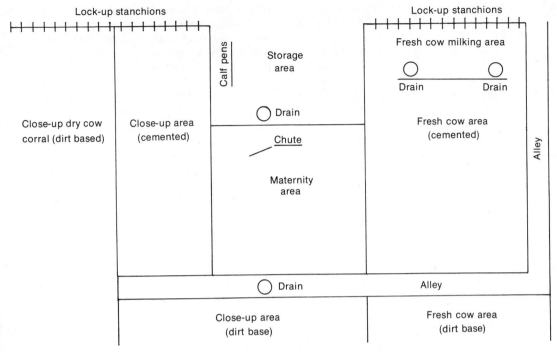

Figure 1. Schematic diagram of calving area. The close-up area, maternity area, storage area and fresh cow area all have sloped cement floors with good drainage and are covered by a single 20 foot high wood framed aluminum roof. The cemented portion is partially bedded with straw.

in an effort to reduce the incidence of coliform mastitis during the periparturient period.

Cows in the close-up areas should have the hair on their udders and flanks clipped. This practice helps to insure clean udders at the time of nursing by the calf and will also allow better udder sanitation after the cow reaches the milking strings.

Maternity Area

The maternity area should be an exceptionally clean area where the cow can calve with minimal contamination of the calf, the exposed fetal membranes and the cow's udder.

The cow should be brought into this area when it is apparent that parturition has started and should be removed after the calf is standing and has nursed. Because of the need for sanitation and the number of cows calving each day, it is often impractical to hold cows and calves in this area longer than several hours.

The calving area should be approximately 2400 square feet. In practice a pen measur-

ing 40 by 60 feet works well. Because of the need for continuous cleaning, such an area should be paved and sloped and have adequate drainage. It should be covered by a roof, preferably about 20 feet high, and have a windbreak. A chute for restraining the cow in cases of assisted deliveries should be located within the maternity area. Water hydrants should be convenient for hosing down the area.

The maintenance of the area should allow for 24-hour calving. In practice this is best accomplished by alternating the bedding and cleaning of each half of the maternity area. While one end is bedded with straw for use by cows that are calving, the other half is left unbedded. After the straw becomes contaminated with use, it is scraped out and the area hosed down and left unbedded until needed (when the alternate end is in need of cleaning). Thus, only one-half of the area of the maternity pen is in use at one time. The use of straw as a bedding material appears to work quite well and is recommended. Sawdust or shavings are less desirable because of their tendency to adhere to the wet calf, especially to its mouth and nose.

Because this area is paved, it may be unwise to bring in older cows with a history of milk fever or locomotor problems. For such cows and for cows that refuse to accept the paved surface and/or confinement, an alternative maternity area is advisable. A small, flat, well-maintained pasture would be ideal. If such an area is not available, allowing cows to calve in the close-up corral is a possible alternative. This practice, however, can be a serious breach of disease control in the case of the brucellosis-infected herd.

The restraint facilities within the maternity area should consist of a funnel chute along one of the perimeters with a head-catching front gate. The facilities should be designed so that a single person can confine the cow suitably for obstetrical procedures. In addition, the footing for this area should not be slick or slippery. The sides to the chute should open on either side and be such that they can be used like a squeeze chute. These side gates should be hinged from the front for maximum versatility and convenience. In the event that the cow goes down, the gates can be opened for easy access to the cow. The head gate, in addition to having a head-catching stanchion-like arrangement, should also be hinged to allow forward exit of the cow when open. At the rear of the cow, another gate should be situated in the side of the chute to allow easy access to and from the cow for obstetrical procedures. Such a chute is not only convenient and safe for the operator but also can make the difference between success and failure in the handling of many calving problems.

Once the cow has calved and the calf is standing and has nursed, the cow and calf can be separated. If the number of other cows calving at this time is few, the cow and calf should be left together as long as possible up to 12 hours. If, on the other hand, many cows are calving at the same time in the maternity area, prompt removal is necessary.

Care of the calf before removal from the maternity area includes: (1) trimming the navel with a clean pair of scissors; (2) tying the navel off if necessary to prevent excessive hemorrhage; (3) disinfection of the navel, preferably with 7 per cent iodine sprayed on and then massaged into the umbilical vessels and surrounding hair manually; (4) identification of the calf and (5) neonatal calf vaccination.

The vaccination of day-old calves with oral or intranasal vaccines has been widely practiced with variable results. It appears that such practices are very beneficial in selected herds with specific problems. The use of live vaccines, killed bacterins or hyperimmune serums should be considered in herds with calf morbidity and mortality problems as one part of calf health management only, not as a panacea to overcome unsound husbandry practices.

The colostrum feeding of the calf in the maternity area should vary according to individual circumstances. Cows with clean, nursable udders that have not leaked excessive amounts of colostrum during the close-up period should be allowed to nurse their calves. Calves from cows that have been leaking large amounts of colostrum, usually high production cows, are to be fed 2 quarts of colostrum obtained from other cows. A nipple bottle should be used for such feeding. If the maternity area has been overcrowded such that the cows and bedding are unacceptably soiled, prompt removal of the calf and bottle feeding of colostrum are advised.

Fresh Cow Area

The fresh cow area serves to collect cows from the maternity area and hold them until their milk is suitable for sale for human consumption. This area is the source of colostrum for the calf-raising program. It also serves as an intensified management area where fresh cows can be given special attention as needed before placing them back with the milking herd.

The fresh cow area should be dirt-based as much as possible to provide good footing for the cows. The population density for such a corral should be only half that of the milking strings. This prevents the rapid build-up of filth and contamination and allows the surface of the area to remain more acceptable for longer periods of time.

This group of cows should have its own milking facilities apart from the milking facilities of the rest of the herd. Flat-barn type construction with stanchions and bucket milking machines is preferable to herringbone-type parlors with milk pipelines. With the former type of milking confinement, better sanitation and observation are possible for both the milking and the treatment of fresh cows.

The sanitation and maintenance of the

milking equipment for this fresh cow group require special mention. Too frequently, in the author's experience, the milking equipment of the fresh cow area suffers from more neglect than the milking equipment in the regular milking area. It is imperative that rubber parts be properly maintained. Routine bacteria counts of the fresh cow milk are advisable, both from the viewpoint of udder health and calf health. Unless a sound wash-up procedure and milking machine maintenance program are adopted, bacteria counts will greatly exceed the bulk tank level. This should be recognized as being inconsistent with good management of the periparturient cow and neonatal calf.

If this fresh cow milking area is also used to milk the "hospital string," another precaution should be realized. That is, fresh cows are to be milked first, mastitis cows last. Too frequently, a common fresh cow and hospital string results in seemingly unsolvable mastitis problems in the herd, which teat-dipping and dry cow treatment are unable to prevent.

The milking time procedure for milking fresh cows should start with hosing off the rear quarters and udder of the cows, followed by a period for the cow to drip dry. Only after the udders are clean and dry and the cows foremilked should the milking machine be attached. Extra effort is usually required to clean udders on fresh cows. Failure to milk clean, dry udders with clean milking equipment is conducive to coliform mastitis. Because of the relatively few cows in a fresh cow string and the increased susceptibility to mastitis as this time, it is advisable to sanitize the milking cluster and hands between cows. This is best accomplished by use of clear rinse water first, followed by sanitizing solution at bactericidal concentration. It is important that the sanitizer not be overloaded with milk so that this procedure becomes an infection process rather than a disinfection process. Postmilking teat-dipping at the time of milking machine removal is recommended.

Milk produced from the fresh cow string belongs in one of three categories and should be segregated accordingly as: (1) first milking colostrum, (2) fresh cow milk and (3) mastitis milk. The first two categories are for use in the calf program, and the third category is waste milk not recommended for the calf program.

The subject of milking out fresh cows deserves mention. It is not advisable to completely milk out fresh cows prone to milk fever or cows recovering from milk fever. Such a procedure often results in unnecessary milk fever or relapses. In practice, these cows should be hand foremilked for only the first several milkings to monitor the secretion until the cow's feed consumption is approaching normal. Teat-dipping of these cows is recommended. The only justification for milking out such cows is as part of the treatment for mastitis, if present. On the other hand, first calf heifers and cows with no history of milk fever should be milked out enough to relieve pressure on the udder, allowing the teat sphincters to close. This should be started with the first milking. Persistent intramammary pressure causes the teats to remain full and the teat sphincters partially open. The likelihood of coliform mastitis in fresh cows is lessened if the intramammary pressure is reduced by milking of the cow.

The nutrition of the fresh cow string should approach that of the heavy-producing milk strings. If the cows are alrady accustomed to concentrate feeding before calving, introduction of higher levels of concentrate usually poses no problem. Unfortunately, fresh cows do not consume as much feed as would be desirable. Frequent feedings of good quality fresh feed should be emphasized. In practice, this group of cows most often has feed left from one feed to the next, and unless it is frequently cleaned up, such feed will become less palatable and will further contribute to the fresh cow's normal underintake.

Before the cow leaves the fresh cow area of the calving area, treatments for retained placentae, metritis, mastitis and other disorders should be completed and recorded, both on the cow herself and on her individual cow record for later reference. Appropriate codes frequently used include RP for retained placenta, OB for dystocia, T with date beside it for treatment and OK if no abnormalities occurred in the fresh cow area.

Calf Holding Area

This part of the calving area is intended to hold the calf from the time it leaves its mother until it is removed to the calf raising area. The area need contain only enough disinfectible pens to hold one-half to one full day's calf crop.

The pens in this area need to be situated away from drafts in cool weather and away from direct sunshine in hot weather. Both the pens themselves and the area they are placed in should be designed for daily cleaning and disinfecting. Elevated metal pens with removable rubber mat bases work well here. Ideally, there should be partitions between calves in these pens to prevent calf-to-calf contact. Twice daily pick-up of calves in this area is recommended. Calf handling facilities ideally should minimize or eliminate calf-to-calf contact during the entire preweaning period.

A refrigerator for storing 2-quart nipple bottles filled with colostrum should be located in this area. Also, hot water should be available for warming colostrum prior to feeding. A hot plate capable of heating a bucket of water can work equally well to warm the colostrum prior to feeding.

COLOSTRUM MANAGEMENT

Good dairy management includes a colostrum management program that is capable of utilizing all colostrum to best advantage. Provisions must be made for obtaining and storing both first-milking colostrum and other fresh cow milk if maximum efficiency and calf health are to be achieved.

A colostrum management program starts with vaccinations of the dam and includes observation of the dry cow udder before calving, the first colostral feeding of the calf and the subsequent use of colostrum in calf nutrition.

The ideal situation is to have a vigorous, unassisted newborn calf nurse its mother within an hour of birth, provided that the following conditions are met: (1) the cow has not leaked excessive amounts of colostrum prior to calving, (2) the calf's environment is clean, (3) the cow is clean, (4) the cow does not have mastitis and (5) the cow is capable and allows the calf to nurse her. Obviously, on large dairies all of these conditions are not always possible. Thus, a satisfactory alternative to natural suckling should be available when needed.

The basis for such alternative colostrum feeding lies in obtaining acceptable colostrum. Two kinds of colostrum should be maintained: (1) the first milking colostrum

from nonleaking cows and (2) other nonmastitic fresh cow milk.

On large dairies the first milking colostrum can be pooled in 10-gallon milk cans, agitated and then decanted into clean 2-quart nipple bottles for immediate refrigeration or freezing. If refrigeration is utilized, the bottles should be dated and unused bottles discarded after several days. Alternatively, they can be used by mixing the contents into the milk fed to older calves. The other fresh cow milk can best be utilized by storage in small refrigerated bulk tanks. Bacteria count estimation, using a cotton swab and blood agar or MacConkey agar, should frequently be done to determine the efficiency of the sanitation and refrigeration.

The 2-quart nipple bottles filled with first milking colostrum are used for those calves that do not have ample opportunity to nurse their dams within an hour of birth for any of the previously mentioned reasons. These bottles should be warmed to body temperature in a hot water bath before feeding. The nipple should have a hole small enough that effort is required by the calf to obtain the colostrum, as opposed to a hole that runs freely, to minimize the likelihood of inhalation pneumonia. In the author's opinion, use of the nipple bottle appears to be preferable to use of an esophageal feeder for this purpose.

In practice, enough first milking colostrum can be obtained to feed 2 quarts of it twice daily to all heifer calves for 3 days. The calves can then feed the fresh cow milk twice daily, at least through the first week of life. The remaining fresh cow milk can be used in conjunction with milk replacers to feed older calves. Although globulin absorption is greatly reduced after the calf is 24 hours old, the local action of the antibody in the intestine and excellent nutritive value of colostrum justify maximum utilization of all nonmastitic fresh cow milk.

It has been the author's experience that such a colostrum management program causes no difference in preweaning calf mortality for those calves bottle fed colostrum shortly after birth versus those calves naturally obtaining first milking colostrum.

CONCLUSION

The foregoing specialized management procedures and facilities for the health management of the periparturient cow and calf have been developed for or adopted by existing large commercial dairy herds. The impetus for such management was the need to reduce animal health losses resulting from the stress of animal concentration. The resulting programs represent a balance between economic considerations, such as labor, construction and feed costs, and logical application of scientific research. For properly designed facilities, these management practices represent the most practical and profitable approach to dairy herd management. For other existing facilities that are not suitable for direct application of these practices, an awareness of them and their rationale may be of assistance in the trouble-shooting of herd health problems arising when less thorough management fails.

Principles of Colostrum Feeding

MAARTEN DROST

University of Florida, Gainesville, Florida

Early ingestion of colostrum is essential for the newborn calf. The protective effects associated with the transfer of colostral immunoglobulins have been amply demonstrated, both in the field and experimentally. The composition of first-milk colostrum changes rapidly to that of normal milk during the first 3 days of lactation (Table 1).

The calf should consume at least 6 per cent of its body weight in colostrum within 6 hours after birth. If the calf is reluctant to nurse, the colostrum should be given by stomach tube. Slightly bloody colostrum can safely be fed to calves if it is otherwise normal. Grossly abnormal colostrum, such as from a cow with acute mastitis, must be discarded. Providing adequate amounts of colostrum will not necessarily prevent diarrhea, but it will aid in the prevention of subsequent septicemia. Immunoglobulins (Ig) are absorbed from the intestine for only a short time after birth, and the efficiency of absorption decreases linearly with time. Furthermore, "shut down" is different for each class of immunoglobulin.[4] IgG can be absorbed for 27 hours and IgA for 22 hours, but IgM is absorbed for only 16 hours. Thus, a calf that nurses for the first time at 10 to 12 hours of age could still acquire high levels of IgG and IgA, but little IgM. As a consequence, such calves are very susceptible to colibacillosis.[2]

A mistaken prognosis would be given for the latter group of calves if a test were used such as the sodium sulfite turbidity test, which measures total immunoglobulin levels. In reality, this rarely happens. However, this simple test, which can be used under field conditions for detecting total immunoglobulin levels in the serum of cattle, is very useful in determining whether or not a calf has received colostrum.

After ingestion, a minimum of 3 hours is required to reflect immunoglobulin levels in the serum, whereas maximum serum levels are not reached until 24 hours of age. Hence, the sodium sulfite turbidity test will give deceptively low values in a calf that is 3 to 5 hours old.

TABLE 1. *Approximate Composition of Colostrum and Normal Holstein Milk**

Constituent	First-Milk Colostrum (per cent)	2nd and 3rd Day Colostrum (per cent)	Milk (per cent)
Fat	6.0	3.5	3.50
Nonfat solids	22.3	12.5	8.80
Protein	18.8	7.5	3.25
Immune globulins	13.1	1.0	0.09
Lactose	2.5	4.0	4.60

*From Appleman, R. D. and Otterby, D. E.: Agriculture Extension Service, University of Minnesota Fact Sheet, Dairy Husbandry No. 9, 1973.

RAPID FIELD TEST FOR SERUM IMMUNOGLOBULINS

1. Place 0.1 ml of calf serum into a glass tube (e.g., 6 × 100 mm, thin-walled).
2. Add 1.9 ml of 18 per cent sodium sulfite solution (anhydrous sodium sulfite formula weight 126.04). Dissolve 18 gm of sodium sulfite in 100 ml of distilled water.
3. Mix well by inverting the tube several times.
4. Score the turbidity from 0 (no change) to 4 (dense precipitate). Adult bovine serum may be used for reference as a score of 4.

If mixtures are allowed to sit overnight, the precipitate will settle out, giving a check on the original relative scoring. The test provides an excellent method for monitoring the overall colostrum feeding program.[7] There is a positive correlation between high sodium sulfite test scores and survival, particularly under poor hygienic conditions.

The results of the test must also be interpreted with some caution, as some calves (as many as 30 per cent in one study)[6] remain agammaglobulinemic despite receiving early colostrum. Agammaglobulinemia or hypogammaglobulinemia also occurs if the calf receives food other than first-milk colostrum initially, which affects the ability of the small intestine to absorb the antibodies. Occasionally cows are milked prior to freshening. In these cases, the milk produced after freshening provides no better disease protection than ordinary milk. Other factors that affect the globulin-absorptive efficiency of newborn calves are: (1) the age at which colostrum is first ingested, (2) the amount of globulin ingested and (3) the effect of the presence of the dam. Calves left with their dam attain significantly higher serum immunoglobulin concentrations than do calves removed from their dam shortly after birth, even when allowance is made for variations in the time of feeding and globulin intake.[5]

CONTINUED COLOSTRUM FEEDING

Apart from its function of conferring passive immunity, colostrum contains high levels of fat-soluble vitamins and all of the essential amino acids, which act as a valuable nutritional source for the rapidly growing calf. Colostrum also has a slight laxative effect.

Dairy cows produce an average of 50 kg of colostrum during the first six milkings after parturition (when it is not normally deemed fit for sale). This is an amount sufficient to feed a calf for about 3 weeks. It may be stored by refrigeration or freezing. Frozen colostrum should be thawed in cold water, as heating denatures the protein.

FERMENTED COLOSTRUM

Excess colostrum from the first 3 days may be stored in covered 70- to 80-liter plastic garbage cans in which it will naturally ferment (sour) in 3 to 5 days. Mastitic, extremely bloody or other abnormal colostrum should not be used. Milk from cows treated with antibiotics at or after freshening should not be included. Stored colostrum should be stirred daily to promote desirable fermentation. Colostrum from more than one cow may be combined and fermented, provided the cows have calved within 1 or 2 days of each other. Do not add fresh colostrum to already fermented material. If pooling is desirable, ferment the colostrum first and then add it to the older fermented product. The colostrum may be used as it is souring.

The newborn calf should be allowed to nurse or should be fed colostrum from its dam as soon as possible after birth. If fermented colostrum is available, it may be fed the second or third day. A few feedings may be required before the calf begins to like the fermented colostrum. Nipple pail or bottle feeding will make the adjustment easier. Fermented colostrum is high in solids, hence, it is usually diluted 1:1 with water. The fermented colostrum should be thoroughly mixed before the amount to be fed is removed from the can. Warm water will allow for a better dispersion of the fat. If the colostrum is diluted with equal parts of water, it is fed at the rate of 10 per cent of body weight. If it is fed undiluted, the amount shoud be reduced. Calves may be switched from milk to fermented colostrum to milk.

NEONATAL ISOERYTHROLYSIS IN CALVES

Hemolytic disease of the newborn calf may occur in calves ingesting colostrum from cows that have previously received a blood transfusion or, more commonly, from those that were immunized against anaplasmosis or babesiosis. At present, commercial anaplasmosis vaccine is made from the pooled red blood cells of cattle infected with *Anaplasma marginale*. These cells are harvested at the peak of parasitemia when maximum numbers of erythrocytes include the intracellular *Anaplasma* bodies. The vaccinated cow produces antibodies to erythrocyte antigens in the vaccine that are foreign to her. At the time of parturition these maternal antibodies are passed on to the calf through the colostrum. If the calf inherits from its sire one or more erythrocyte antigens that react with the maternal antibodies, a hemolytic crisis may develop. Steps should be taken to prevent neonatal isoerythrolysis in calves from cows vaccinated against anaplasmosis. It is not wise to rely on simple crossmatching of the erythrocytes of the calf and the serum or colostrum of the dam, because such tests do not reveal the hemolytic process. An accurate test to determine the presence of offending antibodies requires the use of (1) serum or colostrum of the dam, (2) erythrocytes of the calf and (3) specific complement.

A safe procedure is to remove calves from their dam at birth and feed them colostrum for 2 days from cows that have not been immunized with a blood-derived vaccine. There is no effective treatment in peracute cases. Afflicted calves should be kept as quiet and undisturbed as possible. If transfusion therapy is contemplated, thoroughly washed red blood cells from the dam are recommended, in view of the fact that such red blood cells possess no isoantigenic determinants that will react with the offending isoantibodies.

REFERENCES

1. Appleman, R. D. and Otterby, D. E.: Using colostrum to raise dairy calves. Agriculture Extension Service, University of Minnesota Fact Sheet, Dairy Husbandry No. 9, 1973.
2. Logan, E. F. and Penhale, W. J.: Studies on the immunity of the calf to colibacillosis. Vet. Rec., *89*:633, 1971.
3. Otterby, D. E., Johnson, D. G. and Polzin, H. W.: Fermented colostrum or milk replacer for growing calves. J. Dairy Sci., *59*:2001, 1976.
4. Penhale, W. J., Logan, E. F., Selman, I. E., Fisher, E. W. and McEwan, A. D.: Observations on the absorption of colostral immunoglobulins by the neonatal calf and their significance in colibacillosis. Ann. Rech. Vet., *4*:223, 1973.
5. Selman, I. E.: The absorption of colostral globulins by newborn calves. Ann. Rech. Vet., *4*:213, 1973.
6. Staley, T. E., Jones, E. W. and Bush, L. F.: Maternal transport of immunoglobulins to the calf. J. Dairy Sci., *54*:1323, 1971.
7. Stone, S. S. and Gitter, M.: The validity of the sodium sulfite test for detecting immunoglobulins in calf sera. Br. Vet. J., *125*:68, 1969.
8. Stormont, C.: Neonatal isoerythrolysis in domestic animals. A comparative review. Adv. Vet. Sci. Comp. Med., *19*:23, 1975.

Fetal Immunization Procedures

GABEL H. CONNER

Caldwell Veterinary Medical Center, Caldwell, Idaho

INTRODUCTION AND BACKGROUND INFORMATION

The relatively new concept of immunizing a fetus offers a number of interesting challenges and opens many avenues for basic, as well as applied, research. Ten years ago the immunological capabilities of a bovine fetus were unknown. Today, knowledge concerning *in utero* vaccination has advanced to the point that such a procedure is conceivably practical for prevention of colibacillosis in neonatal calves.

Much of the pioneering work in vaccination of the bovine fetus has been done by scientists at Michigan State University[1,2] and in Australia.[3] The foregoing studies dealt primarily with immunity of the bovine fetus to *Escherichia coli*. Since the cost of research using pregnant cattle is high, there have been limitations on the number of studies. Consequently, questions are unanswered, and the potential uses of prenatal immunization have not been fully realized. For example, the degree of heterogenetic protection resulting from *in utero* injection of a single type of organism, the fetal response to organisms other than *E. coli* and reovirus or the effect of antigenically stimulating a prenatally vaccinated calf are but a few of the important unanswered questions.

Initial immunization studies on ovine fetuses demonstrated that unborn lambs produced antibodies following intracardiac injection of *Brucella* organisms from midgestation (80 days prenatally) to near birth. If unborn lambs were given a second antigenic stimulus (*Brucella* organisms) *in utero,* they developed serum antibody concentrations as high as those attained when adult sheep were given primary and secondary stimulation. When secondarily stimulated at birth, neonatal lambs responded rapidly with high levels of antibody.

The unborn lamb also produced antibodies against *Brucella* organisms when antigen was deposited in amniotic fluid. This was an oral vaccination, since amniotic fluid is constantly being swallowed by the fetus. Secondary responses were elicited in fetal lambs when a booster vaccination was adminsitered intra-amniotically following a primary intra-amniotic vaccination.

The unborn calf is also capable of mounting an antibody response when vaccinated orally (amniotic fluid) with an *E. coli* organism.[2] Not only did fetal calves develop antibodies against *E. coli*, but fetal lambs responded to *E. coli* antigen in a similar manner.

Gay[3] also demonstrated that calves vaccinated prenatally with *E. coli* (some were vaccinated intramuscularly, some intra-amniotically) had antibodies against *E. coli* at birth.

GESTATIONAL AGE OF FETAL IMMUNOCOMPETENCE

The age at which the bovine fetus displays immunological competence has not been extensively studied. The immunological response to some antigens is dependent upon the gestational age at which the fetus is exposed. For example, ovalbumin does not induce any response in fetuses 4 months of age; however, it does elicit an antibody response at 5 months. A list of antigens to which the bovine fetus is known to respond immunologically, and at what age, appears in Table 1.

PROTECTION AT BIRTH

The presence of humoral antibodies at birth is significant only if the newborn is protected against a challenge exposure.

TABLE 1. *Immunological Responses of the Bovine Fetus to Antigens—Earliest Gestational Age Reported*

Antigen*	Antibody Production by Fetus	Gestational Age (days)
Ferritin[4]	+	135
Ovalbumin[4]	neg	135
Anaplasma marginale[5]	+	141
Leptospira Sarkoebing[5]	+	162
Parainfluenza-3 virus[5]	+	163
Ovalbumin[4]	+	165
Bovine viral diarrhea–mucosal disease virus[5]	+	190
Escherichia coli (026)[2]	+	231
Campylobacter fetus[5]	+	235
Chlamydial agent[5]	+	243
Reovirus[2]	+	257
Blue tongue virus[5]	+	282 (term)
Brucella abortus[5]	+	282 (term)

*Numerical superscripts refer to appropriate references listed at end of article.

Calves that were prenatally vaccinated (amniotic fluid) with *E. coli* were protected against an oral challenge dose of live *E. coli* organisms (homologous strain) given at birth.[2] Although totally deprived of colostrum, these calves were normal, healthy animals during the 6-week observation period. The same dose of oral challenge organisms given to five calves not vaccinated *in utero* resulted in death within 2 to 10 days. Similar results were obtained in prenatally vaccinated lambs.[2]

Recent studies in which calves were prenatally vaccinated with reovirus (Scourvax = reo) or a combination of reovirus and *E. coli* showed the presence of serum antibodies against reovirus at birth.[1] Although this was a pilot study involving six animals, results indicated that the fetus produced antibodies within 8 days after vaccination. There was also evidence indicating that *E. coli* in the immunizing inoculum augmented the production of antibody against reovirus.

Gay[3] has reported heterogenetic antibody or protection. In one of his reports, he noted that calves had antibodies against several serotypes of *E. coli* even though a single serotype was used in the prenatal immunizing inoculum. One such calf (vaccinated for the longest period before birth) had antibodies against a *Salmonella* organism. Another study in which challenge exposures were used indicated that *in utero* vaccination with a single serotype of *E. coli* could result in heterogenetic protection against neonatal colisepticemia.

The fact that a fetus reponds to an antigenic stimulus by production of a broad-spectrum antibody is probably significant. The breadth of protection resulting from vaccination with a single type of organism has not been determined by challenge exposures. The effect of using two immunizing organisms is unknown.

LOCAL IMMUNITY

Calves vaccinated prenatally have protection against challenge exposures even though some have no detectable humoral antibodies. At birth, calves vaccinated prenatally with *E. coli* have antibody-producing cells (IgG, IgM and anti-*E. coli*) in the mucosa of the duodenum, jejunum and ileum and in the jejunal lymph node. This local cellular immunity may explain protection in the absence of humoral antibody. One calf given an oral dose of antigen at birth had more immune-producing cells (also found in the spleen) than calves not receiving a booster at birth. The heterogenicity of the antibodies produced at the local cellular level is not known.

INDICATIONS AND APPLICATIONS

A known indication for prenatal immunization is protection of calves against colibacillosis, an enteric disease that kills many calves. Since this disease affects calves before they develop their own defensive mechanisms, protection at the time of birth is of great value.

Potentially useful applications of prenatal vaccination are dependent upon expanded research efforts; however, it appears feasible that the procedure could provide protection against diseases for which there are presently inadequate or unsatisfactory immunization methods available. For example, viral diseases such as bovine viral diarrhea or infectious bovine rhinotracheitis might be prevented by fetal vaccination. Postnatal vaccination for these diseases is not always effective and if given at the wrong time can result in abortions or fetal aberrations. There are at least two viruses (reovirus and coronavirus) that are responsible for enteric disorders of the newborn calf. Although it

may be possible to immunize the neonatal calf against these diseases, prenatal vaccination would be more effective because protective antibodies would be present at the time of birth.

If there is heterogenetic protection, as has been reported in calves vaccinated prenatally, this phenomenon would increase the interest in and significance of the technique.

VACCINATION PROCEDURE

The ovine fetus requires 15 days following injection of *Brucella* organisms to achieve maximum antibody levels. A similar time period is required for maximum levels in lambs stimulated at birth. Antibody that was protective against colisepticemia appeared in the serum of colostrum-deprived calves at 10 to 14 days after birth. Based upon these two reports, the bovine fetus should be vaccinated at least 14 days prenatally for maximum antibody production at birth. Since the gestation period in cows may be somewhat variable, fetal vaccination 3 to 4 weeks before the anticipated date of birth is suggested. Although the fetus is capable of mounting antibody responses considerably earlier than 4 weeks before birth, the level of antibody at birth may be lower if antigenic stimulation occurs too early in the gestation period.

The fetus is intra-amniotically vaccinated by injection through the dam's right flank, where the fetus is closest to the abdominal wall as determined by ballottement. Care is taken to avoid abomasal or duodenal areas. Aseptic techniques are used throughout the vaccination procedure. Following clipping of hair and scrubbing the skin with a surgical antiseptic, a local anesthetic is infiltrated into the subcutaneous tissue, abdominal muscles and peritoneum at the proposed injection site. A stab incision is made in the skin, through which a 12-gauge hypodermic needle, 5 cm long, is inserted into the peritoneal cavity. This short needle serves as a cannula for passage of a 16-gauge needle, 25 to 30 cm long, which is directed toward the uterus and gently pushed through the uterine wall and fetal membranes until the fetus is touched, but not pierced. The presence of the needle in the amniotic cavity may be confirmed by aspirating amniotic fluid prior to the injection; however, on rare occasions fluid cannot be aspirated. The volume of bacterial antigen injected is 2 to 3 ml, containing approximately 2×10^{10} cells per ml. With one assistant, the vaccination can be performed in 5 minutes.

The occurrence of premature birth of some calves vaccinated *in utero* against colibacillosis has prevented widespread field use of the technique. Field experiences are in contrast to the experimental results, in which there have been only four abortions in approximately 90 cows vaccinated *in utero*. The reason for abortions in the field has not been determined.

Because a commercial bacterin was not available for prenatal immunization against colibacillosis, the immunizing inoculum was prepared in laboratories at Michigan State University. Although the same organism, *E. coli* 026:K60, was used for the experimental studies, an *E.coli* organism isolated from any acute, on-the-farm case of bovine colibacillosis would serve for preparation of the bacterin. It is important that the incubated organisms be adequately washed so that there is no free endotoxin in the preparation to be injected intra-amniotically. A suggested procedure for preparation of the bacterin is to seed the organism on bottles of trypticase soy agar and incubate for 20 to 24 hours at 37° C. The growth is then washed twice with sterile saline solution and examined by bacteriological culture techniques to determine purity. The cells are then killed by adding 0.4 per cent formalin, and the mixture is incubated in a shaking water bath (37° C) for 18 to 24 hours. The formalin-killed cells are washed twice with sterile saline, and a cell count is obtained. The suspension is then diluted with sterile saline containing 0.002 per cent thimerosal to the desired concentration of approximately 1.5 or 2×10^{10} cells/ml, stored at 4° C and used within 20 days.

REFERENCES

1. Conner, G. H., and Carter, G. R.: Response of the bovine fetus to reovirus. Vet. Med./Small Anim. Clin., *70*:1463, 1975.
2. Conner, G. H., Richardson, M., and Carter, G. R.: Prenatal immunization and protection of the newborn: Ovine and bovine fetuses vaccinated with *Escherichia coli* antigen by the oral route and exposed to challenge inoculum at birth. Am. J. Vet. Res., *34*:737, 1973.
3. Gay, C. C.: In utero immunization of calves against colisepticemia. Am. J. Vet. Res., *36*:625, 1975.
4. Gibson, D. C., and Zemjanis, R.: Immune response of the bovine fetus to several antigens. Am. J. Vet. Res., *34*:1277, 1973.
5. Kendrick, J. W., and Osburn, B. I.: Immunologic response of the bovine fetus to inactivated infectious bovine rhinotracheitis-infectious putular vulvovaginitis virus. Am. J. Vet. Res., *34*:1567, 1973.

Examination and Interpretation of Findings of the Postpartum Reproductive Tract in Dairy Cattle

ERICH STUDER
Carnation Research Farm,
Carnation, Washington

DAVID A. MORROW
Michigan State University,
East Lansing, Michigan

The prevention and treatment of reproductive tract disorders are extremely important for maintenance of a profitable calving interval and offer the veterinarian a challenge and an opportunity to perform a valuable service.

Veterinary practitioners usually examine cows 20 to 40 days postpartum since uterine involution is complete sometime between 25 and 50 days.[2, 3, 5] Almost all cows acquire some uterine infection postpartum.[1, 3] Studies indicate that 85 to 93 per cent of cows have uterine infections 2 weeks postpartum, but only 5 to 9 per cent are infected by 46 to 60 days.[1, 3] There is no doubt that specific diseases such as brucellosis, leptospirosis, vibriosis and trichomoniasis have an adverse effect on reproduction; however, the importance of nonspecific genital tract infections on fertility rates in cows is not as clear. It would be extremely helpful to the bovine fertility practitioner to be able to ascertain with some degree of accuracy whether a cow requires uterine infusion. Not only are un-

TABLE 1. *Comparison of Gross Genital Tract Rating with Histological Inflammatory Rating in Postpartum Cows*

Factors Evaluated	Number	Correlation	Significance
Gross right horn versus right horn inflammatory rating	104	0.27	<0.01
Gross left horn versus left horn inflammatory rating	103	0.32	<0.01
Purulent exudate rating versus right horn inflammatory rating	104	0.36	<0.01
Purulent exudate rating versus left horn inflammatory rating	103	0.42	<0.01

necessary treatments an added expense, but some medications are of little value or even detrimental.[8] Depending on when infusions are made, the normal estrous cycle may be altered. Solutions irritating to the endometrium that are infused 3 to 5 days after ovulation shorten the cycle, whereas infusions made between days 14 and 17 delay the next estrus. Another disadvantage is the recent demonstration that intrauterine medications are rapidly absorbed into the bloodstream. This may cause adulteration of milk, thereby making it unacceptable for sale. For these reasons it would be helpful to positively identify cows that definitely require treatment. Although some theriogenologists indicate that endometritis may be detected by gross examination of the genital tract, it is generally agreed that the diagnosis of endometritis on the basis of rectal examination alone is not always reliable.[5]

EVALUATING THE POSTPARTUM REPRODUCTIVE GENITAL TRACT

In a recently completed study,[7] there was a highly significant positive correlation between results of genital tract examination *per rectum* and the presence of purulent exudate with histopathology ratings of both uterine horns (P <0.01) (Table 1). The gross purulent exudate rating was also directly correlated with bacterial isolation (r=0.44, P <0.01) (Table 2).

A grading system such as the following is helpful in interpreting and recording gross genital tract findings:

Vagina:
V1. Mild inflammatory changes in vagina.
V2. Moderately severe inflammatory changes in vagina.
V3. Severe inflammatory changes in vagina.

Cervix:
C1. 3.75 to 5.0 cm in diameter with a slightly roughened and thickened feeling, with or without reddening on vaginal examination.
C2. 5.0 to 7.5 cm in diameter with definite rough, irregular shape, with or without reddening on vaginal examination.
C3. Size greater than 7.5 cm in diameter, usually with reddened and lacerated appearance on vaginal examination.

Uterus:
U1. 2.5 to 3.75 cm in diameter with slight thickened feeling.
U2. 3.75 to 5.0 cm in diameter with definite thickened feeling; longitudinal grooves and nodularity from enlarged caruncles are palpable, and the uterine lumen contains fluid in some instances.
U3. Greater than 5.0 cm in diameter; grooves and caruncles are readily palpable, with some fluid usually being palpable in the lumen.

TABLE 2. *Comparison of Gross Genital Tract Rating with Bacterial Isolation in Postpartum Cows*

Factors Evaluated	Number	Correlation	Significance
Purulent exudate rating versus bacterial isolation	106	0.44	<0.01
Gross right horn versus bacterial isolation	106	0.22	<0.05
Gross left horn versus bacterial isolation	106	0.17	≦0.05

Each uterine horn should be evaluated separately and identified as right horn (RH) or left horn (LH) after the grading of the uterus.

Purulent Discharge:

P1. Small clumps of white exudate.

P2. From 10 to 30 ml of purulent exudate.

P3. More than 30 ml of purulent exudate.

The grades for the vagina, cervix and uterus are based on individual interpretation. The vaginal change V1 is characterized by hyperemia, small hemorrhagic areas (bruises), small lacerations and sometimes small lumps of necrotic fat perivaginally. On the other extreme, the grade V3 is characterized by larger masses of necrotic fat, major bruised hemorrhagic areas and major tears with purulent exudate.

The grading of the cervix is somewhat more objective since the size can be measured indirectly. The normal circumference is less than that of the circle formed by touching the tip of the first finger to the distal phalangeal joint of the thumb (3.75 cm in diameter). On vaginal examination the cervix must appear normal. The grade C1 ranges from the upper limit of normal (3.75 cm in diameter) to the diameter of a circle formed when the tips of the first finger and thumb still meet (5 cm in diameter). When palpated, the cervix may feel slightly roughened or thickened, especially on the posterior part. Also, the cervix may or may not be reddened on vaginal examination. The C2 grade ranges from the upper limit of C1 to the point at which the first fingertip and tip of the thumb are about 2.5 cm apart (7.5 cm in diameter). The cervix definitely feels rough and irregular. On vaginal examination the cervix is frequently red and inflamed, although older cows may have a C2 grade without showing inflammation. The C3 grade is anything greater than C2 (7.5 cm in diameter). Vaginal examination reveals that the cervix is often found to have a reddened and bruised appearance.

The uterine grades are also based on indirect measurements and texture of the uterine wall. Just as with the cervix, the extent to which the first finger meets the thumb determines the uterine condition. The texture of the U1 uterine horn is slightly thickened and roughened, whereas the U2 horn has a definitely thickened

feeling, with palpable longitudinal grooves and nodules (incompletely regressed caruncles). The lumen of the uterus may contain some fluid. In the U3 grade, grooves and caruncular lumps may be readily palpable, and some fluid is usually present in the lumen.

To critically evaluate the uterus, the examiner must retract the organ upon the pelvic floor and carefully palpate each uterine horn to its extremity. Examination of all discharges massaged from the vaginal floor and visual inspection of the vagina and cervix by vaginal speculum will add much information to the genital tract palpation.

Immediately after parturition the uterus is a large, flabby sac measuring nearly a meter long and weighing about 9 kg.[4] This sac rapidly decreases in size and weight because of vasoconstriction and muscular contraction. Some fluid can be detected by examination *per rectum* from 7 to 10 days postpartum in most cows. Excessive putrid, brownish, bloody-colored fluid is associated with retained placenta and delayed regression of caruncles, resulting in metritis. Normal longitudinal grooves are palpable on the uterine surface during this early postpartum period. From days 10 to 14 the previously pregnant horn decreases from 12 to 14 cm originally to 7 or 8 cm in diameter.[4] By 30 days postpartum the reproductive tract is palpable in the pelvic canal in all primiparous and most pluriparous cows. The length of the uterine horns is reduced to half by day 15 and to a third by day 30.[4] The diameter of the uterine horns 1 month postpartum should be less than 2.5 cm, approximately one-third of the uterine length from the bifurcation in young cows and no more than 3.75 cm in older cows.

The cervix is palpable *per rectum* craniad to the pelvis 5 to 7 days postpartum. It is large and has a fluctuating consistency. Gradually the size decreases from about 12 cm to 6 to 8 cm at 10 days postpartum, while the consistency becomes firmer.[4] In cows with normal parturitions the cervix will have involuted to 2.5 to 4.0 cm in diameter by postpartum day 30.

Abnormal parturition and postpartum disease, milk fever, ketosis, retained placenta, metritis and displaced abomasum can delay involution by 5 to 10 days, depending on severity. Age and parity must, of course, be considered in evaluating the size of uterine horns since the time required for involution of the uterus and cervix increases directly with parity. Animals rated C1 and U1 are usually normal on bacteriological and histological examination at 30 days postpartum and do not require treatment.

Expansion of the genital tract evaluation may be accomplished by inspection of cervical mucus during estrus. Cows with completely clear estrual mucus do not require treatment in spite of minor cervical enlargements. Cows with purulent vaginal discharges in spite of normal cervical and uterine ratings should be treated, based on the location and severity of infection. Mucus can usually be readily massaged from the vagina by rectal manipulation during estrus.

EVALUATION OF THE OVARIES

The ovaries are examined and the findings recorded as shown in Table 3.

At 30 days postpartum, most properly fed cows have had at least one estrus. The average interval at first estrus following parturition was found to be 15 and 34 days for cows with normal and abnormal calvings, respectively.[5] The first cycle following an early ovulation is approximately 17 days in length. Since many of these early heats with ovulations are unobserved, standing estrus may be observed in only 20 to 30 per cent of cows with corpora lutea at the time of the 30-day examination. Normal corpora lutea will probably be present in 60 to 65 per cent of cows with functional

ovaries, cystic corpora lutea in 20 to 25 per cent and cystic follicles in 15 to 20 per cent. A cystic corpus luteum is a smooth, spherical, fluctuating mass that develops after ovulation and contains a fluid-filled central cavity. It is frequently larger than a normal corpus luteum and is differentiated from a luteal cyst by the rosette of luteal tissue at the site of ovulation. Luteal cysts, anovulatory (luteinized) follicles, are almost always associated with anestrus, as are cystic follicles during early postpartum. Cystic follicles are present more often in high-producing cows and in those that experienced an abnormal parturition. Since about half the cows with early cysts recover spontaneously, treatment is not recommended until 3 weeks prior to breeding or when nymphomania is present. The finding of a normal corpus luteum in the absence of pregnancy or pyometra indicates that a cow is having normal estrous cycles.

The practitioner is constantly presented with anestrous cows with a normal uterus and functional corpus luteum. The anestrous condition is due to observational failure by herd personnel. It is important for the fertility practitioner to be competent in identifying ovarian structures in order to predict the stage of the estrous cycle. Based on ovarian findings, the response of the uterus and the characteristics of the mucus, fairly accurate prediction of the next estrus can be made (see Table 3). A detailed description concerning palpable characteristics of these structures is found in a previous publication.[6] Skill in predicting estrus can best be obtained by examining a few cows daily throughout several estrous cycles and by visually examining ovarian structures both before and after slaughter.

RECOMMENDATIONS

The number of days postpartum at which examination is made is important for interpretation of findings. The following recommendations can be made when a gross genital tract grading system, such as the one outlined in this article, is used at 30 days postpartum:

1. C1 and U1 rated animals are usually normal on bacteriological examination and do not require treatment.

2. Cows with grades C2 and U2 should be examined by using a vaginal speculum

TABLE 3. *Recording Ovarian Findings*

Finding	Days in Estrous Cycle
F –Follicle	Estrus
OVD–Ovulation depression	1–2
CH1 –Soft, developing corpus luteum less than 1 cm in diameter	2–3
CH2 –Soft, developing corpus luteum 1 to 2 cm in diameter	3–5
CH3 –Soft, developing corpus luteum more than 2 cm in diameter	5–7
CL3 –Fully developed corpus luteum	8–17
CL2 –Firm corpus luteum 1 to 2 cm in diameter	18–20
CL1 –Hard corpus luteum less than 1 cm in diameter	Estrus to middle of the subsequent cycle

to investigate for inflammation or pus. Many older cows with a C2 and U1 grade do not require treatment.

3. A U2 grade at 30 days postpartum is frequently associated with pus, and an animal so rated should be treated by uterine infusion.

4. Evaluation of the genital tract may be expanded by inspection of cervical mucus during estrus. Cows with clear estrual mucus do not require treatment in spite of minor cervical enlargements. Cows with purulent vaginal discharges despite normal cervical and uterine ratings should be treated, based on the location and severity of the infection. Mucus can usually be rapidly massaged from the vagina by rectal manipulation during estrus.

5. The practitioner must become competent in identifying ovarian structures and must be able to examine cows on a regular basis. Estrus can most accurately be predicted when ovarian findings are combined with determination of uterine response, characteristics of mucus and history of previous examinations.

REFERENCES

1. Elliot, L., McMahon, K. J., Gier, H. T. and Marion, G. B.: Uterus of the cow after parturition bacterial content. Am. J. Vet. Res., 29:77, 1968.
2. Gier, H. T. and Marion, G. B.: Uterus of the cow after parturition: Involutional changes. Am. J. Vet. Res., 29:83, 1968.
3. Johanns, C. J., Clark, T. L. and Herrick, J. B.: Factors affecting calving interval. J.A.V.M.A., 151:1692, 1967.
4. Morrow, D. A.: Postpartum ovarian activity and involution of the uterus and cervix in dairy cattle. Scope, XIV 2, 1969.
5. Morrow, D. A., Roberts, S. J., McEntee, K. and Gray, H. G.: Postpartum ovarian activity and uterine involution in dairy cattle. J.A.V.M.A., 149:1596, 1966.
6. Studer, E.: Palpation of the genital tract for prediction of estrus in the cow. Vet. Med., 70:1337, 1975.
7. Studer, E. and Morrow, D. A.: Relationship of postpartum genital tract examination per rectum to endometrial biopsy and uterine culture results. J.A.V.M.A., 172:489, 1978.
8. Ulberg, L. C., Black, W. G., Kidder, H. E., McDonald, L. E., Cassida, L. E. and McNutt, S. H.: The use of antibiotics in the treatment of low fertility cows. J.A.V.M.A., 121:436, 1952.

Use of Gonadotropin-Releasing Hormone and Prostaglandins in Postpartum Cows

JACK H. BRITT

North Carolina State University, Raleigh, North Carolina

In order for a beef or dairy cow to produce the most offspring during her life in a herd, she should calve first at about 2 years of age and then again every 12 months or less until she is culled.[1, 6] This sort of calving pattern in dairy cows will also result in the most milk produced per day of herd life.[1] Unfortunately, this goal is seldom realized because the interval from calving to subsequent conception is prolonged beyond that which will result in yearly calving intervals. In dairy cows, first ovulation occurs about 3 weeks after calving, and first estrus is normally observed 3 weeks later. About 15 per cent of dairy cows manifest abnormal ovarian activity (ovarian follicular cysts and ovarian luteal cysts) during the first 2 months postpartum, and this can result in delayed conception. In addition, about 50 per cent of the expected heats in dairy cattle are undetected, causing further delay in the interval from calving to conception. In suckled cows, the period of anestrus is prolonged, especially in cows that make inadequate gains in body weight during the last trimester of pregnancy and the first 2 months postpartum.[6] Thus, treatments given to initiate normal estrous cycles during the first month postpartum and those given to induce ovulation at a preset time should result in opportunities to manage reproductive performance in cattle so that yearly calving intervals can be achieved.

Discovery of a naturally occurring decapeptide that caused release of luteinizing hormone (LH) when injected into laboratory and domestic species led to the availability of gonadotropin-releasing hormone (GnRH), a synthetically prepared product identical to the natural decapeptide. GnRH appeared to be useful for inducing LH release and subsequent ovulation in early postpartum cows. Similarly, the discovery that prostaglandin-$F_{2\alpha}$ ($PGF_{2\alpha}$) was a potent luteolytic agent led to the availability of another naturally occurring compound considered potentially useful for inducing corpus luteum (CL) regression and subsequent estrus in diestrous cows.

TREATMENT OF EARLY POSTPARTUM DAIRY COWS WITH GnRH

Endocrine and ovulatory responses were studied after GnRH treatment in early postpartum dairy cows.[2, 3] In the first experiment, 20 lactating Holstein cows were given 100 μg of GnRH or saline on day 14 postpartum. Blood samples were collected from a jugular vein on a schedule designed to detect changes in LH and progesterone levels, and changes in ovarian structures were monitored by rectal palpation.

Blood LH levels peaked about 4 hours after GnRH treatment on day 14 postpartum but did not change during a 6-hour period after treatment with saline (Fig. 1). One of 10 cows given GnRH ovulated on day 9 postpartum, the remaining nine cows ovulated on day 15, 1 day after treatment. Two of 10 cows given saline ovulated by day 15 postpartum (Fig. 2). Two cows given saline developed ovarian follicular cysts and had not ovulated by day 65 postpartum. Another

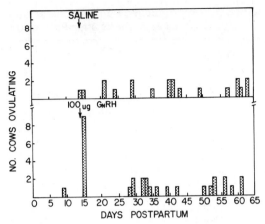

Figure 2. Number of cows ovulating after administration of GnRH or saline on day 14 postpartum. Ten Holstein cows were treated in each group. (From Britt, J. H., Kittok, J. and Harrison, D. S.: J. Anim. Sci., *39*:915, 1974.)

saline-treated cow developed a luteal cyst and failed to manifest normal estrous cycles prior to day 65. On the average, saline-treated cows had 2.0 ± 0.4 ovulations prior to day 65, compared with 3.1 ± 0.1 ovulations for cows given GnRH.

Blood progesterone concentration during the 3 weeks after GnRH treatment was similar to that observed during normal estrous cycles. All cows given GnRH exhibited similar profiles in blood progesterone concentration, suggesting that the CL formed after GnRH-induced ovulation was capable of normal function. Thus, GnRH treatment at 2 weeks postpartum in dairy cows resulted in an ovulatory surge of LH, ovulation and establishment of regular estrous cycles that continued for at least 2 months postpartum.

In a second experiment either 200 μg of GnRH or saline was given to 204 Holstein cows between 8 and 23 days postpartum during biweekly visits to each of four commercial dairy herds.[2] The incidence of ovarian follicular cysts, reasons for culling and fertility of cows remaining in the herds were compared. Fewer GnRH-treated cows developed ovarian follicular cysts following treatment compared with their saline-treated herdmates (Table 1). There were no differences between the two groups in incidence of uterine infection or anestrus after treatment. The rate of culling was similar between the two groups, but more saline-treated cows were culled for infertility. Since fewer GnRH-treated cows had to be culled for infertility, more low milk produc-

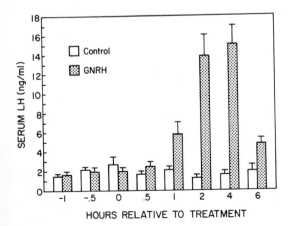

Figure 1. Serum LH after administration of GnRH (100 μg) or saline to Holstein cows on day 14 postpartum. (From Britt, J. H., Kittok, J. and Harrison, D. S.: J. Anim. Sci., *39*:915, 1974.)

TABLE 1. *Reproductive Performance of Cows Given Saline Solution or GnRH at 2 Weeks after Parturition*

Number	Saline Solution		GnRH (200 μg IM)	
	TOTAL	AVERAGES OR SUBTOTALS	TOTAL	AVERAGES OR SUBTOTALS
I. No. cows treated:	98		106	
A. No. pregnant and remaining in herds		70		72
B. No. culled for various reasons		28		34
II. No. cows culled:	28		34	
A. Culled as repeat breeder		10		6
B. Culled for cystic ovaries		6		3
C. Culled for injury or disease		4		4
D. Voluntary culls (low milk production)		8		21
III. No. cows pregnant and remaining in herds:	70		72	
A. Days from calving to first observed estrus		63 ± 4		67 ± 4
B. Days from calving to first insemination		86 ± 4		89 ± 4
C. Days from calving to conception		120 ± 7		118 ± 6
D. Inseminations per conception		1.7 ± 0.1		1.8 ± 0.1
E. Conception rate at first insemination (%)		55		56
IV. No. cows with ovarian follicular cysts:		15		6
A. Eventually conceived		9		3
B. Eventually culled		6		3

ers were available for culling. Similar percentages of cows were culled from each group for reasons of injury or disease. Thus, early postpartum treatment with GnRH reduced the incidence of abnormal ovarian activity and decreased the percentage of cows culled for infertility. These results provide evidence that GnRH may be a useful prophylactic for improving reproductive performance in dairy cows.

In addition to its effect in reducing abnormal ovarian activity in postpartum dairy cows, GnRH has been shown to be an effective treatment for cows with ovarian follicular cysts. When given at a dosage of 100 μg to cows with ovarian follicular cysts, GnRH was as effective as human chorionic gonadotropin (HCG; 10,000 IU) in causing luteinization of the cystic follicle and establishing regular estrous cycles. Thus, GnRH may be useful both as a prophylactic for preventing cystic ovaries and as a treatment of choice for cows diagnosed as having this condition. GnRH may be preferable to HCG for use in cattle since it acts at the pituitary to release LH and, because of its low molecular weight, is less likely to result in the formation of antibodies.

TREATMENT OF SUCKLED BEEF COWS WITH GnRH

Results from studies in suckled beef cows suggest that GnRH is less effective in initiating ovulation while the cow is nursing a calf. In an experiment with Holstein-Angus cows that were suckling calves, GnRH (200 μg IM) caused ovulation and establishment of regular estrous cycles in six of eight cows treated at 1 month postpartum. In these studies we noted that the first estrous cycle after GnRH treatment was frequently of 10 to 15 days' duration, compared with subsequent cycles averaging about 20 days. Therefore, we gave another 14 cows a second injection of GnRH 2 weeks after the first treatment. This regimen resulted in establishment of estrous cycles by 60 days postpartum in 13 of 14 GnRH-treated cows, compared with establishment of cycles in five of eight cows given two injections of saline. In these studies with suckled beef cattle, GnRH treatment always resulted in an increase in blood LH concentration, but this was not always followed by an ovulation. Possibly those cows that failed to ovulate had no mature ovarian follicles that were capable of ovulating in response to the LH stimulus.

In order for GnRH treatment to be most effective in initiating early postpartum estrous cycles in beef cattle, cows should be fed so they gain 0.2 to 0.4 kg per day during the last trimester of pregnancy and 0.1 to 0.2 kg per day after calving.[6] With this sort of feeding regimen, ovarian activity is enhanced and more cows should have ovarian follicles capable of ovulating in response to the surge of blood LH induced by GnRH treatment.

USE OF PROSTAGLANDINS IN POSTPARTUM CATTLE

Once estrous cycles have been established in postpartum cattle, cows with a functional corpus luteum are in a physiological state to allow induction of luteolysis and subsequent estrus by a single treatment with prostaglandin-$F_{2\alpha}$ or one of its analogs.[4,5] However, prostaglandins are not effective in inducing estrus during the first 4 or 5 days following ovulation (before the CL is fully functional) or during the follicular phase of the estrous cycle (days 17 to 21). In order to have all cows in a physiological state that will allow induction of estrus with prostaglandin treatment, it is necessary to administer a second dose of prostaglandin 10 to 12 days after the initial injection. At the time of this second treatment, those cows that responded to the initial injection, as well as those that were in early or late stages of an estrous cycle initially, will have a functional corpus luteum. Thus, all should respond to the second prostaglandin treatment. After the second injection, a majority of cows will begin estrus between 48 and 72 hours, and most will ovulate between 72 and 96 hours.[4, 5]

An alternative to administering two injections of prostaglandin 12 days apart is to give progesterone or a synthetic progestogen for 1 week and then administer prostaglandin on the last day of treatment with the progestational agent.[5] With this system, those cows in the early stages of an estrous cycle initially will be in diestrus at the time of prostaglandin treatment and those that were in the late stages of an estrous cycle initially will be inhibited from expressing estrus until the progestational agent is withdrawn.[5] With either the double injection of prostaglandin or the system utilizing a progestational agent in combination with prostaglandin, the cattle have to be handled at least twice for treatments to be administered.

Since synchrony of ovulations is precise in a group of cows after two prostaglandin injections or after administration of progesterone for 7 days in combination with prostaglandin, insemination can be at a fixed time following treatment. A single insemination at 80 hours after the second prostaglandin injection resulted in conception rates similar to those in nontreated animals bred at estrus.[4] Giving two inseminations, the first at 72 hours and the second at 96 hours,

also resulted in fertility similar to that in cows bred at estrus.[5] Thus, use of prostaglandins eliminates the need to check cows for estrus at the time of the initial insemination. Furthermore, cows that fail to conceive at the fixed-time insemination return to estrus at a more predictable time, so that detection of estrus in those cows can be scheduled in advance.

MODEL FOR CONTROL OF OVULATION IN GROUPS OF DAIRY COWS

In most dairy herds, calvings occur the year round, so the breeding period is not restricted as with beef cattle herds. In such a situation, use of prostaglandins may offer an opportunity to manage reproduction in groups of cows rather than handling each cow individually. A model for such a system is shown in Figure 3. With this system, all cows that calve in a given 3-week period are treated as a group.[1] Twelve days after the last calving date for a group, all cows are given a single injection of GnRH to assure that estrous cycles are initiated in all cows in the group. Ten and 22 days following the GnRH injection, each cow is given prostaglandin-$F_{2\alpha}$ or its analog, and then each is inseminated at 80 hours following the second dose of prostaglandin. Cows that do not conceive to the timed insemination should exhibit their next estrus during the time of induced estrus for cows calving during the subsequent 3-week interval. Pregnancy diagnosis via rectal palpations is conducted about 35 days after the initial

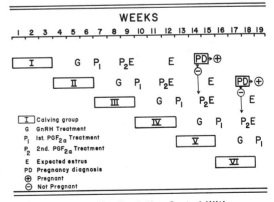

Model For Ovulation Control With GnRH and PGF$_{2\alpha}$ In Dairy Cows

Figure 3. Model for control of ovulation in groups of dairy cows. See text for details of procedures. (From Britt, J. H.: J. Dairy Sci., *60*:1345, 1977.)

artificial insemination, and cows found to be nonpregnant are grouped with those individuals receiving their second $PGF_{2\alpha}$ treatment in order to resynchronize ovulations. With this scheme, detection of estrus and inseminations are limited to a 3-day period every 3 weeks.

To work best, such a scheme should be conducted by a central organization that would provide technical supervision, GnRH and PGF treatments, semen and inseminations. In addition, the central organization might provide computerized reproductive management records and pregnancy diagnosis service.

Although application of these procedures in dairy cows is not yet sanctioned by the United States Food and Drug Administration, it seems plausible to expect that such a regimen will be used to manage reproduction in dairy cows in the future.

REFERENCES

1. Britt, J. H.: Strategies for managing reproduction and controlling health problems in groups of cows. J. Dairy Sci., *60*:1345, 1977.
2. Britt, J. H., Harrison, D. S. and Morrow, D. A.: Frequency of ovarian follicular cysts, reasons for culling, and fertility in Holstein-Friesian cows given gonadotropin-releasing hormone at two weeks after parturition. Am. J. Vet. Res., *38*:749, 1977.
3. Britt, J. H., Kittok, R. J. and Harrison, D. S.: Ovulation, estrus and endocrine response after GnRH in early postpartum cows. J. Anim. Sci., *39*:915, 1974.
4. Hafs, H. D., Manns, J. G. and Drew, B.: Onset of oestrus and fertility of dairy heifers and suckled beef cows treated with prostaglandin $F_2\alpha$. Anim. Prod., *21*:13, 1975.
5. Roche, J. F.: Fertility in cows after treatment with a prostaglandin analogue with or without progesterone. J. Reprod. Fertil., *46*:341, 1976.
6. Wiltbank, J. N.: Management programs to increase reproductive efficiency of beef herds. J. Anim. Sci. (Suppl. I), *38*:58, 1974.

Prostaglandin Therapy in Cattle with Unobserved Estrus

BRAD SEGUIN

University of Minnesota, St. Paul, Minnesota

Failure to observe estrus is one of the major factors decreasing reproductive efficiency in dairy herds in which artificial insemination (AI) breeding programs are used. Recent studies indicate that up to 40 per cent of estrous periods frequently are not detected. It has also been reported that of those cows that farm personnel are unable to detect in estrus, the majority (probably $\geq$ 90 per cent) are usually cycling normally. Upon examination *per rectum,* mature corpora lutea (CL) are frequently detected in these cows, as mature CL's are present during 60 to 65 per cent of the estrous cycle. Reexamination, typically in 2 to 4 weeks, frequently also reveals the presence of a mature CL. Changes in location of the CL and knowledge of the rarity of "persistent" CL's lead one to conclude that the cow has "cycled" but that estrus has gone undetected. Convincing farm personnel of this is often difficult, and emphasizing the need for improved estrous detection procedures is frequently unrewarding. Indeed, some studies have shown that extraordinary measures such as constant observation may be needed to allow detection of estrus in some cows. Thus, these cows are cycling but are not being detected (unobserved estrus) and must be differentiated from cows that are functionally anestrous because of ovarian atrophy.

The recent development of and experimentation with the potent luteolytic agent prostaglandin-$F_{2\alpha}$ ($PGF_{2\alpha}$) and some of its analogs such as cloprostenol (CP) have given indications of potential solutions for dealing with cows with unobserved estrus. The average intervals to estrus, release of luteinizing hormone (LH) and ovulation in normal cows given $PGF_{2\alpha}$ during the luteal phase of the estrous cycle are approximately 72, 72 and 96 hours, respectively. Fertility at the estrus following administration of $PGF_{2\alpha}$ and CP has been equivalent to that of controls when treated cows were inseminated based upon observed signs of estrus or by appointment. Administration of these luteolytic agents to cows with unobserved estrus may prove to be more satisfactory than the previously used management and therapeutic approaches.

UNOBSERVED ESTRUS

For the purposes of this discussion, unobserved estrus is defined as the absence of detected estrus (1) at the time of desired first insemination, resulting in delayed first insemination, or (2) after 35 days following insemination of cows found to be nonpregnant upon pregnancy examination. In trials designed to test the use of CP as a treatment for cows with unobserved estrus, a normal reproductive tract and the presence of a mature CL (as indicated by palpation *per rectum*) were also required. The requirement for the presence of a mature CL is critical for the success of $PGF_{2\alpha}$ or CP administration, as their mechanism of action is via the induction of luteolysis, which is followed by the onset of estrus. These products will not induce or stimulate estrus in cows that do not have a mature CL at the time of treatment. Cows that are anestrous because of ovarian atrophy associated with high milk production, low energy intake or nursing stimulation will not respond to $PGF_{2\alpha}$ or CP.

TREATMENT WITH PROSTAGLANDIN

Use of $PGF_{2\alpha}$ or CP in cows with unobserved estrus may not improve the detection rate of estrus. In one trial in which cows with unobserved estrus were treated with saline or a luteolytic dose of CP (500 μg IM) and given equal chances to exhibit estrus (i.e., 21 days of observation), the incidence of detected estrus did not differ between groups (Table 1). Cows given CP were in estrus sooner after treatment, however, than were controls; 66 per cent of those treated with CP were inseminated within 5 days of treatment versus 13 per cent for controls. Farm personnel in this trial were given basic information about CP and the anticipated results, but they did not know which cows received which treatment. Conception rates (i.e., number of cows palpated as pregnant of those inseminated) were similar for the two groups. Apparently, factors that create the unobserved estrous condition initially will remain following CP treatment. As with general heat detection efficiency, detection efficiency following CP administration will vary among farms, being influenced by several management-related factors. Perhaps as use of $PGF_{2\alpha}$ and CP in cattle becomes

more common and possibly as increased individual attention is provided for treated cows 3 to 5 days after treatment, the percentage of treated cows detected in estrus may increase.

Insemination by appointment without dependence on observed signs of estrus may be a more effective method for breeding cows treated with $PGF_{2\alpha}$ or CP for unobserved estrus. Table 2 presents results from anoth-

TABLE 1. *Estrus and Fertility in Dairy Cows with Unobserved Estrus Treated with Cloprostenol or Placebo*

	Treatments	
Cows Treated	CLOPROS-TENOL*	SALINE
No. treated	98	83
Per cent inseminated:		
In 5 days	66†	13†
In 21 days	74	66
Conception rate	44%	44%
Per cent of total pregnant:		
In 5 days	31†	5†
In 21 days	33	29

*500 μg of cloprostenol given intramuscularly.
†$(P < 0.01)$.

TABLE 2. *Reproductive Performance of Dairy Cows Treated for Unobserved Estrus with Cloprostenol and Inseminated at Estrus or by Appointment*

	Cloprostenol* and Artificial Insemination	
Cows Treated	AT ESTRUS	AT 72 AND 96 HOURS
No. treated	78	87
Per cent inseminated:		
In 5 days	60†	98(87% per schedule)†
Conception rate	40%‡	59%‡§
Per cent of total pregnant:		
In 5 days	24†	55†

*500 μg of cloprostenol given intramuscularly.
†$(P < 0.01)$.
‡$(P < 0.05)$.
§For those bred per schedule.

er trial using CP to treat cows with unobserved estrus, in which inseminations based upon observed estrus were compared with inseminations by appointment at 72 and 96 hours after treatment. Results from the group inseminated at estrus were similar to previous results for similarly handled animals (see Table 1). Many cows ($\approx$ 40 per cent) were not detected in estrus following treatment and thus were not inseminated. Nearly all cows scheduled to be inseminated by appointment were inseminated within 5 days of treatment. Fertility for the cows inseminated at estrus was lower than that for cows inseminated at 72 and 96 hours after treatment. The reduced fertility for cows inseminated at estrus may also reflect problems with heat detection. Efficacy of the double inseminations (72 and 96 hours) by appointment is indicated by the acceptable conception rate that resulted — 59 per cent of cows were palpated pregnant. Combining respective insemination and conception rates to obtain the proportion of treated cows that conceived within 5 days of treatment reveals that a substantial advantage is realized for inseminating cows with unobserved estrus treated with $PGF_{2\alpha}$ or CP by appointment (at 72 and 96 hours after treatment) rather than by observed signs of estrus (see Table 2).

The relative advantage of double appointment inseminations at 72 and 96 hours compared with single appointment insemination in cows treated for unobserved estrus remains to be determined. Such comparisons in beef and dairy cattle that were inseminated following double injection schemes for $PGF_{2\alpha}$ and CP have produced variable re-

sults. It appears that conception rates are usually 5 to 10 percentage points higher for cows inseminated twice by appointment (72 and 96 hours) than for those inseminated once by appointment (72 or 80 hours) following two injections of $PGF_{2\alpha}$ or CP. An additional factor to consider is the greater apparent variability in the onset of estrus following an initial injection as opposed to a second injection. The apparent spread in time of breeding in dairy cows treated on the previously discussed trials (see Tables 1 and 2) for unobserved estrus and inseminated at estrus may indicate that two inseminations by appointment are preferable to one (Table 3).

CONCLUSION

Prostaglandin-$F_{2\alpha}$, cloprostenol and possibly other similar analogs should prove to be effective treatments for cows with unobserved estrus (provided a mature CL is present at the time of treatment). Successful application of these products to the treatment of cows with unobserved estrus is critically dependent upon accurate identification of a mature CL by rectal palpation. A significant proportion of cows (30 to 40 per cent) may still be difficult to detect in estrus if insemination is to be based upon observed signs of estrus. Inseminating cows by appointment after treatment with these products appears to be a feasible alternative to the problems associated with the heat detection. With AI by appointment, the need for heat detection is eliminated, virtually all cows are inseminated soon after treatment, labor requirements are probably reduced and, based on the previously discussed trial utilizing appointment inseminations at 72 and 96 hours after treatment, conception rates may be higher. Most importantly, by combining insemination and conception rates, the percentage of treated cows that become pregnant within 5 days of treatment is likely to be substantially greater when inseminations are by appointment (72 and 96 hours) rather than based upon observed estrus.

TABLE 3. *Distribution of Breeding in Dairy Cows Treated for Unobserved Estrus and Assigned to Be Inseminated at Estrus**

Days after Treatment	No. Bred	Per Cent of Total
1	2	2
2	9	8
3	41	34
4	38	32
5	20	17
6	4	3
7	5	4
Total:	119	

*Treated with cloprostenol (500 μg IM).

REFERENCES

1. Hafs, H. D.: Ovulation Control and Release of Hormones with Prostaglandin $F_{2\alpha}$ in Cattle. VIIIth International Congress on Animal Reproduction and A. I. Krakow, Poland, July, 1976.

2. King, G. J., Hurnik, J. F. and Robertson, H. A.: Ovarian function and estrus in dairy cows during early lactation. J. Anim. Sci., *42*:688, 1976.
3. Seguin, B. E., Gustafsson, B. K., Hurtgen, J. P., Mather, E. C., Refsal, K. R., Wescott, R. A. and Whitmore, H. L.: Use of the prostaglandin $F_{2\alpha}$ analog (cloprostenol, ICI 80, 996) in dairy cattle with unobserved estrus. Theriogenology, *10*:55, 1978.
4. Weaver, L. D. and Schultz, R. H.: Synchronization of estrus and ovulation in dairy cows using clopros-tenol. Presented at the 72nd Annual Meeting, American Dairy Science Association, June, 1977, Ames, Iowa.
5. Williamson, N. B., Morris, R. S., Blood, D. C. and Cannon, C. M.: A study of oestrous behaviour and oestrus detection methods in a large commercial dairy herd. Vet. Rec., *91*:50, 1972.
6. Zemjanis, R., Fahning, M. L. and Schultz, R. H.: Anestrus — The practitioner's Dilemma. Scope (Upjohn), *XIV*:14, 1969.

Initiation of Lactation in Barren, Nonlactating Cows and Heifers

K. LARRY SMITH

Ohio Agricultural Research and Development Center, Wooster, Ohio

INTRODUCTION

Infertility is an acknowledged problem in the management of dairy cattle. All too often the situation arises in which pregnancy has not been achieved and either the cow is not lactating or the level of production is such that drying-off is indicated. The cost of maintaining a barren, nonlactating dairy cow necessitates management decisions as to whether or not to retain the cow and to continue efforts toward achieving pregnancy or to cull immediately and avoid further monetary loss. Such management decisions are easily made with low-producing cows but are somewhat more difficult with cows of above average production potential or of high value from a genetic standpoint.

The ability to economically cause lactogenesis within a relatively short time period would provide both veterinarians and herdsmen with an alternative management practice when dealing with the infertile cow. Smith *et al.*[2] and Smith and Schanbacher[3, 4] have reported a 7-day series of 17β-estradiol and progesterone injections that causes initiation of substantial lactation within a 3-week period. Although the technique appears to work equally well in adult cows and heifers with no previous lactation experience, practical application is somewhat inhibited owing to variability in the number of treated animals that respond and variability in the subsequent level of production. In general, lactation will be initiated in 60 per cent of treated cows, and these cows will produce at a level of 60 to 70 per cent of anticipated milk yield. An additional factor is that the availability of 17β-estradiol and progesterone is limited to research purposes until Food and Drug Administration (FDA) approval is obtained. Given these limitations, the following is a detailed description of the technique of hormone induction of lactation for veterinarians who may wish to apply such therapy.

HORMONES AND DOSAGE

The dosage of 17β-estradiol was 0.05 mg/kg of body weight per injection, and that of progesterone was 0.125 mg/kg of body weight per injection. A series of 14 injections at 12-hour intervals was made (see Table 2), and the ratio of injected 17β-estradiol to progesterone was 1:2.5.

FORMULATION OF INJECTABLE 17β-ESTRADIOL AND PROGESTERONE STOCK SOLUTION

The amount of stock solution required can be calculated or determined from Table 1. The storage life of the stock solution is now known, and generally only that quantity that will be used within 1 or 2 months is made up. The stock solution contains 20 mg/ml of 17β-estradiol and 50 mg/ml of progesterone (ratio 1:2.5). The powdered hormones were weighed out separately to the nearest milligram and added via a

TABLE 1. *Amounts of 17β-Estradiol, Progesterone and Injectable Stock Solution Required to Induce Lactation in Cows Weighing 800 to 2000 Pounds*

Body Weight (lb)	Stock Solution per Injection* (ml)	Total Volume of Stock Solution Required† (ml)	Total Amount of Hormone Required	
			17β-ESTRADIOL (mg)	PROGESTERONE (mg)
800	0.9	12.6	252	630
1000	1.1	15.6	308	770
1200	1.4	19.6	392	980
1400	1.6	22.4	448	1120
1600	1.8	25.2	504	1260
1800	2.0	28.0	560	1400
2000	2.3	32.2	644	1610

*Stock solution contains 20 mg of 17β-estradiol and 50 mg of progesterone per ml absolute ethanol.
†Fourteen injections at 12-hour intervals.

small glass funnel to a serum bottle (generally 100 ml). The injection vehicle was absolute ethanol. The required volume of ethanol was measured in an appropriate-sized graduated cylinder and slowly added via the glass funnel to the serum bottle containing the powdered hormones. The bottle was then *tightly* stoppered with a rubber stopper to prevent evaporation of the absolute ethanol. The bottle was then held under a stream of hot tap water and agitated vigorously until all crystals of the hormones were dissolved.

The stock solution was stored at room temperature in the absence of direct sunlight or fluorescent lighting. If the storage temperature drops below approximately 10° to 15° C or if the bottle is refrigerated, the hormones will crystallize out of solution. Should this occur, place the bottle in a stream of hot tap water and shake vigorously until all hormone crystals are redissolved. *The stock solution should be observed before each injection to insure that all hormones are in solution.* This is particularly true in cooler climates during winter months.

INJECTIONS

Formulation of the 17β-estradiol and progesterone stock solution as just described allows the following computation for injection volume. The body weight in kilograms divided by the factor 400 equals the milliliters per injection. Thus, 600 kg ÷ 400 = 1.5 ml per injection. Likewise the body weight in pounds divided by the fac-

tor 880 equals the milliliters per injection. Thus, 1320 pounds ÷ 880 = 1.5 ml per injection.

Table 1 shows the milliliters of stock solution per injection for body weights from 800 to 2000 lb. In addition, Table 1 permits easy determination of the total volume of stock solution as well as total quantities of 17β-estradiol and progesterone required to induce lactation.

The 17β-estradiol and progesterone injections are made subcutaneously in the area on the upper part of the rib cage posterior to the scapula. Injections are alternated from side to side of the animal, and an attempt is made to allow at least a 3- to 5-cm space between injection sites. A 3- or 2.5-ml. syringe with a 1.5-inch, 18-gauge needle is used for injection, and an attempt is made to make injection volumes accurate to the nearest 0.1 ml.

Twelve to 24 hours following most injections, a nodule approximately 1.0 to 1.5 cm in diameter can be palpated beneath the skin. These nodules persist for various periods of time but in general are completely gone by 2 or 3 weeks. No complications such as necrotic skin, loss of hair, change in hair color or infection have been observed following the injection of the absolute ethanol-hormone complex. It is theorized that following the injection, the steroid hormones precipitate rapidly in the more aqueous media of the subcutaneous tissue, and, in effect, a small implant is formed.

In preliminary experiments, the subcutaneous injections were made in the region of the neck and on occasion would result in large nodules approximately 5 cm in diameter. Such injection sites were subjected to more rubbing on stanchions and posts than those made on the upper part of the rib cage. Intramuscular injections did not result in the initiation of lactation. In addition, previous findings indicate that: (1) the exact amount (milligram per kilogram of body weight) of hormone injected, (2) the exact ratio of 17β-estradiol to progesterone injected, (3) the actual number of injections made and (4) the need for exact 12-hour intervals between injections are not absolutely critical factors with regard to subsequent success or failure to induce lactation. However, *no alteration* in these parameters has been reported to improve the technique, either by reduced variability or increased production. In addition, field trials have shown that precise body weights are not absolutely required and that it is sufficient to obtain an accurate estimation of body weight by someone skilled in the art or by use of weight tapes.

PRETREATMENT CONSIDERATIONS

Research observations reported indicate that the 17β-estradiol and progesterone treatment cannot be used to augment an existing lactation. In addition, field trial experience has shown a high degree of unresponsiveness when the injection series was begun with dry periods of less than 30 days. Considerable data suggest that approximately 30 days are required to achieve full involution. Thus, we suggest that all cows have at least a 30-day dry period before initiating treatment.

To avoid possible complications due to mastitis, all quarters should be observed for signs of clinical infection prior to the start of treatment. If signs of infection are observed or the cow has a previous history of mastitis, all quarters should be treated with an approved "dry cow" infusion product.

All cows should be pregnancy checked by rectal palpation prior to the start of treatment. Farm records alone are not sufficient. Field experience has shown that many dairymen will have declared the animal not pregnant but continued to house the cow with a bull or to have continued artificial insemination. Treatment of pregnant animals results in abortion and in general a less than desirable lactation response.

Existing records and palpation data should be used to determine if the cow is cycling. If cyclic activity is occurring, it is recommended that treatment begin 4 to 7 days after standing heat. If palpation and farm records indicate a lack of cyclic activity, treatment can begin at any time.

Some thought and consideration should be given to housing treated cows with other cattle during the injection series and for a period of 2 to 3 weeks following treatment. Most treated animals will exhibit increased estrous behavior as a result of the injections, and precautions should be taken to avoid possible injury to the treated animal as well as to her herdmates.

An additional housing consideration relates to research results showing that circulating prolactin levels are sensitive to photoperiod. Increased photoperiod results in higher serum prolactin levels, and higher serum prolactin levels are in general associated with a more desirable treatment response. Likewise, decreased photoperiod results in decreased serum prolactin levels, and lower serum prolactin levels have been associated with a less than optimum response. Although there are no experimental data to support the concept, practical field experience has suggested a less than optimum response when photoperiod has been dramatically decreased during treatment. On a practical basis, a dramatic decrease in photoperiod may be imposed if during the summer months the animal is removed from a pasture and housed in a poorly lighted structure during the treatment to initiate lactation.

CHRONOLOGY OF TREATMENT EVENTS

In order to discuss the sequence of events, the day of first 17β-estradiol and progesterone injection is referred to as experimental day 1 (Table 2). Previous experience has shown that experimental day 21 serves as a useful reference point as the day that regular twice daily milking is begun. Thus, a period of 21 days is considered to be required to initiate lactation.

As shown in Table 2, the 17β-estradiol and progesterone injections are made twice daily on experimental days 1 through 7. Whether attempting to induce lactation in

TABLE 2. *Time Sequence of Events during Induced Lactation*

Experimental Day	17β-Estradiol and Progesterone Injection		Reserpine Injection	Secretion Accumulation	First Milking	Estrous Activity
	AM	PM				
1	X	X				
2	X	X				X
3	X	X				
4	X	X				
5	X	X				
6	X	X				
7	X	X				
8			X			
9						
10			X			
11						
12			X	X		
13				X		
14			X	X		X
15				X		X
16				X		X
17				X	X	X
18				X	X	X
19				X	X	X
20				X	X	X
21				X	X	X

heifers or cows, little or no change in the appearance of the mammary gland is noted while the hormones are being injected. Reserpine injections were made by Collier *et al.*[1] on experimental days 8, 10, 12 and 14 (see later discussion).

First indications of a successful induction of lactation are generally associated with changes in teats. In heifers, marked growth of teats is often observed between experimental days 8 and 14. In adult animals, teats will become somewhat turgid and at times will feel noticeably warm to touch. These changes are generally observed prior to noticeable udder growth in heifers and secretion accumulation in adult animals.

In the majority of animals, secretion accumulation, and thus major increase in udder size, is first noted about experimental day 14. However, this can vary from experimental day 10 to 20. The rapid increase in udder size that occurs is often accompanied by edema in heifers, but edema is seldom observed in adult animals.

A major decision with regard to hormone-induced lactations is when to start milking. If prior to experimental day 21 the gland fills with secretion and appears distended, regular twice daily milking should be initiated. On this basis, the earliest we have started milking was experimental day 12. Prior to experimental day 21 an additional guideline used is leakage of milk from teats. If this is observed, milking is begun. If at day 21 there has been a definite increase in udder size but the gland does not appear to be filled, regular milking should be started. On the other hand, if by day 25 little or no change in the appearance of the gland has occurred, experience has shown that the attempt to initiate lactation was probably a failure. Our experience has been that cows or heifers exhibiting marginal or no udder change by experimental day 25 will not produce satisfactorily even if milked three times daily.

Increased estrous activity (Table 2) is sometimes observed on experimental day 2 or approximately 24 hours following the first hormone injection. Generally, treated cows are reasonably quiet for the remainder of the injection period and for 7 to 10 days after the last hormone injection. The increased estrous activity will generally reappear by experimental day 14 in most animals. The duration or extent of this activity is highly variable among treated cows. Some cows will be highly active for 2 to 3 weeks.

LACTATIONS

Most reported data would indicate that the 17β-estradiol and progesterone treatment will successfully initiate lactation in approximately 60 per cent of treated cows[3] and heifers[4] and that these lactations in cows will average approximately 70 per cent of the yield from previous lactations. The actual magnitude of lactations is highly variable, but cows of the Holstein breed can be expected to produce between 4500 and 7000 kg of milk per 305 days. Lactations in excess of 9000 kg per 305 days have been reported from field trials. The most rapid increase in milk production occurs during the first 1 to 2 weeks of the lactation. As might be expected, the more rapid the increase in production, the better the subsequent lactation.

Peak lactation is seldom achieved prior to 30 days; it is more likely to occur at 60 to 90 days but may not occur until after 100 days. Although the length of lactation depends somewhat upon the level of daily production achieved, most hormone-induced lactation cows are capable of lactating for 305 days.

The potential success of the treatment can be assessed as follows: If the assumption is made that 60 per cent success is an accurate estimation of the average 17β-estradiol and progesterone treatment capabilities, the probability of having all failures in a group of three randomly chosen animals is 0.064. Thus, the treatment should initiate at least one successful lactation in a group of three treated cows 94 per cent of the time.

Reasons for variability are not fully understood, but considerable evidence has suggested that low serum prolactin levels in 17β-estradiol and progesterone-treated cows were associated with poor response and less productive lactations. In this regard, Collier *et al.*[1] have reported that the addition of a series of reserpine injections (5 mg IM per injection) (Table 2) caused significant elevation of serum prolactin levels, substantially reduced treatment variability and increased milk yield. In their study,[1] reserpine-treated groups produced 76 to 98 per cent more milk than

control groups, and all reserpine-treated animals lactated successfully. Certainly these data are encouraging and require further investigation; however, reserpine is not a commonly used drug in cattle, and caution may be advisable, particularly as regards dosage (see Treatment Complications).

The first secretion obtained from hormone-induced lactation cows is colostrum, and the change in composition to normal milk occurs over a 2- to 4-day period. It is not uncommon to obtain 9 to 15 kg of colostrum at first milking. There is no reason to believe that such colostrum cannot be fed to calves. There have been no reports of significant compositional differences between milk from hormone-induced lactation cows and normal parturient cows. Likewise, hormone levels do not appear to be markedly elevated in hormone-induced lactation cows, and the mammary gland does not appear to be a major excretory pathway for the injected 17β-estradiol and progesterone.

TREATMENT — OVARIAN INTERACTION AND SUBSEQUENT REPRODUCTIVE PERFORMANCE

During treatment and until experimental day 30 or 40, the vulva is enlarged, the uterus is turgid and mucus is discharged. Rectal palpation of ovaries on experimental day 21 generally reveals that they are smooth and devoid of either corpora lutea or follicles. These findings suggest that the 17β-estradiol and progesterone treatment causes inactivity of ovaries and prevents the occurrence of normal estrous cycles for a period of 30 to 60 days. On occasion a definite corpus luteum or follicles have been detected on day 21, and our experience has been that these animals fail to lactate successfully. The recurrence of normal cyclic activity is highly variable among cows but is often observed between experimental days 40 and 70. The ovaries should be examined by rectal palpation at weekly intervals beginning about experimental day 21. Such data will help to determine whether subsequent observed estrous activity is the result of (1) the hormones injected, (2) development of cystic follicles or (3) normal follicle development and ovulation. The cow should be bred at the first indication of normal estrous activity. There is no need to wait 45 to 60 days after lactation has begun, as is recommended following normal parturition.

A number of research reports have indicated that cystic follicles may develop about experimental day 40, and field observations have indicated that cows showing persistent estrous activity beyond experimental day 30 to 40 will most likely have cystic follicles present on ovaries. Luteinization of follicles and estrous cycles of normal length have been achieved following treatment with human chorionic gonadotropin (HCG). Standing estrus is usually observed 2 to 3 weeks after HCG treatment. It is recommended that breeding occur at this time.

Collectively, research results show that 60 per cent of the 17β-estradiol and progesterone-treated cows conceive during the induced lactation and have a normal pregnancy. These results are very encouraging, considering that such cows were regarded as "problem breeders" during their previous normal lactation. Clearly, research shows that subsequent reproductive performance is not impaired in induced lactation cows. There is no indication that subsequent pregnancy can be achieved by any one standard therapy regimen. Instead, each cow should be considered as an individual case and appropriate therapy applied as indicated once lactation has been initiated.

TREATMENT COMPLICATIONS

The following pathological conditions have been observed in one or more cows during or after treatment to initiate lactation:

1. Depressed feed intake. This condition generally appears in all animals between experimental days 1 and 21. An occasional animal may become anorectic.

2. Constipation. The condition is variable among animals and generally occurs during the period of depressed feed intake.

3. Ataxia. An occasional cow may appear to have difficulty in rising from a recumbent position and may seem to have impaired mobility of the rear legs. Our experience has been that the condition is temporary, is noted between experimental days 5 and 30 and is often associated with overweight cows.

4. Parturient paresis. One case has been diagnosed and verified by blood chemistry studies. It occurred in an aged Jersey cow.

5. Cystic follicles. Cystic follicles have been variously reported to occur in 30 to 60 per cent of treated cows.

6. Abortion. If pregnant cows are treated, they will abort. Our experience has been that cows pregnant more than 120 to 150 days will have successful lactations, whereas cows pregnant less than 60 to 80 days will either not lactate or lactate poorly.

7. Development of hematomas. A small percentage of the cows treated have developed hematomas in the area of the brisket, posterior ribs or flank. Such hematomas may represent impaired clotting mechanisms. They have generally been associated with overweight animals and were thought to have resulted from a bruise. Impaired function has been noted in only one animal. Similar hematomas have been observed in untreated herdmates but at an apparently reduced incidence.

8. Reserpine complications. Collier et al.[1] have reported that side reactions following reserpine injection were labored breathing, nasal congestion and drowsiness on the afternoon following the third and fourth injections. They report that approximately one-fourth of the animals were sedated moderately and refused to rise on the afternoon following the fourth reserpine injection. By 48 hours after the last reserpine injection, the side reactions were no longer apparent in their experimental animals. All animals used by Collier et al.[1] were of the Holstein breed, and it is not known whether breed differences with regard to dosage of reserpine or sensitivity to reserpine exist. Our experience would indicate that reserpine injections should be discontinued if animals are sedated and refuse to rise 12 to 18 hours following a second or third injection. The effects of the reserpine injections would appear to be cumulative and have on occasion resulted in the death of the animal.

SUMMARY

The technique of hormone-induced lactation as originally described by Smith et al.[2] and Smith and Schanbacher[3, 4] has been described in detail. Clearly, substantial milk production can be initiated in barren, nonlactating cows and heifers, and approximately 60 per cent of animals injected with 17β-estradiol and progesterone to initiate lactation can subsequently become pregnant. However, there is variability in the degree of response among treated animals. A series of reserpine injections has been reported to substantially reduce the 17β-estradiol and progesterone treatment variation.

At the present stage of development, the technique of hormone-induced lactation should be viewed as an option when major reproduction problems are encountered and not as a supplement to pregnancy. Thus, the first objective for hormone-induced lactation is to attempt to establish a profitable level of milk production, and the second objective is to get the animal pregnant as rapidly as possible. In this way the animal is returned to the normal herd management procedures with a minimum loss of profit from both milk and offspring.

REFERENCES

1. Collier, R. J., Bauman, D. E., and Hays, R. L.: Effect of reserpine on milk production and serum prolactin of cows hormonally induced into lactation. J. Dairy Sci., *60*:896, 1977.
2. Smith, K. L., Muir, L. A., Ferguson, L. C., and Conrad, H. R.: Selective transport of IgG₁ into the mammary gland: Role of estrogen and progesterone. J. Dairy Sci., *54*:1886, 1971.
3. Smith, K. L., and Schanbacher, F. L.: Hormone induced lactation in the bovine. I. Lactational performance following injections of 17β-estradiol and progesterone. J. Dairy Sci., *56*:738, 1973.
4. Smith, K. L., and Schanbacher, F. L.: Hormone induced lactation in the bovine. II. Response of nulligravida heifers to modified estrogen-progesterone treatment. J. Dairy Sci., *57*:296, 1974.

Laparoscopic Examination of the Cow's Reproductive Tract

ROBERT F. ROWE
University of Wisconsin, Madison, Wisconsin

Reproductive dysfunction or infertility in the cow is still one of the most difficult diagnoses to make. Short of an exploratory laparotomy to actually visualize the reproductive organs, we still must depend upon rectal palpation to "see" anatomical abnormalities that may impair fertility. Yet palpation of the bursa, fimbria and oviduct, which under ordinary circumstances is difficult, is impossible in some of the valuable repeat breeder cows that we are asked to examine.

Use of the laparoscope will never replace rectal palpation as the chief tool for diagnosing reproductive disorders. However, it has become an extremely useful device in helping to assess the prognosis of repeat breeder cows; in locating anatomical abnormalities of the ovary, bursa or oviduct; in assessing adhesions that may have developed from previous intra-abdominal surgery; in utilizing repeated observation of the ovary to note ovulation and formation of the corpus luteum and in carrying out research projects dealing with reproductive physiology.

For example, we have used the laparoscope in conjunction with our nonsurgical embryo collection projects. Palpation of the superovulated donors to accurately estimate the number of corpora lutea (CL) becomes extremely difficult when six or more CL's are present on an ovary. However, using the laparoscope, accurate counts of the CL numbers have been obtained.

EQUIPMENT

The laparoscope used in our laboratory is the Wolfe fiberoptic 130° 10-mm lumina telescope. Information concerning the light source and accompanying equipment is found in Appendix B.

TECHNIQUE

The cow should be held off feed and water for 24 to 48 hours to reduce the size of the rumen and have the intestines fairly empty. Observation of the reproductive tract can be achieved without insufflation of the abdominal cavity; however, inflation of the abdomen with a compressed gas (oxygen, carbon dioxide or air) allows more rapid location of the uterus and ovaries and forces intestines, mesocolon and omentum away from the pelvic inlet. Caudal elevation can also be of great assistance in allowing abdominal contents to gravitate away from the pelvis and permitting easier visualization of the reproductive tract.

Animals are restrained in a squeeze chute, and a 4–square-inch area is clipped in the central portion of the paralumbar fossa. After thorough cleaning and disinfecting, two areas 2 to 4 inches apart are infiltrated with 5 to 10 ml of a suitable local anesthetic. Two small 1-cm incisions are made through the skin only.

The Verres needle is introduced through the subcutaneous tissues, muscle layers and peritoneum into the abdominal cavity. Compressed gas is forced into the abdomen until both paralumbar areas are distended. The Verres needle is withdrawn, and the 10-mm trocar sleeve is introduced through one incision; the 6-mm trocar sleeve is introduced through the other. Following removal of the trocars, the telescope and manipulating rod are introduced into the abdomen, and observation is begun.

DISCUSSION

It should be remembered that the left kidney is freely movable and is frequently displaced toward the right paralumbar fossa by the rumen. For this reason placement of the Verres needle is usually preceded by insertion of an arm into the rectum of the cow and palpation of the paralumbar fossa as the needle is inserted. This will also prevent insufflation of the mesocolon, cecum or omentum, which can make observation of the reproductive tract impossible.

Using the endoscope alone makes it difficult to view the entire surface of the ovaries and the oviduct. Thorough examination is

accomplished by using a blunted rod or grasping forceps to move the ovary and bursa. The manipulating rod used in our laboratory is a 5-mm stainless steel rod, 75 cm in length, and we prefer it to the Jacobs-Palmer grasping forceps with blunt jaws because it is less traumatic and can be used from the contralateral as well as the ipsilateral side. The rod is strong enough to lift and visualize heavy postpartum uterine horns.

Practical experience with the laparoscope is necessary for placement of the instrument and quick identification and examination of the ovaries, oviducts and uterus. One may use either side of the animal to view the reproductive tract; however, approaches depend upon the anatomical structures of that side. On the left side one must be aware of the position of the rumen, whereas on the right side the position of the cecum and omentum must be considered. Usually the manipulating rod is inserted ipsilateral to the laparoscope, but it has been possible to manipulate from the contralateral side of the cow.

We feel that this technique is especially valuable for determining anatomical causes of repeat breeders. Several of the differential diagnoses that could be ruled out by use of the laparoscope are adhesions blocking the oviduct, delayed or premature ovulation and abnormalities of the bursa or oviduct.

In summary, we feel that the fiberoptic laparoscope is a tool that can be used successfully to assist in field problems of repeat breeders and infertility in cattle.

REFERENCES

1. Seeger, K.: Laparoscopic investigation of the bovine ovary. Vet. Med./Small Anim. Clin., *72*:1037, 1977.
2. Wishart, D. F. and Snowball, J. B.: Endoscopy in cattle: Observation of the ovary in situ. Vet. Rec., *92*:139, 1973.

Physical Examination of the Reproductive System of the Bull

LESTER LARSON

*American Breeders Service, DeForest,
Wisconsin*

The proper examination of the bull for adequacy of reproductive function is a unique procedure for the veterinarian in that it demands a combination of proficiencies rarely required. It is necessary to employ a goodly amount of (1) clinical competence, (2) animal psychology, (3) patience, (4) common sense, (5) knowledge of clinical pathology and, in some cases, (6) athletic prowess coupled with raw courage.

Since standard anatomy texts generally treat anatomy of the bull's reproductive organs in a cursory manner, it seems justified to bring together in this article some of the available anatomical illustrations showing in detail the genital organs of the bull.

Through the generosity of Erik Blom and N. O. Christensen,[7] their classic anatomical illustrations of the bull's genital organs have been made available for this book (see Figures 2 to 9 and Figure 11). It is the wish of these highly respected Danish colleagues that these illustrations be superbly reproduced in the veterinary literature of North America in commemoration of Paul H. Winther, the artist, now deceased, whose skill has captured so precisely the anatomical details of these structures.

This article places major emphasis on the examination of the mature dairy bull. An effort will be made to point out differences between beef and dairy bulls from the point of view of the examiner. The underlying clinical principles, however, remain the same regardless of the kind of bull or the intended purpose of the examination.

PREPARATION

Restraint. This requirement takes on unusual significance when, as in the examination of a mature bull, one is required to perform all observations and manipulative procedures with all of the bull's faculties intact. These faculties may include an intense desire to demolish veterinarians or to be at a place different than the location at which the examination is scheduled to take place. These desires are often enforced with 2000 to 3000 pounds of a highly coordinated neuromusculoskeletal system.

It is patently obvious that application of restraint to a fractious 2500-pound bull must be on the veterinarian's, rather than a bull's, terms. There is little doubt of the outcome if bull mentality is applied to bull restraint.

In the absence of adequate facilities, competent handlers and a bull accustomed to being restrained by a nose ring, which is often the case, the principles of good restraint for mature bulls must be all the more fully utilized.

The bull should be secured in a roomy box or tie stall by anchoring the head to a structural beam or post with a strong halter, neck chain or neck strap, preferably through a stanchion or headgate. One handler must remain at the bull's head. A light but strong rope is attached to the nose ring and half-hitched to a structure directly forward of the bull, so that the rigging that actually secures the head tightens before the nose tie as the bull pulls back. With one hand on the nose ring and one on the rope to prevent the half-hitch from slipping, the bull's attention can usually be adequately maintained. The nose ring may be quickly released to prevent tearing of the muzzle if the bull becomes excessively fractious.

The bull must be afforded the opportunity to gain confidence in the examiner. The degree of the bull's nervousness will determine the time requirement for the bull's realization that the upcoming ordeal is not painful. It is *absolutely essential* that physical contact is achieved between bull and examiner and that the bull's initial sensation to the contact is pleasurable. Approach is best made slowly, deliberately and with the hand extended toward the shoulder area while talking in tones of kindness and confidence. The move into contact is made only as the bull's cowering subsides. Essentially, all bulls react favorably to rubbing or currying over the withers and dorsal neck area, given enough time. It may take 10 to 30 minutes to reach this "end point," but it is the time best spent during the entire examination.

With this state of restraint achieved, the examination can usually proceed uninterrupted if reinforcement is provided by continuing verbal and body-contact reassurance. Sudden moves and loud noises must be completely avoided by all participants.

Identification. The examining veterinarian has an important responsibility as a neutral party to check personally for agreement between the bull's permanent identifying marks and the official written record. This is particularly necessary so that blood obtained for typing can be correctly identified.

The subject of blood typing is discussed in detail in Section XIV. Suffice it to say here that access to the immunological identification of the red blood cell–associated antigens of cattle is an absolutely essential initial point of reference for determining the facts in all animal identification disputes.

THE EXAMINATION

Health History and General Physical Examination

Other than to point out factors particularly pertinent to the examination of a large bovine male and, especially, to attempt to categorize clinically the potency-impairing diseases of the neuromusculoskeletal system, it is not within the scope of this article to elaborate on the classic approach to general physical examinations. The following outline lists the components of special significance in the general examination of the bull.

History of Disease

The breeding history and general physical examination must be utilized to determine the presence of recessive genes in the bull, which, if brought together with other similar genes from a female, would create lethal, semilethal or economically undesirable conditions in offspring (see page 410).

Systems Review

Integument and Body Wall. Bulls with umbilical, inguinal or other hernias or with surgically repaired hernias may not be justifiably recommended for use in breeding.

Lymphatic System. During palpation of internalia (pelvic and abdominal genital organs), the iliac and deep inguinal lymph nodes are especially accessible for detailed examination.

Circulatory System. Typically, the thickness of the body wall in large bulls makes meaningful cardiac auscultation difficult. Characterizing the pulse by direct palpation of distal aortic, iliac or hypogastric arteries is easily accomplished. This enables one to recognize minimal pulse aberrations, which are rare.

Digestive System. Detailed examination of the oropharyngeal cavity by visual inspection or palpation, or both, and examination by palpation of the abdominal digestive organs within reach via the rectum are always a necessary part of a complete examination of the digestive system.

Urinary System. Full attention should be given the urinary organs by the examiner, either before or after conducting the detailed examination of the internalia.

Locomotor (Neuromusculoskeletal and Hooves, NMSH) System. Liberty is taken to use this systems conglomeration in order to more easily emphasize the significance that these individual body systems, in consort, play in determining a bull's potency, that is, the function of his semen delivery system. The semen delivery system can loosely be divided into two components: the penis with its support systems, which is a marvel of efficiency, and the NMSH system, which is unsound in many ways and fails all too often.

Through genetic improvement of cattle for production, larger animals have been developed without necessarily providing a system for locomotion and coition that is proportionately stronger. Therefore, situations arise at coitus that require the pelvic limbs of a bull to support upwards of 3000 pounds while engaging in highly coordinated movements. It cannot be overemphasized, therefore, that veterinarians examining bulls for adequacy of reproductive function must critically evaluate NMSH.

Conformation

The examiner must be fully aware, as an anatomist, of limb-hoof conformation traits that are functionally sound and therefore contribute to the bull's longevity and usefulness. The veterinarian will, thereby, readily recognize the significant conformation defects. Pertinent questions such as the following must be answered:

1. Are the angles of the tarsal joints proper (Fig. 1D), i.e., not excessively small and "sickle-hocked" (Fig. 1E) or excessively large and "posty" (Fig. 1F)?

2. Do the axes of the stifle, tarsal and fetlock joints approximately intersect single right and left sagittal planes (Fig. 1A), or are the pelvic limbs rotated laterally so a "cow-hocked" trait is evident (Fig. 1C)? Are the pelvic limbs rotated medially, resulting in a "bow-legged" attitude (Fig. 1B)?

3. Do the axes of the joints of the forelimbs approximately intersect single right and left sagittal planes, or is there excessive outward rotation (supination) with consequent "toeing out"?

4. Is the slope of the pasterns (angle of metatarsophalangeal, metacarpophalangeal joints) proper as in Figure 1D and not too "weak" as in Figure 1F or too straight?

5. Are the hooves of adequate size consistent with age? Are the shape and placement of the hooves upon the third phalanx such that:

   a. Adequate weight-bearing surfaces are present?

b. The medial and lateral hooves are symmetrical in size and shape?

c. The axial hoof walls are flat, parallel to and equidistant from the sagittal plane in which the limbs are located and that they are in close apposition to each other?

d. The anterior and abaxial hoof walls, together with the bulbs of the heels, form hooves of medium length with adequate width and depth of the heel, rather than hooves that are long and narrow with shallow heels? Such hooves many times are associated with weak pasterns and turning axially of the distal abaxial hoof wall, forming the so-called corkscrew or scissor hooves.[15]

6. Is the gait that of a well-coordinated animal?

Evaluation of conformation of hooves is often complicated by gross horn overgrowth because of neglect.

Pathology. Limb conformation defects resulting in dysfunction are by definition pathological conditions. Defects of a lesser degree may be termed blemishes, when dysfunction is not a consequence of the lesion.

It is not the intent here to discuss the

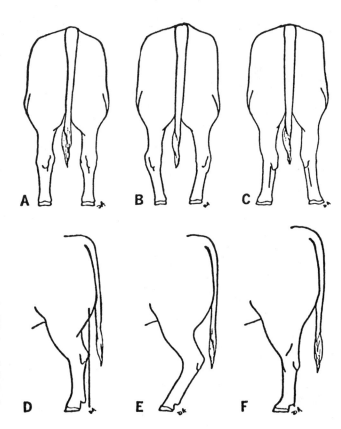

Figure 1 Normal and abnormal conformation characteristics of rear limbs of bulls. *A* and *D*, Normal. *B*, "Bow-legged," medial rotation, narrow base. *C*, "Cow-hocked," lateral rotation, wide base. *E*, "Sickle-hocked," angle of tarsus small. *F*, "Post-leg," angle of tarsus large, and "weak pastern," angle of metatarsophalangeal joint reduced. (From Ott, R. S.: Vet. Med./Small An. Clinician, November, 1976, 1592–1595.

TABLE 1. *Incidence of Degenerative Diseases of Rear Limbs in Bulls**

Disease	Mature (>5 years) Experience of 1588 bull-years	Immature (<5 years) Experience of 2556 bull-years	500 Mature Dairy Bulls Examined Prepurchase	205 Mature Beef Bulls Examined Prepurchase
Progressive posterior paralysis	3.8%/year	0.2%/year	0	0
Postiness	0.7%/year	1.0%/year	2%	0
Spastic syndrome	3.2%/year	0.5%/year	5%	0

*Degenerative disease not initially or primarily arthritic. Data based on 76% dairy and 24% beef experience.

pathological conditions of NMSH, which are so superbly handled in the book by Greenough *et al.*[15] However, in case of the potency-impairing degenerative disease conditions of the rear limbs that are not primarily arthritic and are most frequently observed in mature bulls, there are nomenclature contradictions that need to be rectified.

A summary of extensive clinical-pathological experiences clearly identifies three such disease entities of rear limbs: (1) progressive posterior paralysis, (2) "postiness" and sequelae and (3) spastic syndrome[18] (Table 1). A fourth, closely related condition, spastic paresis or Elso heel, although not a disease of mature bulls, will be discussed briefly from the standpoint of differential diagnosis. Unfortunately, the terms progressive posterior paralysis, spastic syndrome and "crampy" have been applied to a combination of rear limb diseases.[3] It is proposed that the term progressive posterior paralysis be reserved for the disease for which the description follows and for which the term itself is highly descriptive.

PROGRESSIVE POSTERIOR PARALYSIS. This is a clinically specific paralyzing disease of older bulls. It is rarely seen in bulls under 6 years of age and is generally characterized by a slow onset with signs of ataxia. Impairment seems to be exclusively of motor and proprioceptive function. Skin esthesia usually remains intact.

Typically, the bilateral partial paralysis worsens perceptibly from week to week, as though there is progressive destruction of motor nerve fibers, or neurons, in the spinal cord. Given adequate time, the bull usually becomes fully paralyzed in the rear limbs. The disease may reach a plateau for many months at certain levels of severity. Apparent improvement, which occurs rarely, seemingly is by compensation through learning rather than by an improvement in neurological function.

Occasionally, other structures whose nerve supply is from lumbosacral segments of spinal cord are affected. The terminal rectum and anus may become paralyzed so that fecal evacuation is by abdominal press. The urinary bladder may lose capacity to contract reflexly so that urination is by spillover. Tail muscles may become fully or partially paralyzed.

Spondylosis deformans as part of nutritional hypercalcitoninism may well be a contributing cause. Bone spicules encroaching upon the vertebral canal have been observed on rare occasions at necropsy in affected bulls. In most cases, however, no such specific lesions are evident.[22] Other more subtle etiologies that are degenerative in nature at the central nervous system level, may also cause this defect.

As Table 1 shows, progressive posterior paralysis has a relatively high incidence among older bulls. The distribution among breeds, both beef and dairy, appears to be quite uniform. The average age of 66 affected bulls was 9.8 years. Only five were below 7 years of age.

"POSTINESS" ("POST-LEG"). This defect (Fig. 1*F*) in severe form is the direct cause of more rear limb pathology than any other abnormal conformation trait in mature bulls. In this condition the anatomical system (peroneus tertius and gastrocnemius muscles) that causes hock and stifle joints to flex or extend together is so structured that joints remain in perpetual extension. Postiness nearly always becomes evident bilaterally, often by 1 to 3 years of age.

The primary condition, a conformation defect, must be differentiated from acquired, secondary postiness, which may develop in older bulls either unilaterally or bilaterally. This appears to be a voluntary (reflex?) pain-sparing action on the part of the bull as a result of degenerative arthritis of the stifle joint. Localized hyaline cartilage destruction is usually associated with secondary postiness but is not common in primary postiness.

In essentially all cases of primary postiness, the following sequelae occur at varying rates and degrees of severity. Pain is evidenced by the affected animal's shifting of weight-bearing from limb to limb. The first signs of pain may be accompanied by or preceded by increased synovial fluid in the tarsal joints. Later, as tarsitis becomes chronic, there is often development of osseous periarthritis, which, together with local edema, results in a rather post-like limb largely devoid of the normal angles, depressions and protuberances of the tarsus. Often, degenerative processes occur in the stifle joints as sequelae to lesions of the tarsus. Primary postiness rarely improves. Typically, the degenerative processes initiated by the primary fault continue unabated but at varying rates. Rarely does a bull whose tarsus is too straight remain functionally normal throughout life.

Only 2 of 37 bulls with primary postiness cited in Table 1 were of beef breeds, even though beef bull experience constitutes 24 per cent of the total bull-years cited.

As with other conformation defects, the inheritance of these tendencies is complex. In the case of primary postiness, which is usually so functionally debilitating, veterinarians should maintain a strong position against employing such bulls in extensive breeding programs.

SPASTIC SYNDROME ("CRAMPINESS," "STRETCHES," NEUROMUSCULAR SPASTICITY). This is a disease of mature dairy and dual-purpose cattle. It is characterized by intermittent bilateral tonic spasms of skeletal muscle groups in the standing animal. Early in the course of the disease or in cases in which signs are slight, the rear limb muscles only may be involved either unilaterally or bilaterally. Anterior progression of muscular contractions usually occurs. Such progression may vary in rate but involves all axial and trunk muscles. In the severest form, all muscles appear to be involved in contractions, causing an appearance of opisthotonos.

Spasms do not occur during recumbency but are most prominent on arising, while the bull is adapting to weight-bearing. Pain stimuli from limbs severely aggravate the signs. These and other clinical observations strongly suggest that the primary defect in this disease involves the highly complex myotatic-postural reflex system.

The aggravation of muscle contractions by pain and adaptation to weight-bearing is more readily explained if an assumption is made that spastic syndrome is the result of impaired spinal cord connections and interpretations of the afferents of the myotatic reflex, resulting in abnormally increased efferents. That is, both pain stimuli and stimulation of muscle spindle fibers by stretching, such as in weight-bearing, increase afferent stimuli. In the case of bulls with functionally abnormal cord connections, as in spastic syndrome, increased afferent stimuli result in abnormal, highly exaggerated efferent stimuli and characteristic involuntary contractions of skeletal muscles.

It has been frequently observed that some bulls, usually younger animals, show typical signs of spastic syndrome only in the presence of severely painful hoof lesions such as traumatic or infectious laminitis. This has been interpreted to mean that such bulls have latent spastic syndrome, which may surface as frank disease with advancing age. Thus, an indicator, of sorts, exists for latent spastic syndrome.

The average age of the 55 bulls from which data are cited in Table 1 was 7.6 years. Twelve of the animals were less than 5 years of age, while only one was under the age of 3 years.

Although the beef bull experience is 24 per cent of the total bull-years cited, not a single case of spastic syndrome has been observed in beef bulls.

The mere fact that spastic syndrome is a disease exclusively of dairy and dual-purpose cattle suggests heritability in some form. A familial occurrence of the disease has been reported.[15] In an extensive statistical study,[3] conclusions were drawn that suggested inheritance for spastic syndrome ("crampy") by a single recessive factor with incomplete penetrance. However, in this study precise diagnoses were apparently not available, and bulls were included in the survey whose afflictions were variably descriptive of progressive posterior paralysis and polyarthritis in addition to spastic syndrome ("crampy"), the disease under consideration. Accurate conclusions concerning inheritance of a tendency for a single disease simply cannot be drawn from source material that includes at least three disease entities.

Semen from the 55 bulls with spastic syndrome (Table 1) has been sold for use in artificial insemination (AI). Conservatively

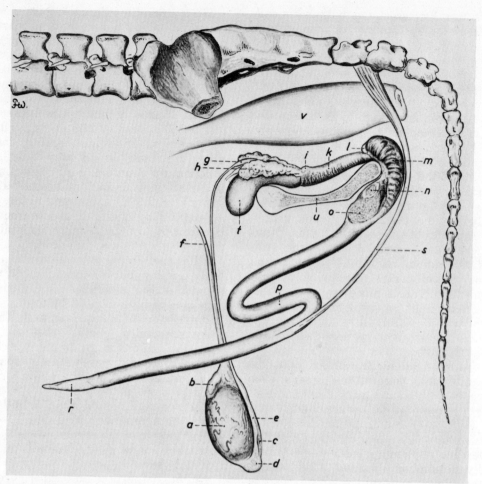

Figure 2. General view of genital organs of bull, left testis and spermatic cord have been removed. (a) Right testis, (b) head of epididymis, (c) body of epididymis, (d) tail of epididymis, (e) right ductus deferens, (f) mesorchium, (g) right ampulla ductus deferentes, (h) left vesicular gland, (i) body of prostate, (k) pelvic portion of urethra with urethralis muscle, (l) left bulbourethral gland, (m) left bulbospongiosus, (n) left crus penis (cut), (o) left ischiocavernosus (cut), (p) penis with sigmoid flexure, (r) glans penis, (s) retractor penis, (t) urinary bladder, (u) symphysis pelvis and (v) rectum. (From Blom, E. and Christensen, N. O.: Skandinavisk Veterinartidskrift, 1947, 1–45.)

estimated, more than 100,000 female offspring have been sired by them. In spite of a feedback system designed to ferret out and report unusual offspring, records show no such reports for spastic syndrome in offspring of these bulls. It is apparent, therefore, that neither the incidence nor severity of spastic syndrome among daughters of afflicted bulls has warranted reporting by herd owners.

Over a 25-year period the following working hypothesis has been found very useful in confronting the question of heritability of spastic syndrome. Since the expression of the disease is variable and is modified by factors such as age, standing position and pain and since definitive evidence for inheritance following a predictable pattern is

lacking, the mode of inheritance is considered to be highly complex and therefore difficult to elucidate. Consequently, bulls with spastic syndrome are handled on an individual basis. Whenever signs of the disease occur at a relatively young age, are uncomplicated by pain and are typical, severe and worsening, the problem is self-limiting in that potency impairment is or will soon be complete. All such bulls should be held out of extensive breeding programs. In cases in which onset of spastic syndrome occurs in older bulls (often associated with pain of arthritis or other painful limb afflictions and therefore amenable to treatment with analgesic drugs), the disease is handled as though it has no ramifications beyond the specific bull involved. Potency is maintained with pain-relieving drugs such as phenyl-butazone.

SPASTIC PARESIS (ELSO HEEL). This disease has some clinical signs[14] and part of its name in common with spastic syndrome. Therefore, it seems appropriate to consider spastic paresis briefly from a standpoint of differential diagnosis. Spastic paresis is most common in European Friesian cattle. It is uncommon in the United States but has been reported in Holstein, Ayrshire, Angus and Beef Shorthorn breeds. Clinical signs are most frequently unilateral. Onset is rare after 1 year of age, but it may occur within a few weeks of birth. The disease is characterized and explainable by chronic contraction of gastrocnemius and superficial digital flexor muscles. As a result, hock and stifle joints are typically maintained in near full extension, holding the fibular tarsal bone and its os calcis in close apposition to the distal tibia. Partial separation of the os calcis from the fibular tarsal bone gives an increased area of reduced radiopacity at its epiphyseal plate.

Tremulous muscle contractions are present in the affected limb, especially on arising. The limb appears shorter, may not touch the ground, often swings in a pendulous manner and usually points caudomedially. Symptomatic surgery, in which either the achilles tendon or branches from the tibial nerve to the gastrocnemius muscle are interrupted, usually gives marked relief.

Sire-daughter matings provide firm evidence that spastic paresis is not transmitted by a simple recessive mechanism.[10]

It has been determined that calves with spastic paresis display deviations from normal of some components of cerebrospinal fluid. The most significant deviation may be a substantial reduction of homovanillic acid, the main metabolite of the neurotransmitter dopamine.[11]

SPECIAL EXAMINATION OF THE REPRODUCTIVE ORGANS

Internalia

The pelvic and abdominal genital organs constitute the internalia (Figs. 2 to 9).

The *vesicular glands* are readily examined by palpation on the anterior floor of the pelvic cavity. They converge posteriorly along with the ampullae ductus deferentes at the anterior end of pelvic urethral muscle at the point at which the body of the prostate gland is palpable. The vesicular glands lie just lateral to the ampullae ductus deferentes (Figs. 2, 6, 7). Their normal consistency is yielding and meaty, and their lobulated outlines are readily discernible.

Pathology of the vesicular glands is restricted nearly exclusively to hypoplasia and aplasia, which are rare,[17] and infectious conditions, which may be acute or chronic. Acute seminal vesiculitis may show all the signs of localized pelvic peritonitis. On palpation pain may be severe, and the affected glands may be found markedly enlarged and firm. Fibrin exudation upon the peritoneum with subsequent organization may occur. Purulent exudate is consistently present in semen.

Chronic seminal vesiculitis, which may or may not follow an acute phase, is associated with persistent or intermittent purulent exudate in semen. Usually localized or gener-

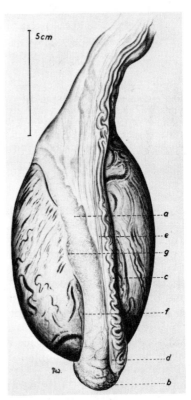

Figure 3. Left testis and epididymis from a 2-year-old bull, caudomedial view. (a) Body of epididymis, (b) tail of epididymis, (c) ductus deferens, (d) ligament of tail of epididymis (cut), (e) mesorchium (cut), (f) testicular bursa and (g) part of epididymis attached to testis, no testicular bursa is formed. (From Blom, E. and Christensen, N. O.: Skandinavisk Veterinartidskrift, 1947, 1–45.)

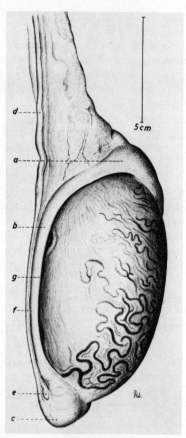

Figure 4. Right testis and epididymis from 3-year-old bull, caudolateral view. (*a*) Head of epididymis, (*b*) body of epididymis, (*c*) tail of epididymis, (*d*) ductus deferens, (*e*) ligament of tail of epididymis (cut), (*f*) mesorchium (cut) and (*g*) testicular bursa. (From Blom, E. and Christensen, N. O.: Skandinavisk Veterinartidskrift, 1947, 1–45.)

alized fibrosis and enlargement with loss of lobulation are present, but pain on palpation ordinarily is absent (Fig. 9).

In young beef bulls under ranch conditions, the incidence of seminal vesiculitis has been found to be 2.4 per cent.[8] Under conditions of an AI stud, the annual incidence was determined to be 1.3 and 0.7 per cent for bulls more than 1½ and less than 1½ years of age, respectively. Incidence was proportionately distributed among beef and dairy bulls.[18]

In young group-housed bulls, seminal vesiculitis in some cases appears to be contagious. Transmission may be retrograde as a result of urethral contamination during homosexual activity. In most such cases, resolution occurs spontaneously but slowly. In older bulls, which more commonly are af-

flicted with chronic seminal vesiculitis, cure is rarely possible.

Etiological agents that have been reported are nonspecific opportunistic pathogens such as streptococci, staphylococci, actinobacilli, corynebacteria, mycoplasmata and chlamydia or specific pathogens such as *Brucella abortus*, *Mycobacterium bovis* and *Mycobacterium paratuberculosis*.

Surgical removal of offending vesicular glands has been performed with varying degrees of success, but, mostly, results have been poor.

The *ampullae ductus deferentes* are readily palpable in their entirety. They lie in the urogenital fold between the vesicular glands (Figs. 2, 6, 7). Their junction with the pelvic urethra at the body of the prostate may be dorsal to vesicular glands, as in Figure 6, or intermediate or ventral. Rarely do ampullae show hypoplasia or aplasia. If present, such anomalies are usually associated with defects of the other derivatives of the wolffian ducts. The incidence of segmental aplasia of the wolffian ducts has been reported as 0.56 per cent on necropsy specimens[5] and 0.1 per cent on clinical specimens.[8]

Clinically, ampullitis is not readily recognized; however, in bulls with a high incidence of seminal vesiculitis an equal or greater incidence of infection in the ampullae was found at necropsy.[1] Müllerian cysts are rather commonly encountered in the urogenital fold of the interampullar space. Extremely rarely, a uterus masculinus is found in the same location.

The *prostate gland* is composed of the palpable *body* and nonpalpable *pars disseminata,* which lies deep to the pelvic urethralis muscle (Figs. 2, 6, 7, 8). Inflammatory processes have been identified at necropsy, but not clinically, in 43 per cent of bulls with a high incidence of seminal vesiculitis.[1]

The *bulbourethral glands* (Figs. 2, 6, 7) are not palpable, being imbedded under the bulbospongiosus. Thus, disease of these glands, determined clinically, has not been reported. However, at necropsy of bulls with a 49 per cent incidence of seminal vesiculitis, 15 per cent showed bulbourethral adenitis.[1] A significant anatomical aspect of the bulbourethral glands is the urethral recess (Fig. 7), which is formed in the dorsal wall of the urethra at the ischial arch by a fold of urethral mucosa. The excretory ducts of the bulbourethral glands enter the urethra upon the free end of this mucosal fold. Because of

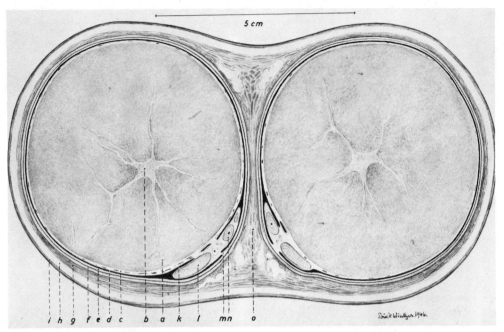

Figure 5. Dorsal section through the scrotum and testes. The section passes approximately through the middle of the body of the epididymis. (*a*) Testis, (*b*) mediastinum testis, (*c*) tunica albuginea with vessels, (*d*) tunica vaginalis visceralis, (*e*) tunica vaginalis parietalis (vaginal cavity is between *d* and *e*), (*f*) spermatic fascia, (*g*) dartos, (*h*) and (*i*) skin, (*k*) testicular bursa, (*l*) body of epididymis, (*m*) mesorchium, (*n*) ductus deferens with mesoductus and (*o*) scrotal septum. (From Blom, E. and Christensen, N. O.: Skandinavisk Veterinartidskrift, 1947, 1–45.)

its location and structure, the urethral recess forms an obstruction to passage of a sound or catheter into the urinary bladder via the urethra.

The *inguinal rings* are easily palpable at a point 12 to 18 cm ventral to the deep inguinal lymph nodes. If the opening is too large, i.e., transmits three or more fingers, the animal is predisposed to inguinal hernia. Hereditary implications of enlarged inguinal rings may be of greater significance than the abnormality itself in an individual bull. Incidences of enlarged inguinal rings of 0.15 per cent[8] and 0.11 per cent [18] have been observed.

Externalia

Scrotum and Testes

Examination of the scrotum and testes is by visual inspection and palpation. The tunica dartos should be fully relaxed in warm weather, revealing a scrotal "neck" that is trim and is free of fat and of varicoceles of the pampiniform plexus. The scrotal abaxial contour should be convex (Fig. 10), and the relaxed scrotal wall should be thin and pliable. Adhesions involving visceral and parietal layers of tunica vaginalis propria should not exist between testes asnd scrotum.

The normally suspended testis hangs in the scrotum so that the body of the epididymis is located caudomedially and the head of the epididymis lies on the proximoanterolateral surface. Thus, the view of the left testis in Figure 3 is from the caudomedial aspect (see also the body of the epididymis and the ductus deferens in Figure 5).

Rarely, there is malformation of the scrotum by differential growth of the scrotal wall or septum. Typically, the former results in an abbreviated caudal scrotal wall, so that the testes are unilaterally or bilaterally held in a near horizontal position. This condition seems mainly restricted to young beef bulls. A shortened scrotal septum results in a midventral scrotal cleft. In older bulls the scrotum, if unpigmented, seems uniquely susceptible to "blood warts," which are varicose dilatations of scrotal veins.[16]

Ventral scrotal scab formation as a sequela to scrotal frostbite is substantial evidence that super-cooling of the testis has occurred and that resultant transitory (at best) testicular degeneration has taken place.[12]

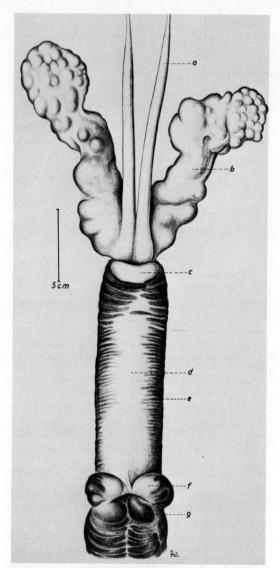

Figure 6. The internal genital organs of a 3 1/2 -year-old bull with typical dorsal position of the ampullae ductus deferentes. The superficial layer of bulbospongiosus has been dissected off to show the bulbourethral glands. (*a*) Ampulla ductus deferentis, (*b*) vesicular gland, (*c*) body of the prostate, (*d*) pelvic portion of urethra, (*e*) urethralis, (*f*) right bulbourethral gland with deep bundles of bulbospongiosus (*g*). (From Blom, E. and Christensen, N. O.: Skandinavisk Veterinartidskrift, 1947, 1–45.)

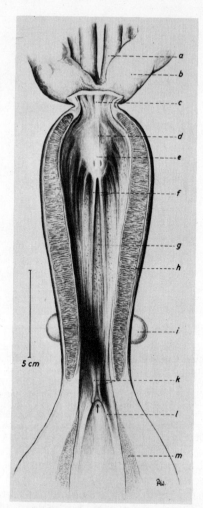

Figure 7. The proximal part of urethra opened ventrally. (*a*) Ampulla ductus deferentis, (*b*) vesicular gland, (*c*) neck of bladder, (*d*) urethral crest, (*e*) colliculus seminalis with ejaculatory orifices, (*f*) frenula of colliculus seminalis, (*g*) excretory orifices from pars disseminata of prostate, (*h*) urethralis, (*i*) bulbourethral gland loosened and moved laterally, (*k*) excretory ducts from bulbourethral glands distended by injection of plaster of Paris, (*l*) the free distal border of the mucosal fold forming urethral recess into which the arrow points and (*m*) corpus spongiosum. (From Blom, E. and Christensen, N. O.: Skandinavisk Veterinartidskrift, 1947, 1–45.)

The normal left testicle with the epididymis and proximal ductus deferens is well illustrated in Figure 3. Note that testicular length is roughly 2× its diameter.

The mean testicular size in mature bulls, both beef and dairy, when expressed as length and diameter, is approximately 14 to 16 cm × 7 to 8 cm. Expressed as scrotal circumference (SC), testicular size in such bulls is 41 to 44 cm (Table 2). Normal consistency of the testes is that of being turgescent yet resilient.

Testicular hypoplasia has been determined to be heritable in Swedish Highland cattle. An association has been made between testicular hypoplasia and autosomal secondary constrictions, as determined by

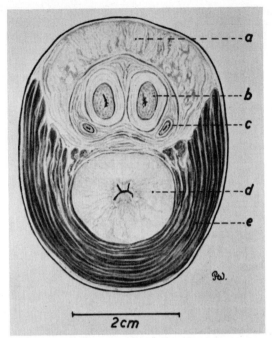

Figure 8. Cross section through pelvic urethra at level of body of prostate, with typical dorsal position of the ampullae ductus deferentes. (*a*) Body of prostate, (*b*) ampulla ductus deferentis, (*c*) excretory ducts of vesicular glands, (*d*) neck of bladder and (*e*) urethralis. (From Blom, E. and Christensen, N. O.: Skandinavisk Veterinartidskrift, 1947, 1–45.)

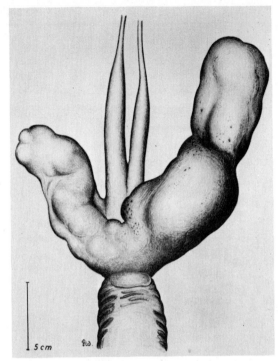

Figure 9. Ampullae, ductus deferentes and vesicular glands of a 4- to 5-year-old bull. Brucellar inflammation of the right vesicular gland and the left ampulla ductus deferentis is present. Note enlargement and lack of lobulation of the right vesicular gland. (From Blom, E. and Christensen, N. O.: Skandinavisk Veterinartidskrift, 1947, 1–45.)

cytogenetic studies. By definition, testicular hypoplasia connotes both small size and spermatogenic malfunction. The latter, if slight, is often indistinguishable on histological examination from testicular degeneration, to which bulls with slight degrees of testicular hypoplasia are particularly susceptible. The difference between these two conditions may, thus, under some circumstances, be only of definition or underlying cause, and the diagnosis must be based upon history, clinical findings and evaluation of repeated semen samples. Incidence has been reported to be 0.2 per cent,[6] 1.3 per cent[8] and 0.3 per cent,[18] depending on populations studied.

Cryptorchidism is of extremely low frequency in bulls. Two comprehensive studies reveal a near identical incidence of 0.1 per cent.[6, 8] Evidence for heritability has been cited.[23]

Figure 10. Scrotal configurations. *A*, Flat-sided scrotum associated with moderate-sized testes. *B*, Normal scrotum. Testes are usually large. *C*, Short, ventrally tapered scrotum, often associated with small testes. (From Cates, W. E.: Observations on scrotal circumference and its relationship to classification of bulls. Proceedings of the Annual Meeting of the Society for Theriogenology. Cheyenne, Wyoming, September 1975.)

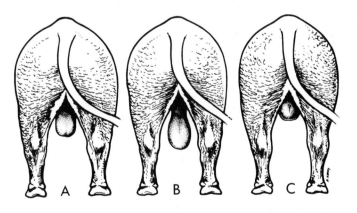

TABLE 2. *Changes in Testicular Size in Holstein and Angus Bulls with Age*

	Scrotal Circumference			
	Holstein		Angus	
AGE IN MONTHS	NO. OF MEASUREMENTS	MEASUREMENT (cm)	NO. OF MEASUREMENTS	MEASUREMENT (cm)
6–12	371	30.0 ± 3.3*	3	33.5 ± 3.1*
12–18	696	34.9 ± 2.4	19	36.1 ± 3.0
18–24	597	37.4 ± 2.2	19	40.1 ± 4.0
24–30	510	39.1 ± 2.9	43	40.0 ± 2.7
30–36	488	40.1 ± 2.3	37	39.5 ± 3.2
36–42	466	40.8 ± 2.7	38	40.6 ± 2.5
42–48	431	41.2 ± 2.5	18	40.5 ± 3.1
48–54	375	41.6 ± 2.5	25	40.3 ± 3.1
54–60	361	41.7 ± 2.9	8	39.7 ± 2.5
60–72	616	42.1 ± 2.7	16	40.0 ± 2.3
72–84	307	42.6 ± 2.7	21	41.0 ± 2.4
84–96	219	42.6 ± 3.9	21	41.1 ± 2.9
96–108	158	43.3 ± 2.5	23	42.1 ± 2.3
108–120	116	43.5 ± 2.6	18	42.1 ± 2.3
120–132	82	43.9 ± 2.7	12	41.6 ± 2.0
132–144	62	43.5 ± 2.8	8	40.0 ± 2.9
144–156	30	43.1 ± 2.6	6	40.3 ± 2.1
156–168	16	41.5 ± 2.7	3	41.0 ± 3.0
168–180	6	41.8 ± 3.9	1	39.0 ±
Total	5909		339	

*Mean ± standard deviation. (From Coulter, G. H., Larson, L. L. and Foote, R. H.: J. Anim. Sci., *41*:1383, 1975.)

Testicular degeneration is the partial or complete failure of the spermatogenic epithelium to proceed normally with spermatogenesis. It may be transitory or permanent. As the degree of degeneration increases, palpable and tonometric testicular flaccidity and the numbers of spermatocytes, spermatogonia and malformed spermatozoa in ejaculated semen increase as well. In gradual testicular degeneration, such as in aging, there is concurrent fibrosis of the seminiferous tubules. The products of degeneration become calcified. With rapid but permanent degeneration, fibrosis takes place after the degenerative process, and the connective tissue itself may become calcified.[16]

Etiological factors regarded as significant in testicular degeneration are (1) elevation of testicular temperature, whether caused by local or environmental factors; (2) supercooling, such as occurs in scrotal frostbite; (3) circulatory ischemia to the testes, whether due to trauma or to degenerative vascular lesions; (4) congenital occlusion of efferent tubules — as spermatogenesis commences at puberty, back pressure and edema of the testes cause megalotestis and complete testicular degeneration; (5) autoimmunity; (6) toxins; (7) gonadotropin deficien-

cies — actual difference between testicular degeneration due to gonadotropin deficiency and testicular hypoplasia may be only a matter of degree and (8) viral infection.

Orchitis-periorchitis is usually unilateral. An incidence of 0.45 per cent has been reported in an extensive survey of young ranch beef bulls,[8] and an annual incidence of 0.12 per cent has been recorded in bulls maintained under conditions of an AI stud.[18] If source infection is hematogenous, a testis is infected first, but periorchitis often eventually occurs. If infection is retrograde via the ductus deferens, the corresponding epididymis is usually injected first. Often periorchitis, which also involves the peritoneum, is primary. In acute cases, classic inflammatory signs are present, followed by testicular degeneration, which ordinarily is complete. In no instance is the prognosis other than poor. Unilateral castration has been used to retain function of the contralateral gland.

Brucella abortus (including Strain 19), *Corynebacterium pyogenes,* streptococci and other bacterial opportunists are among the etiological agents for orchitis-periorchitis. Figure 11 illustrates an eventual lesion in which adhesion about the distal testis and tail of the epididymis has occurred. Rarely, abscessation is a final outcome.

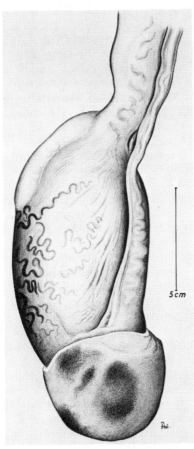

5 cm

Figure 11. Right testis and epididymis of a 2 1/2-year-old bull. Inflammation of the tail of the epididymis caused by *Corynebacterium pyogenes*. The inflamed-organized tunica vaginalis parietalis adheres to the tail of the epididymis. (From Blom, E. and Christensen, N. O.: Skandinavisk Veterinartidskrift, 1947, 1–45.)

Testicular tumors diagnosed clinically are extremely rare.[18] However, at necropsy a considerable incidence of primary testicular tumors in aging bulls has been reported.[16]

Hydrocele, the accumulation of transudate within the processus vaginalis, has been observed but is extremely infrequent in bulls.[17]

Hematocele, traumatically induced by testicular rupture in group-housed bulls, is the most common traumatic disease of the scrotum and testes in bulls so maintained.[18] Typically, there is extreme distention of the affected scrotum. Resolution is by organization of the blood clot with complete fibrosis, resulting in acquired monorchism.

The variability of fertility among bulls with normal potency, i.e., semen delivery system function, is dependent upon the number of normal sperm produced in the testes and made available to the tails of the epididymides, from which final delivery is made at ejaculation. In turn, the total number of sperm ejaculated is related to the adequacy and amount of the parenchymal mass of the testes and the functional normalcy of the efferent ducts and epididymides.

Thus, clinicians, after determining that all components of the scrotum and its contents are present and free of obvious abnormalities, have at their disposal only the characteristics of size and consistency with which to substantiate data regarding fertility/infertility derived from laboratory findings on collected semen.

Scrotal circumference (SC) is the most easily reproducible single measurement of testicular mass[24] (see page 335 for the technique for determining SC). Table 2 is very useful to the clinician, as it gives SC averages for Holstein and Angus bulls at age increments of 6 months between age 6 and 180 months. Other studies are in close agreement with these findings.

As a clinical guideline in interpretation of SC data, especially if obtained prior to sexual maturity, a scrotal circumference that is more than one standard deviation less than average indicates a marked deficiency in testicular mass. At two standard deviations less than average, a clinical diagnosis of "hypoplasia" is mandatory.

Slight asymmetry in testicular size is very common. If size ratio exceeds 60:40, unilateral hypoplasia may not be adequately reflected by scrotal circumference. Obviously, scrotal circumference for unusually spherical or elongated testes must be modified by an appropriate decreasing or increasing factor, respectively, to reflect testicular mass accurately.

Within limits, the degree and significance of testicular turgescence, flaccidity and fibrosis can be readily determined by palpation by experienced clinicians. However, correct diagnosis can be made with assurance in the absence of semen evaluation only in cases of testicular degeneration that are severe and acute or those that are severe and chronic with fibrosis. In cases in which degeneration is moderate and acute or is moderate and chronic with fibrosis, there must be supporting data concerning semen quality for a definitive diagnosis.

A more precise measure of testicular consistency may be obtained with a tonometer. If used properly, a highly repeatable number that characterizes the degree of turgescence will be obtained. Consistently high relationships have been found between tonometer ratio and semen quality as determined in the laboratory.[13] Used in conjunction with palpation, this instrument provides useful points of reference for the clinician. Testicular degeneration with fibrosis will, obviously, give a false high tonometer reading for which the correct interpretation is possible only after careful palpation.

Epididymis

An epididymis (Figs. 2, 3, 4, 5) is palpable in its entirety. The head is easily recognized as a flattened structure, more firm than the testis, on the proximoanterolateral surface of the testis (Fig. 4). The body is readily exposed for palpation by raising the contralateral testis. The tail is composed of the terminal epididymal tubule and mostly, but not always, protrudes well beyond the ventral limits of the testis.

The epididymis is a single, tightly convoluted tube, 30 to 35 m in length, whose diameter increases as it progresses through the arbitrary segments designated head, body and tail. Most pathology of this structure, therefore, is related to nonpatency, the etiology of which may be segmental aplasia, trauma or infection with cicatrix formation.

Spermatocele is often a sequela to epididymal occlusion for whatever reason. It is a cystic dilation of an epididymis, with accumulation of inspissated sperm immediately proximal to the occlusion. Since efferent ducts of the testes have the capability of resorbing noncellular products of the seminiferous tubules, back pressure and resultant testicular degeneration are delayed. Congenital occlusion of efferent ducts, however, results in rapid back pressure producing a large, markedly turgescent testis with complete testicular degeneration at the time of onset of spermatogenesis.

Eventually, most spermatoceles develop into spermatic granulomas as the epididymal wall degenerates and permits direct contact of sperm with epididymal stroma, whereupon a granulomatous reaction is elicited.[16] These, plus inflammatory lesions, constitute the vast majority of palpable conditions of the epididymis.

Penis and Prepuce

The penis and prepuce (Figs. 12, 13, 14) are best examined at the time of semen collection with an artificial vagina. Penile protrusion for examination may also be accomplished with an electroejaculator or with regional anesthesia of the pudendal nerves. When visual observation of the penis and free preputial membrane is not possible, these structures are readily palpable.

Failure of full penile development, especially in bulls with "paunchy" abdomens or in bulls that fail to properly flex vertebral joints at penile intromission, results in impotency due to inadequate penile protrusion.

Other forms of impotency caused by failure of normal penile protrusion are:

1. Lack of erection with normal mounting. This is extremely rare (annual rate of 0.02 per cent).[18]

2. Congenital persistence of the penile frenulum. This is found most frequently in Beef Shorthorn and polled beef bulls.[8]

3. Phimosis caused by adhesions as a result of (a) traumatic, physical or chemical injury; (b) nonspecific balanoposthitis, e.g., caused by filth and/or trauma or (c) specific balanoposthitis, such as in infectious pustular balanoposthitis (IPB).

4. Large penile papillofibromata.

5. Penile fracture with a hematoma and its organization.

Avulsion of the free preputial membrane at the fornix during intromission into an artificial vagina, usually with copious preputial hemorrhage, is by far the most common preputial injury among bulls in AI. Successful surgical repair is readily achieved in the standing bull under pudendal nerve block, provided early closure is possible.

A deviated or corkscrew penis created by abaxial tensions at erection by the apical ligament (Fig. 12) results in impotency at coitus but, usually, not for service of an artificial vagina.

Patency of the tunica albuginea of the glans penis with blood loss at erection (a very difficult lesion to handle surgically) creates a situation in which ejaculated semen is consistently contaminated with blood.

In bulls of Brahman breeding, pendulous prepuce, coupled with chronic eversion of free preputial membrane, predisposes such

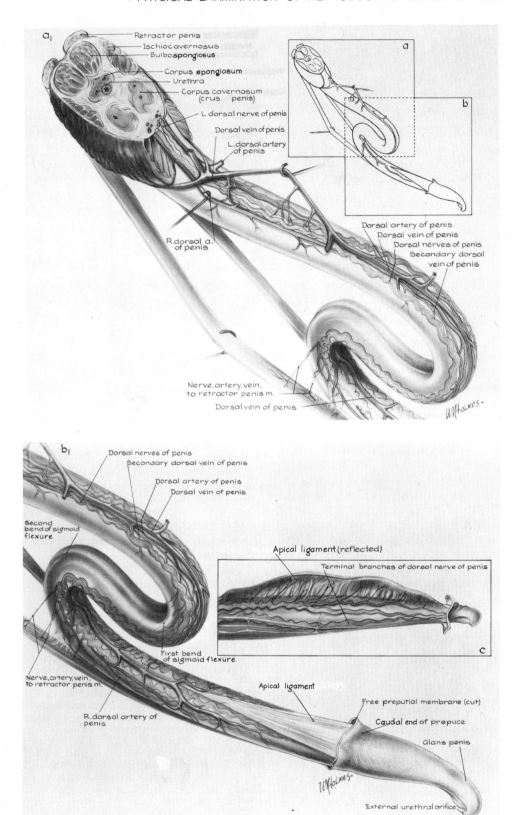

Figure 12. Penis of bull. (From Larson, L. L. and Kitchell, R. L.: Am. J. Vet. Res., *19*:853, 1958.)

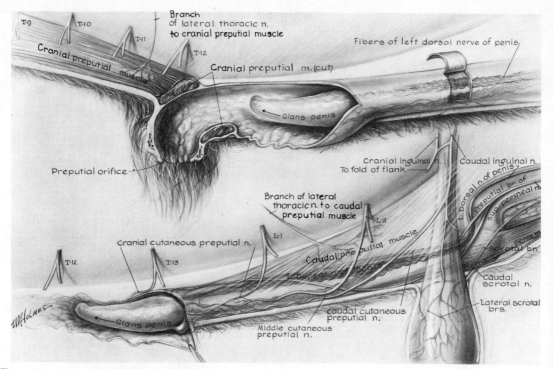

Figure 13. Nerve supply to the distal parts of the external genitalia of the bull. (From Larson, L. L. and Kitchell, R. L.: Am. J. Vet. Res., *19*:853, 1958.)

animals to paraphimosis as a result of the vicious circle of trauma, edema, increased trauma and increased edema. This conformation defect frequently requires surgical correction in order to maintain potency of the affected bull. Polled bulls, however, which tend to have chronically everted free preputial membranes but a sheath that is not pendulant, do not seem to have an increased incidence of traumatic preputial disease.

CLINICAL ASPECTS OF SEMEN COLLECTION

The technical considerations of semen collection and semen evaluation will be covered in detail on page 345. An attempt will be made here to discuss briefly the art of semen collection under other than ideal circumstances, and to point out the unqualified usefulness of semen collection via the artificial vagina (AV) in the clinical interpretation of potency-related neuromusculoskeletal function.

The employment of the AV makes collection of a physiological semen sample as a

"biopsy" for study of spermatogenic membrane an extremely simple procedure. Also, it creates a confrontation between bull and veterinarian, enabling clinical evaluation of nonspermatogenic components of bull fertility, namely, potency and libido, the interrelationships of which are depicted in the following outline.

BULL FERTILITY — fertility in the larger sense.*

---

*Effective bull fertility, obviously, is equally dependent upon normal spermatogenesis, normal potency and freedom from venereal or semen-borne pathogens. Availability for ejaculation and delivery of spermatozoa in optimal numbers and of superb fertilizing capacity has no fertility value unless the spermatozoa can readily be delivered at coitus of through AI to a site in a fertile cow/heifer at which their capacity to fertilize may be realized. Conversely, vigorous libido coupled with virile potency contributes nothing to effective bull fertility other than to insure the proper delivery of the spermatozoa. Likewise, if high quality semen is produced and properly delivered but becomes contaminated with pathogens from a diseased bull, the resultant infertility may be as complete as though fertilization had not occurred. It is important in all fertility/infertility contemplations to be able to conceptualize the interrelationships of the male and female fertility components, which together make up the actual, expressed, fertility.

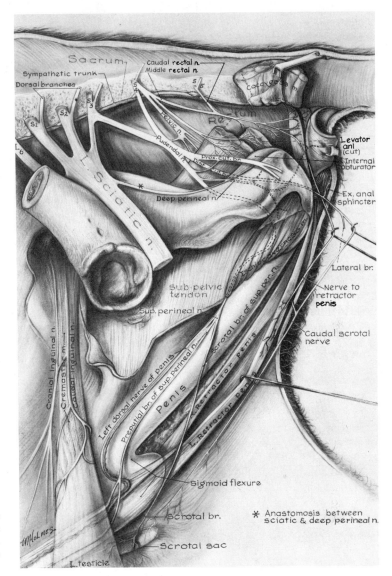

Figure 14. Nerve supply to the proximal parts of the external genitalia of the bull. (From Larson, L. L. and Kitchell, R. L.: Am. J. Vet. Res., *19*:853, 1958.)

Spermatogenesis — capacity to produce optimal numbers of sperm with high fertilizing capability.

Potency — ability to readily deliver sperm to anterior vagina, natural or artificial. This requires:

A. Physiological and physical soundness of the tubular components and accessory glands of the genital system.

B. Integrity and coordination of the neuromusculoskeletal system and hooves (NMSH).

C. Libido — sexual desire:
1. Innate libido — genetically conferred.

2. Environmental modifiers of innate libido:
   a. Painful disease of NMSH.
   b. Nutrition—malnutrition or obesity.
   c. Age.
   d. Poor management practices that have produced pain or anxiety at coitus or at semen collections or that have resulted in sexual exhaustion.

Freedom from infectious agents — which if present in the bull may impair fertility in cows/heifers similarly infected at coitus or from AI with contaminated semen.

Semen collection with an electroejaculator reveals partial information concerning spermatogenesis and essentially no information regarding potency.

Leading, Restraint and Safety

All bulls must be considered extremely dangerous with but few individual and breed exceptions. The safest and most suitable means of leading bulls is to use two 15 to 25-foot light and flexible, yet strong, ropes of ⅝-inch braided nylon. One, for restraining, should be bowline-tied around the horns or neck and then passed through a strong nose ring. The other, for leading, may be tied directly to the nose ring.

It is an illusion that mature aggresive bulls can be safely handled with a bull staff. A staff requires the handler to be much too close to a bull's head. Should the bull make a fast move or lower his head so that control is lost, the staff can become a deadly instrument for impaling, entangling or flailing the handler.

Under no circumstances must one get caught in a corner from which there is no escape when a bull attacks.

English beef bulls are usually not aggressive; neither are they usually accustomed to being handled by ropes. With such bulls, the practical solution may be to use no restraint, or at most a rope halter, on a bull broken to a lead.

"Mount" Animal and Semen Collection Site

A cow in estrus, obviously, is most suitable as a "mount." But an in-heat cow is seldom available when needed. Therefore, substitution with a sturdy, nonestrous cow that is easy to handle is often necessary.

Suitable breeding chutes are rarely available for confining the "mount" animal. Characteristically, chutes on farms or ranches have been built for natural mating. Some have been modified for semen collection by people unfamiliar with hazards of semen collection with an AV. Such stocks generally are constructed with maximum emphasis on bull-escape prevention. Chute side panels and approach alley walls are high, and openings for the person handling the AV are small and in the wrong location and often are perfectly designed to enhance to the ultimate degree the arm-breaking hazard for the semen collector. In most cases the procedure is safer, and opportunity for success is greater, at an improvised collection site than in an improperly constructed chute-alley.

The desirable elements of an improvised collection site are: (1) sidewise and back and forth movement of the "mount" must be restricted; (2) the ground surface must not be excessively smooth, slippery, rough or muddy; (3) there must be space available for freedom of movement and escape by the collector and (4) bull handlers must be able to maintain a fence between themselves and the bull. One arrangement that provides most of these desirable elements is to halter-tie a "mount" snugly into a corner of a sturdy board fence that is readily available to the bull.

In this set-up, the fence on the far side from the collector serves to prevent the "mount" from moving excessively away from the collector and also serves as a safety rail for the bull handlers. It is often necessary to hand-hold a nose-lead in the "mount's" nares to keep attention away from what must seem to the nonestrous cow as an impending disaster.

An assistant on the "mount's" near side can be very useful in preventing excessive "mount" movement toward the collector by firmly holding the end of a blunt stick or bar into the "mount's" midthorax.

With "mount" and collection site thus arranged and the collector ready with a properly prepared AV in hand, the bull is brought in with a lead rope, while the restraining rope is being paid out from a hitch around a strong post or plank. The handlers must always maintain at least a 20-foot distance from a bull's head unless working over a sturdy fence.

In order to obtain a physiological ejaculate, it is essential that the bull be restrained from mounting until his penis is partially erect and a flow of seminal fluid from accessory sex glands is well underway. During this period of 5 to 10 minutes of "teasing," it is well not to permit direct nuzzling of the vulva of the nonestrous "mount." This is in an effort to delay full realization by the bull that the cow is nonestrous. During this preparatory period, the veterinarian-collector must utilize every opportunity to evaluate the bull for lameness, coordination, gait, conformation and intensity of libido.

At the moment when the bull shows partial erection, i.e., the glans penis protrudes from its prepuce or the glans penis distends the prepuce near its orifice, and there is liberal dripping of seminal fluid, along with display of willingness to mount, the handlers should, on the veterinarian's command, give the bull freedom but should keep the restraining rope anchored. They should be especially watchful for a fast move by the bull toward the collector. The attendant at the "mount's" head should, at the same time, place some tension on the nose-lead while the blunt stick or bar is being placed more snugly into the mid-seventh to eighth intercostal space by a person so assigned.

To avoid natural intromission, as the bull mounts the collector moves in quickly, but quietly, from a point lateral to and slightly behind the bull.

The penis is gently deflected laterally toward the collector with near cupped hand on the distal sheath.*

As the bull makes probing movements with his penis, the artificial vagina is placed in direct line with the diverted penis, which is permitted to probe the AV. If consistency, temperature, lubrication and pressure of the artificial vagina closely approximate the bovine vagina, the bull will typically enter his penis deeply and forcefully into the AV. Ejaculation with semen emission occurs within 1 second of the time that intromission commences. The bull should be permitted to retract his penis from the AV voluntarily. Frequently this is not done prior to dismounting, in which instance it may be necessary to follow the bull down, with the AV remaining on the penis, as dismounting occurs. At this point also, bull handlers must be especially alert to prevent the bull from making a pass at the collector.

Evaluative observations regarding a bull's potency are best made during the act of semen collection. Was libido intense, adequate or subnormal? If apparent libido was subnormal, could this be attributed to low innate libido or to normal libido, environmentally modified, as previously described?

*It may be desirable not to permit the bull to find the AV at first mounting but to allow him to make repeated probings with the penis diverted away, so the "mount" is not contacted. This is termed a false mount. Such precoital stimulation has the advantage of increasing sperm numbers in a prospective ejaculate and permitting closer scrutiny by the veterinarian of the erected penis and of the bull's mounting behavior. The obvious disadvantage of a false mount is that if a bull is not accustomed to mounting without attaining ejaculation, the opportunity for obtaining a subsequent semen collection may be lost, especially if conditions for collection are less than optimal.

Is the bull an athlete? Was mounting accomplished readily without the bull's partially supporting his weight by employing his head and neck in order to "slide" onto the "mount"? A bull's need for such support may be evidence of pain in vertebral, pelvic or limb joints. Was the "mount" animal firmly grasped with the bull's forelimbs? Was intromission vigorous, and was it made without hesitation? If not, could the failure be attributed to an improperly prepared AV or to the imperfect coordination by the collector of the bull's probing movements with accessibility of the AV for the bull's "finding"?

The evaluation of properly collected semen is discussed elsewhere. It cannot be overemphasized, however, that semen is at its highest quality the moment it leaves the external urethral orifice. It is, therefore, axiomatic that meaningful semen evaluation is impossible unless semen is ejaculated into, and maintained in, an environment that closely simulates that from which sperm cells were ejaculated. Semen must be handled out of direct sunlight, at body temperature and in an environment free of filth and deleterious foreign ions. Microscopic examination of the semen must not be unduly delayed.

EXAMINATION FOR SPECIFIC INFECTIOUS DISEASES OF BULLS

The subject of venereal or semen-borne diseases of bulls, as well as other (emerging?) diseases of special concern in examination of bulls, such as bluetongue, bovine leukemia, chlamydial infections, Q fever, and the ubiquitous pathogens, has recently been reviewed.[2] Therefore, cursory discussion only seems indicated here, with emphasis on testing methods for bulls.

Bovine Tuberculosis. Full consideration must be given to tuberculosis in the health evaluation of bulls. Not only can *Mycobacterium bovis* be transmitted from an infected bull to contact cattle via the usual respiratory-alimentary route, but in the case of urogenital tuberculosis, the infection can be transmitted at coitus and by artificial insemination.

The insidious nature of bovine tuberculosis and the inherent inaccuracy of the intradermal test when applied diagnostically to a single animal demand employment of additional testing methods in order to be certain that the animal is disease-free.

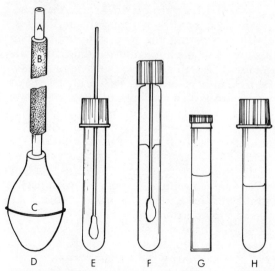

Figure 15. Apparatus and media used in preputial sample collection, transport and culture. *A*, Plastic sampling pipette 81 cm × 6 mm OD × 3 mm ID. *B*, Stainless steel tube 62 cm × 1 cm OD × 8 mm. ID. *C*, Rubber bulb, 1 ounce capacity. *D*, Sampling device assembled. Plastic envelope not shown. *E*, Sterile plastic vial with swab. *F*, Modified Stuart's carrier medium with inoculating swab in place. *G*, Sterile physiological saline in 8 ml plastic tube for *T. foetus* sample transport. *H*, Thyoglycollate medium in plastic vial for *T. foetus* culture.

In addition to the intradermal test (preferably comparative cervical) of the bull in question, it is important to obtain a complete history about herd additions, outside contacts by the bull and recent herd test results. If recent and frequent complete herd tests have not been done, such testing often is essential in arriving at a diagnosis for the bull.

Bovine Brucellosis. A battery of effective serological tests are available for determining the brucellosis status of cattle. Of particular interest in bulls is the need to determine whether or not infection of the genital organs has occurred, resulting in liberation of infective organisms in semen. It has been established that the semen plasma tube agglutination test identifies genital infection with discharge of purulent material and infectious organisms in the semen earlier and with higher titer than do serological tests. Bulls with negative serological findings but which were shedding brucella organisms in semen have been identified.[4, 21]

The semen plasma tube test, therefore, is most critical and meaningful in determining the brucellosis disease status of bulls of semen-producing age and must be a part of every bull examination, along with appro-

priate serological brucella tests, herd disease history evaluation and herd test results for the disease.

Bull calves should not be vaccinated for brucellosis with Strain 19 vaccine. Vaccination may destroy bull's fertility by infecting genital organs, and Strain 19 may be shed in semen from the infected organs.

Bovine Vibriosis and Bovine Venereal Trichomoniasis. These, the well-established, true venereal diseases of cattle, are amply described on pages 479 and 482. Diagnosis in the bull depends largely upon obtaining an adequate sample from the fornix-glans penis area of the prepuce (Figs. 12 and 13). Unless the bull has had at least 4 days without sexual activity to permit population build-up of organisms lost at coitus or semen collection, opportunity for obtaining a reliable sample is reduced. Necessary assurance that these infectious agents are not present in the genital organs of bulls may be achieved only if adequate preputial specimens are obtained and competently examined on three or more occasions during a 3 to 4-week period.

A sampling system has been developed that enables a veterinarian to readily obtain, at a single attempt, useful samples for examination for both *Campylobacter fetus* (var. *venerealis*) and *Trichomonas foetus*.

The sample collecting device (Fig. 15*D*) is composed of a plastic disposable preputial sampling pipette (Fig. 15*A*) that is gas sterilized in a plastic envelope* and a sterile stainless steel tube (Fig. 15*B*) that has been aseptically placed onto the pipette so that both are contained within the envelope. A 1-ounce rubber bulb (Fig. 15*C*) is attached to the exposed end of the plastic pipette. Thus, a plastic pipette is used to aspirate the smegma sample, the steel tube forms a protective sheath for the plastic pipette and the plastic envelope maintains asepsis.

To obtain the sample the entire unit is first passed to within approximately 10 cm of the glans penis, with the plastic pipette fixed so that its tip is located 10 to 12 cm back from the distal end of the steel sheath. Then the steel sheath is used to break through the plastic envelope and is held in place, separated 8 to 10 cm from the glans penis, as the plastic aspirating pipette is brought to the area of the preputial fornix.

The actual technique for picking up smegma from the recesses of the convoluted skin

---

*Edwards Agri-Supply, Inc., Baraboo, Wisconsin.

of the glans and fornix is by aspiration. While diligently and firmly massaging the glans with one hand, the rubber bulb is compressed and released successively with the other hand. This is done while simultaneously moving the aspiration pipette back and forth with its tip in close apposition with, and sometimes lightly scraping, the glans and fornix area. Fifteen to 30 such strokes are required to obtain a good sample.

Prior to removal from the prepuce, the plastic pipette is withdrawn into the steel sheath to the approximate position on entry. The entire device is removed, maintaining this configuration until *immediately* prior to transfer of the sample.

The portion of the sample (1 to 3 drops) destined to be cultured for *Campylobacter fetus* (var. *venerealis*) must first be aseptically expelled into the bottom of a sterile vial (Fig. 15*E*). The remainder, for use with the *T. foetus* sample, is flushed into 3 to 4-ml sterile physiological saline in an 8-ml test tube (Fig. 15*G*). This inoculum should be sufficient to create marked turbidity of the saline. If direct microscopic examination for *T. foetus* is not to be conducted, the sample may be gently flushed directly into the upper layer of *T. foetus* culture medium (Fig. 15*H*).

C. fetus (var. *venerealis*) samples are best transported to the laboratory in modified Stuart's (SBL) carrier medium (Table 3). This medium permits samples to remain useful for culture for up to 48 hours.[9] Inoculation into Stuart's medium should be done *immediately* after collection and is best accomplished by absorbing the sample onto the sterile swab (Fig. 15*E*) and then stab-inoculating it to a depth of 4 to 5 cm, where the swab should remain until removed at the laboratory (Fig. 15*F*). Stuart's medium is best maintained at refrigerator temperature, especially after inoculation. Laboratory culture procedures for *C. fetus* (var. *venerealis*) have been competently described.[10]

TABLE 3. *Modified Stuart's (SBL) Carrier Medium**

Method	For Approx. 1000 ml	For Approx. 500 ml
1. *Ingredients*		
Bacto agar	8 gm	4 gm
Difco Laboratories		
Detroit, Michigan		
Thioglycollic acid	0.5 ml	0.25 ml
Cat. #A–319		
Fisher Scientific Co.		
P.O. Box 171		
Itasca, Illinois		
Sodium glycerophosphate	10 gm	5 gm
Cat. #3532		
Eastman Kodak Co.		
Rochester, New York		
Calcium chloride, laboratory grade	10 ml	5 ml
(1 per cent in water)		
Cat. #C–81		
Fisher Scientific Co.		
Cysteine hydrochloride	0.025 gm	0.013 gm
Cat. #C–562		
Fisher Scientific Co.		
Methylene blue (0.1 per cent in distilled water)	2 ml	1 ml
Cat. #6A–766		
Fisher Scientific Co.		
Prepare by dissolving 0.1 gm in 1 ml	950 ml	475 ml
ethyl alcohol, then make up to 100 ml		
with distilled water		
Distilled water		

2. Adjust pH to 7.2

3. Heat to boiling. Dispense 10 ml portion into medium-sized glass and screw cap tubes. Place caps on loosely. Evacuate atmosphere and replace with N_2 four times in desiccator jars. Quickly tighten screw caps and autoclave at 10 lb/sq in for 20 minutes.

*For transport of preputial samples.

TABLE 4. *Thioglycollate Broth Medium**

Method	For Approx. 1000 ml	For Approx. 500 ml
1. Mix (dissolve):		
A. Fluid Thioglycollate Medium, Dehydrated Difco Laboratories Detroit, Michigan	29.8 gm	14.9 gm
B. Distilled water	1000 ml	500 ml
2. Autoclave for 20 minutes, cool to 56°C		
3. Add, using aseptic technique:		
A. Fetal calf serum Cat. #614 Gibco Diagnostics Madison, Wisconsin	100 ml	50 ml
B. Aqueous suspension of procaine penicillin (200,000 units/2 ml) and dihydrostreptomycin sulfate (0.5 gm/2 ml)	4.5 ml	2.25 ml
4. Inactive medium and serum for 30 minutes at 56°C		
5. Add, aseptically, Fungizone (amphotericin B, 20 μg/ml)	2 ml	1 ml
6. Dispense 5 ml, aseptically, into sterile 17 × 100 mm clear plastic tubes with cap		
7. Incubate overnight so contaminating bacteria will be revealed by growth.		
8. Refrigerate until used. Do not store more than 30 days prior to use		

*For *T. foetus* culture.

The *T. foetus* sample, which has been placed into sterile saline, must be maintained at room temperature and must be permitted to settle for at least 1 hour. Centrifugation is contraindicated. For direct microscopic evaluation remove 1 or 2 drops of sediment with a sterile pipette and spread onto one-half of a microscopic slide. Do not coverslip. Examine this entire sample systematically at 100× in reduced light. Proper examination will take more than 10 minutes. Repeat. The entire remainder of the sedimented sample is then layered onto thioglycollate culture medium (Table 4 and Fig. 15*H*).[19] A drop from the bottom of a culture tube is examined for the presence of *T. foetus* after 24 to 48 hour and 72 to 96-hour incubation at 37°C. If present in culture, the protozoa will be numerous. This is in contrast to directly examined samples, which require a higher degree of diligence and technical competence in order to find and recognize *T. foetus*.

The morphological identifying features of *T. foetus* are its size (6 to 8 × 10 to 25 microns), its spindle or pear shape and its continual motility characterized by an undulating membrane. There are three anterior and one posterior flagella. The characteristic continual motility, size and spindle shape are recognizable under 100× magnification in reduced light. The details of the undulating membrane and number of flagella are best recognized in an organism showing reduced motility examined at 400×.

Leptospirosis. The definitive immunological test in cattle for identification of species-specific antibodies is the blood serum microscopic agglutination (MA) test.[19] This method ordinarily identifies specific antibodies at 8 days following infection. The highest titer is usually reached in 3 to 4 weeks and may remain high for several months before declining.

Since the hazard for venereal transmission exists largely from urine contamination of semen in shedder bulls, it is imperative that bulls with significant titers be further tested for the presence of leptospires in urine[19] or be monitored by additional MA testing for stabilization or regression of titer.

The incidence of various *Leptospira* species varies with locality. Generally *L. pomona, L. hardjo, L. grippotyphosa, L. canicola* and *L. icterohaemorrhagiae* are the species for which MA testing is indicated in the United States.

Infectious Bovine Rhinotracheitis/Infectious Pustular Vulvovaginitis/Infectious Pustular Balanoposthitis (IBR/IPV/IPB). Clinically, in bulls, the highly characteristic pustular ulcers of the preputial-penile membrane are pathognomonic. The virus, during the clinical course of IPB, is highly contagious and readily infects the vulva-vagina on contact in susceptible females.

As is characteristic for preputial herpes viral infections, a latent infection remains, presumably for life. Generally, thereafter, antibody titers are remarkably persistent. Substantial research evidence is accumulating that in spite of persistent infection, shedding of the virus in semen rarely occurs except under conditions of stress or as a result of repeated administration of corticosteroids. Under these conditions, recrudescence of the virus may occur without clinical signs of disease. Testing for presence of IPB virus in semen may be done with a tissue culture-serum neutralization method. Modified live virus vaccination via the nasal route at 4 to 6-month intervals apparently prevents all shedding of the virus from the genital tract of bulls.[20]

Johne's Disease (Paratuberculosis). In addition to its classic form, this has now been well established as a disease deserving of major concern among veterinarians examining bulls for genital health. *M. paratuberculosis* has been isolated from the genital organs, except the testes, and from semen of six of six bulls that showed clinical evidence of the disease.

Negative fecal culture along with a history of negative herd of origin for the disease are indicated prior to moving the bull into a new herd and into extensive service.

DIAGNOSIS AND PROGNOSIS

In undertaking the assignment of the examination of a bull for normalcy of reproductive function, the veterinarian assumes the responsibility for arriving at and communicating to his client in writing the diagnoses and prognoses for the various aspects of the examination. All determinations of unusual

risks in placing a bull in service and the options open to the client must be thoroughly explained.

The veterinarian must take an especially hard line on holding out of service those bulls with infectious genital diseases, pathological conformation traits and conditions that are known to be heritable in a predictable manner.

REFERENCES

1. Ball, L., Young, S. and Carroll, E. J.: Seminal vesiculitis syndrome: Lesions in genital organs of young bulls. J. Vet. Res., *29*:1173, 1968.
2. Bartlett, D. E., Larson, L. L., Parker, W. G. and Howard, T. H.: Specific pathogen free (SPF) frozen bovine semen: A goal? Proc. 6th Technical Conference on Artificial Insemination and Reproduction. National Association of Animal Breeders, Milwaukee, Wisconsin, Feb., 1976.
3. Becker, R. B., Wilcox, C. J. and Pritchard, W. R.: "Crampy" progressive posterior paralysis in mature cattle. Bulletin 639, University of Florida, Gainesville, Fla., 1966.
4. Bendixen, H. O. and Blom, E.: Undersogelser over Forkomsten of Brucellose hos tyre specielt med Henblik paa Betydningen vad den Kunstige Insemination. Maanedsskr, Dyrl., *59*:61, 1947.
5. Blom, E.: Segmental aplasia of the wolffian duct in the bull. Reprinted from: Scritti in onore di *Telesforo Bonadonna,* Milano, Apr., 1972.
6. Blom, E. and Christensen, N. O.: A systematic search for abnormalities in testis-epididymis in pedigree bulls in Denmark. Studies on pathological conditions in the testis, epididymis, and accessory sex glands in the bull. VII. Communications from The State Veterinary Serum Laboratory, Copenhagen, Denmark. 514 (Separatum) Royal Veterinary and Agricultural University, Yearbook, 1972, pp. 1–36.
7. Blom, E, and Christensen, N. O.: Studies on pathological conditions in the testis, epididymis and accessory sex glands in the bull. Skand. Vet., 1–45, 1947.
8. Carroll, E. J., Ball, L. and Scott, J. A.: Breeding soundness in bulls — A summary of 10,940 examinations. J.A.V.M.A., *142*:1105, 1963.
9. Clark, B. L., Duffy, J. H. and Monsborough, M. J.: A method for maintaining the viability of *Vibrio fetus* var. *venerealis* in samples of preputial secretions collected from carrier bulls. Aust. Vet. J., *48*:462, 1972.
10. Dawson, P. L. L.: The economic aspect of spastic paresis of the hind legs of Friesian cattle. Vet. Rec., *97*:432, 1975.
11. DeLey, G. and DeMoor, A.: Bovine spastic paralysis: Cerebrospinal fluid concentrations of homovanillic acid and 5-hydroxyindoleacetic acid in normal and spastic calves. Am. J. Vet. Res., *36*:227, 1975.
12. Faulkner, L. C., Hopwood, M. L., Masken, J. F., Kingman, H. E. and Stoddard, H. L.: Scrotal frostbite in bulls. J.A.V.M.A., *151*:602, 1967.
13. Foote, R. H., Larson, L. L. and Hahn, J.: Can fertility of sires used in artificial insemination be improved? AI Digest, *20*:6, 1972.

14. Formston, C. and Jones, E. W.: A spastic form of lameness in Friesian cattle. Vet. Rec., *68*:624, 1956.

15. Greenough, P. R., MacCallum, F. J. and Weaver, A. D.: Lameness in Cattle. Philadelphia and Toronto, J. B. Lippincott Co., 1972, pp. 132, 135, 426.

16. Jubb, K. V. F. and Kennedy, P. C.: Pathology of Domestic Animals. 2nd Ed. Vol. 1. New York and London, Academic Press, 1970, pp. 445, 450–452, 458, 460–463.

17. Larson, L. L. and Kitchell, R. L.: Neural mechanisms in sexual behavior. II. Gross neuroanatomical and correlative neurophysiological studies of the external genitalia of the bull and ram. Am. J. Vet. Res., *19*:853, 1958.

18. Larson, L. L., Bartlett., D. E. and Parker, W. G.: Disease incidence in bulls: I. When examined for use in A. I. II. In environment of a large stud. Proc. VII International Congress on Animal Reproduction and Artificial Insemination, June, 1972, pp. 1473–1478.

19. Lyle, W. E., Brown, L. N., Bryner, J. H., Hanson, L. E., Kirkbride, C. A. and Larson, A. B.: Recommended uniform diagnostic procedures qualifying bulls for the production of semen. Proc. 77th Annual Meeting, USAHA, Oct., 1973, pp. 455–473.

20. Schultz, R. D., Hall, C. E., Sheffy, B. E. and Bean, B. H.: Current status of IBR-IPV infection in bulls. Proc. 80th Annual Meeting, USAHA, Miami, Florida, Nov., 1976, pp. 159–168.

21. Smith, G. F. and Monroe, J. B.: The testing of bulls for *Brucella abortus* infection with some reference to A.I. stud experience. Report of the Production Division of Milk Marketing Board, 1956, p. 120.

22. Thomson, R. G.: Vertebral Body Osteophytes in Bulls. Supplement to Pathologia Veterinaria, *6*. New York, S. Karger, 1969, p. 18.

23. Wheat, J. D.: Cryptorchidism in hereford cattle. J. Heredity, *52*:244, 1961.

24. Willett, E. I. and Ohms, J. I.: Measurement of testicular size and its relation to production of spermatozoa by bulls. J. Dairy Sci., *40*: 1559, 1957.

Breeding Soundness Evaluation in Bulls

PETER JOHN CHENOWETH
Texas A&M University,
College Station, Texas

LESLIE BALL
Colorado State University, Fort Collins, Colorado

INTRODUCTION

Veterinarians often examine bulls for breeding soundness before purchase or use. This procedure is more commonly followed in the beef than in the dairy industry, although some dairy bulls are screened for use in artificial insemination (AI) organizations. Beef bulls may have lower overall reproductive capacity than dairy bulls. One AI organization rejected a significantly higher proportion of yearling beef than yearling dairy bulls because of inadequate reproductive capability. However, the selection criteria used by the AI industry are more stringent than those used routinely by practitioners in the field.

PURPOSE OF BREEDING SOUNDNESS EXAMINATION

A complete assessment of the bull's reproductive capacity should be attempted within the limitations imposed by cost, time and facilities. Ideally, it should include a detailed, systemic examination for general health and soundness, as well as for specific reproductive system disease, and an assessment of libido and mating ability.*

This article is concerned with examination for reproductive soundness, using the seminal evaluation system advocated by the Society for Theriogenology. Some special investigative procedures are also reviewed.

METHODS OF BREEDING SOUNDNESS EXAMINATION

Physical Examination of Bulls

The general health of a bull should be observed before applying more detailed tests. A breeding bull should be sound in all respects. Any factor that lowers the efficiency of a bull can affect reproductive performance. A history of diseases and problems should be obtained whenever possible because diseases that affect sperma-

---

*When practicable, a bull should be observed with one or more females in estrus to detect deficiencies in libido or mating ability. This procedure may reveal physical defects that are not detected by physical examination.

togenesis may affect seminal quality months after the original condition has subsided. Physical conditioning of the bull should be evaluated; bulls that are either too fat or too thin may have unsatisfactory reproductive performance.

Following the physical examination, the reproductive organs and semen should be examined thoroughly.

Seminal Collection and Evaluation

Semen may be collected from bulls by artificial vagina, electroejaculation or massage of the internal reproductive organs. Other methods are less effective.

Breeding soundness evaluations have traditionally included the assessment of spermatozoal motility, percentage of live spermatozoa, spermatozoal morphology, seminal pH and spermatozoal concentration. Recently, scrotal circumference has become part of the evaluation. In the field, the measurement of some of these criteria is less precise and dependable than desired. Also, some criteria for evaluating seminal quality are more highly correlated with fertility than are others. These latter criteria have been incorporated into a new scoring system advocated by the American Society for Theriogenology.

Spermatozoal Motility

Correlations between spermatozoal motility and fertility have been reported, but most of these come from AI centers that have optimal conditions for motility evaluation. Such conditions are not common in the field. Motility estimates can be adversely affected by environmental factors such as heat and cold, as well as by the osmolarity and chemical composition of diluents.

Motility can be evaluated in many ways; however, field methods must be kept simple. Evaluation of gross and individual motility are two methods commonly used by practitioners in the field. Photographic techniques and other methods that require excessive time or expensive equipment are unsatisfactory. Motility can be assigned a maximum value of 20 of a possible 100 points whether assessed grossly or individually (Table 1).

Gross Motility. Gross motility (mass activity) can be classified as very good, good, fair or poor (Table 1). A drop of fresh, undiluted semen is placed on a prewarmed slide protected from wind and cold. Hanging-drop preparations are probably most satisfactory but are more difficult to prepare. Observation is made using low-power microscopy. Both concentration and rate of individual motility affect visualization of gross motility. Concentrated semen with good motility appears more active than thin semen with similar motility. Such variations cause poor repeatability of gross motility estimations made under field conditions. Attempts to classify gross motility in thin seminal samples should be avoided; thin semen should be evaluated by rate of motility of individual spermatozoa.

Rate and Percentage of Individual Motility. Motility of individual spermatozoa can be evaluated in a diluted sample using high-power microscopy (Table 1). As with gross motility estimations, precautions should be taken to protect the semen from adverse environmental stresses. In addition, the diluent can have adverse effects on semen. For example, spermatozoa are inactivated after a short time in physiological saline; if such a diluent is used, the sample should be observed as soon as possible after mixing. Buffered egg yolk-citrate diluents are used in bull studs for this purpose, but their perishable nature generally prevents their usage in the field. Buffered 2.9 per cent sodium citrate solutions are satisfactory but are also subject to bacterial degradation. Thus, it is important to use freshly prepared diluent and to read the motility as soon as possible after mixing the semen with it.

A drop of diluent is placed on a prewarmed (38° C) slide, and a small amount of semen is added to and mixed with it. Some skill is required to estimate the proper amount of semen to place with the diluent. Either too much or too little semen makes the sample difficult to evaluate.

A coverslip is placed over the mixture, and the rate of individual spermatozoal motility is estimated (Table 1). It is important to evaluate only spermatozoa that are progressively motile. When motility is poor and other seminal quality criteria are normal, urine contamination or poor handling techniques should be suspected.

TABLE 1. *Scoring System for Seminal Characteristics and Scrotal Circumference of Bulls*

Factors Evaluated	Classification			
	VERY GOOD	GOOD	FAIR	POOR
Spermatozoal motility:				
Individual	Rapid linear	Moderate linear	Slow linear to erratic	Very slow to erratic
Gross	Vigorous swirls	Slow swirls	No swirls (generalized oscillation)	Laborious movement (sporadic oscillation)
Score	20	12	10	3
Spermatozoal morphology:				
Primary abnormalities (%)	<10	10–19	20–29	>29
Total abnormalities (%)	<25	26–39	40–59	>59
Score	40	25	10	3
*Scrotal circumference:**				
Age in months:				
12–14	>34	30–34	<30	<30
15–20	>36	31–36	<31	<31
21–30	>38	32–38	<32	<32
Over 31	>39	34–39	<34	<34
Score	40	24	10	10

*Refers to Tables 2 and 3.

Percentage of Live Spermatozoa (Live-Dead Ratio)

The percentage of live spermatozoa can be estimated by determining the percentage of motile spermatozoa in a coverslip preparation (see previous discussion) or by counting the percentage of spermatozoa that are not stained by a supravital (live-dead) stain. This estimation, employing either technique, has low repeatability and little relationship to fertility when performed under field conditions. Consequently, it is not used in the new scoring system.

Spermatozoal Morphology

Excessive numbers of abnormal spermatozoa have been correlated with lowered fertility in most species. Morphological counts are obtained by staining smears of spermatozoa with appropriate stains. For field usage, supravital stains such as Blom's or Hancock's (both employing nigrosin and eosin) or fine suspensions of India ink are effective. Methods for preparation and use of such stains have been described in the literature. The most common method involves counting and classifying 100 or more spermatozoa in several fields, employing oil immersion microscopy (approximately 1000× magnification).

Classification Systems for Spermatozoal Morphology

A relatively simple classification system for spermatozoal morphology has been used in which spermatozoa are classified as normal or as having primary or secondary abnormalities. Primary abnormalities (abnormal head and midpiece shapes, abaxial attachment of midpieces and tightly coiled tails) are considered to be caused by faulty spermatogenesis. Secondary abnormalities (separated heads, distal droplets and bent tails) are considered to result from malfunction of the excurrent duct system. However, in reality the pathogenesis of these abnormalities is not so clear-cut. Albeit, this system is simple to apply and has proved useful in the rapid field assessment of semen. Another method is classification of spermatozoa into major and minor categories. Major defects are those with proven association with infertility; minor defects have not been positively correlated with infertility. Some abnormalities encountered in bull semen are shown in Figures 1 and 2.

The numbers of primary spermatozoal abnormalities remain more constant in repeated ejaculates than the numbers of secondary abnormalities and in general are considered to be more serious. If primary abnormalities exceed 18 to 20 per cent of the spermatozoal population, reduction of fertility may occur. Spermatozoal morphology can be assigned a maximum value of 40 points of a possible 100 points of the total score in the new scoring system (Table 1).

Seminal pH

Semen collected from bulls or rams by electroejaculation has a higher and more variable pH than that collected by artificial vagina. The pH is also increased in urine-contaminated semen, which usually shows decreased motility. When an otherwise satisfactory seminal sample has poor spermatozoal motility, appropriate pH paper might be used to test for urine contamination. Otherwise, pH is not an important factor in the evaluation of semen in the field and is not part of the new scoring system.

Spermatozoal Concentration

Assessment of concentration of spermatozoa is important in AI studs. However, this criterion has poor correlation with the fertility of bulls whose semen is collected sporadically, as is done under field conditions. Furthermore, electroejaculation increases variability in spermatozoal concentration. Consequently, field estimations of spermatozoal concentration are of little value in assessing the reproductive capability of bulls. This assessment is not included in the new scoring system.

Scrotal Circumference

Scrotal circumference, testicular size and seminal production are highly correlated, especially in bulls less than 3 years of age.

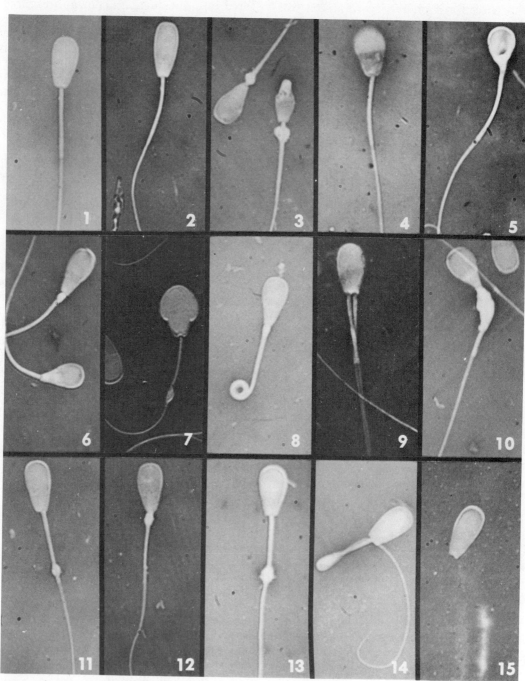

Figure 1. Bovine spermatozoal abnormalities (phase contrast microscopy): (*1* and *2*) Normal bovine spermatozoa; (*3*) proximal droplets, head defects; (*4*) large head; (*5*) round head; (*6*) pyriform head, proximal droplets; (*7*) head defect, distal droplet; (*8*) coiled tail; (*9*) double midpiece; (*10*) swollen midpiece, pyriform head; (*11*) abaxial midpiece, distal droplet; (*12*) proximal droplet; (*13*) distal droplet; (*14*) simple bent tail with distal droplet and (*15*) separated head.

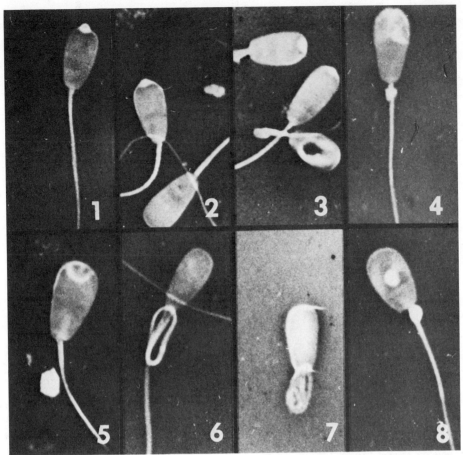

Figure 2. Bovine spermatozoal abnormalities (phase contrast microscopy): (*1* and *2*) *Knobbed acrosomes;* (*3*) knobbed acrosomes, midpiece defect; (*4*) ruffled acrosome, proximal droplet; (*5*) folded acrosome; (*6*) double bent tail (bent midpiece); (*7*) coiled midpiece and tail and (*8*) proximal droplet (dense spot on sperm head is probably an artifact).

Thus, measurement of scrotal circumference can give a relatively accurate estimation of a young bull's ability to produce spermatozoa. Scrotal circumference is probably also the best measurement for evaluating the spermatogenic capability of 4- to 5-year-old bulls, although the correlations are not as high as in younger bulls. Scrotal circumference measurements are not useful in old bulls because senile changes may decrease the amount of seminiferous epithelium without decreasing testicular size. Testicular size is moderately heritable in bulls; selection for this trait should increase semen production in bull populations. Scrotal circumference measurements are highly repeatable whether taken by the same or different technicians.

Methodology

To measure scrotal circumference, the testicles are first retracted into the lower part of the scrotum (Fig. 3). Special care should be taken, particularly in cold weather, to pull the testicles down far enough into the scrotum to eliminate scrotal wrinkles, otherwise, measurements are inaccurate. The thumb and fingers should be placed on the sides rather than on the front and back of the scrotum so that separation of the testicles does not occur (Fig. 3). The scrotal tape is looped and slipped over the scrotum and testicles and contracted snugly around their greatest diameter for the measurement.

Testicular Growth Patterns

Testicular growth is fairly rapid in Holstein bulls until they are 4 years of age, when it becomes much slower. However, testicular size is more highly correlated with bull weight than with age. Similar testicular growth patterns probably occur in beef breeds. The testes of bulls of some

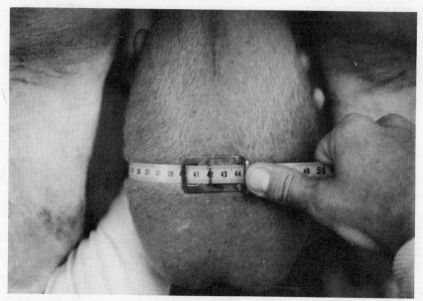

Figure 3. Correct method for measurement of scrotal circumference.

beef breeds grow more slowly than others. Thus, breed differences should be taken into consideration in evaluating scrotal circumference measurements. The standards used in the new scoring system (see Table 1) were developed mostly with information obtained from performance-tested Angus, Hereford and Charolais bulls. Bulls of *Bos indicus* breeding generally mature slowly (Table 2), so these standards are invalid for them. Consideration should also be given to slower maturing *Bos taurus* breeds and to the body condition and weight of the bull.

Preliminary data are presented comparing scrotal circumference measurements of bulls of various ages (Tables 2 and 4) and weights (Table 3).

Young bulls with relatively small testicles also have relatively small testicles when they are mature. Thus, an accurate prognosis of potential spermatozoal production could probably be established for most bulls when they are young. Most yearling beef bulls of *Bos taurus* breeding should have a scrotal circumference of at least 30 cm. However, more work is needed to establish standards for the different breeds under different environmental conditions. Scrotal circumference measurements are converted to a score that may be assigned a maximum of 40 points of a possible 100 points in the new scoring system.

Semen Scoring Systems

The objective of a semen scoring system is to standardize semen quality evaluations. The new system recommended by the Society for Theriogenology is based on spermatozoal morphology, relative scrotal circumference and spermatozoal motility (see Table 1). Each criterion is evaluated and given a numerical score. These scores are then combined. A bull with a score of 60 or more should generally be classified as satisfactory, 30 to 59 as questionable and less than 30 as unsatisfactory when applying this system. Some flexibility is necessary for bulls that are either very young or convalescing. Many old bulls with marginal semen quality should be culled because of senescence. This scoring system applies to seminal quality criteria only. Additional tests are necessary to evaluate the physical capability and libido of a bull.

Special Tests

Cytogenetic Evaluation*

Cytogenetic investigations have not often been a part of the breeding soundness examination. However, techniques for cytogenetic evaluation have been well de-

*Written by Richard A. Bowen.

TABLE 2. Average Scrotal Circumference (SC) of Different Breeds of Beef Bulls Compared by Age

Age in Months	SC and No.	Angus*	Charolais*	Horned Hereford*	Polled Hereford*	Simmental*	Limousin*	Santa Gertrudis*	Average	Brahman†
<14	SC	34.8	32.6	33.0	34.8	33.4	30.6	34.0	33.1	21.9
	No.	(125)	(240)	(244)	(15)	(65)	(68)	(71)	(828)	(73)
14 < x < 17	SC	35.9	35.4	32.2	34.2	36.5	31.7	35.3	35.0	27.4
	No.	(73)	(294)	(44)	(75)	(9)	(13)	(27)	(535)	(34)
17 < x < 20	SC	36.6	34.5	34.1	34.9	—	32.0	35.5	35.3	29.4
	No.	(271)	(226)	(62)	(181)		(3)	(72)	(815)	(260)
20 < x < 23	SC	36.9	34.9	36.2	34.9	—	33.9	36.7	36.0	31.4
	No.	(125)	(66)	(9)	(71)		(5)	(63)	(339)	(16)
23 < x < 26	SC	36.7	34.6	33.4	34.8	36.0	—	36.5	35.4	31.7
	No.	(161)	(55)	(79)	(57)	(2)		(40)	(394)	(21)
26 < x < 30	SC	36.3	36.2	33.8	35.0	—	—	36.4	35.6	33.5
	No.	(9)	(19)	(10)	(15)			(15)	(68)	(2)
30 < x < 36	SC	36.6	37.11	35.2	35.6	—	—	38.3	36.0	34.7
	No.	(55)	(15)	(85)	(12)			(12)	(179)	(9)
36 plus	SC	38.2	38.1	34.0	36.4	37.2	35.5	40.5	36.4	36.7
	No.	(68)	(29)	(87)	(20)	(4)	(4)	(12)	(224)	(22)

*Data from Colorado State University and University of Missouri.
†Data from Texas A & M University.

TABLE 3. *Average Scrotal Circumference (SC) Measurements of Different Breeds of Beef Bulls Compared by Weight**

Weight in Pounds	SC and No.	Angus	Charolais	Horned Hereford	Polled Hereford	Simmental	Limousin	Average
400 < × < 900	SC No.	35.2 (5)	30.4 (26)	30.8 (38)	30.9 (9)	33.5 (7)	29.2 (32)	30.6 (117)
900 < × < 1000	SC No.	33.1 (10)	30.8 (22)	32.9 (41)	32.9 (7)	32.1 (24)	32.4 (14)	32.3 (118)
1000 < × < 1100	SC No.	36.4 (37)	31.8 (65)	34.3 (28)	34.6 (13)	33.9 (25)	30.1 (4)	33.7 (172)
1100 < × < 1200	SC No.	36.8 (75)	32.9 (85)	35.4 (12)	34.1 (56)	36.2 (7)	33.0 (2)	34.6 (237)
1200 < × < 1300	SC No.	37.3 (122)	33.8 (106)	35.6 (22)	35.2 (108)	– 	– 	35.5 (358)
1300 < × < 1400	SC No.	37.5 (77)	35.2 (64)	36.2 (13)	35.4 (89)	38.1 (4)	– 	36.1 (247)
1400 < × < 1500	SC No.	37.6 (30)	35.6 (43)	36.7 (5)	35.7 (21)	– 	– 	36.3 (99)
1500 < × < 3000	SC No.	40.0 (8)	37.7 (39)	– 	36.8 (9)	– 	– 	37.9 (56)

*Data from Colorado State University and University of Missouri.

fined, and there is evidence that cytogenetic abnormalities are associated with infertility in cattle. Use of this technique is limited in the field because sophisticated equipment and extensive training are required.

Some cytogenetic abnormalities cause problems in the carrier; others in the offspring. Robertsonian translocations are found in several breeds of cattle and are

Table 4. *Age and Scrotal Circumference – Dairy Breeds*

Breed	Number	Average Age (mo)	Average Scrotal Circumference
Mixed dairy*	8	13.4	31.7
Holstein†	59	15.5 (13–18)	34.9
	54	21.5	37.1
	52	27.5	38.7
	54	33.5	39.3
	208	Mature	42.0
Mixed dairy*	267	Mature	41.0
Jersey*	41	Mature	38.5

*Adapted from Willett and Ohms: J. Dairy Sci. *40:* 1559, 1957. The data presented above were modified from the footnoted citations.

†Adapted from Hahn *et al.;* J. Anim. Sci., *29:*41, 1969.

thought to be associated with infertility. However, their occurrence and significance in the cattle population are unknown. Chromosomal abnormalities have also been associated with testicular hypoplasia in bulls.

Practitioners should be aware that cytogenetic evaluation is available for bulls. Cytogenetic evaluation should be used for valuable bulls, especially those going to artificial insemination centers. Unnecessary effort and expense would be avoided by bull studs if bulls with cytogenetic defects could be identified before purchase. Cytogenetic tests would decrease dissemination of defects to progeny. Aside from demonstrating cytogenetic defects in potential breeding bulls, screening programs could increase fundamental knowledge of bovine cytogenetics and provide a sounder foundation for genetic consultation.

Immunological Factors*

The immune system developed phylogenetically to provide protection against invasion by foreign pathogens. However, the

---

*Written by Thomas J. Reimers.

immune system can turn against its host and cause destruction of its own tissues. This phenomenon is generally referred to as autoimmunity. In recent years, the possible relationship between autoimmunity and reproductive problems has stimulated interest among many scientists.

Reduced fertility caused by immunological factors has been described in man and domestic animals and induced experimentally in laboratory animals. The male has been most extensively studied. However, the extent to which testicular function is adversely affected by the immune system under natural conditions is unknown.

There are two components of the male reproductive tract that are capable of eliciting an autoimmune reaction. The first component includes antigens of the testes, epididymides and spermatozoa. The second includes the accessory sex glands and fluids. Semen contains both antigenic components.

Autoallergic aspermatogenesis can be induced experimentally and is characterized by progressive loss of germinal epithelium. Shedding of spermatozoa, spermatids and spermatocytes in areas of the seminiferous tubules occurs in mild reactions. In severe cases, all germinal cells may be lost.

Several naturally occurring immune-like reactions similar to the experimentally induced conditions have been observed. Epididymitis, scrotal trauma and vasectomy often incite an autoimmune sensitization caused by release of antigens from the reproductive tract. Traumatic injury to one testis can result in damage, apparently of an immune origin, in the contralateral testis.

There has been much interest in autoimmunity as a possible source of infertility in humans. Although much work remains to be done, tests can now be applied to detect which bulls possess antibodies to their own spermatozoa.*

REFERENCES

1. Carroll, E. J.: Reproductive soundness in beef bulls. Bovine Pract., Nov., 1971, p. 20.
2. Carroll, E. J., Ball, L. and Scott, J. A.: Breeding soundness in bulls — A summary of 10,940 examinations. J.A.V.M.A., *142*:1105, 1963.
3. Blom, E.: The ultrastructure of some characteristic sperm defects and a proposal for a new classification of the bull spermiogram. Atti. del VII. Simposio Inter. die Zootechia, 1972, p. 125.
4. Elmore, R. G., Bierschwal, C. J. and Youngquist, R. S.: Scrotal circumference measurements in 764 beef bulls. Theriogenology, *6*:485, 1976.
5. Hackett, A. J. and Macpherson, J. W.: Some staining procedures for spermatozoa. A review. Can. Vet. J., *6*:66, 1965.
6. Hahn, J., Foote, R. H. and Seidel, G. E., Jr.: Testicular growth and related sperm output in dairy bulls. J. Anim. Sci., *29*:41, 1969.
7. Harasymowycz, J., Ball, L. and Seidel, G. E., Jr.: Evaluation of bovine spermatozoal morphologic features after staining or fixation. Am. J. Vet. Res., *37*:1053, 1976.
8. Society for Theriogenology: A compilation of current information on breeding soundness evaluation and related subjects. Journal Vol. VII, 2nd Ed., 1976.
9. Wiltbank, J. N., Rowden, W. W. and Ingalls, J. E.: Relationship between measures of semen quality and fertility in bulls mated under natural conditions. Univ. of Nebraska Res. Bull. 224, 1965.

*We would like to thank Larry Johnson for his technical and photographic assistance with this article.

Puberty in the Bull

EDWARD C. MATHER
Michigan State University,
East Lansing, Michigan

INTRODUCTION

Puberty has been described as that time when the bull's sexual organs are functionally developed, sexual instincts are prominent and reproduction is possible. By this definition, most bulls have reached puberty and are capable of paternity at somewhat less than 1 year of age. It must be kept in mind that at this time the bull's full reproductive capacity has not been established and that sexual maturity will continue.

The young bull has received increased attention by the cattle industry in recent years. In most cases, this is a result of the desire to have good young bulls put into maximum production as early as possible. Evaluation of the young (puberal) bull has been encouraged by progeny testing programs and by the increased number of breeding soundness examinations being performed on young bulls used for pasture breeding programs.

Because of this increased attention being given the young bull, it is useful to recognize the complexity involved in sexual maturity. One needs to know that the attainment of sexual maturity includes much more than the ejaculation of the first mature, motile sperm cell.

An evaluation of breeding soundness, as described in other articles in this section, must therefore be conducted with a knowledge of what factual determinations can be made at a particular age, what predictions might be made and what the limitations are of the evaluation. The judgments that one must make in declaring that a bull is sound not only require a knowledge of disease but of age, characteristics of the breed, nutrition, environment and the methods used to make the evaluations.

CHANGES ASSOCIATED WITH PUBERTY

Behavioral and Endocrine Changes

It is the opinion of most authors that sexual desire or libido is genetically determined but can be modified by various environmental factors. It is extremely difficult to evaluate libido and mounting ability in the Indian breeds (Bos indicus) since these breeds copulate rapidly and usually do so at night. European dairy breeds represent the other end of the spectrum, typified by aggressive, uninhibited exhibition of libido. Comparatively, the European beef breeds exhibit an intermediate behavior. Even with the difficulty of comparing libido between breeds, it appears that there is a difference in onset of behavioral activity and that early onset is positively correlated with the more sexually aggressive breeds. Also, great variation occurs in the onset of sexual desire among bulls within breeds.

It has been shown that variation in the rearing of bulls has a significant effect on the onset of sexual behavior. Bulls raised with other bulls or heifers develop sexual instincts at an earlier age than bulls raised in separate quarters.

Studies on pituitary follicle-stimulating hormone (FSH), hypothalamic luteinizing-releasing hormone (LRH) and plasma luteinizing hormone (LH) production indicate that the onset of puberty commences at 2 months and should be qualitatively completed by 10 months in Holstein bulls. As a result of these studies and others, it appears that production of testicular androgens may trigger and coincide with a biphasic pattern of testicular development that begins with an accelerated growth period from 2 to 4 months and another at 6 to 9 months. The second period of pubertal development is typified by the external physical and sexual manifestations of puberty and the onset of spermatogenesis.

Anatomical Changes

The size of the testicles increases most rapidly between 16 and 32 weeks of age, after which testicular growth continues but at a slower rate and is correlated more with body weight. The establishment of spermatogenesis is a long and progressive process with several identifiable stages. Gonocytes are found in the center of the sex cords in the newborn bull calf. They divide by mitosis and give rise to spermatogonia at about 8 weeks of age. The prepuberal period is marked by the differentiation of spermatogonia. With the onset of puberty, the differentiated cells undergo maturation and the first cells are released. Following puberty, there is an increase in spermatogenic yield as the testes continue to grow. Quantitative development of the seminiferous tubules and spermatogenic process is a gradual process, with not all tubules developing simultaneously. In English breeds, seminiferous tubule development is completed only qualitatively by 10 to 11 months. Sperm production continues to increase to maturity. Conversely, the interstitial tissue is present at birth, and its functional activity can be measured by serum androgen determinations and by development of the accessory sexual glands. Little additional quantitative development of the interstitial tissue occurs after puberty.

It is often difficult to clinically differentiate between partial testicular hypoplasia and delayed testicular development since both processes might exhibit abnormal semen characteristics such as increased head abnormalities and protoplasmic droplets and decreased motility and sperm numbers. Repeated physical and semen examinations, an evaluation of management procedures and environment and a thorough knowledge of breed differences are necessary before a sound judgment can be made. Differentiation between the two conditions is useful since it has been shown that although both delayed testicular development and testicular hypoplasia may be genetically influenced, delayed testicular development may also result from faulty nutrition and management.

It has been shown that sperm can be stored for a long time in the cauda epididymidis without losing their fertilizing ability, but one often overlooks other equally important functions of the epididymal duct. As the sperm pass through the epididymal duct, they undergo both a morphological and a physiological maturation process. Not until they have passed through the majority of the epididymal duct and reached the cauda epididymidis have the sperm reached full functional ability.

In a normal bull, the epididymis will have undergone development and attained maturity in ample time to receive spermatozoa from the testis. It appears very probable that delayed development of the epididymis may result in increased morphologically defective sperm in the ejaculate. The most commonly recognized defect would involve the increased presence of protoplasmic droplets. It is also possible, however, that cells that have not undergone proper development within the testis may not complete their maturation in the epididymal duct, even though the duct developed normally. The semen picture may then mistakenly appear to be associated with a defect in epididymal development.

Secretions from the vesicular glands (seminal vesicles) are recovered by 6 months of age. The glands are responsive to circulating androgens and continue to grow through puberty and until a bull is 4 to 6 years of age. They also continue to become more lobulated and their secretion more voluminous. Removal of the glands in the bull reduces semen volume but does not appear to reduce sperm number or fertilizing ability. Since seminal vesiculitis is a common disease entity, one should be aware of the normal size of the glands in reference to the age of the bull.

The penis of the newborn bull calf is without a sigmoid flexure and is completely adhered to the prepuce. The sigmoid flexure begins to develop at about 12 weeks and becomes more pronounced with age. The penis increases in length by 2 to 5 times by the onset of puberty and continues to increase in length following puberty. Congenitally, development of a short penis is sometimes observed and should be considered a serious fault. Separation of the penis and prepuce starts at 4 weeks and is usually completed by 32 weeks. Penile separation can be retarded by low levels of nutrition and can be accelerated by androgen administration. Since separation of the penis and prepuce is influenced by circulating androgens, early castration will often arrest the process. A persistent penile frenulum, which is a failure in the separation process, is not unusual in young breeding-age bulls, but the relationship of this condition to hormonal deficiencies has never been clarified.

Much has been written about the correlation of scrotal size to testicular production. It has been shown that there is good correlation between body weight and testicular size; however, whether age may be the more important factor to correlate with testicular production (since age and body weight correlate very well) has not yet been determined.

It has been shown that scrotal circumference, spermatogenesis and steroidal activity are higher in bulls maintained on high-energy diets, compared with low-energy diets, from 3 to 8 months of age. In actuality, instead of the high-energy diets promoting testicular development, the low-energy diets may have reduced such development. On the other hand, many producers are of the impression that "over-fitting" of bulls at the time of puberal development may jeopardize their future breeding capabilities.

It has also been shown that frequent (6 times per week) ejaculation of bulls from puberty to 2 years of age is not deleterious to semen traits, weekly sperm output or testis growth and that the frequent ejaculation yielded 3.3 times more motile sperm per week than ejaculation that occurred once weekly. The same workers have shown that 83 per cent of the ejaculates from Holstein bulls were acceptable for freezing by 13 to 24 weeks after puberty, or at about 15 months of age. A slightly smaller percentage of beef bulls produced ejaculates acceptable for freezing at this age. Since there is great variation among bulls within breeds, it should be remembered that sufficient insemination units can be obtained from many bulls at a much younger age.

REFERENCES

1. Abdel-Raouf, M.: The postnatal development of the reproductive organs in bulls with special reference to puberty. Copenh. Acta Endocrinol. (Suppl.), *49*:9, 1960.
2. Abdel-Raouf, M.: Sexual behaviour and semen picture of bulls of the Swedish Red and White breed between the ages of 9 and 15 months. Nord. Vet. Med., *17*:318, 1965.
3. Almquist, J. O. and Amann, R. D.: Reproductive capacity of dairy bulls. XI. Puberal characteristics of postpuberal changes in production of semen and sexual activity of Holstein bulls ejaculated frequently. J. Dairy Sci., *59*:986, 1976.
4. Ashdown, R. R.: Adherence between penis and sheath in beef calves at the time of castration. J. Agr. Sci., *58*:71, 1962.
5. Coulter, G. H., Larson, L. L. and Foote, R. H.: Effect of age on testicular growth and consistency of Holstein and Angus bulls. J. Anim. Sci., *41*:1383, 1975.
6. Gustafsson, B.: Luminal contents of the bovine epididymis under conditions of reduced spermatogenesis, luminal blockage and certain sperm abnormalities. Acta Vet. Scand. (Suppl.), *17*:1, 1966.
7. Humphrey, J. D. and Ladds, P. W.: Quantitative histological studies of changes in the bovine testis and epididymis associated with age. Res. Vet. Sci., *19*:135, 1975.
8. MacMillan, K. L. and Hafs, H. D.: Pituitary and hypothalamic endocrine changes associated with reproductive development of Holstein bulls. J. Anim. Sci., *27*:1614, 1968.

Libido and Mating Ability in Bulls

PETER JOHN CHENOWETH

Texas A&M University,
College Station, Texas

INTRODUCTION

Beef bulls are often exposed to a breeding soundness examination (BSE) prior to their use in natural mating programs. This examination has traditionally emphasized a physical examination of the genital system as well as examination of a seminal sample. The procedures recommended for this examination are described on page 330. Assessment of libido and mating ability is usually not undertaken despite recommendations that it should be considered. It was shown by Blockey[2] that failure to incorporate a testing procedure such as his serving capacity test could result in numbers of substandard bulls passing the BSE.

Information is lacking on breed differences in the mating behavior of bulls, particularly in relation to natural breeding. There is evidence that beef bulls in artificial insemination centers require different stimulus patterns for optimal sperm harvest than do dairy bulls and may have more prolonged reaction times than the latter group. Breed differences in mating behavior among bulls of European breeds have been reported, and references have been made to a "sexual sluggishness" in Zebu bulls. The overriding influence of genetic factors on the expression of libido and mating ability of bulls have been well documented.[1]

There does not appear to be a significant relationship between sex drive and seminal characteristics in bulls; therefore, it would be possible for bulls of low libido to have good seminal quality and vice versa.

TESTING PROCEDURES

The simplest way to determine if a bull has adequate libido is to observe him in a restricted area with one or more females that are in heat. This can also help detect disabilities that prevent him from mating properly. It may be useful to spend some time observing the bull in the breeding pasture, although most workers consider that sporadic observations of this nature are usually not very helpful. These types of observations will not give results that can be used to assess a bull quantitatively, nor will they provide a controlled basis for comparisons between bulls.

Quantitative and comparative studies of libido and mating ability in range beef bulls have been hampered by the lack of a simple, repeatable testing method. A technique for assessing libido and mating ability in artificial insemination (AI) bulls was developed in Sweden in the 1950's. These workers employed a nonestrous cow restrained in a service bail as the stimulus object. Three attempts were made to collect semen with an artificial vagina over a 10-minute period. The reaction of the bull to the cow, his approach to service and his behavior in completing service into the artificial vagina were scored. Libido was treated quantitatively. This scheme was modified for use with young, untrained beef bulls in Australia.[4] Here, a 5-minute test was employed in which individual bulls were each exposed to a female in a small, easily observed pen. Further modification[3] resulted in the use of ovariectomized heifers in which estrus had been induced and an expanded scoring system utilizing 11 categories for libido and four for mating ability. The procedures employed for this test were as follows:

The examination for libido and mating ability was conducted in a small yard (approximately 200 to 300 square meters) suitable for easy surveillance. Bulls were admitted individually and were allowed exactly 5 minutes with a prepared heifer. The criterion for selection of a heifer was that she would stand while other heifers mounted her. All reactions and movements of the bull during the test were recorded on magnetic tape. When this was replayed, libido was scored as follows:

0 = Bull showed no sexual interest.

1 = Sexual interest showed only once (e.g., sniffs at perineal region).

2 = Positive sexual interest in female on more than one occasion.

3 = Active pursuit of female with persistent sexual interest.

4 = One mount or mounting attempt. No service.

5 = Two mounts, or mounting attempts. No service.

6 = More than two mounts or mounting attempts. No service.

7 = One service followed by no further sexual interest.

8 = One service followed by sexual interest, including mounts or mounting attempts.

9 = Two services followed by no further sexual interest.

10 = Two services followed by sexual interest, including mounts, mounting attempts or further services.

Each bull was tested twice on separate days, and the poorer result of the two was discarded.

Separate categories were used to describe mating ability as follows:

Groups 1 = Bulls that served satisfactorily.

Group 2 = Bulls that made mounting attempts that did not culminate in service. This was due to inexperience, faulty mating technique or pathological factors.

Group 3 = Bulls that mounted but did not achieve service because of lack of cooperation by the female. This often reflected factors such as lack of confidence by the bull or low libido.

Group 4 = Bulls for which there was no record of mating ability because of lack of sufficient activity for an assessment to be made.

This testing procedure proved of value with young bulls, particularly those of *Bos indicus* derivation, as it enabled a score to be given that was not dependent upon service. When 56 2-year-old bulls were assessed by this system prior to their use in controlled mating trials, the correlation between the libido score and pregnancy rate was $r = 0.32$, whereas the correlation between their semen score and pregnancy rate was $r = 0.13$ (unpublished data). This showed that the libido score, in these bulls, was considerably more effective in predicting pregnancy rate than was the quantitative assessment of seminal quality. However, a disadvantage for routine use of this procedure in beef herd bulls was that considerable time and effort were necessary to prepare the heifers.

A serving capacity test for beef bulls was developed recently that seems to avoid this problem.[2] The procedure for this test follows:

1. Nonestrous cows were placed in service crates.

2. Bulls were sexually stimulated prior to their exposure to the test by allowing them to watch other bulls mount the restrained cows for 10 or more minutes.

3. Bulls were admitted to the yard containing the restrained cows at the bull-to-female ratio of 5:2 or 5:3.

4. The duration of the yard test was 40 minutes.

5. The number of services performed by each bull during that period was recorded as his serving capacity score.

This test was applied to 75 bulls (aged 2 to 5 years) that were then mated in groups with heifers at a bull-to-female ratio of 1:5. The heifers had been ovariectomized and induced to show estrus. It was found that the serving capacity scores of groups of bulls were highly correlated with their performance under simulated pasture mating conditions.

Recent trials at the San Juan Basin Experiment Station, Hesperus, Colorado, compared both the libido score and serving capacity tests on yearling bulls. The overall repeatability of both, when used as recommended, was similar. However, a large number of bulls did not complete a service in the 30-minute serving capacity tests, and thus relative information about their sexual behavior was lacking. It was concluded, at least with yearling bulls, that a more descriptive assessment system that was not dependent on service (such as the libido score) would provide more information on individual bulls. Some features of the serving capacity test such as prestimulation of the bulls and the use of nonestrous females restrained in service crates were considered to constitute valuable improvements that should be retained in the testing procedure.

Other studies with these same bulls showed that a single measurement of testosterone or luteinizing hormone concentration in the peripheral blood had little relationship to the libido score or serving capacity score. Also, measurements of scrotal circumference and seminal quality were not significantly related to libido or serving capacity, confirming previous findings.[2] This illustrates the importance of assessing all of these factors for best bull selection and usage.

CONCLUSION

Practitioners should be aware that bulls vary considerably in libido and mating ability and that the major influence on these factors in young bulls is genetic.

Libido and mating ability assessment can contribute to fertility prognosis in younger beef bulls destined for natural service. Although not a practical proposition for all

bulls undergoing routine examination for breeding soundness, certain groups of bulls, such as young bulls coming off feeding trials and sale bulls of registered breeders, should be considered for such an assessment.

Several procedures for evaluating sex drive in bulls are described. These procedures all have advantages and disadvantages. They do provide a means of quantitating sex drive so that comparisons can be made between bulls. If a quantitative assessment is not necessary, it is of value to observe the actions of a bull placed in a restricted area with one or more estrous females. Most bulls should attempt a service within 5 to 10 minutes unless the female is nonreceptive or the bull's attention is diverted. Old bulls may have slower patterns of excitation. One advantage of pre-exposing young bulls to receptive females in a controlled situation is that it can give them greater breeding confidence and competence when they are initiated into the breeding pasture.

Libido tests in bulls have applications apart from fertility prognosis. Accurate assessment of the sex drive of bulls could be of value in studies investigating hormonal and environmental influences on this trait. Evaluations of the results of fertility and estrous detection trials should include such an assessment of the entire or teaser bulls employed. The use of high-libido bulls in mating programs with selected groups of "problem" females, such as first calf heifers, could markedly increase the latter's conception rate at first estrus.

REFERENCES

1. Bane, A.: Sexual functions of bulls in relation to heredity, rearing intensity and somatic conditions. Acta Agric. Scand., *4*:95, 1954.
2. Blockey, M. A. de B.: Studies on the social and sexual behaviour of bulls. Ph.D. thesis, University of Melbourne, Victoria, 1975.
3. Chenoweth, P. J.: Consideration of Behavioural Aspects of the Natural Breeding Bull. Proceedings Annual Meeting of Society for Theriogenology, Lexington, Kentucky, 1976.
4. Osborne, H. G., Williams, L. G. and Galloway, D. B.: A Test for libido and serving ability in beef bulls. Austral. Vet. J., *47*:465, 1971.

Semen Collection by Electroejaculation and Massage of the Pelvic Organs

LESLIE BALL

Colorado State University, Fort Collins, Colorado

Ejaculation is a two-phase process. First, semen is expelled from the ampullae and vasa deferentia into the urethra (emission phase). Second, it is propelled through the urethra by forceful contractions of the urethral muscles (ejaculatory phase). The nerves associated with both processes have different origins and locations in the pelvic cavity. The emission process is controlled by lumbar sympathetic (hypogastric) nerves. These terminate in the region of the ampullae and seminal vesicles in the bull and when stimulated alone cause emission of semen into the pelvic urethra and subsidence of erection. The nerves causing erection and ejaculation ramify more posteriorly in the region of the pelvic urethra and originate from the sacral plexus (pelvic splanchnic nerve and internal pudendal nerve).

ELECTROEJACULATION

Some problems in electroejaculation are related to the location of the emission and ejaculation nerves. Many other nerves are located nearby. For example, the sciatic and obturator nerves innervate the heavy muscles of the thighs and legs. These motor nerves are often stimulated at the same time as the nerves causing emission, erection and ejaculation. Smaller electrodes, such as finger- or hand-held electrodes, effectively decrease the amount of stimulation of these adjacent nerves. However, such electrodes are too small to stimulate both the emission and ejaculation nerves simultaneously. Therefore, the electrodes must be moved back and forth between the nerves as stimuli are applied. The operator of the electrodes is also unable to observe the penis since he must stand behind the bull.

Stimulation of nerves other than those associated with penile erection and seminal emission and ejaculation can be decreased by covering two electrodes of four-electrode probes with electrical tape or, more effectively, by using probes that have three ventral longitudinally oriented electrodes. Such probes stimulate erection, emission and ejaculation with minimal stimulation of the adjacent motor nerves of the rear limbs. The probe is placed in the rectum and attended by an assistant who is also able to push forward on the sigmoid flexure of the penis if necessary to obtain protrusion of the penis during stimulation.

Technique of Electroejaculation

It is important to use the proper techniques when collecting semen from bulls with the electroejaculator. Adequate restraint is necessary for good results. The bull should be restrained from excessive movement in any direction. Some bulls attempt to lie down during stimulation. This can be prevented by passing a belt or heavy doubled rope under the bull's brisket, tying it securely to each side of the restraining chute or alleyway. The prepuce should be clipped carefully before electroejaculation is begun to assure collection of a clean semen sample when penile protrusion does not occur. Proper stimulation will usually elicit protrusion.

Most ejaculators have power step controls and stimulator controls. The power step control limits electrical potential (power) and current to the bull by steps, whereas the stimulator control allows variable application within the limits of each power step. The power step control is initially set low (step 1 or 2), and the stimulator control knob is rotated in increasing increments until the maximum stimulus within the power step is obtained. Several stimuli are given after the maximum level is reached; then the power step control is turned to the next higher level and the process is repeated. The bull may move and show uneasiness in the beginning, but if rhythmic stimulation is continued, he will usually settle down. Increases in stimulus strength ideally should be made without breaking the stimulation rhythm. The stimulator control should be operated smoothly and fairly rapidly when increasing and decreasing the stimulation. The bull should be held on stimulus for 2 to 3 seconds but should not be allowed off stimulus longer than approximately 0.5 second. Failure to follow this procedure results in loss of penile erection or failure of protrusion and also in poor quality semen samples. Too rapid stimulation causes excessive discomfort and equally poor results. Stimulation that is too slow is less discomforting but also is less effective.

Clear pre-ejaculatory fluids begin to drip from the penis as a first indication that ejaculation will occur soon. When these fluids begin to turn turbid, collection should begin. When they turn relatively clear again, ejaculation is usually completed. Semen should be collected in a calibrated tube attached to a director cone immersed in a water bath maintained at about 38° C to prevent cold shock to the spermatozoa.

The penis of many bulls develops the "corkscrew" configuration during electroejaculation. This is not abnormal unless it occurs during natural service before intromission. Urination also occurs occasionally during electroejaculation and is probably related to pain or possibly to increased stimulation of the pelvic nerves associated with urination. This can be decreased by applying stimuli in as gentle a manner as possible and by using probes that decrease stimuli to adjacent nerves that are not involved in the ejaculatory process.

Studies of semen quality criteria comparing semen collected by electroejaculation (EE) and artificial vagina (AV) indicate some consistent differences. Concentration is higher in semen collected by AV, and volume is greater when semen is collected by EE. Total numbers of spermatozoa per ejaculate remain the same. These differences appear not to affect the freezability or fertility of semen.

Failure to collect semen by electroejaculation may be due to faulty technique or to bull factors such as poor response to the electric current or lack of semen production. The latter condition is often associated with small testes. Either faulty technique or failure of the bull to respond to stimulation should be suspected when the testes are of normal size and no semen is collected. When failure of semen collection occurs on an initial attempt, it is worthwhile to rest the bull

for at least 10 minutes and then try again. Different patterns of stimulation will sometimes elicit ejaculation during subsequent attempts.

OTHER METHODS OF SEMEN COLLECTION

If repeated attempts to collect semen by electroejaculation are unsuccessful, manual massage of the pelvic genitalia is indicated. Each of the vesicular glands and then the ampullae and pelvic urethra are stroked repeatedly after the bull is rested. These organs can often be lifted from the floor of the pelvis and stroked between the fingers and thumb. The stroking is repeated until a sufficient quantity of semen is collected from the tip of the slightly protruded but flaccid penis or from the prepuce.

When this method also fails, the bull should be classified as either a questionable or an unsatisfactory potential breeder, depending on the results of the physical examination. If the bull has testes of normal size, he would usually be classified as questionable. If he has small or hypoplastic testes, he should be classified as an unsatisfactory potential breeder.

In some instances, semen can be collected by AV when other methods fail. Notwithstanding occasional failure, semen can be collected more consistently by EE than by AV in young beef bulls. In one study, semen was collected 86 per cent of the time with AV and 100 per cent with EE. In another study, semen was collected by AV 54 per cent of the time within 10 minutes after introduction of trained young beef bulls to a "bait" steer. By contrast, semen was collected 97.5 per cent of the time in the same bulls using the electroejaculator. Thus, EE is the method of choice for untrained bulls when small quantities of semen are desired or for certain other bulls that are intractable or from which it is difficult to collect semen with an AV. Collection of semen by AV is discussed in Physical Examination of the Bull, page 322.

REFERENCES

1. Austin J. W., Hupp, E. W. and Murphree, R. L.: Comparison of quality of bull semen collected in the artificial vagina and by electroejaculation. J. Dairy Sci., 44:2292, 1961.
2. Ball, L.: Electroejaculation. *In* Klemm, W. R. (ed.):

Applied Electronics for Veterinary Medicine and Animal Physiology. Springfield Ill., Charles C Thomas, 1976, p. 394.

3. Carrol, E. J., Ball, L. and Scott, J. A.: Breeding soundness in bulls — A summary of 10,940 examinations. J.A.V.M.A., *142*:1105, 1963.
4. Easley, G. T.: A hand electrode for the electroejaculation of bulls. Bovine Pract., *5*:12, 1970.

5. Goodwin, D. E.: The collection of semen from Aberdeen Angus bulls by massage of intrapelvic organs. J.A.V.M.A., *157*:831, 1970.
6. Semans, J. H. and Langworthy, O. R.: Observation on the neurophysiology of sexual function in the male cat. J. Urol., *40*:836, 1938.

Evaluation of Frozen Semen

W. E. BERNDTSON
AND B. W. PICKETT

Colorado State University, Fort Collins, Colorado

Although an individual can be reasonably confident that semen from a reputable artificial insemination (AI) organization is of high quality, semen may be damaged while in storage, during shipment or by mishandling in the field.[1, 5] Whenever the quality of frozen semen is in question or fertility is depressed, a portion from each ejaculate should be evaluated by experienced personnel.

The best measure of fertility is the percentage of pregnancies or the number of inseminations per live calf.[6] Unfortunately, unless at least 30 cows are bred to an individual ejaculate, the possibility of an error in predicting fertility will be accentuated.[3] Also, the conditions under which the semen is used must be considered, as fertility is influenced by many factors in addition to seminal quality. Since information regarding fertility is often too costly and time-consuming to obtain, some laboratory test, or tests, is generally required. The ideal method should be rapid, inexpensive, simple, objective and reliable. No ideal test has been developed to date.[3, 6, 8] The tests that are available can be used to eliminate samples that are of obvious poor quality. However, the fact that a sample may meet or exceed minimum standards for these tests does not insure high fertility.

Under most circumstances the practitioner would be ill-advised to evaluate frozen semen because: (1) suitable equipment will generally be lacking, (2) inexperienced personnel do not know what results to expect from assessment of a frozen semen sample, (3) most procedures are subjective and therefore should be performed by experienced individuals who make such assessments routinely and (4) information that is important for a proper evaluation may be known only by the semen processor. For the latter reason, the organization that processed the semen will usually be most qualified to perform such an evaluation. However, if for some reason it is suspected that the processor may be unable to perform an unbiased evaluation, the semen should be sent to another reputable organization for testing.

In most semen processing organizations, each ejaculate is evaluated for volume, spermatozoal concentration, the percentage of progressively motile spermatozoa (the percentage of spermatozoa swimming in a progressive, forward manner) and the rate of motility (speed of forward movement) immediately after collection. Spermatozoal morphology of selected samples is also examined at regular intervals. On the basis of these measurements, the ejaculate will be discarded or processed so that each inseminate contains the desired number of motile spermatozoa. In general, about one-half to two-thirds of the motile spermatozoa will be rendered immotile by freezing and thawing. Thus, each inseminate must contain sufficient spermatozoa prior to freezing to compensate for this loss, and motility must be determined after freezing to insure that both an adequate percentage and an adequate total number of motile spermatozoa are available after thawing.

We believe that semen returned from the field for evaluation should be assessed for the percentage of progressively motile spermatozoa, rate of motility and number of motile spermatozoa per inseminate. Additional tests may be used under special circumstances.

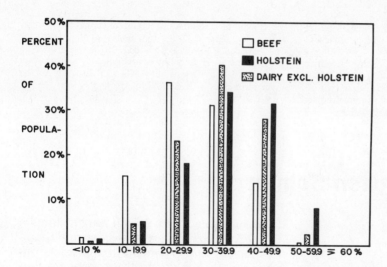

Figure 1. Frequency distribution of annual average postfreeze progressive motility in percent (mature bulls). (Adapted from Elliott, F. I.: Proc. Twentieth Ann. Conv. N.A.A.B., 1967.)

ASSESSMENT OF QUALITY OF FROZEN SEMEN

Motility

We have adopted 20 per cent progressively motile spermatozoa as the minimum acceptable motility for frozen semen. However, because motility estimations are made subjectively, a different minimal standard may be required by other organizations. In addition, the spermatozoa must show a reasonable rate of forward movement. Inexperienced personnel often expect much greater motility from a frozen sample. For example, complaints have been received from some farm owners, veterinarians and so forth that frozen semen contained less than 50 per cent motile spermatozoa.[6] The distribution of post-thaw motilities for a large population of bulls at one artificial insemination (AI) organization is summarized in Figure 1. Definite differences in mean post-thaw motility existed among beef, non-Holstein dairy and Holstein bulls. More important, less than 10 per cent of all semen samples had post-thaw motility that exceeded 50 per cent regardless of breed, even though these bulls had been selected for fertility.[2]

Post-thaw motility is influenced by thawing procedures.[1, 7] Whereas iced water is widely accepted as ideal for thawing semen in ampules,[5] seminal processing organizations have not adopted uniform thawing procedures for semen in straws.[1] Rapid thawing of semen in straws is clearly beneficial to post-thaw motility. Nonetheless, many procedures that do not result in maximum mo-

tility have been advocated by some organizations[1] because they are simple and more convenient for the inseminator or because fertility has not been depressed by such procedures in all studies. Presumably the latter resulted because the inseminates contained a sufficient number of motile spermatozoa after thawing to overcome differences in fertility due to thawing method. Unfortunately, samples that meet the minimum standards for motility when thawed rapidly may fail to do so when thawed slowly. Thus, any evaluation of motility of spermatozoa in straws must be qualified by stating that samples did or did not meet minimal standards when thawed by a specific method.

Number of Motile Spermatozoa per Inseminate

To properly evaluate a sample of frozen semen about which the evaluator has no prior information, the number of motile spermatozoa per inseminate must be determined. However, once this is done, it still may be impossible to know if too few or too many sperm are present for *maximum reproductive efficiency*, since the optimal number of spermatozoa depends upon the breed and the fertility level of each bull.[9] This is illustrated in Figures 2 and 3. In the first study (Fig. 2), 57,130 cows were bred to Holstein bulls. When averaged for all bulls, the nonreturn rate (NR) was lower for inseminates containing 5 million motile spermatozoa compared with 10 or 15 million motile spermatozoa after thawing. The bulls

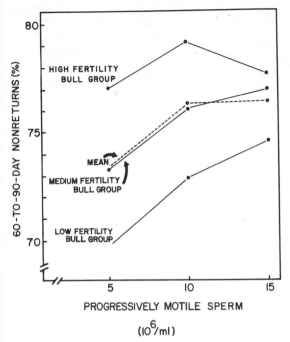

Figure 2. Nonreturn rate as affected by the number of motile spermatozoa after thawing and the fertility level of Holstein bulls. (From Sullivan, J. J.: Proc. Third N.A.A.B. Tech. Conf. A.I. Reprod., 1970.)

spermatozoa was increased from 5 to 10 million. A further increase to 15 million spermatozoa resulted in 1.7 and 0.9 percentage-point improvements in the fertility of the low- and medium-fertility groups and a 1.5 percentage-point decrease in the high-fertility group. Similar results were obtained for 5230 Angus and Hereford services to dairy cows, except that fertility was greater with inseminates containing 10 million spermatozoa, regardless of the fertility level of the bull (Fig. 3).

We have concluded that for most bulls each inseminate should contain at least 10 million motile spermatozoa after thawing, regardless of how semen is packaged.[7] However, AI organizations that can monitor the fertility of each bull may utilize fewer than 10 million motile spermatozoa if this results in greater fertility. Such information will be known only by personnel at the processing organization, who are most qualified to perform the evaluation. The influence of the method of thawing on post-thaw motility will also be reflected in the number of motile spermatozoa per inseminate.

were also divided into low (72.6 per cent NR), medium (75.4 per cent NR) and high (77.9 per cent NR) fertility groups. Fertility of each group increased when the number of

Acrosomal Integrity

Many routine evaluations of frozen semen now include examination of the integrity of the spermatozoal acrosome.[8] Since the acrosome is involved in the fertilization process, it has been postulated that spermatozoa with deteriorated or damaged acrosomes are unlikely to be capable of fertilization. Furthermore, a relatively high positive correlation has been reported for acrosomal integrity and fertility of Holstein bulls.[8] Evaluation of acrosomal integrity requires highly specialized equipment and is more time-consuming than the evaluation of motility. Also, the relationship between acrosomal integrity and fertility of semen from beef bulls has not been reported. However, this technique may be useful when applied in addition to the aforementioned tests and is likely to be employed more extensively in the future.

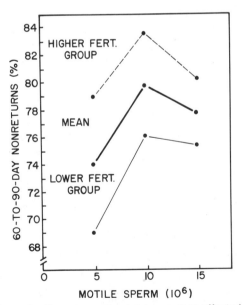

Figure 3. Nonreturn rate of dairy cows as affected by the number of motile spermatozoa after thawing and the fertility level of semen from Angus and Hereford bulls. (From Sullivan, J. J.: Proc. Third N.A.A.B. Tech. Conf. A.I. Reprod., 1970.)

METHODS USED TO EVALUATE FROZEN SEMEN

The following procedures apply specifically to the evaluation of frozen semen submitted to our laboratory for evaluation. A mini-

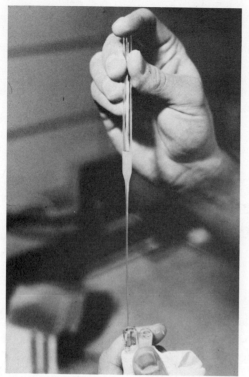

Figure 4. Mix the semen thoroughly before evaluation.

liness, adjustment and proper temperature. All material in contact with the semen, except the thawing baths, should be at 38° C. Two ampules or straws are removed from the liquid nitrogen, thawed, thoroughly dried and opened (to be described in the following article). Semen in ampules is thoroughly mixed with a Pasteur pipette (Fig. 4). Because of the higher spermatozoal concentration, semen from each straw is diluted to a final volume of 1.0 ml with warm extender (Fig. 5) and gently mixed. A small drop of semen is then placed on each end of a slide (Fig. 6) maintained on a warming plate and is covered in a manner that prevents air bubbles from being trapped (Fig. 7).

Separate slides are prepared with semen from each ampule or straw. The slide is then placed in a stage incubator at 38° C. (Fig. 8). Semen at both ends of each slide is viewed under phase-contrast microscopy at approximately 480 magnifications. Motility is estimated to the nearest 5 per cent, and the rate of motility is recorded as 0, 1, 2, 3, 4 or 5. If motility differs by 10 percentage points or more between the two ampules or straws, a third sample is thawed and evaluated.

mum of three ampules or five straws is required for such an evaluation.

Motility

The thawing bath, slide warmer, stage incubator, ampule holder, phase-contrast microscope and all glassware that will be in contact with the semen are checked for clean-

Number of Motile Spermatozoa per Inseminate

If the sample meets minimal standards for spermatozoal motility, the number of motile spermatozoa per inseminate must then be determined. For this, one additional ampule or three additional straws are removed from the liquid nitrogen, and their contents are thawed. The volume per inseminate is deter-

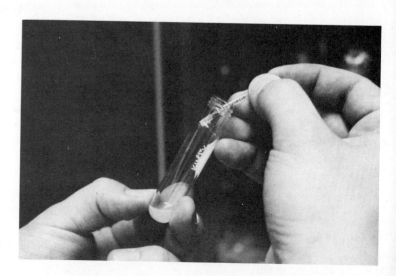

Figure 5. Mix the contents of each straw with additional extender.

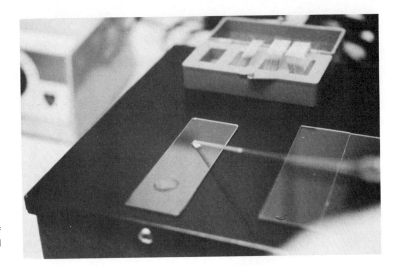

Figure 6. Place a small drop of semen on each end of a prewarmed microscope slide.

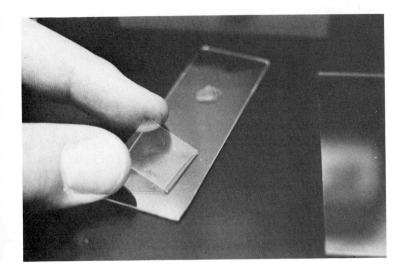

Figure 7. Cover each drop with a cover slip.

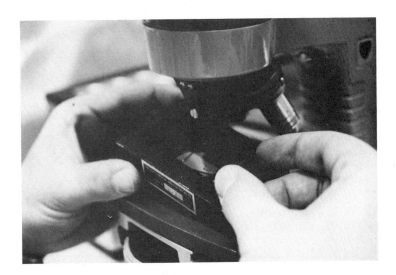

Figure 8. Place the microscope slide in a stage incubator.

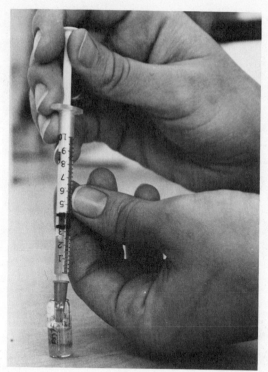

Figure 9. Carefully measure the volume of the inseminate.

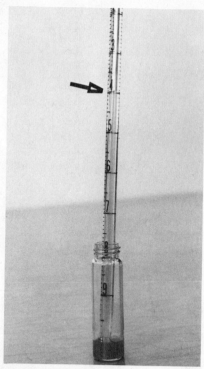

Figure 10. Extremely careful measurements must be made for accuracy.

mined by aspirating the contents of one ampule or the pooled contents of three straws into a graduated syringe (Fig. 9). The contents of three straws are pooled to improve the accuracy of the determination because of the smaller volume contained in most straws.

Spermatozoal concentration is determined by hemocytometry. The pooled contents of semen from the straws used for determination of inseminate volume or of ampules used both for motility and volume determination are utilized. This semen is thoroughly mixed, and an aliquot (approximately 1.0 ml) is removed and diluted in a solution containing 10 per cent formaldehyde and 0.9 per cent sodium chloride. The dilution ratio depends upon the inseminate volume, which usually is inversely related to the spermatozoal concentration and the type of extender utilized. A 1:10 or 1:20 dilution is used for egg yolk or milk extenders, respectively, when the semen is packaged in 1.0-ml ampules. Dilution should be increased by a factor of two or four if 0.5-ml or 0.25-ml straws are used. Dilution is accomplished by pipetting semen into a screw-capped vial containing the appropriate volume of diluting fluid. For accurate pipetting, semen should be drawn into the pipette, taking spe-

cial precautions not to exceed the volume needed (Fig. 10), and excess semen should be wiped from the outer surface of the pipette (Fig. 11). After expelling the contents into the diluting fluid, the inside of the pipette

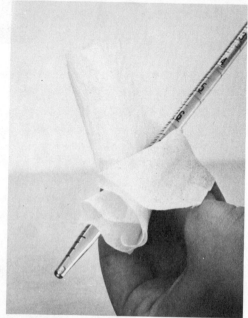

Figure 11. Wipe the excess semen from the outer surface of the pipette.

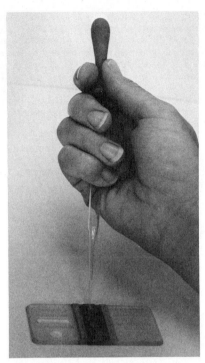

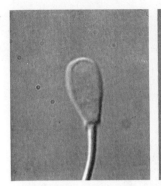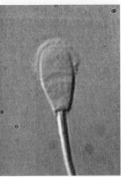

Figure 13. Spermatozoa with intact (left) and degenerating (right) acrosomes.

Figure 12. The hemocytometer chamber is filled, using a Pasteur pipette.

should be rinsed by drawing fluid into the pipette three times. The sample is then mixed by inverting 10 times, the hemocytometer chamber is filled by using a Pasteur pipette (Fig. 12), the specimen is allowed to settle for three to five minutes and the spermatozoa are counted. The number of motile spermatozoa per inseminate is calculated as follows:

Number of motile sperm per inseminate =

$$\frac{\text{Number of sperm/ml} \times \text{inseminate volume}}{\% \text{ motility}} \times 100$$

Acrosomal Integrity

The integrity of spermatozoal acrosomes is evaluated in our laboratory as an added test when it is suspected that semen may be of low fertility but the sample meets minimal standards for motility and number of motile spermatozoa per inseminate. The procedure for assessing acrosomal integrity involves the examination of spermatozoa in wet seminal smears under differential-interference phase-contrast microscopy.[8] When viewed in this manner, normal, intact and degenerating acrosomes can be observed, as in Figure 13.

The procedures for preparing semen for acrosomal evaluation are identical to those employed when semen is to be evaluated for motility. However, the sample is incubated at 37° C, and aliquots are removed for evaluation after 0, 2, 4 and 8 hours. The aliquots may be used without further processing or may be diluted with two volumes of 0.2 per cent glutaraldehyde in phosphate-buffered saline (the latter procedure is currently restricted to semen in egg yolk-sodium citrate extender).[4] Slides are then prepared as for evaluation of motility. One hundred sperm are examined in each of two fields, and the percentage of spermatozoa with intact acrosomes is determined. The semen is maintained at room temperature during evaluation. This reduces the rate of motility and allows better observation of the acrosome when motile spermatozoa are present. Alternatively, if the aliquots of semen are diluted in the glutaraldehyde solution, the acrosome is fixed, and the samples can be stored for at least 29 days before evaluation.[4] This procedure is convenient, it arrests motility and thereby permits better observation of the acrosome than when spermatozoa are motile and it allows randomization and coding of samples to insure objectivity. However, very few laboratories have the equipment and personnel required to perform this evaluation.

In conclusion, whenever there is doubt with respect to the quality of frozen semen, it should be evaluated prior to use as a part of the overall herd management program.

REFERENCES

1. Berndtson, W. E., Pickett, B. W. and Rugg, C. D.: Procedures for field handling of bovine semen in plastic straws. Proceedings Sixth N.A.A.B. Tech-

nical Conference on Artificial Insemination and Reproduction, 1976, pp. 51–60.

2. Elliott, F. I.: Comparative history of dairy and beef semen production. Proceedings Twentieth Annual Convention N.A.A.B., 1967, pp. 109–115.

3. Erb, R. E., Ehlers, M. H., Mikota, L. and Schwarz, E.: The relation of simple semen quality tests to fertilizing capacity of bull semen. Wash. Agr. Exp. Sta. Tech. Bull. No. 2, 1950.

4. Johnson, L., Berndtson, W. E. and Pickett, B. W.: An improved method for evaluating acrosomes of bovine spermatozoa. J. Anim. Sci., *42*:951, 1976.

5. Pickett, B. W.: Factors affecting the utilization of frozen bovine semen for *maximum reproductive efficiency.* A.I. Digest, *19*(2):8, 1971.

6. Pickett, B. W.: Evaluation of frozen bovine semen. Bovine Practit., Nov., 1971, pp. 12–17.

7. Pickett, B. W., Berndtson, W. E. and Sullivan, J. J.: Influence of seminal additives and packaging systems on fertility of frozen bovine spermatozoa. J. Anim. Sci., Suppl. (in press).

8. Saacke, R. G. and White, J. M.: Semen quality tests and their relationship to fertility. Proceedings Fourth N.A.A.B. Technical Conference on Artificial Insemination and Reproduction, 1972, pp. 22–27.

9. Sullivan, J. J.: Sperm numbers required for optimum breeding efficiency in cattle. Proceedings Third N.A.A.B. Technical Conference on Artificial Insemination and Reproduction, 1970, pp. 36–43.

Procedures for Handling Frozen Bovine Semen in the Field

B. W. PICKETT AND
W. E. BERNDTSON

Colorado State University, Fort Collins, Colorado

There is little doubt that most of the fertility problems associated with the use of frozen semen are due to improper handling or deposition of semen by the technician (inseminator). The suggestions contained in this article are designed to minimize the reduction in fertility resulting from improper handling techniques for frozen semen packaged in ampules or straws. The problems caused by technicians' errors have been discussed elsewhere.[4]

MAINTAINING TEMPERATURE OF FROZEN SEMEN

The key factor enabling the successful long-term storage of frozen bovine spermatozoa is low temperature.[7] It appears that the temperature of the semen should be maintained at −130° C or lower at all times for *maximum reproductive efficiency.*[1-3, 5, 8, 10] Although liquid nitrogen (LN), which has a temperature of −196° C, is the storage medium used for transportation of semen, there are numerous opportunities for exposure of frozen semen to elevated temperatures from the time of freezing at the central artificial insemination (AI) organization to the time of thawing for deposition in the cow.

When semen is delivered by common carrier, the unit in which the semen is received must contain LN. Just being frozen is not acceptable. Unless there is at least a measurable amount of LN in the unit, the shipment should not be accepted. If there is no LN present, the temperature should be determined before LN is added. If the temperature has risen above −80° C, the semen should not be used to breed cows because the fertility may have been greatly reduced.

Transfer of Semen

In many cases, the first opportunity for improper handling comes when the semen is delivered to or picked up by the technician or rancher. Semen can be exposed to elevated temperatures when it is transferred from one tank to another. If the transfer is made at a central storage area or truck, the field unit should be filled with LN before the semen is transferred. Thus, the semen is immediately submerged in LN when the transfer occurs.

The relatively large surface area and the small volume of extended semen contained in most straws are conducive to rapid heat exchange. Therefore, changes in seminal temperature occur more quickly within straws than within ampules during exposure to elevated temperature. This is illustrated in Figure 1. In this study, semen was removed from LN and exposed to ambient conditions. Rates of warming were related to the surface-area-to-volume ratio, since the seminal temperature rose more quickly

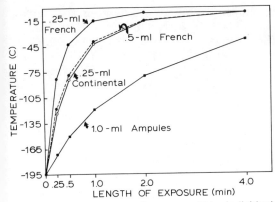

Figure 1. Temperature of semen within individual straws held by forceps, or ampules clipped to metal canes (racks), during exposure to ambient (20 ± 0.6° C). conditions. (Each curve represents the mean of five replicates. The curve for ampules is a mean of the temperature of semen within the top and bottom ampules on the same rack). (From Berndtson et al.: Proc. Sixth N.A.A.B. Tech. Conf. A.I. Reprod., 1976.)

in the post-thaw motility of spermatozoa within straws than within ampules. The most dramatic loss in motility was in 0.25-ml French straws. For example, after 1 minute of exposure, no loss of motility was evident for spermatozoa within 1.0-ml ampules, whereas 81.5 per cent of the motile spermatozoa in 0.25-ml French straws were rendered immotile.

It is obvious that individual straws must never be exposed to ambient conditions, such as during transfer to other storage tanks and so forth, without additional protection. AI organizations must package straws for distribution and field storage in protective devices that are conducive to minimizing damage from mishandling. Some systems of packing ampules and straws for shipment are shown in Figure 3.

Plastic goblets are effective in reducing temperature changes within straws during

within the long, slender 0.25-ml French straws than within the shorter, greater diameter Continental straws containing the same volume of extended semen. More importantly, the temperature rose at a faster rate within each type of straw than within ampules. The importance of this finding cannot be overstated. In this same study, semen was exposed for 0, 0.25, 0.5, 1.0, 2.0 or 4.0 minutes, immediately plunged back into LN and subsequently thawed and evaluated for the percentage of progressively motile spermatozoa, which is a reasonably reliable measurement of fertility. The results are presented in Figure 2. As expected, less exposure was required to produce a reduction

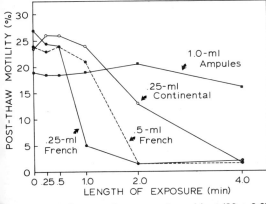

Figure 2. Influence of exposure to ambient (20 ± 0.6° C) conditions on the post-thaw motility of spermatozoa within individual straws or ampules on racks. (Semen in straws was thawed in water at 37° C, whereas ampules were thawed in iced water). (From Berndtson et al.: Proc. Sixth N.A.A.B. Tech. Conf. A.I. Reprod., 1976.)

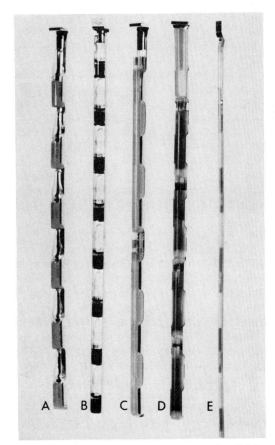

Figure 3. Methods of packaging semen for distribution. Left to right: (A) 1.0-ml ampules on a rack, (B) 0.5-ml ampules on a rack, (C) 0.5-ml French straws in goblets on a rack, (D) 0.25-ml Continental (United States) straws in goblets on a rack and (E) 0.25-ml Continental (United States) straws in a plastic retriever.

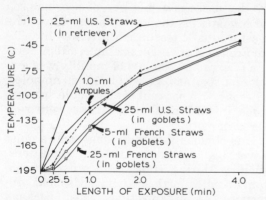

Figure 4. Influence of packaging in goblets or other protective devices on seminal temperature during exposure to ambient (20 ± 0.6° C) temperature. (Each goblet contained five 0.25-ml Continental (United States) or 0.5-ml French straws or ten 0.25-ml French straws. Goblets did not contain liquid nitrogen (LN) at the start of exposure. Each curve represents the mean of five replicates.) (From Berndtson *et al.*: Proc. Sixth N.A.A.B. Tech. Conf. A.I. Reprod., 1976.)

exposure to ambient conditions. In this same study, straws were placed in goblets clipped to metal racks for exposure. Changes in the temperature of semen within straws placed in goblets were virtually identical to those within ampules (Fig. 4). Temperature changes would have been further minimized if the goblets had contained LN at the start of exposure,. The 0.25-ml Continental straws were also placed in Continental "plastic tubes with metal retrievers" for exposure. These devices were less effective than plastic goblets in minimizing changes in seminal temperature (Fig. 4).

In this study, no significant loss of motility was observed when spermatozoa, in ampules or in straws placed in goblets, were exposed to ambient conditions for 1 minute. However, one must not conclude that semen packaged in this manner can be safely exposed for up to 1 minute. Damage can be expected any time the temperature of semen rises above −130° C. Since the rate of warming is influenced by many factors, including the ambient temperature, length of exposure, wind velocity and intensity of solar radiation, rates of warming will vary. Thus, the only realistic recommendation is that *straws should be distributed and transferred while in goblets or some similar device, preferably containing LN, and that the transfers should be completed as quickly as possible, away from wind and sunlight.*

It is also recommended that when ampules are transferred from one storage unit to another, the unit receiving the semen should be full of LN. Under these conditions, the temperature will return to −196° C more rapidly following exposure if the ampules are placed directly in LN, as opposed to LN vapor. It is desirable to cool semen quickly after exposure, but it is better to prevent the temperature from rising during exposure. Straws in goblets filled with LN are not subjected to elevated temperatures until the LN has boiled away. For this reason, it is preferable that the unit from which the straw is removed be filled with LN prior to the transfer, if the straws are maintained in goblets or other devices that hold LN.

Exposure of Semen during Removal

Semen may also be exposed to damaging temperatures each time it is raised into the neck of a field unit to permit removal of an individual straw or ampule. The temperature within the neck of a typical field unit is much higher toward the top of the tank (Fig. 5). Since spermatozoa will be damaged at these temperatures, the canister containing the semen should be raised no higher than absolutely necessary, and the individual straw or ampule should be removed for thawing as quickly as possible.

One need not be nearly as concerned about the temperature of semen within the straw or ampule being removed as with the temperature of other semen remaining in the same canister or goblet. This semen is exposed to elevated temperatures each time another insemination unit is removed. The damage from exposure to elevated temperatures is additive. Further, unless sufficient

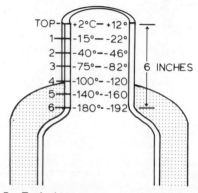

Figure 5. Typical temperature range in the neck of a LN field storage unit. (Adapted from Saacke, R. G.: Proc. Eighth N.A.A.B. Conf. A.I. Beef Cattle, 1974.)

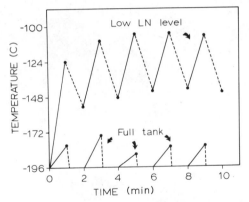

Figure 6. Influence of level of LN on the temperature of semen during repeated exposure to the neck of a field storage unit. Figure depicts temperatures for semen within 0.5-ml French straws (five straws/goblet). (Pickett *et al.*: Proc. Tenth N.A.A.B. Conf. A.I. Beef Cattle, 1976.)

time is allowed between exposures to permit the semen to cool completely, higher temperatures will be reached during subsequent exposures. This is illustrated in Figure 6. In this study, semen in straws, placed in goblets on metal racks, was raised to the neck of a typical field unit. The rack was held in the neck for exactly 1 minute, returned to the tank for 1 minute and the procedure immediately repeated for five consecutive exposures. When the tank contained 14 cm of LN (low level), the temperature rose quickly during the first minute of exposure. Moreover, the semen failed to cool completely within 1 minute upon return to the tank. Thus, higher temperatures were reached during subsequent exposures. More than 10 minutes were required for the temperature to reach $-196°$ C upon return of the semen to the tank after the fifth exposure. When the tank was full of LN, the goblets contained LN at the start of each exposure. Thus, increases in temperature were minimized, and the semen cooled to $-196°$ C almost immediately upon return to the tank.

It is obvious that the seminal temperature reached during exposure to the neck of a field storage unit depends upon the height to which semen is raised, length of exposure, level of LN in the tank and the interval between exposures. Therefore, *semen should be raised no higher than necessary to facilitate removal of a straw or ampule for thawing, and removal should be executed as quickly as possible.* Since under normal circumstances it is impossible to maintain a high LN level at all times, *inseminators must be instructed to allow more time between exposures when the LN level is low.*

To further reduce the possibility of exposure, an accurate inventory of the number and location of straws or ampules should be maintained at all times. Semen should not be packed in the tank in a manner that will impede rapid removal. With a little practice and the proper arrangement of tank and thaw box, removal can be accomplished in 3 to 5 seconds. If more time is required, the proper arrangement has not been established, or there is some unnecessary obstruction to removal of the semen. Thus, the longer that specific ampules or straws are carried by a technician, the greater the opportunity for repeated exposure. Fertility of the uppermost samples in the tank would be expected to be lowered if the semen had been improperly handled and frequently exposed to elevated temperatures.

THAWING AMPULES AND STRAWS

The procedures for thawing ampules and straws are different, and several excellent reviews have appeared.[1, 4-7, 9] The following are our recommendations:

Procedures for Handling Semen Packaged in 1.0-ml Ampules

Note: Glass ampules have generally been designed to contain 0.5 or 1.0 ml of extended semen (Fig. 7). Although the techniques for handling semen in 0.5- and 1.0-ml ampules

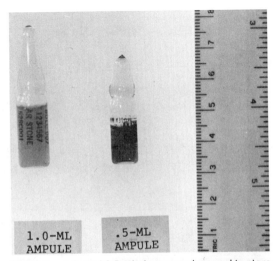

Figure 7. 1.0- and 0.5-ml glass ampules used to store frozen bovine semen.

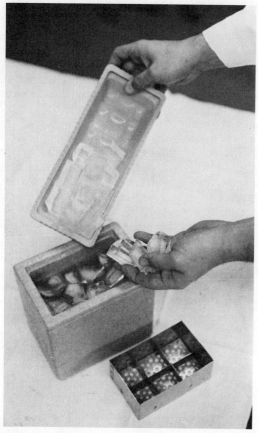

Figure 8. Preparation of thawing bath for 1.0-ml ampules.

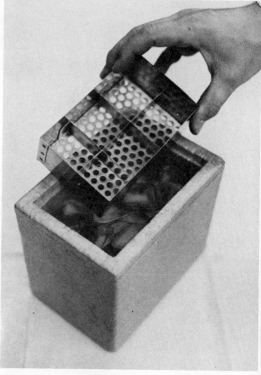

Figure 9. Thawing container used to thaw 1.0-ml ampules of frozen bovine semen.

are similar, the following techniques apply specifically for semen in 1.0-ml ampules.

Prepare an iced-water bath by placing several ice cubes in at least 0.5 liter of clean, fresh water in an insulated container (Fig. 8). This volume of water will prevent a sig-nificant decrease in temperature when several ampules are thawed at once. The bath should be prepared 30 minutes before use or stirred rapidly for 5 minutes.

The thawing container (Fig. 9) is designed to (1) keep the ice cubes separated from the thawing ampules and (2) keep the ampules separated from each other as they are thaw-ing. This arrangement will permit easy, rapid removal of the thawed ampules with-

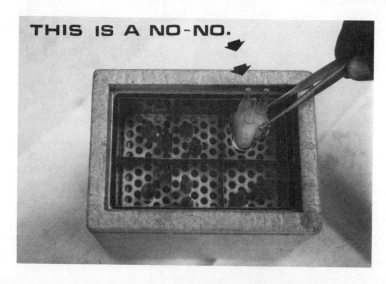

Figure 10. Thaw ampules to prevent them from freezing together.

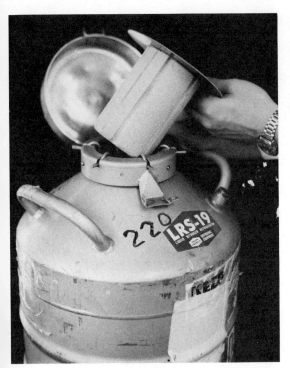

Figure 11. Removal of the lid from the LN storage unit.

out interference by the ice cubes and will prevent the ampules from freezing to the ice cubes or to each other. Freezing of an ampule to the ice cubes or to other ampules (Fig. 10) reduces the rate of thawing.

Remove the lid from the LN storage unit containing the semen to be used (Fig. 11), and identify the canister holding the ampules that are to be used (Fig. 12). Next lift the proper canister *no higher than the frost line* in the neck of the LN storage unit (Fig. 13). With the thumb and forefinger, quickly grasp the upper tip of the rack holding the ampules. *Note:* The top of the tin racks will be labeled with the bull's code, and each ampule on a rack will be labeled with the bull's name, registration number, code number, date of freezing and the code number of the organization that processed the semen. *Identify the ampule before use.*

Remove the ampule as quickly as possible (Fig. 14) and place it in the thawing container. If ampules are in bulk storage, a long grasping device will be essential for removing them from the storage unit (Fig. 15).

Prepare the insemination device by connecting a syringe to an insemination catheter (Fig. 16).

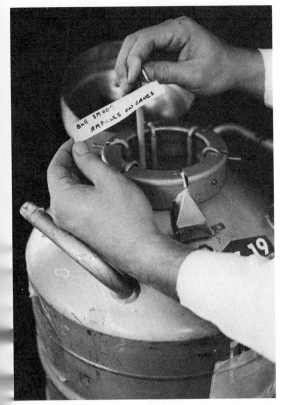

Figure 12. Identify the canister that contains the ampules to be thawed.

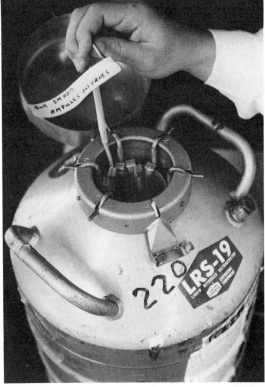

Figure 13. Lift the canister no higher than the frost line in the neck of the LN storage unit.

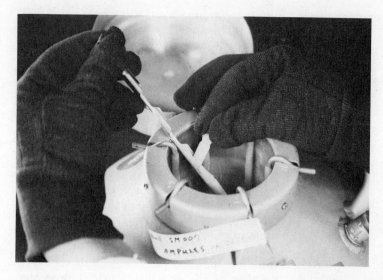

Figure 14. Remove the ampules as quickly as possible.

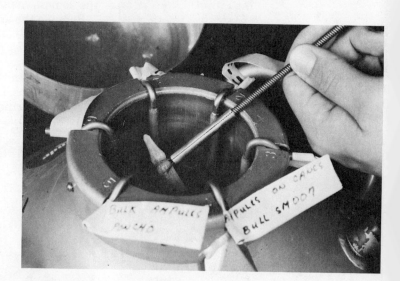

Figure 15. Removing ampules from bulk storage.

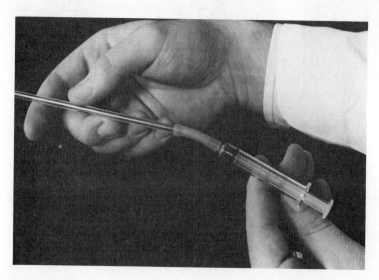

Figure 16. A syringe is attached to the catheter with a small piece of rubber tubing.

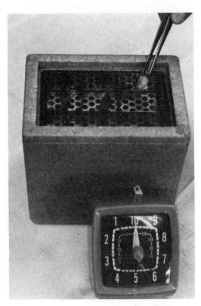

Figure 17. Allow the ampule to thaw for 10 minutes before removal.

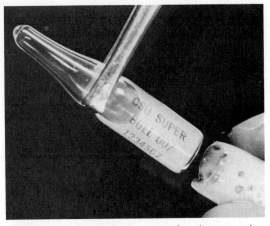

Figure 18. Remove the ice coat after the semen has thawed.

Allow 10 minutes for the ampule to thaw. *Note:* Do not disturb the ampule while it is thawing by removing the coat of ice. After thawing for 10 minutes, remove the ampule from the thawing bath (Fig. 17), remove the ice coat (Fig. 18) and dry the ampule thoroughly (Fig. 19).

Score the ampule (Fig. 20) and snap off the top portion (Fig. 21). Some ampules are pre-scored. *Note:* Ampules should always be opened in the upright position.

Insert the insemination catheter slowly, withdrawing semen as the catheter is lowered into the ampule (Fig. 22). *Note:* The catheter and ampule should be held in an

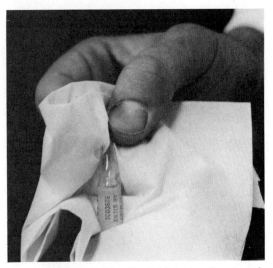

Figure 19. Water is spermicidal; dry the ampule thoroughly before opening.

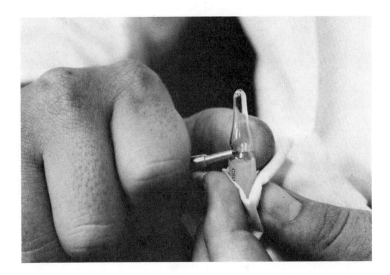

Figure 20. Scoring an ampule.

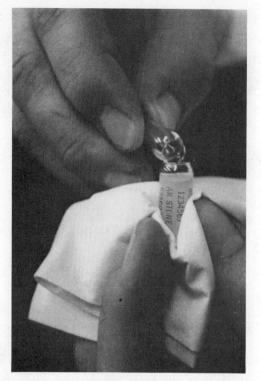

Figure 21. Removing the top portion of the ampule.

upright position and all the semen withdrawn without breaking the liquid column within the catheter (Fig. 23).

Inseminate the cow. Deposit the semen into the posterior portion of the body of the uterus (Fig. 24). A steady, 5-second squeeze should be used to expel the semen. *Note:* Count, do not guess at 5 seconds.

Withdraw the catheter and inspect it to be certain that the maximum amount of semen was placed in the cow (Fig. 25). Dispose of the catheter, keeping the syringe for further use.

Note: For maximum reproductive efficiency, semen should be used immediately after thawing.

Procedures for Handling Semen Packaged in 0.25-ml Continental (U.S.) Straws

Note: The proper handling procedures for semen packaged in straws depend upon the type of straw (Fig. 26). Inseminators must be aware that 0.25-ml and 0.5-ml French straws are not handled in exactly the same

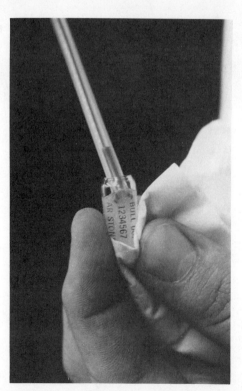

Figure 22. Aspirate semen as the catheter is lowered.

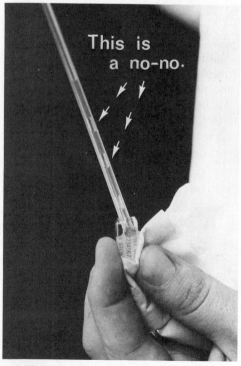

Figure 23. When removing semen, do not break the liquid column in the catheter.

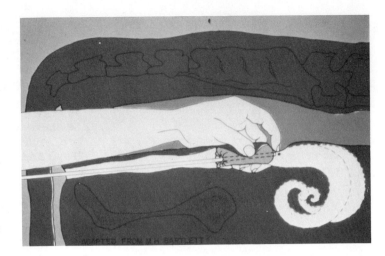

Figure 24. The proper site of semen deposition in the cow.

manner as 0.25-ml Continental (U.S.) straws. Thus, one must learn to identify the various types of straws if the semen is to be properly handled.

Prepare a thawing bath containing water at 35° C (Fig. 27). An electrically heated, thermostatically controlled bath is recommended.

Remove the lid from the LN storage unit containing the semen to be used (see Figure 11). Identify the canister holding the 0.25-ml U.S. straws that are to be used (Fig. 28). Lift the proper canister *no higher than the frost line* in the neck of the LN storage unit (Fig. 29).

With the thumb and forefinger, quickly grasp the upper tip of the rack holding the straws (Fig. 30) and lower the canister back into the tank. *Note:* The 0.25-ml U.S. straws will be in plastic goblets (five straws per goblet). The plastic goblets will be on tin racks (four full goblets per rack, with one empty goblet at the top of the rack). In other words, there will be 20 straws on a full rack. The top of the tin racks will be labeled with the same information as is provided for ampules.

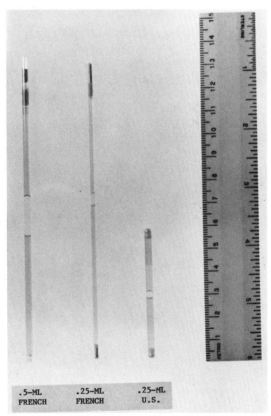

.5–ML FRENCH   .25–ML FRENCH   .25–ML U.S.

Figure 26. Types of straws commonly used to package semen in the United States.

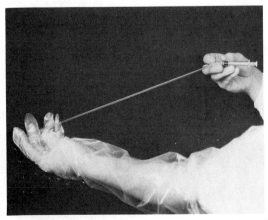

Figure 25. Inspect the catheter to be certain that all semen was placed into the cow.

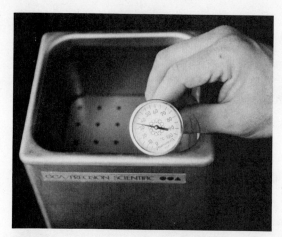

Figure 27. A water bath maintained at 35° C is used to thaw semen in straws.

Remove the empty plastic goblet at the top of the rack with a pair of tweezers (Fig. 31). With the same pair of tweezers, grasp an individual straw and remove it from the plastic goblet, *keeping the straw below the frost line in the neck of the storage unit at all times* (Fig. 32). At the same time, lower the rack to the bottom of the canister within the storage unit.

Immediately transfer the straw from the storage tank to a bath containing water at 35° C (Fig. 33). The 0.25-ml U.S. and 0.5 ml French straws should be held in the water for *exactly* 12 seconds, whereas 0.25-ml French straws should be submersed for 6 seconds. *Note:* Do not linger with the straw in the neck of the LN storage unit or in the

air. *Note:* Before attempting to remove semen from the storage unit, make sure that the thawing bath is at 35° C.

Remove the straw from the thawing bath immediately after the proper thawing time has passed to prevent excessive warming of the semen. After removing the straw from the thawing bath, carefully dry the straw with a clean tissue (Fig. 34). Inspect the straws and discard any with cracks or defective seals.

With a pair of sharp scissors, carefully clip one end of the straw. Make sure that the clipped end of the straw has a straight, clean cut with no jagged edges (Fig. 35). Place the straw (clipped end first) into the funneled end of the plastic insemination sheath (Fig. 36). *Note:* The insemination device is composed of four parts: a plastic sheath, a plastic button-like locking device, a metal plunger and a metal sleeve that slides over the plunger (Fig. 37). Other devices are available for use with French straws.

Place the metal sleeve, with plunger and locking device in place, into the funneled end of the plastic insemination sheath, and guide the straw and the plunger to the opposite tip of the sheath (Fig. 38). Apply gentle pressure to the metal sleeve to seat the straw.

Twist the plastic locking device into the funneled end of the insemination sheath, thus locking the straw in place within the insemination device (Fig. 39).

Inseminate the cow. Expel the semen slowly by pushing on the plunger with the

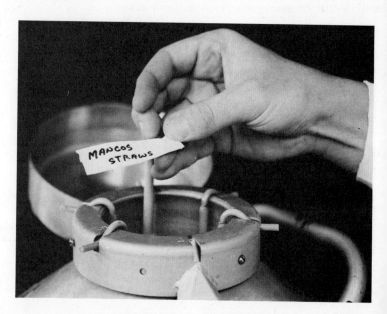

Figure 28. Identify the canister that contains the straws to be thawed.

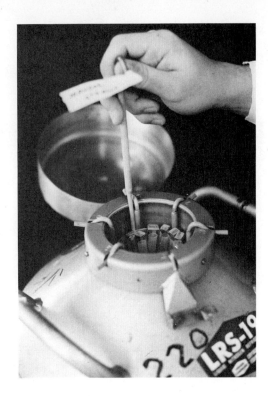

Figure 29. Lift the canister no higher than the frost line in the neck of the LN storage unit.

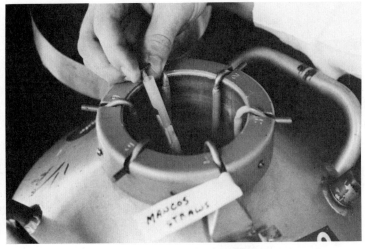

Figure 30. The rack holding the straws is held with the thumb and forefinger.

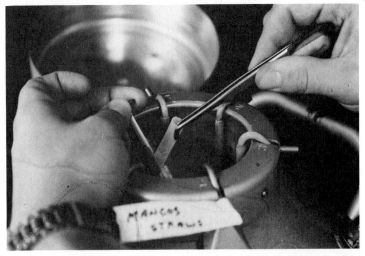

Figure 31. Empty goblets are removed with tweezers.

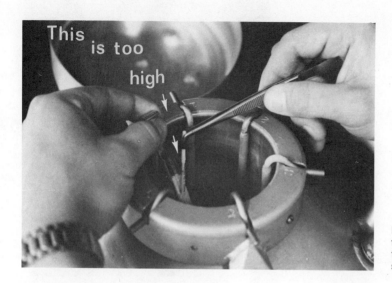

Figure 32. Only the straw to be thawed should be raised higher than the frost line in the neck of the LN storage unit.

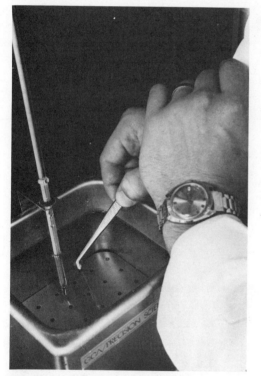

Figure 33. Thaw the straw in a water bath maintained at 35° C.

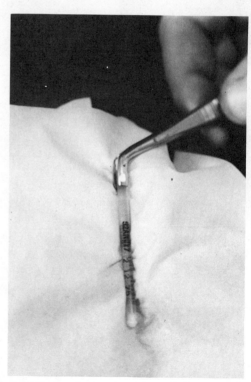

Figure 34. Dry the straw, then inspect for cracks or defective seals.

thumb while holding the remaining portion of the insemination device between the first and second fingers (see Figure 24).

Withdraw the insemination device. Inspect it to insure that all the semen was placed in the cow (Fig. 41). Discard the outer plastic sheath. Keep the two-part metal plunger and the plastic locking device for further use. *Note: For maximum reproductive efficiency,* semen should be used immediately after thawing.

Several precautions must be observed to avoid reducing fertility with warm water thawing techniques. The temperature of the semen must be prevented from reaching excessive levels; i.e., the thawing time must be carefully controlled. Figure 41 shows the mean post-thaw motility of spermatozoa immediately after exposure to temperatures of 35 to 60° C for 5 minutes. When the temperature of the semen was elevated above 45° C, motility declined precipitously. However, the possibility that temperatures below

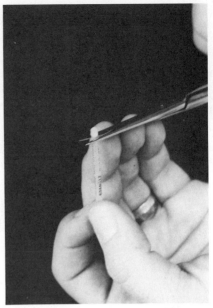

Figure 35. Clip one end of the straw with a sharp instrument.

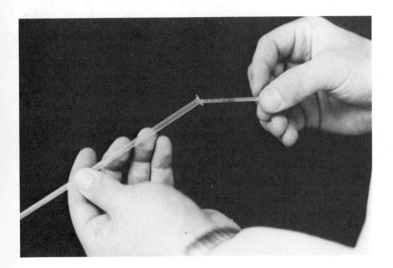

Figure 36. Loading the insemination sheath.

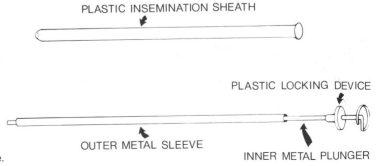

PLASTIC INSEMINATION SHEATH

PLASTIC LOCKING DEVICE

OUTER METAL SLEEVE

INNER METAL PLUNGER

Figure 37. The insemination device.

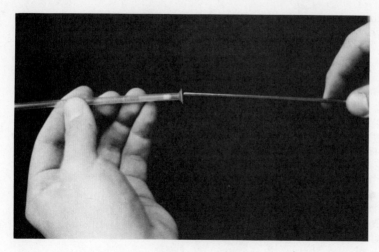

Figure 38. Insert the plunger into the disposable sheath.

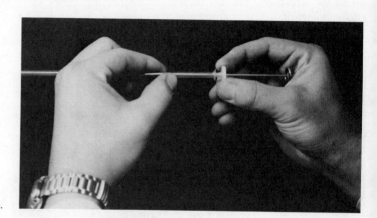

Figure 39. Lock the straw in place.

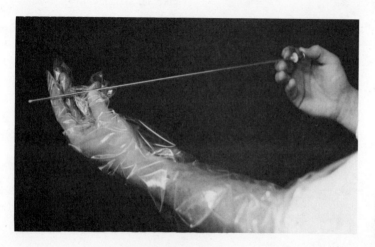

Figure 40. Inspect the insemination device to be certain that all semen was placed into the cow.

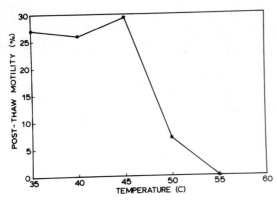

Figure 41. Effect of 5-minute exposure to water at different temperatures on post-thaw motility of spermatozoa in straws. (From Berndtson *et al.*: Proc. Sixth N.A.A.B. Tech. Conf. A.I. Reprod., 1976.)

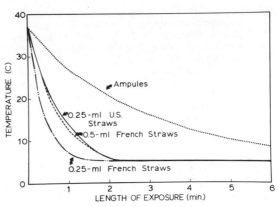

Figure 42. Cooling rates for semen in various packages during exposure to air in a cold room maintained at 5° C (41° F). (From Berndtson *et al.*: Proc. Sixth N.A.A.B. Tech. Conf. A.I. Reprod., 1976.)

45° C might be detrimental to fertility must be considered, in spite of the motility observations. For example, it is known that elevated temperatures can cause a transient stimulation of motility, which is followed by a rapid decline in survival. Also, it has been shown that when rabbit spermatozoa were exposed to temperatures of 38 to 40° C for 3 hours before insemination, no effects were observed on fertilization rates, but fertilization by spermatozoa exposed to temperatures of 40° C was followed by high rates of embryonic mortality.[11] Thus, when spermatozoa are exposed to temperatures higher than those of the female reproductive tract, fertility may be reduced. If thawing temperatures above 37° C are employed, the exposure of the straws to these temperatures should be timed to prevent excessive warming of the spermatozoa. Since the geometry of the straw will influence thawing rates, thawing times have been established for each size and type of straw.

Another potential hazard with the use of warm water thawing is cold shock. Figure 42 shows the rates of cooling observed when 1.0-ml ampules, 0.25-ml Continental straws and 0.25- or 0.5-ml French straws were removed from a 37° C water bath and exposed to the air in a 5° C coldroom. Although rapid rates of cooling of semen occurred within each package, the smaller diameter straws cooled more rapidly. Therefore, avoid conditions that will reduce the temperature of the thawed semen.

Remember, most poor fertility results with frozen semen are due to improper handling or deposition of the semen, or both, by the inseminator.

In addition, the following must also be kept in mind.[9]

1. Deal with reputable semen processing organizations so that you will have confidence in their product.

2. Follow the proper recommendations for handling and inseminating semen.

3. Keep up to date regarding new developments.

4. Avoid experimentation on your own — *Follow instructions.**

REFERENCES

1. Berndtson, W. E., Pickett, B. W. and Rugg, C. D.: Procedures for field handling of bovine semen in plastic straws. Proceedings Sixth N.A.A.B. Technical Conference on Artificial Insemination and Reproduction, 1976, pp. 51–60.
2. Larson, G. L. and Graham, E. F.: Effects of low temperatures in storage of bovine semen. A.I. Digest, *6*(12):6, 1958.
3. Meryman, H. T.: Mechanics of freezing in living cells and tissues. Science, *124*:515, 1956.
4. Pickett, B. W.: Factors affecting the utilization of frozen bovine semen for *maximum reproductive efficiency*. A.I. Digest, *19*(2):8, 1971.
5. Pickett, B. W. and Berndtson, W. E.: Preservation of bovine spermatozoa by freezing in straws: A review. J. Dairy Sci., *57*:1287, 1974.
6. Pickett, B. W., Berndtson, W. E. and Rugg, C. D.: Semen handling in the field. Proceedings Tenth N.A.A.B. Conference on Artificial Insemination of Beef Cattle, 1976, pp. 54–75.

*Portions of the data used in this article were adapted from a publication in the CHAROLAIS BULL-O-GRAM, the Proceedings of the Tenth N.A.A.B. Beef Artificial Insemination Conference and the Sixth N.A.A.B. Technical Conference on Artificial Insemination and Reproduction.

7. Pickett, B. W., Berndtson, W. E. and Sullivan, J. J.: Techniques for processing and packaging bovine semen. Proceedings Sixth N.A.A.B. Technical Conference on Artificial Insemination and Reproduction, 1976, pp. 34–50.

8. Pickett, B. W., Martig, R. C. and Cowan, W. A.: Preservation of bovine spermatozoa at −79 and −196° C. J. Dairy Sci., 44:2089, 1961.

9. Saacke, R. G.: Concepts in semen packaging and use. Proceedings Eighth N.A.A.B. Conference on Artificial Insemination of Beef Cattle, 1974, pp. 11–19.

10. Stewart, D. L.: Observation on the fertility of frozen semen stored at −79° C and −196° C. V. Inter. Congr. Anim. Reprod. and Artif. Insem., 4:617, 1964.

11. Ulberg, L. C. and Burfening, P. J.: Embryo death resulting from adverse environment on spermatozoa or ova. J. Anim. Sci., 26:571, 1967.

Genital Surgery of the Bull

DONALD F. WALKER
Auburn University, Auburn, Alabama

HEMATOMA OF THE PENIS

The term "hematoma of the penis" would ordinarily indicate that any situation resulting in blood being trapped in or around the penis fits this diagnosis. However, by general understanding and usage, the condition is much more specific and refers to a rent that occurs in the tunica albuginea as the result of a breeding accident that lets the blood, normally encased in the corpus cavernosum penis (CCP) under the high pressure of erection, explode into the surrounding tissues of the penis. The term "rupture of the tunica albuginea" would be a more accurate diagnosis for the malady, as considered in the following writing.

Rupture of the tunic occurs in all breeds of bulls with moderate frequency and with little predisposition. The accident is believed to occur at the time of the breeding lunge. When the penis is improperly inserted into the vagina or meets an unnatural obstruction, severe downward bending of the penis and consequent tearing of the tunica albuginea are produced. This tear almost invariably occurs on the dorsum of the penis at the distal flexure. At the time of the breeding lunge the pressure in the penis is normally greater than 10,000 mm of mercury (200 pounds per square inch). With this in mind, the damage to the tissues surrounding the penis when the rupture occurs is quite understandable. The CCP is not filled with blood in the bovine except during erection. Consequently, it does not continue to bleed following the rupture, and the volume of blood in the hematoma depends upon successive attempts at coitus following the original rupture.

Diagnosis

Hematoma of the penis is characterized by a large, firm swelling just anterior to the scrotum. Frequently there is a prolapse of the prepuce, which tends to confuse the diagnosis. The prolapse results from the compression of the lymphatic and venous drainage by the hematoma. The prepuce and the sheath are often discolored and blotchy, particularly during the first week (Fig. 1). The prepuce may become contused and lacerated secondarily.

Diagnosis is chiefly based upon palpation. The firm hematoma is noted to surround the penis uniformly, and the distal flexure is indistinguishable. Swelling as a result of preputial laceration is located more anteriorly and is soft in the phlegmonous state. In cases of abscessation following preputial laceration, the swelling is usually fluctuant and located off to one side, separate from the body of the penis. Paracentesis is to be avoided as a diagnostic procedure, as it may provide a means of contaminating the hematoma.

Conservative Treatment

Spontaneous resorption of the hematoma and healing of the tunica albuginea occur in many of the cases following supportive treatment. The indication for surgical procedure and the factors involved in making the decision to operate or to take the conservative course will be discussed later. In the course of natural healing, a vesicular bed forms around the hematoma. This is accompanied by a moderate amount of fibrosis of the elastic tissue, which has been mutilated at the time of the trauma. There is a remod-

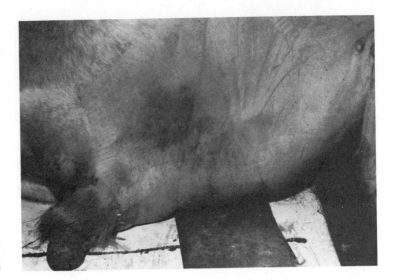

Figure 1. Hematoma of the penis with secondary preputial prolapse and blotchy cutaneous discoloration of the sheath. (From Walker, D. F. and Vaughan, J. T.: Bovine and Equine Urogenital Surgery. Philadelphia, Lea & Febiger, 1980.)

eling of the torn edges of the tunica albuginea, and granulation tissue is present until healing occurs. Forced movement of the tissue by sexual stimulation during the first 3 weeks tends to promote fibrosis and retard the normal healing process. Therefore, complete removal from sexual excitement is advised for a period of 30 days. This is contrary to earlier opinions that advocated keeping the bull with an estrogenized cow to provide exercise and prevent adhesions.

The healing process may require 60 to 90 days, depending upon the size of the hematoma and the nature of the tear in the tunic. Moderate exercise by manual extension of the penis can be done after 30 days. This is not mandatory, as most bulls will exercise the penis of their own accord. The area of fibrosis in the vicinity of the distal flexure may persist for several months, which may keep the bull from copulating normally (Fig. 2A). This fibrosis is often misinterpreted as being adhesions (Fig. 2B). Patience and understanding must be instilled in the client at the onset when dealing with hematoma of the penis.

The suggested regimen for conservative treatment is as follows: Remove the bull from the herd and isolate him from animals that might produce sexual stimulation. The hematoma and debilitated tissue provide excellent media for metastatic infection and consequent abscess formation. Therefore, administer antibiotics for 1 week following the original rupture. The use of proteolytic enzymes to aid in the reduction of the hematoma is of controversial value. Those opposed to their usage do not believe that

enough benefit is derived to justify the expense. The use of hot packs, water sprays and ultrasound therapy tends to shorten the resorption time of the hematoma, but these also increase the amount of fibrosis in the damaged tissue with the ultimate return to service being immaterially affected.

Thirty days after occurrence manually extend the penis. Note the sensation of the free portion of the penis. If bilateral nerve damage has occurred, it can be ascertained at this time. Test the sensation by pinching the penis or by using electrical shock. Lack of sensation at this time indicates that bilateral nerve damage has occurred and that the bull will not be able to breed, nor will he serve the artificial vagina with no sensation to stimulate ejaculation. Earlier attempts to determine complete nerve damage may be misleading. Palpation of the damaged area and the ability to extend the penis at this time indicate the remaining time required for the bull to copulate.

Surgical Procedure

The ideal time for surgical procedure is about 5 days after occurrence. By this time the tissue has recovered from the original shock and the healing process is beginning, but the vascularity and granulation tissue are at a minimum. When surgical repair is delayed beyond 10 days, exteriorization of the penis becomes more difficult, as does exposure of the rent in the tunica albuginea. Place the bull on antibiotic therapy as soon as possible prior to surgery. In cases of prolapse of the prepuce, place a tube in the

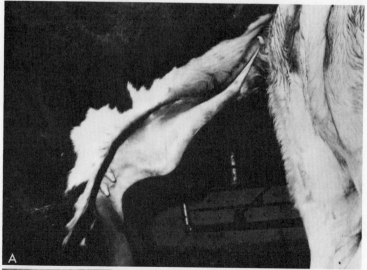
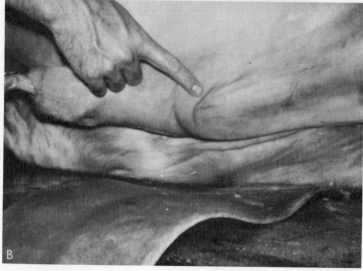

Figure 2. Incomplete penile extension following hematoma. *A*, Incomplete extension due to fibrosis at the distal flexure of the penis following hematoma of the penis. *B*, Adhesions of the elastic tissue of the penis to the subcutaneous tissue. (*B* from Walker, D. F. and Vaughan, J. T.: Bovine and Equine Urogenital Surgery. Philadelphia, Lea & Febiger, 1980.)

prepuce and wrap it with elastic tape, as described in the section on preputial prolapse.

Remove the bull from feed and water 48 hours prior to repair, in preparation for general anesthesia. It is possible to do the operation under tranquilization and infiltration analgesia, but asepsis and delicate dissection down to the ruptured tunic can both be accomplished much more easily under a general anesthetic. Table the bull on his right side. Administer gas anesthesia and elevate the left leg to give adequate exposure to the surgical site.

Prepare the surgical site on the left side of the penis well into the inguinal area. Drape the site, leaving the oblique section just anterior to the rudimentary teats for the skin incision, which should be about 20 cm long on an oblique line over the hematoma, ending at the midline. Such an incision gives maximum exposure to the hematoma and allows exteriorization of the distal flexure of the penis. Deepen the incision through the subcutis until the dark-colored hematoma is visible, without actually cutting into it (Fig. 3*A*). Control all subcutaneous bleeders and apply towels to the wound edge in the usual manner. With a scalpel incise the final layers of the tissue into the hematoma.

Manually remove the hematoma from around the penis (Fig. 3*B*). At this time do not try to remove the portions of the hematoma trapped in the tissue. Exteriorize the penis through the surgical wound (Fig. 3*C*). Some difficulty may be encountered owing to that portion of the hematoma trapped in the elastic layers. Success is achieved with care and perseverance. Note the retractor penis muscle as it becomes adjacent to the penis. This marks the ventral side of the penis and the ventral portion of the distal flexure. The rent in the tunica albuginea is located on the dorsum of the penis at the distal flexure. Carefully dissect through the layers of the elastic tissue of the penis on the dorsal midline. Note the vessels and nerves in the deepest layer (Fig. 3D). Identify these and cut between them, exposing the tunic and the rent. Pay particular attention to the dorsal nerves. Reflect them along with the deepest layers of the elastic laminae to either side, fully exposing the rent. Debride the torn edges of the rent with a scalpel (Fig. 3E).

Close the tunica albuginea with synthetic No. 1 gut (Dexon), using a simple continuous or bootlace pattern (Fig. 3F). Make sure that the edges of the tunic are in tight apposition. Remove any frayed edges of the elastic la-

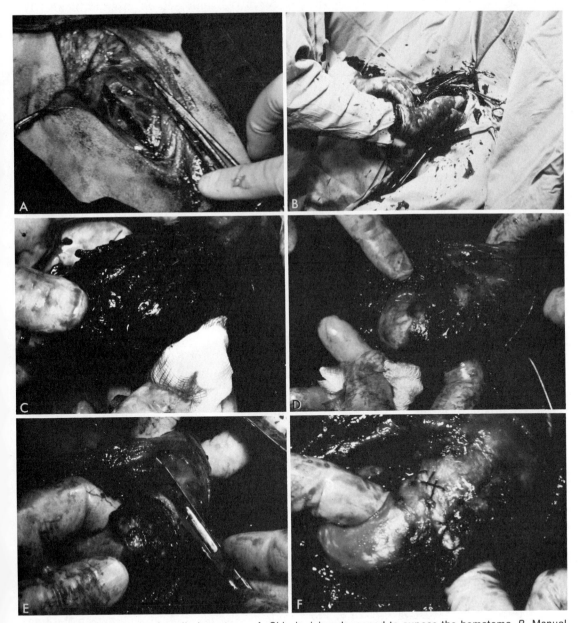

Figure 3. Surgical repair of penile hematoma. A, Skin incision deepened to expose the hematoma. B, Manual removal of the hematoma. C, Exteriorization of the penis and blood-filled layers of the elastic tissue. D, Exposure of the rent in the tunica albuginea and reflection of the dorsal vessels and nerves. E, Débridement of the edge of the rent. F, Bootlace sutures in place in the tunic bringing the edges into tight apposition.

minae and remove all loosened portions of the entrapped hematoma; then close with a few interrupted 00 gut sutures. Return the penis to its normal position, and flush the cavity with tepid (43°C) saline containing a 10 per cent povidone iodine (Betadine) solution. This process flushes out many of the small fragments of the broken-down hematoma and controls seeping hemorrhage. At this time instruct an assistant to grasp the free portion of the penis and extend it to the maximum with firm traction. Close the subcutaneous tissue with 0 gut suture; then close the skin with a nonabsorbable suture.

Postoperatively, administer injectable antibiotics for 5 days. Keep the bull from sexual excitement for 30 days. Remove skin sutures on the tenth day. Some swelling may occur shortly after the surgical repair as the space formerly occupied by the hematoma fills with serum. Attempts to prevent this by installing drains usually lead to eventual contamination and abscess formation. The seroma is regressing by the tenth day. After 30 days manually extend the penis and check the sensitivity, as previously described. Return the bull to service 60 days following surgery.

Complications

Several complications may arise either in the surgically or the conservatively handled cases. These include abscessation, adhesions, nerve damage, shunt formation and recurrence. Prevention of abscessation has been previously mentioned. Abscesses ultimately terminate as extensive adhesions. The ability to repair these adhesions depends upon the amount of destruction that they have produced in the elastic layers.

Adhesions may also occur along the retractor penis muscles when their sheaths have been severely damaged. Minor adhesions are often self-corrected. Some temporary swellings may occur as a result of breakdown of adhesions when the bull is put back into service. This must be differentiated from recurrence.

Latent nerve damage may occur. The bull may have had several successful breeding attempts and then develop an analgesia of the penis. The normal tortuous tracks of the nerves may lose their elasticity and thus become torn in the thrust of breeding. For this reason a delay in return to service is advisable in very valuable animals to permit complete reorganization of the tissue.

The subject of shunt formation will be discussed under that specific heading.

Recurrence of the hematoma is common. This may be due to the aggressive breeding habits of the bull or may result from poor healing of the tunica albuginea. Fewer cases of recurrence are noted when proper surgical closure of the tunica has been performed.

Surgical Indication

The decision to operate or to take the conservative approach is often difficult. The magnitude of the hematoma does not reflect the damage done to the tunica albuginea, but naturally those with large swellings will be longer in the resorbing process unless surgically treated. In cases with prolapse of the prepuce, correction provides a faster recovery. The chief concerns are often nonpathological. The availability of equipment for aseptic surgery is a factor.

The value of the bull must be sufficient to warrant the surgical expense, bearing in mind the surgical advantages, which are shorter recovery period, less likelihood of recurrence and less likelihood of shunt formation. Surgical repair is the best approach to the recurring case. When surgery is done, it is not simply to remove the hematoma. The primary objective is to form a neat closure of the torn tunica albuginea.

DEVIATIONS OF THE PENIS

Deviations of the penis can occur as a result of trauma to either the prepuce or the penis with subsequent scar formation, but the most common deviations occur spontaneously and insidiously as a result of a problem basically stemming from the apical ligament of the penis. These latter types will be considered in the following writing.

The apical ligament of the bovine penis originates from fibers issuing from the midline of the tunica albuginea on the dorsum about 25 cm from the distal tip. These fibers fan out over the penis and encase the distal extremity. In a mature bull, the ligament is about 3 mm thick in its central portion. It has a firm attachment near the ventral portion on the left side but has a very loose attachment on the right side. There is an interposing layer of fascia between the ligament and the tunic, more marked in the proximal portion. The apparent physiological purpose of the apical ligament is to ele-

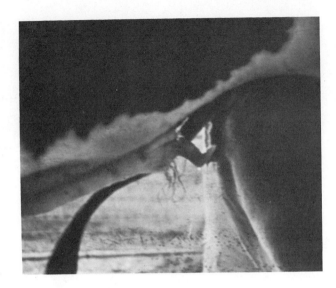

Figure 4. Spiral deviation of the penis.

vate the distal portion of the penis and hold it straight during erection. When the apical ligament is experimentally cut, the erected penis bends down sharply and to the right.

Diagnosis

Spiral deviation is evident during erection when the ligament slips off to the left side of the penis, giving it a left-handed corkscrew appearance. This phenomenon can be observed in normal bulls during masturbation, occurring with full engorgement and extension of the penis. By using a transparent artificial vagina, the deviation can be seen in many bulls at the time of the ejaculatory lunge. When the cause is pathological, the penis spirals before the entrance thrust into the vagina can be attempted (Fig. 4). Once the condition begins, it becomes progressive-

ly worse. It is not uncommon to have the malady occur before the penis clears the prepuce in advanced cases. Spiral deviation of the penis is frequently observed when ejaculation is produced by the electroejaculator, but this does not necessarily indicate that the penis will deviate during normal coitus. Diagnosis of spiral deviation should not be based on this observation alone. The electroejaculator offers a means by which the penis can be studied during erection once the malady has been discovered during normal breeding.

Ventral deviations occur when the apical ligament is insufficient and does not hold the penis straight during erection (Fig. 5). Cavernosal shunts result in an incomplete erection, which may be confused with ventral deviations (Fig. 6), and a differential diagnosis must be made between the two by

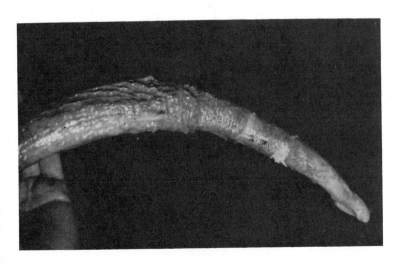

Figure 5. Ventral deviation of the penis.

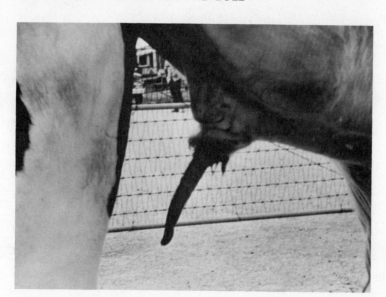

Figure 6. Flaccid penis caused by cavernosal venal shunt. (From Walker, D. F. and Vaughan, J. T.: Bovine and Equine Urogenital Surgery. Philadelphia, Lea & Febiger, 1980.)

careful observation during breeding or with the electroejaculator. When the problem is due to a shunt, the penis is somewhat flaccid. A more exacting diagnosis can be made with a cavernosogram. Palpation reveals a thin apical ligament that can be detected with experience.

Surgical Procedure

Several surgical techniques have been performed to correct penile deviations. Only two will be discussed. The first is the use of strips harvested from the apical ligament and implanted to fix the ligament to the dorsum of the penis, thereby preventing the spiral deviation. The second technique utilizes fascia lata, which is planted between the apical ligament and the tunica albuginea. This latter method is used primarily for ventral deviation, as the fascia adds support to the apical ligament. It is also the current choice for correcting spiral deviations. However, the procedure is more time-consuming and necessitates a second incision to obtain the fascia. On two known occasions cavernosal venal shunts have formed when the strip technique was done, but in spite of this, the surgeon may wish to employ this method because of its simplicity.

Strip Technique. When using the strip technique, withhold feed and water for 48 hours prior to the surgical procedure. Table the bull on his right side, clip the preputial hairs, manually extend the penis and thoroughly scrub it and the prepuce. Either gas anesthesia or local block may be used. If possible, avoid tranquilizers, as the penis may protrude from the sheath following surgery, subjecting the incision to contamination or trauma. For a local block inject 5 ml of Xylocaine (Lidocaine) across the dorsum at the preputial orifice while extending the penis. This is approximately 30 cm posterior to the glans penis. The dorsal nerves lie just superior to the tunica albuginea and supply sensation to the free portion of the penis and the prepuce. Scrub the surgical site and inject the analgesic agent while holding the penis in extension with towel forceps in the tip of the tunica albuginea, carefully avoiding the corpus spongiosum penis and the urethra (Fig. 7). Drape the area and replace the forceps with a sterile pair.

Incise the dorsum of the penis on the midline from a point 3 cm distal to the tip, extending the incision proximally for 20 cm through the skin. Continue through the subcutaneous tissue and through the free portion and the elastic layers in that part of the incision that involves the prepuce until the white fibrous apical ligament is exposed. Visually examine the ligament and determine the center of the fan-like fibers, which frequently has been displaced to the left side of the penis. Make an incision through the midline of the apical ligament without regard to the exact dorsum of the penis (Fig. 8*A*). Begin at the plane of loose fascia separating the ligament and the tunic; then extend the incision in both directions to the attachments. Avoid cutting across the fibers. Remove the loose areolar tissue, covering the tunica albuginea on the dorsum of

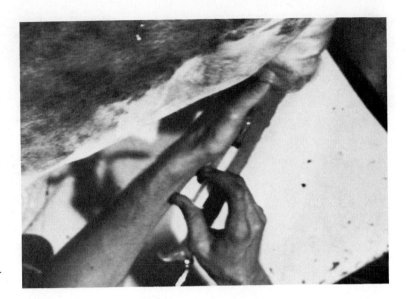

Figure 7. Technique for blocking dorsal nerves of the penis.

the penis by curettement or dissection to insure adhesions of the ligament through the tunica.

Cut a 2-mm thick strip from each edge of the apical ligament produced by the incision (Fig. 8B). Begin at the distal end and leave the strips attached to the proximal end. Now close the incision and the apical ligament with No. 0 chromic gut (Fig. 8C). An important step in the surgical procedure is to be sure that the central portion of the apical ligament is over the exact midline of the penis. Fix it in this position by catching the superficial portion of the tunic with some of the sutures. To accomplish this when the ligament has been shifted to the left, pull the ligament to the right as far as necessary. These stay sutures must hold only until the strips are implanted and are not intended as permanent fixation. Examine the strips and remove any fascia that might carry blood vessels. It is currently hypothesized that vessels carried into the CCP at the time of implanting the strips become functional and lead to the cavernosal venal shunts that have been observed on rare occasions.

Thread one of the strips into a large-eyed, full-curved needle at a point 1 cm lateral to the attached end of the strip. Pass the needle through the apical ligament into the tunic and back through the ligament in a direction parallel to the long axis of the penis (Fig. 8D). Care must be taken to reflect the exposed elastic layers of the prepuce laterally to exclude them. This process is repeated at 2-cm intervals until the entire strip has been implanted, ending as close to the tip of the penis as possible. Apply a pair of hemostatic forceps to the end of the strip while the companion strip is being implanted in a similar manner. Now, while applying traction to the strips to assure their tautness, transfix them together with No. 0 chromic gut. Secure the resulting tag ends of the strip to the apical ligament with the same suture material.

Accomplish closure of the area by first suturing the deepest elastic layers of the prepuce with No. 000 gut, using a continuous pattern (Fig. 8E); then close the epithelium of the prepuce and penis with simple sutures of No. 0 gut. In this last closure place the first suture at the juncture of the free portion of the penis and the prepuce; then work in both directions with sutures placed about 4 mm apart. Apply liquid nitrofurazone (Furacin) to the penis (Fig. 8F) and return it to its normal retracted position. No aftercare is necessary. In 10 days extend the penis for examination and removal of sutures. Keep the bull sexually quiet for 30 days before he makes a breeding attempt.

Fascia Lata Implant Technique. When executing the fascia lata implant for ventral deviations or as an alternate approach for spiral deviation, prepare the bull and the penis as described for the strip technique. A gas anesthesia is preferred, as the procedure requires a longer period of time and there are two surgical sites. In addition, shave and surgically prepare a site proximal to the patella for harvesting the fascia lata. Make an incision through the skin and superficial fascia lata laterally

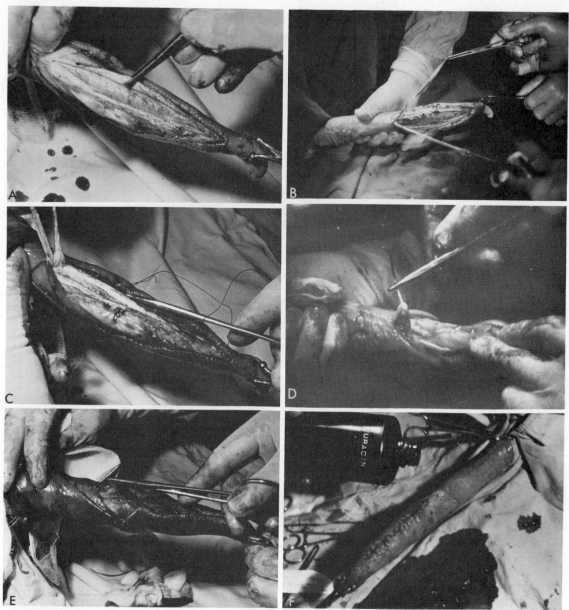

Figure 8. Technique for correction of spiral deviation. *A*, Incision through the apical ligament exposing the tunica albuginea. *B*, Strip cut from edge of the apical ligament. *C*, Closure of the apical ligament. *D*, Implantation of the strip into the tunica albuginea. *E*, Closure of the skin with interrupted sutures. *F*, Complete closure, medication in process. (*A* and *C* from Walker, D. F. and Vaughan, J. T.: Bovine and Equine Urogenital Surgery. Philadelphia, Lea & Febiger, 1980.)

over the vastus lateralis muscle about 15 cm long, starting about 5 cm above the patella and running in the direction of the tuber coxa (Fig. 9*A*). Superficial fascia lata is not used because it is too thin and a much thicker material is available from the deep layer covering the vastus lateralis. Remove a rectangular portion about 12 cm long and 2 cm wide and place this in a normal saline bath until the implantation site has been prepared. Close the wound in the fascia lata of

the vastus lateralis with No. 1 Dexon. Use the same material to close the incision in the superficial layer. Now close the skin wound with a cutaneous interlocking pattern of 0.6-mm Vetafil or similar nonabsorbable suture.

Incise the skin and apical ligament of the penis down to the tunica albuginea as described in the foregoing procedure. Dissect the apical ligament free from the tunic laterally in each direction from the middorsal line about 1.5 cm (Fig. 9*B*). Be aware of two rather large veins on the right ventral portion of the penis that are the exhaust veins of the corpus spongiosum and must not be cut. They will not be encountered unless the dissection is carried too far around the penis on the right side. The dorsum of the penis is now ready for the fascia lata overlay. Remove the overlay from the saline bath and dissect away any fragment of muscle or loose fascia that might be present (Fig. 9C). With No. 0 Dexon, suture it into place on the tunica albuginea, stretching it in all directions and trimming it to fit. Specifically, anchor the proximal edge first with four interrupted sutures as far up under the apical ligament as possible (Fig. 9D). Place four sutures on the distal end, keeping it under tension. Suture laterally along the edge at 1-cm intervals. Close the apical ligament over the fascia patch with No. 0 Dexon; then close the elastic tissue and the skin as previously described.

Aftercare is minimal. Do not allow the bull to breed for 60 days. In experimental cases in which this technique was employed, the patch was well implanted in 2 weeks and by 2 months was well blended with both the apical ligament and the tunica albuginea. The use of synthetic material for the patch has often resulted in rejection. Fascia lata is far superior. Currently under study is the use of fascia recovered from cadavers stored in 70 per cent alcohol or frozen. This has not been used extensively enough to recommend it at the present time, but it makes an operation much more appealing to the client, as the wound over the vastus lateralis is unnecessary.

PENILE PAPILLOMATOSIS

Penile papillomatosis is a condition commonly observed in young bulls reared together. Papillomas often persist until the bull becomes of breeding age, at which time they present a copulatory and fertility problem. Papillomas are usually located on the free portion of the penis and rarely on the prepuce (Fig. 10). They are generally of a subepithelial nature and are covered with epithelium when they become chronic.

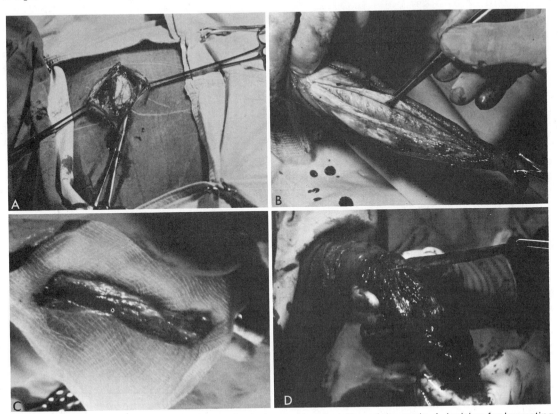

Figure 9. Fascia lata implant for correction of spiral or ventral deviation of the penis. *A*, Incision for harvesting fascia lata. *B*, Apical ligament incised. *C*, Fascia lata cleaned, ready for implant. *D*, Fascia lata sutured at proximal end. (*B* and *C* from Walker, D. F. and Vaughan, J. T.: Bovine and Equine Urogenital Surgery. Philadelphia, Lea & Febiger, 1980.)

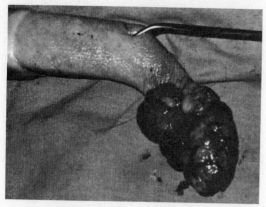

Figure 10. Penile papillomatosis.

When this happens, they become permanent and do not desquamate, as do papillomas on the body surface. In some cases they become so massive that the penis cannot be extended through the preputial orifice.

Etiology and Transmission

The condition is caused by a host-specific papovavirus. It is spread to the penis of a young bull from other bulls that develop body warts on the neck and shoulder region, and particularly from those that develop them around the tailhead. The bull becomes infected by riding warty animals in a homosexual manner.

Diagnosis

Papillomatosis of the penis is usually called to the client's attention by hemorrhage from the prepuce. This may be observed in the young bull but is more common after the bull is turned with the cows. Frequently it is first noticed when breeding soundness examinations are made on bulls prior to sale or service. Diagnosis is confirmed by visual examination and identification of the characteristic warty growth on the free portion of the penis. True neoplasms of the penis have never been observed by the author. On occasion, chronic forms may be completely epithelialized, leaving a pendulous mass attached to the penis. These have been mistakenly identified as biphallus.

Treatment and Surgical Procedure

The simple administration of wart vaccine generally fails to bring about a spontaneous regression. This is probably due to the protection that these growths receive in the pre-

putial cavity, and, consequently, they do not desquamate in the manner that they do on the body of the animal. At least the regression is so slow that from a practical standpoint surgical removal is indicated in order to put the bull into service at a reasonable time. Wart vaccines should be administered at the time of surgery to aid in the prevention of other warts developing afterwards. The surgical procedure is very simple and should be done with a cutting instrument rather than with cautery or cryosurgical techniques that leave slow-healing wounds. The operation can be complicated when the base of the papilloma is near the urethra, requiring care not to open the urethra and produce a fistula. Table restraint is more convenient for the surgeon, but the procedure can be done in the chute.

Manually extend the penis and secure it with towel forceps placed in the terminal portion of the tunica albuginea. Produce analgesia by blocking the dorsal nerves of the penis with 5 ml of Lidocaine placed across the dorsum of the penis and on the tunica albuginea at the level of the preputial orifice. The subcutaneous ringblock proximal to the papilloma is satisfactory. Remove the pendulous papilloma by cutting at its base with a pair of surgical scissors. Remove a small portion of the epithelium at the base and pick up and ligate significant bleeders. Close the opening in the epithelium with No. 0 gut. Apply liquid Furacin to the area and return the penis to its retracted position. Administer wart vaccine. The bull will be ready for use in 3 weeks. Because of the use of gut sutures, no further care is required.

PERSISTENT FRENULUM

Persistent frenulum is an inherited congenital anomaly of bulls, characterized by an attachment of the prepuce to the free portion of the penis along the ventral median raphe (Fig. 11). The attachments may be singular or multiple. It is observed chiefly in Angus and Shorthorn cattle or in their crossbreeds. Persistent frenulum produces an inability to breed in most bulls, except the crossbreeds of Bos Indicus cattle such as Santa Gertrudis and Brangus, if the prepuce is of sufficient length to permit full extension without deviation when the attachment is present. In these animals the attachment is occasionally torn loose on breeding.

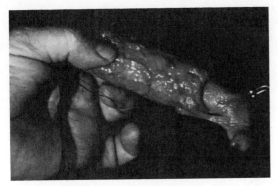

Figure 11. Persistent frenulum.

Surgically the attachment can be cut very simply. On occasion the tissue band may carry blood vessels large enough to require ligation. The basic preparation and procedure are similar to those described for papillomatosis.

CAVERNOSAL VENAL SHUNTS

Cavernosal venal shunts are vessel connections between the corpus cavernosum penis and the exterior circulation of the penis. They may exist as shunts between the corpus cavernosum penis and the corpus spongiosum penis on rare occasions. When they exist in sufficient magnitude, they cause an inability to erect the penis. Cavernosal venal shunts can be congenital or traumatic in origin. The corpus cavernosum penis is normally a closed system in which the blood that produces erection enters the spongy bulbs of the crus of the penis and is pumped into the corpus cavernosum penis by the ischiocavernosus penis muscle to a normal erection pressure of 200 to 400 pounds per square inch (10,000 to 20,000 mm of mercury). Upon relaxation the blood passes back out through the same vessels to the general circulation.

The erection blood system is entirely independent of the nutritional systems. It is also independent of the system associated with the corpus spongiosum penis. The congenital shunts are believed to occur when the nutrient vessels in the distal portion of the penis become confluent with the spaces in the corpus cavernosum. The shunts may be insufficient in size in young bulls to prevent a certain amount of erection, but they apparently become larger as time passes, making it impossible for sufficient pressure to develop for erection. The heritability of this anomaly is unknown at the present time. Bulls with the anomaly have been known to have had a few successful copulations early in life.

Traumatic shunts occasionally develop when the tunica albuginea is damaged, exposing the corpus cavernosum penis. Known examples are hematoma of the penis and lacerations of the penis. Such shunts have also been observed following the surgical procedure for deviation of the penis, when tissue strips or nonabsorbable sutures were placed completely through the tunic. Traumatic shunts respond more favorably to surgery than congenital shunts, as they represent a specific area that can be located, removed and closed well. Congenital shunts are often multiple and occur over a large area of the penis, making it difficult to locate all the leaks.

Diagnosis

A complaint of the client is that the bull is unable to copulate. Symptoms to be considered in the differential diagnosis are juvenility, ventral deviations, thrombosis of the corpus cavernosum, fibrosis of the retractor penis muscles, penile adhesions and penile analgesia. The final diagnosis is made by cavernosogram.

A tentative diagnosis can be made by physical examination. When observing the bull in a breeding situation, the penis is usually extended but is too flaccid to reach the vulva. Flaccidity helps differentiate this disorder from ventral deviation, juvenility and penile analgesia but does not eliminate the diagnosis of thrombosis. The degree of flaccidity is difficult to assess by observation. Examination of the penis with the bull in a chute permits the testing of penile sensitivity. Hypertrophy of the superficial vessels may be evident if the condition has persisted for some time. This resembles varicose veins.

If the shunt exists in the distal portion of the penis, a severe blushing will appear when erection is produced with the electroejaculator (Fig. 12). If one grasps the penis below the preputial orifice to restrict the venous return during erection, petechial hemorrhages will occur in the epithelium that are due to subjecting the small vessels to high pressure.

To make cavernosograms, lay the bull down on his right side on the surgical table. Extend the penis and in this case hold it in

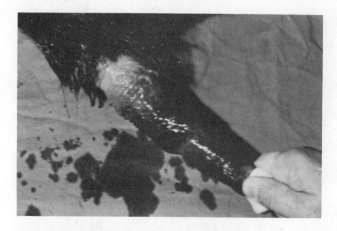

Figure 12. Superficial hemorrhage as observed when distal shunts are present.

extension by placing a towel forceps, secured to the apical ligament, near the tip rather than in the tunica albuginea. Surgically prepare the penis. In most cases in which a shunt is suspected following a hematoma of the penis, it is necessary to pull the penis away from the body as well as to extend it. To accomplish this with the penis in extension, pass a double strand of heavy Vetafil through the skin between the body of the penis and the retractor penis muscle and then through the skin on the opposite side. Tie the suture into a large loop that will serve as a handle to apply traction while taking the serial radiographs (Fig. 13A). The radiologist may choose to take a scout film at this time to be assured of proper exposure.

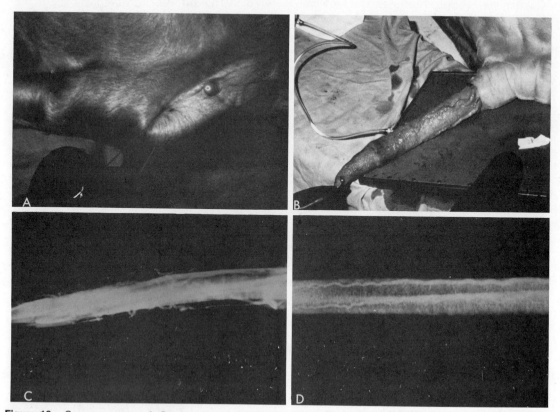

Figure 13. Cavernosogram. *A,* Suture around retractor penis muscle, allowing traction of the penis away from abdominal wall. *B,* Apparatus in place for injecting contrast media and taking radiographs. *C,* Radiograph with contrast media in the external vessels of the penis. *D,* Normal penis with smooth outline of corpus cavernosum penis; ventral canals of the penis visible. (*A* and *B* from Walker, D. F. and Vaughan, J. T.: Bovine and Equine Urogenital Surgery. Philadelphia, Lea & Febiger, 1980.)

Insert an 18-gauge needle at a 45° angle into the central portion of the CCP about 4 cm from the distal end. Attach a 10-ml syringe filled with normal saline and adjust the needle position until a free flow is established. Replace that syringe with a 30-ml syringe filled with contrast material (Conray 60). Place a Venotube-20 between the needle and the syringe to remove the surgeon from the radiation area (Fig. 13*B*).

Have four cassettes identified and ready. Place the first cassette under the penis, inject 5 ml of the contrast material and shoot as quickly as possible. While an assistant replaces the first cassette with the second, continue to inject another 15 ml. Rotate the distal end of the penis 90° and shoot again. Continue injecting up to 25 ml while the third cassette is placed as far distal as possible and the penis is pulled away from the body. This shot should include the distal flexure of the penis, which is marked by the Vetafil suture loop. Shoot as quickly as possible. Make the fourth shot after all the media has been injected. When the shunt is expected in the distal portion of the penis, all four shots can be taken in this area.

A positive diagnosis can be made if the vessels outside the tunica albuginea contain contrast material (Fig. 13*C*). The point of leakage can be roughly ascertained by comparing the radiographs. Do not be confused by the deep vessels of the penis, which are canals that lie within the CCP (Fig. 13*D*). If a shunt exists between the CCP and the corpus spongiosum penis (CSP), the CSP will demonstrate the contrast medium in a characteristic pattern. In this case the veins exterior to the penis are also evident, as there is a direct drainage into them near the distal end of the penis from the CSP. The possibility of contrast medium entering the exterior vessels after it has passed up through the normal vessels has not been investigated, but this should not present any problem when serial radiographs are taken and comparisons of directional flow are made.

Surgical Procedure

The surgical approach obviously varies according to the position of the shunt. In those that occur at the distal flexure of the penis as a result of hematoma, prepare the bull and make the skin incision to expose the penis as described for hematoma of the penis repair. The general area of the shunt is determined by palpation of a fibrous area on the dorsum of the penis (Fig. 14*A*). Carefully cut through the elastic laminae to expose this area. Open the lamellae and reflect them laterally until the vessels become visible. Inject an indicator dye, consisting of 10 per cent methylene blue solution used for nitrate poisoning and 90 per cent sterile saline solution, into the corpus cavernosum penis. Utilize the same technique as described for injecting the contrast medium for cavernosograms. As dye flows through the shunt, find the exact location of the leak (Fig. 14*B*).

Note that the leak occurs from several small vessels rather than from an isolated

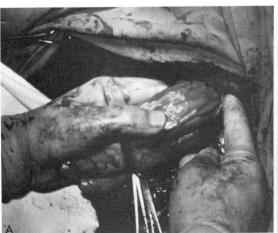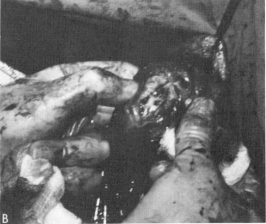

Figure 14. Surgical correction of shunt at the distal flexure of the penis. *A,* Palpation of fibrous point, indicating probable location of the shunt. *B,* Dissection carried to the tunica albuginea and dye indicating the location of the leak.

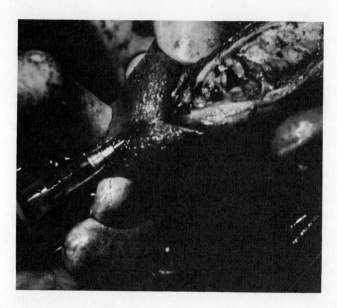

Figure 15. Reflection of the apical ligament, with dye being injected to show multiple leaks of distal shunts.

single vein. Dissect out the area stained with the dye and close the edges of the tunica albuginea with a No. 1 Dexon suture. Replace the penis in its normal position. Suture the subcutaneous tissue and then the skin in the conventional manner. The bull will be ready for a breeding attempt in about 30 days.

When shunts occur on the distal portion of the penis, they generally are under the apical ligament of the penis. Prepare the bull and make the same approach as described for correction of the ventral deviation of the penis. After reflecting the apical ligament from the tunica albuginea, inject the CCP with diluted methylene blue solution. If the shunt has originated from a single laceration, the involved area will be small. Dissect this by making a longitudinal elliptical incision through the tunica around the involved area. Close the incision tightly with No. 1 Dexon.

Congenital shunts are multiple, making it impossible to remove each one surgically (Fig. 15). Cauterize each one with a sharp-pointed electrode. Air can be used rather than methylene blue, in which case the shunts are discernible by bubbles issuing from the leaks. After all of them have been cauterized, cover the area with a patch from the fascia lata of the vastus lateralis, using the same technique employed in correction of ventral deviation. Close the apical ligament and skin in the same manner.

URETHRAL FISTULAE

Fistulae of the urethra from traumatic causes may occur on the free portion of the penis. They result in a variable degree of infertility when bulls are used for natural service, but present no problem when bulls are used for artificial insemination. Infertili-

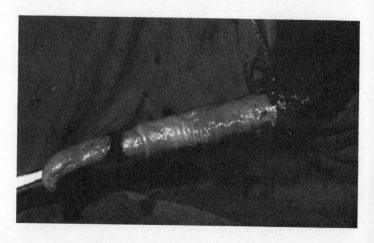

Figure 16. Penile hair ring.

ty is due to an inefficient deposition of semen to the cervical area.

The fistulae can occur from any type of trauma that causes a laceration into the lumen of the urethra. They often result from hair rings that roll up on the penis and cause a pressure necrosis to the urethral wall (Fig. 16). The degree of infertility caused by the fistula and whether or not to recommend surgical correction must be considered by the veterinarian. The decision to operate should be based upon known reduction of conception rates and by a breeding soundness examination to eliminate other possible causes for lowered fertility. The more proximal and extensive fistulae are more likely to be significant.

Surgical Procedure

Although the surgical procedure is relatively simple, urethral fistulae are very difficult to close successfully. Repeated surgical attempts are often necessary before achieving complete closure. The forceful urinary blast produced by the bulbospongiosus muscle makes it difficult to prevent leakage, and dehiscence is common. Because of the rather delicate nature of the procedure, best results are obtained when the bull is tabled.

Extend the penis, apply towel forceps, surgically scrub and administer a local block to the dorsal nerves. Note the line along which the epithelium of the penis and the mucosa

of the urethra have healed to form the fistula (Fig. 17A). Carefully separate the two tissues along this line and reflect them for a distance of 5 mm. Place a No. 12F catheter up the urethra to a point 5 cm above the fistula. First close the urethra over the catheter with simple interrupted sutures spaced 2 mm apart, utilizing 000 gut with the swaged-on, atraumatic needle; then close the epithelium with closely spaced nonabsorbable sutures and remove the catheter (Fig. 17B). The purpose of the catheter was to function as a stint during the closure, and it does not materially aid the healing process (Fig. 17C). Examine the penis in 10 days to determine the efficacy of the correction.

PREPUTIAL PROBLEMS

Preputial problems of the bull are primarily of traumatic origin. The major exception is a balanoposthitis produced by the infectious bovine rhinotracheitis (IBR) virus (Fig. 18). It presents many typical manifestations due to the anatomical variations, severity and type of trauma, depth of laceration, virulence of contaminating organisms and duration before treatment. The anatomical variations are the pendulous sheath found in Bos Indicus breeds and their crosses and the eversion of the prepuce in animals with incomplete or missing retractor prepuce muscles.

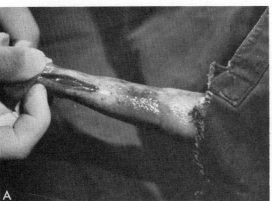

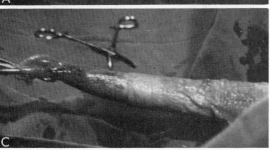

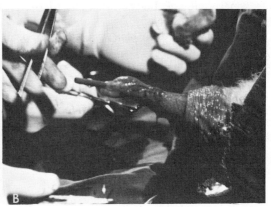

Figure 17. Urethral fistula and its surgical closure. *A*, Original fistula; note line of demarcation between penile epithelium and urethral mucosa. *B*, Closure of the urethral mucosa completed and closure of the penile skin in progress. *C*, Completed closure, after which the catheter will be removed.

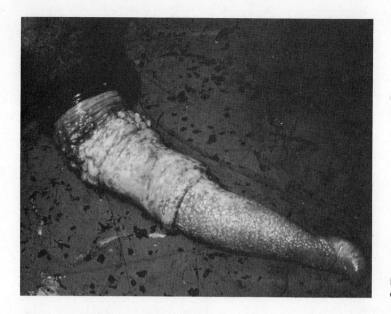

Figure 18. Balanoposthitis produced by IBR virus.

Preputial Lacerations

Lacerations of the prepuce are the most common malady affecting the genitals of bulls. The exact etiology of the lacerations is not entirely clear. An increase in incidence has been noted in bulls breeding in brushy pastures, leading to the conclusion that lacerations occur from dragging the extended prepuce through rough material. Preputial lacerations have been observed occurring during coitus.

Most lacerations are longitudinal and on the ventral side of the prepuce. The fact that some bulls with poorly developed retractor prepuce muscles tend to evert the prepuce does not particularly predispose them to the deep longitudinal lacerations. This does affect the prognosis in secondary manifestations of the trauma, however. These bulls are much more subject to contusions of the prepuce and balanoposthitis, which occur secondarily to minor trauma.

Anatomy of the Prepuce

When the penis is in its nonextended position, the preputial cavity is formed. The sheath is the external hair-covered portion and the prepuce is the denuded epithelial tube extending from its junction with the sheath at the preputial orifice posteriorly to its attachment to the penis, leaving the free portion of the penis extending into the preputial cavity.

Surrounding the prepuce and separating it from the sheath are a series of thin, elastic laminae. These laminae continue posteriorly over the penis to their origin in the inguinal area. The precise manner in which these elastic layers function in extension and retraction of the penis is not well understood. In general, these layers undergo both compression and extension, as well as lineal folding during the process. Consequently, damage to them at the time of laceration is of major importance in the prognosis and healing time required before the bull is again serviceable.

The protractor prepuce muscles originate near the umbilicus as slips from cutaneous trunci muscles. They circumscribe the preputial orifice and attach to the skin of the sheath. Their primary purpose is to serve as a constrictor of the preputial orifice rather than to pull the prepuce forward as the name implies.

The retractor prepuce muscles originate in the inguinal area from a divided attachment, both medial and lateral to the cord. They pass anteriorly as well-defined muscle bodies to their interlacing attachment into the elastic layers of the prepuce over an area of about 8 cm just posterior to the preputial orifice. They do, in fact, bring about a retraction of the anterior portion of the prepuce, but complete retraction of the prepuce is dependent upon the elastic nature of the laminae surrounding the prepuce and, to a greater extent, upon the contractions of the retractor penis muscle.

Contraction of the protractor prepuce

muscle also augments a closure of the preputial orifice, along with the retractor prepuce muscles. Their common action also tends to elevate the sheath.

An inherited congenital modification of the retractor prepuce muscles occurs. The modification may include a complete absence of only one muscle or a great reduction in the amount of muscle tissue present. This anomaly is associated with the poll gene of cattle and is the apparent reason that some bulls, particularly those without horns such as Angus or Polled Herefords, habitually evert the proximal portion of the prepuce when at rest (Fig. 19).

Some of the Bos Indicus breeds of cattle or their crossbreeds have pendulous sheaths. This is part of the loose hide syndrome. When trauma occurs to the prepuce, gravitational edema becomes much more pronounced and requires special care and consideration. Circumcision is often required in these animals following preputial problems.

Many lacerations of the prepuce that only involve the epithelium and do not penetrate into the elastic layers heal spontaneously. Others that involve only the superficial layers of the deep tissue will heal uneventfully if the bulls are removed from service. When the elastic tissue is exposed to microbial or urine contamination, fibrosis with loss of elasticity results. Then when erection

and extension occur, the wound widens and deepens, exposing more tissue in the process, and thereby becomes self-aggravating with repeated breeding attempts. If the lacerations extend completely through the elastic layers of the prepuce and into those surrounding the penis, a spreading of the contamination will result posteriorly when the penis is retracted. This often results in a phlegmon in varying amounts of necrosis (Fig. 20).

When necrosis occurs, the prognosis becomes grave because even after the process subsides, the tissue lost because of the necrosis results in an inability to properly extend the penis, at least for a considerable period of time. Phlegmons with necrosis become severe in cases in which urine is expressed into the tissues surrounding the prepuce.

Lacerations with prolapse of the prepuce are very common in bulls that do not have retractor prepuce muscles. When the laceration becomes visible, it appears at first glance to be transverse, but this is due to the gaping edges of the wound and the partial retraction of the prepuce (Fig. 21).

Nonsurgical Treatment of Preputial Lacerations

Fresh lacerations are seldom observed. Even when they are, it is doubtful that they should be sutured, particularly if they are

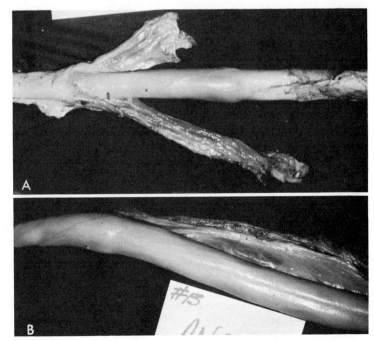

Figure 19. Difference in the development of the retractor prepuce muscles. *A*, Retractor penis muscle of a horned Hereford bull's penis. *B*, Vestiges of the retractor penis muscle of an Angus bull's penis.

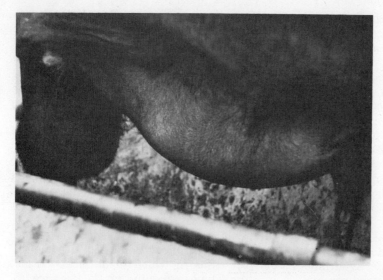

Figure 20. Phlegmon of the sheath following severe preputial laceration.

deep, because of spreading of infection or trapping of a hematoma. Treatment is aimed at prevention of necrosis, minimizing and localizing infections and eliminating latent abscess formation.

When treating bulls with lacerations in which the prepuce has returned to the normal retracted position, separate the animal from the cow herd as soon as possible to minimize self-aggravation and spread of contamination. Administer general antibiotics daily until all signs of swelling have subsided. Place the bull in a chute. Clip the preputial hairs and flush the preputial cavity with 60 ml of liquid Furacin daily (Fig. 22). After 2 or 3 days when the wound has organized, this treatment may be preceded with a hydrogen peroxide flush to assist in the removal of necrotic material. Solutions containing a proteolytic enzyme may be used. Betadine solutions are often used advantageously if organisms resistant to Furacin are present. No serious attempt should be made in the first 2 weeks to extend the penis and visually examine the laceration. It is permissible to examine the area by digital palpation, however.

The length of treatment time is variable, depending upon the severity of the laceration and the complications present. The usual case is treated for 10 days. After treatment keep the bull sexually quiet for an additional 30 days. At this time examine the penis and prepuce by manual extension. If the penis can be extended and the prepuce unfolds properly, the bull can be returned to service. If moderate stenosis is still present, it will be necessary to rest the bull for an additional time. If the prepuce has healed improperly, reconstruction can be considered at this time. If stenosis is severe, a modified circumcision may be required to remove the stenotic portion.

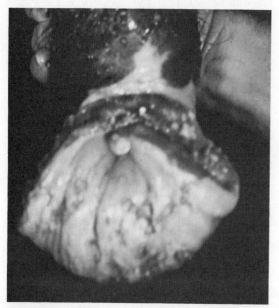

Figure 21. Longitudinal laceration of the prepuce with a prolapse depicting transverse appearance. (From Walker, D. F. and Vaughan, J. T.: Bovine and Equine Urogenital Surgery. Philadelphia, Lea & Febiger, 1980.)

Lacerations with Prolapse

Lacerations complicated by prolapse of the prepuce are common in Polled and Bos Indicus bulls. Circumcision is often indicated in the Bos Indicus bulls when there is a tenden-

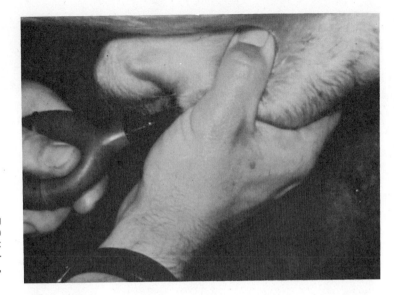

Figure 22. Technique for flushing the prepuce with medication. (From Walker, D. F. and Vaughan, J. T.: Bovine and Equine Urogenital Surgery. Philadelphia, Lea & Febiger, 1980.)

cy to develop chronic fibrosis associated with the prolapse (Fig. 23). In the Bos Tarus breeds that lack sufficient preputial length to permit circumcision, the first consideration is conservative treatment and the salvage of as much prepuce as possible. Even when circumcision is considered necessary, the preoperative treatment is conservative until all edema and infection have subsided to assure a successful termination.

Conservative Treatment. The regimen for conservative treatment is as follows: Place the bull in a chute. Clip the preputial hairs and scrub the exposed prepuce thoroughly with Betadine. Mechanically remove any debris and necrotic tissue present (Fig. 24A). Prepare a tube to put into the preputial cavity for draining urine with a 12-cm-long piece of gum rubber or plastic tubing that is 1 cm in diameter, and wrap tape around it 2 cm from one end to form an enlargement. Place this end inside the preputial cavity. Cover the exposed portion of the prepuce and the laceration with an antibiotic ointment (Fig. 24B). Then bandage securely with elastic tape (Elastikon) to completely cover the prepuce and at the same time retain the drain tube (Fig. 24C). Administer parenteral antibiotics if there is any indication that the infection has migrated proximally into the elastic tissue of the prepuce.

Rebandage and treat the lesion at 48-hour intervals until there is healthy organization of the wound (Fig. 24D). When treatment has been initiated before there is extensive damage, the prepuce can be reduced to its

normal position within a few days. It is usually advisable to keep the preputial orifice bandaged with the tube in place for several days after the prolapse has been replaced to prevent recurrence. Cases that require an operation can be repaired at this stage.

A modified surgical procedure is often adaptable to chronic cases in European breeds of cattle in which exuberant granulation tissue has developed and replacement is impossible. After conditioning the wound by bandage for a few days and eliminating in-

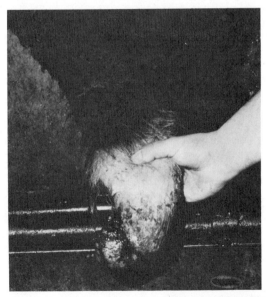

Figure 23. Laceration of the prepuce with chronic fibrosis in a Bos Indicus bull.

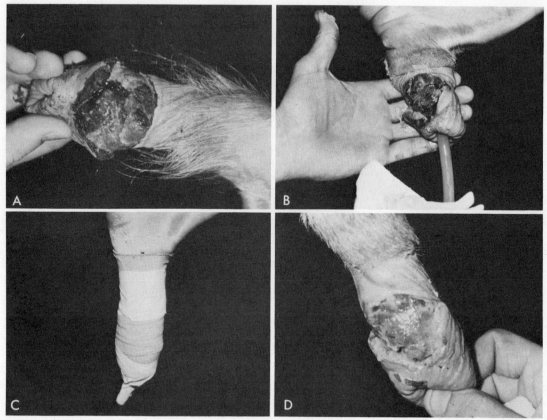

Figure 24. Nonsurgical treatment of preputial laceration with prolapse. *A,* Lesion cleaned. *B,* Lesion medicated and urine relief tube in place. *C,* Prepuce under bandage. *D,* Appearance 3 days later. (*C* from Walker, D. F. and Vaughan, J. T.: Bovine and Equine Urogenital Surgery. Philadelphia, Lea & Febiger, 1980.)

fection, debride the granulation and fibrous tissue along the wound edges sufficiently to allow replacement. Now treat the bull with ointments and close the orifice with a purse-string suture or the taping technique for 5 to 10 days.

In extremely chronic cases the wound may heal along the wrong axis, leaving a pendulous portion of prepuce (Fig. 25). The fibrosis may have disappeared and the prepuce becomes retractable. The pendulous portion may be confused with papillomatosis, but careful examination reveals a greatly shortened prepuce. The shortening may be so severe that in order to have sufficient prepuce for the bull to breed, the surgeon must use reconstructive surgery and salvage a portion of the prepuce that is in the pendulous mass. As a general criterion to making this judgment, the usable prepuce must be twice as long as the free portion of the penis.

Reconstructive Surgery. Administer general anesthesia with the bull in right lateral recumbency on the surgical table. Extend and thoroughly scrub the penis and prepuce. Examine the healed scar, which will be in the form of a cross (Fig. 26*A*). Incise through the epithelium along the transverse line of the scar and remove all

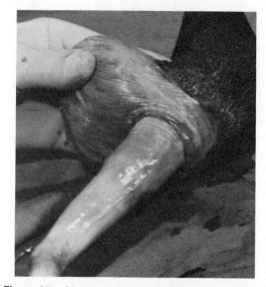

Figure 25. Chronic case of laceration of the prepuce with wound healed on the wrong axis. (From Walker, D. F. and Vaughan, J. T.: Bovine and Equine Urogenital Surgery. Philadelphia, Lea & Febiger, 1980.)

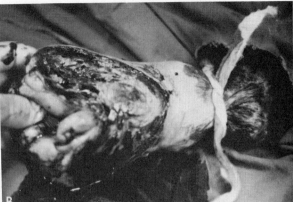

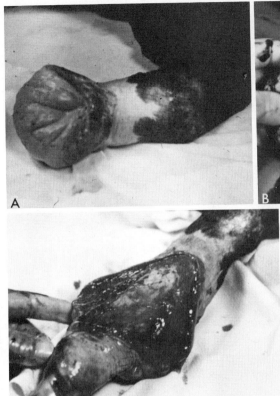

Figure 26. Reconstruction surgery of the prepuce. *A,* Prolapsed prepuce with laceration prepared for surgery. *B,* Appearance following removal of fibrous tissue. *C,* Penis extended through the prepuce to re-establish normal preputial length.

fibrous tissue present in the elastic layers of the prepuce (Fig. 26*B*). Apply tension to the free portion of the penis to gape the incision and lengthen the prepuce as much as possible. The pendulous mass should now be almost completely reduced. Carefully ligate all bleeders (Fig. 26*C*). As efficiently as possible close the elastic tunic longitudinally with a simple interrupted suture of 00 Dexon. Close the epithelium along the longitudinal axis with a bootlace pattern of 0 Dexon or No. 1 gut. A cicatricial contraction has a tendency to reduce the diameter of the prepuce.

It may be impossible to replace the penis because of the tautness of the prepuce following suturing if the closure is made with the penis in full extension. To avoid this problem, put the suture pattern in so that both free ends of the suture are at the distal end of the prepuce. Leave the sutures lax. Replace the penis into the prepuce as well as the proximal portion of the incision. Then pull the free ends of the sutures to close the incision and tie. Suture a 12-inch section of 1-inch Penrose drain to the free portion of

the penis by placing five interrupted 0 gut sutures through the drain tube, which has been placed over the distal end and skin of the penis. It may be necessary to take this step before suturing the prepuce. Trim the Penrose drain so that about 4 cm hang from the preputial orifice when the penis is in full retracted position.

It is usually unnecessary to close the preputial orifice with purse-string or tape sutures in these cases. In the event that the epithelium of the prepuce cannot be pulled completely around the penis, flush the cavity daily for 5 days with Betadine solution. Keep the bull sexually quiet for 60 days before a breeding attempt is made. Manual extension and examination may be done after 2 weeks.

Contusions of the Penis and Prepuce

Contusions of the free portion of the penis and prepuce often occur when bulls tred on the flaccid extended penis. These bulls have

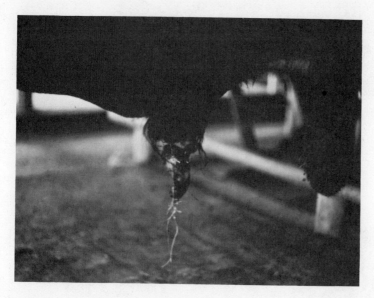

Figure 27. Contusion of the penis and prepuce.

a swollen penis in a paraphimosis position (Fig. 27). Treated conservatively they usually respond favorably.

Place the bull in a squeeze chute. Clip the preputial hairs and wash and cleanse the extended penis and prepuce. Cover the area with a protective antibiotic ointment and place a 2-inch stockinette over it, allowing this to hang 3 cm below the distal end of the penis. Wrap the penis with Elastikon tape, starting above the stockinette on the hairline. Do not cover the tip of the penis and urethral orifice distally, as these are covered with the stockinette alone.

Leave this bandage in place for 4 days. Remove it and apply ointment daily until the penis naturally retracts into the prepuce. This process usually requires about 10 days, depending upon the severity of the trauma. An excellent ointment for this purpose is prepared by melting 500 gm of lanolin and then stirring in 60 ml of scarlet oil and 2 gm of tetracycline powder.

Chronic Preputial Prolapse

Chronic preputial prolapse is a condition in which the everted prepuce has become indurated and fibrotic following lacerations or continued contusions. It is often associated with multiple small abscesses and a phimosis. Bulls that habitually evert the prepuce and those with pendulous sheaths are predisposed. Circumcision is usually indicated, particularly in the Bos Indicus breed in which the prepuce apparently hypertro-

phies in length, so that even if conservative treatment brings about relief, the condition recurs.

Circumcision

Several techniques for circumcision have evolved over the years, and the choice of procedure is often a personal matter involving the surgeon's experience and equipment and the value of the bull. The two chief surgical problems involved are hemorrhage control and postoperative stenosis (Fig. 28).

Two techniques will be discussed in this writing, the classic resection in anastomosis and a simplified technique using a plastic ring, which can be done as a field procedure. In either case the prepuce is treated and bandaged, as described under conservative treatment, for several days prior to surgery to reduce the edema, fibrosis and infection. Proper management greatly increases the prognosis and shortens the postoperative healing period.

Resection and Anastomosis. Table the bull and utilize gas anesthesia. Closely clip or shave the hair from the distal portion of the sheath and the preputial orifice. The prepuce may be somewhat stenotic, but extend the penis as far as possible with towel forceps placed in the tip of the tunica albuginea. Thoroughly scrub and prepare the entire prepuce and penis. Apply a tourniquet around the prepuce and penis proximal to the area to be resected. A section of sterile Penrose drain wrapped tightly and tied does a satisfactory job (Fig. 29A).

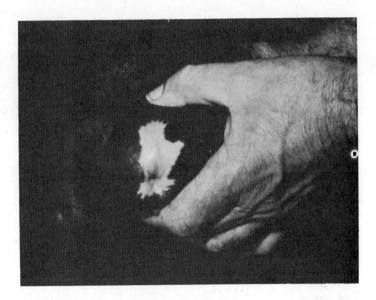

Figure 28. Preputial stenosis.

Carefully examine the portion of the prepuce to be removed. This should contain all of the pathological portion but should leave a sufficient amount of prepuce for normal function (approximately twice the length of the free portion of the penis). In Bos Indicus bulls the portion removed should be 10 to 15 cm long.

Make a circumscribing incision through the epithelium of the prepuce at the ascertained point distal to the preputial orifice. Deepen this through several layers of the elastic tissue until it has a relatively normal appearance. Do not invade the layers common to the penis. Now make the distal circumscribing incision in a similar manner. Connect the two transverse incisions with a longitudinal incision and remove the section of prepuce along their common layer of elastic tissue (Fig. 29*B*).

The major vessels can be detected by close examination without removing the tourniquet. Take up all of these with forceps and ligate with 0 gut. There will be 20 to 30 of these vessels, and the process is greatly expedited by the use of electrocautery (Fig. 29*C*). Remove the tourniquet and ligate or cauterize any bleeders that were missed. The area must be free of bleeders. Flush the area with warm saline containing 10 per cent Betadine solution to wash away fibrin clots and aid in the control of seeping hemorrhage. Extend the penis to straighten out the prepuce, and then push it back until the circumscribing incisions are in apposition.

Close the incision with two layers of suture, one in the elastic tissue and one in the epithelium. Use 0 gut with a simple interrupted pattern in the elastic layers. Place one suture at each quadrant; then fill in the area between. Again extend the penis to check its function. Close the skin of the penis with simple interrupted and mattress sutures used alternately. This process results in an edge-to-edge pattern with little interference in circulation (Fig. 29*D* and *E*). Apply a section of Penrose drain to the free portion of the penis with interrupted gut sutures to carry the urine away from the incision line during the healing period (Fig. 29*F*). Apply liquid Furacin to the penis and prepuce, and return it to its retracted position. Prevent prolapsing of the prepuce by taping the preputial orifice (Fig. 29*G*). This technique has been found superior to a purse-string suture. Some edema of the prepuce may be evident from the fifth to the fourteenth day during the healing process. When this has begun to subside, remove the tape and the Penrose drain. The suture line can be examined by digital palpation at this time, but do not make a vigorous attempt to extend the penis until the third week (Fig. 29*H*). Prevent coitus for 60 days postsurgically.

Ring Technique. Before beginning this procedure prepare a tube 5 cm long and 4 cm in diameter with 1-mm holes drilled through the wall, spaced 5 mm apart around the center. This can be prepared from polyvinyl chloride (PVC) pipe or black plastic plumber's pipe. Round the ends so that there are no sharp protrusions, and place the tube in a cold sterilization solution. It is more con-

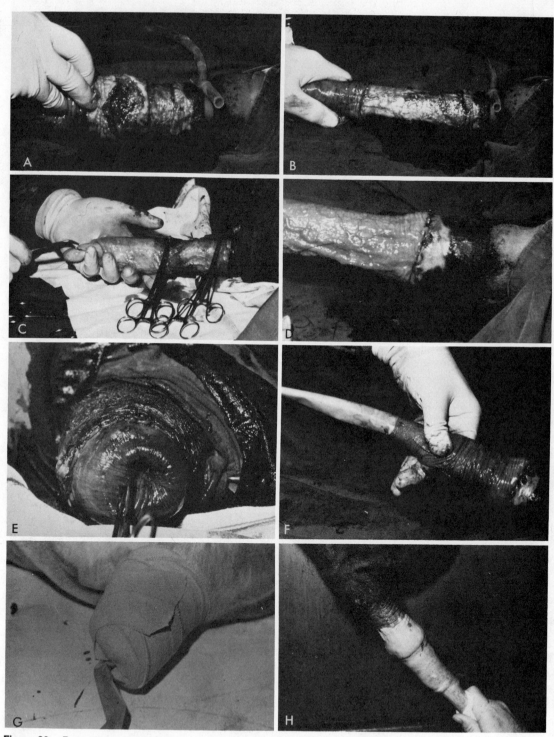

Figure 29. Resection and anastomosis of the prepuce. *A*, First circumscribing incision proximal to the pathological portion to be removed. Note tourniquet in place. *B*, Pathological portion removed. *C*, Hemorrhage controlled. *D* and *E*, Skin sutures of alternate mattress and simple interrupted pattern in place. *F*, Penrose drain in place. *G*, Preputial orifice taped to prevent prolapse. *H*, Appearance of the healed wound 30 days postsurgically. (*A*, *B*, *C*, *D*, *E*, and *H* from Walker, D. F. and Vaughan, J. T.: Bovine and Equine Urogenital Surgery. Philadelphia, Lea & Febiger, 1980.)

venient to perform this technique on a table, but it can be done with the bull cast on the ground in clean surroundings.

Accomplish anesthesia by blocking the dorsal nerves of the penis as previously described. Thoroughly wash and prepare the prepuce and penis (Fig. 30*A*).

Leave the prepuce in the prolapsed position, insert the plastic ring into the cavity and position it so that the holes in the ring are at the desired point of amputation. Thread 0.6-mm Vetafil in a 4-inch, half-curved needle without cutting it from the

roll. The Vetafil container serves the purpose of a bobbin, making it unnecessary to handle a long, awkward length of suture material. Pass the needle into the lumen of the prepuce and tube. Pass it out through one of the holes and remove it from the suture (Fig. 30*B*).

Double the suture material between the ring and the bobbin, and thread the double suture through the needle eye. Pass the needle into the lumen, locate the adjacent hole, pass it out through the prepuce and remove the needle, leaving the free end of the suture

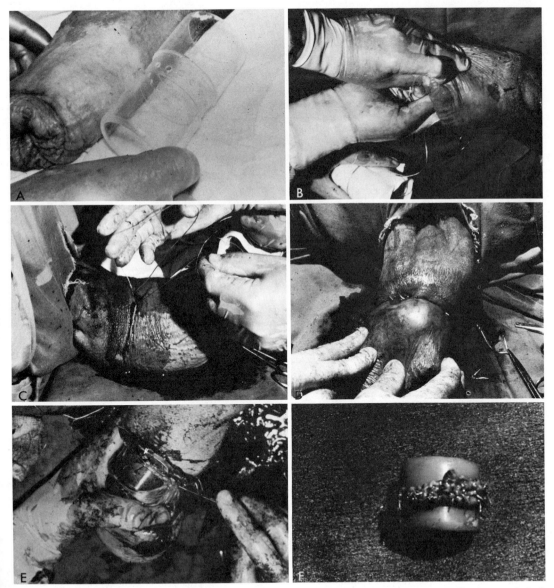

Figure 30. Ring technique for circumcision. *A*, Prepuce conditioned for surgery and plastic ring ready to be placed into the preputial cavity. *B*, Needle placed through ring and prepuce. *C*, Suturing technique. *D*, Sutures in place. *E*, Amputation of the fibrotic portion of the prepuce. *F*, Ring after removal, with necrotic tissue and sutures attached. (*B*, *C*, *D*, and *E* from Walker, D. F. and Vaughan, J. T.: Bovine and Equine Urogenital Surgery. Philadelphia, Lea & Febiger, 1980.)

and a loop (Fig. 30C). Very tightly tie the free end to the side of the loop from which it is continuous to form a ligature. Cut the simple interrupted suture above the knot, and there is now a new free end through the same hole. Repeat the process through the next hole. Continue this pattern completely around the prepuce, and overlap two holes (Fig. 30D).

Amputate the prepuce 3 mm distal to the suture line (Fig. 30E). There will be no hemorrhage if all sutures have been tightened sufficiently. Extend the end of the penis through the lumen of the tube, and attach a Penrose drain, 20 cm in length. Let the penis retract into its normal position, and flush 30 ml of liquid Furacin through the lumen of the tube. Replace the prolapsed portion of the prepuce to its retracted position, and apply elastic tape around the orifice to maintain it in this position. Trim the Penrose tube to the desired length.

Remove the tape retainer after 2 weeks, grasp the edge of the tube and withdraw it from the preputial cavity. The epithelium may not be completely healed, but by this time the sutures have necrosed through the prepuce and the tube is free. Through the holes in the tube note a ring of necrotic tissue and all the sutures in place (Fig. 30F). Leave the Penrose drain on the penis for a few more days, and flush the preputial cavity with Betadine solution or liquid Furacin.

Thirty days postsurgically, extend the penis manually. Some constriction at the site of amputation may still be present. If so, wait an additional 30 days before attempting to use the bull for breeding.

SURGICAL PREPARATION OF ESTRUS-DETECTOR BULLS

Many factors have developed in the past decade that have greatly increased the demand for aids in detection of estrus in cows. Artificial insemination has reached a high plateau of acceptability in the beef cattle industry, as well as in the dairy industry. Mechanization of livestock rearing, which removes man from contact with the animals throughout the day, and increasing herd sizes have brought about the necessity for finding means of detecting estrus other than personal observation. Increased labor costs make it very expensive to hire personnel solely for this purpose.

Mechanical devices such as heat patches are a great aid but do not provide the efficiency to satisfy the majority of breeders. Androgenized cows or steers have proved themselves to be very effective but have failed to gain popularity over bulls prepared as heat detector animals. This is probably due to the complexity of initiating and maintaining the androgenation and the failure of laymen to trust the unnatural. For these reasons the demand for estrus-detector bulls is currently at a high level.

Preparation of heat-detector bulls would be rather simple if it involved only sterilization of the bull. Popular opinion and practices also dictate that the bull's penis must not enter the vagina to prevent disease transmission and lower conception rates.

Preparation of heat-detector bulls involves some technique to prevent extension of the penis plus an epididymectomy or vasectomy as a fail-safe measure to prevent conception in the event that the technique for preventing penile extension fails. A multitude of techniques have been proposed to prevent coitus, but it is not within the scope of this article to present them all in detail. Some guidelines to aid veterinarians in their selection of a technique will be presented.

First and foremost the selected technique must be absolutely safe. In several court cases veterinarians were held liable for estrus-detector bulls that brought about conception in the cows. The technique must be as simple and inexpensive as possible and must elicit no pain afterward during the breeding attempt or the bulls will soon lose interest. It should not produce preputial stenosis to the point of urine accumulation and the eventual formation of calculi, which in turn necrose through the preputial epithelium and lead to infections. The technique must not interfere with micturition. Healing should be fast, require little or no care and leave no abnormal tissue exposed to infection. The postsurgical rest period should be as short as possible for the convenience of the client.

Surgical Procedure

Two methods will be presented. The translocation of the penis technique is currently employed on a wide scale with excellent results. The greatest objection is the involved surgical procedure. The second technique, originated by Dr. Robert Hudson and favored by the author, is based on the principle of placing an artificial thrombus in the CCP to prevent erection and is free of secondary complications.

Penile Translocation. There have been numerous modifications of this procedure. The following method locates the transplanted preputial orifice just above the flank on the left side. After selecting a vigorous, healthy, young bull, administer a heavy tranquilizer and cast or table him on his right side. Closely clip or shave and prepare the ventral area of the abdominal wall, including the preputial orifice. Also prepare an area above the fold of the left flank. Inject procaine, outlining the area to be removed above the flank as well as along the midline from the scrotum to the preputial orifice (Fig. 31*A*). Then encircle the preputial orifice with a ring block.

Remove a circular section of skin 4 cm in diameter 3 cm above the flank fold. Also remove a similar section of the cutaneous trunci muscle immediately below, exposing the abdominal tunic (Fig. 31*B*). Ligate the bleeders and cover with a surgical sponge until later.

Starting at a point on the midline 8 cm anterior to the scrotum, make a longitudinal incision through the skin to a point 2 cm from the preputial orifice (Fig. 31*C*). Make a circumscribing incision around the preputial orifice through the skin (Fig. 31*D*). Grasp the penis and surrounding elastic tissue through the longitudinal incision. By blunt dissection and traction, free the penis, prepuce and surrounding tissue from the abdominal fascia to the preputial orifice. Two large veins, one on either side (Fig. 31*E*), will be encountered at the approximate level of the posterior termination of the prepuce. Double ligate these and incise.

Continue the dissection anteriorly until the penis, prepuce and preputial orifice are completely free. A second area of hemorrhage is encountered when the prepuce is dissected free from its anterior attachment. Ligate all major bleeders (Fig. 31*F*).

With a Knowles forceps or similar instrument, force a tunnel from the flank incision through the subcutaneous tissue to a point anterior to the scrotum. With the forceps through the tunnel grasp the preputial orifice and withdraw it up the tunnel until it is exteriorized (Fig. 31*G*). Straighten out the prepuce and suture the subcutaneous tissue of the preputial orifice to the cutaneous trunci muscle by first placing an interrupted

0 gut suture at each quadrant of the circle and then filling in between with sutures. Follow this with a similar suture pattern of nonabsorbable material, closing the circular skin wound. Manually extend the penis through its new mooring to assure proper function (Fig. 31*H*).

Close the longitudinal incision with nonabsorbable, interlocking sutures, starting at the posterior portion. Some surgeons catch the fascia over the abdominal tunic with some of the sutures to prevent serum accumulation (Fig. 31*I*). Do not completely close the wound by leaving the circular portion open for drainage, and cover the surgical site with an antibiotic powder such as furazolidone (Topazone) (Fig. 31*J*).

Although it is probably unnecessary with this technique, many surgeons also do an epididymectomy in all procedures, except the penile amputation technique, to be absolutely sure that the bull does not bring about conception. Remove the sutures after 2 weeks, and the bull is ready for use.

Corpus Cavernosal Block. This technique can be done with the bull standing in a chute and under an epidural anesthesia. Special material needed is an acrylic substance (Technoviz soft formula).

Prepare the area posterior to the scrotum for surgery. Make a 15-cm skin incision starting just proximal to the posterior edge of the scrotum and extending it posteriorly and dorsally on the midline (Fig. 32*A*). Deepen the incision through the subcutaneous tissue and dense layer of fascia, exposing the penis and retractor penis muscle. Grasp the penis and surrounding elastic layers and exteriorize it through the skin incision. Palpate the urethral groove and note the dorsal vessels of the penis on the opposite side (Fig. 32*B*).

Insert a 14-gauge needle through the tunica albuginea on the lateral side of the penis into the CCP. Attach a 10-ml syringe filled with sterile saline, and adjust the needle position until a free flow is established into the CCP. Maintain the needle in this exact position and remove the syringe. Instruct an assistant to fill a second 10-ml plastic syringe with a fresh mixture of Technoviz solution and powder. This mixture should be about 1 to 1. Immediately inject 5 ml of the mixture into the CCP (Fig. 32*C*). It sets up almost immediately following the injection and can be palpated within the CCP. When you are satisfied with the injection, remove the needle. If it becomes prematurely

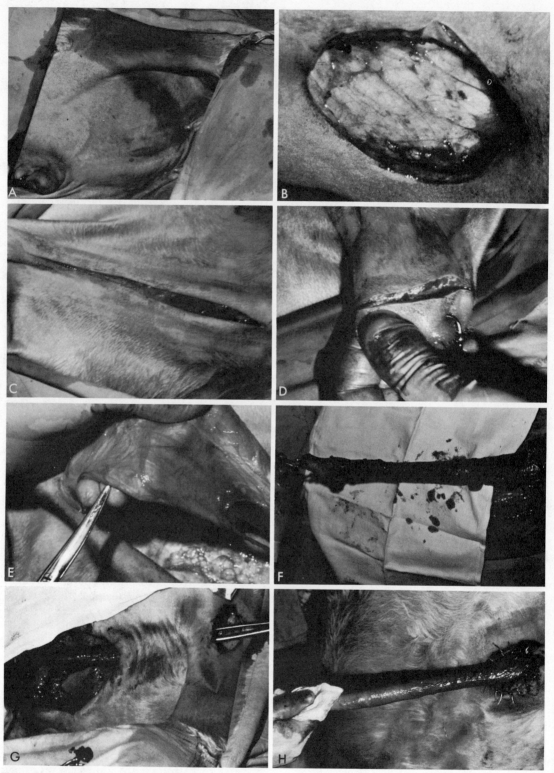

Figure 31.   Translocation of the penis technique for estrus-detector bull preparation. *A*, Bull prepared for surgery. *B*, Circular area of skin and cutaneous trunci muscle removed. *C*, Skin incision anterior to the scrotum. *D*, Circumscribing incision around the preputial orifice. *E*, Penis and elastic tissue dissected free; scissors point to large vein to be ligated. *F*, Penis completely dissected free. *G*, Exteriorization of the penis through the tunnel. *H*, Extension of the penis through its new mooring.

Figure continued on opposite page.

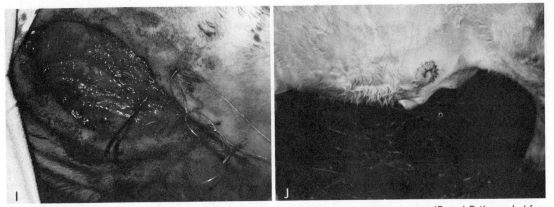

Figure 31 *(Continued).* *I,* Closure of the ventral incision. *J,* Postoperative appearance. (*B* and *D* through *J* from Walker, D. F. and Vaughan, J. T.: Bovine and Equine Urogenital Surgery. Philadelphia, Lea & Febiger, 1980.)

clogged, a second attempt may be necessary.

A temporary retaining suture is placed into the penis using 0.6-mm Vetafil. To accomplish this, pass the suture through the skin 2 cm lateral to the wound edge; then take a bite into the lateral wall of the penis through the tunica albuginea about 2 cm above the point where the retractor muscle becomes confluent with the penis (Fig. 32*D*). Now pass the suture back through the skin 1 cm above or below the original point of entry

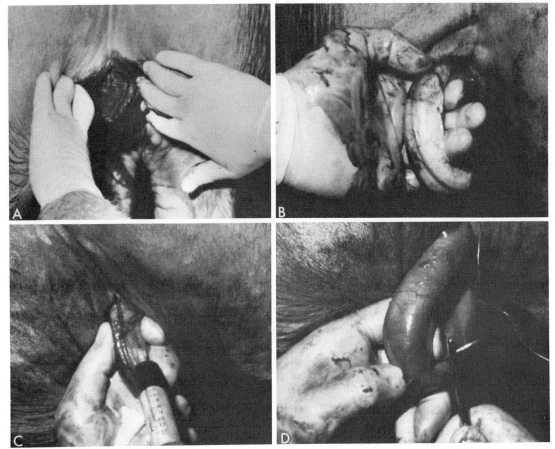

Figure 32. Corpus cavernosal block technique for preparation of estrus-detector bulls. *A,* Skin incision. *B,* Exteriorization of the penis. Note the urethral groove. *C,* Injection of the acrylic into the CCP. *D,* Technique for placing the temporary retaining suture.

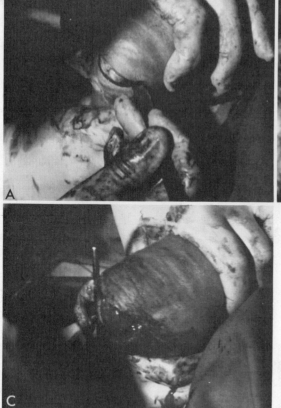
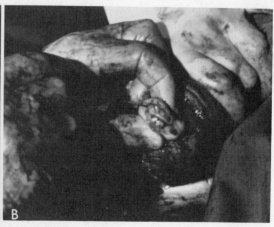

Figure 33. Technique for epididymectomy. *A*, Skin incision. *B*, Incision through the tunica vaginalis. *C*, Ligation of the body of the epididymis and the vas deferens at separate levels.

and tie. This suture will keep the penis from protruding. It can be left in place indefinitely but is only required for about 10 days.

Close the skin incision in the conventional manner and after 10 days remove the skin sutures. Perform an epididymectomy as a safety measure. The bull is ready for use in 2 weeks.

EPIDIDYMECTOMY. Epididymectomy is preferred over vasectomy because of its simplicity and being less prone to error and resultant recannulization. Surgically prepare the scrotum, giving particular attention to the fundus. Inject a local anesthetic solution subcutaneously over the caudal epididymis of both testes.

Make a 3 cm-skin incision over the tail of the epididymis while forcing the testes to the most ventral portion of the scrotum (Fig. 33A). Deepen this incision through the vaginal tunic until the epididymis pops through (Fig. 33B). Grasp it with a forceps and dissect it loose from the testicle until the body of the epididymis and the vas deferens are well exposed. Apply a ligature around

the body of the epididymis and incise below the ligature. Now apply traction to the vas deferens and place a ligature around it as far proximal as possible (Fig. 33C). Again incise ventral to the ligature, removing the caudal epididymis. Remove the remaining epididymis in a similar manner; no skin sutures are required. It may be prudent to place the surgical specimen in a vial of formalin marked with the bull's identification number and store it to be examined in case of controversy. Do not suture the skin wound. Semen remaining in the ampullae will not be viable after 3 weeks.

REFERENCES

1. Ashdown, R. R.: The angloarchitecture of the sigmoid flexure of the bovine corpus cavernosum penis and its significance in erection. J. Anat., *106*:403, 1970.
2. Ashdown, R. R. and Comb, M. A.: Experimental studies on spiral deviations of the bovine penis. Vet. Rec., *82*:126, 1967.
3. Ashdown, R. R. and Pearson, H.: Correction of corkscrew penis. Vet. Rec., *93*(2):30, 1973.
4. Ashdown, R. R. and Smith, J. A.: The anatomy of

the corpus cavernosum penis of the bull and its relation to spiral deviation of the penis. J. Anat., *104*:153, 1969.

5. Aubry, H. N. and Butterfield, R. M.: The structure and function of the muscles of the prepuce of the bull. J. Anat., *106*:192, 1970.
6. Beck, C. C.: Vasectomy vs. caudal epididymectomy. VM/SAC, *68*:1015, 1973.
7. Boyd, C. L. and Hanselka, D. V.: Implantation of a silicone prosthesis for correction of bovine penile deviation. J.A.V.M.A., *161*:275, 1972.
8. Farquharson, J.: Fracture of the penis in the bull. Vet. Med., *47*:175, 1952.
9. Johnson, L. and Williams, E. I.: Surgical disorders of the genital tract in the bull. Oklahoma Vet., *22*(4):2, 1970.
10. Larsen, L. H. and Bellenger, C. R.: Surgery of the prolapsed prepuce in the bull; Its complications and dangers. Austral. Vet. J., *47*:349, 1971.
11. Lewis, J. E., Walker, D. F., Beckett, S. D. and Vachon, R. I.: Blood pressure within the corpus cavernosum penis of the bull. J. Reprod. Fertil., *17*:155, 1968.
12. Long, S. E.: Eversion of the preputial epithelium in bulls at artificial insemination centres. Vet. Rec., *84*:495, 1969.
13. McEntee, K.: Fibropapillomas of the external genitalia of cattle. Cornell Vet., *40*:304, 1950.
14. Olson, C., Robl, M. G. and Larson, L. L.: Cutaneous and penile fibropapillomatosis and its control. J.A.V.M.A., *153*:1189, 1968.
15. Sisson, S. and Grossman, J. D.: The Anatomy of the Domestic Animals. 4th Ed. Revised. Philadelphia, W. B. Saunders Co., 1953.
16. Walker, D. F.: Deviations of the bovine penis. J.A.V.M.A., *145*:677, 1964.
17. Walker, D. F.: A method of circumcision in the bull. Auburn Vet., *22*(2):56, 1966.
18. Walker, D. F.: Preputial disorders and deviation of the penis in the bull. VI International Conference on Cattle Diseases, Philadelphia, 1970, pp. 322–326.
19. Walker, D. F. and Vaughan, J. T.: Bovine and Equine Urogenital Surgery. Philadelphia, Lea and Febiger, 1979.
20. Weissenberg, Y. and Cohen, R.: The preparation of teaser bulls by surgical deflection of the penis. Rufuah Veterinarith, *28*:31, 1971.
21. Wenkoff, M. S.: Problems associated with teaser bulls prepared by the Pen-O-Block method. Can. Vet. J., *16*:181, 1975.
22. Williamson, W. B.: Methods of estrus detection. Vet. Rec., *91*(3):50, 1972.
23. Young, S. L.: Impotence in bulls due to vascular shunts from the corpus cavernosum penis. J.A.V.M.A., *171*:643, 1977.

Seminal Vesiculitis in Bulls

ALAN D. McCAULEY
Via Pax Inc., Elizabethtown, Pennsylvania

INTRODUCTION

Seminal vesiculitis is a disease condition affecting both dairy and beef bulls. The seminal vesicles are paired structures and are the major accessory sex glands in the bull. These glandular organs have a lobular surface and lie on each side of the posterior portion of the dorsal surface of the bladder. The apical ends of these glands are partially covered by the peritoneum of the urogenital fold. The size of the seminal vesicles varies somewhat among individual animals, and there is generally asymmetry between the seminal vesicles themselves in a given animal. In adult bulls the seminal vesicles may measure 12 cm in length, 5 cm in width and 3 cm in thickness. The excretory duct of each seminal vesicle opens into the colliculus seminalis lateral to the opening of the ductus deferens. Although once thought to be reservoirs for sperm, in actuality, the seminal vesicles of the bull usually do not contain spermatozoa but function as the major source of seminal plasma.

The inflammatory process of seminal vesiculitis generally results in inflammatory cells being discharged into the semen. This inflammatory process may not be restricted to the seminal vesicles only. Inflammatory lesions may be present in the epididymides, ampullae, prostate, bulbourethral glands and urethra, with extension into or from the urinary bladder, ureters and kidneys. Because of the complexity of the inflammatory process in many bulls, workers at Colorado State University have labeled this condition the seminal vesiculitis syndrome.

The fertility of bulls with seminal vesiculitis may or may not be altered, depending on the organism and the circumstances involved. Bulls with this condition may be capable of settling cows fairly well when used naturally but have semen with poor freezability when put into artificial insemination (AI) service.

The incidence of seminal vesiculitis is highly variable. Figures encountered may range from less than 1 per cent to greater than 10 per cent of all bulls. Seminal vesiculitis may occur in bulls of all ages; however, the condition is most common in young bulls and appears to be related to puberty and subsequent sexual aggressiveness.

ETIOLOGY

A wide variety of micro-organisms including bacteria, viruses, chlamydiae and mycoplasmas may be involved in the seminal vesiculitis syndrome. In regions plagued with brucellosis, *Brucella abortus* is the most common agent. In areas where brucellosis is controlled, *Corynebacterium pyogenes,* which causes a suppurative vesiculitis, is most often diagnosed. Other bacteria isolated from bulls with seminal vesiculitis include *Streptococcus* spp., *Pseudomonas* spp., *Escherichia coli, Proteus mirabilis, Mycobacterium paratuberculosis* and *Actinobacillus actinoides.* Viruses that have been associated with seminal vesiculitis include the "Epivag" group and entero-like, rheo-like and papova-like viruses. A chlamydial agent has been isolated from the semen and epididymal tissues of bulls having seminal vesiculitis with unsatisfactory semen quality. *Mycoplasma bovigenitalium* and *Mycoplasma bovis* have also been found to cause the seminal vesiculitis syndrome. Too frequently the etiology is not determined because of either inadequate culture attempts and procedures or the fact that the inciting agent may no longer be present.

The pathogenesis of seminal vesiculitis is not completely understood. Some investigators have suggested that it results from an ascending infection via the urethra. Frequent urethral flushing during urination makes this route of infection unlikely under natural field conditions. Seminal vesiculitis has been shown to result secondary to orchitis or epididymitis by means of a descending infection. It is frequently associated with urinary tract infections and may be secondary to this inflammatory process. The seminal vesiculitis syndrome most likely results from hematogenous spread of the involved agent from concurrent lesions outside the genitourinary tract or by other humoral routes via the various body orifices. Often an affected bull will have a history of septicemia, pneumonia or omphalophlebitis as a young calf. Homosexual activity among young bulls may increase the likelihood of infectious agents entering hematogenously via the oral, nasal, ocular or genital routes. Certain bulls with seminal vesiculitis may have mild inflammatory lesions throughout the urogenital tract. Parsonson has suggested that this may be a form of an immune reaction initiated by an infectious process. Also, as in the case of certain pneumonic processes, an agent such as a virus or mycoplasma may set the initial stage for eventual secondary bacterial invasion of the seminal vesicles.

Several predisposing factors have been pinpointed by veterinarians working with the seminal vesiculitis syndrome. As mentioned previously, age is certainly a factor in that the syndrome generally occurs in young bulls. Aged bulls are not usually affected with seminal vesiculitis unless it is of the persistent chronic type or results from metastasis from another diseased organ such as the bladder or kidney. Young bulls that are on a high nutritional plane appear to be more susceptible to seminal vesiculitis. Bulls that are housed in groups in which homosexual activity flourishes also may be predisposed to this disorder. Stress of any kind is also likely to play a role in the initial states of the syndrome.

COURSE OF DISEASE

The course of the seminal vesiculitis syndrome is highly variable but usually involves an acute stage followed by spontaneous remission. In these cases the inflammatory process is likely to be initiated by a viral or mycoplasmal infection and may be asymptomatic. As mentioned earlier, an immune reaction may follow this type of initial infectious process. If there is no secondary bacterial invasion, the seminal vesiculitis will undergo spontaneous remission and with time the vesicles may return to a normal state. However, if there is secondary bacterial takeover or if the vesiculitis originated as a primary bacterial infection, spontaneous remission is less likely to occur. In general, with bacterial involvement the acute stage passes to the chronic state. When vesiculitis becomes chronic, the seeding of adjacent areas from chronically infected bacterial foci within the vesicles becomes a likely possibility. Thus, bacterial ampullitis, prostatitis, bulbourethritis, epididymitis, orchitis, urethritis, cystitis and/or pyelonephritis are possible sequelae.

DIAGNOSIS

The outward manifestations of this condition may vary from the usual asymptomatic type to the infrequent severe form, which resembles acute localized peritonitis. With this latter form, the bull may be anorectic, have decreased rumen activity, stand with his lumbar area arched and be somewhat reluctant to move. There may be pain on defecation, a lack of normal vigor during the breeding act or complete loss of libido. Body temperature may range from 39.4 to 41.1° C, especially if there is bacterial involvement.

Although many bulls with this syndrome have glands that seem normal on palpation, rectal examination during an acute episode of seminal vesiculitis may reveal glands that feel enlarged and swollen, with evidence of a loss of lobulation. The bull may show evidence of pain as the vesicles are palpated rectally. With severe bacterial involvement, adhesions of the vesicles to surrounding structures may be felt. In chronic cases, rectal examination may reveal firm, thickened, fibrotic areas within the vesicles. With secondary ampullitis the ampullae may feel thickened, enlarged or asymmetrical. In cases of suppurative vesiculitis, areas of abscessation may be felt within the glands and/or surrounding structures. Abscessed glands can fistulate to the rectum, bladder, peritoneal cavity or skin surface in the area of the ischiorectal fossa or flank.

Examination of the semen is quite revealing and frequently is used to detect the asymptomatic case. In general 50 to 80 per cent of bulls with seminal vesiculitis have semen of questionable or substandard quality. The presence of leukocytes, mostly neutrophils, within the ejaculate is a constant finding except in some long-standing chronic cases. Variable numbers of primary and secondary spermatozoal defects are present. These increase as the inflammation of the epididymides and testes increases. The motility of the ejaculate is usually reduced and the pH elevated.

Culture of the semen to identify the causative agents is not satisfactory because of contamination from the preputial cavity. Culture of the seminal vesicular fluid itself is of much greater diagnostic significance, as it is not contaminated by the preputial flora. A technique for the collection of this fluid is as follows: The bull is well restrained in a chute and may be mildly tranquilized if necessary. The phenothiazine-derivative tranquilizers tend to give the best penile relaxation. Promazine hydrochloride (0.2 mg per pound) or acepromazine (2.0 mg per 100 pounds) may be used intramuscularly for best results. Rapid intravenous injection of these two agents may lead to cardiovascular collapse. One should wait 10 to 15 minutes after intramuscular injection for the desired effect. Xylazine, which produces less satisfactory penile relaxation, may be used in a low total dose, such as 10 to 20 mg intravenously. This intravenous dose of xylazine will be effective in several minutes. The preputial orifice is clipped free of long hair and wiped clean. The pelvic portion of the penis is massaged rectally by an assistant with one hand, and the sigmoid flexure is pushed forward with the other hand. This massaging action will generally stimulate protrusion of the penis. If this method is unsuccessful, the penis may be protruded with the aid of an electroejaculator. As the penis is protruded, it is grasped with an unfolded 4- by 4-inch piece of sterile gauze. The penis is then wrapped with 2 or 3 feet of 4-inch sterile gauze roll, which is held firmly in place by a second assistant to stabilize the penis and divert it laterally. The bull should be well restrained during this procedure to avoid quick movement and resultant trauma or laceration of the penis. The glans penis is rinsed with a 1:1250 benzalkonium chloride (Roccal) solution followed by physiological saline. This rinsing process is repeated four times.

After the first assistant applies tail restraint to the bull, the main operator inserts a 20-cm length of Silastic medical grade tubing (1.57 mm internal diameter and 2.42 mm external diameter) into the external urethral orifice until 5 cm remains visible. Fluid may be allowed to flow freely from the tubing into a sterile test tube, or a syringe with a blunted needle can be connected to the tubing to aspirate vesicular fluid. The first assistant stimulates fluid flow by massaging the seminal vesicles and pelvic urethra rectally. Ten to 20 ml of fluid can easily be obtained in this manner. The tip of the penis is again rinsed and the gauze removed. The shaft of the penis is carefully examined for gauze remnants and is rinsed with saline. A less satisfactory alternative method for seminal fluid collection is to collect the fluid into a Whirl-Pak sterile plastic bag as it is sprayed from the protruded erect penis during stimulation with an electroejaculator. The seminal vesicular fluid is examined grossly. Flakes of pus may be obvious on initial examination. Some samples that appear very clear upon collection will form a small amount of flocculent debris upon standing for a few minutes. The fluid is cultured, and cytological examination is performed. Serological testing of the fluid for commonly involved agents such as *Brucella abortus* is recommended.

TREATMENT

The prognosis and response to treatment of seminal vesiculitis are also highly variable. Most favorable results occur in those cases that undergo spontaneous remission and return to normal by virtue of time. Long-term antibiotic therapy has previously been recommended as a means of treatment, but, in general, the response to such therapy has not been good. Culture and sensitivity testing should be done to be sure that a proper antibiotic is being used. High doses at the correct dosage interval for 2 weeks or longer are probably necessary to be effective. It is not known whether minimal inhibitory concentrations of antibiotics can be attained in the glandular parenchyma or vesicular fluid, and this requires thorough investigation. One 1500-pound Holstein bull with *Escherichia coli* seminal vesiculitis was treated at the Large Animal Clinic at Cornell University with 3 gm of oxytetracycline every 8 hours for 8 days without a favorable response. Negative culture results were obtained on repeated samples following antibiotic therapy, but inflammatory cells were still abundantly present in the semen.

This same bull was later treated with tylosin, as it was thought that mycoplasmas might have been involved in this particular case. Tylosin was given at twice the recommended dose at a 12-hour dosage interval for 2 weeks. Negative culture results were again obtained from the vesicular fluid on repeated samples but the inflammatory cells in the semen persisted. During the administration of oxytetracycline, blood and seminal fluid were collected for antibiotic concentration studies. Unfortunately the antibiotic assays have not been performed at the time of

this writing. It is possible that an immune reaction may have accounted for the persistence of the inflammatory cells in the absence of the infectious *E. coli* agent that had originally been grown in pure culture repeatedly before antibiotic therapy was instituted. Immunosuppressive drugs may be of value in cases such as this, but their use has not been reported. Several months following the two intense courses of antibiotic therapy, *E. coli* organisms in pure culture were again isolated repeatedly from the seminal fluid of this bull.

It was also interesting that semen morphology was markedly altered during both antibiotic regimens. There were approximately 50 per cent detached heads in samples collected 7 to 10 days after initiation of each course of antibiotic therapy. The morphological findings gradually returned to normal over a 1-month period following the termination of each antibiotic course.

In cases in which spontaneous regression has not occurred and in which antibiotic therapy has not been successful, surgical correction should be considered. Of course, this method is feasible only when the lesion is restricted to the seminal vesicles and when extensive adhesions are not present. Presurgical preparation includes keeping the bull off bulk feed for 48 hours and off water for 24 hours. The bull is well restrained in a chute, very lightly tranquilized and given an epidural anesthetic. The rectum is emptied, and the anus is closed with a purse-string suture pattern using nonabsorbable suture material. Local anesthetic is infiltrated deep into the pararectal area through the ischiorectal fossa. A crescent-shaped pararectal skin incision is made outside the zone of the anal sphincter muscles. The tissues are separated by blunt dissection down to the area of the seminal vesicle. The anterior pole of the vesicle may be adherent to the peritoneum, and if so, the adhesions must be gently broken down. The ampullae must be identified, and care should be taken not to traumatize them during the dissecting procedure. By blunt and sharp dissection the seminal vesicle is freed to the base, where it joins the pelvic urethra. Using a wire saw écraseur, the vesicle is removed as close to the pelvic urethra as possible. A few 0 gut sutures will obliterate the pararectal dead space. The skin is sutured and the purse-string suture removed.

It is again wise to culture the seminal

vesicle and do antibiotic sensitivity testing on all isolates. Vigorous antibiotic therapy is recommended prior to surgery and for 2 weeks or longer following surgery. Histopathological examination of the excised seminal vesicle is advisable. In cases of unilateral involvement, this procedure may halt the problem. If there is bilateral involvement, a second surgical procedure on the opposite side 6 weeks following the first procedure is necessary. Vigorous antibiotic therapy is again maintained, as previously mentioned. It is *not* advisable to attempt bilateral removal at one time by means of surgical entrance from one or both sides because of excessive swelling and danger of damage to the ampullae and colliculus seminalis. The bull may be collected 14 days after either surgical procedure and semen examination performed to evaluate the results of surgical intervention.

PREVENTION

Managerial considerations are most important in the prevention of seminal vesiculitis. The prevention of calfhood diseases such as septicemia and pneumonia is critical. Young bulls should be fed on a good nutritional plane but not to excess. If possible, bulls should be loose-housed in individual pens. All forms of stress on young breeding bulls should be minimized around the time of puberty.

The seminal vesiculitis syndrome is an important, complex entity. Because bulls with seminal vesiculitis may transmit certain reproductive pathogens via the venereal route, the prevention, diagnosis, treatment and control of seminal vesiculitis in breeding bulls (whether used naturally or for artificial insemination) are imperative.

REFERENCES

1. Ball, L., Griner, L. A. and Carroll, E. J.: The bovine seminal vesiculitis syndrome. Am. J. Vet Res., *25*:291, 1964.
2. Ball, L., Young, S. and Carroll, E. J.: Seminal vesiculitis syndrome: Lesions in genital organs of young bulls. Am. J. Vet. Res. *29*:1173, 1968.
3. Lein, D. H.: Male bovine urogenital Mycoplasmosis. Ph.D. thesis, University of Connecticut, Storrs, Conn., 1974.
4. Roberts, S. J.: Veterinary Obstetrics and Genital Diseases. 2nd Ed. Ann Arbor, Mich., Edward Bros., Inc., 1971, pp. 68–91.

Health Management of Bulls Used in AI

DAVID E. BARTLETT

American Breeders Service,
DeForest, Wisconsin

INTRODUCTION

Breeding of cattle by artificial insemination (AI) is practiced to some extent in almost all countries of the world, developed and underdeveloped, in which cattle are raised. From several thousand to many million inseminations may be made annually, involving a small percentage to virtually 100 per cent of various countries' cattle populations. A total of approximately 90 million inseminations are made worldwide.

Application of AI varies widely. At times, AI is used intraherd, with semen collected and kept a few days in liquid form at 1 to 2° C. At other times, AI may utilize semen that has been preserved, frozen and stored in a liquid nitrogen refrigerator at −190° C for an indefinite period of time, varying from several months to several years. When desired, the frozen semen may be transported thousands of miles from the site of sperm collection to the site of insemination.

At its technological best, the AI process can be an effective and positive force in cattle improvement, delivering to recipient females: (1) genes that are highly selected and known to improve subsequent generations by imparting sound, economically important genetic characteristics; (2) semen that is free of pathogenic organisms, which, if present, might harm the female recipient's reproductive system, impair or destroy her general health and, potentially, result in secondary transmission of similar infections to her herdmates; and (3) sperm cells of sufficient number and adequate quality to achieve a maximal probability of fertilization and normal pregnancy.

Whether or not AI fulfills its potential is a direct function of the technical competence and diligence invested in AI's implementation. In this article, discussion of these factors is limited to consideration of the infectious disease aspects of AI.

As a practical, working concept based upon numerous research studies, it seems reasonable to expect that micro-organisms contaminating bovine semen will survive processing, freezing and storage, at least as well as sperm cells survive these procedures. Furthermore, intragenital deposition of infectious material seems to result quite consistently in disease transmission. The United States has no federal regulations governing interstate movement of semen and only the states of Washington, Virginia, Montana, Mississippi and Wisconsin control intrastate movement. Thus, those involved in collecting, processing, freezing, storing and distributing bovine semen for use in AI must be responsible for defining, electing and following their own policies. They may either (1) take all active measures commensurate with the technical capabilities of the day or (2) ignore the potentials for disease transmission and hope for the best.

There are numerous examples of semen-borne infectious diseases (as well as genetic diseases) having occurred incident to AI under field conditions. In fact, some of these may be considered as classics in veterinary medicine. Additionally, there is an impressive mass of experimental and supportive evidence related to the behavior of specific pathogens under conditions of semen collection, processing, storage and "insemination." For example, under certain conditions, organisms such as foot and mouth and IBR/IPV/IBP viruses have been shown to be shed in the semen of infectious bulls, to remain well preserved along with frozen spermatozoa and, subsequently, to infect inseminated females. Blue tongue virus is shed in semen and is transmitted venereally. Individual bulls with genital lesions of tuberculosis and brucellosis have transmitted these infections to customers' herds and to many cows following routine AI. *Trichomonas foetus* is unaffected by antibiotics employed in semen processing, and *Campylobacter fetus* has been transmitted via frozen semen

despite treatment with 500 mg of penicillin and 500 units of streptomycin. Leptospira organisms shed from the kidneys may contaminate semen and still survive following frozen semen processing.[1]

The average bull in use by AI organizations in the United States produces about 5000 units of frozen semen per year. However, the top semen-producing bulls may yield more than 100,000 units of frozen semen per year. It follows that insemination with each unit of frozen semen is, in effect, one "animal contact." With frozen semen, the aggregate of contacts from a single collection of semen may occur over several years and at locations that may be statewide, nationwide or worldwide.

CONTROL

Semen-Borne Pathogens

In a recent review of semen-borne pathogens[1] and methods for their control, classification into four control-related lists was proposed, as follows:

1. The Specific Pathogen Free (SPF) list.
2. The Control by Surveillance List.
3. The Control by Sanitation/Hygiene List.
4. The Control by Antibiotics Additives List.

The Specific Pathogen Free (SPF) List. This list is divided into two parts: Part A (Table 1), which is comprised of diseases definitely not present in the territory of the semen's origin, and Part B (Table 2), which is comprised of those diseases amenable to programmed test and retest procedures that periodically validate the SPF status.

The Control by Surveillance List. This list (Table 3) includes those diseases (mostly viruses) that are widespread within the cattle population and are so difficult to diagnose and control that establishing and maintaining SPF status for a population of bulls is at present neither technologically possible nor realistic. Control is exercised by clinical and laboratory monitoring of the individual bull and, in some instances, of the individual ejaculate. If monitoring reveals that significant contamination has occurred, collection of semen should cease at once and recently frozen semen in storage should be discarded.

TABLE 1. *The Specific Pathogen Free (SPF) List — Part A*

Etiological Agent	Objective	Control
Virus of foot and mouth	SPF	All are subject to national official programs and declarations
Virus of rinderpest	SPF	
Mycoplasma mycoides (contagious pleuropneumonia)	SPF	

The Control by Sanitation/Hygiene List. This listing (Table 4) includes those vagrant micro-organisms that are ubiquitous in the environment of cattle. Such organisms may be pathogenic, nonpathogenic, of very low pathogenicity or opportunistic.

The Control by Antibiotic Additives List. This list (Table 5) still includes *Campylobacter fetus* var. *venerealis* and *Leptospira* spp. However, these organisms have been advanced to the Specific Pathogen Free (SPF) List, Part B, in bull populations under other than technically delinquent management. It should be noted that there is no precise, positive evidence to indicate that use of antibiotics in processed frozen bovine semen is effective for pathogens other than *C. fetus* var. *venerealis* and *L. pomona*.

A discussion of the specific venereal and AI-related aspects of each of the previously listed diseases and/or etiological agents, with citations for relevant background literature, appears elsewhere.[1]

Other Disease Entities

In addition to established, semen-borne pathogens, several other disease entities must be considered in the health management of a population of bulls used for AI, not because of disease transmission potential in-

TABLE 2. *The Specific Pathogen Free (SPF) List — Part B*

Disease Entity	Objective	Diagnostic Method	Test Frequency While in: PRE-ENTRY AND ADMITTANCE	RESIDENCE	Disease Treatable in Bulls?
Mycobacterium bovis	SPF	Comparative cervical Intradermal	2×–>60 days	2× yearly	No
Mycobacterium paratuberculosis	SPF	Fecal culture Intradermal: (presumptive, while awaiting culture results)	1×	1× yearly	No
Brucella abortus	SPF	Blood serum Semen plasma: tube agglutination	2×–>60 days 2×–>60 days	2–3× yearly 2–3× yearly	No No
Leptospira: pomona hardjo canicola icterohaemorrhagiae grippotyphosa	SPF	Blood serum: microagglutination lysis	2×–>60 days	2–3× yearly	Yes
Campylobacter fetus var. *venerealis*	SPF	Smegma: culture	3–6× weekly	2–4× yearly	Yes
Trichomonas foetus	SPF	Smegma: direct microscopic culture	3–6× weekly	2–4× yearly	Yes

TABLE 3. *The Control by Surveillance List*

Etiological Agent	Objective	Diagnostic Method	Test Frequency While in:		Disease Treatable in Bulls?
			PRE-ENTRY AND ADMITTANCE	RESIDENCE	
Virus of IBR/IPV/IPB*	Informative	Blood serum: microagglutination lysis Semen: culture of individual ejaculates	– –	– –	No
Virus of bovine virus diarrhea	Informative	Clinical awareness Blood serum: serum neutralization micro-titer-cell culture	–	–	No
Virus of parainfluenza₃	Informative	Clinical awareness Blood serum: hemagglutination inhibition	–	–	No
Virus of fibropapillomatosis	Informative	Clinical awareness Blood serum: immunodiffusion	–	–	No
Virus of blue tongue	Informative	Blood serum: complement fixation	As indicated	As indicated	No
Virus of bovine leukemia	Informative	Blood serum: immunodiffusion complement fixation	As indicated	As indicated	No
Chlamydia†	Informative	Clinical awareness	–	–	No
Coxiella burnetii (Q fever)	Informative	Clinical awareness	–	–	No

*Virus of infectious bovine rhinotracheitis, infectious pustular vulvovaginitis, infectious pustular balanoposthitis.
†Chlamydia (Bedsonia/Miyagawanella):
   Agent of psittacosis-lymphogranuloma-venereum group.
   Agent of psittacosis-lymphogranuloma-trachoma group (epizootic enzootic sporadic bovine abortion, genital bedsoniasis).

TABLE 4. *The Control by Sanitation/Hygiene List*

Etiological Agent	Objective	Control
Pseudomonas aeruginosa	Minimized possibility of entry into semen and/or extender	Control is possible only by establishing and enforcing procedures designed to consistently assure the lowest level of entry of listed and similar organisms into the semen and its extender, beginning with ejaculation of the semen, continuing through all laboratory procedures and ending with sealing of the semen in its package and then freezing
Corynebacterium pyogenes	–	
Staphylococcus spp.	–	
Streptococcus spp.	–	
Escherichia coli	–	
Mold, yeast, fungi		

TABLE 5. *The Control by Antibiotic Additives List*

Etiological Agent	Objective	USAHA Recommendations*
Campylobacter fetus var. *venerealis*†	Bactericidal	Present justification for antibiotic additives rests upon (1) "fail safe" value against *C. fetus* var. *venerealis* and *Leptospira pomona* and (2) "expectation" value against a host of miscellaneous, unknown, possible or probable antibiotic-sensitive organisms. Some are designated or implied in Table 4, The Control by Sanitation/Hygiene List
Leptospira spp.†	Bactericidal	
Mycoplasma bovogenitalium and *agalactiae*‡	Bacteriostatic	
Miscellaneous unknown antibiotic sensitive organisms(?)	Bactericidal	

*Subcommittee on AI of USAHA Committee on Infectious Diseases of Cattle recommends:
"Immediately after semen is collected, before cooling and before addition of extender, for each milliliter of semen must be added 2000 micrograms of dihydrostreptomycin and 1000 units of polymyxin B sulfate contained in 0.02 ml distilled water.

Prior to cooling semen to 5°C, each milliliter of extender added must contain 2000 micrograms of dihydrostreptomycin, 1000 units of polymyxin B sulfate, and 500 units of penicillin.

In fully extended semen, final concentration of antibiotics for each milliliter must be not less than 1000 micrograms dihydrostreptomycin sulfate, 500 units polymyxin B sulfate, and 500 units of penicillin."

†SPF procedures should supersede control by antibiotics.
‡Final concentrations of Lincomycin (300 mg) and Spectinomycin (150 mg), if included, have been found to be bacteriostatic, not bactericidal.

cident to AI but rather for protection and preservation of the health value of the bulls *per se* as producers of semen.

Programmed measures against both external and internal parasitism are essential. Test and treatment procedures for anaplasmosis are also essential and readily accomplished.

Continuing clinical surveillance is in order for all other infectious diseases that affect cattle, ranging from anthrax to clostridial infections, listeriosis, malignant catarrhal fever and rabies to vesicular stomatitis. Also, clinical observations should be maintained for all diseases indigenous to the geographical area.

Programmed immunizations employing killed antigens against clostridial infections, fibropapillomatosis, leptospirosis and vibriosis might be indicated, based on local clinical experiences and circumstances.

Specific judgment is indicated relative to IBR/IPV/IPB vaccine. A high incidence of elevated titers, ranging from 25 to 40 per cent in dairy bulls and much higher in beef bulls, is to be expected in inbound and resident bulls, reflecting their prior immunization* or field exposure. To elevate the immunity of serologically positive bulls and reduce

---

*The number of doses of IBR/IPV/IPB vaccine approved annually by USDA approximates the number of calves born annually in the United States.

the possibility of their shedding of virus, it has been recommended that populations of bulls used in AI be repeatedly vaccinated against IBR. However, repeated tissue culturing of the semen for either reimmunized bulls or bulls with low titers in regular AI use has not revealed the presence of virus. A limitation to the repeated use of IBR vaccine for all bulls is that regulations of some countries importing bovine semen require certification of the serologically negative status of each bull from which semen is derived.

Immunization against brucellosis using Strain 19 vaccine is contraindicated for bulls used in AI. It has been shown that Strain 19 organisms may localize in the internal male genitalia and be shed in the semen.

In countries where foot and mouth disease is present, bulls are routinely vaccinated against this disease. Bulls receiving foot and mouth vaccine shed virus in their semen subsequent to vaccination. Obviously, semen from such bulls should not be transported to countries free of foot and mouth disease.

DISEASE PREVENTION PROCEDURES

Bulls used in AI are typically gathered from widespread sources, since the search for desirable sires has become not only nationwide but continent- and worldwide. No other bovine herds have such frequent introduction of new herdmates from such diverse origins with such variety of microbiological milieus as have bull studs used in AI.

Disease prevention for bulls used in AI involves five steps, beginning with establishing the health status of the herd of origin of each new bull. A competent, comprehensive on-the-farm or on-the-ranch examination of each prospective bull and his herdmates is therefore the first step in disease prevention. Transportation to the bull center in a contact-free, cleaned and disinfected vehicle is the second step.

Retention for 6 to 10 weeks in a secure admittance or quarantine facility is the third step, during which continuous close observation, a programmed series of diagnostic tests and indicated treatment and prophylactic procedures should be carried out to further establish the individual bull's disease-free status.

The fourth step involves resident membership on premises with a herd maintained

exclusively for producing semen for AI. Semen-producing populations of bulls must be isolated from all other cattle and protected, insofar as possible, from fomites. The bulls must also be protected from other animals of all species capable of carrying bovine disease. The herd must be under continuous surveillance by veterinarians who are alert to the expected as well as the unexpected. In addition to daily clinical observations, scheduled procedures of testing and retesting to probe for the unexpected and to establish disease-free status are essentials.

The fifth and final step should be the routine necropsy of as many animals as possible in order that conditions not previously recognized clinically may be revealed.

REFERENCE

1. Bartlett, D. E., Larson, L. L., Parker, W. G. and Howard, T. H.: Specific Pathogen Free Semen (SPF) Frozen Bovine Semen: A Goal? Proceedings, Sixth N.A.A.B. Annual Technical Conference on Artificial Insemination and Reproduction. Milwaukee, Wisc., 1976.

Congenital Defects Affecting Bovine Reproduction

HORST W. LEIPOLD and STANLEY M. DENNIS
Kansas State University, Manhattan, Kansas

INTRODUCTION

Congenital defects are present in all cattle breeds and are caused by genetic or environmental factors or by their interactions. Many defects have no clearly established cause. Although more than 80 inherited diseases in cattle have been identified throughout the world, there is little information on the majority of these disorders. Many more defects undoubtedly exist and await identification. Congenital bovine defects require different methods of control than those for infectious or toxic diseases.

Definitive etiological knowledge of the broad spectrum of congenital defects is scarce, and more research and field studies

are needed to clarify involvement of genetic and environmental factors. Many bovine congenital defects have not been studied genetically, and with time and additional study, more may prove to be inherited. Present knowledge suggests one-quarter to one-third of such defects are inherited, one-sixth are induced by viruses and the remainder are due to other environmental agents.

Cattle breeders and veterinarians are prime sources for advancing our knowledge of congenital defects by identifying and reporting defective calves. Practitioners should be familiar with the common defects in the breeds in their area and should be vigilant concerning new defects that are emerging. Many defective calves are encountered as obstetrical problems.

Genetic variation is a tool of cattle breeders. Along with favorable variations, there are unfavorable variations resulting in disease. Genetic defects may spread insidiously through breeds until these traits become economically disastrous and difficult to control. It is therefore essential that genetic defects be recognized early to prevent spread. Many breed associations and artificial insemination (AI) centers have programs for monitoring and controlling undesirable genetic traits.

IDENTIFYING CONGENITAL DEFECTS IN CATTLE

Definition and Classification

Congenital defects are defined as abnormalities of structure or function that are present at birth. They may affect a single anatomical structure or function, an entire system, parts of several systems or both a structure and a function.

Congenital defects may be lethal, semilethal or nonlethal. They are usually classified by the body system that is primarily affected.

Nature and Effect

A defective calf is an adapted survivor from a disruptive event at one or more stages in the complexly integrated process of embryonic or fetal development. Susceptibility to injurious agents varies with the stage of development and decreases with age. Before day 14 (period of preattachment), the zygote or embryo is resistant to teratogens but susceptible to genetic mutations and chromosomal aberrations. During the embryonic period (days 14 to 42), the embryo is highly susceptible to teratogens, but this decreases with embryonic age as the critical periods for the various organs are passed. The fetus (day 42 plus) becomes increasingly resistant to teratogenic agents with age, except for the later differentiating structures such as the cerebellum, palate and urogenital system.

The most frequently encountered congenital defects in cattle involve the skeletal, central nervous and muscular systems. Common bovine defects include arthrogryposis, cleft palate, hydrocephalus and syndactyly (Figs. 1 to 6).

Although economic losses due to congenital defects are less than those caused by infectious, chemical and nutritional agents, they may be economically important to individual cattle owners. With the increasing use of artificial insemination, defects are no longer rare, and all are important. Collectively, congenital defects cause economic losses by increasing perinatal calf mortality, decreasing maternal productivity and decreasing the value of viable defective calves and their relatives.

Frequency

The frequency of the various congenital defects in cattle is difficult to assess. Because congenital defects are caused by hereditary and environmental factors, the frequency of individual defects and the total number of defects vary among breeds, geographical areas and season. Frequencies are not easily obtained, as many defects are detected only by necropsy. Some defects go unnoticed, and others are not reported for economic or other reasons. Some may be seen so rarely as to defy accurate account-

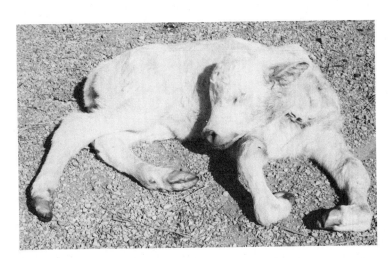

Figure 1. Arthrogryposis in a neonatal calf. Note the bilateral symmetrical contracture of the joints.

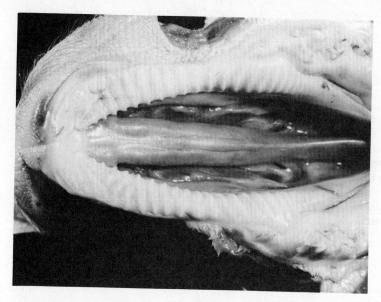

Figure 2. Cleft palate in the arthrogrypotic calf depicted in Figure 1.

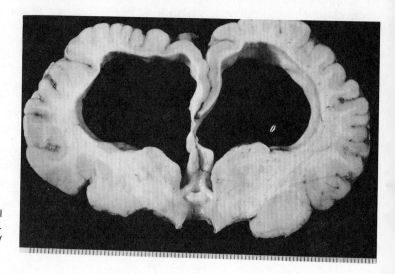

Figure 3. Cross section of internal hydrocephalus in a neonatal calf. The lateral ventricles are markedly dilated.

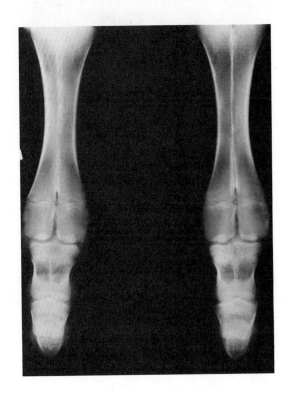

Figure 4. Radiograph of front legs of a neonatal syn-dactylous calf.

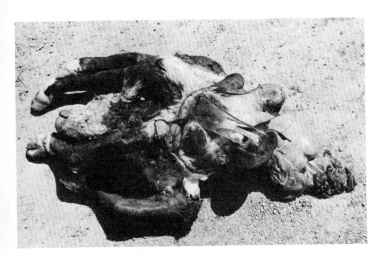

Figure 5. Schistosomus reflexus — a common cause of dystocia due to a defective calf.

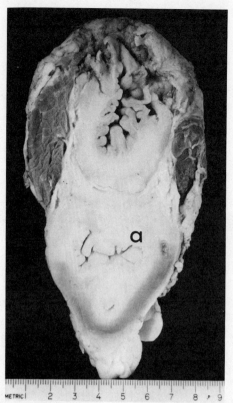

Figure 6. Cross section of vestibule and rectum of a cow with rectovaginal constriction (RVC). Note hypoplastic vestibule (*a*).

ing, and frequent reporting of other defects may reflect interest of the observers rather than a high incidence.

Review of reported congenital defects in cattle and other domestic animals reveals that skeletal anomalies are the most common. Skeletal defects are more easily recognized than other anomalies, such as internal defects. The known incidence of various defects is, therefore, partly dependent on the frequency with which they are reported.

It is estimated that 0.5 to 1.0 per cent of all calves born are defective. The reported incidence ranges from 1 in 100 to 1 in 500, with 40 to 50 per cent being born dead.

Causes

As mentioned previously, congenital defects in cattle are caused by genetic or environmental factors or by their interaction. Some are inherited and others are suspected of being so but the inheritability of the majority is unknown. Differentiation of the cause is often difficult because it usually ex-

erted its effects some 8 months before the defect was recognized.

Genetic

Genetic defects are pathophysiological results of mutant genes or chromosomal aberrations occurring in any environment. Except for chromosomal aberrations, genetic defects are recognized only when they occur in characteristic intragenerational familial frequencies and intergenerational patterns. Chromosomal aberrations, that is, variations in the normal number of chromosomes or structural abnormalities of individual chromosomes, have received little attention in cattle.

All genetic defects have their counterparts in environmentally induced phenocopies. The problem is to recognize which are genetic and which are environmental.

Environmental

Only a few environmental factors have been incriminated as being teratogenic for cattle. In general, environmentally induced defects do not follow familial patterns but rather seasonal patterns or known or suspected maternal stress. They are produced in any genotype during the appropriate critical period during embryogenesis.

Plant Teratogens. Ingestion of lupines has resulted in arthrogryposis or crooked calves. Other plants incriminated or suspected as being cattle teratogens include *Senecio* and related plants, *Indigofera spicata, Cycadales, Blighia,* locoweeds, *Papaveraceae, Colchicum, Vinca* and tobacco and related plants.

Viruses. Certain prenatal virus infections have been found to be teratogenic for cattle: bovine virus diarrhea virus resulting in cerebellar hypoplasia, blue tongue virus causing hydranencephaly and recently Akabane virus resulting in arthrogryposis-hydranencephaly syndrome.

Others. The following have been incriminated or suspected of being teratogenic in cattle: iodine deficiency, hyperthermia, drugs, irradiation, fetal hypoxia, maternal age and aging of ova.

Specific Defects

Congenital defects reported in cattle are summarized in Table 1, which is divided into
Text continued on page 436

TABLE 1. *Congenital Defects of Cattle Classified by Body System*

Defect	Description	Etiology	Frequency	Diagnosis	Associated Defects
1. Congenital Defects of the Entire Skeletal System:					
Dwarfism	Disturbance of longitudinal epiphyseal growth; appositional bone growth is normal. Abnormal head	Genetic, autosomal recessive	Rare	X-ray of lumbar vertebrae, short stature	May be affected with internal hydrocephalus
Osteogenesis imperfecta	Fragile bones, reduced bone mass	Genetic, simple autosomal recessive	Rare	X-ray, histological examination	None
Osteopetrosis	Continuous formation of chondro-osseous matrix, lack of resorption and remodeling of bones. Born dead	Genetic, autosomal recessive	Common	X-ray, necropsy	Short lower jaw, dam may have hydramnios
Acroteriasis (congenital "amputated")	Involves entire skeleton, amputation of all four legs, defects of facial skeleton, cleft palate and short lower jaw	Genetic, autosomal recessive	Rare	External examination and x-ray	Vertebral column, eye defects
Porphyria (pink tooth)	Metabolic defect. Teeth and bone store porphyrin, giving characteristic brown appearance	Genetic, simple autosomal recessive	Common	Clinical examination	Photosensitivity
2. Congenital Defects of the Facial Skeleton:					
Cleft palate without associated defects	Median cleft due to nonclosure of hard palate	Unknown	Rare	Clinical examination	None
Cleft palate associated with arthrogryposis	Complete nonclosure of hard palate. Permanent joint contracture present at birth	Simple autosomal recessive. Other cases are sporadic	Common	Necropsy examination	Hypoplasia of patella

Table continued on following page

TABLE 1. Congenital Defects of Cattle Classified by Body System (Continued)

Defect	Description	Etiology	Frequency	Diagnosis	Associated Defects
Cleft palate associated with crooked legs	Variable degrees of cleft palate, varying degrees of joint contracture	Maternal ingestion of lupine between days 40 and 70 of pregnancy	Common	Necropsy, external examination	Variable
Short lower jaw	Shortened mandible	Unknown	Common	External examination	None
Prognathism	Shortened upper jaw and protruding lower jaw	Possibly genetic	Uncommon	External examination	None
Campylognathia	Curved jaw	Unknown	Rare	External examination	None
Agnathia	Aplasia of mandible	Possibly genetic	Uncommon	External examination, x-ray	Other mandibulo-facial defects
Craniofacial dysplasia	Deficient ossification of frontal sutures, convex profile of nose, short lower jaw	Incompletely dominant with incomplete penetrance	Rare	External examination	Macroglossia, patent ductus arteriosus
3. Congenital Defects of the Axial Skeleton:					
Scoliosis	Lateral deviation of vertebral column	Unknown	Rare	External examination	May have arthrogryposis, may occur without associated defects
Kyphosis	Dorsal deviation of vertebral column	Unknown	Rare	External examination	May be associated with other musculoskeletal defects
Kyphoscoliosis	Dorsal and lateral deviation of vertebral column	Genetic and environmental causes	Common	External examination	Frequently associated with arthrogryposis
Torticollis	Twisted neck, also referred to as wryneck	Genetic and environmental causes	Fairly common	External examination	None

Defect	Description	Cause/Genetics	Frequency	Diagnosis	Central nervous system (CNS) defects
Short spine	Reduction and fusion of vertebrae and ribs from 13 to 6 or 7	Genetic, simple autosomal recessive	Rare	External examination	Central nervous system (CNS) defects
Atlanto-occipital fusion	Fusion of first cervical spine to occipital bones. Hypoplasia of dens of axis	Unknown	Rare	X-ray, necropsy	Spinal cord defect
Perosomus elumbis	Agenesis of lumbosacral and coccygeal vertebrae with blind ending vertebral canal and spinal cord in thoracic area	Unknown	Fairly common	External examination and necropsy	CNS defects
Tail absent	Agenesis of coccygeal vertebrae	Nongenetic environmental cause unknown	Common	External examination	None in most cases, other calves have microphthalmia
Wrytail	Kink between coccygeal vertebrae	Genetic, simple autosomal recessive	Rare	External examination	None

4. Congenital Defects of Appendicular Skeleton:

Defect	Description	Cause/Genetics	Frequency	Diagnosis	Central nervous system (CNS) defects
Polymelia	Duplication of one or more limbs	Unknown	Uncommon	External examination and x-ray	None
Polymelia, heterotopic	One or two supernumerary limbs attached to various regions, e.g., thoracomelia if attached to thorax	Unknown	Uncommon	External examination	None
Abrachia	Agenesis of both front limbs	Unknown	Uncommon	External examination	None
Monobrachia	Agenesis of one front limb	Unknown	Uncommon	External examination	None
Monopodia	Agenesis of one hind limb	Unknown	Uncommon	External examination	None
Micromelia	All parts of appendicular skeleton present but hypoplastic	Unknown	Uncommon	External examination and x-ray	None

Table continued on following page

TABLE 1.   *Congenital Defects of Cattle Classified by Body System (Continued)*

Defect	Description	Etiology	Frequency	Diagnosis	Associated Defects
Peromelia	Agenesis of distal appendicular parts	Unknown	Uncommon	External examination and x-ray	None
Phocomelia	Agenesis of proximal appendicular parts, whereas distal parts are developed	Unknown	Uncommon	Clinical examination and x-ray	None
Tibial hemimelia	Agenesis of both tibias	Genetic, simple autosomal recessive	Common	External examination	Brain hernia, ventral abdominal hernia, male—cryptorchid; female—nonunion of müllerian ducts
Ectrodactyly	Partial or complete absence of digits	Possibly genetic	Rare	External examination and x-ray	None or arthrogryposis
Adactyly	Complete or partial lack of development of digits	Genetic, simple autosomal recessive	Rare	External examination and x-ray	None
Polydactyly	Development of additional digits on one or more limbs	Unknown, genetic cases have been described	Common	External examination and x-ray	None
Syndactyly	Fusion or nondivision of functional digits	Genetic, simple autosomal recessive with incomplete persistence and varying degrees of manifestation	Common	External examination and x-ray	Hyperemesis
Brachydactyly	Short stature of calf caused by shortness of metacarpal and metatarsal bones	Possibly genetic	Rare	External examination and x-ray	None

5. Congenital Defects of the Muscular System:

Arthrogryposis	Permanent joint contracture present at birth	Genetic, simple autosomal recessive. Sporadic cases occur. Needs careful analysis	Common	Clinical examination, necropsy	Cleft palate, kyphoscoliosis
Double muscling	Fine neck and head. Bulging muscles in back and hind quarters. Deep creases between muscles. Absence of fat	Genetic, simple autosomal. Other hereditary modes are currently being investigated	Common in some breeds	Inspection at slaughter	Abnormalities of bone and reproductive systems, dystocia

6. Congenital Defects of the Cerebrum:

Agenesis of corpus callosum	Absence of corpus callosum	Unknown	Rare	Necropsy	Absence of septum pellucidum and other CNS defects
Anencephaly	Absence of cerebral hemispheres. Nonclosure of anterior portion of neural tube and failure of closure of cranium, pons, medulla and cerebellum. Eyes present	Unknown	Rare	Necropsy	Acrania, cranioschisis craniorachischisis totalis, cleft palate, absence of pituitary, taillessness, atresia ani
Arhinencephaly	Absence of olfactory bulbs, tracts and nerves	Unknown	Rare	Necropsy	Aprosopia, atresia of nostrils, cleft palate, encephalomeningocele, internal hydrocephalus, cerebellar hypoplasia, Arnold-Chiari malformation, facial-digital syndrome, aplastic pituitary (prolonged gestation)

Table continued on following page

TABLE 1. *Congenital Defects of Cattle Classified by Body System (Continued)*

Defect	Description	Etiology	Frequency	Diagnosis	Associated Defects
Encephalo-(meningo)cele	Herniation of meninges and/or cerebral tissue through a cranial defect, usually in frontal region	Unknown	Common	Necropsy	Agnathia, cleft palate, cranioschisis, spinal cord defects, cerebellar defects, eye defects, arthrogryposis, atresia ani
Exencephaly	Exposure of brain from a defectively developed cranium	Unknown	Rare	Necropsy	Acrania, cervical spina bifida
Hydranencephaly	Cerebral tissue replaced by thin fluid-filled bags	Unknown, blue tongue virus	Uncommon	Necropsy	Arthrogryposis, cerebellar hypoplasia, spinal dysraphism, meningocele
Hydrocephalus, internal	Accumulation of excessive amount of CNS fluid within lateral and other ventricles of brain, leading to dilation of lateral ventricles	Genetic, simple autosomal recessive, environmental causes possible	Common	Necropsy	More common associated defects are cleft palate, eye defects, cerebellar defects, spinal cord defects, myopathy, arthrogryposis, heart defects
Micrencephaly	Abnormally small brain, small and reduced number of gyri	Possibly genetic	Rare	Necropsy	Micrognathia, agenesis of corpus callosum, pachygyria, enlarged third cerebral ventricle, arthrogryposis

7. Congenital Defects of the Cerebellum:

Defect	Description	Etiology	Frequency	Diagnosis	Associated Defects
Cerebellar hypoplasia	Cerebellum absent or small, smooth surface, cross section reveals small and narrow cortex and folia. Cerebral hemispheres and brain stem normal	Possibly genetic, as a simple autosomal recessive trait	Rare	Necropsy and histological examination	None

Cerebellar atrophy	Cerebellum reduced in size. Mild to severe depletion of cortical layers and narrow, fiber-depleted streaks to large, irregular cavities in the folial white matter of cerebellum	BVD-MD virus	Rare	Necropsy and histological examination	Ocular lesions: cataract, retinal degeneration, hypoplasia and neuritis of optic nerves. Also fetal mummification, mandibular brachygnathia, skin defects
Cerebellar ataxia and hypomyelinogenesis congenita	CNS grossly normal. Histological changes consist of diffuse spongy appearance	Genetic, simple autosomal recessive	Rare	Histological examination	None
Hereditary neuraxial edema	CNS grossly normal, sometimes brain appears pale and swollen. Histological examination reveals spongy vacuolation of long axis of myelinated fibers in white and gray matter	Genetic, simple autosomal recessive	Rare	Histological examination	None
Arnold-Chiari malformation	Herniation of tongue-like processes of cerebellar tissue through the foramen magnum dorsal to anterior cervical spinal cord. Associated with displacement of medulla oblongata, pons and fourth cerebral ventricle	Unknown	Rare	Necropsy	Spina bifida of lumbar spinal column

8. Genetic Spastic Diseases:

Spastic paresis	Spastic contracture of muscles and extension of stifle and tarsal joints of one or both hind limbs. Progressive, varies in severity and time of onset from 3 to 6 months of age or as late as 2 years	Genetic influences and environmental factors play a role	Common	Clinical examination	None

Table continued on following page

TABLE 1. *Congenital Defects of Cattle Classified by Body System (Continued)*

Defect	Description	Etiology	Frequency	Diagnosis	Associated Defects
Spastic syndrome	Chronic progressive disease characterized by intermittent spastic contractures of muscles of both hind limbs. Straight rear limbs and weak hocks. No CNS lesions	Genetic, simple autosomal recessive with incomplete penetrance	Common	Clinical examination	None
Spastic lethal (neonatal) syndrome	Spasms and incoordination involving all four limbs, present at birth or developing later. No pathological lesions. Affected calves cannot stand. Sudden touch and noise will precipitate spasms	Genetic, simple autosomal recessive	Rare	Clinical examination	None
Epilepsy	True epilepsy is a convulsive state without definitive CNS lesion	Dominant	Uncommon	Clinical examination	None
Congenital tremor	Tremor of forelimbs. No lesions in CNS	Unknown	Uncommon	Clinical examination	None
Doddlers	Muscle spasm, convulsion, nystagmus, incoordination. Calcification of small vessels and neurons of the brain stem and cerebellum	Possibly genetic	Uncommon	Clinical examination	None
Ataxia and stagger	Twenty-five calves were affected with ataxia, incoordination and stagger. No anatomical lesion was discovered except for one calf with cerebellar hypoplasia	Unknown	Uncommon	Clinical examination	None

9. Congenital Defects of the Spinal Cord:

Spina bifida	Dorsal vertebral laminae not closed, with or without associated spinal cord defects	Possibly genetic, autosomal recessive or dominant gene with low penetrance and variable expressivity	Uncommon	Necropsy	Arthrogryposis, kyphoscoliosis, lordosis, cleft diaphragm, spinal dysraphism, meningomyeloschisis, perosomus elumbis, myopathy, a single (fused) kidney, aplasia of one uterine horn, atresia ani, taillessness
Spinal dysraphism	Varying lesions of segmental nature. Hydromyelia, dilation of central spinal canal and syringomyelia, defined as cavitation of spinal cord tissue	Unknown, possibly genetic	Uncommon	Necropsy and histological examination	Spina bifida. Arnold-Chiari malformation, calf. Cerebellar agenesis, arthrogryposis hydranencephaly, internal hydrocephalus, cleft palate, facial-digital syndrome

10. Hereditary Storage Diseases of the Central Nervous System:

α-Mannosidosis (pseudolipidosis)	Deficiency of mannosidase results in accumulation of oligosaccharides in neurons, reticuloendothelial system and other cells. Characterized clinically by ataxia, incoordination, head tremor, failure to thrive, aggressive behavior. Onset 6 to 12 months of age	Genetic, simple autosomal recessive	New Zealand and Australia common, recently diagnosed in United States	Clinical examination, histological examination, blood biochemistry for α-mannosidase	Moderate internal hydrocephalus

Table continued on following page

TABLE 1. Congenital Defects of Cattle Classified by Body System (Continued)

Defect	Description	Etiology	Frequency	Diagnosis	Associated Defects
GM-gangliosidosis	Deficiency of β-galactosidase resulting in accumulation of GM-gangliosides in neurons. Clinical signs in calves are swaying of hind quarters, reluctance to move, stiff gait, failure to thrive.	Genetic, simple autosomal recessive	Uncommon	Clinical examination and histological examination, enzyme studies	None
Neuronal lipodystrophy	History of blindness intermittent circling, periodic convulsions, coma. Histological lesions consist of eosinophilic granules in cytoplasm of neurons, macrophages	Familial	Uncommon	Clinical examination, histological examination	None

11. Congenital Defects of the Eye:

Defect	Description	Etiology	Frequency	Diagnosis	Associated Defects
Exophthalmos	Protrusion of eyeballs. Initial sign is impaired vision	Simple autosomal recessive	Rare	Clinical examination	None reported
Strabismus	Deviation of eyeballs from proper axis	Simple autosomal recessive	Rare	Clinical examination	None
Anophthalmia	Absence of one or both eyes	Unknown	Rare	Clinical examination	Some animals have no tails
Microphthalmia	One or both eyeballs are abnormally small	Unknown	Common	Clinical examination	Tailless, high ventricular septal defect
Microphthalmia associated with other ocular defects and internal hydrocephalus	Usually bilateral reduction of size of eyeballs with internal hydrocephalus	Simple autosomal recessive	Common	Clinical examination	Myopathy, cerebellar hypoplasia, optic nerve hypoplasia, retinal detachment, cataracts
Glaucoma	Increased intraocular pressure	Autosomal dominant	Rare	Clinical examination	Cataracts, lens luxated

Defect	Description	Inheritance	Frequency	Diagnosis	Associated findings
Entropion	One or both eyelids turned inward. Leads to conjunctivitis and corneal lesions	Possibly genetic	Rare	Clinical examination	None
Ectropion	One or both eyelids turned outward	Possibly genetic	Rare	Clinical examination	None
Distichiasis	Double row of eyelids	Unknown	Uncommon	Clinical examination	None
Dermoid	Skin-like appendage on eyelids, conjunction, nictitating membrane or cornea. Same color as eyelid, contains hair	Possibly genetic	Common	Clinical examination	None
Corneal edema	Mild corneal edema and cloudiness present at birth. Condition progresses with age and may lead to blindness	Possibly genetic, simple autosomal recessive	Rare	Clinical examination	None
Heterochromia iridis	Multi-colored iris	Genetic, may be autosomal recessive, others dominant	Rare	Clinical examination	Deafness, coloboma
Albinism, complete	Lack of pigment, ocular structures pink	Simple autosomal recessive	Rare	Clinical examination	Enzyme deficiencies
Albinism, incomplete	Gray to blue irides, skin is white or may have a few pigmented spots	Autosomal dominant	Rare	Clinical examination	Deafness, coloboma of optic disc
Chédiak-Higashi syndrome	Gray iris, color reduction in skin	Simple autosomal recessive	Rare	Clinical examination, blood smears to demonstrate intracytoplasmic inclusions in leukocytes	Susceptible to infection
Cataract	Lens opacity of one or both eyes	Genetic	Common	Clinical examination	Usually a single defect. Other calves may have multiple ocular defects

Table continued on following page

TABLE 1. *Congenital Defects of Cattle Classified by Body System* (Continued)

Defect	Description	Etiology	Frequency	Diagnosis	Associated Defects
Retinal dysplasia	Nonattached retina that is dysplastic	Genetic, others considered environmental	Rare	Clinical examination	May have internal hydrocephalus, myopathy and other defects
Coloboma of optic disc	Defect occurs in ventral position at optic disc, characterized by hypoplasia of sclera, choroid, retinal thinning and gliosis	Genetic cause most likely	Rare	Ophthalmological examination	None

12. Congenital Defects of the Heart and Large Vessels:

Defect	Description	Etiology	Frequency	Diagnosis	Associated Defects
Ectopia cordis cervicalis	Heart located outside thoracic cavity, usually in ventral neck area, and covered by skin	Possibly genetic	Common	External examination	Abnormalities of ribs and large vessels
Ectopia cordis sternalis	Fissure in sternum, heart located outside thorax, not covered by skin	Unknown	Uncommon	External examination	Sternum has fissure, large vessels abnormal
Ectopia cordis abdominalis	Heart located in abdominal cavity	Unknown	Uncommon	Clinical examination	Large vessels abnormal
Cor triloculare biventriculare	Three-chambered heart, one atrium and two ventricles. Calves die within hours to days after birth	Unknown	Uncommon	Necropsy	Vascular defects, arthrogryposis
Cor triloculare biatriatum	Three-chambered heart, two atria and one ventricle. Calves survive a few days after birth	Unknown	Uncommon	Necropsy	Vessels abnormal
Cor biloculare	Two-chambered heart. Calves usually born dead	Unknown	Uncommon	Necropsy	Multiple defects of bones and muscles

Defect	Description	Cause	Frequency	Diagnosis	Other
Patent foramen ovale	Persistence of foramen ovale, opening between right and left atrium, usually partially covered by membrane	Unknown	Common	Clinical examination, necropsy	About half the animals may have patent ductus arteriosus
Ventricular septal defect	Ventricular septal defects are common and provide an opening between right and left ventricle. May vary in location in ventricular septum	Possibly genetic	Common	Clinical examination, necropsy	May be single isolated defect or may have abnormalities of blood vessel, microphthalmia, taillessness
Tetralogy of Fallot	High ventricular septal defect, stenosis of pulmonary artery, dextraposition of aorta and hypertrophy of right ventricle	Unknown	Rare	Clinical examination	None
Patent ductus arteriosus	Persistence of fetal vessel from pulmonary artery to aorta that shunts blood away from lung	Unknown	Common	Clinical examination	May have patent foramen ovale
Common aortic trunk	Failure of separation of common trunk of aorta and pulmonary artery	Unknown	Rare	Clinical examination, necropsy	None
Persistence of right aortic arch	Encircling of esophagus by pulmonary artery, aorta, ligamentum ateriosum and trachea	Unknown	Uncommon	Clinical examination, necropsy	None
Left cardiac hypoplasia	Hypoplasia of aorta and left ventricle. Calves die shortly after birth	Possibly genetic	Rare	Clinical examination, necropsy	Atrial septal defect and patent ductus arteriosus
Valvular hematocysts	Blood-filled cysts at the margins of the atrioventricular valves, measuring up to 1.0 cm in diameter	Unknown	Common	Usually no clinical signs	None
Endocardial fibroelastosis	Abnormal diffuse thickening of endocardium in left ventricle, hypertrophy of left ventricle. Death in late neonatal period	Unknown	Rare	Necropsy	May have other vessel and heart defects

Table continued on following page

TABLE 1. *Congenital Defects of Cattle Classified by Body System (Continued)*

Defect	Description	Etiology	Frequency	Diagnosis	Associated Defects
13. Congenital Defects of the Intestinal System:					
Atresia ani	Rectum ends blindly in a cul-de-sac or opens into urinary bladder, urethra or vagina. Distended abdomen, no feces around anal area	Unknown	Rare	Clinical examination	Defects of urogenital system, or tailless or spinal dysraphism of lumbar spinal cord. May have no associated defects. Some calves may have atresia coli
Atresia of rectum	Rectum ends blindly in cul-de-sac, more extensive than atresia ani. Distended abdomen, no feces at anal area	Unknown	Rare	Clinical examination	None. Older calves may have urogenital defects, skeletal defects
Atresia coli	Rectum and anus usually patent. Passage of some meconium. Distended abdomen. Location of atresia is variable	Unknown	Rare	Clinical examination, laparotomy, necropsy	May have no other defect, or may have atresia ani, skeletal defects, urogenital defects.
Atresia of ileum	Ileum ends blindly	Possibly genetic	Uncommon	Necropsy	None
14. Congenital Defects of the Skin:					
Epitheliogenesis imperfecta	Discontinuity of squamous epithelium, epithelial defects of circumscribed areas (1 to 2 cm) in areas distal to carpus and tarsus, muzzle, nostrils, tongue, hard palate, cheeks, esophagus, forestomach. One or more claws may be defective, ears may lack epithelium	Genetic, simple autosomal recessive	Common	Clinical and histopathological examinations	Lesions may involve jaw, anus and vagina

Defect	Description	Genetics	Frequency	Diagnosis	Treatment
Congenital ichthyosis	Severe skin defect, variable in degree. Characterized by large scales of horn on skin. Separated by deep fissures. Lethal	Genetic, simple autosomal recessive	Uncommon	Clinical examination	None
Collagenous tissue dysplasia	Collagenous tissue dysplasia (dermatoparaxis, skin fragility) is characterized by skin fragility, resulting in severe laceration with nominal trauma and delayed skin healing. Histological and ultrastructural studies disclose lack of mature collagen fibers	Genetic, simple	Rare	Clinical examination	None
Acantholysis	Shedding of epidermis, leaving ulcers in oral mucosa. Skin of carpus, phalanges, coronary border and hooves may separate	Genetic, simple autosomal recessive most likely	Rare	Clinical and histological examinations	None
Lethal hairlessness	Calves die shortly after birth. Hair present only on muzzle, eyelids, ears, tail and perineum; otherwise naked	Genetic, simple autosomal recessive	Rare	Clinical examination and genetic analysis	None
Semi-hairlessness	Affected calves are viable. Have fine, thin, curly hair coat. Skin is patchy, wrinkled and scaly	Genetic, simple autosomal recessive	Rare	Clinical examination and genetic analysis	None
Hypotrichosis with anodontia	Completely hairless at birth, may develop a fine short hair coat later in life. Teeth missing. Calves do not thrive	Genetic, sex-linked recessive	Uncommon	Clinical examination and genetic analysis	None
Viable hypotrichosis	Completely or partially hairless at birth. May develop patches of hair later	Genetic, simple autosomal recessive	Rare	Clinical examination and genetic analysis	None and genetic
Hypotrichosis with missing incisors	Patches of short hair at birth loacted on face and neck. Later hair coat is normal. Agenesis of four to six incisor teeth.	Genetic, possibly a dominant trait	Uncommon	Clinical examination and genetic analysis	None

Table continued on following page

TABLE 1. Congenital Defects of Cattle Classified by Body System (Continued)

Defect	Description	Etiology	Frequency	Diagnosis	Associated Defects
Streaked hairlessness	Affected calf lacks hair development; vertical streaks involving lip, lateral abdominal and leg areas	Genetic, dominant sex-linked gene	Uncommon	Clinical examination and genetic analysis	None for females, apparently lethal to males
15. Congenital Defects of the Body Cavities:					
Schistosomus reflexus	Severe closure defect of thorax and abdominal cavities with exposure of viscera	Unknown	Common	Clinical examination	Spinal column defective and twisted
Abdominal fissure	Variable degrees of opening in ventral abdominal wall with herniation of organs	Unknown	Uncommon	Clinical examination	None
Umbilical hernia	Hernia involving umbilical area and covered by skin	Incomplete dominant, other cases are recessive, sporadic	Common	Clinical examination	None
16. Congenital Defects of the Female Reproductive System:*					
Vulva and vagina:					
Atresia	Vulva nonpatent	Unknown	Rare	External examination	Associated with atresia ani
Cloaca	Failure of vulva and vestibule to separate from the urogenital sinus	Unknown	Common	External examination	Associated with majority of cases of atresia ani
Rectovaginal constriction	Stenotic vestibule and anus	Possibly recessive	Common in Jersey cows, possibly Friesians	Rectal and vaginal examinations	Anal stenosis in bulls and cows
Persistent hymen	Persistent hymen strands	Genetic	Relatively common	Vaginal examination	Associated with white heifer disease or freemartinism

*Includes only reported congenital defects and excludes the following conditions that may be genetic or have a hereditary susceptibility but are also caused by other factors: vaginal and uterine prolapse, abnormal fertility (ranging from reduced fertility to sterility), embryonic resorption and cystic ovaries (follicular and luteal cysts).

Defect	Description	Inheritance	Frequency	Diagnosis	Effect on oviducts / associated
Dysplasia of Müllerian ducts:					
Segmental aplasia (white heifer disease)	Part or all of the vagina, cervix or uterus may be missing	Recessive	Not uncommon	Rectal examination	Oviducts rarely involved and usually normal. Mucovagina, mucocervix and mucometra
Uterus unicornis	Segmental aplasia of one horn	Recessive	Rare	Rectal examination	None
Uterus didelphys	Double uterus resulting from failure of the Müllerian ducts to fuse	Unknown	Rare	Rectal examination	Double cervix
Double cervix	Failure of the Müllerian ducts to fuse in the cervical region	Unknown	Rare	Rectal examination	None
Ovaries:					
Aplasia	One or both ovaries missing	Unknown	Rare	Rectal examination	Usually associated with other more extensive defects
Hypoplasia	One or both ovaries smaller than normal	Recessive	Common	Rectal examination, breeding records	Usually nil. Freemartinism
Mammary glands:					
Aplasia	One or more quarters missing	Unknown	Rare	External examination	None
Hypoplasia	One or more quarters smaller than normal	Unknown	Rare	External examination	Freemartinism
Agenesis of a teat	Missing teat	Unknown	Rare	External examination	None
Polythelia	Supernumerary teats, caudal type most common	Unknown	Relatively common	External examination	None
Synthelia	Fused teats	Recessive	Relatively common	External examination	None
Intersexuality:					
Hermaphroditism	Internal genitalia and gonadal tissue of both sexes. External genitalia are intermediate	Unknown	Rare	External and internal examination	None

Table continued on following page

TABLE 1. *Congenital Defects of Cattle Classified by Body System (Continued)*

Defect	Description	Etiology	Frequency	Diagnosis	Associated Defects
Pseudohermaphroditism	Male variety more common	Unknown	Relatively common	External and internal examination	None
Freemartinism	Vagina nonpatent, small vulva, uterus cord-like, ovaries hypoplastic	Inconclusive	Relatively common	External and internal examination	Usually co-twin to a male

17. Congenital Defects Usually Resulting in Dystocia:*

Defect	Description	Etiology	Frequency	Diagnosis	Associated Defects
Asymmetrical twins:					
Holoacardius acephalus	Small nonviable twin with a trunk, two hind legs and no heart, neck or head	Unknown	Rare	External examination	Many
Amorphus globosus	Rounded, edematous structure having no general body form	Unknown	Rare	External examination	Many
Conjoined twins:					
Anterior or posterior types	Various combinations	Unknown	Not uncommon	External examination	Many, depending upon attachment
Hematic mummification	Usually occurs between fourth and sixth months of gestation	Recessive	Not uncommon	External examination	None
Fetal dropsy	Edematous fetus	Recessive	Not common	External and internal examination	Milder form may be associated with edema of the hind legs
Hydramnios	Slowly developing edema due to viscid amniotic fluid	Recessive	Not common	Usually diagnosed at parturition by syrupy, viscid amniotic fluid and small defective calf	Defective calf

*Other defective calves such as schistosomus reflexus and those with arthrogryposis are listed in Sections 5 and 15, respectively.

Prolonged gestation	Two types recognized. One with a large nonviable calf and the other with a small defective fetus with cranial anomalies	Recessive	Not common	Based on the appearance and size of the calf, the length of gestation and associated lesions	First type has hypoplastic adrenals. The second is associated with adenohypophyseal aplasia

18. Congenital Defects of the Male Reproductive System:

Scrotum:					
Aplasia	Missing scrotum	Unknown	Rare	External examination	Usually associated with pseudo-hermaphroditism
Partially to completely divided scrotum	Partial to complete lack of fusion of the two scrotal pouches	Unknown	Not common	External examination	Hypospadias
Scrotal hernia	Unilateral or bilateral displacement of small intestines	Unknown	Not common	External examination	None
Testes:					
Aplasia	One or both testes missing	Unknown	Not common	External and internal examination	Commonly associated with incomplete twinning
Cryptorchidism	Incomplete descent of one or both testes	Recessive	Common	External and internal examination	None, or other defective syndromes
Polyorchidism	More than two testes	Unknown	Rare	External and internal examination	Usually part of incomplete twinning
Hypoplasia	One or both testes smaller than normal	Recessive with incomplete penetrance	Common	Palpation, semen examination, evaluation of breeding records	None
Abnormal spermatozoa	Various abnormal spermatozoa	Many are thought to be hereditary	Common	Semen examination	None, or various conditions

Table continued on following page

TABLE 1. *Congenital Defects of Cattle Classified by Body System (Continued)*

Defect	Description	Etiology	Frequency	Diagnosis	Associated Defects
Epididymis:					
Segmental aplasia	Part or all of the epididymis, vas deferens or seminal vesicles may be missing	Recessive	Not common	Palpitation, semen examination, breeding performance	Spermatic granuloma aspermia if bilateral
Spermatic granuloma	Granulomatous reaction to extravasation of spermatozoa	Unknown	Common	Palpitation, histological examination	May or may not be associated with aplasia
Paradidymis	Small gray nodule or nodules of a few convoluted tubules from the mesonephros located in the anterior part of the spermatic cord	Unknown	Common, found in 25 to 46 per cent of calves	Incidental finding at necropsy	None
Uterus masculinis	A small blind pouch arising in the prostate and opening into the seminal colliculus. Remnant of the distal portion of the Müllerian duct	Unknown	Common, found in 24 to 44 per cent of bulls	Incidental necropsy finding	None
Seminal vesicles:					
Segmental aplasia	Part or all of both lobes may be missing, usually unilateral	Recessive	Not common	Palpation	Usually associated lack of part or all of epididymis and vas deferens
Hypoplasia	One or both lobes smaller than normal	Unknown	Not common	Palpation	None, or other Wolffian duct defects
Duplication	Doubling of the seminal vesicles	Unknown	Not common	Palpation	None, or other Wolffian duct defects

Penis:				
Short penis	Smaller than normal	Possibly recessive	Not common, seen more in Herefords and Guernseys	Palpation and service behavior	Usually none
Corkscrew penis	Penis spirals counterclockwise ventrally and to the right	Unknown	More common in younger bulls	Service	Usually none
Rainbow deviation	Ventral deviation	Unknown	Not common	Observation of service	Usually none
Persistent frenulum	Persistence of the fold beneath the glans penis to prepuce	Unknown, suspected to be hereditary	Not common	Examination and observation of service	Penile
Diphallia	Penile duplication	Unknown	Rare	Examination	Usually scrotal duplication
Hypospadias	Abnormal ventral opening in the extrapelvic urethra due to incomplete closure of the genital folds	Possibly recessive	Not common	External examination	Bifid scrotum. Regarded as a mild form of pseudohermaphroditism
Epispadias	Dorsal opening in the penile urethra	Unknown	Rare	Careful examination of penis, evaluation of breeding records	None, or other penile and scrotal defects
Pseudohermaphroditism	See Section 16				
Spastic paresis	See Section 8				

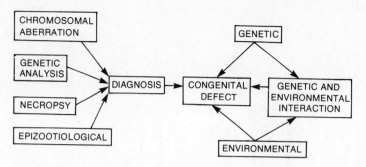

Figure 7. Diagrammatical presentation of the factors involved in diagnosing congenital defective calves.

sections according to the principal body system involved.

Factors Influencing Diagnosis of Congenital Defects

As diagnosis of bovine congenital defects is complex, various limiting factors need to be considered first (Fig. 7).

Defects Not Reported. Defective calves are frequently not reported unless they are unusually bizarre or several defective births have occurred. Nonreporting is a major difficulty limiting our knowledge of congenital defects in cattle. Cooperation of breeders by reporting all defective calves to the appropriate cattle associations and AI centers is essential for controlling or eliminating undesirable genetic traits.

Professional Knowledge. Limited knowledge and incomplete examination have led to defective calves being mistaken for premature births or abortions. Practitioners should be familiar with the more common cattle defects and, if in doubt, should seek specialized assistance. Practitioners are required to advise breeders about control measures, which may require altering herd management or breeding programs, depending on whether they consider the congenital defect to be environmentally or genetically induced. Veterinarians, both practitioners and laboratory diagnosticians, should always be cognizant of their roles in preventive teratology.

Inadequate History. Too often defective calves are submitted for diagnosis with little history being supplied. Diagnostic judgment and documentation of congenital defects require information on the geographical region, gestation season, feeding and management practices, types of pastures, presence of poisonous or teratogenic plants, vaccinations, stresses and any sickness or medication during pregnancy.

Breeding Records. Diagnosis of genetic defects is handicapped by lack of or inadequate records. This restricts genetic analysis, which requires enumerating normal and defective calves and recording their familial relationships. Most known genetic defects in cattle follow a simple autosomal recessive pattern.

Classification and Terminology. Lack of a standardized system for classifying birth defects makes comparisons in the literature difficult. This deficiency interferes with exchange between the various disciplines and with accumulating readily retrievable data on congenital birth defects. Consequently, many reports are virtually lost in the literature. For easy reference and to facilitate interdisciplinary comparisons, it is recommended that congenital defects be classified by the body system that is primarily affected.

Differentiation of Genetic Defects. Genetic defects arise from mutant genes and tend to run in families. Mutant genes become evident over two or more generations by one of four major hereditary patterns: dominant, incomplete dominant, recessive and overdominant. These patterns involve certain characteristic ratios of normal and defective progeny that form the basis for accurate genetic diagnosis. Most known genetic defects in cattle are caused by autosomal recessive genes. Characteristics of recessive mutations are that defective calves come from normal-appearing parents and usually occur in small numbers. Recessive genes are carried generation after generation by normal carriers or heterozygotes and are insidiously perpetuated. The difficulty of identifying normal-appearing carriers makes control virtually impossible. Genetic defects may also be polygenic.

Diagnosis of a genetic origin for a single defective calf is impossible without an adequate breeding record. Even when several congenital defects occur in a herd, differentiation between a genetic or environmental cause may be difficult.

Differentiation of Chromosomal Aberrations. Although chromosomal aberrations have been known in cattle for some time, they have not achieved the diagnostic significance that they have in man.

Genetic-Environmental Interaction. Even though little understood, the complex interaction between genetic and environmental factors is slowly gaining prominence as knowledge of congenital defects is increased.

Etiological Agents. Identifying etiological agents of bovine congenital defects is often difficult for several reasons. In many cases, there is no clearly established cause. The first question is whether the defect is genetic or environmental. Even with several calves with similar defects, it is not easy to incriminate or eliminate the possibility of disease, plant or drug teratogens or nutritional deficiencies as the causative agent. When defective calves are restricted to a single herd or region, environmental factors are usually investigated first.

Confirmation. Most genetic defects are due to recessive genes. Diagnosis can be confirmed by test matings resulting in the predictable occurrence of defective and normal progeny. When the number of defective calves is small and test matings are not possible, it is difficult to determine the mode of transmission, and a tentative diagnosis is usually made on the basis of contributing evidence.

Recessives can also be detected by reporting all defective animals; this is efficient and easier to organize than test matings.

Suspected plant teratogens can be tested by feeding trials with pregnant cows or laboratory animals in early pregnancy.

BASIC GENETIC PRINCIPLES

Cattle breeders use genetic recombination or mutation in an effort to improve their cattle. Unfavorable variation can result, however, which causes undesirable productive traits as well as genetic diseases.

Genes are units of inheritance that determine growth and development within environmental limits. In using genetic variation to improve their livestock, animal breeders are concerned with the action of a single gene, gene pairs or multi-gene inheritance. Analyzing genetic defects is based on the fact that: (1) genetic diseases are passed by genes from parents to offspring and (2) mating closely related animals increases the probability of offspring receiving a copy of the same desirable or undesirable gene. To determine if a disease is caused by genetic action, offspring have to be classified as normal or abnormal, and family relationships must be established. Most genetic defects are caused by simple inheritance (one pair of genes), and, for the most part, the defective gene is recessive to the normal gene (normal gene dominates the effect of the defective gene).

Diagnosing genetically caused congenital defects is based on the fact that genetic diseases run in families; i.e., they occur in typical intergenerational patterns and intragenerational family frequencies. This requires classifying normal and abnormal calves and identifying their familial relationships. Various statistical methods are used to analyze such data. Confirming the genetic nature and pattern of a congenital defect can be obtained by test matings. The recessive genetic pattern is the commonest and involves only two kinds of calves: normal or defective. Among the normal calves are a few that can transmit the disease and most that cannot. Although mating two defective parents produces only defective calves, most defective animals do not reproduce. Therefore, most defective calves are born to normal-appearing parents, although most normal parents cannot transmit the disease. Each normal parent producing a defective calf transmits one of the two abnormal genes necessary to produce defective offspring.

When homozygous normal cattle are mated with other homozygous normal cattle or even with normal-appearing carriers, they produce only normal calves. When normal-appearing cattle that produced a defective offspring are mated repeatedly, 25 per cent of their offspring will be defective and 75 per cent normal. Moreover, two of every three normal calves from such parents also carry a hidden abnormal gene that they, too, can transmit to offspring just as their parents transmitted a recessive gene to them. Thus, recessive defects are "carried" from generation to generation by normal-appearing carriers or heterozygotes. The defects are exposed only when heterozygous cattle are mated to other heterozygotes and defective calves appear. Eliminating defective offspring usually keeps the frequency of recessive defects low.

Other simple inheritance patterns include dominance, incomplete dominance and overdominance.

Dominant is the opposite of recessive. With dominant inheritance, the normal cattle breed true but the abnormal animals may produce both normal and abnormal calves. With dominant genetic diseases, the defective calves are readily recognized, and the gene can be easily eliminated.

Incomplete dominance creates three kinds of cattle: normal, slightly abnormal and severely abnormal. The normal and the severely abnormal cattle breed true. Slightly abnormal cattle that are mated to each other produce 25 per cent normal, 50 per cent slightly abnormal and 25 per cent severely abnormal calves. The disease is easily controlled by eliminating all abnormal calves.

Overdominance is similar to incomplete dominance in that three kinds of cattle are recognized: normal, superior and abnormal. The normal and abnormal animals breed true. Mating superior cattle produces 25 per cent normal, 50 per cent superior and 25 per cent defective calves. The superior cattle usually are selected as replacements in preference to the normal animals because the person selecting does not know that 25 per cent of the offspring from like mates will be defective. Overdominant traits are difficult to control because all superior animals also carry the undesirable gene, and owners are reluctant to choose inferior breeding animals. Few traits, however, show overdominance.

Few characteristics are sex-linked. Some reports describe chromosomal aberrations. Congenital defects may also be inherited in a polygenic manner (many genes involved).

DIAGNOSING CONGENITAL DEFECTS IN CATTLE

For accurate diagnosis of congenital defects in cattle, the following standardized procedures are recommended.

Reporting Defects. As mentioned previously, continual efforts should be made to have breeders report all defective calves. This will require the constant cooperation of veterinarians, AI centers, animal scientists and cattle breed associations. Monitoring congenital defects by cattle breed associations and AI centers will provide information on the frequency of various defects and on changing incidences.

Recording All Defective Calves. All defective calves should be thoroughly examined and documented.

History. The following history should be obtained and carefully evaluated: breed, geographical region, time of year, type of pasture, soil type, exposure to or suspected exposure to teratogenic plants, feeding and management practices, type of breeding, previous breeding records, maternal medical and vaccination records, disease status of herd, periods of stress, drugs administered, congenital defects observed previously and any history of similar congenital defects in neighboring herds.

Necropsy. Defective calves should be subjected to a standardized necropsy, and all lesions should be documented by photographs. This should be carried out by the practitioner or the regional diagnostic laboratory or by a specialist. Defects should be classified by the body system primarily involved.

Serum samples should be taken whenever possible and checked for bovine virus diarrhea, blue tongue, and other viral antibodies. Sections of spleen, liver and brain should be taken for possible virus isolation if a viral teratogen is suspected and if the defective calf has little autolysis. Virus isolation is difficult, as most viruses are labile and have disappeared by birth. Serological and fluorescent antibody techniques are more reliable when a viral teratogen is suspected.

Sections of brain, spinal cord, lungs, liver, kidneys and other appropriate tissues should be collected and fixed in 10 per cent buffered neutral formalin for histopathological examination.

Chemical Teratogens. The history should be carefully evaluated for any possible exposure to chemical or plant teratogens, especially during mating and embryogenesis. If necessary, the ranch should be revisited and the pastures checked for possible plant teratogens.

Chromosome Examination. With live defective calves, leukocytes and various tissues should be collected for culture and examination for possible chromosomal aberrations.

Genetic Analysis. Breeding records should be examined for characteristic intra- and intergenerational hereditary patterns of genetic disease. Analysis should proceed along several lines: segregation analysis with full-sib families and compatibility

TABLE 2. *Simple Hereditary Defects in Cattle*

Genotype of Animal	Appearance of Animal Based on Inheritance Patterns			
	RECESSIVE	DOMINANT	INCOMPLETE DOMINANT	OVERDOMINANT
A_1A_1	Normal	Normal	Normal	Normal
A_1A_2	Normal	Abnormal	Weak	Super
A_2A_2	Abnormal	Abnormal	Abnormal	Poor

analysis of close and distant relatives. Several methods may be used to test results of segregation analysis and to search for inbreeding.

Differential Diagnosis. Congenital defects must be differentiated from embryonic mortalities, abortions, premature births, stillbirths and neonatal deaths.

Diagnosis. Etiological diagnosis of defective calves is made after carefully considering the results of all the criteria of the standardized approach just discussed.

Confirmation. Confirmation of a genetic defect and mode of inheritance is possible by trial matings between suspected carriers or close relatives. As mentioned before, suspected plant teratogens can be tested by feeding trials with pregnant laboratory animals or cows in early pregnancy.

TESTING SUSPECTED CARRIER BULLS

The four major hereditary patterns commonly encountered in defective calves are summarized in Table 2. There is usually no need to test for a dominant trait since it is easily recognized. It may be necessary to test a bull to determine whether it is homozygous normal or heterozygous for a simple autosomal recessive gene. If the bull is of standard phenotype (not abnormal or surgi-

cally corrected for a defect), one or more of the following tests may be required:

Bred to Unknown Population. The resulting offspring are carefully monitored, and any abnormal calves are recorded. If specified defects occur or if the number of specific defective calves exceeds a predetermined threshold, the bull is regarded as being a heterozygote and is removed from service.

Bred to Daughters. A suspected bull may be bred to his daughters, and the results are summarized in Table 3. This procedure is expensive and time-consuming and is usually only employed for problem defects.

Bred to Known Heterozygotes. A bull may be tested for a specific defect by being bred to cows that are heterozygous for the defect. The probability of the bull being heterozygous is given in Table 3.

Bred to Homozygous Abnormals. Another method of testing bulls is by breeding them to homozygous abnormals if they can be raised to breeding age (Table 4).

The commonly used sire testing procedures are summarized in Table 4. Although they all have the disadvantage of being expensive and time-consuming, they are much cheaper than trying to eliminate a genetic defect after it has insidiously spread throughout a given cattle population. Remember, there are no minor defects when AI is used. A bull that is siring defective calves of unknown cause should immediately be

TABLE 3. *Probability of Bull Not Carrying an Undesired Recessive Gene**

No. of Offspring	Known Carrier Matings†	Sire-Daughter Matings‡
8	0.90	0.66
12	0.97	0.80
16	0.99	0.88
22	0.99+	0.95
40	0.99+	0.99

*If no abnormal calves are produced.
†Checks for only one recessive trait.
‡Checks for all recessive traits.

TABLE 4. *Sire Testing Procedures*

Procedure	Offspring Needed to Reach Probability Level of		
	0.05	0.01	0.001
Homozygous abnormals	5	7	10
Heterozygotes	10	16	24
Father-daughters	22	35	52
Matings to offspring of known heterozygotes	22	35	52

removed from service. Bulls with any defect should not be used.

Embryo transfer alone or in conjunction with preterminal cesarean section offers promise for being the method of choice for testing bulls for simple autosomal recessive defects. It has the additional advantage of being less expensive and less time-consuming.

WHAT SHOULD VETERINARIANS DO?

Practitioners should be familiar with the more common cattle defects, particularly those known to occur in the breeds in their area. When consulted about defective calves, they should attempt to diagnose the defect and determine if it is known to be hereditary. Veterinarians should ask the following questions:

1. Were the defective calves sired by the same bull?
2. Did other bulls on the ranch sire any abnormal calves?
3. Were the dams of the defective calves related?
4. Was inbreeding practiced?

If the answers indicate that the defect is genetic, they should recommend disposal of the bull and its offspring.

If these answers are inconclusive, they should also try to determine whether the dams were sick or stressed during early pregnancy or if the dams were vaccinated or exposed to possible teratogens during this period. If negative, the veterinarian should then seek specialized help.

PREVENTION OF CONGENITAL DEFECTS

Determining whether congenital defects are genetically or environmentally induced is important, as this dictates the control measures. It is essential to recognize genetic defects early in order to control their insidious spread. The difficulty of identifying heterozygotes makes control of recessive defects extremely difficult.

To minimize the effects of defective calves, it is recommended that:

1. An accurate diagnosis should be established.

2. If not, all congenital defects should be regarded as genetic until proved otherwise.
3. Defective calves should not be bred.
4. All newborn defective calves should be disposed of.
5. If the defect is environmentally induced, the management program should be adjusted.
6. If in doubt, specialized assistance should be sought.
7. All defective calves should be reported to cattle breed associations or AI centers.

IMPROVING KNOWLEDGE OF CONGENITAL DEFECTS

Breed associations, AI centers and veterinarians should actively encourage cattle breeders to report rather than hide defective calves. Many breeders still routinely destroy such animals. It is unfortunate that these calves are not reported and made available for research. The more we know, the better we can control congenital anomalies. Research and control of congenital defects depend primarily upon individual cattle breeders.

With the changing demands within the cattle industry and the importation of new breeds in recent years, new inherited defects will emerge in the new breeds and their crosses. It is hoped that complete records of such defects will be kept by the breed associations and AI centers and that appropriate cases will be available for diagnosis and research.

Expanding the knowledge of congenital defects in cattle will result mainly from the availability of numerous, adequately described reports containing detailed clinico-pathological examinations and genetic analyses. This will require the continual cooperation and effort by cattle breeders, veterinarians, breed associations, AI centers and animal scientists. Adopting standardized classification and terminology and diagnostic procedures should improve descriptions, diagnoses and interdisciplinary exchange of information. This, in turn, should improve knowledge and diagnosis of congenitally defective calves in the future.

REFERENCES

1. Greene, H. J., Leipold, H. W., Huston, K. and Dennis, S. M.: Congenital defects in cattle. Irish Vet. J., 27:37, 1973.

2. Guffy, M. M. and Leipold, H. W.: Radiologic diagnosis of economically important genetic defects in cattle. J. Am. Vet. Radiol. Soc., *18*:109, 1977.
3. Jolly, R. D. and Leipold, H. W.: Inherited diseases of cattle — a perspective. N. Z. Vet. J., *21*:147, 1973.
4. Leipold, H. W., Dennis, S. M. and Huston, K.: Congenital defects in cattle: Nature, cause and effect. Adv. Vet. Sci. Comp. Med., *16*:103, 1972.
5. Leipold, H. W., Dennis, S. M. and Huston, K.: Syndactyly in cattle. Vet. Bull., *43*:399, 1973.
6. Roberts, S. J.: Veterinary Obstetrics and Genital Diseases. Published by the author, Ithaca, New York, 1971, p. 49.

Effects of Climate on Bovine Reproduction

WILLIAM W. THATCHER
University of Florida, Gainesville, Florida

HERIBERTO ROMAN-PONCE
Instituto Nacional de Investigaciones, Mexico City, Mexico

ENVIRONMENTAL ASSOCIATIONS WITH REPRODUCTIVE PERFORMANCE

Seasonal climatic effects on reproductive performance influence herd management efficiency and management programs and are becoming even more important as tropical, subtropical and arid areas of the world take on an even greater role in supplying man's food. The veterinarian's understanding of thermal stress effects on reproductive physiology, endocrinology and overall animal performance is essential for providing proper recommendations for treatment and management of cattle during periods of thermal stress.

Suppression of conception rates in conjunction with monthly increases in adverse climatic conditions is well documented. In a large commercial dairy herd of 600 cows managed under a subtropical climate of Western Mexico, Ingraham et al.[2] demonstrated that as the temperature humidity index (THI) (Fig. 1) increased during monthly periods of high temperature and humidity, conception rates declined. Comparable periods of seasonal infertility occur in arid areas such as Arizona. Seasonal or monthly associations of climatic measurements with fertility may not be so apparent or may even be opposite from expected when nutrients available to the animal are also seasonally controlled. For example, in certain geographical locations, periods of high temperature and humidity may occur during the rainy season when nutrient availability or quality is increased or no longer limited. Consequently, a clear, direct effect of climatic parameters on cattle fertility is masked by an increase in available nutrients. Nutrition serves a permissive role, allowing reproductive processes to occur. Both environmental and management conditions need to be appraised when evaluating seasonal changes in fertility.

Of practical importance is whether specific climatic parameters near the time of insemination can be identified and quantitatively related to fertility on a service-to-service basis. Climatological indices have been developed for prediction of summer milk production losses within various geographical areas of the United States, but comparable indices have not been developed for fertility rates. A study of various climatic parameters in conjunction with

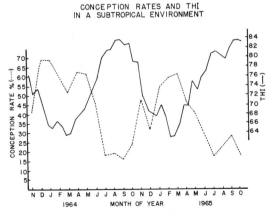

CONCEPTION RATES AND THI
IN A SUBTROPICAL ENVIRONMENT

Figure 1. Association of temperature humidity index (THI) with conception rate. (From Ingraham, R. H., Gillette, D. D. and Wagner, W. D.: J. Dairy Sci., *57*:476, 1974.)

fertility would identify climatic factors that may be modified to improve reproductive efficiency within certain geographical areas. Both maximum environmental temperature the day after insemination and solar radiation the day of insemination (Fig. 2) had negative curvilinear relationships with conception rate in the subtropical environment of Gainesville, Florida.[4] Estimates of these climatic effects were based on 3500 to 5000 services over a 10-year period and were adjusted for various management and cow effects such as inseminator, breed of cow, month of service, service number and age of cow. These auxiliary influences are also important for the veterinarian to recognize when coping with reproduction. Marked differences in conception rate were detected among inseminators, which emphasizes the importance of periodic retraining of inseminators. When specific climatic factors such as maximum temperature or solar radiation were evaluated, month-to-month differences in conception rates no longer occurred. This indicated that normal monthly effects were most likely related to climatological factors to a greater degree than nutritional and management factors in the Florida Experiment Station herd. This type of characterization done under fairly uniform management conditions indicated that reducing incident solar radiation may improve conception rates.

These climatic measurements represent changes in the animal's microenvironment that are related to conception rates. However, uterine temperature associations with fertility have also been detected and indicate that the temperature of the embryo's microenvironment, i.e., the uterus, is also critical, as would be expected. A rise of 0.5°C above mean uterine temperature on the day of or day after insemination was associated with decreases in conception rates of 12.8 and 6.9 per cent, respectively.[4] Uterine temperature measurements were taken close to the time of ovulation and fertilization. Periods of temperature associations with fertility may vary, depending upon the intensity and duration of heat stress and the acclimation of animals to their environment. Nevertheless, certain climatic measurements and uterine temperature are associated with variability in conception rates.

MANAGEMENT SYSTEMS TO REDUCE THERMAL STRESS AND IMPROVE REPRODUCTIVE AND LACTATIONAL EFFICIENCY

Arizona workers have been successful in lowering air temperature 9.8 to 12°C on a large-scale basis in commercial dairy herds by use of evaporative cooling. Both milk production and fertility are improved in cows exposed to cooled shades.[3] However, environmental conditions in tropical and subtropical areas are not ideally suited for evaporative cooling, owing to high relative humidity. Two alternative management systems studied by our laboratory have been air conditioning and a shade management system.

Daily total air conditioning or partial air conditioning during different times of the day allowed for gradient increases up to 9.4 per cent in production of 4 per cent fat-corrected milk.[4] If cows were either cooled during daylight hours (5:30 AM to 7:30 PM) or cooled throughout a 24-hour period, conception rates were higher (Table 1). However, benefits of increased milk production and fertility were not great enough to pay for the expense of operating the unit. Nevertheless, this study conducted with 208 cows documents the fertility response of cattle to air conditioning, in that a seasonal period of infertility was partially alleviated. The milk production and reproductive responses of these cows to environmental modification set a practical upper limit of achievement or a goal to be obtained using less costly structures to modify the environment.

As mentioned, solar radiation was a climatic factor that was quantitatively relat-

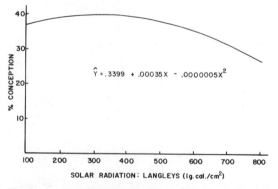

Figure 2. Association of solar radiation on the day of insemination with conception rate.

TABLE 1. *Milking Performance and Reproductive Efficiency of Air Conditioned Dairy Cows*

Treatment	Number of Cows	4% Fat Corrected Milk[*] (lb)	Total Services	Conception[†] (%)
Outside 24 hours	52	31.34	89	28.1(22.6)[‡]
Outside 5:30 AM to 7:30 PM Inside 7:30 PM to 5:30 AM	53	31.89	81	28.4(19.0)
Inside 5:30 AM to 7:30 PM Outside 7:30 PM to 5:30 AM	52	32.95	55	40.0(41.9)
Inside 24 hours	51	34.30	80	38.8(40.0)

[*]Differences among treatments $P < .01$.
[†]Differences among treatments $.10 < P < .25$.
[‡]Parentheses contain per cent conception for first summer of study ($P < .025$).

ed to conception rates (Fig. 2). Since solar radiation contributes to the animal's heat load, we were interested in determining whether a simple shade structure would improve dairy cattle performance by reducing net solar radiation. A shade structure of 2400-square feet was built to accommodate 30 to 33 cows. The lower truss chords of the gable roof were 12 feet above the floor. The 26-gauge sheet metal roof was painted white, and the underside was covered with a 1.5-inch layer of polystyrene tongue-and-grooved insulation board. The structure was oriented east-west to provide maximum shading efficiency for the cows. The floor was 4-inch reinforced concrete with a 2 per cent slope that was cleaned once daily with three 300-gallon dump tanks. A sweeptrough type of feeder combined with a continuous California-style head gate was located along the full length on the north side. A drinking facility was installed on the south side. East of the shade structure was a Bermuda grass sod area of 5 acres with no artificial or natural shade, to which the cows had free access. North of the shade was a separate but comparable sod area with similar water and feeding facilities and no artificial or natural shade. Cows managed in this area served as a no-shade control group.

Reproductive efficiency and milk production were monitored during the summers of 1974 (beginning August 28, 1974) using 39 cows and 1975 (beginning May 25, 1975) using 77 cows. Cows were assigned randomly to either the shade management treatment or the no-shade control manage-

ment group. The major climatological parameter that differed appreciably between the two experimental areas was black globe temperature. The average difference in black globe temperature (measured over 32 days) between areas was 8.3°C, and this difference was greatest (about 12°C) during midday. Black globe temperature integrates the effects of net radiation, dry bulb temperature and wind speed. Since no major differences were detected for dry bulb temperature, dew point temperature or wind speed, a reduction in net solar radiation is likely to be the important difference between shade and no-shade areas. Shade cows had lower ($P<.01$) respiration rates per minute (54 versus 82) and rectal temperatures (38.9 versus 39.4°C) than no-shade cows. This is also reflected when the respiration rate was measured every 2 hours for a 24-hour period in six cows under the shade structure and in the no-shade control area (Fig. 3). The improved physiological well-being of the shade-managed cows resulted in a 10.6 per cent greater mean daily milk yield. The lactation curves for the two groups differed ($P<.01$) in that the shade-managed cows were more persistent (Fig. 4). These types of production responses during the hot summer months in a subtropical environment are similar to the production trends of dairy cows exposed to evaporative cooling in Arizona.[3]

Conception rate to all services was higher for cows exposed to shade (44.4 versus 25.3 per cent) (Table 2). It was interesting that 25 per cent of the services for

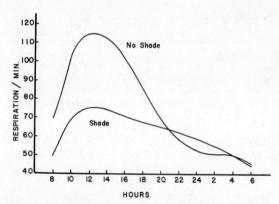

Figure 3. Respiration rates of cows exposed to a shade structure and no shade.

cows in the no-shade treatment group resulted in pregnancies. Apparently some cattle have the inherent ability to reproduce under adverse environmental conditions. Results of this experiment indicate that providing shade plus feed, water and an adjacent pasture area (for cattle to radiate their heat load during the evening and night hours) will alter the animal's microenvironment, lower respiration rates and rectal temperatures, and improve milk yield and reproductive performance.

USE OF SHADE MANAGEMENT MODEL TO EVALUATE HORMONAL CHANGES DURING ESTROUS CYCLE

Mechanisms by which thermal stress suppresses fertility have been the subject of intense investigation across many spe-

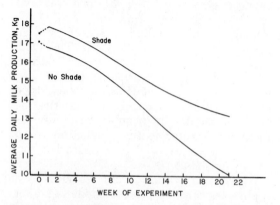

Figure 4. Lactation curves of cows exposed to shade or no shade.

cies. A clear, well-documented answer to this question is not yet available for cattle. The responses of the animal to thermal stress that decreases fertility probably are multifold, interrelated and difficult to classify simply as a direct temperature effect, a hormonal imbalance, a nutritional effect, a nervous system response or a biochemical effect. Undoubtedly the "infertility heat stress syndrome" is due to a combination of these factors that compromise the well-being of the zygote and/or embryo in its oviductal or uterine microenvironment.

A logical hypothesis is that thermal stress alters the hormonal balance of the animal, which interferes with reproductive processes culminating in a successful pregnancy. Research results to date are not consistent in documenting the various hormonal responses to thermal stress. This probably reflects differences between environment control chamber studies and field experiments; intensity of thermal stress and its duration (acute, chronic, diurnal); sensitivity of experimental designs; and hormonal procedures for quantification.

We have followed daily changes in plasma hormone levels (estradiol, estrone, luteinizing hormone, progesterone and corticoids) throughout the estrous cycle of five shade-managed and four no-shade–treated lactating dairy cows. The nine cows were a subsample of 66 cows assigned at random to the shade and no-shade protocol during the summer of 1976. Increased experimental manipulation of all cows for various physiological studies reduced the treatment milk yield difference to 6 per cent. However, additional management data were collected. Concentrate intake was held constant by design, and forage was offered *ad libitum*. Shade cows consumed 9 per cent more forage daily on a group basis during the summer. All cattle for all treatments drank significantly more water during the daylight hours of 8:30 AM to 5:00 PM (0.69 gallon/hour) than during the evening and night hours of 5:00 PM to 8:30 AM (0.58 gallon/hour). Throughout the summer no-shade cows drank 20 per cent more water than shade cows during a 24-hour period (0.67 versus 0.56 gallon per hour; P<.01). Per cent conception to all services was higher for the shade treatment group (38 per cent versus 14 per cent; P<.05) as reported for 1974 and 1975. Consequently, environmental conditions in 1976 between

TABLE 2. *Reproductive Performance of Shade Experiment for Years 1974 and 1975*

Factors	Shade	No Shade
Number of services	54	75
Number of cows pregnant	24	19
Per cent conception	44.4	25.3*
Total services/total pregnancies	2.25	3.95
Number of early embryo deaths	0	2

*P < .005.

treatments caused differential physiological, fertility and lactational responses.

Plasma samples were collected from indwelling jugular catheters with minimal disturbance to the cycling cows after they had adapted to their environments. Mean estrous cycle length for the cows was 21.0 days ± 0.9 day, and there was no difference between treatments. Daily hormonal concentrations were analyzed in two graphic phases. The curves (Figs. 5 to 7) represent the least squares regressions, using day as a continuous independent variable. The individual day point estimates are the least squares means for each treatment day of the experiment, utilizing day of estrous cycle as a discrete variable.

Hormonal concentrations differed significantly between treatments, with plasma concentrations of progesterone, luteinizing hormone (LH) and corticoids being higher for no-shade cows during the estrous cycle. Although plasma progesterone concentrations were higher (P<.01) in the no-shade cows, they were well within the concentrations documented in the literature. In fact,

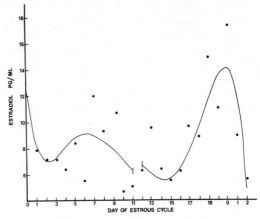

Figure 6. Plasma estradiol concentrations during the estrous cycle of shade- and no–shade-treated cows.

they tended to be lower, and perhaps this is a consequence of a general thermal stress (Fig. 5). These changes reflect periods of corpus luteum development, maintenance and regression. Associated with the higher progesterone levels of no-shade cows was a higher basal concentration of mean LH throughout the entire estrous cycle (5.4 versus 3.9 ng/ml). LH is the luteotropic hormone in the bovine and may contribute to the higher progesterone concentrations in the no-shade cows. With daily sampling only once per day, no inference can be made as to whether there is a difference in magnitude of the preovulatory surge of LH on day 21 in this experiment.

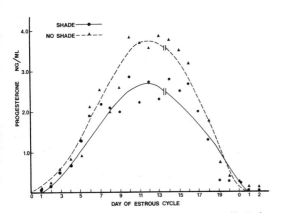

Figure 5. Plasma progesterone concentrations during the estrous cycle of shade- and no-shade-treated cows.

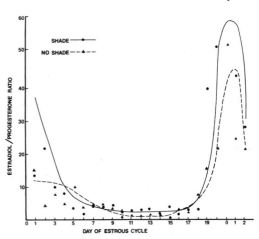

Figure 7. Plasma estradiol (pg) to progesterone (ng) ratio during the estrous cycle of shade- and no-shade–treated cows.

We also failed to detect a systematic difference in plasma estradiol concentration between treatments. The overall pooled regression for plasma estradiol is presented in Figure 6. The proestrous rise in plasma estradiol concentration (days 17 to 21) was less for the no-shade cows but not of sufficient magnitude to alter treatment concentrations across the entire cycle. A smaller rise in proestrous estradiol levels of heat-stressed heifers (32 versus 21°C) also was detected in our laboratory when the hormonal changes were monitored every 6 hours in an environmental chamber.[5] The estradiol-to-progesterone ratio is probably critical in controlling blood flow to the reproductive tract. The estradiol (pg)-to-progesterone (ng) ratio was lower for the no-shade treatment group during the proestrous, estrous and metestrous phases (P<.05) (Fig. 7). This difference may cause a suppressed blood flow to the reproductive tract of the no-shade–treated cows. The significance of this effect will be discussed later.

The transitory hormonal concentrations among the two treatment groups indicated that thermal stress of the magnitude observed in this study was not inhibiting the recurrence of estrous cycles. The fall in progesterone levels associated with corpus luteum regression and the proestrous rise in estradiol levels were sufficient to trigger a preovulatory surge of LH and induce estrus followed by ovulation in each cow.

In the present study, a significant increase in basal plasma corticoid concentration was detected in no-shade cows throughout the entire estrous cycle (13.0 versus 8.7 ng/ml). Furthermore, a comparably managed group of no-shade cows had a lower corticoid response to adrenocorticotropic hormone (ACTH) after an intravenous injection compared with shade cows (P<.01) (Fig. 8). This difference in response also has been detected in two other experiments in our laboratory. Apparently, the adrenals of chronically heat-stressed lactating cows are not as responsive to an ACTH challenge. This may be due to a previous chronic daily period of adrenal stimulation such that a greater number of adrenal ACTH receptors are occupied. The adrenal may then be less capable of responding to an acute exogenous ACTH challenge. Endogenous adrenocortical hypersection has been identified as having

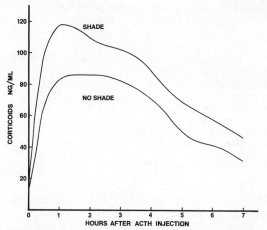

Figure 8. Plasma corticoid response to ACTH in cows exposed to shade and no shade.

counteractive influences on estrogen actions such as expansion of the uterine microcirculation. Consequently, increased plasma corticoid concentrations and a decreased estradiol-to-progesterone ratio may contribute to a decreased uterine blood flow during periods of thermal stress.

Cattle in southern parts of the United States during warm and hot months have shorter heat periods and less intense estrous behavior.[4] Consequently, accurate estrous detection for proper timing of insemination becomes a management problem. This may result in missed heats or possibly in detecting heats but inseminating cattle too late for ideal conception rates. Prostaglandin-$F_2\alpha$ appears to work effectively in heat-stressed cattle,[5] and it may be an effective management tool in synchronizing estrous behavior during the summer periods or in managing animals to avoid breeding during the summer months.

These hormonal studies indicate that either under carefully controlled environmental conditions or under practical field conditions transitory hormonal concentrations are not altered sufficiently to prevent heat-stressed animals from cycling. However, the subtle increase in peripheral plasma hormonal concentration, which ultimately supplies the uterus of no-shade–treated cows, may alter blood flow as previously suggested. The general increased concentration of plasma hormones in no-shade–stressed cows may reflect changes in water movement between tissues and the vascular bed or altered clearance rates of hormones. More detailed studies are needed to evaluate changes in water metabolism of thermal-stressed lactating cows under these types of practical experimental conditions.

UTERINE TEMPERATURE AND UTERINE BLOOD FLOW INTERRELATIONSHIPS

As previously described, uterine temperatures at the time of insemination are related to conception rates in the bovine. Various workers have reported direct adverse temperature effects on early developing embryos and spermatozoa. Consequently, factors controlling uterine temperatures in cattle are of paramount importance. Figure 9 shows variations in uterine serosa and aortic blood temperatures of a Guernsey cow in association with air temperature during a 40-hour period of continuous temperature recordings in a stanchion barn. Uterine temperature was always higher than that of the arterial blood supplying the uterus. After air temperature rises, there is a delay during which both aortic blood and uterine temperatures increase. Of interest is the observation that uterine temperature appeared to increase at a greater rate than aortic blood temperature and reached a temperature peak of greater than 40°C. Uterine temperatures of this magnitude are sufficiently high to decrease early embryo survival. The relative changes in temperature difference between the uterus and aortic blood are an indirect measurement of changes in uterine blood flow of the cow.[1] An increase of the temperature difference indicates a decrease in uterine blood flow. Temperature changes shown in Figure 9 suggest that uterine blood flow may decrease during thermal stress periods when aortic blood temperatures are elevated.

An experiment was designed to test this hypothesis directly using the shade versus no-shade treatment models previously described. Blood flow transducers were surgically implanted around a segment of one miduterine artery in three ovariectomized Brown Swiss dairy animals. Uterine blood flow (ml/minute) could then be recorded directly. Each cow received a series of intra-

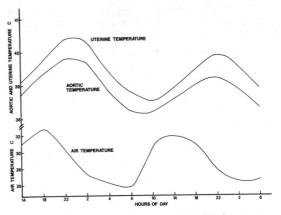

Figure 9. Uterine serosa and aortic blood temperatures recorded continuously over a 40-hour period.

venous injections of estradiol (200 μg) to elevate uterine blood flow. The subsequent increase in flow was then measured. Each cow received a minimum of two injections under both environments so that there was a total of seven blood flow responses in cows under the shade structure and seven in cows under no-shade conditions.

At approximately 45 minutes after estradiol injection, uterine blood flow started to increase from 45 ml/minute, and peak flows (130 to 170 ml/minute) were obtained between 3 and 3.5 hours (Fig. 10). Re-

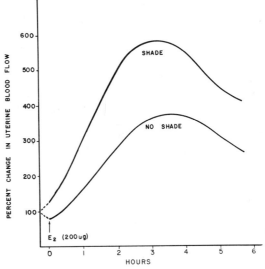

Figure 10. Uterine blood flow response after estradiol injection of cows exposed to shade and no shade.

sponses of cows to estradiol under the shade structure were characterized by a greater rate of increase in uterine blood flow and a higher peak than responses of the same cows exposed to no shade. Shade-treated cows had an overall percentage change of 412 per cent, whereas the change for no-shade–treated cows was only 287 per cent. Results of this experiment indicate that thermal stress conditions, which are known to reduce fertility under practical farm conditions, also suppress uterine blood flow responses to estradiol injection. Apparently the animal's attempt to thermoregulate under thermal stress conditions decreases uterine blood flow.

Additional studies are now needed to determine whether the subtle hormonal differences due to thermal stress alter uterine blood flow during the estrous cycle and early pregnancy. A thermal stress-induced reduction in uterine blood flow may further elevate uterine temperatures. Fertilized ova, developing embryos and spermatozoa deposited into the reproductive tract are sensitive to elevated temperatures. Decreases in uterine blood flow may also affect availability of water, nutrients and hormones to the uterus. Such thermal-stressed responses may contribute to the higher rate of embryo death during early pregnancy.

We are not aware of any drug therapy that will reduce the rise in temperature of the reproductive tract during a period of thermal stress that does not interfere with the intricate hormonal balance necessary to maintain pregnancy or affect the animal's ability to thermoregulate.

Additional studies are needed to determine the minimal periods necessary for environmental modification to increase reproductive rates under practical farm conditions. However, it is clear that practical systems of environmental modification and management can be recommended by the veterinarian that will improve milk production and conception rates during periods of seasonal infertility induced by thermal stress.

SPECIFIC RECOMMENDATIONS

The following are specific recommendations to maximize reproductive rates during periods of thermal stress:

1. Provide access for cattle to a system of environmental modification (type depends on location) that reduces exposure to environmental climatic factors known to reduce fertility.

2. Provide ready access to water and feed within the modified environment.

3. Allow cattle free access to loafing areas away from the environmental structure so they can more effectively radiate their heat loads during the evening and night hours.

4. Place intensive management efforts on obtaining greater frequency and accuracy of heat detection and proper timing of insemination, since intensity of estrous behavior is reduced.

5. Incorporate a system of pregnancy diagnosis *per rectum* in order to maintain intensive management awareness such that reproductive efficiency is maximized.*

---

*The authors acknowledge the capable and imaginative input of Dr. F. C. Gwazdauskas, a former student whose research contributed to this manuscript.

REFERENCES

1. Gwazdauskas, F. C., Abrams, R. M., Thatcher, W. W., Bazer, F. W. and Caton, D.: Thermal changes of the bovine uterus following administration of estradiol-17β. J. Anim. Sci., *39*:87, 1974.
2. Ingraham, R. H., Gillette, D. D., and Wagner, W. D.: Relationship of temperature and humidity to conception rate of Holstein cows in subtropical climate. J Dairy Sci., *57*:476, 1974.
3. Stott, G. H. and Wiersma, F.: Response of dairy cattle to an evaporative cooled environment. Proceedings International Livestock Environment Symposium. ASAE SP–0174:88, 1974.
4. Thatcher, W. W.: Effects of season, climate and temperature on reproduction and lactation. J. Dairy Sci., *57*:360, 1974.
5. Thatcher, W. W. and Chenault, J. R.: Reproductive physiological responses of cattle to exogenous prostaglandin $F_2\alpha$. J. Dairy Sci., *59*:1366, 1976.

The Role of Nutrition in Dairy Cattle Reproduction

DAVID A. MORROW

Michigan State University, East Lansing, Michigan

Nutritional deficiencies and imbalances are frequently implicated as the cause of infertility in cattle. If the ration is having an adverse effect on fertility, it is frequently deficient in more than one nutrient which makes it difficult to evaluate the effects of a specific nutrient on fertility. The clinical signs observed with a deficiency of a specific nutrient are variable, depending on the degree of the deficiency. For example, a moderate energy shortage reduces fertility, whereas a severe deficiency results in anestrus.

The purpose of this article is to summarize the available research information on the role of nutrition in dairy cattle reproduction. This information is designed to aid the practitioner in recognizing and correcting nutritionally related field reproductive problems.

ENERGY

Puberty

There is a close relationship between energy intake and onset of puberty in both females and males. When 102 Holstein heifer calves in a Cornell University study were fed at the rate of 62, 100 or 146 per cent of digestible nutrients, the onset of puberty occurred at 20, 11 and 9 months, respectively. Despite these wide age differences, heifers on all three levels of nutrition weighed approximately 600 pounds at the onset of puberty. These data suggest that body weight is more important than age in determining the time of first estrus.

When 24 Holstein bull calves were fed at the rate of 70, 100, 115 and 130 per cent of digestible nutrients, the average age at the onset of semen production was 61, 45, 41 and 44 weeks, respectively, in this Pennsylvania State University study. Comparable figures for body weight at the onset of semen pro-

duction were 523, 643, 675 and 748 pounds, respectively. The average motile sperm output per ejaculate at 80 weeks of age for the 70 per cent group was only one-half as large as that for the 130 per cent group. The level of energy intake had no effect on sperm output after 112 weeks of age. The libido decreased after 156 weeks of age in the group receiving 130 per cent of the National Research Council recommended total digestible nutrient (TDN) allowances. There were no differences in fertility that could be attributed to the level of energy intake.

The clinical signs observed with an energy deficiency are a delay in the onset of estrus in small, thin heifers with inactive ovaries. This condition is most frequently observed in late fall or winter when feed supplies are likely to be in short supply. The condition can be treated by free choice feeding of high quality forages in the form of pasture, hay, haylage or corn silage. The addition of 5 pounds of grain daily will increase growth and decrease the time required for the onset of puberty. The level of feeding does not affect estrous activity after the heifers begin to cycle unless severe restrictions occur.

Heifers should be maintained on a ration that will provide for daily gains of approximately 1.5 pounds per day. These heifers should exhibit estrus before 12 months of age and reach a breeding weight of 750 pounds by 14 months. It is important that heifers be gaining weight for 30 days before and after breeding for optimum fertility. The weights of calves from heifers are approximately the same regardless of age and body condition at parturition. Heifers should reach 1200 pounds and calve at 24 months of age to minimize calving difficulty.

Postpartum Reproduction

The clinical signs of infertility related to an energy deficiency in cows include inactive ovaries, repeat breeding and decreased progesterone production by the corpus luteum. Severe emaciation may result in abortions.

In an Israeli study with 14 cows on low and high levels of nutrition, the cows that conceived on first service gained weight and had higher progesterone levels during the previous cycle, whereas cows that did not conceive lost weight and had lower progesterone levels during the same period.

Plasma luteinizing hormone (LH) and progesterone levels were studied in six heifers on 62 per cent and 100 per cent of Morrison's TDN allowance. A progressive increase in plasma LH levels occurred from the first to third estrous cycle in heifers on the low energy intake, and there was a concurrent decrease in plasma progesterone levels ($P<0.01$). These results show that ovarian hypofunction under conditions of restricted energy intake is due to a reduced ability of ovarian tissue to respond to LH rather than to reduced circulating levels of LH.

In a 3-year liberal concentrate feeding study with 50 cows, cows fed up to 20 pounds of grain daily prepartum and ad libitum for 6 weeks postpartum had a longer calving interval ($P<0.01$) than cows fed up to 6 pounds of grain daily prepartum and a maximum of 20 pounds postpartum. The liberally fed cows also had more cystic follicles, abortions and services per conception ($P<0.05$).

The effects of average and high nutrition (i.e., 150 per cent concentrate of the average group) on reproductive performance in 393 calving intervals were reported in a Wisconsin study. The intervals to first postpartum ovulation and estrus were shorter in the average group ($P<0.05$). The occurrence of retained placenta and metritis was lower in the average than in the high nutrition groups.

High milk production can also have an adverse effect on fertility. In a Cornell study with 204 cows, the interval from calving to conception and services per conception increased as milk production increased. These effects were especially pronounced in cows producing more than 7272 kg of milk.

Similar results were observed in a recent study of 125 New York dairy herd improvement (DHI) herds. In this study, cows producing at levels that exceeded their herdmates by more than 907 kg had a lower first service conception rate (36 per cent versus 54 per cent) and were open longer (133 versus 108 days) than the cows producing up to 907 kg less milk than their herdmates. The actual complete lactation production of these two groups of cows was 8270 and 6042 kg, respectively. Reproductive performance in high producing cows within any one herd appeared to be impaired in comparison to that observed in lower producing herdmates.

It is well known that high producing dairy cattle are in negative energy balance during early lactation because they cannot consume enough feed to meet the nutrient requirements for high levels of milk production. Tissue energy stores are mobilized and weight losses occur during the several weeks preceding, and sometimes including, the period during which the cow should be inseminated and become pregnant. Factors associated with this negative energy balance, weight loss and their associated stresses have been suggested as causes of reproductive failure.

Conception rates are higher in cows gaining weight at time of service than those losing weight. In one English study, 98 cows gaining weight had a first service conception rate of 78 per cent, whereas the rate was 16 per cent in 81 cows losing weight. In a United States study, 814 cows with a net gain in weight during the 30- to 90-day postpartum period had a first service conception rate of 64 per cent, whereas the conception rate was only 46 per cent ($P<0.01$) in the 358 cows losing weight during this period.

The greatest problem with weight loss usually occurs in the high producing 2-year-old heifer that is using nutrients for growth in addition to maintenance and lactation. A New Zealand study of 1028 anestrous 2-year-old heifers reported that 85 per cent had inactive ovaries at 60 days postpartum compared with only 47 per cent of 808 cows at 4 years of age.

Cows must be in good physical condition at calving for best postpartum reproductive performance. Cows in poor condition have delayed onset of estrus and reduced fertility, whereas excessively fat cows are predisposed to the fat cow syndrome.

Although it is practically impossible to prevent high producing cows from losing weight during peak lactation, they should be fed high quality forages free choice, and challenge feeding of grain is recommended. In challenge feeding, cows receive a small amount of grain 10 to 14 days prior to calving, with grain increased at the rate of 2 pounds per day or to appetite following calving until the cow peaks in milk production. This method of feeding challenges the cow to maximum production and minimizes weight loss. An additional 2 to 4 pounds of grain should be fed during the first and second lactation to allow for growth.

PROTEIN

Clinical signs of infertility associated with a protein deficiency include a delay in the onset of puberty, an increase in the number of days open and a decrease in appetite. As a result of the latter sign, it may be difficult to separate a protein deficiency from a concurrent energy deficiency; however, it is generally believed that an energy deficiency has a much greater effect on reproduction than a protein deficiency.

Protein is essential for proper fetal development and function of the reproductive organs. Delayed sexual maturity is observed in heifers fed diets inadequate in protein. A protein deficiency in lactating cows results in emaciation and low milk production. Bulls consuming a 2 per cent protein diet exhibited anorexia and weakness along with decreased libido and decreased sperm per ejaculate.

In an Oregon study with 45 high producing cows, highest fertility was achieved when the ration contained 12.7 per cent crude protein. An increase in the dietary protein had a negative influence on reproductive parameters.

Urea is frequently incriminated as a cause of lowered fertility in dairy cattle. The effects of urea feeding were evaluated in 85,281 calving intervals and 3157 herd year observations in Michigan DHI herds. Daily urea intake averaged 81 gm in 1709 herd year observations. There were no differences in the calving interval and the number of cows sold for sterility between the urea and nonurea fed herds.

In a Purdue University study, Holstein heifers were fed 0, 145, or 290 gm of urea daily in a blended ration for several lactations. The cows on the highest urea intake had an increased abortion rate for first pregnancy, greater incidence of retained placenta at second calving and increased calving intervals, whereas there was a decrease in ovarian cysts and gestation length compared with controls (P<0.05). Heifers receiving 145 gm of urea performed as well as controls. This level is similar to current recommendations and would be equivalent to concentrate containing 2 per cent urea. It was concluded that heifers should not be fed more than 30 to 40 gm of urea daily during the first gestation to avoid abortions. Cows can consume greater quantities of urea when it is included in a blended ration fed free choice rather than when it is fed in the concentrate twice daily only.

The protein content of hay crop forages and corn silage is highly variable. It is essential that forages be tested in order to determine the actual available protein content. The total ration for lactating cows should contain 12 to 16 per cent protein, depending on the level of production. The feeding of either inadequate or excess dietary protein many impair reproductive performance. The circumstances under which dietary protein affects reproduction in high producing cows need additional research.

VITAMINS

The vitamin needs of dairy cattle are frequently met by a combination of rumen and tissue synthesis and natural feeds. Commercial concentrates and minerals frequently contain supplemental vitamins. As a result, the probability of infertility due to a vitamin deficiency is greatly reduced.

Vitamin A

The clinical signs of infertility associated with a vitamin A deficiency in cattle include (1) delayed onset of puberty, (2) abortion or birth of weak, blind, incoordinated calves, keratinization and degeneration of the placenta, retained placenta and metritis in the female and (3) suppressed libido in the male. Deficient cows have normal estrous cycles, ovulate and conceive with normal early fetal development.

Vitamin A maintenance requirements in bulls and lactation requirements in cows are adequate for preventing infertility. Vitamin A deficiency can develop in colostrum-deprived calves or in cattle fed forages damaged by weather, overheated in storage or maintained in storage for a long period of time.

Injectable vitamins A, D and E were administered alternately to 957 milk cows at drying off and at parturition in a Cornell study. Each injection contained 2,500,000 USP units of vitamin A, 500,000 USP units of vitamin D_2 and 250 IU of vitamin E.

There were no positive effects observed on any of the 26 measures of production and reproduction studied.

Lactating and nonlactating dairy cows require 1500 IU of vitamin A activity per pound of total ration dry matter. This includes carotene as well as preformed vitamin A. One mg of carotene equals 400 IU of vitamin A in dairy cattle rations. A recommended daily vitamin A supplementation for dairy cows is 30,000 to 50,000 IU.

Vitamin D

This vitamin is essential for proper calcium and phosphorus absorption, normal bone growth and prevention of rickets. A vitamin D deficiency reduces fertility by suppressing the signs of estrus and by delaying the onset of estrus. However, massive doses of vitamin D are toxic.

The effect of 43,000 IU of vitamin D_3 daily on postpartum reproductive performance was studied in 58 cows receiving 100 or 200 gm of calcium and 80 to 100 gm of phosphorus daily. First estrus and conception occurred 12 and 35 days earlier, respectively, in the group receiving the vitamin D supplementation compared with the controls ($P<0.05$); however, uterine involution was delayed by vitamin D supplementation. The advisability of supplementing rations with high levels of vitamin D needs further documentation.

The vitamin D requirement for lactating dairy cows is 150 IU per pound of dry matter in the ration. A recommended daily vitamin D supplementation for dairy cows is 6000 to 12,000 IU.

Vitamin E

There is no documented evidence that indictates that vitamin E alone is essential for reproduction in cattle.

MINERALS

Minerals are the nutrients frequently implicated in infertility in cattle. The large number of interrelationships that exist in the absorption and utilization of minerals makes it difficult to delineate relationships between a specific mineral and fertility. Since some clinical signs may be produced by a deficiency of more than one mineral and since several minerals may be deficient simultaneously, it is frequently difficult in the field to pinpoint a direct relationship between infertility and a specific mineral.

Calcium

A deficiency of this mineral is believed to have an indirect effect on reproduction in cattle. Limited data indicate that the uterus of cows fed 200 gm of calcium and 43,000 IU of vitamin D involuted to normal 8 days earlier than for cows fed 100 gm of calcium and 43,000 IU of vitamin D daily. The calcium intake is important for preventing milk fever, and there is an increased incidence of dystocia and retained placenta in cows with milk fever. The first service conception rate in 2454 normal cows was 42 per cent, but it was reduced to 30 per cent in 297 cows with retained placenta whereas services per conception increased from 2.7 to 3.4 because of retained fetal membranes.

Although there has been a great deal of interest in the dietary Ca:P ratio, studies with both heifers and cows have failed to show a relationship between fertility and this ratio. The concentration of minerals in the diet is more important than the ratio. The amount of phosphorus and vitamin D must also be considered.

The calcium content of 498 Michigan forages ranged from 0.6 to 2.8 per cent. The calcium content of the ration for the high producing cow should be at least 0.6 per cent of the total dry matter and should be 0.37 per cent for the dry cow. The ratio of calcium to phsophorus should be between 1.5:1 and 2.3:1.

Phosphorus

The mineral most frequently associated with infertility in cattle is phosphorus. Diets low in protein and energy are also frequently deficient in phosphorus. The effects of a phosphorus deficiency on fertility are variable, depending on the degree of deficiency. A severe deficiency can delay the onset of puberty and postpartum estrus because of inactive ovaries, whereas a moderate deficiency may be associated with repeat breeding. The clinical impression that there is a relationship between phosphorus intake and the development of cystic follicles needs further documentation. The calves of phosphorus-deficient dams may be stillborn or weak, but abortions do not occur.

In a study with 27 dairy heifers on a phosphorus-deficient diet, the blood phosphorus level was 3.9 mg/100 ml, whereas it was 6.6 mg/100 ml in 26 heifers receiving phosphorus supplementation. The number of services per conception declined from 2.8 to 1.3 with phosphorus supplementation in these 53 heifers.

The phosphorus content of forages is determined primarily by the phosphorus level in the soil. The phosphorus content of 498 Michigan forages varied from 0.12 to 0.54 per cent. Approximately 35 per cent of these forages were deficient in phosphorus for animals that derived a majority of their dry matter intake from these rations. Yearling heifers and dry cows are two groups of animals frequently on all forage ration and as a result may have mineral deficiencies.

Mineral supplements commonly used in balancing dairy cattle rations are listed in Table 1. High phosphorus supplements are used for rations high in legumes and high calcium supplements for rations high in corn silage. These supplements and trace mineralized salt are added at the rate of approximately 1 per cent each to the grain ration. The phosphorus content of the ration for the high producing cow should be at least 0.4 per cent of the total dry matter and should be 0.26 per cent for the dry cow.

Iodine

Iodine exerts its influence on fertility in cattle by its action on the thyroid gland. The basic interaction between low levels of thyroid function and reproduction appears to be an impairment of ovarian activity. Toxic levels of iodine can cause abortions.

An iodine deficiency in the diet of pregnant cows can cause the premature birth of dead or weak calves affected with goiter. Estrous detection and fertility improved in cattle supplemented with iodine, compared with controls in iodine-deficient areas.

Iodine toxicity can also result in abortions. A herd of 70 Michigan dairy cows received approximately 12,000 mg of supplemental iodine daily for a 1-month period. This is approximately 3000 times the recommended daily requirement of 4 mg. Abortions occurred in 13 cows, a majority of which were in the first trimester of pregnancy.

In iodine-deficient areas the inclusion of 0.01 per cent potassium iodide in salt is recommended to meet the minimum requirements of animals. Allowances must be made for variations in forages and the presence of goitrogenic substances in feeds such as soybean meal. The level of iodine in the ration must be increased when utilizing feeds containing goitrogenic substances. The dietary iodine content for high producing cows should be 0.5 parts per million (PPM) of the total dry matter.

Copper

An increase in retained placenta, inactive ovaries, delayed estrus and infertility has been attributed to a copper deficiency in dairy cattle according to some studies, whereas others report no benefit from copper supplementation. The dietary content for high producing cows should be 10 PPM of the total dry matter intake.

TABLE 1. *Mineral Supplements Commonly Used in Balancing Dairy Cattle Rations*

Supplement	Calcium (%)	Phosphorus (%)	Ca:P Ratio
Monosodium phosphate	0	22	—
Dicalcium phosphate	26	20	1:3
Sodium tripolyphosphate	0	25	—
Defluorinated phosphate	25	10	2:5
Bone meal	30	14	2:2
Limestone	38	0	—

Manganese

Silent estrus, infertility, abortions and birth of calves with deformed or twisted legs are the clinical signs reported for cows with a manganese deficiency. The dietary manganese content for high producing cows should be 40 PPM of the total dry matter intake.

Cobalt

A delay in the onset of puberty and postpartum estrus as well as anemia are the effects reported for a cobalt deficiency in unthrifty animals with a depraved appetite. The dietary cobalt content for high producing cows should be 0.10 PPM of the total dry matter intake.

Zinc

The reported signs of a zinc deficiency included a delay in testicular development in the young bull or testicular atrophy in the adult. Reduced fertility is also reported for the female. Parakeratosis is also common. The dietary zinc content for high producing cows should be 40 PPM of the total dry matter intake.

Selenium

This essential element is an integral component of the glutathione peroxidase enzyme. The signs of a deficiency include a decrease in the fertilization rate, an increase in retained placenta and muscular dystrophy.

In England a trial compared the results of three different dry period treatments on the incidence of retained placenta in dairy cattle. Either no selenium was given or 15 mg of selenium or 680 IU of vitamin E and 15 mg of selenium were injected intramuscularly 28 days prior to the projected calving date. The percentages of cows calving in which the placentae had to be manually removed were 26.5, 0 and 7 per cent, respectively.

The injection of 50 mg of selenium and 680 IU of vitamin E 20 days prepartum reduced the occurrence of retained placenta from 51 per cent in 80 control cows to 9 per cent in 133 treated cows in a selenium-deficient area of Ohio. Prevention of retained placenta was achieved by consumption of 0.1 PPM of selenium daily during the dry period. It was concluded that retained placenta, when not caused by infectious agents, was an expression of selenium deficiency in dairy cows. The selenium content of the ratio of high producing cows should be 0.1 PPM of the total dry matter.

It is also important to feed the dry cow a balanced ration according to nutrient requirements and to provide a sanitary calving area free of pathogenic organisms to prevent retained placenta and postpartum metritis.

CONCLUSIONS

Maximum reproductive performance is achieved when a ration balanced for energy, protein, vitamins and minerals is fed to meet the animal's nutrient requirements for growth, maintenance, lactation and gestation (Table 2).

The ration that is having an adverse effect on reproductive performance is usually deficient in more than one nutrient, which makes it difficult to evaluate the effect of a specific nutrient on fertility. The clinical signs observed are variable, depending on the degree of deficiency.

A majority of the nutritionally related reproductive problems in cattle can be prevented by the following procedures:

1. Balance ration for energy, protein, vitamins and minerals based on results of laboratory analysis and feed to meet nutrient requirements.

2. Give high priority to the feeding program used before puberty, before and after breeding and before and after calving to maximize fertility.

3. Practice challenge feeding to meet nutrient requirements during peak lactation.

4. Feed 20 per cent and 10 per cent above maintenance during first and second lactation, respectively, for growth.

5. Teamwork between the dairyman, nutritionist and veterinarian is essential for high fertility, production and profits.

TABLE 2. *Recommended Nutrient Concentrations in Dry Matter of Daily Cattle Diets and Toxic Amounts**

Nutrient	Units	Milking Cow	Dry Cow	Toxic or Maximum	Amount/Cow per Day†
Protein	%	13–16	11	—	6–7 lb
Energy NE$_l$	Mcal/lb	0.65–0.8	0.6	—	30–35 Mcal
ME	Mcal/lb	1.07–1.31	1.01	—	—
TDN	%	63–75	60	—	29–34 lb
Crude fiber	%	15–17	17	—	7 lb
Acid detergent fiber	%	20–22	23	—	9 lb
Crude fat	%	2	2	—	0.9 lb
Minerals:					
Ca	%	0.7	0.4	—	0.32 lb
P	%	0.35	0.25	0.5	0.16 lb
Mg	%	0.2	0.16	2	0.09 lb
K	%	0.8	0.8	5	0.36 lb
NaCl	%	0.46	0.25	5–9	0.21 lb
S	%	0.2	0.17	0.35	0.09 lb
Fe	PPM	100	100	1000	2 gm
Co	PPM	0.1	0.1	10	2 mg
Cu	PPM	10	10	80	200 mg
Mn	PPM	40	40	1000	800 mg
Zn	PPM	40	40	500	800 mg
I	PPM	0.5	0.25	50	4 mg
Mo	PPM	?	?	6	—
Se	PPM	0.1	0.1	3–5	2 mg
F	PPM	?	?	30	—
Vitamin A	IU/day	40,000–50,000		+++	—
Vitamin D	IU/day	5,000–20,000		+++	—
Vitamin E	IU/day	100–400		?	—

*Adapted by Thomas, J. W.: From Nutrient requirements of dairy cattle. Washington, D. C., National Academy of Sciences, 1978.

†Assuming a DM intake of 45 lb and producing about 60 lb of milk (1 PPM = 0.0001%).

REFERENCES

1. Anon. Nutrient requirements of dairy cattle. National Academy of Sciences, Washington, D.C., 1978, pp. 1–76.
2. Fielden, E. D.: The anoestrus syndrome. Proceedings of the Veterinary Services Council Postgraduate Course on Reproduction of Cattle and Pigs, Hamilton, N.Z., 1976, pp. 11–20.
3. Folman, Y., Rosenberger, M., Herz, Z. and Davidson, M. The relationship between plasma progesterone concentration and conception in postpartum dairy cows maintained on two levels of nutrition. J. Reprod. Fertil., *34*:267, 1973.
4. Julien, W. E., Conrad, H. R., Jones, J. E. and Moxon, A. L.: The prevention of retained placenta with supplemental selenium. J. Am. Dairy Sci. Assoc., *59*:1954, 1976.
5. Morrow, D. A.: Phosphorus deficiency and infertility in dairy heifers. J.A.V.M.A., *154*:761, 1969.

Nutrition and Reproductive Processes in Beef Cattle

THOMAS G. DUNN
University of Wyoming, Laramie, Wyoming

INTRODUCTION

Beef cattle herds in most parts of the world are managed under extensive conditions rather than intensive conditions typical of most dairy herds; therefore, the majority of the diet of the beef cow herd is obtained from forage. Thus, the beef cattleman must manage his herd and forage production to maximize benefit from his forage resources so that a minimum of supplemental feed is required. This article will discuss some nutritional practices that influence the reproductive performance of male and female beef cattle. The objective is not to provide a short course in nutrition but to provide some insight into how nutrition influences reproduction in beef cattle. Additional information on nutrition of beef cattle may be obtained from the several textbooks listed in the References section of this article. A most essential reference source is *Nutrient Requirements of Beef Cattle* of the National Research Council (NRC).[10]

DEFINITION OF TERMS

It is first necessary to review the meaning of some nutrition terms. The energy content of a ration is most important, since energy usually makes up the greatest portion of the diet. *Gross energy* (GE) is a measure of the heat of combustion of a feedstuff. This determination is made in a bomb calorimeter and is expressed as kilocalories per gram (kcal/gm), megacalories per kilogram (Mcal/kg) or British Thermal Units per pound (BTU/lb). *Digestible energy* (DE) is a measure of the energy absorbed by an animal and is the difference between gross energy of the feed and gross energy of the feces. Since some energy is lost through urine and combustible gases (especially in ruminants), *metabolizable energy* (ME), which accounts for these energy losses, becomes a more useful measurement. *Heat increment* or *specific dynamic effect* represents the difference between absorbed energy and energy that is actually captured by the metabolic processes of the animal. For example, if glucose is oxidized to generate adenosine triphosphate (ATP), 44 per cent of the gross energy of a molecule of glucose is converted to high-energy phosphate compounds, and the remainder (56 per cent) is lost as heat. Other processes contributing to specific dynamic effect include: mastication, the work of moving food through the gastrointestinal tract and the heat of fermentation in the rumen. When heat increment is deducted from ME, the difference is *net energy* (NE). Net energy therefore is the energy that is available to the animal for useful purposes such as maintenance, growth, fattening, milk production and reproduction.

Net energy is a useful method of measuring energy content of feed and is being used more often in ration formulations in the United States. One major shortcoming of the net energy concept is that each feedstuff has a specific net energy value for a specific function. For example, alfalfa hay at midbloom (NRC feed reference no. 1-00-063) has 1.99 Mcal ME per kilogram. When utilized for maintenance (NE_m), it has 1.17 Mcal/kg net energy. Such hay has 1.21 Mcal/kg for milk production (NE_1), 0.48 Mcal/kg for gain (NE_g) and 0.28 Mcal/kg NE for fetal growth.

Another major shortcoming of the net energy concept is that there have not been many net energy determinations of feeds since this involves costly digestion trials. Most of the net energy values are estimated from other energy measurements such as total digestible nutrients (see following paragraph), DE or metabolizable energy. Although formulations using the net energy concept are quite efficient since the ration can be formulated for a specific function for specific kinds of cattle (e.g., 1.1 kg/day gain for 400-kg steers), sufficient information is not available for using net energy formulations for grazing, reproducing beef cows. In such situations, the net energy content of the forage is difficult to determine, and, moreover, the net energy requirements for reproduction in beef cattle have not been determined.

Another system frequently used to estimate the energy content of feeds in the United States is the *total digestible nutrients* (TDN) system. The percentage of TDN in a feed equals the percentage of digestible crude protein plus the percentage of digestible crude fiber plus the percentage of digestible nitrogen-free extract plus 2.25 (per cent digestible ether extract). TDN values can be converted to DE values by the relationship: 1 kg TDN = 3.6155 Mcal DE.[9]

Following energy, protein is the most important nutrient (in quantity) in the diet. The *crude protein* (CP) content of a feedstuff is estimated from the nitrogen (N) content of the feedstuff. The percentage of CP equals the percentage of N times 6.25. This calculation makes use of two assumptions that are not altogether correct. First, it assumes that all N present in a feed is protein. This is usually the case except for young, actively growing plants in which considerable N is present in the form of nitrates, amides and amino acids. The second assumption is that all proteins contain 16 per cent nitrogen. This value varies from 15.7 to 18.9 per cent. Although the value of 16 per cent is not totally accurate, it is a sound estimate of the N content of proteins in most feeds.

Nonprotein nitrogen (NPN) is a term used to describe sources of N that are not proteins. The most common source of NPN is urea, which may be used in certain diets to replace a portion of the crude protein. Urea is converted to ammonia in the rumen and is then utilized by rumen micro-organisms for synthesis of microbial protein, which is then utilized by the ruminant animal.

Digestible protein (DP) is the difference between CP consumed and CP excreted in the feces.

The vitamin A content of feeds is important, especially during the winter and periods of drought. The vitamin A content is usually estimated from the amount of β-carotene in the feed. β-carotene in plants is converted to vitamin A by the animal. The international standards for vitamin A are based on the rate at which a rat converts β-carotene to vitamin A (1 mg of β-carotene is equivalent to 1667 IU of vitamin A for the rat). In contrast to rats, cattle have a much lower rate of conversion (1 mg of β-carotene is equivalent to about 400 IU of vitamin A for cattle).

The mineral content of feeds is usually expressed as a percentage. For bulls, cows and replacement heifers, the most important mineral is ordinarily phosphorus (P). These animals consume a diet consisting mainly of forage, which usually contains more than adequate calcium (Ca). On the other hand, P content of forages is usually marginal to low. In certain areas of the United States, other minerals are not present in sufficient quantities in forage. Some examples of mineral deficiencies by region are: iodine in the Great Lakes region and the Northwest; copper in Florida and the Coastal Plains region of the southeastern United States; and cobalt in Florida, the Great Lakes region and New England. In addition, mineral deficiencies may occur in small areas and under unusual circumstances in other regions of the United States. Selenium is an interesting mineral, as it may be deficient in forages of certain areas, whereas it is present in toxic amounts in the forages of other regions (e.g., eastern Montana, western Dakotas, and eastern Wyoming and Colorado). Salt should be provided free-choice to all animals, as most feeds are very low in sodium and chloride.

NUTRITION OF THE BEEF BULL

The nutrient requirements of the beef bull will be discussed in two sections: nutrition necessary for the occurrence of puberty and nutritional preparation for the breeding season.

Puberty in the Male

Puberty in the bull is marked by the first appearance of motile spermatozoa in an ejaculate. There are two limiting factors that determine the onset of puberty in bulls — age and weight. No matter how old a bull is, he will not reach puberty until he attains a threshold weight. Conversely, regardless of weight, he will not attain puberty until he has reached a certain threshold age. The critical weights and ages for Hereford and Angus bulls appear to be about 700 lb and 45 weeks of age. Charolais bulls are somewhat heavier and younger, reaching puberty at about 800 lb and 41 weeks of age. Crossbred bulls tend to reach puberty at a younger age and lighter weight than do their straightbred contemporaries. Unfortunately, information on the threshold weights and ages is not available for the larger Continental breeds that have rapidly gained popularity in the American beef industry.

Formulation of Rations

If the weight and age at which puberty occurs are known, a ration can be formulated to provide the necessary nutrients to insure the necessary growth during a particular time period. For example, if a Hereford bull calf weighed 440 lb when weaned at 150 days of age, he can be expected to reach puberty at about 45 weeks (315 days) of age and at 700-lb body weight. This means that during the 165 days following weaning, the bull must gain 260 lb, or 1.58 lb/day.

A ration that is adequate for the young bull at weaning will not be adequate 100 days later since the animal will be (or should be) 160 lb heavier by then. Probably the best solution is to formulate a ration that can be expected to produce the desired weight gain (1.58 lb/day) when the animal weighs 570 lb (midway between weaning and puberty). The nutrient requirement tables appearing in the NRC publication[10] do not show requirements for a 570-lb bull calf. The necessary requirements were extrapolated from those for growing and finishing steer calves and yearlings. This was accomplished by finding the requirements necessary for a 441-, 551-, 661- and 772-lb steer to gain 1.6 lb/day. These requirements were calculated by interpolation of the values given for a 1.5 and 2.0 lb/day gain. Next, the requirements necessary for a 700-lb animal to gain 1.6 lb/day were calculated by interpolation of the values calculated for 661- and 772-lb steers. Finally, the requirements for a 570-lb bull calf to gain 1.6 lb/day were estimated by interpolation of the values for 441- and 700-lb animals. From the preceding calcula-

tions, the 570-lb Hereford bull calf would require 14.2 lb of dry matter (DM), 9.81 lb of TDN, 0.89 lb of DP, 18 gm of Ca, 17 gm of P and 14,855 IU of vitamin A to gain 1.6 lb/day.

It is well to remember several "rules of thumb" for formulating diets. First, balance the ration for energy (TDN), since this is the major portion of the diet. Second, utilize forage to the maximum extent, since forages are almost always less expensive than concentrates and also are usually homegrown. For the problem at hand, assume that alfalfa hay is the most plentiful and cheapest forage and that corn is the most plentiful and cheapest concentrate. The nutrient composition of midbloom alfalfa hay and corn is obtained from the NRC[9] and is shown in Table 1.

Using the requirement for TDN (9.81 lb/day), one can calculate the amount of corn and alfalfa hay that must be fed to meet the TDN requirement. There are two methods that can be used to solve the problem — the Pearson square method or the use of simultaneous equations. Simultaneous equations will be used for this example. The equations are set up as shown, in which X equals the amount of DM from alfalfa hay and Y equals the amount of DM from corn. The sum of these two feedstuffs equals the minimum DM requirement (14.2 lb/day). In the second equation, the amount of TDN in alfalfa hay plus the amount of TDN in corn are set equal to the amount of TDN required (9.81 lb/day):

$$X + Y = 14.2$$
$$0.55X + 0.91Y = 9.81$$

Solve the first equation for either X or Y (it was solved for X in this example) and substitute this value in the second equation:

TABLE 1. *Composition of Alfalfa Hay and Corn**

Ingredient	DM (%)	DP (%)	TDN (%)	Ca (%)	P (%)	β-Carotene (mg/lb)	Vitamin A† (IU/lb)
Midbloom alfalfa hay (1-00-063)‡	89.2	12.1	55.0	1.35	0.22	15.1	6047
Corn (4-02-931)‡	89.0	7.5	91.0	0.02	0.35	0.9	363

*From National Research Council (NRC): Nutrient Requirements of Domestic Animals. No. 4. National Academy of Sciences, Washington, D.C., 1976.
†Calculated from β-carotene (1 mg of β-carotene = 400 IU of vitamin A for cattle).
‡NRC feed reference number.

TABLE 2. *Example Ration to Meet Requirements for a 570-lb Bull Calf to Gain 1.6 lb/day*

Item	DM (lb)	TDN (lb)	DP (lb)	Ca (gm)	P (gm)	Vitamin A (IU)
Requirements	14.2	9.81	0.89	18	17	14,855
Ration (as fed):						
9.7 lb alfalfa (1-00-063)*	8.64	4.75	1.05	53	7	52,246
6.25 lb corn (4-02-931)*	5.56	5.06	0.42	1	9	2,018
Totals	14.20	9.81	1.47	54	16	54,264

*NRC feed reference number.

$$X = 14.2 - Y$$
$$0.55(14.2 - Y) + 0.91Y = 9.81$$

The second equation is then solved for Y:

$$Y = 5.56$$

This value for Y is then substituted into the original equation and that equation is solved for X:

$$X + 5.56 = 14.2$$
$$X = 8.64$$

The solution to the pair of simultaneous equations shows that 5.56 lb of DM from corn plus 8.64 lb of DM from alfalfa hay will meet the TDN requirement. To convert the DM values to "as fed" values, divide each DM value by the percentage DM:

5.56 lb/0.89 = 6.25 lb corn
on an as-fed basis
8.64 lb/0.891 = 9.7 lb alfalfa hay
on an as-fed basis

The next step is to determine if the amounts of corn and alfalfa hay that will meet the TDN requirement will also meet the requirements for the other nutrients. This comparison is shown in Table 2.

The ration formulated from alfalfa hay and corn will meet all the requirements for the growing bull calf except the phosphorus requirement. Meeting this requirement can be accomplished by feeding a salt:sodium tripolyphosphate mixture (50:50) or a commercial high-phosphorus:low-calcium supplement free choice.

The quantities of alfalfa hay and corn shown in Table 2 can also be used to calculate the quantities of these feeds that will be required for the 165-day feeding period. These calculations show that about 1600 lb of alfalfa hay plus 1030 lb of corn will be required for the bull calf during the 165-day period from weaning until the bull is expected to reach puberty.

Obviously, feeding the ration shown in Table 2 during the entire 165-day period will not accomplish the desired goal. During the early part of the feeding period, the bull calf would receive too much feed, and he would not receive enough feed during the latter part of the feeding period. Consequently, the ration should be adjusted periodically during the feeding period. Some examples of rations are shown in Table 3 for the bull at the beginning, middle and end of the feeding period.

Not only is it essential to provide adequate feed for the beef bull to attain puberty, but the young bull should be provided a diet that will insure adequate postpubertal growth. Either inadequate energy intake or inadequate protein intake will retard the growth and development of the reproductive tract, especially the testes. Since sperm output is directly related to testicular size in young bulls, small testes mean low sperm output. A decreased sperm output may mean fewer pregnant cows.

Preparation for the Breeding Season

Many beef producers are keenly aware of the reproductive failures associated with

TABLE 3. *Example Rations (Using Alfalfa Hay and Corn) for Bull Calves of Various Weights to Gain 1.6 lb/day*

Item	DM (lb)	TDN (lb)	DP (lb)	Ca (gm)	P (gm)	Vitamin A (IU)
440-lb bull:						
Requirements	12.9	8.46	0.86	19	17	13,000
Ration (as fed):						
10.22 lb alfalfa hay (1-00-063)*	9.11	5.01	1.10	56	9	55,088
4.26 lb corn (4-02-931)*	3.79	3.45	0.28	0	6	1,376
Total supplied by ration	12.90	8.46	1.38	56	15	56,464
570-lb bull (from Table 2):						
Requirements	14.2	9.81	0.89	18	17	14,855
Ration (as fed):						
9.7 lb alfalfa (1-00-063)*	8.64	4.75	1.05	53	7	52,246
6.25 lb corn (4-02-931)*	5.56	5.06	0.42	1	9	2,018
Total supplied by ration	14.20	9.81	1.47	54	16	54.264
700-lb bull:						
Requirements	15.6	11.15	0.92	17	16	16,710
Ration (as fed):						
9.5 lb alfalfa hay (1-00-063)*	8.46	4.65	1.02	52	8	51,158
8.0 lb corn (4-02-931)*	7.14	6.50	0.54	1	11	2,592
Total supplied by ration	15.60	11.15	1.56	53	17	53,750

*NRC feed reference number.

malnutrition in the cow herd. Unfortunately, too few producers are aware that beef bulls also need nutritional preparation prior to the breeding season. In western range country and other beef-producing areas of the United States, beef bulls are often allowed to fend for themselves from the end of one breeding season to the beginning of the next season. Since the spermatogenic process requires about 60 days for completion, the minimum amount of time that must be allocated for preparing bulls for the oncoming breeding season is 60 days. A more sensible arrangement would be to maintain bulls in a thrifty condition during the nonbreeding season so that when the breeding season begins, the producer is assured that his bulls will be ready to service cows immediately.

Formulation of Rations

As with nutrient requirements for other classes of cattle, the requirements for bulls are found in the NRC reference.[10] The requirements are given for bulls varying in weight from 660 to 2200 lb. The requirements for a 1500-lb bull and two example rations are shown in Table 4.

Feeding 31.9 lb of alfalfa hay (described in Table 1) would meet all requirements of the bull. Although both the Ca and P furnished by the ration are more than adequate, the Ca:P ratio is 6.2:1, which is typical of all-forage rations. A Ca:P ratio greater than 4:1 is detrimental to the animal, since the excess Ca appears to prevent absorption of P from the gut. This problem can be alleviated by feeding a salt:sodium tripolyphosphate mixture free choice.

Also as shown in Table 4, feeding 33 lb of mountain meadow hay (ration number 2) would not meet the protein requirement for the bull. The ration was made adequate in protein by supplementing the mountain meadow hay with 2 lb of cottonseed pellets. Supplementation with 2 lb of cottonseed pellets not only meets the protein requirement for the bull but also adds 11 gm of P. The Ca:P ratio is therefore 64:30, which is within the acceptable range. The same results could be accomplished with a commercial high-protein supplement with added phosphorus. When feeding mountain meadow hay, it is not a good idea to use a commercial protein supplement that contains urea.

The example for ration number 2 in Table 4 does not show the vitamin A content of the ration. This does not mean that mountain meadow hay does not contain β-carotene, it simply means that such information was not included in the NRC reference.[10] Mountain meadow hay is similar to any other hay. If is green and leafy, it probably contains ade-

TABLE 4. *Dietary Requirements and Example Rations for a 1500-lb Beef Bull*

Item	DM (lb)	TDN (lb)	DP (lb)	Ca (gm)	P (gm)	Vitamin A (IU)
Requirements	28.40	15.60*	1.32	23	23	50,000
Example rations:						
1. 31.9 lb alfalfa hay (1-00-063)†	28.40	15.60	3.44	174	28	171,735
2. 33.0 lb mountain meadow hay (1-03-181)†	27.90	14.23	0.81	72	22	
2.0 lb cottonseed oil meal pellets (5-01-621)†	1.83	1.37	0.66	1	11	
Total supplied by ration No. 2	29.73	15.60	1.47	73	33	

*From Table 2B in NRC publication.[10] The value given in Table 1B of this publication is excessive.
†NRC feed reference number.

quate β-carotene. If it is straw-colored and weathered, it probably does not contain adequate vitamin A.

The preceding example (ration number 2, Table 4) illustrates a common practice among cattlemen — that of trying to winter bulls on large amounts of low-quality roughage. Semen production is decreased when bulls are fed diets deficient in protein. Consequently, such a practice will result in lower sperm output at the start of the breeding season. Since the spermatogenic process requires 60 days, the availability of abundant green forage, although high in protein content, may be too late to insure adequate sperm production early in the breeding season. Such inadequate sperm production may mean a low conception rate for cows showing heat early in the breeding season. If these cows fail to become pregnant early in the breeding season, they will wean lighter calves the following year because the calves will be younger at weaning. As discussed later in this article, suckling beef calves gain about 1.6 lb/day. If a calf is 21 days younger at weaning because its mother failed to become pregnant on first service, it would be about 34 lb lighter at weaning (1.6 lb/day × 21 days).

Whereas inadequately nourished bulls are often a problem, the converse can also be true. Producers should remember that overly fat bulls will probably be reluctant to travel the pastures in search of cows in heat. Moreover, such bulls often have less than normal libido. A middle of the road course thus seems to be most appropriate. Bulls should be in thrifty, healthy condition, neither overly thin nor overly fat.

Vitamin and Mineral Supplementation

One often hears about the use of wheat germ oil as a cure-all for reproductive problems in bulls. Wheat germ oil is an excellent source of vitamin E, which is essential for reproduction in the male rat. However, there is no evidence to show that giving vitamin E supplements to bulls increases any measure of reproductive performance. Apparently, vitamin E is present in natural feeds in adequate amounts for normal reproduction.

Vitamin A is essential for adequate reproductive performance in bulls because this vitamin is necessary to maintain the integrity of the seminiferous epithelium. Other symptoms of vitamin A deficiency (e.g., night blindness) appear before abnormal sperm cells begin to appear; thus, warning signals of impending problems are broadcast. Once sperm production is affected, however, several months are required for the bulls to regain normal sperm production when the animals are fed a diet adequate in vitamin A. Ordinarily, vitamin A deficiencies do not present a problem except in drought years or when bulls are maintained for long periods on badly weathered forage (e.g., being maintained during long winters on cured, standing-range forage). Almost all hay that is of good quality and has some green color will contain adequate carotene to meet the bull's requirement. If such forage is not available, many commercial supplements are available that will supply the daily requirement of vitamin A.

Although little information is available concerning the effect of different mineral deficiencies on sperm production of bulls, it seems best to follow general guidelines for mineral supplementation that are peculiar to a given geographical area. As previously mentioned, the mineral that is most likely to be deficient in the grazing or forage-fed animal is phosphorus. One should remember that forages are usually low in P, whereas grains are usually fairly adequate in P content. In order to formulate an adequate mineral supplement, it is essential to know the mineral content of the forage that animals are consuming. This information is often scarce, although agricultural extension personnel can usually provide some information on the mineral content of forages in a particular area. Providing supplemental P can be accomplished by feeding a salt-mineral mixture free choice. A mixture that has worked well at the University of Wyoming is 50 lb of sodium tripolyphosphate, 50 lb of loose salt and 10 lb of cottonseed oil meal.[13] Cottonseed oil meal serves two functions: it helps prevent the salt-mineral mixture from caking, and it improves the palatability of the mixture. Monosodium phosphate can be substituted for sodium tripolyphosphate in this mixture, depending upon the price of the two phosphorus sources. Phosphorus can also be incorporated into range cubes up to 2 per cent of the supplement without adversely affecting the palatability of the supplement. Commercial mineral supplements high in P and low in Ca can also be purchased.

I do not recommend the use of high-Ca, low-P mineral supplements because most forages are high in calcium. Providing additional Ca in an attempt to supplement P often increases the Ca:P ratio beyond 4:1. As previously mentioned, when the Ca:P ratio exceeds 4:1, the excess Ca decreases absorption of P from the digestive tract, thereby creating a P deficiency in spite of adequate levels of P in the diet.

It is very difficult to make general recommendations concerning trace minerals, since trace mineral problems are regional in nature. Probably the best suggestion is to contact local agricultural extension personnel to determine if trace mineral problems exist in a particular area. If such problems are not present, there is little to be gained by providing trace mineral supplements. Commercial mineral supplements and formula feeds generally are fortified with trace minerals.

NUTRITION OF THE BEEF FEMALE

In all areas where beef cows are bred during a finite breeding season, one of the major goals of a cow-calf or cow-yearling operation is to have a high percentage of calves born early in the calving season. A quick look at the economics of a cow-calf operation shows the importance of having a high percentage of early births. The gross income from a cow-calf operation is as follows: Gross income = (number of calves sold) × (weaning weight of calves) × (price per lb).

The number of calves sold is dependent upon several factors including size of the available feed resource for the cow herd. The two most important factors that decrease the number of calves sold are failure of cows to become pregnant and neonatal losses.[1] Of lesser importance are abortions and calf losses from 2 weeks of age until weaning.

The weaning weight of a calf then becomes important in determining the gross income from a cow-calf operation. Weaning weight is dependent upon three factors, as follows: Weaning weight = (birth weight) + (average daily gain from birth to weaning) × (age at weaning).

When this equation is examined, one can quickly see that there are two factors that must be manipulated to increase weaning weight — average daily gain and age at weaning. Average daily gain can be increased primarily by increasing the milk production of the dam or by creep feeding. Increasing milk production usually involves a long selection procedure or changing the breed of dam. One factor that the cow-calf operator can alter quickly is average age at weaning. As shown in Table 5, age has little effect on the average daily gain of calves. From 106 to 252 days of age, the average daily gain of some 19,330 calves ranged from 1.52 to 1.59 lb/day. Thus, the average daily gain for most calves is nearly constant prior to weaning. Therefore, the most important factor affecting the weaning weight of the calves is the age at weaning.

In order to increase age at weaning, a calf must be born early in the calving season. To do this, its mother must conceive early in the breeding season and must, therefore, also come into heat early in the breeding season. Thus, having a large number of cows in heat early in the breeding season is required. This

TABLE 5. *Age and Weaning Weight for 20,192 Wyoming Calves**

Weaning Age (days)	No. Calves	Weaning Weight (lb)	Average Daily Gain (lb/day)
105	54	263	1.87
106–126	123	260	1.59
127–147	589	292	1.59
148–168	2107	322	1.56
169–189	5103	360	1.59
190–210	6507	385	1.56
211–231	3892	418	1.56
232–252	1009	438	1.52
253–273	637	451	1.48
274–294	109	453	1.37
294	62	449	1.26

*From Schoonover, C. O.: University of Wyoming, unpublished data, 1977.

is one of the major problems a cow-calf operator faces, i.e., how to get a large percentage (at least 90 per cent) of his cow herd in heat during the first 21 days of the breeding season. In my opinion, three things *must be done* to accomplish this goal:

1. Replacement heifers *must* be bred to start calving at least 20 and preferably 30 days before the older cows.

2. Cows *must* be in thrifty condition (not thin) at calving time.

3. Cows *must* weigh at least as much 24 hours after calving as they did 100 days prior to calving. This means a weight gain of 100 to 150 lb during the last trimester of gestation. Most, if not all, of this weight gain will be from the fetus, fetal membranes, uterine growth and fetal fluids.

How nutrition affects each of these goals will be discussed in the following section.

Puberty in the Female

The first question that one is likely to ask is why heifers should be bred to start calving 30 days before the older cows. The major reason is to prevent heifers from becoming late calvers for their second and succeeding calves. As there are 365 days in a year and the average gestation length for cows is about 285 days, the difference between 365 and 285 is 80 days. This means that a beef cow has 80 days in which to recover from the previous calving and become pregnant with her next calf if she is to maintain a yearly calving interval. If a cow is to conceive by 80 days after calving, she must show heat by 80 days after calving. The data shown in Table

6 indicate that about 90 per cent of mature cows had shown estrus by 80 days after calving but only 68 per cent of first-calf heifers had shown estrus by 80 days after calving. This means that at least 30 per cent of the first-calf heifers will not be able to maintain a yearly calving interval. First-service conception rates vary from 55 to 80 per cent. To insure that a cow will conceive and maintain a yearly calving interval, she should be afforded more than one opportunity to conceive within the 80-day limit. If a cow is to have the opportunity for two services, she must show heat by 60 days after calving. The data in Table 6 show that about 70 per cent of mature cows had shown heat by 60 days after calving but less than 50 per cent of the first-calf heifers had shown heat.

If the breeder "buys" additional time for his first-calf heifers by calving them ahead of older cows, there will be a greater percentage of the first-calf heifers that will show

TABLE 6. *Cows and Heifers Showing Estrus after Calving**

Days after Calving	Percentage Showing Estrus	
	FIRST-CALF HEIFERS	MATURE COWS
40	15	30
50	24	53
60	47	72
70	62	82
80	68	89
90	79	94

*From Wiltbank, J. N.: J. Anim. Sci., *31*:755, 1970.

heat early in the breeding season. If the heifer nursing her first calf is in heat early in the breeding season, she will be likely to be an early calver for the remainder of her productive life. Work in Montana has clearly shown that heifers that calved early their first time had a higher lifetime production than heifers that calved late the first time.[8] Therefore, it seems important to breed yearling heifers to calve 30 days earlier than the older cows.

If a cattleman wishes to breed heifers so that they will calve 30 days ahead of the older cows, the heifers must have reached puberty (exhibited first heat) prior to or during the breeding season. As previously discussed for bulls, there are two limiting factors within each breed that determine the age at puberty — weight and age. No matter how old a heifer is, she will not reach puberty until she has achieved a threshold weight. On the other hand, regardless of how heavy a heifer is, she will not reach puberty until she reaches a threshold age. Some target weights for the occurrence of puberty for several breeds are shown in Table 7.

Formulation of Rations

Using the same approach utilized previously for bulls, the following example ration can be formulated. Assume that a 440-lb Hereford heifer calf was weaned on November 1. If the calving season for the older cows starts on April 1, the breeding season for the older cows will have to begin on June 20. To calve first-calf heifers 30 days ahead of the older cows, the breeding season for the heifers must start on May 20. Using the target weight data from Table 7, the heifer

TABLE 7. *Target Weights for Occurrence of Puberty in Different Breeds and Crosses of Beef Females*

Breed	Target Weight at Puberty (lb)
Hereford	650
Angus	600
Black Baldie	600
(Angus × Hereford crossbred)	
Simmental crosses	725
Charolais crosses	700
Jersey crosses	500

weaned on November 1 will have to gain 210 lb to weigh 650 lb by May 20. The time interval from November 1 until May 20 is 200 days. The heifer must therefore gain 210 lb in 200 days or have an average daily gain of 1.05 lb/day. The requirements and example rations using alfalfa hay and corn silage for heifers of various weights are shown in Table 8. The rations shown in Table 8 will provide all the nutrients required for growing heifers to gain 1.1 lb/day. In each ration, however, the Ca:P ratio exceeds 4:1, which is typical of all-forage diets. Again, this problem can be alleviated by feeding a salt-sodium tripolyphosphate mixture free choice.

As most cattlemen are aware, not all heifer calves weigh the average amount. Using the preceding example, if one assumes that 440 lb is the average weight for a pen of heifers, there will be heifers that weigh more than 440 lb and heifers that weigh less than 440 lb. If the rations are formulated for the "average" heifer, some heifers will be getting more feed than they need (the heavier heifers do not have to gain as much weight between November 1 and May 20). On the other hand, some heifers will not receive enough feed to reach the target weight of 650 lb by May 20. By obtaining individual weights, the heifers can be divided into two groups — those heavier than the average and those lighter than the average. The average weights of each group can then be calculated and rations formulated to achieve the average daily gain necessary for each group to reach the target weight by May 20 (see work by Varner et al.[12])

The Pregnant Female

The most critical period of time in the productive life of the beef female is the last trimester of gestation plus the first 60 days of lactation. Nutrition during this 5-month period is crucial for satisfactory reproductive performance of the beef female.

Adequate nutrition during the last trimester of gestation becomes important for two reasons: First, malnutrition during the last trimester of gestation reduces the ability of the offspring to grow and increases the incidence of neonatal mortality. Second, cows that are in thin condition at calving time have an extended interval from calving to the first postpartum estrus. Calves that are weak and light reduce the gross income

TABLE 8. *Example Rations for Replacement Heifers of Various Weights to Gain 1.1 lb/day*

Item	DM (lb)	TDN (lb)	DP (lb)	Ca (gm)	P (gm)	Vitamin A (IU)
440-lb heifer:						
Requirements	13.2	7.70	0.77	14	13	13,000
Ration (as fed):						
11.4 lb alfalfa hay (1-00-063)*	10.2	5.61	1.23	62	10	61,608
10.7 lb corn silage (3-08-154)*	3.0	2.10	0.15	4	3	
Total supplied by ration	13.2	7.71	1.38	66	13	61,608
550-lb heifer:						
Requirements	14.3	8.60	0.81	13	13	14,000
Ration (as fed):						
12.8 lb alfalfa hay (1-00-063)*	11.4	5.20	1.15	58	10	57,380
10.4 lb corn silage (3-08-154)*	4.8	3.40	0.24	6	5	
Total supplied by ration	16.2	8.60	1.39	64	15	57,380
660-lb heifer:						
Requirements	16.3	9.90	0.88	14	14	16,000
Ration (as fed):						
11.2 lb alfalfa hay (1-00-063)*	10.0	5.50	1.21	61	10	60,400
22.6 lb corn silage (3-08-154)*	6.3	4.41	0.31	8	6	
Total supplied by ration	16.3	9.91	1.52	69	16	60,400

*NRC feed reference number.

for the current year, whereas cows that have an extended interval from calving to first heat will produce light calves the following year because the calves will be younger at weaning, hence reducing the gross income from the next year's calf crop.

The growth of the fetal calf is greatest during the last trimester of gestation. In spite of the economic importance of cattle, only a few studies have been made of the intrauterine growth rate of the bovine fetus. An excellent study by Ferrell *et al.*[7] has provided some needed information. By slaughtering cows at different stages of gestation, the authors acquired sufficient data to derive equations that mathematically describe the growth of the fetus, conceptus (fetus plus fetal fluids and fetal membranes) and the gravid uterus (conceptus and uterus). Their data indicate that uterine growth precedes fetal membrane growth, which, in turn, precedes fetal growth. In other words, the machinery must be installed before production can be initiated.

As shown in Table 9, weight of the gravid uterus increased from 37.7 lb at 180 days of gestation to 144.4 lb at 280 days of gestation, which is an increase of nearly 100 lb in 100 days or an average daily gain of almost 1 lb/day. Weight of the fetus increased more than 70 lb during the last trimester of gesta-

tion (from 13.1 lb at day 180 to 84.7 lb at day 280). During the last 20 days of gestation, the weight of the gravid uterus increased 31 lb or an average daily gain of 1.57 lb/day. During this same period, the fetal calf gained 19.4 lb or nearly 1 lb/day.

Formulation of Rations

Since the gravid uterus is rapidly increasing in weight during the last trimester of gestation, the nutrient requirements of the dam also increase. The data in Table 10 show the rate at which protein and energy were deposited in the gravid uterus as well as the increased nutrient intake over maintenance requirements necessary to meet the demands of the gravid uterus.

The NRC recommendations[10] do not indicate the changing nutrient requirements as shown in Table 10 but reflect an average requirement for the last trimester of pregnancy. Formulating a ration for pregnant females is not difficult if the animals are maintained in drylot. However, very few beef cow herds are maintained in drylot during the last trimester of gestation. Most herds obtain at least some forage from grazing winter range, meadow aftermath or other crop residues. These animals may receive supplemental harvested forage, grain

TABLE 9. *Predicted Weights of Gravid Uterus, Conceptus and Fetus during Last Trimester of Gestation**

Length of Gestation (days)	Gravid Uterus[a] (lb)	Conceptus[b] (lb)	Fetal Membranes[c] (lb)	Fetal Fluids[d] (lb)	Fetus[e] (lb)
180	37.7	30.6	2.4	15.1	13.1
200	50.5	41.7	3.1	17.3	21.3
220	66.8	56.2	3.9	19.6	32.7
240	87.4	74.8	4.8	22.4	47.6
260	113.0	98.4	5.7	27.4	65.3
280	144.4	127.6	6.7	36.2	84.7

*Calculated from equations presented by Ferrell, C. L., Garrett, W. N. and Hinman, N.: J. Anim. Sci., *42*:1477, 1976.

[a]Uterine wt $= 1.639e^{(0.02 - 0.00001431)}$

[b]Conceptus wt $= 1.035e^{(0.0217 - 0.0000161t)}$

[c]Membrane wt $= 0.0906e^{(0.0236 - 0.0000294t)t}$

[d]Fluid wt = conceptus wt − (membrane wt + fetal wt)

[e]Fetus wt $= 0.0129^{(0.0512 - 0.0000707t)t}$

or commercial supplements. During this period, feed costs per animal are higher than during other times of the year. Hence, it is important to have sufficient knowledge of the available forage resources to be able to make economical decisions concerning the use of supplemental feed.

Since most of the ration will be furnished by a combination of grazed material plus harvested forage, it is essential to know the nutrient composition of this material. This information is difficult to obtain from feed analyses tables such as those in the NRC publication.[10] Some states have forage analyses programs similar to the one operated by the University of Wyoming whereby ranchers can have forage samples analyzed. The results of the forage analyses can be used to formulate a supplemental feeding program for their cattle. If this service is available, I recommend that cattlemen make use of it. Results from Wyoming's program clearly indicate that there simply is

not an "average" forage.[14] The quality of forage depends upon weather, fertilization rates, irrigation rates, stage of maturity at harvest and other factors. For example, the crude protein content of dry-land meadow hay varied from 6.00 to 12.56 per cent in 32 different samples from Wyoming. This wide range further stresses the need for individual forage analyses for each cattle operation.

As an example, let us formulate a winter supplemental feeding program for a cow herd in north-central Wyoming. The feeding program will be designed for 1000-lb mature cows during the last trimester of gestation. Assume that the cows consume about 5 lb of meadow aftermath (3 per cent CP and 30.0 per cent TDN on an as-fed basis) per day. The following homegrown, harvested forages are available: grass-legume hay (about 75 per cent grass, 11.65 per cent CP and 61.4 per cent TDN on an as-fed basis) and grass hay (7.3 per cent CP, 0.19 per cent P, 38.8 mg carotene/lb and 57.31 per cent

TABLE 10. *Protein and Energy Deposition in Gravid Bovine Uterus and Additional Nutrients Required during Pregnancy**

Day of Gestation	Deposited in Gravid Uterus		Additional Nutrients in Ration	
	PROTEIN (lb/day)	ENERGY (kcal/day)	DIGESTIBLE PROTEIN (lb/day)	TDN (lb/day)
190	0.07	263	0.17	1.15
220	0.12	457	0.30	1.99
250	0.21	752	0.50	3.27
280	0.34	1167	0.81	5.08

*Ferrell, C. L., Garrett, W. N. and Hinman, N.: J. Anim. Sci., *42*:1477, 1976.

TDN on an as-fed basis). The animal requirements and the example ration are shown in Table 11.

This diet will be more than adequate for a 1000-lb cow during the last trimester of gestation, except for phosphorus. This assumes, of course, that the animal will be able to obtain 5 lb of meadow aftermath each day. Such an assumption is tenuous at best since the amount of meadow aftermath consumed will be governed by the amount of snow cover, weather conditions and the amount of aftermath available. Moreover, this does not allow for the deterioration of the meadow aftermath. Toward spring, the crude protein content is likely to be 1 to 2 per cent instead of 3 per cent. This ration, however, insures that the cows will receive the daily requirements, since 15 lb of the grass hay meets the protein, energy and vitamin A requirements of the cow. The meadow aftermath therefore provides a bit of "gravy." Again, the necessary phosphorus can be supplied in a salt-mineral mixture.

As the cow herd progresses toward calving and in view of the data presented in Table 10, the cows should be fed more of the grass hay to meet the increasing requirements of the growing conceptus.

The many uncertainties involved in wintering the cow herd suggest that formulating a ration and then sticking to it throughout the winter, whatever the circumstances, are not advisable. A more sound approach is to determine a ration, based on the available forage and supplemental feed if necessary, that will meet the requirements of the pregnant cow during the last trimester of gestation. If possible, all the cows, or at least a representative sample, should be individually weighed at about the start of the last trimester. These cows should then be weighed monthly to determine if they are gaining or losing weight. Remember, a weight gain of 100 lb will be entirely utilized by the gravid uterus — the cow herself will gain nothing. The amount of feed can then be adjusted according to the gain of the animals during the last trimester.

Few producers have the capability to weigh cattle either individually or in lots; therefore, cow weight gains will often have to be monitored by changes in cow condition. This can be particularly difficult because cows often lose condition before the cattleman notices the change. By the time the change is noticed, it is often too late to prevent a large weight loss during the last trimester of gestation.

Heifers pregnant with their first calves present a special problem during the last trimester of gestation. These animals have several demands placed upon them. They are young and thus still growing, and they must nourish the fetal calf, prepare for lactation and maintain their body functions. These animals must not be wintered with the older cows during the last trimester of gestation because they are too small to compete for their fair share of feed. Thus, during this time pregnant heifers should be separated from the older cows so that they will receive the amount of feed allocated to them.

Effects of Maternal Malnutrition

What are the consequences of maternal malnutrition during the last trimester of gestation? Let me introduce a term, *net weight change*, which is the weight change in the cow that occurs from the beginning of the last trimester of gestation (90 to 100 days prior to calving) until 1 day after calving. If a cow has a positive net weight

TABLE 11. *Example Ration for a 1000-lb Mature Cow during Last Trimester of Gestation*

Item	Crude Protein (lb/day)	TDN (lb/day)	P (gm/day)	Vitamin A (IU/day)
Requirements for 1000-lb cow	1.06	9.4	15	23,000
Ingredients of diet:				
5 lb meadow aftermath	0.15	1.50	—	—
15 lb grass hay				
(described in text)	1.10	8.60	13	232,800
Totals	1.25	10.10	13	232,800

change, she has produced a calf plus the associated fetal membranes and fluids and has gained some weight herself. On the other hand, if a cow has a negative net weight change, she has utilized her body tissues to provide nutrients for the developing conceptus. The data from three different experiments[2, 4, 5] show that if a cow utilizes her body stores to provide nutrients for the developing fetus, the fetus will be smaller at birth and at weaning. The data also show that the rate of gain from birth to weaning is lower for calves from mothers that lost excessive amounts of body weight during the last trimester of gestation.

There are at least two possible explanations for the decreased ability to grow. First, and most likely, is that cows that are malnourished during the last trimester of gestation produce less milk during lactation than adequately nourished cows. In Corah's study,[4] however, heifers with the greatest net weight loss (−119 lb) produced slightly more milk than heifers with a smaller (−35 lb) net weight loss (11.0 versus 10.6 lb milk/day). The other explanation is that maternal malnutrition during the last trimester of gestation inhibits the ability of the fetus to grow. The preweaning gains of calves from malnourished dams were lower in Nebraska (206 versus 219 lb),[5] Montana (280 versus 300 lb)[2] and Wyoming (262 versus 286 lb).[4] Since small calves are also small yearlings (C. C. Kaltenbach, University of Wyoming, unpublished results and C. O. Schoonover, University of Wyoming, unpublished results), it seems likely that the adverse influence of maternal malnutrition on the ability of a calf to grow may carry over to yearling cattle.

In another experiment, Corah et al.[4] demonstrated that many of the adverse effects of maternal malnutrition could be reversed by feeding a high level of energy during the last 30 days of gestation. One of the interesting results of this experiment was the discovery that more calves from malnourished mothers were affected by neonatal calf diarrhea than from mothers that received a high-energy intake during the last 30 days of gestation (52 per cent versus 33 per cent incidence of scours). Not only were more calves affected with scours but the mortality was also greater in calves born to malnourished mothers (19 per cent versus 0 per cent). The net result was that all calves born to dams fed the high-energy ration during the last 30 days of gestation survived, whereas only 71 per cent of the calves born to malnourished mothers survived.

In a study from Idaho, Bull et al.[3] have shown that the incidence of "weak calf syndrome" is related to the protein intake of cows during the last trimester of gestation. Herds with a high-protein intake had a 0.6 per cent incidence of weak calf syndrome, whereas herds with a low-protein intake had an incidence of 9.8 per cent.

Beef females that fail to gain at least the weight of the conceptus (about 100 to 150 lb) during the last trimester of gestation are likely to have calves that are lighter at birth and more susceptible to disease and that do not grow as well as calves born to adequately nourished cows.

Not only does maternal malnutrition affect the weight of calves produced during the current year but it also decreases the weight of calves produced the following year because malnourished cows usually have an extended interval from calving to first estrus. As discussed previously, the interval from calving to conception must be less than 80 days if a cow is to maintain a yearly calving interval. If a cow is to have two opportunities to conceive and maintain a yearly calving interval, she must be in heat by 60 days after calving. Large net weight losses during the last trimester of gestation were highly correlated with decreased percentages of cows that had shown heat by the start of the breeding season.[2, 4, 6, 16] In fact, cows with large net weight losses often fail to show estrus at all during the breeding season. This is especially true for cattle with Brahman breeding.

As feeding programs are highly dependent upon economic conditions, it is necessary to estimate the loss of production caused by maternal malnutrition during the last trimester of gestation. This estimate can then be used to determine if some level of supplemental feeding during gestation will be economically feasible. The data shown in Table 12 are an attempt to predict calf production for 2 years starting with 2-year-old heifers that were adequately nourished compared with those that were malnourished during the last trimester of gestation. I have made several assumptions while making these estimations:

1. The heifers were adequately fed during the last trimester of their second pregnancy.

TABLE 12. *Projected Calf Production from 2-Year-Old Heifers Malnourished during Last Trimester of Gestation Compared with Production from Adequately Nourished Heifers**

Location and Nutrition Level[†]	Calf Production, First Year			Calf Production, Second Year				Projected Total Calf Production (lb)
	WEANING WEIGHT (lb)	PROJECTED CALVES WEANED (no.)	CALF PRODUCTION (lb)	PRO-JECTED CALVES BORN (no.)	PRO-JECTED CALVES WEANED (no.)	PROJECTED WEANING WEIGHT (lb)	PROJECTED CALF PRODUCTION (lb)	
Nebraska:								
Adequate	397	87	34,587	97	87	360	31,320	65,907
Malnourished	372	80	29,738	93	83	343	28,469	58,207
Difference	25	7	4,849	4	4	17	2,851	7,700
Montana:								
Adequate	363	87	31,581	97	87	360	31,320	62,901
Malnourished	339	80	27,120	97	87	329	28,623	55,743
Difference	24	7	4,461	0	0	31	2,697	7,158
Wyoming:								
Adequate	354	87	30,798	97	87	360	31,320	62,118
Malnourished	325	80	26,000	90	80	358	28,640	54,640
Difference	29	7	4,798	7	7	2	2,680	7,478

*Based on 100 cows over a 2-year period.
†Sources of data: *Nebraska*: Dunn, T. G., Wiltbank, J. N., Ingalls, J. E. and Zimmerman, D. R.: Proc. West. Am. Soc., Anim. Sci., *16*:V, 1965; Dunn, T. G., Ingalls, J. E., Zimmerman, D. R. and Wiltbank, J. N.: J. Anim. Sci., *29*:719, 1969; *Montana*: Bellows, R. A., Varner, L. W., Short, R. E. and Pahnish, O. F.: J. Anim. Sci., *35*:185, 1972; *Wyoming*: Corah, L. R., Dunn, T. G. and Kaltenbach, C. C.: J. Anim. Sci., *41*:819, 1975.

2. Weaning weights for the first year were taken from experimental data.

3. The number of calves weaned the first year was calculated from the data obtained from R. A. Bellows,[1] which showed a 13 per cent loss from pregnancy diagnosis to weaning. Corah *et al.*[4] found that 7 per cent more calves born to malnourished dams died than similar calves born to adequately nourished dams. The survival rate for the malnourished group has therefore been reduced by 7 percentage points compared with the adequately nourished group (Table 12).

4. Calf production for the first year is the product of projected calves weaned and their weaning weight.

5. In calculating projected calves born the second year, I assumed that only pregnant cows are carried into the winter and that they experience a 3 per cent loss from abortions prior to calving. Since a certain percentage of cows did not show estrus during the breeding season in the malnourished groups, the number of calves born has been reduced by the percentage of such cows that failed to show estrus.

6. The projected calves weaned reflects 10 per cent loss from birth to weaning.[1]

7. The projected weaning weight for the second calf crop was estimated as follows: (a) The weaning weight for calves born to ade-

quately nourished dams was estimated from the data shown in Table 5. (b) Since maternal malnutrition extends the postpartum interval (interval from calving to first heat), the weaning weight of the second calf crop born to malnourished dams was reduced to reflect the effect of the extended postpartum interval. This was accomplished by reducing the weaning weight used in 7(a) by the product of 1.56 lb/day (average daily gain for these calves) and the difference in days for the postpartum interval between adequately nourished heifers and malnourished heifers.

8. Projected calf production for the second year is the product of calves weaned and weaning weight.

9. The total projected calf production is the sum of calf production for the first year and calf production for the second year.

The projections from Table 12 show that heifers that have a large net weight loss during the last trimester of their first gestation are likely to produce from 70 to 77 lb less calf over a 2-year period than heifers that do not have a net weight loss. With this information available, plus the current calf prices and current feed prices, a cattleman has a reasonable opportunity to project profit or loss from a supplemental feeding program.

The Postpartum Suckled Female

The major goal of the cattleman is to have a large percentage (at least 50 per cent) of his calves born during the first 21 days of the calving season. In order to achieve this goal a large percentage (at least 90 per cent) of cows must show heat during the first 21 days of the breeding season and have a high conception rate at first service (at least 60 per cent). In general, the plane of nutrition prior to calving influences the length of the postpartum interval and thereby the percentage of cows that are in heat early in the breeding season. The plane of nutrition following calving affects conception rate at first service.

Unfortunately, dramatically increasing the plane of nutrition following calving has little influence on the length of the postpartum interval if cows are thin at calving time. It appears that they must regain a certain body condition before resuming estrous activity. It is difficult, therefore, to shorten the postpartum interval with heavy feeding after calving. Only early weaning or allowing calves to suckle only once daily seems to be effective in shortening the postpartum interval. Under most management situations, weaning calves or allowing them to suckle only once daily is not the treatment of choice. Therefore, it appears that a proper nutritional program during the last trimester of gestation is a more sound solution to the problem of an extended postpartum interval.

Formulation of Rations

The most dramatic change in the nutrient requirements of the beef female occurs at calving, when she must begin nursing her offspring. This change becomes especially important for heifers nursing their first calves since they not only must provide nutrients for milk production and maintenance but also must provide for continued growth and finally for reproduction for the next calf crop. The current NRC publication[10] lists two sets of requirements for cows nursing calves for the first 3 to 4 months of lactation. One set is for cows of average milking ability, and one set is for cows of superior milking ability. The requirements given for *cows of average milking ability* (11 lb/day) *should be ignored* since the levels of most nutrients are inadequate to support satisfactory re-

production. The requirements listed for cows of superior milking ability (22 lb/day) should be used *only for mature cows of average milking ability*.

The energy requirements for cows of superior milking ability[10] are inadequate for heifers that are nursing their first calves. Heifers that weigh 1000 lb or less should receive at least 15 lb of TDN per day (24.62 Mcal DE). Heavier heifers should receive at least 16 lb of TDN per day (26.26 Mcal DE).

It is difficult to formulate a ration for cows that are nursing calves because the dietary intake necessary for adequate reproduction is dependent upon many factors. The condition of the cow at calving time certainly must be considered. Cows that are thin at calving are more likely to have an extended postpartum interval, whereas cows that are in good condition will have a shorter interval. Consequently, cows that are thin at calving time will require more feed after calving than will similar cows that are in good condition. The age and milking ability of the cow also influence the postpartum nutrient requirements. For example, heifers that are nursing their first calves have a greater requirement for both energy and protein than do mature cows of similar body weight.

Few cow herds are maintained under drylot conditions following calving; consequently, the majority of their diet is made up of grazed forage. This further complicates the problem because the amount of nutrients in the grazed forage must now be estimated. This is an especially difficult process and is best done by collecting forage samples for chemical analyses with animals equipped with esophageal fistulae — not the sort of animal found on the average range or pasture. Probably the next best method is to follow the weight gains of the animals or weight gains of a sample of animals. In general, the following guidelines can be used: cows that lose weight following calving have a lower first-service conception rate than cows that gain weight after calving. If the weight loss after calving is severe, cows will not show estrus at all. Cows that are in good condition after calving will attain satisfactory reproduction by gaining 0.5 to 1 lb/day. Cows that are thin at calving will probably have to gain in excess of 2 lb/day in order to achieve a satisfactory pregnancy rate for the following calf crop. An example ration that should produce 0.5 to 1 lb/day gain for a mature, suckled cow is as follows:

Assume that a 992-lb mature cow of average milking ability and in good condition at calving requires 14.1 lb TDN and 1.6 lb DP daily (NRC publication[10] for cows of superior milking ability). Twenty-eight and 4/5 lb of alfalfa hay (1-00-063, NRC feed reference number) would provide adequate TDN and more than adequate DP, vitamin A and calcium. The diet would be deficient in P, which again could be provided with a salt-sodium tripolyphosphate mixture. If the cow is fed 28.8 lb of alfalfa hay, it means that she must consume about 2.9 per cent of her body weight in roughage. However, some animals may not be able to consume that much roughage.

Since feeding 28.8 lb of alfalfa hay provided more than adequate protein (nearly twice as much DP as needed), it would be appropriate to seek a high-energy feed to supplement the alfalfa. This is especially true if the supply of alfalfa is limited. The requirements for the cow are shown in Table 13 plus an example ration using corn to supplement alfalfa (first example ration shown). Again, this ration is deficient in P, which can be supplemented free choice. The ration is also deficient in DM, which suggests that the cows would be hungry. If this is the case, the animals can be fed straw or other low-quality roughage as a "filler."

The second example ration shown in Table 13 presents a slightly different problem. Native mountain meadow hay is low in protein, so it is necessary to find a feed that will supplement both protein and energy. In this case, commercial breeder pellets were chosen. As shown in Table 13 (second example ration) feeding 23 lb of native hay plus 4.5 lb of breeder pellets meets most of the requirements for the lactating beef cow except phosphorus. Also notice that the second example ration was balanced by using CP instead of DP, since only the CP content of the breeder pellets was known. The amounts of Ca and P provided by the breeder pellets were estimated, but this information is available on the feed tags.

The rations shown in Table 13 would provide well for cows in drylot. They may not be practical rations except during periods when cows cannot consume any forage by grazing (e.g., early spring in the northern United States). In spring-calving herds, the cows will consume some forage by grazing, depending upon the climatic situation. Early spring forage, although high in nutrient content, is also high in moisture. Cattle must therefore graze huge quantities to obtain sufficient dry matter. In most instances, cows can obtain sufficient spring forage to meet their protein needs but cannot consume enough to meet their energy needs. The cattleman then is faced with providing an energy supplement for his cow herd.

Energy Supplementation

Often, the most inexpensive energy supplement would be some form of hay. Unfortunately, when green spring forage is available, cattle become very reluctant to

TABLE 13. *Requirements for 992-lb Suckled Cow of Average Milking Ability and Example Rations to Meet Requirements**

Item	DM (lb)	CP (lb)	DP (lb)	TDN (lb)	Ca (gm)	P (gm)	Vitamin A (IU)
Requirements	24.9	2.71	1.59	14.1	45	42	36,000
Example ration No. 1 (as fed):							
20 lb alfalfa hay (1-00-063)†	17.80		2.16	9.80	109	18	107,762
5.3 lb corn (4-02-931)†	4.73		0.35	4.30	–	8	1,718
Total supplied by ration	22.53		2.51	14.10	109	26	109,480
Example ration No. 2 (as fed):							
23 lb native hay (1-03-181)†	21.37	1.94		10.90	34	29	
4.5 lb commercial breeder pellets, 20% protein, estimated 80% TDN	4.07	0.81		3.26	11	11	
Total supplied by ration	25.44	2.75		14.16	45	40	

*Based on cow's being in good condition at calving.
†NRC feed reference number.

consume dry roughage. This means that some form of concentrate should be provided to meet the energy requirements of suckled cows. Several commercial feed companies sell some form of "breeder" pellets or cubes. These supplements are high-energy supplements with minimum levels of protein. In addition, many firms add supplemental phosphorus to their formula feeds. These cubes have an advantage in that they do not require specialized equipment for feeding. On the other hand, the pellets or cubes are usually expensive.

An economical method of supplementing energy is to simply use some form of ground or rolled grain, e.g., corn, milo, barley or oats. Although grain has a cost advantage, it has disadvantages in that it requires troughs or feed bunks for feeding. Grain is also seldom sacked, as are formula feeds. For some operators who are equipped to handle bulk feed, this is an advantage. For those who do not have such equipment, feeding bulk grain can be a problem.

The quantity of energy supplement required is inversely related to the moisture content and quantity of the spring forage. For example, on a native range in Wyoming, moisture content of native forage was 68 per cent in late May and 69 per cent in June.[11] Esophageal fistula samples of native forage collected on a range near Cheyenne, Wyoming, averaged 13.88 per cent CP and 53 to 55 per cent TDN in May and June.[9] In late May, a 1000-lb mature cow of average milking ability would have to consume 61 lb of native range forage per day to meet her protein requirements and 80 lb to meet her TDN requirements. If we assume that the cow consumes 61 lb of native forage, she would receive adequate protein but would receive only 10.7 lb of TDN. In order to meet her requirement, she would need an additional 3.4 lb of TDN. The following amounts of various supplemental feeds would provide the needed amount of TDN: 4.2 lb corn (NRC feed reference number 4-02-931), 4.6 lb barley (NRC feed reference number 4-00-549), 4.8 lb milo (NRC feed reference number 4-04-444), 5.0 lb oats (NRC feed reference number 4-03-309) or 4.7 lb commercial breeder pellets (80 per cent TDN). One frequent mistake in providing an energy supplement to suckled cows grazing early spring forage is to provide too little supplement. Although 1 or 2 lb/head/day may be adequate for a protein supplement during the winter for dry, pregnant cows, this pro-

vides less than half of the supplemental energy required by suckled cows.

If at all possible, the cattleman should keep his first-calf heifers segregated from the older cows until the spring forage is abundant enough so that supplemental energy is no longer required. First-calf heifers are usually smaller than older cows and consequently are not able to successfully compete for supplemental feed. The net result is that the animals that have the greatest requirement for supplemental feed (the first-calf heifers) receive less than they should, and the animals with a lower requirement for supplemental feed receive more than they need.

Providing supplemental feeds on southwestern desert ranges in the United States has often produced lower calf crops than in unsupplemented herds. The apparent explanation is that the supplemented cows quit foraging and wait for the supplemental handout. This does not mean that the animals do not require supplemental feed; it only means that some usable system must be devised to deliver the supplement without disrupting grazing behavior.

There is no question that providing supplemental energy is necessary on early spring native ranges because the forage is not sufficiently abundant to meet the needs of the suckled cow. Such a cow simply cannot spend enough hours grazing to gather the quantity of forage that she needs. There are other alternatives to providing supplemental energy. One is to postpone the calving season until more abundant forage is available. In other words, calve in May instead of April. This may not be a feasible solution if the cattleman must sell calves at a particular time in the fall. On the other hand, it may be quite feasible for a cow-yearling operation.

Another solution that holds much promise is the use of introduced grass species to provide early spring grazing. In the high plains region, crested wheatgrass provides excellent early spring grazing. This introduced grass provides adequate forage about 2 to 3 weeks earlier than does native shortgrass range. For example, near Cheyenne, Wyoming, the protein content of esophageal samples from a crested wheatgrass pasture averaged 17.8 per cent protein in May and June compared with 13.8 per cent protein for native range.[9] In addition to providing excellent early pasture, crested wheatgrass is easily established.

The Dry, Pregnant Female

The least critical period in the productive cycle of the beef cow is that period from the time the calf is weaned until the start of the third trimester of gestation. During this time, cows usually can afford some weight loss. It is during this period that cows can effectively make use of aftermath feeds and crop residues. If it is necessary to provide supplemental feed to the cow herd, the lowest quality feed should be used during this time.

SUMMARY

Forage must constitute the greatest part of the diet of beef cattle. By recognizing the nutrient requirements of beef cattle at particular times during their productive cycle and by being aware of the quality and quantity of the forage resource at particular times of the year, the cowman can match the forage resource to the requirements of his beef cattle herd so that the maximum benefit can be obtained. This procedure will reduce the requirement for supplemental feed, which should increase the net profit from the beef cattle herd.

I am convinced that there are three very important items that require the strict attention of the producer:

1. Replacement heifers should be fed to reach puberty early so they can be bred to calve 20 to 30 days earlier than the older cows.

2. The most important period of the reproductive cycle of the beef cow is the last 90 days of gestation (last trimester) plus the first 60 days after calving. Beef cows must gain the weight of the conceptus during the last trimester of gestation if they are to wean heavy calves and conceive early in the breeding season for the next calf crop.

3. Bulls should receive the careful attention that one-half of the calf demands. Bulls should be nutritionally prepared for the start of the breeding season at least 60 days in advance of the first day of the breeding season.

REFERENCES

Literature Cited

1. Bellows, R. A.: Personal communication.
2. Bellows, R. A., Varner, L. W., Short, R. E. and Pahnish, O. F.: Gestation feed level, calf birth weight and calving difficulty (abstr.). J. Anim. Sci., *35*:185, 1972.
3. Bull, R. C., Loucks, R. R., Edmiston, F. L., Hawkins, J. N. and Stauber, E. H.: Nutrition and weak calf syndrome in beef cattle. University of Idaho College of Agriculture Current Information Series No. 246, 1974.
4. Corah, L. R., Dunn, T. G. and Kaltenbach, C. C.: Influence of prepartum nutrition on the reproductive performance of beef females and the performance of their progeny. J. Anim. Sci., *41*:819, 1975.
5. Dunn, T. G., Wiltbank, J. N., Ingalls, J. E. and Zimmerman, D. R.: Dam's energy intake and milk production and calf gains. Proc. West. Sect. Am. Soc. Anim. Sci., *16*:V, 1965.
6. Dunn, T. G., Ingalls, J. E., Zimmerman, D. R. and Wiltbank, J. N.: Reproductive performance of 2-year-old Hereford and Angus heifers as influenced by pre- and post-calving energy intake. J. Anim. Sci., *29*:719, 1969.
7. Ferrell, C. L., Garrett, W. N. and Hinman, N.: Growth, development and composition of the udder and gravid uterus of beef heifers during pregnancy. J. Anim. Sci., *42*:1477, 1976.
8. Lesmeister, J. L., Burfening, P. J. and Blackwell, R. L.: Date of first calving in beef cows and subsequent calf production. J. Anim. Sci., *36*:1, 1973.
9. Marshall, B. M.: Summer range grass utilization by beef cattle. M.S. thesis, University of Wyoming, Laramie, Wyoming, 1976.
10. National Research Council (NRC): Nutrient Requirements of Domestic Animals, No. 4, Nutrient requirements of beef cattle. National Academy of Sciences, NRC, Washington, D.C., 1976.
11. Schoonover, C. O., Smith, G. E., Inloes, G. and Richardson, B.: Moisture content of grasses grazed by cattle. Proc. West. Sect. Am. Soc. Anim. Sci., *19*:367, 1968.
12. Varner, L. W., Bellows, R. A. and Christensen, D. S.: A management system for wintering replacement heifers. J. Anim. Sci., *44*:165, 1977.
13. Waggoner, J. W.: Personal communication.
14. Waggoner, J. W. and Radloff, H. D.: Wyoming hay — its nutrient content. Wyoming Beef Cattle Fact Sheets, MP 37.5, Wyo-102, 1977.
15. Wiltbank, J. N.: Research needs in beef cattle reproduction. J. Anim. Sci., *31*:755, 1970.
16. Wiltbank, J. N., Rowden, W. W., Ingalls, J. E., Gregory, K. E. and Koch, R. M.: Effect of energy level on reproductive phenomena of mature Hereford cows. J. Anim. Sci., *21*:219, 1962.

Textbooks on Animal Nutrition

1. Church, D. C. (ed.): Digestive Physiology and Nutrition of Ruminants, Vol. 2, Nutrition. O and B Books, 1215 NW Kline Place, Corvallis, Oregon, 1971.
2. Church, D. E. (ed.): Digestive Physiology and Nutrition of Ruminants, Vol. 3, Practical Nutrition. O and B Books, 1215 NW Kline Place, Corvallis, Oregon, 1972.
3. Church, D. C. (ed.): Digestive Physiology and Nutrition of Ruminants, Volume 1, Digestive Physiology. 2nd Ed. O and B Books, 1215 NW Kline Place, Corvallis, Oregon, 1975.

4. Church, D. C. (ed.): Livestock Feeds and Feeding. O and B Books, 1215 NW Kline Place, Corvallis, Oregon, 1977.
5. Church, D. C. and Pond, W. G.: Basic Animal Nutrition and Feeding. O and B Books, 1215 NW Kline Place, Corvallis, Oregon, 1974.

6. McDonald, P., Edwards, R. A. and Greenhalgh, J. F. D.: Animal Nutrition. 3rd Ed. Oliver and Boyd Croythorn House, 24 Ravelston Terrace, Edinburgh EH4 eTJ, Scotland, 1973.
7. Maynard, L. A. and Loosli, J. K.: Animal Nutrition. 6th Ed. New York, McGraw-Hill Book Co., 1969.

Effects of Urea on Bovine Reproduction

R. E. ERB and C. J. CALLAHAN
Purdue University, West Lafayette, Indiana

INTRODUCTION

About 100 years ago it was established that cattle and other ruminants could utilize urea and other dietary nonprotein nitrogen (NPN) compounds to synthesize body proteins. In 1940, urea was approved for use as a feed ingredient in ruminant rations in the United States. In 1973, urea replaced 4 to 5 million tons of soybean meal. Worldwide, protein is a major limiting nutrient for animal production, especially for those ruminants maintained on either low-quality forages or crop residues. In addition, human beings will require increased quantities of edible plant proteins in the future, which precludes increased use of NPN and nonedible plant proteins in the diets of animals.

Ruminants depend upon the population of micro-organisms in the rumen to obtain energy from lignocellulose complexes of plants in order to obtain amino acids for synthesis of body proteins from dietary protein and NPN.[1] Urea can replace at least 99 per cent of dietary protein-nitrogen in purified diets of cattle for several years without having a severe detrimental effect upon growth, milk production or reproduction. Function is about two-thirds normal. Although such studies establish an upper limit of safety and utilization, they do not define variables encountered when natural feedstuffs are used under an infinite number of practical conditions. Moreover, purified diets used in the studies were balanced for known essential nutrients, whereas practical diets may have gross imbalances. Although research on urea as a nutrient has been extensive,

effects on reproduction were not included in a majority of studies.

Various NPN compounds are normal constituents in biological fluids of ruminants, even when none are actually fed to the animals. Ammonia results from degradation of dietary protein and NPN compounds.[1] Breakdown of urea to ammonia and carbon dioxide is mediated by microbial urease. Most rumen bacteria prefer free ammonia to amino acids for synthesis of microbial proteins. Utilization of ammonia from urea or proteins in the rumen depends upon available carbohydrate (about one part urea to four parts carbohydrate). However, the rate of release of ammonia from urea is about fourfold greater in the rumen (80 mg/hr/100 ml of rumen fluid) than the release that occurs from fermentation reactions on complex carbohydrates.[1] This limits the amount of urea that can be utilized at one time without excessive absorption of ammonia through the rumen wall. Absorbed ammonia may be reconverted to urea by the liver and recycled to the rumen or excreted in urine. When protective mechanisms are overcome, ammonia toxicity results (ammonia would be about 80 mg/100 ml of rumen fluid and more than 0.6 mg/100 ml of peripheral blood).

TOLERANCE TO UREA

Factors Affecting Tolerance. Acute and subacute signs of urea toxicity seldom, if ever, occur if guidelines for feeding urea are followed. Major causes of toxicity are errors in formulation, incomplete mixing and otherwise careless handling of urea. However, under practical conditions other factors affect tolerance dramatically. These are (1) fasting or low intake of low-quality roughage and/or water, (2) diets based on forage that varies from very low to high available carbohydrate, (3) failure to increase dietary urea gradually to permit adaptation when the amount to be fed is relatively high for conditions listed in factors 1 and 2 and (4) methods of feeding.

Tolerance Levels. Since urease is highly active and always present in rumen contents, the rate of conversion of urea to ammonia should be rapid, independent of the factors just listed. Absorption of ammonia from the rumen is a function of (1) rate and quantity of ammonia released, (2) availability of carbohydrate to support rapid fermentation and (3) viable microbial mass to utilize carbohydrate and ammonia. Under least favorable conditions, as little as 100 gm of urea at one time could be fatal to an unadapted fasted animal. Prior adaptation of fasted animals to urea could increase tolerance by 30 to 50 per cent. Under the most optimal conditions (high-energy rations fed free choice), tolerances for adapted animals may be up to five-fold higher than for the least favorable conditions. Within any nutritional regimen, upper nontoxic levels of urea exceed quantities that can be utilized economically for productive purposes. This is so even when urea replaces all protein-nitrogen, as in purified diets.

Abortion. Studies showed that toxicity induced one time in pregnant beef cows, followed by treatment with acetic acid to prevent death, had no effect on the fetuses or on subsequent reproductive efficiency of the cows.[5] However, the abortion rate at first calving was 19 per cent for one group of Holstein heifers that were fed urea at a rate of 45 per cent of ration nitrogen up to midpregnancy and 15 per cent thereafter. There were no abortions in two groups fed either one-half as much urea or no urea. Heifers fed urea but not aborting had shorter gestation periods.[2] Abortions were not observed when high-urea rations were not fed until the end of first pregnancy rather than prior to the first pregnancy or during subsequent years.[2] Currently, there is no evidence that dietary urea causes abortion in cows after the first pregnancy.

LONG-TERM FEEDING — BLENDED RATIONS

Trials. Rations in two trials were high in energy and were isocaloric and isonitrogenous among treatments.[2] The rations were primarily corn silage and meadow crop silage (ratio 4.4:1), ground corn and supplemental nitrogen from urea or soybean meal. The rations were balanced for known nutrient requirements, including minerals and vitamins. Total rations were blended and group-fed free choice once daily. On a dry matter basis, lactation rations contained 46 per cent concentrate mixture and 54 per cent silage mixture. After adaptation to urea, trial 1 heifers in groups 1, 2 and 3 consumed 0, 95 and 191 gm/day of urea (0, 22 and 45 per cent of ration nitrogen) from first inseminations to midpregnancy; 0, 34 and 68 gm/day after midpregnancy and 0, 145 and 290 gm/day during the first lactation. Urea nitrogen in lactation rations was 0, 18, and 36 per cent of ration nitrogen, and urea was 0, 0.9 and 1.8 per cent of total ration dry matter. Trial 1 was continued until diagnosis of the third pregnancy. In trial 2, heifers were adapted to group 1 and group 3 lactation rations just prior to first calving and were continued on their respective rations for four consecutive lactations.[2]

General Performance. Urea intake of group 2 animals equaled or exceeded amounts fed in natural diets to lactating dairy cows by workers other than those in the study through at least one lactation. All were in agreement that this level of feeding had no effect on milk production, general health, reproduction or calf survival. However, decrease in daily yields of milk, fat and protein on high-urea rations (group 3) averaged 8, 6 and 13 per cent respectively, for four lactations, a result consistent with short-term trials.[1] High-urea rations had no effect on the growth of heifers and the general health of heifers and cows, including the incidence of clinical mastitis (treated cases), positive California mastitis test scores or concentrations of somatic cells in milk.

Effects on Reproduction. Apart from abortions among heifers on high-urea rations (group 3) during trial 1 (see preceding section on abortion), high levels of dietary urea had no serious long-term effects on reproduction. Some differences were noted, but, as discussed later, they were not repeatable between experiments or between years of the same experiment.[3]

Dietary urea had no effect on ovarian function during any year, as indicated by regularity of cycles, frequency of ovulations without estrus, re-establishment of cycles postpartum, incidence of cystic ovaries and conception rates based on total services per conception. Other studies are in agreement (for review, see reference 2). Average intervals between calvings were significantly longer for high-urea (group 3) animals during trial 2 but not during trial 1. The intervals were not excessively long in any group of either trial (385 to 420 days). The percentage of cows open more than 6 months was somewhat higher for those fed high-urea rations.[2] Rates of retention of fetal membranes for more than 24 hours did not differ significantly, except at end of the first year of trial 2 when rates were 0 per cent for no-urea intake and 44 per cent for high-urea feedings. The latter contributed to a higher rate of postpartum metritis, which may have caused the longer calving intervals for cows fed high-urea rations (group 3) during trial 2.

Failure to find repeatable year-to-year differences in reproductive parameters may indicate variations due to other factors or prolonged adaptation to high levels of urea.

Effects on Endocrine Functions. Hormonal studies were done only during trial 1. In general, the results supported the concept of prolonged adaptation to high-urea levels, which seemed to continue through the second pregnancy.

High levels of dietary urea had no effect on concentrations of progesterone and luteinizing hormone (LH) in blood plasma 1 to 18 days after first insemination of heifers, but excretion of estradiol in urine was decreased, especially among those not pregnant following first insemination. Later, during first pregnancy, heifers fed high levels of urea had higher concentrations of progesterone and lower concentrations of total estrogen in blood plasma. However, the rather substantial differences between dietary groups could not be related to premature births among heifers that were fed urea. During second pregnancy, those on high-urea rations had higher concentrations of both progesterone and total estrogen in blood plasma and excreted more estrogen in urine at calving than those fed no urea (group 1). No clear hormonal differences were noted among groups 0 to 18 days after insemination for the third pregnancy.

In a short-term study, heifers fed high-urea rations (145 to 240 gm/day) had smaller corpora lutea at midcycle and their excised corpora lutea synthesized less pro-

gesterone *in vitro* compared with heifers that were not fed any urea.

Even though hormonal differences attributable to dietary urea were observed,[3] these seemed to equalize among groups within 2 years. In a practical way, if high levels of dietary urea, as in group 3, do have an adverse effect on reproduction, differences would be expected during the first year but not during successive years of feeding urea continuously in blended high-energy rations.

GUIDELINES

General Guidelines. Controlled research studies regarding effects of urea on reproduction are inadequate to establish upper limits of daily intake that assure absence of undesirable effects on reproduction under varied practical conditions. Data for lactating dairy cows fed high-energy rations support a general conclusion that moderate amounts of urea (up to at least 227 gm/day for adapted animals) have no short- or long-term effects on reproduction.[1, 2, 3, 4] Unfortunately, data on reproduction are minimal and inadequate to support recommendations when urea is used to supplement low-quality roughages that are high in fiber and deficient in digestible energy, protein and often other nutrients.

However, there is no reason to believe that the limits recommended for efficient utilization of urea for maintenance, growth and lactation of breeding-age cattle would affect reproduction adversely. Unfortunately, there is no simple approach to determining how much urea can be fed because of many variables, including daily requirements for dietary protein, daily intake of feed by individual cattle and the crude protein and energy levels in rations.

Because of varied conditions under which dietary urea is fed, no single guideline is satisfactory. However, if one or more guidelines are applied, it is unlikely that unsafe levels would be fed to adapted cattle, even though other variables may affect efficient utilization of urea (Table 1).

Four guidelines are suggested as follows:

1. Provide no more than 25 per cent of total nitrogen in ration from urea nitrogen.

2. Use no more than 0.5 per cent urea in dry matter of all-roughage rations that are lower than 65 per cent in total digestible

TABLE 1. *Approximate Guidelines for Rations Ranging from 45 to 80 Per Cent Total Digestible Nutrients (TDN)**

Total Ration Dry Matter (% TDN)	Maximum CP from Plant Protein plus Urea (% CP)	Maximum Urea in Total Ration Dry Matter (%)	Maximum Urea in Total Ration Dry Matter (gm/lb)	Increase in CP from Urea (%)	Remarks
45	6.5[a]	0.5	2.27	1.4[b,c]	All roughage
50	7.2	0.5	2.27	1.4	All roughage
55	8.0	0.6	2.72	1.7	d
60	8.7	0.7	3.18	2.0	d
65	9.4	0.8	3.63	2.2	d
70	10.2	0.9	4.09	2.5	e
75	10.9	1.0	4.54	2.8	e
80	11.6	1.0	4.54	2.8	e

*Note limitations on crude protein (CP), which are dependent on level of TDN. Guidelines apply to beef and dairy cattle, even though cow herds managed for beef production tend to utilize low-energy rations, as compared with high-energy rations for dairy cows.

[a]About 70 per cent of CP is utilized when CP is about 14.5 per cent of TDN (1:7 ratio) and urea supplies no more than 25 per cent of nitrogen in total ration. Utilization decreases as ratio decreases to 1:6, but additional urea that is equivalent to about 1.5 per cent CP may be 40 to 70 per cent utilized (see footnote c).

[b]One gram of urea/lb of dry matter increases CP 0.62 per cent for urea containing 45 per cent N ($0.62 \times 2.3 = 1.4$ per cent). CP from 1 gm of urea/lb dry matter = per cent N in urea × protein equivalent/gm of N ÷ grams in 1 lb or $45 \times 6.25 \div 454 = 0.62$ per cent.

[c]If per cent CP from urea plus per cent natural CP in ration exceeds maximum per cent CP shown in column 2, urea should be reduced to avoid its poor utilization. Increase maximum per cent CP shown in column 2 about 1.5 per cent (6.5 per cent to 8 per cent or 11.6 per cent to 13.1 per cent) if decreased utilization of urea is economical, as compared with supplemental plant protein, and provided that the guideline limits for levels of urea are not exceeded.

[d]If grain is used to increase TDN of total ration, restrict urea to 0.5 per cent of roughage dry matter plus 5 gm of urea/lb of grain consumed. Include grain-equivalent in silages such as corn silage.

[e]Blended rations fed free choice. Total intake of urea/day should not exceed 227 gm (0.5 lb). This limit is exceeded if dry matter consumption by individuals is more than 50 lb/day (23 kg/day).

nutrients (TDN), up to a maximum of 1.0 per cent in dry matter of rations containing more than 70 per cent TDN (see column 3, Table 1).

3. Use no more than 3 per cent urea in grain-mix consumed up to 15 lb/day (14 gm of urea/lb, which would represent about 50 per cent of nitrogen when blended into ground corn). When grain-mix consumption exceeds 15 lb/day, as is common for lactating dairy cows, base calculations on the total dry matter consumed, as in guideline 2. The rate of intake decreases as urea is increased in the grain-mix.

4. If grain-mix is used to increase the TDN of roughage, restrict urea to 0.5 per cent of dry matter plus 5 gm of urea/lb of grain consumed (footnote d, Table 1).

Practical Limits. Application of the guidelines indicates that daily limits of urea vary from 23 gm/day to 46 gm/day when intake of forage (45 to 65 per cent TDN) by 1000-lb cattle is limited to 1 to 2 per cent of body weight. The upper limit is about 227 gm (0.5 lb) or urea per day for lactating dairy cows consuming about 50 lb of dry matter in rations containing more than 70 per cent TDN (Table 1).

Two field studies utilizing lactating dairy cows have been reported. One study compared Holstein cows in one herd for 18 months. The maximum daily intake of urea by any individual was 170 gm (85 gm fed twice daily in a concentrate containing 6.3 gm of urea/lb or 1.4 per cent urea). Cows fed urea had a similar rate of milk production as compared with herdmates fed no urea, and services per conception averaged 1.6 and 1.9, respectively. Ryder *et al.*[4] reported 3157 herd-year observations (5-year period) from Michigan Dairy Herd Improvement Association herds. Among the 3157 herd-year observations, 1709 animals were fed urea (range 9 to 370 gm/day). Milk production was similar among groups. The correlation between length of calving interval and level of dietary urea was very low (r = 0.01). Cows sold because of sterility averaged 2.15 per cent in herds fed no urea and 2.42 per cent in herds fed urea. The difference of only 0.27 per cent was statistically significant but probably has no practical significance. Results from long-term feeding of urea in high-energy rations reported by Erb *et al.*[2, 3] are in general agreement. However, the latter results suggest that reproductive efficiency may be reduced if urea constitutes 1.8 per cent of the dry matter, compared with 0 per cent or 0.9 per cent urea. Based on the foregoing data, it appears unlikely that daily intakes of up to 227 gm of urea in high-energy rations (daily intake of 50 lb of dry matter containing 1 per cent urea) would affect reproduction in lactating dairy cows.

The amounts of urea that can be utilized increase as supplemental energy from low-protein cereal grains or molasses is increased in diets of poor-quality forage. Limited or no utilization of urea nitrogen may occur if intake of poor-quality forage is limited severely. Efficient utilization of limited urea occurs generally for submaintenance (acceptable weight loss) if poor-quality roughage satisfies appetite. Maintenance of or moderate gains in weight occur generally as supplemental energy from low-protein concentrates is increased. Although the amount of urea that can be utilized increases as fermentable carbohydrate is increased, the extent and efficiency of utilization of urea are limited by the crude protein and TDN in the ration before urea is added.[1] These limitations are illustrated in Table 1 along with calculations for estimating the crude protein equivalent of urea (footnotes, Table 1).

Precautions. Supplemental urea must be mixed uniformly into whatever carrier is used, including commercial supplements, silages, grain mixtures or blended complete rations fed free choice. Feeding practices should insure regular intake of feedstuffs to avoid overconsumption of urea at one meal, even by cattle adapted to urea. Daily rates of no more than 50 gm of urea should be consumed during one meal by cattle on low-energy roughages or no more than one-half the daily intake by dairy cows fed concentrate containing urea only when being milked. Intake of urea at one time is not critical when blended high-energy rations are fed free choice at least daily because of frequent eating (12 or more times each day).

Natural diets of forage, excluding whole plant corn silage, normally would contain 7 to 10 per cent crude protein before the addition of urea and would also contain 50 to 60 per cent TDN. Therefore, the addition of urea to such rations may be unnecessary, poorly utilized or not utilized at all (see column 2, Table 1). Pregnant and nonlactating beef cows require about 6.5 per cent crude protein for maintenance and up to about 10 per cent when nursing calves. In addition requirements for younger cattle are 1 to 2 per cent higher to support growth. Therefore, urea fed with most natural forages may not be required even if utilized, especially for mature, nonlactating beef cattle. Corn silage is a special kind of forage because it also contains variable amounts of corn grain. Urea may be added to corn silage at ensiling (0.5 per cent of wet weight when dry matter is about 33 per cent). This would increase the protein equivalent of the corn silage by about 2.8 per cent. Overfeeding corn silage to nonpregnant yearlings and cows can result in overconditioning whether or not the silage contains urea. Overconditioning is counterproductive to good reproduction and subsequently may cause decreased milk production in heifers. An opposite problem may exist under range conditions because energy is often the major deficiency.

Data from a majority of experiments under range conditions providing marginal nutrition indicate that there is more improvement in reproductive efficiency from supplemental energy than from supplemental protein. Although the reason is unknown, such results suggest that increasing dietary protein (plant protein nitrogen and/or urea nitrogen) without increasing dietary energy is counterproductive and may even decrease reproductive efficiency. In any case, urea should not be fed if its inclusion either increases crude protein above dietary requirements or results in poor utilization due to interacting effects of energy and crude protein in natural diets (Table 1). Failure to recognize the latter restrictions may be the major factor regarding overuse of urea and even use of supplemental protein from other sources.

SUMMARY

Controlled research with urea-adapted lactating dairy cows fed high-energy balanced rations indicates no effect on reproduction when the intake of urea by individuals averages as much as 227 gm/day (0.5 lb). Moreover, daily intakes that are 50 per cent higher may or may not decrease reproductive efficiency. Similar reproductive comparisons from controlled research cannot be made when urea is used to supplement protein in diets low in energy and crude protein (cornstalks, cereal straws, matured grasses) or when more urea is used than can be utilized. Overuse of urea is uneconomical and also should be avoided because of the potential for affecting reproduction adversely. Currently, it can only be assumed that reproduction probably is unaffected by supplemental urea if guidelines for its efficient utilization are followed. The simplest guideline is use of 0.5 per cent urea in roughage plus 5 gm of urea for each pound of high-energy grain mix consumed daily when nonurea crude protein is 1 to 2 per cent below dietary requirements (maintenance, growth or lactation of beef cattle). Also, the latter guideline may be applied to dairy cattle if the grain-equivalent in silages is considered as a portion of total concentrates consumed daily.

On this basis, the recommended daily intake of urea may be less than 23 gm for unpalatable low-quality, all-roughage diets and up to 227 gm per day for high-energy rations. This range of urea intake (23 to 227 gm) is considered safe when diets are otherwise balanced to approximate nutrient requirements under the conditions applied.

REFERENCES

1. Board on Agriculture and Renewable Resources — Subcommittee on Nonprotein Nitrogen: Urea and other nonprotein compounds in animal nutrition. National Academy of Sciences, Washington, D.C., 1976.
2. Erb, R. E., Brown, C. J. Jr., Callahan, C. J., Moeller, N. J., Hill, D. L. and Cunningham, M. D.: Dietary urea for dairy cattle. II. Effect on functional traits. J. Dairy Sci., *59*:656, 1976.
3. Erb, R. E., Garverick, H. A., Patton, R. S., Randel, R. D., Monk, E. L., Udo-Aka, M. I., and Callahan, C. J.: Dietary urea for dairy cattle. IV. Effect on reproductive hormones. Theriogenology, *5*:213, 1976.
4. Ryder, W. L., Hillman, D. and Huber, J. T.: Effect of feeding urea on reproductive efficiency in Michigan Dairy Herd Improvement Association herds. J. Dairy Sci., *55*:1290, 1972.
5. Word, J. D., Martin, L. C., Williams, D. L., Williams, E. I., Panciera, R. J., Nelson, T. E. and Tillman, A. D.: Urea toxicity in the bovine. J. Anim. Sci., *29*:786, 1969.

Bovine Genital Vibriosis

ALVIN B. HOERLEIN
Colorado State University,
Fort Collins, Colorado

DEFINITION

Bovine genital vibriosis is a venereal disease of cattle caused by *Campylobacter fetus* ss. *fetus* and is characterized by temporary infertility of the female. It is transmitted from infected to noninfected animals during the act of breeding. The disease is widespread and is the most important cause of infertility in cattle.

CLINICAL SIGNS

The chief clinical sign of the infection is the return to estrus in the infected female. Death of the fetus occurs so early that no exudate is noted. Abortions are infrequent. The interval between exposure and recovery is variable. Pregnancy may result in some animals after two or three estrous cycles, and if left with the bulls, most females will be pregnant within 9 months after infection occurred. This variable interval until recovery in individual animals in the herd results in a prolonged calving season. Pregnancy examinations after the breeding season will reveal a great variation in the age of the fetuses. Pregnancy rates in seasonally bred herds will vary from 30 to 85 per cent, depending on many factors associated with the carrier rates, susceptible animals, immune status and management procedures.

PATHOGENESIS

The ability to diagnose vibriosis depends on a thorough understanding of the pathogenesis of the disease in the individual animal and its means of transmission through the herd. The infected bull deposits semen and vibrios in the area of the cervix during breeding. The ovum is fertilized after the initial exposure to infection. Bacteria multiply in the cervix and by 7 to 14 days can be found in the oviducts. The fertilized ovum is destroyed early, probably by direct action of the organisms as evidenced by the observation that more than half of the susceptible heifers return to estrus at the normal interval. In breedings subsequent to the initial exposure, fertilization may not occur since it has been shown that the organisms can adversely affect the cilia of the epithelial lining cells of the oviducts. From 3 weeks to 3 months after exposure, most susceptible heifers will have large numbers of bacteria in the cervical mucus. Eventually almost all infected cattle will conceive if repeatedly bred and will give birth to normal calves. Some cows having normal pregnancies will still carry the infection after parturition. There is a measure of convalescent immunity in female cattle that have recovered from the infection. When subsequently rebred, they become reinfected as evidenced by the temporary presence of *C. fetus* in the cervical mucus, but fertility is not affected. If the cow is rebred to noninfected bulls for 2 or 3 years before being rebred by an infected bull, convalescent immunity will have almost disappeared. It appears that the cow must receive an annual booster infection to maintain a reasonable level of immunity.

The bull contracts the disease from infected females during breeding. The organisms grow in the crypts of the penis and prepuce, but do not enter the deeper tissues. A bull may be transiently infected or infected for years. More permanent infections are found in older bulls, probably because they have more and deeper penile and preputial epithelial crypts. Bulls develop no convalescent immunity from infection since they can be reinfected even after the organisms are removed by treatment. In beef cattle herds in which bulls do not get very old, it is thought that most of the herd carry-over of the infection from one year to the next is from carrier cows. Most beef bulls appear to eliminate the infection during the nonbreeding season. The bull is not affected directly by the infection, but in infected herds of susceptible cattle the burden of repeat breeding may overtax his breeding capacity, resulting in temporary infertility or refusal to breed cattle in estrus.

DIAGNOSIS

Tentative Diagnosis

A thorough understanding of the pathogenesis of the disease makes it possible to evaluate the varying patterns of herd infertility encountered so that a tentative diagnosis of vibriosis can be made. The classic disease characterized by repeat breeding, delayed conception and eventual development of convalescent immunity is not seen often, since this requires that all of the bulls be infected from the beginning of breeding and that all of the females be susceptible. If this situation exists, a 20 to 30 per cent pregnancy rate after 60 days of breeding may be expected.

In most herds the initial introduction of the infection results in a small number of infected cattle the first year with an increasing number being infected in subsequent years. It may take years before a problem is recognized. In fact, many herds have been infected for years and have annual pregnancy rates of 70 to 85 per cent. The degree of infertility may be known only after study of calving records. A prolonged calving season is an excellent indication of infection. Although all cattle are susceptible to infection, the usual herd will have a mixed population at the beginning of each breeding season. Only a few of the cattle infected the previous year will be carrying the infection. Most of the bulls in seasonally bred beef herds will not be carrying the vibrio organisms. The cows previously infected will have a varying degree of convalescent immunity. Thus, variable patterns of infertility can be expected from herd to herd.

In beef cattle herds in the western United States, the highest pregnancy rates are usually found in the heifers, since it is common practice to breed them separately to young bulls that have not been previously exposed to infection. The lowest pregnancy rates are often found in those young cows being bred in the cow herd for their second calf by the older herd bulls.

Vibriosis is seldom spread in dairy herds in which artificial insemination is used exclusively. However, in many dairy herds, bulls are used to breed heifers and those cows not pregnant after several inseminations. An examination of the herd history and breeding management is essential to lead to a tentative diagnosis of vibriosis.

Confirmed Diagnosis

The tentative diagnosis of vibriosis is most easily confirmed by culture and identification of the organism from a freshly aborted fetus. Unfortunately, under most conditions of husbandry in beef cattle herds, the small number of aborted fetuses either are not found while fresh enough for examination or are destroyed by predators.

The bacteriological examination of cervicovaginal mucus is the most practicable method of diagnosis of vibriosis in an infected herd. Cervical mucus can be easily collected and cultured in the laboratory for *C. fetus*. The techniques have been well tested and described in detail.[2] Success will be enhanced by the selection of those animals for sampling that are most likely to be infected, based on an understanding of the pathogenesis of the disease. Almost all susceptible, nonpregnant animals will have positive results from 3 weeks to 3 months after initial exposure, and five to ten mucus samples collected from females in midcycle are adequate to establish diagnosis. At 6 months after initial exposure, about 20 per cent of the nonpregnant cattle still have positive results, so that 20 or more animals need to be sampled for a reliable diagnosis. The animals should be selected from those bred for the first time by the older bulls in the cow herd, since the heifers being bred the first time to young bulls may not have been exposed. The older cows may have convalescent immunity and quickly clear the organism from the genital tract. The sampling of pregnant or postpartum cows is rarely successful in demonstrating *C. fetus*. If the mucous samples cannot be cultured within 6 hours, the plastic collection pipettes should be frozen on dry ice immediately after collection for transport to the laboratory. An ordinary freezer should not be used. A single positive culture of *C. fetus* indicates herd infection.

Immunological methods of diagnosis have limited value. Blood serum agglutinins are of no value in the diagnosis of vibriosis. Cervicovaginal mucous agglutinins are present in some infected animals for a short time and have been used to a limited extent. However, only a few laboratories have the capability of running these tests. It is generally more difficult to obtain samples for this test than to collect cervicovaginal mucus for culture. One of the great limitations, especially in beef cattle herds in which the stage of the estrous cycle is not known, is the contamination of the mucus with blood serum from postestrous bleeding or rough manipulation. The presence of blood serum results in false positive reactions. The fluorescent antibody technique has limited value since the fluorescent antiserums are not specific for the venereal strains of *C. fetus* and do not differentiate the intestinal strains that are common in the feces of cattle. If the intestinal strains of *C. fetus* contaminate the vagina, false positive tests will result. However, these tests may have limited value as a screening procedure.

Diagnosis in the Bull

The *C. fetus* carrier state in the bull can be determined by bacteriological culture and identification of the organism in semen, preputial smegma or washings from an artificial vagina. Preputial samples are preferred since they are easier to obtain and the organisms are generally more numerous. There are relatively few laboratories that can provide competent bacteriological service because the procedures are difficult and require considerable experience. A positive culture is conclusive, but infected bulls may yield numerous negative cultures.

Diagnosis of vibriosis in bulls is most easily accomplished by breeding virgin test heifers. Cervicovaginal mucus from the test-mated heifers is examined bacteriologically in 3 weeks. Artificial insemination stud bulls that are not used for natural breeding can be similarly tested by collecting preputial smegma and introducing it into the cervix of virgin test heifers. Pooled samples of preputial smegma from several bulls can be inoculated into a single virgin heifer for a screening test. If results are positive, each bull can then be tested separately.

CONTROL AND PREVENTION

Exclusive use of artificial insemination with semen from noninfected bulls is an efficient method of controlling the spread of vibriosis. Although this procedure can be utilized in most dairy herds, it is useful in only a few beef cattle herds. It is difficult to obtain satisfactory reproductive rates in most beef cattle herds without using bulls in natural service following the artificial insemination period. Such bulls can therefore perpetuate the disease in the herd.

The best method for control of vibriosis in herds in which exclusive artificial insemination is impractical is the vaccination of all the female cattle. Oil adjuvant bacterins with high cell content of immunogenic strains of *C. fetus* ss. *fetus* have given adequate protection against the infertility of vibriosis. For best results one should vaccinate 30 to 90 days before the onset of breeding. Since both vaccinal and convalescent immunity wane with the passage of time, annual revaccination is required to maintain maximal reproductive rates. Revaccination of cows in beef cattle herds at weaning time has been shown to be effective, even though several months will elapse before the next beeding season. Because vaccinal antibody titers decrease rapidly, it was concluded in one study that booster vaccinations should be given approximately 10 days before breeding to provide maximum protection during the breeding season. Since the oil adjuvant vaccine became available in 1965, no vibrio-infected herds that were properly vaccinated have been found with less than 90 per cent pregnancy rates.

The vaccination of bulls has not been recommended, but recent research in Australia and Belgium suggests that the carrier state in bulls may be modified by vaccination. In these countries, vaccination of bulls with vaccines containing sufficient antigen was effective in decreasing the infertility observed in herds with vibriosis. A bull vaccination program should be approached with caution until additional research demonstrates its value.

The infection can be effectively eliminated in bulls by antibiotic treatment. Dihydrostreptomycin is used in a dosage of 10 mg/lb of body weight injected subcutaneously, and 5 gm of 50 per cent solution of the same antibiotic is applied locally to the penis and prepuce. After bulls are cured by antibiotic treatment, they are still susceptible to reinfection. Antibiotics have not been of value in treatment of the infected female, although vaccination will hasten recovery from the infection.

REFERENCES

1. Carroll, E. J. and Hoerlein, A. B.: Diagnosis and control of bovine genital vibriosis. JAVMA *161*:1359, 1972.
2. Hoerlein, A. B.: Vibriosis. *In* Gibbons, W. J., Catcott, E. J. and Smithcors, J. F. (eds.): Bovine Medicine and Surgery. Evanston, Ill., American Veterinary Publications, 1970, pp. 91–104.

Trichomoniasis in Cattle

BRUCE ABBITT

Tex. Vet. Med. Diag. Lab., College Station, Texas

DEFINITION

Trichomoniasis is a venereal disease of cattle, characterized primarily by early embryonic loss (infertility) and occasionally by abortions and pyometra. The etiological agent is a protozoan, *Trichomonas foetus* (Fig. 1).

OCCURRENCE

In the United States, the incidence is difficult to ascertain because of the nonreportable status of the disease. However, the author's experience would support the opinion that the disease is probably endemic in some areas, occurs sporadically in many others and is generally underdiagnosed. Even though sporadic in occurrence, outbreaks frequently result in severe economic loss.

PATHOGENESIS

In most cases, initial service by an infected bull will result in the female contracting the disease. The protozoan localizes in the secretions of the vagina, uterus and oviduct and initially does not interfere with conception.[17] A mucopurulent discharge associated with vaginitis or endometritis, or both, occurs in some but not all cases. The discharge is often of small quantity and therefore seldom observed. The vaginitis itself may or may not be grossly observable.

Embryonic wastage may be due to the inflammatory response detectable in the uterus of heifers approximately 50 days' postservice by an infected bull.[17] Once infected, females remain infertile for 2 to 6 months, regardless of the method of service, i.e., use of a noninfected bull or artificial insemination (AI). This infertility may be the result of several episodes of early embryonic loss or perhaps one episode of embryonic loss followed by a period of failure of conception or nidation due to an inflamed uterus. After a variable period of infertility, females become immune and will conceive and carry to term, even though bred by infected bulls. The duration of this immunity as well as the pathogenesis of reinfection varies with the individual cow.[1] The cow occasionally carries the infection throughout a normal gestation.[14, 15] However, this is unusual, and the incidence of this postpartum infection decreases over time postpartum, and, perhaps most importantly, over the number of postpartum estrous periods. The possibility of chronically infected or carrier females does, however, markedly affect procedures for eradicating trichomoniasis in the herd. Palpable postcoital pyometra and abortion are fairly unusual manifestations of trichomoniasis infection that are reported to occur relatively more frequently in chronically infected herds.

Trichomoniasis is asymptomatic in the male. The protozoan localizes in the secretions of the epithelium lining the penis, prepuce and anterior portion of the urethra.[16] Empirical evidence indicates that once exposed, bulls older than 4 year of age tend to become permanent carriers, whereas younger bulls either spontaneously recover or do not contract the disease.[5, 10] However, the author has observed young infected Brangus and Santa Gertrudis bulls that failed to recover spontaneously. Therefore, on a herd basis, trichomoniasis is manifested by infertility, the severity of which depends on the immunological status of the herd and factors related to the method of introduction of the infection. In the simplest case, if an infected bull is introduced into a uniformly susceptible group of cows, a few cows conceive and calve normally, whereas the majority go through a 2- to 6-month period of infertility characterized primarily by abnormally long interservice intervals. Introduction of trichomoniasis into the same herd via an infected cow midway through

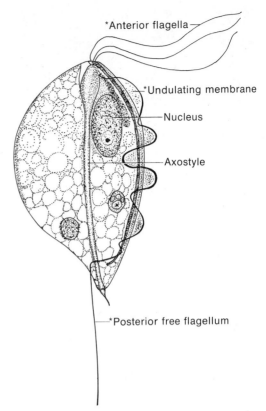

Anterior flagella

Undulating membrane

Nucleus

Axostyle

Posterior free flagellum

Figure 1. *Trichomonas foetus*: approximate size 10 to 25 μg in length by 5 to 10 μg in width. (*Can be seen without staining.)

the breeding season results in a somewhat different clinical picture. The presence of infected and noninfected bulls in a large herd further confuses the issue. However, a period of infertility in the susceptible females is common to any method of introduction. Chronic herd infection is typified by a marked reduction in reproductive efficiency due to continual reinfection of a percentage of the cows.

DIAGNOSIS

A tentative diagnosis is often based on clinical symptoms after systematic exclusion of other common etiologies for herd infertility. Chief among the latter are inadequate nutrition, vibriosis and bull infertility. Definitive diagnosis depends on the isolation of the *T. foetus* organism. The protozoan occurs in great numbers, both in the fluids associated with trichomonad-induced abortion (amniotic, abomasal, pharyngeal and so forth) and in fluids associated

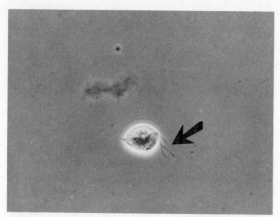

Figure 2. Photomicrograph taken at 400× under phase contrast microscopy and enlarged to 560×. Arrows point to the three anterior flagella.

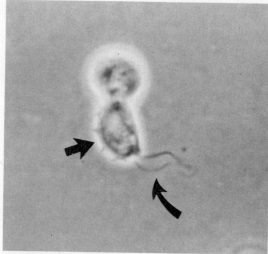

Figure 3. Photomicrograph taken at 1000× under phase contrast microscopy and enlarged to 1400×. Arrows point to the undulating membrane and two visible anterior flagella. Second structure in field is tissue debris.

with pyometra. These fluids are often examined microscopically* for conclusive proof of herd infection. However, as these conditions occur infrequently, microscopic evaluation of preputial smegma following centrifugation or culture is the most common method of diagnosis. Samples of smegma can be collected by several methods:

1. *Douche:* The sheath is infused with approximately 200 ml of physiological saline solution (PSS). The preputial opening is then occluded while the trapped fluid is massaged and then re-collected. This fluid is centrifuged (2000 rpm for 10 minutes) and the sediment examined microscopically.*

2. *Swab:* A cotton swab is used to obtain a sample of smegma from the fornix of the bull's prepuce. The swab is rinsed in 5 to 10 ml of PSS, which is then centrifuged (2000 rpm for 10 minutes) and the sediment examined microscopically.*

3. *Pipette:* An AI pipette or trichomonad pipette is introduced into the fornix of the bull's prepuce, and smegma is collected by scraping and aspirating. Vigorous scraping combined with alternating positive and neg-

ative pressure using a rubber bulb or syringe will aid in the collection of a suitable sample. The epithelial cells and smegma that accumulate in the pipette are mixed with 5 to 10 ml of PSS, centrifuged (2000 rpm for 10 minutes) and the sediment examined microscopically.*

The douche method is reportedly the most efficient of these three techniques.[8] However, in bulls known to be infected, the pipette method used in conjunction with culture media has been shown to be at least 97 per cent accurate,[4] which is superior to any of the methods used alone. The author has

---

*In each case, the sediment, fluid or culture medium is examined at 40 to 100× magnification under coverslip for the trichomonads, which move in an irregular, jerky manner associated with continual rolling. In preparations of sediment, movement of tissue debris in association with individual trichomonads is all that is generally observable under low power. Confirmation in each case is by examination at 400× magnification, at which time the undulating membrane and flagellae can be seen coming in and out of view as the organism moves and rolls. See Figure 1 and associated photomicrographs (Figs. 2 to 4).

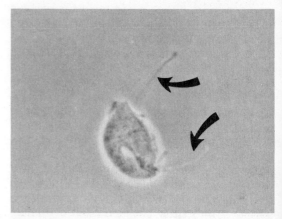

Figure 4. Photomicrograph taken at 1000× under phase contrast microscopy and enlarged to 1400×. Arrows point to the three anterior flagella and trailing posterior flagella.

used the pipette method in conjunction with culture in a modified Plastridge medium (Diamond's medium)[6] (Table I) and found the combination to be very effective. Only one of 30 samples taken from bulls known to be infected was negative. A positive sample was obtained from this bull on the third of three samples taken at weekly intervals.

Using this combination procedure, a test tube containing 10 ml of the Diamond's medium is inoculated by layering preputial smegma on its surface. The anaerobic, motile trichomonads swim to the bottom and multiply, leaving competitive bacteria to multiply in the upper layers. If the smegma is accidentally mixed with the culture media, a subsample can be taken from the first tube and layered on a fresh column of media. If necessary, the inoculated media can be refrigerated for 24 hours prior to incubation. The medium is incubated at 38° C and evaluated at 24 and again at 48 hours if negative on first reading. Evaluation is by microscopic examination* of fluid pipetted from the *bottom* of the test tube. Bacterial overgrowth, as indicated by cloudiness of the normally clear media, begins at the top of the column and approaches the bottom by 48 hours of incubation. Samples should be evaluated before the cloudiness reaches the bottom of the test tube. Positive samples will generally have large numbers of trichomonads present by 24 to 48 hours of incubation.

Culturing cervicovaginal mucus (CVM) may also be a valuable diagnostic aid. This method proved to be extremely accurate in a group of 20 heifers experimentally infected by allowing service with an infected bull and then cultured weekly for up to 100 days postinfection.[17] These samples were taken in both pregnant and nonpregnant heifers without regard to the stage of the estrous cycle in the nonpregnant group. As such, the efficacy of sampling during various stages of the estrous cycle was not evaluated. Earlier attempts to isolate *T. foetus* organisms from the vagina of cows with and without the use of culture media indicated increased efficiency of sampling during estrus. The author has found that CVM samples cultured in Diamond's media may be valuable as an indicator of impending embryonic loss, as approximately 50 per cent of pregnant females (average 81 days' postservice) with positive cultures subsequently aborted. These results indicate that culture of CVM samples

TABLE 1. *Preparation of Diamond's Medium (100 ml)*

Ingredient	Gm
Trypticase peptone	2.0
Yeast extract	1.0
Maltose	0.5
L-cystine hydrochloride	0.1
L-ascorbic acid	0.02
Distilled water to make 90 ml	–
K_2HPO_4*	0.08
KH_2PO_4*	0.08

1. Mix all ingredients and check to see if pH is 7.2 to 7.4. If not, adjust pH with NaOH or HCl.

2. Add 0.05 gm of agar and autoclave for 10 minutes at 121°C.

3. Cool to 49°C and aseptically add 10 ml of inactivated (56°C for 30 minutes) bovine serum,* 100,000 units of penicillin G (1 ml of a stock solution prepared by adding 10 ml of sterile H_2O to 10^6 units of penicillin G) and 0.1 gm of streptomycin in sulfate (0.5 ml of stock solution prepared by adding 5 ml of sterile H_2O to 1 gm of streptomycin sulfate).

4. Aseptically dispense 10 ml per sterile 16 × 125 mm screw cap vial. Check for sterility by incubating 24 hours at 37°C

*Original media as reported by L. S. Diamond did not contain K_2HPO_4 or KH_2PO_4, were adjusted to a pH of 6.8 to 7.0 and contained 10 ml per 100 ml of inactivated sheep serum. All asterisks refer to slight modifications in media. The modifications are a result of experience in field and laboratory use of the media in conjunction with the diagnosis of *Trichomonas foetus* by Dr. C. P. Hibler of the Pathology Department, College of Veterinary Medicine and Biomedical Sciences, Colorado State University, Fort Collins, Colorado 80523.

may be a reliable method of diagnosis in the individual cow. However, more work is required before this technique can be recommended as a method for reliably identifying infected cows.

CONTROL

The prognosis for the infected herd is generally good provided control measures can be adequately implemented. Details involving the implementation of control measures for a specific herd will vary. The clinician must base control measures on both a knowledge of the epidemiology of the disease and the particular herd situation. Proven control methods generally fall into five broad categories:

1. Depopulation of infected animals is often of limited value because of economic

considerations but should be considered when the disease is not widespread or relatively few animals are involved.

2. AI is also effective and ofteri used on a percentage of the affected cows. However, a total change from natural service to AI is often impractical because of managerial or economic factors, or both. If natural service is resumed, consideration should be given to possible carrier animals and some form of surveillance initiated.

3. The herd can be separated into two groups, one containing exposed cows, the other unexposed cows in a quarantine system. Heifers and purchased unexposed cows can be added to the unexposed group, while allowing natural attrition to eliminate cows in the exposed group. This method is potentially effective but is generally not practical because of the difficulty and potential hazard involved in maintaining an infected herd in isolation.

4. Cows bred to suspect or infected bulls, or both, can be sexually rested before rebreeding. Following successful calving, cows are not bred until at least 90 days have elapsed following calving. Allowing two normal estrous periods has also been recommended prior to rebreeding. However, accurate observation for estrus is difficult in many herds, in which case this procedure is impractical. This extended postpartum interval in conjunction with normal estrous periods will decrease the likelihood of a cow carrying the infection into the next breeding season. The author also feels that a thorough physical examination of the genitalia in conjunction with a culture examination may also be beneficial prior to rebreeding. A surveillance system for detecting trichomoniasis should also be initiated following the resumption of breeding. This method has limited appeal because of economic factors associated with delay of breeding until 90 days postpartum.

5. A method combining sexual rest and isolation is also reported to be effective.[2] Following successful calving, a 90-day postpartum interval and no less than two normal estrous periods, cows in the infected group are moved into the clean group. Regardless of the method of breeding, all cows in the infected group would go through this procedure prior to introduction into the clean group.

6. A method of selective culling combined with the use of young bulls is also effective under field conditions.[4] Cows failing either

to conceive or to calve before the next breeding season are culled. Breeding is limited to bulls younger than 4 years of age that have been tested for trichomoniasis prior to use. This procedure is repeated for several years, with the progress of the herd monitored by testing the bulls for trichomoniasis after each breeding season. The possibility of maintaining a low level of trichomoniasis in a herd using this method requires continual surveillance for trichomoniasis, especially if older bulls are again used for breeding. This method may not be effective in certain breeds such as Brangus and Santa Gertrudis cattle, since the author has observed young bulls of these breeds to be chronically infected.

In general, control methods involving natural service require culling of infertile cows because they may serve as foci of infection. In addition, after the breeding season, bulls should be pastured separately from cows, as infected cows may abort, come into estrus and serve as foci of infection. Infected bulls should be isolated from noninfected bulls, as the homosexual activity of bulls may spread trichomoniasis. Surveillance for trichomoniasis in conjunction with any of the control programs should include both astute observation of the cows for abnormal estrous periods and periodic culture examination of the breeding bulls. Successful control generally depends on educating the herdsmen as to the *exact* pathogenesis of the disease and then giving them technical assistance and advice in choosing control measures that are appropriate for their herds.

INDIVIDUAL TREATMENT

The prognosis for treatment of the individual bull is generally good. Because of their ability to recover spontaneously, treatment of bulls less than 4 years of age should begin with a period of several weeks of sexual rest. For bulls that require treatment, treatment regimens fall into two broad categories, systemic and local.

Systemic Treatment

Dimetridazole (1,2-dimethyl-5-nitroimidazole) is effective orally at 50 mg/kg of body weight daily for 5 days.[11] The drug can be administered via boluses, as a drench or mixed in the feed. Use of dimetridazole as a feed additive should be tempered by the knowledge that resistant strains of trichomonads may develop when subtherapeutic levels are used.[12] Bulls often either do not like the drug in their ration or tend to go off feed for several days following the initial dosage and therefore consume subtherapeutic amounts. Rumen stasis is frequently observed during or following treatment of bulls on high concentrate rations. This can generally be prevented by feeding a diet high in roughage for several days before and during treatment. Dimetridazole is also effective when given intravenously in dosages ranging from 10 mg/kg of body weight daily for 5 days to 50 to 100 mg/kg of body weight in a single intravenous injection.[13]

Dimetridazole is soluble only in relatively low pH solutions, and, in fact, the vehicle reportedly used was 10 to 20 per cent sulfuric acid. Response to injection of these acidic solutions (13 to 27 ml/100 kg body weight) varied among bulls. Some showed no response, but others experienced respiratory difficulty, ataxia, recumbency for up to 15 minutes and weakness for periods of up to 2 days. Although these effects were transitory, they were manifestations of severe interruption of homeostasis. The author prefers forced oral treatment, as it assures adequate dosage without the risk involved with intravenous therapy.

Metronidazole (1-β-hydroxyethyl-2-methyl-5-nitroimidazole) is reported to be effective when given intravenously at dosages ranging from 75 mg/kg of body weight for three successive injections at 12-hour intervals to 10 mg/kg of body weight given once daily for 2 days.[9] Trichomonads that became resistant to dimetridazole were also resistant to metronidazole, a chemically similar compound.[12] Neither of these drugs is approved for use in the bovine species in the United States.

Local Treatment

Local treatment involves use of trichomonacidal compounds applied via massage or douche onto the penis or prepuce and in some instances the anterior portion of the urethra. Compounds that have been used include acriflavine[7, 18] (a mixture of 2,8-diamino-10-methyl-acridinium chloride and 2,8-diaminoacridine), a proprietary compound, Boboflavin Salbe, containing trypaflavine,[2, 18] the compound p.p.-diguanyl-

diazdaminobenzene diaceturate[7] and metronidazole.[9] In addition to producing either inconsistent or unproven results, local treatments also have the disadvantage of being somewhat difficult and time-consuming to administer. For these reasons, systemic treatments are now preferred. Local treatment should not be totally ignored because of the possibility of development of dimetridazole-resistant strains of trichomonads.

A treated bull should not be used for breeding until cultures have been performed both immediately following treatment and at least three times thereafter at weekly intervals beginning 45 to 60 days later. The second series of cultures is theorized as necessary, as the number of surviving protozoa may be too low to detect immediately posttreatment.

Treatment of individual cows has not been thoroughly studied because of their propensity for spontaneous recovery and the lack of a reliable method of testing for infection.

PREVENTION

Trichomoniasis can be prevented by adequate screening, testing and isolation procedures for all additions to an established herd. Prior to use, bulls, unless virgin, should be tested by culture methods at least three times at weekly intervals. As testing procedures for individual cows are not well established, additions to established herds should be limited to animals from familiar herds or to virgins. All other female additions should be tested by culture prior to entering the herd. Ideally, in addition, they would be handled in one of the following ways: Pregnant females should be isolated from bulls until 90 days postpartum and until another culture examination has been performed. Open cows following breeding by AI or natural service should be isolated from all bulls until calving and a 90-day postpartum period have elapsed and another culture examination has been performed. Bulls used on these cows should be tested for trichomoniasis prior to use on clean cows.

REFERENCES

1. Bartlett, D. E.: Trichomonas foetus infection and bovine reproduction. Am. J. Vet. Res., *8*:343, 1947
2. Bartlett, D. E.: Further observations on experimen-

tal treatments of trichomonas foetus infection in bulls. Am. J. Vet. Res., *9*:351, 1948.

3. Bartlett, D. E. and Dikmans G.: Field studies on bovine venereal trichomoniasis effects on herds and efficacy of certain practices in control. Am. J. Vet. Res., *10*:30, 1949.

4. Clark, B. L., White, M. B. and Banfield, J. C.: Diagnosis of trichomonas foetus infection in bulls. Aust. Vet. J., *47*:181, 1971.

5. Clark, B. L., Parsonson, I. M., White, M. B., Banfield, J. C. and Young, J. S.: Control of trichomoniasis in a large herd of beef cattle. Aust. Vet. J., *50*:424, 1974.

6. Diamond, L. S.: The establishment of various trichomonads of animals and man in axenic cultures. J. Parasit., *43*:488, 1957.

7. Fitzgerald, P. R., Johnson, A. E. and Hammond, D. M.: Treatment of genital trichomoniasis in bulls. JAVMA, *143*:259, 1963.

8. Fitzgerald, P. R., Hammond, D. M., Miner, M. L. and Binns, W.: Relative efficacy of various methods of obtaining preputial samples for diagnosis of trichomoniasis in the bulls. Am. J. Vet. Res., *49*:452, 1952.

9. Gasparini, G. Vaughi, M. and Tardani, A.: Treatment of bovine trichomoniasis with metronidazole (8823 R.P.). Vet Rec., *75*:940, 1963.

10. Ladds, P. W., Dennett, D. P. and Glazebrook, J. S.: A survey of the genitalia of bulls in Northern Australia. Aust. Vet. J., *49*:335, 1973.

11. McLoughlin, D. K.: Dimetridazole, a systemic treatment for bovine venereal trichomoniasis. I. Oral administration. J. Parasit., *51*:835, 1965.

12. McLoughlin, D. K.: Drug tolerance by Tritrichomonas fetus. J. Parasit., *53*:646, 1967.

13. McLoughlin, D. K.: Dimetridazole, a systemic treatment for bovine venereal trichomoniasis. II. Intravenous administration. J. Parasit., *54*:1038, 1968.

14. Morgan, B. B.: Bovine Trichomoniasis. Minneapolis, Burgess Publishing Co., 1964, pp. 1–150.

15. Morgan, B. B.: Studies on the trichomonad carrier-cow problem. J. Anim. Sci., *3*:437, 1944.

16. Parsonson, I. M., Clark, B. L. and Duffy, J. H.: The pathogenesis of *Tritrichomonas foetus* infection in the bull. Aust. Vet. J., *50*:421, 1974.

17. Parsonson, I. M., Clark, B. L. and Dufty, J. H.: Early pathogenesis and pathology of Tritrichomonas fetus infection in virgin heifers. J. Comp. Path., *86*:59, 1976.

18. Thorne, J. L., Shupe, J. L. and Miner, M. L.: The diagnosis and treatment of Trichomoniasis in bulls. Proceedings of 92nd Annual Meeting AVMA, 1955, pp. 374–377.

Effects of Leptospirosis on Bovine Reproduction

LYLE E. HANSON

University of Illinois, Urbana, Illinois

Leptospirosis is an economically important disease that is widespread in cattle and other domestic animals and in wildlife throughout the world. The disease causes serious economic losses in the cattle industry, primarily owing to its effects on milk production and reproduction. The causative agents are members of the genus *Leptospira* of micro-organisms, and the various members are identified antigenically as serotypes (serovar). Serological surveys indicate that the cumulative reactor rates for cattle in the United States vary between regions from 5 to 20 per cent.[1]

Leptospirosis is a disease that can be caused by any one of many pathogenic leptospiral serotypes. In the United States, six serotypes belonging to five serogroups isolated from cattle have been associated with clinical illness. The serotypes are *canicola, grippotyphosa, hardjo, icterohaemorrhagiae,* *pomona* and *mini szwajizak,* with the serotypes of *hardjo* and *pomona* most commonly associated with bovine leptospirosis.[1] The organisms are motile spirochetes with long, tightly spiraled filaments that are usually hooked at either end. As these organisms are not stained by analine dyes, darkfield microscopy is usually used to visualize live organisms and to observe their unique spinning. The many leptospires are classified by antigenic characteristics into serogroups and serotypes, as biochemical tests are inadequate for differentiation. Free-living, nonpathogenic leptospires that are morphologically similar to pathogenic organisms can be readily isolated from surface waters. Therefore, caution should be exercised in diagnosis to avoid confusing the nonpathogenic from the pathogenic members.

PATHOGENESIS

Leptospiral infections are usually contracted during exposure of the skin and mucous membranes to surface waters of ponds and streams contaminated by urine from domestic animals or wildlife that are shedding pathogenic leptospires. *Hardjo* and *mini szwajizak* serotypes are apparently limited to cattle in the United States, as no infections have been detected in wildlife. *Pomona,* although primarily transmitted between cattle and swine, is also widely distributed in some common wildlife species. *Grippotyphosa,* a serotype that is primarily enzootic in wildlife, occasionally infects cattle, causing costly herd infections. *Canicola,* most commonly found in dogs and occasionally carried in wildlife, has been responsible for disease in cattle. *Icterohaemorrhagiae,* a serotype that is enzootic in Norway rats, occasionally causes disease in cattle.

Venereal transmission can occur from infected semen or urine during breeding when one of the animals is in either the acute or the shedding stage.[3] Although arthropod transmission has been verified, it is not a common mode of infection because of the brief leptospiremic periods in most cattle. Food chain transmission occurs in some wildlife, and possibly in swine, but is unlikely in cattle because of their feeding habits.

Leptospires multiply rapidly in the liver and spleen, causing clinical signs after an incubation period of 5 to 7 days. Acute leptospirosis is first evident by elevated body temperature and anorexia. In severe infections, the acute phase is associated with various signs and lesions. Some lesions indicate that a toxin is produced in acute leptospiral infections that causes necrosis of hepatic cells, kidney tubular epithelial cells and capillary endothelial cells. The resulting increased capillary permeability is responsible for release of plasma and erythrocytes into tissues. Secretion of yellow, clotted milk containing blood clots followed by marked agalactia is probably also due to toxin action. Encephalitis, which has been reported in an occasional severe infection, is associated with the presence of leptospires in the brain tissue. Death, although more common in calves, occasionally occurs in adults and is primarily due to kidney failure.

During the leptospiremic stage, leptospires migrate to the kidneys and brain and in the pregnant cattle to the uterus. Leptospires pass from the maternal placenta into the uterus and infect the fetus.[4] The effect on the fetus varies with the stage of gestation, the serotypes involved and the virulence of the organisms. Infections during the first two-thirds of the gestation

period generally do not cause death of the fetus. However, infections initiated during the last third often cause fetal death, resulting in abortions and stillbirths. In addition, some calves that appear normal at birth and grow normally may also shed leptospires in their urine for a relatively short period without showing recognizable signs or lesions caused by the infection.

The fetal calf is immunologically competent to produce leptospiral antibodies to leptospiral infections as early as 153 days of gestation. The presence of leptospiral agglutinins in the aborted or stillborn calves is of diagnostic importance. These agglutinins indicate a fetal response, as the maternal antibodies cannot pass the placental barrier.[1]

Leptospiral infection causes moderate lesions in the uterus of the pregnant animals, which apparently contributes to the abortions and infertility.[4] *Hardjo* and *mini szwajizak* serotype infections cause few abortions but are frequently associated with long-term sterility problems.[1]

CLINICAL SIGNS

Leptospiral infections may cause both acute and chronic signs that vary in intensity from subclinical to severe and occasionally result in the death of calves and adult cattle. The acute disease is usually initiated by an elevation in body temperature, which persists from a few hours to several days. The milk of lactating cattle becomes yellow, viscous and sometimes blood-tinged during the period of the acute disease and is followed by an agalactia that persists from 5 to 14 days. Most cattle return to normal milk production; however, some cows fail to return to normal production during the affected lactation period.[2] Although agalactia is not readily recognized in beef cattle, it may become apparent by the presence of weak calves that do not receive adequate nutrition.

Cattle affected with severe acute infections also show malaise, anorexia, icterus, hemorrhages on mucous membranes, conjunctivitis, hemoglobinuria and pneumonia. Occasionally, deaths occur in adult cattle due to the combined effects of hepatitis and kidney failure. Some cattle show abnormal behavior as a result of encephalitis.[2]

Abortion and stillbirths are the most obvious signs and therefore are most frequently associated with leptospirosis in cattle. As the fetuses are expelled in 1 to 4 weeks following the initial acute infection, the cow may appear normal at the time of the delivery and usually is serologically positive. Calves that are born infected often are weak and succumb to either leptospirosis or secondary infections.

Relapses occur in some animals, causing several febrile responses and malaise.[2] Infertility is often observed in herds endemically infected with *hardjo* and *mini szwaji-zak*.[1]

Orchitis has been demonstrated in bulls during the acute stage of infection, but there is no indication that these infections persist for extended periods in the testicles that are shedding leptospires in the semen.[3] Urine shedding can result in contamination of semen for 1 to 3 months following acute infections.

LESIONS

Leptospiral infections produce the most marked lesions in the liver and kidneys. During the acute stage, gross examination in severe cases can reveal yellow coloring of the mucous membranes and various visceral tissues. Focal necrosis and hemorrhages occur in the liver and kidneys. As the disease persists in the kidneys, white infarcts of varying size are scattered throughout the renal cortex.

Lesions are usually evident in kidneys of calves and adult cattle. In the acute stage, petechial and ecchymotic hemorrhages are usually present but vary in distribution and intensity. If hepatic lesions are extensive, icterus is also often present along with the hemorrhages. Histological examination will demonstrate capillary damage, tubular necrosis and tubular casts. If the disease becomes chronic, the lesions of tubular necrosis and glomerular degeneration become more prominent. Interstitial accumulation of lymphocytes, plasma cells and fibroblasts may become so extensive that large areas of the kidney tubules and glomeruli are replaced. Glomeruli in affected areas of the kidney may develop a thickening of the Bowman's capsule and a degeneration of the capillary tufts, greatly reducing filtration and resulting in atrophy of the affected glomeruli.[1]

The uterus of cattle infected with lepto-spires appears little changed in gross appearance, although some edema is evident. However, on histological examination, tissue changes are apparent in both nongravid and gravid uterine tissues of infected cows. In the pregnant cow, the primary lesions in the uterus are degenerative, and proliferative changes occur in the cotyledons. Retained placenta is commonly associated with some leptospiral infections.[4]

DIAGNOSIS

Diagnosis of leptospirosis based entirely on clinical observations is usually not possible because of the great variation in signs. Therefore, diagnosis should be determined by correlation of clinical signs with laboratory procedures.[5]

Although blood and urine analyses are frequently utilized in small animal medicine, the tests are seldom definitive. Changes in specific gravity have been associated with chronic stages of the disease.

Serological testing is the most frequently used laboratory procedure in the diagnosis of leptospirosis.[2] Macroscopic (plate) and microscopic agglutination (MA) tests are the principal procedures used for detection of leptospiral antibodies. Agglutinins appear in the sera several days following the onset of acute signs and persist from several weeks in a few cattle, to 1 to 2 years in most cattle and to as many as 8 years in some animals. As abortions and stillbirths occur 1 to 4 weeks following the acute disease, positive reactions generally are detected in the sera of the dam at that time. An MA titer of 1:100 or greater or a plate agglutination titer of 1:40 or greater is accepted as diagnostically significant. With *hardjo*, titers as low as 1:10 on the plate test are accepted as significant.[5] No one titer can be equated with an infection because the procedure measures the antibody concentration, which indicates the immune response rather than the extent of the disease. Agglutinins may not be present in all cattle throughout the entire urine-shedding period, as localization of lepto-spires in kidney or brain tissues may not stimulate systemic responses. Because of individual variations in antibody responses, serum from at least 10 per cent of a herd should be tested and the results evaluated with consideration given to the herd problem.[5]

Serum neutralization tests and growth inhibition tests are used for evaluation of the protective immunoglobulin IgG response, which is not measured by the agglutination tests. The time required for the tests and the costs involved preclude use of these procedures in routine diagnosis and limit their use to research situations.

Demonstration of leptospires in cattle urine by darkfield examination, in kidney tissues of hamsters following inoculation with cattle urine or in special bacteriological media after cultivation is used for final diagnosis in special cases. The most appropriate procedure for field use is collection of urine in sterile containers and immediate inoculation of suitable media with 0.1 ml of the test urine. The media can be returned to a laboratory without incubation, either by courier or through the mail.

Tissues collected during a necropsy of a suspect case can be used for histological examination, animal inoculation or culture in special media. Leptospires can be observed in tissues with silver staining when large numbers of organisms are present. The Warthin-Starry procedure is most commonly used. Kidney tissue provides the most consistent source of viable leptospires. Brain, kidney and liver are the most suitable tissues for either animal inoculation or propagation in media. If inoculations cannot be made immediately, tissues should be held under refrigeration but not frozen. Fetal calf tissues usually have undergone too much autolysis for persistence of viable organisms at time of abortion; therefore, tissues from weak calves are better sources of viable leptospires. Blood should be collected, when possible, from aborted or stillborn calves, as detection of leptospiral agglutinins indicates a response of the fetus to the organisms.[1]

Observation of organisms in the urine by darkfield microscopy is possible, but recognition of the typical motility of the organisms is necessary before their presence can be confirmed. Fluorescent microscopy can also be used with suspect urine and tissues, but, again, caution is required as nonspecific fluorescence is common in tissue preparations.

TREATMENT AND CONTROL

Strict separation of cattle from swine and fencing of cattle areas from streams, ponds and marshes will reduce contact with potentially contaminated water. However, the wide host reservoir range of some serotypes that involve many species of wildlife makes it virtually impossible to avoid all possible exposure to leptospires in surface waters.

Prophylactic medication of cattle by administration of oxytetracycline or chlortetracycline has been demonstrated to be effective. Continuous administration is not recommended because of the cost of the medication, the danger of developing resistant bacterial flora and the excretion of the antibiotics in the milk of lactating cattle.

Parenteral administration of 12.5 mg/lb of body weight of dihydrostreptomycin to cattle with acute leptospirosis is recommended for several days.[1] Administration of dihydrostreptomycin to cattle with persisting high antibody titers has not effectively reduced the serological response.

The most economical control procedure is the periodic vaccination of cattle with bacterins containing the leptospiral serotypes present in the geographical region.[1] As all commercial leptospiral bacterins are inactivated whole-cell preparations, they can be administered alone or in combination with antibiotics.[1] The resistance developed by cattle following vaccination is due to the moderate, relatively short-term IgM response measured by the agglutination test and a substantial and much longer-termed IgG response measured by neutralization tests. The resistance is substantial for up to 6 months, with a gradual decline during the next 6 months. Vaccination should be conducted annually in low-risk (closed) herds and every 6 months in high-risk (open) herds. Multivalent leptospiral bacterins are recommended in areas where a variety of serotypes are present or in open herds that receive periodic additions from other herds.

Sterility problems related to endemic *hardjo* herd infections usually decrease following vaccination with a specific bacterin. The improvement may be due to transduction of IgG from the serum into the uterus, resulting in elimination of the uterine infection.

Persistent serological titers in bulls have not been associated with transmission, as leptospires are shed for short periods from semen and for no longer than 12 months in urine. However, in an effort to provide more protection from venereal transmission, the Leptospirosis Committee of the United

States Animal Health Association has recommended only constant retesting of low-titered bulls followed by medication and inoculation of four hamsters from three separate urine collections 90 days following medications. If all hamsters develop neither titers nor infections, the bulls can be considered safe for breeding.[5]

PUBLIC HEALTH ASPECTS

All serotypes of *Leptospira* pathogenic to cattle can also cause disease in man. Transmission from cattle to man is most likely from spattered urine in milking parlors or by urine-contaminated streams or pond water. Although relatively small numbers of cases in humans have been reported in the United States, New Zealand and Australia have reported relatively high transmission of bovine leptospiral infections to man. Aborted and stillborn calf tissues and placental membranes often contain leptospires during acute outbreaks. Therefore, cattle owners should be informed of the zoonotic potentials of leptospirosis.

RECOMMENDATIONS

1. Obtain serological or bacteriological confirmation of cases clinically suggestive of leptospirosis to identify the responsible serotype.

2. Administer streptomycin at the rate of 12.5 mg/lb of body weight to cattle to reduce acute clinical illness.

3. Vaccinate cattle in open herds every 6 months or cattle in closed herds annually with a multivalent bacterin containing serotypes endemic in the region.

4. Fence cattle away from ponds and streams to reduce exposure to leptospiral organisms endemic in domestic animals and wildlife.

5. Inform cattle owners of the public health significance of leptospirosis.

REFERENCES

1. Hanson, L. E.: Bovine leptospirosis. J. Dairy Sci., *59*:1166, 1976.
2. Roberts, C. S.: Leptospirosis. *In* Gibbons, W. J., Catcott, E. J. and Smithcors, J. E. (eds): Bovine Medicine and Surgery. Wheaton, Ill., American Veterinary Publications, Inc., 1970.
3. Sleight, S. D., Atallah, O. A. and Steinbauer, D. J.: Experimental *Leptospira pomona* infection in bulls. Am. J. Vet. Res., *25*:1663, 1964.
4. Smith, R. E., Reynolds, I. M. and Clark, G. W.: Experimental leptospirosis in pregnant ewes. VII. Pathogenesis of fetal infection and mechanism of Abortion. Cornell Vet., *60*:40, 1970.
5. Stoenner, H. G.: Report of the committee on leptospirosis. Proc. U. S. Anim. Hlth. Assoc., *17*:142, 1975.

Effects of Infectious Bovine Rhinotracheitis on Reproduction

ROBERT F. KAHRS
University of Florida,
Gainesville, Florida

Infectious bovine rhinotracheitis (IBR), a herpesvirus infection with widespread geographical distribution, produces a diversity of clinical manifestations, some of which have profound effects on reproduction in both male and female cattle.

ETIOLOGY

IBR virus is sometimes called the IBR-IPV virus. It has physical, biochemical, epidemiological and immunological properties of the herpesvirus group with which it is classified. The virus grows readily in a wide variety of cell cultures, producing distinctive cytopathological changes that serve as a basis for virus isolation, virus titration and neutralization tests for determining the presence of antibody in serums. This ease of laboratory manipulation has expedited studies on pathogenicity, epidemiology, diagnosis and vaccine technology and helps to make IBR one of the most "fashionable" of cattle diseases.

EPIDEMIOLOGY

As mentioned, IBR shares the epidemiological traits of the herpesvirus group. These include easy transmission by exteriorization of large quantities of virus in respiratory, ocular and reproductive secretions of infected cattle. In addition, the virus is perpetuated in populations by latent infections, which are occasionally reactivated accompanied by shedding of virus. Cattle are believed to be the principal reservoir, although goats and mule deer can be infected. Antibody prevalence studies indicate that the virus is widely distributed among cattle populations, and unless they are extremely isolated, cattle raised for breeding purposes have a high probability of eventual exposure.

PATHOGENICITY AND PATHOLOGY

Initial exposure and primary infection may result in a variety of clinical signs and lesions or in a mild inapparent or unobserved infection. The characteristic mucosal lesions are typified by adherent, whitish, necrotic material raised above the mucosal surface. These lesions, frequently referred to as plaques, result from coalescence of discrete pustules and consist of leukocytes, fibrin and necrotic epithelial cells. Intranuclear inclusion bodies are a histological feature. The lesions may appear at the site of inoculation or at other target organs after systemic distribution by macrophages. When these lesions are predominant in the respiratory tract, the principal manifestation is the upper respiratory disease. When they mostly involve mucosal surfaces of the reproductive tract, the manifestation is an infectious balanoposthitis in the male and infectious pustular vulvovaginitis (IPV) in the female. Focal necrosis is the classic lesion found in the parenchyma of body organs. Fetuses and newborn calves are more likely to suffer serious systemic effects than are mature animals. Following primary infection, a latent infection may develop that endows the animal with the potential for infrequent or intermittent shedding of virus (see page 503).

Abortion can occur following or concurrently with inapparent infection, respiratory disease, conjunctival infection or IPV. The principal clinical signs and diagnosis of each form will be discussed briefly.

FORMS OF IBR

IBR as a Respiratory Disease

The respiratory form of IBR is manifested by elevated temperature, reduced appetite, rapid respiration and upper respiratory dyspnea. Occasionally, blockage of the upper airways is adequate to result in open mouth breathing.

Affected cattle may have profuse nasal discharge that is clear in the early stages and later becomes mucopurulent. There is hyperemia of the nasal turbinates and sometimes of the muzzle, which explains the nickname "red nose" that is often applied to IBR.

Careful examination of the visible portions of the nasal mucosa frequently reveals adherent, white, necrotic debris that results from the coalescence of pustules. These lesions, although not pathognomonic, are very highly suggestive of IBR.

Some cattle with respiratory IBR have conjunctivitis and excess ocular secretions that change from clear to mucopurulent as the disease progresses. Usually, auscultation with a stethoscope reveals no abnormal lung sounds other than an increased vesicular murmur (the resonant sound of normal breathing) or referred sounds due to occlusion of the upper air passages. If râles or other lung sounds are heard, the clinician is advised to suspect another respiratory disease (particularly pulmonic pasteurellosis) or other complications.

The mortality rate in respiratory IBR is low unless secondary bacterial infections, superimposed viral infections or other complications occur. Occasionally, a severely infected animal will suffocate from mucopurulent material in the trachea.

When respiratory IBR is present in a herd containing pregnant cattle, abortions may begin while clinical signs are present in the herd and may continue for 90 to 100 days. Most fetuses are aborted during the last 4 months of gestation, and the belief exists that fetuses are more susceptible during late gestation. This may be true. However, the difficulty of finding small aborted fetuses and the variable exposure-abortion interval make us question whether this represents true susceptibility or an artifact of observation.

IBR Conjunctivitis

Inflammation of the conjunctiva accompanies the classic respiratory form of IBR. Occasionally, in outbreaks in which respiratory signs are not evident, conjunctivitis appears as the principal manifestation of IBR infection. Such outbreaks may be misdiagnosed as pinkeye or may be missed because of occurring simultaneously with pinkeye. The diagnosis of IBR conjunctivitis is suggested when the opacity of the cornea appears to originate at the corneoscleral junction (limbus). In contrast, classic pinkeye, caused by the bacterium *Hemophilus bovis,* produces a corneal opacity that originates in the center of the cornea and spreads centrifugally.

In our experience, the abortion rates have been high in herd outbreaks that are manifested primarily as conjunctivitis. Sometimes a cluster of aborted fetuses occurs, and it is learned from the history that the herd experienced an outbreak of "a peculiar form of pinkeye" a month or two earlier. When the abortions are subsequently identified as IBR by virus isolation, histopathological examination or fluorescent antibody assay, the diagnosis of IBR conjunctivitis is arrived at retrospectively.

The diagnosis of IBR conjunctivitis is strengthened by finding pustules or plaques of white, necrotic debris on the conjunctiva. Such conjunctivae are frequently edematous and painful, and affected cattle object to the careful conjunctival examination needed to see these lesions. The significance of isolation of IBR virus from the conjunctivae of cattle with ocular disease must always be regarded with some skepticism in light of knowledge that IBR virus can exist as a latent infection with reactivation by stressors such as might be associated with outbreaks of other eye conditions.

Infectious Pustular Vulvovaginitis (IPV)

The disease known as IPV is caused by the IBR virus.

The viruses isolated from both locations (i.e., the reproductive tract and respiratory tract) are immunologically similar and should be regarded as identical until technology is developed that enables workers to distinguish strains with a predilection for reproductive mucosa from biotypes with an affinity for the respiratory tract. Although IPV is usually not observed during respiratory outbreaks (and vice versa), occasionally both respiratory IBR and IPV occur simultaneously when nose-to-vulva contact is common. This observation fosters the belief that the etiologies of these two "diseases" are similar and that the location of the lesions is determined primarily by the route of inoculation.

IPV is usually first noticed because of the unusual tail position. The owner observes that the cow's tail fails to return to the normal relaxed position after defecation or urination, suggesting pain in the perineal area. Frequently, IPV is accompanied by edema and mucopurulent discharge from the vulva. Internal examination reveals pustules or plaques of white, necrotic material on the walls of both the vulva and vagina and pools of mucopurulent, usually odorless material on the floor of the vagina.

Infectious pustular vulvovaginitis can be transmitted by natural breeding and in some cases probably by the sniffing habits of cattle. In one epizootic outbreak, a dog with a habit of licking the vulva of cattle as they lay in stanchions was implicated epidemiologically as being the mode of transmission.

The differential diagnosis of IPV should be prefaced by the admonition that not all pustular or necrotic lesions in vulva or vaginal mucosa are caused by this virus. Necrotic vaginitis (secondary to parturition injuries), sadism and application of caustic materials must be considered. In addition, every clinician should be familiar with the disease known as granular vaginitis, which produces elevated granular lesions on the vulvar mucosa. These lesions sometimes have a brownish or off-orange color and can be found in many normal cattle. They are probably a hypoplasia of lymphoid follicles in the mucosa. The individual lesions are smaller than those produced by IPV and do not increase in size on subsequent days. Furthermore, they are usually not associated with mucopurulent discharge or discomfort.

Other causes of pustular vulvovaginitis that must be considered before unequivocally making a clinical diagnosis of IBR etiology are the disorders caused by mycoplasmas that have occasionally been associated with similar lesions and the disease known as catarrhal vaginitis of cattle. Examination of the vulvar mucosa is frequently neglected as a diagnostic aid in respiratory IBR because vulvar lesions are frequently not severe enough to produce discomfort or otherwise attract attention. When these lesions are found, they add evidence that IBR is the disorder that the clinician is dealing with.

Bulls that are bred to cows with IPV can acquire the infection and develop a severe balanoposthitis with lesions similar to those seen in IPV. Such bulls can transmit the disease during breeding. The shedding of virus from these lesions into semen is a definite hazard. If the semen is frozen, the viral activity is preserved. The artificial insemination industry is also concerned with IBR contamination of semen from bulls with latent infections (see page 503).

IBR ABORTION

In order for abortion to result from IBR, the female must be both pregnant and susceptible at the time of primary infection. Under field conditions, with cattle of various stages of gestation and susceptibilities and with variations in the severity of exposure, about 25 per cent of pregnant cattle may abort following an outbreak. In experimental situations with known seronegative animals inoculated with large doses of virus, higher percentages of abortions are reported. Most fetuses aborted as a result of IBR are in the last third of gestation when expelled. Fetuses exposed at any time during gestation can be aborted. Although the interval between exposure and abortion is sometimes prolonged, abortion can follow infection by a few days. That is, fetuses may be expelled while clinical IBR is present in the herd or shortly thereafter, or abortion may be delayed for as long as 100 days.

Occasionally, fetuses exposed in late gestation are carried to term. These may be dead at birth or may succumb within a few days with lesions of fatal systemic IBR (to be discussed).

Fetuses aborted because of IBR are usually dead *in utero* for several days before expulsion. This explains the presence of autolysis, the brownish-stained, friable tissues and the fluid in both body cavities as well as the lack of obvious gross lesions. Such fetuses are frequently reported as being too

decomposed for adequate diagnostic workup. Gross lesions are difficult to find under these conditions, but astute pathologists can find focal necrosis and intranuclear inclusions in the autolyzed fetal liver and adrenal.

Diagnosis of IBR Abortion

Fetuses aborted as a result of IBR usually have no characteristic gross lesions other than indistinct petechiation throughout and marked autolysis manifested as brownish-stained tissue discolorations and serosanguineous fluids in both body cavities. Some diagnosticians suggest that finding fetuses in this autolyzed condition is highly suggestive of IBR. However, this condition can result from retention of a fetus *in utero* following death from a number of reasons, and other reasons for a diagnosis of IBR must be found.

To diagnose abortion, the entire placenta and fetus should be submitted refrigerated to the laboratory, enabling the diagnostician to do a complete workup for a variety of abortifacient agents. The virus of IBR can sometimes be isolated from the fetal liver, adrenal, kidney, placenta and other tissues. Likewise, virus can be demonstrated in these areas by fluorescent antibody assay.

The focal necrosis and inclusions in the fetal adrenal and liver can be found after careful histopathological search. Serological examination of fetal cardiac blood or of fluids found in body cavities has not been a productive means for the diagnosis of IBR. It is speculated that the fetal disease is so acute that the fetus dies before it can respond immunologically with antibody.

Some clinicians attempt to base a diagnosis of IBR abortion on paired serological tests on the dam. This approach is productive only if the fetus is aborted in the early stages of the disease. Usually by the time the fetus is aborted, the dam's antibody titer is elevated at a high enough level that a further rise is not demonstrable when a second (convalescent) sample is collected.

EFFECTS OF IBR ON FERTILITY

Reports, which have not been substantiated by controlled studies, suggest that a period of temporary infertility follows intramuscular vaccination or natural infection of

IBR. The credibility of such speculation is enhanced by the finding that large doses of IBR virus inoculated into the uterus cause a mild endometritis and temporary failure of conception. For this reason, the prohibition concerning intramuscular vaccination of pregnant cattle should be extended to cover the period 1 month prior to breeding.

FATAL SYSTEMIC IBR IN NEONATES

The birth of a healthy calf capable of surviving to maturity culminates the reproductive process, and thus the fatal systemic form of IBR that sometimes appears in neonatal calves is encompassed in the field of theriogenology. Fetuses that acquire primary IBR infection in late gestation or calves that acquire the infection shortly after birth sometimes experience an acute febrile form of IBR that usually terminates fatally. Such fetuses or calves have respiratory distress and may have necrotic lesions on the mucosa of the mouth, the tongue, the esophagus and all four stomach compartments. In addition, a diffuse peritonitis is frequently present. Such calves may have diarrhea and may be misdiagnosed as having calf septicemia, but the lesions are so characteristic that they indicate IBR to the experienced pathologist.

IBR ASSOCIATED WITH METRITIS

Belgian workers have isolated a virus resembling IBR from the uterine exudate of postparturient cows delivered by cesarean section. These cows had fever, metritis and mucopurulent uterine discharge, and a crepitant feel to the uterus on palpation *per rectum* was also present. The source of infection was not determined.

TREAMENT OF IBR

Because it is a viral disease, IBR is unaffected by available antimicrobial substances, and treatment is directed toward controlling complications. Therefore, the welfare of patients is maintained by good nursing care, supportive therapy and antibiotics when clinical judgment dictates that bacterial complications are significant. Antibiotic therapy must be evaluated with respect to its value to the patient as weighed against withdrawal times and residue potential.

Infectious pustular vulvovaginitis can be treated locally with soothing antiseptic or antibiotic ointments. By and large, IPV is self-limiting and without complications. In bulls, severe cases of balanoposthitis may produce preputial adhesions. Treatment with antibiotic or antiseptic ointments may be necessary to reduce the likelihood of this sequela.

PREVENTION OF IBR

The prevention or control of IBR is difficult. Preventing exposure by rearing animals in isolation is impractical because of the ubiquity of the virus and the ever-present hazard of virus exteriorization from reactivated latent infections in clinically normal cattle.

Vaccination is currently the most logical means of control. IBR vaccines are obtainable from many manufacturers, come in many combinations and are available for intramuscular or intranasal inoculation.

In using any IBR vaccine, it is important to study the label and package insert for contraindications against vaccinating pregnant cattle and for precautions about vaccinating cattle that are in contact with pregnant cattle. In general, the vaccine should be used on healthy, well-nourished cattle that have not recently been moved or exposed to disease.

To prevent the effects of IBR on reproductive efficiency, it is recommended that cattle be vaccinated well before their first breeding. Since maternal antibody may persist for 4 to 6 months, it is best to vaccinate after 6 months of age and prior to breeding. If carried out in the area where calves are raised, such a program will result in repopulation of herds with partially resistant cattle. The protection induced by vaccine should last for a lifetime in most cattle. Although some animals may lose their vaccine-induced humoral antibody, it will persist in others. In some cases, restimulation may occur by natural exposure or by reactivation of vaccine virus infection. An additional percentage of vaccinated cattle can probably develop an anamnestic response in sufficient time to resist systemic distribution of virus to the fetus following exposure. The duration of immunity is controversial, and contrary to the recommendation just provided, many veterinarians and vaccine producers recommend annual revaccination.

The intramuscular vaccines may be less attenuated than vaccines prepared for intranasal use. The intramusclar vaccines can cause abortion and are contraindicated for use in pregnant animals and in cattle or calves that may come in contact with pregnant animals within 30 days following vaccination. Generally, it is accepted that calves 4 months or older will have lost enough maternal antibody that they can respond satisfactorily to these vaccines. Calves can be vaccinated at an earlier age. However, the conservative clinician who vaccinates before 4 months of age anticipates interference from maternal antibody in a certain proportion of vaccinated calves and therefore repeats the vaccination at a later date prior to breeding.

The intranasal vaccines appear to be more attenuated than those used intramuscularly. Most are approved for use in pregnant animals. Careful scrutiny of all labels and package inserts of each product is necessary because it cannot automatically be assumed that all intranasal vaccines are tested and approved for use in pregnant cattle. The proposed advantages of intranasal vaccines include the induction of local or secretory antibody and the prompt appearance of interferon in nasal secretions. It is suggested that interferon provides early protection and may be of some value in controlling early infection. In addition to eliciting a local immune response, the intranasal vaccines cause a humoral antibody response comparable to that of the intramuscular vaccines. There are suggestions that intranasal vaccines can override low levels of maternal antibody and thus be effective for very young calves. However, the conservative clinician attempting to prevent adverse effects on reproduction will be thinking of lifelong immunity or anamnesis and will not rely on inducing active immunity in calves vaccinated under 4 to 6 months of age. When management situations dictate early vaccination, a second vaccination should be administered before breeding.

Intranasal administration is difficult in mature animals unless restraint is excellent. However, vaccination of younger animals is not quite as difficult. Precautions must be taken to see that restraint is excellent and that both nostrils are inoculated with viable vaccine. In addition, care must be taken to see that the cattle do not blow the vaccine out following its administration.

Because of uncertainty about the duration of immunity and a desire to be on the safe side, most manufacturers usually recommend annual revaccination. Annual revaccination is indicated for the bovine paramyxovirus parainfluenza-3 vaccine, which is usually combined with intranasal IBR vaccines. Also, annual revaccination affords the opportunity to immunize cattle that failed to respond to earlier inoculations. In addition, such vaccination could conceivably "boost" waning vaccine-induced titers, assuring greater protection and higher colostral antibody titers for passage to nursing calves.

The clinician must decide if the advantages of annual revaccination outweigh the expense of vaccination and problems of restraint. In my view, one properly administered vaccination in the lifetime of each animal should be adequate to provide herds with enough herd immunity that catastrophic episodes of IBR abortion can be avoided.

The question of whether to vaccinate purebred bulls for IBR is difficult to answer because of the many ramifications. When all things are considered, the safest course is to avoid vaccination of breeding bulls and purebred bull calves on the farm. This seems feasible because some purchasers of purebred bulls and semen discriminate against seropositive individuals because of their potential for exteriorizing virus from reactivated latent infections. Thus, vaccination may limit the opportunity for sale of a purebred bull for export or to an artificial insemination unit. In a total herd health program involving IBR vaccination, the impact of leaving a few bulls unvaccinated would probably be minimal when regarded on a population basis.

In the management of bull studs, whether or not to use IBR vaccine must be based on the serological status of the bull stud population, the requirements of foreign importers of semen and the disease control philosophies of the management. These considerations must be tempered by the arguments that the virus is virtually ubiquitous and may eventually gain entrance to the stud. The exclusion of bulls because of IBR serotiters constitutes a serious loss of genetic material that may not be justified by the minimal hazard associated with transmission of virus by semen.

Effects of Bovine Viral Diarrhea on Reproduction

ROBERT F. KAHRS
University of Florida, Gainesville, Florida

Bovine viral diarrhea (BVD) is most widely known as a systemic disease producing lesions in gastrointestinal mucosa. However, in animals kept for breeding purposes, its most serious economic impact results from damage to the developing fetus. These reproductive manifestations usually follow inapparent or undiagnosed BVD infections. Thus, the significance of BVD as a reproductive disorder is greatly unappreciated.

The disease is most often clinically manifested in young cattle and can be acute or chronic. It appears sporadically and is characterized by fever, diarrhea and erosions or necrosis of the mucous membranes of the gastrointestinal tract. The erosions may be almost imperceptible or quite severe (resembling rinderpest). When oral erosions are not observed, the disease usually goes undiagnosed. In herd outbreaks with minimal diarrhea or mucosal involvement, BVD is frequently diagnosed as "undifferentiated respiratory disease" because fever, nasal discharge and rapid breathing are prominent signs.

ETIOLOGY

The BVD virus is not definitely classified but may eventually be regarded as a togavirus along with the viruses of hog cholera and equine viral arteritis with which it shares many characteristics. It grows readily in a variety of cell cultures, and many strains produce distinctive cytopathogenic changes. Other strains of the BVD virus are not readily cytopathogenic and require more complicated techniques for identification. Cytopathogenic strains are utilized in neutralization tests for detection of serum antibody.

EPIDEMIOLOGY

Epidemiologically, BVD is characterized by widespread distribution, easy transmission, high antibody prevalence, frequent inapparent or undiagnosed infection and a very variable incubation period. Although sheep and swine can be infected, the epidemiological significance of these infections is not known, and cattle are usually considered the principal reservoir. The presence of chronic persistent infections in a few cattle enhances the efficiency of the bovine species as a reservoir. When susceptible cattle and sheep are infected during pregnancy, a variety of fetal abnormalities can occur, which are usually not evident until months after infection.

The pathogenesis of the disease in postnatal cattle is usually explained by a tendency for the virus to replicate in lymphoid tissues. The resulting lymphoid depletion, leukopenia and profound immunosuppression at the cellular level are manifested by degeneration, necrosis and ulceration of mucosa. In the fetus, hypoplasia or degeneration of ocular and brain tissue occurs.

The virus of BVD is virtually ubiquitous in cattle populations. Even cattle raised under relatively isolated conditions seem to become infected frequently. The consequences of BVD infection in cattle vary from a mild inapparent or undiagnosed infection to an acute or chronic fatal illness. Cattle with fatal infections succumb before the effects on the developing fetus are evident, and those with chronic infections are usually culled. Therefore, the mild inapparent (frequently undiagnosed) infections have the greatest impact on reproduction. This makes the economic loss insidious. Before discussing the effects of BVD on reproduction, the clinical forms of the infection will be reviewed.

FORMS OF BVD

Acute Systemic BVD

The typical textbook case seen today differs from initial descriptions. In early reports, attack rates were high, all ages were affected and most sick cattle survived.[3]

Today (at least in the eastern United States) the disease occurs sporadically and is frequently fatal. Most patients are between

6 and 24 months old. Unless examined carefully, herdmates usually appear normal. When careful examination of the oral mucosa is conducted, mildly affected penmates or herdmates are detected by recognition of sparse mucosal erosions or blunted, reddened buccal papillae.

The typical case is characterized by an elevated temperature, salivation, gingivitis and erosions of the lips, gums and palate. Although not always present, diarrhea is a common finding and is frequently intractable, leading to a severe dehydration that signals death. Rapid respiration occurs, and the animal is leukopenic. In some cases, acute laminitis may be present. Some cattle have hyperkeratosis or partial alopecia, but these are nonspecific signs, as are the corneal opacities that occasionally develop.

Chronic BVD

The chronic form of BVD is the syndrome that many people think of as mucosal disease. It may appear in cattle recovering from recognized acute disease or may be seen in cattle in which no prior evidence of infection was observed. The chronically infected animal is unthrifty; there is loss of weight and failure to grow or gain weight at the same rate as penmates of the same age. Such patients are frequently culled as "poor doers," without an accurate diagnosis being made. This chronic form is frequently manifested by an intermittent diarrhea followed by periods of recovery and relapse. The carefully examined animal with a chronic infection may have any of the lesions seen in the acute form. Erosions heal rapidly, and new erosions may appear throughout the course of the disease, which may be several months. Cattle with chronic BVD may have dry, scruffy skin; lameness; cracking or necrosis of skin in the interdigital spaces and erosions or necrosis around the coronary band. Protracted cases may show overgrowth and malformation of hooves, prompting a diagnosis of chronic laminitis.

Cattle with chronic BVD usually have a persistent infection, and virus may be isolated from blood or from ocular and nasal secretions for prolonged periods. Chronic patients frequently fail to develop detectable circulating antibody. It is speculated that such animals are inept at handling the BVD virus and are incapable of immunological

response of a magnitude sufficient to tip the host-parasite relationship in favor of the animal. With the virus prevailing, the animal's physical state declines, and it eventually dies or is culled.

Mild Clinical BVD

Because the severely ill animals (both acute and chronic cases) are usually removed from herds, it is the mild, undiagnosed and inapparent infections that account for most reproductive losses. Some inapparent and mild cases appear in herds when severe acute or chronic cases are present. In other herd infections, there is only mild diarrhea or "undifferentiated respiratory disease," and the association with BVD is not suspected unless careful examination of the oral mucosa is performed or thorough necropsy or laboratory studies are conducted.

Mild clinical bovine viral diarrhea is characterized by fever and leukopenia, both of which may go undetected. The animal frequently has an increased respiratory rate and a few scattered erosions of the oral mucosa or blunted, reddened buccal papillae. These lesions are hard to find unless the mouth is examined meticulously. Mild BVD cases are usually not fatal unless milk fever, metritis, acute mastitis, peritonitis or another infectous disease is superimposed or occurs concurrently. Because of the mild symptomatology and the similarity to other diseases, these mild cases frequently are not diagnosed. Thus, the vast majority of reproductive damage from BVD is undiagnosed or unreported.

Inapparent BVD Infection

Most commonly, BVD infections are unobserved. Such infections result in a leukopenia, a transient biphasic temperature elevation and occasional oral erosions or blunted buccal papillae. These infections occur in susceptible cattle and may occasionally occur in animals with low levels of humoral antibody, particularly if the antibody is derived from colostrum and is near its point of diminution. Immunologically normal cattle with low levels of actively induced antibody can be expected to elicit an anamnestic response with prompt production of antibody that is adequate to prevent serious clinical disease and dissemination of virus to the fetus.

Postvaccination BVD

All of the forms of BVD infection just discussed can occasionally occur following vaccination with modified live virus (MLV) vaccines. The vaccines are attenuated by serial passage in cell cultures, and the probability of postvaccination reactions other than mild inapparent infection should be relatively low.

When pregnant cattle with no previous experience with the virus are vaccinated, abortion can result, and vaccination of pregnant cattle is clearly contraindicated. When BVD-like disease occurs within a "reasonable incubation period" following vaccination, several explanations are possible. The diagnosis may be inaccurate, the BVD infection may have been acquired before vaccination or the animal may belong to that small population of cattle that are unable to handle the vaccine virus and develop the clinical disease. The same factors that determine why some calves succumb to the natural infection while herdmates experience only a subclinical infection probably explain postvaccination BVD. Some proposed explanations for the occurrence of postvaccination BVD are: innate immunological deficiencies, vaccination of "stressed" animals, vaccination of corticosteroid-treated animals, vaccination of animals subjected to other immunosuppressive influences, the immunosuppressive effect of the vaccine virus itself, "immune tolerance" developed *in utero* during infection of the pregnant dam and, finally, immune paralysis from an excess of antigen.

When investigating postvaccination BVD, the first question the clinician should ask is "why were these cattle vaccinated?" In many cases, the answer is "because BVD was present in the herd." Those who conduct calfhood vaccination programs with BVD vaccine know that eventually some "normal calves" will develop the disease following the vaccination. However, if vaccination of animals of breeding age is avoided, vaccination of other animals should not interfere with reproductive efficiency. If practiced early enough, vaccination should prevent the effects of the natural infection upon reproductive efficiency.

DIAGNOSIS OF BVD

The diagnosis is usually based on clinical signs and lesions in live animals and on necropsy findings. Virus isolation, fluorescent antibody assay for virus and serological examination are additional diagnostic aids.

At necropsy, the typical BVD-infected carcass is thin, dehydrated and soiled with feces. A scruffy hair coat is a frequent finding. Occasionally the mucous membranes of the vulva have erosions at the mucocutaneous junction, and the nasal orifices are usually encrusted. Erosions or ulcerations may be present in the oral mucous membranes, the esophagus (where they may be healed or very hard to find) and in the rumen and abomasum. A characteristic finding is lymphoid depletion, hemorrhage or necrosis of Peyer's patches. An occasional fatal case is observed to have necrotic areas around the skin of the lower limbs, particularly in the area of the coronary band.

The diagnosis can be confirmed by isolation of the virus from the spleen, lymph nodes or bone marrow. These must be harvested aseptically because bacterial contaminants readily overgrow tissue culture systems. In the live animal, virus can be isolated from blood or from nasal or ocular discharges. Some laboratories rely heavily on fluorescent antibody (FA) assay to identify BVD virus in tissues taken at necropsy. However, difficulties with reagents frequently make FA tests an inadequate diagnostic tool.

Serological diagnosis is usually based on a neutralization test performed in cell cultures. In most bovine populations there is a high antibody prevalence from previous infection or vaccination. Thus, a single serum specimen provides inadequate information for diagnosing the disease in an individual animal. Paired serum specimens are useful if the first specimen (taken during the acute stages of the disease) is negative and a second specimen (taken from the same animal 3 to 4 weeks later) is positive, indicating seroconversion around the time of clinical disease. Many animals with acute infections die before the second specimen can be collected, and many with the chronic form fail to have demonstrable humoral antibody. Therefore, serological diagnosis is severely limited.

Early profound leukopenia in most cases is an additional diagnostic aid.

ABORTIONS AND CONGENITAL ANOMALIES FROM BVD

For BVD infection of the developing fetus to occur, the cow or heifer must be *both* pregnant and susceptible at the time of infection. Fetal BVD frequently occurs in herds in which BVD has never been diagnosed. Usually an etiological diagnosis is not obtained because of the obscure nature of the maternal infection. Because of the variable time between maternal infection and abortion or birth of anomalous calves, a variety of pregnancy terminations can occur over many months without arousing suspicion of a common etiology.

Abortion is more likely if the dam is infected in the early months of gestation,[2] but this can also occur following infection at other stages of gestation. Actual expulsion of the fetus can occur close to the time of maternal infection or many months afterward.

The most clearly delineated syndrome resulting from fetal BVD infection is cerebellar degeneration with ocular defects. Ocular and cerebellar defects do not always occur in the same calf; however, their concurrent appearance is highly suggestive of congenital BVD. Affected fetuses may be aborted, but many are carried to term. Individual cases are frequently regarded as curiosities and pass off as genetic defects. However, births of these calves tend to cluster in time, becoming evident with the parturition of cows that were in the middle trimester of pregnancy at the time the BVD infection was active in the herd.

Calves with congenital ataxia from cerebellar deficiency produced by *in utero* BVD infection are usually normal except for ocular and visual deficiencies and motor incoordination. Severely affected calves are unable to rise after birth and eventually die. The mildly affected calf will have difficulty in rising and walking after birth. All reflexes are usually normal, and if hand-fed, such calves frequently accommodate and are able to survive. They may have a head tilt and a stilted basewide gait and may stumble easily. By the time they are several weeks of age, mildly affected calves can appear normal.

In addition to damage to the developing cerebellum, such calves frequently have congenital cataracts, microphthalmia or other ocular defects. The diagnosis of congenital BVD is confirmed by finding an ataxic, partially blind calf with cataracts that has BVD humoral antibody demonstrable in serum collected before nursing and that is shown at necropsy to have cerebellar degeneration.

Aside from abortion and the cerebellar-ocular syndrome, brachygnathia and other musculoskeletal defects and alopecia are occasional sequelae to fetal infection with BVD.

Fetal mummification can also occur after infection of the pregnant cow with BVD. Two cases have been produced experimentally.[1] Mummified fetuses can probably develop following fetal death from many causes. Therefore, the mere presence of a mummified bovine fetus is no assurance that BVD was the cause.

When BVD infection is introduced into a totally susceptible herd, about 25 per cent of pregnancies may be expected to terminate abnormally.

In pregnant sheep used as an experimental model for the bovine syndrome, infection with BVD causes an inapparent infection, but this can be followed by low fertility, fetal death with abortion or mummification, cerebellar hypoplasia, hydrocephalus and congenital malformation of the limbs.[4] Like BVD in cattle, the actual economic impact of this disease remains to be elaborated.

Diagnosis of BVD Abortions and Congenital Anomalies

Serological specimens collected from the dam at the time of abortion or birth of anomalous calves are worthless as a tool for confirming BVD. On the other hand, the detection of BVD antibody in presuckle serums collected from anomalous or stillborn calves or aborted fetuses provides convincing evidence that the fetus was infected *in utero* and supports the hypothesis of BVD etiology. If the calf is ambulatory, the diagnostician must have assurance that it has not nursed and acquired colostral antibody. Serum antibody in a calf that has nursed indicates only that the dam had been vaccinated or exposed to BVD at some time in her life, and like the dam's serum, adds very little to the diagnostic picture. Assurance that the calf had not nursed can be obtained if the calf was dead at birth, if the clinician was present at birth or if the calf was unable to stand up and therefore could not have suckled. In all cases in which presuckle serological studies are to be done, the udder of the dam should be examined for evidence of suckling. This is because the owner will frequently report that the calf has not nursed, but the cow's teats will be clean, wet and covered with foamy milk and saliva or one or two quarters will be slack, indicating that the calf did suckle. Another clue to ascertaining that the neonate did not nurse is a stomach free of milk at necropsy. Specimens for serological testing of anomalous calves and aborted fetuses must be collected with sterile precautions. This is a particular problem in aborted fetuses because they contain many "garden variety" bacteria that overgrow the cell cultures in which the serological tests are performed.

Attempts to isolate virus from aborted fetuses and anomalous calves are usually unsuccessful. Some develop antibody, which neutralizes the virus, and some are heavily contaminated. In addition, some BVD virus strains are noncytopathogenic.

Fluorescent antibody assay on aborted fetuses is a potentially useful diagnostic tool. This procedure should be performed by well-trained, experienced, skillful and patient technologists using high quality reagents. It needs perfecting before significant improvements in the diagnosis of BVD fetal disease can be accomplished.

TREATMENT OF BVD

Specific therapeutic measures are not available for treating BVD. Clinical manifestations are usually treated empirically with supportive therapy. Although fluid therapy, antibiotics and antidiarrheals are used, most veterinarians agree that the outcome of the disease is not greatly influenced by therapeutic regimens and supportive measures. The infections resulting in congenital anomalies are usually unrecognized and thus untreated. By the time abortion occurs or an anomalous calf is recognized, the damage is done.

PREVENTION OF BVD

Rearing cattle in isolation has proved inadequate for preventing infection with BVD virus. Thus, preventive methods are limited to the use of vaccines. Experimental work is under way on the development of an inactivated viral vaccine. However, at this writing, the only commercially available product is the MLV vaccine, which is widely used alone or in combination with infectious bovine rhinotracheitis (IBR) and/or bovine paramyxovirus parainfluenza-3 (BPI-3) vaccines.

Successful immunization requires that the vaccinated animal be infected with the vaccine virus and subsequently responds immunologically. Most findings suggest that previously infected animals usually have enough resistance to ward off fetal BVD infection. Thus, the approach to the control of BVD-induced reproductive disease is vaccination prior to breeding. Any vaccination program should have the objective of preventing totally susceptible herds, which are most likely to have catastrophic reproductive losses. It is unrealistic to expect any procedure to eliminate all abortions and other reproductive disorders.

The maternal antibody acquired from colostrum may persist from 6 to 8 months of age and sometimes longer. A large percentage of calves possess this maternal antibody, which can interfere with successful vaccination. Therefore, vaccination of heifers should be carried out some time after 6 to 8 months of age and before breeding.

Calfhood vaccination programs for BVD can be maintained on an ongoing basis. Although there is some feeling to the contrary, this author feels that one successful vaccination prior to the first breeding is sufficient to markedly reduce the probability of BVD interfering with reproductive efficiency throughout the animal's life.

In addition to being abortifacient, the BVD vaccine has a reputation for inducing postvaccination mucosal disease in a small percentage of vaccinated cattle. Therefore, only healthy, well-nourished, unstressed and socially adjusted heifer calves should be vaccinated. Pregnant cattle should never be vaccinated. The use of MLV-BVD vaccine on lactating animals is also not recommended.

Because the major benefit derived from BVD vaccine is prevention of fetal damage, there appears to be no advantage to vaccinating bulls.

Each veterinarian should evaluate the management scheme on each farm or ranch and make a decision regarding a BVD vaccination program.

REFERENCES

1. Kahrs, R. F.: Effects of bovine viral diarrhea on the developing fetus. JAVMA, *163*:877, 1973.
2. Kendrick, J. W.: Bovine viral diarrhea-mucosal disease virus infection in pregnant cows. Am. J. Vet. Res., *32*:533, 1971.
3. Olafson, P., MacCallum, A. D. and Fox, F. H.: An apparently new transmissible disease of cattle. Cornell Vet., *36*:205, 1946.
4. Ward, G. M.: Experimental infection of pregnant sheep with bovine viral diarrhea-mucosal disease virus. Cornell Vet., *61*:179, 1971.

Current Status of Viral Infections of Bovine Genital Tract

with Emphasis on IBR-IPV Virus

R. D. SCHULTZ

Auburn University, Auburn, Alabama

and B. E. SHEFFY

Cornell University, Ithaca, New York

INTRODUCTION

The bovine herpes viruses (BHV), including infectious bovine rhinotracheitis (IBR) virus and infectious pustular vulvovaginitis (IPV) virus, are known to cause respiratory and genital tract infections in susceptible cattle of all ages.

The classic respiratory infection is characterized by discrete pustules or plaques found on the mucosal surfaces, hyperemia of nasal turbinates, nasal discharge, febrile response, rapid respiration, dyspnea and occasional conjunctivitis.

Infection of the bovine genital tract results in balanoposthitis in the male and infectious pustular vulvovaginitis (coital exanthema) in the female. These infections, like the respiratory infections, are characterized by pustules or plaques on the penis and prepuce or the vulva of the infected animal. The lesions can persist for several days to more than a week. Frequently the penis will be red and painful, the vagina may have an exudate and the animal will demonstrate pain and frequent urination. Respiratory infections are rarely associated with genital forms of the disease, and genital forms of the disease are only occasionally associated with respiratory disease. This observation has led some to believe that slight but significant differences exist between the viruses that infect the respiratory tract and those that infect the genital tract. Also, it has been demonstrated by neutralization kinetic tests and low affinity antibody testing that serological differences may exist for the strains of viruses we collectively refer to as IBR.

BHV infections of cattle present a unique problem in that after the primary respiratory or genital infection, animals remain latently infected, presumably for life. Latent virus can be sporadically reactivated by natural mechanisms or can be consistently reactivated by treatment with adrenocorticotropic hormone (ACTH) or corticosteroids. In bulls used for semen production, the potential for viral reactivation presents a special problem since semen can be contaminated with large quantities of IBR-IPV virus. Shedding of virus can occur in animals that are clinically healthy, in that reactivation of virus in latently infected animals results in mild or no clinically apparent disease, presumably because of the presence of host immune factors such as antibody. The recognition of clinical signs of disease will therefore be of little or no value in preventing virus-contaminated semen from being included in the semen pool for distribution and sale. Virus-contaminated semen presents a potential threat to the cattle population in that IBR-IPV virus can cause infectious pustular vulvovaginitis, endometritis, salpingitis and shortened estrous cycles in susceptible cattle. Spread of the virus to susceptible pregnant cattle in the herd can lead to abortions, and infection of susceptible neonates could potentially lead to a fatal septicemic disease. Because of the threat to the cattle population, some workers have advocated maintaining and collecting only bulls that are serologically negative for IBR virus.

Because of the potential hazards from IBR-IPV virus-contaminated semen, we have been involved in: (1) determining conditions that result in reactivation of virus after primary infection; (2) developing and testing numerous types of IBR vaccines, with an aim at preventing genital infection or genital shedding of virus; (3) examining the effect of virus-contaminated semen on reproductive performance and disease of the female; (4) developing sensitive and accurate techniques to detect virus in semen; (5) developing tests to distinguish between vaccine strains and wild virus and (6) determining the role that serologically positive and serologically negative bulls play in the transmission of IBR virus.

REACTIVATION OF IBR-IPV VIRUS

Several reports have appeared concerning natural reactivation and shedding of IBR virus in semen for periods up to 1 year after initial primary infection. Experiments have demonstrated consistent and repeated shedding of virus after ACTH and corticosteroid treatment of cattle in which primary infection occurred months or years prior to treatment. IBR virus appears to be more readily reactivated by corticosteroids than the herpes viruses of other species or other herpes viruses of this species. Additionally, on rare occasions we have recognized reactivation of IBR virus at parturition, presumably as a result of elevation of endogenous steroid, and reactivation of the virus in conjunction with febrile responses associated with viral or bacterial infections or neoplastic disease. Natural reactivation associated with these conditions has been assumed because the virus was isolated and/or marked increases in viral neutralizing antibody titer occurred. The usual therapeutic doses of corticosteroid used topically or systemically should not lead to reactivation of the virus because the dose is too low, and the duration of treatment is too short. However, the treatment with an equivalent of 10 mg or higher of dexamethasone for 3 days or longer would in general be expected to cause viral reactivation.

The mechanism of viral reactivation is not known. However, the immunosuppressive effect of steroid, particularly on the T cells, may contribute to replication of the virus. It would appear that low levels of neutralizing antibody allow the exteriorization and shedding of the virus. Therefore, maintenance of high antibody titers is recommended.

Caution should be exercised in attempting to recognize viral shedding by the appearance of clinical signs of disease, since such signs may be mild or nonexistent. Therefore, the potential for viral reactivation is always present if serologically positive bulls are maintained. However, a well-managed, low-stress situation greatly reduces the likelihood of reactivation of the virus.

Therefore, we recommend the following: Do not collect semen from a bull with clinical signs of respiratory or genital IBR-IPV infection; do not treat serologically positive bulls with corticosteroid preparations that could activate the latent virus; exercise extreme caution in collecting bulls that are febrile for more than 3 days and maintain a low-stress management situation at all times.

VACCINATION STUDIES

Numerous questions need to be considered when testing vaccines for their efficacy and safety. Special considerations need to be given to vaccination of bulls because of the potential for (1) viral shedding in the semen, (2) the effect that vaccination may have on reproductive performance and semen quality (3) and the potential for reactivation of the vaccine virus. The obvious safety features of a killed viral vaccine led to early studies with inactivated viral vaccine. Inactivated viral vaccine administered in two or more doses resulted in viral neutralization titers similar to titers after live viral vaccine or after inapparent natural infection. However, bulls challenged with virulent virus did not develop signs of clinical disease, but they did become latently infected. When these bulls were later treated with corticosteroid, virus was reactivated and isolated from nasal secretions and the genital tract. Therefore, it was suggested that killed IBR virus vaccine was not effective in preventing infection and development of the latent carrier state.[10] Vaccination with intramuscular vaccines led to latent infection, and after steroid treatment, virus was isolated from the respiratory and genital tracts. The intramuscular vaccine viruses have been demonstrated to cause death and abortion of inoculated fetuses (see section on Cornell Fetal Test) similar to that of wild virus. Therefore, we consider them unsafe and cannot recommend vaccinating bulls with intramuscular vaccine.

An intranasal vaccine for IBR and bovine parainfluenza-3 (BPI-3) has been described. Vaccination with an intranasal IBR and BPI-3 vaccine (Nasalgen IP) provided results suggesting that this vaccine virus may be both safe and efficacious for bulls. Serologically negative bulls were vaccinated intranasally, or intranasally and intrapreputially, with Nasalgen IP. Virus was isolated from the respiratory tract for periods up to 12 days after intranasal vaccination. However, virus was not isolated from the prepuce or the semen at any time after intranasal or intrapreputial vaccination. Steroid treatment of these bulls did not cause the virus to be shed from the prepuce or respiratory tract, suggesting that the virus did not become latent or that virus is not readily reactivated with the corticosteroid regimen used to reactivate intramuscular vaccine virus or wild virus.

Since intrapreputial vaccination did not result in genital tract infection, as determined by the inability to reisolate virus shortly after vaccination, and since it did not produce an increase in immunoglobulin or specific antibody in the preputial washings, intrapreputial vaccination was discontinued. Bulls vaccinated intranasally were divided into three groups. The first group consisted of 9 bulls, the second 10 bulls and the third 9 bulls. Bulls in group I were challenged intranasally with virulent virus 1 month after vaccination, bulls in group II were challenged intranasally and intravenously 3 months after vaccination and bulls in group III were challenged intranasally and intravenously 6 months after vaccination with $1 \times 10^{6.5}$ TCID$_{50}$ of virulent virus. Virus was not isolated from the prepuce during a 2-week period following viral challenge in any of the three groups of bulls. One month after viral challenge, six bulls from group I and all the bulls in groups II and III were treated with corticosteroid. Virus was not isolated from the prepuce of bulls in group I or group II but was isolated from the prepuce

of two bulls in group III. This suggests that protection against reinfection persisted for at least 3 months but for less than 6 months.

A limited number of intranasally vaccinated bulls were challenged intrapreputially with 1×10^7 IPV virus. Animals were resistant to challenge in that no virus replication could be determined, as demonstrated by an inability to isolate virus 7 days postchallenge, and no clinical signs developed.

Our experience for the past 4 years with intranasal vaccination in a stud of approximately 300 bulls indicates that there are no complications associated with the frequent vaccination, antibody titers are being maintained and virus is not being shed in the semen. (See section on Cornell Semen Tests.)

Young bulls are vaccinated when they enter the stud. Older bulls that were serologically positive as a result of infection with virulent virus are also vaccinated. However, a small number of these bulls have been demonstrated to shed virus in the semen for short periods after experimental steroid treatment but have not been demonstrated to shed virus under normal conditions of low-stress management in the stud.

Recently we have tested a new temperature sensitive (TS) IBR vaccine. We found that inoculation of bovine fetuses (see section on Cornell Fetal Test) of various ages with this virus did not result in death or evidence of virus replication, presumably because the fetal temperature restricted the growth of the virus. In a limited number of animals, intranasal vaccination did not result in genital infection, nor did steroid treatment cause virus reactivation in the genital tract. Direct intratesticular and intrapreputial inoculation of the virus resulted in local infection and mild testicular swelling, but no additional lesions or effect on sperm numbers or quantity was observed. The testicular swelling was unilateral, the inoculated testicle returned to normal size within a few days and no evidence of the infection in the uninoculated testicle was noted. These preliminary results are encouraging and demonstrate that this vaccine, like Nasalgen, may be safe for vaccination of bulls. The unanswered question with regard to vaccination of bulls with the TS-IBR mutant is whether or not intranasal vaccination would protect the genital tract, since the virus replicates only at the site of inoculation.

We therefore currently recommend that if vaccination is deemed necessary, administer an intranasal vaccine (Nasalgen IP) every 4 to 6 months.

EFFECT OF VIRUS-CONTAMINATED SEMEN ON REPRODUCTION

The effects of virus-contaminated semen on the female are influenced by at least three factors: (1) the amount of virus in the semen, (2) the strain of virus and (3) the immunological status of the female.

A number of studies have demonstrated that semen can contain viral doses adequate to cause severe vaginitis, endometritis, salpingitis and shortened estrous cycles in serologically susceptible females.

Studies from this Institute (James A. Baker Institute for Animal Health, Cornell University), in which heifers were inseminated with small quantities of virus (200 TCID$_{50}$) in the semen, indicate that neither serologically negative nor serologically positive heifers were adversely affected. Of 25 serologically negative heifers, 19 remained serologically negative after breeding with contaminated semen. A majority conceived after the first breeding and the others after the second or third breeding. Six heifers developed minimal lesions on the vaginal mucosa, and virus was shed from the vaginal tract in all six animals and from the respiratory tract in one of the six animals. Six heifers developed antibody to IBR virus by 14 days postinsemination. One of the six conceived after the first breeding, four of the six after the second breeding and the sixth animal required five services before she settled. One animal in this group aborted, was rebred and had a normal fetus that she carried until slaughtered at 150 days. Of the nine serologically positive heifers included in the study, none developed clinical signs of infectious pustular vulvovaginitis (IPV), six heifers conceived after the first breeding and all conceived after three attempts at breeding. The length of the period between estrous cycles was normal for the 34 heifers.

Strain differences for IBR-IPV virus may lead to certain strains causing more severe genital disease than others. In a limited number of serologically susceptible bulls and heifers, inoculation of the prepuce or vagina with IBR (Nasalgen IP) did not cause clinical signs of balanoposthitis or infectious pustular vulvovaginitis. Therefore, semen contaminated with this vaccine virus would presumably have little or no potential for producing disease. Likewise, inoculation of the prepuce and testicle with a TS mutant of IBR virus did not cause balanoposthitis.

Virus-contaminated semen would be expected to have a less serious effect on immune animals than susceptible animals. However, preliminary results of I. M. Parsonson[6] would suggest that immune animals inseminated with virus-contaminated semen have sequelae similar to susceptible animals. These preliminary findings have not been verified in our own recent studies.

Our recommendation currently would be not to inseminate cattle with semen containing IBR virus that can be detected by the Cornell Semen Tests (see next section).

CORNELL SEMEN TESTS

We have developed an *in vitro* and an *in vivo* test to detect virus-contaminated semen (Table 1).

The *in vitro* test is best used with single ejaculates or pooled ejaculates from the same bull and can be used with raw or extended semen. Because seminal plasma and sperm are toxic for cell cultures, the seminal plasma is treated with trypsin inhibitor, which reduces, but does not always eliminate, the toxicity. The sample is then tested by a standard virus isolation procedure.

The *in vivo* (animal) semen test utilizes pooled semen samples and requires IBR serologically negative calves. Semen samples (0.1 ml of raw semen from each ejaculate) are pooled daily and stored in liquid nitrogen. Daily samples are pooled at the end of the week or end of the month. Ten ml of semen is inoculated intranasally and 10 ml intravenously into one or more IBR-susceptible calves. Serum samples collected at the time of inoculation and 3 and 5 weeks later are tested for the development of IBR neutralizing antibody. Animals are arbitrarily used twice for this test. The advantage of the animal test is the ability to pool samples without reducing the sensitiv-

TABLE 1. *Comparison of the Cornell Semen Tests*

Test Factors	In Vitro Test	In Vivo Test
Cost/ejaculate*	$10.00–$15.00	$1.50–$3.00
Time for results	3 to 4 weeks	4 to 5 weeks
Virus sensitivity (TCID$_{50}$)	Requires 5×10^2 to 5×10^3/ml raw semen	1×10^3 to 5×10^3/ml raw semen
Sample volume required	0.5 ml semen	0.1 ml semen
Total sample that can be tested	0.1 ml/tube	20–40 ml/animal
Use extended or raw	Both	Both
Animals required	None	Susceptible calves
Special provisions and equipment	Tissue culture equipment and techniques	Isolation or barn facility; tissue culture facility
Ability to detect other viruses	All cytopathic viruses	Within limits of sensitivity—all viruses if susceptible animal employed

*Cost for the *in vitro* test is based on individual ejaculates of a single bull to maintain sensitivity, and cost for the *in vivo* test is based on a pool of 50 or more ejaculates, since sensitivity is not affected by pooling.

ty. Pooling samples also results in a marked reduction in the cost of the test. A significant disadvantage is that unless there is a low frequency of positive samples, extensive rechecking of individual samples will be required to determine which bull is shedding virus.

In an attempt to modify the test to use an animal other than cattle, groups of goats, ferrets, rabbits, guinea pigs, rats, hamsters and mice were inoculated intranasally with 200 TCID$_{50}$ of IBR virus or intravenously with 200 TCID$_{50}$ of IPV virus, a dose of virus found to cause infection in susceptible cattle. Only cattle were susceptible to infection with this amount of virus, as determined by the development of serum neutralizing antibody. Therefore, the animal test must employ cattle if sensitivity is to be maintained.

Employing both of the Cornell Semen Tests, we have examined more than 40,000 semen samples from bulls with natural IBR infection and/or bulls vaccinated with Nasalgen.

We recommend that if small numbers of individual ejaculates are to be tested (i.e., for export), use the *in vitro* test. If large numbers of pooled ejaculates need to be tested, use the *in vivo* (animal) test.

CORNELL FETAL TEST

Currently few or no methods are available to differentiate between virulent and attenuated IBR viruses. This results from the fact that *in vitro* characteristics of virulent and vaccine viruses are similar or

identical. One notable exception is the temperature-sensitive mutant of IBR virus recently licensed as an intranasal vaccine. *In vivo* characteristics of certain vaccine strains and virulent virus are similar in that intranasal challenge with virulent virus and intramuscular vaccine can lead to either inapparent infection or mild disease, and development of severe infection is rare. Because of the lack of markers, we decided to use fetal inoculation as a method to distinguish less attenuated vaccine virus or wild virus from more attenuated vaccine viruses.

Fetal inoculation with several intramuscular vaccines and with wild virus resulted in fetal death and abortion 9 to 19 days postinoculation, regardless of the age of the fetus. If abortions occurred during the first 3 days after surgery, they were considered to be due to the surgical manipulation rather than the virus.

Unlike fetuses inoculated with intramuscular vaccine and wild virus, fetuses 90 days or older inoculated with IBR (Nasalgen IP) vaccine alone survived infection, and some developed humoral and cellular immunity to IBR virus. Similarly, fetuses 150 days or older inoculated with IBR virus in Rhivin developed an immune response and survived infection. Fetuses 100 to 255 days of age inoculated with the TS-IBR vaccine survived inoculation. Unlike inoculation with the other IBR intranasal vaccine viruses, with one exception an immune response was not detected, suggesting that the temperature of the fetus restricted the replication of the TS-IBR virus.

The Cornell Fetal Test has been used to

determine the virulence of numerous intranasal vaccines, field isolates and viruses present in the semen or prepuce of experimentally infected or vaccinated bulls that have been steroid stressed in certain of the studies described previously in this article.

We recommend using this test to distinguish between virulent and attenuated strains of IBR virus that are not temperature-sensitive mutants.

ROLE OF BULLS IN TRANSMISSION OF IBR VIRUS

Attempts to maintain a serologically negative stud will eventually fail because the large number of serologically positive bulls dictates eventual acquisition of an actively or latently infected animal. In addition, the virus could be introduced by man. Excluding IBR positive bulls could also result in a loss of outstanding genetic potential. Furthermore, virus-contaminated semen could be collected from serologically negative bulls if the following conditions are present:

1. Susceptible animals may be actively infected and shedding virus before antibody development.

2. Animals with low titers could be recorded as negative in an insensitive serological test used to detect antibody.

3. Some infected animals may develop a cellular immune response without measurable humoral (neutralizing antibody) response.

The likelihood of each of these is low, but cases of each have been recognized during this study.

In an attempt to determine the role that serologically IBR-IPV positive bulls play in the transmission of IBR-IPV virus, we have examined more than 40,000 semen samples over the past 5 years, including samples collected during the time of inapparent infection. In a cooperative study, more than 4000 additional ejaculates were tested independently in a second laboratory. The results of these studies using the *in vitro* and/or *in vivo* semen tests revealed that virus was not isolated by either test from any bull at any time during or subsequent to the mild respiratory infection induced by virulent IBR virus or after repeated vaccination with Nasalgen IP. Contrary to our results in which respiratory infection of bulls was not accompanied by or followed by genital shedding of virus, primary genital infection is associated with virus isolation from the semen during infection and sporadically for a year or more after infection in a small percentage of infected bulls.

Therefore, IBR virus reactivation and shedding is a potential threat when serologically positive bulls are used for production of semen. However, after testing more than 70,000 ejaculates for over 5 years from approximately 300 bulls that developed a mild or inapparent respiratory infection with IBR and that had been vaccinated every 4 months with Nasalgen IP, we conclude that there is *no* reason to suspect that these bulls transmitted IBR-IPV virus.

OTHER BOVINE VIRUSES

Previous unpublished studies at the Baker Institute concerning experimental BVD infections of bulls suggested that this virus was not readily recovered from the semen or prepuce after primary infection and that virus was not isolated from steroid-treated bulls that had recovered from infection with BVD virus. Recently, it was reported and we have also found (using the *in vivo* Cornell Semen Test) that BVD virus could be isolated sporadically from semen of a limited number of bulls after primary infection. Additionally, a clinically BVD-infected bull shed virus in the semen over an extended period of time. Therefore, this virus may occasionally be isolated from semen.

During the present study of IBR-IPV virus, we investigated the possible transmission of PI-3 in the semen. Although certain bulls were serologically positive as a result of infection and all bulls were vaccinated every 4 months with PI-3, this virus was never isolated from semen nor was there any evidence that PI-3 serum-negative animals serologically converted after they were inoculated with pools of semen.

The current evidence would suggest that neither the bovine leukemia virus (BLV) nor the viral genome is present in semen of bulls infected with BLV. However, we are currently attempting to determine if BLV-infected leukocytes in semen serve as a potential source of bovine leukemia virus or other viruses known to persistently infect leukocytes.

Blue tongue virus was reported to be transmitted in the semen. This virus may be intracellular, unlike the viruses discussed above, which are contaminants of semen and present in seminal plasma. Further work is necessary to determine the role of semen as a vector in the transmission of viruses.

REFERENCES

1. Bitsch, V.: IBR virus infection in bulls, with special reference to preputial infection. Appl. Micro., *26*:337, 1973.
2. Davies, D. H. and Duncan, J. R.: The pathogenesis of recurrent infections with IBR virus induced in calves by treatment with corticosteroids. Cornell Vet., *64*:340, 1974.
3. Gillespie, J. H., McEntee, K., Kendrick, J. W. and Wagner, W. C.: Comparison of IPV virus with IBR virus. Cornell Vet., *49*:288, 1959.
4. Kendrick, J. W. and McEntee, K.: The effect of artificial insemination with semen contaminated with IBR-IPV virus. Cornell Vet., *57*:3, 1967.
5. McKercher, D. G., Straub, O. C., Wada, E. M. and Saito, J. K.: Comparative studies of the etiologic agents of IBR and IPV. Can. J. Comp. Med., *23*:320, 1959.
6. Parsonson, I. M.: Personal communication.
7. Parsonson, I. M. and Snowdon, W. A.: The effect of natural and artificial breeding using bulls infected with semen or contaminated with IBR virus. Aust. Vet. J., *51*:365, 1975.
8. Schultz, R. D., Hall, C. E., Sheffy, B. E., Kahrs, R. F. and Bean, B. H.: Current status of IBR-IPV virus infection in bulls. Proc. USAHA, 1976, pp. 63–73.
9. Sheffy, B. E. and Davies, D. H.: Reactivation of a bovine herpesvirus after corticosteroid treatment. Proc. Soc. Exptl. Biol. Med., *140*:974, 1972.
10. Sheffy, B. E. and Krinsky, M.: IBR in extended bovine semen. Proc. 77th USAHA, 1978.
11. Snowdon, W. A.: The IBR-IPV virus: Reaction to infection and intermittent recovery of virus from experimentally infected cattle. Aust. Vet. J., *41*:135, 1965.
12. Todd, J. D., Volenec, F. J. and Paton, I. M.: Intranasal vaccination against IBR: Studies on the early onset of protection and use of the vaccine in pregnant cows. JAVMA, *159*:1370, 1971.

Immunization Program to Maximize Reproductive Performance

R. ZEMJANIS
University of Minnesota, St. Paul, Minnesota

In order to be successful, preventive programs for bovine reproduction have to consider every known cause of infertility, be it infectious or noninfectious. Conception failure, prenatal deaths and congenital abnormalities are well documented manifestations of a number of infectious diseases. Some are primary genital infections such as brucellosis, campylobacteriosis (formerly known as vibriosis) and trichomoniasis. Others affect more than the reproductive system, although often the genitotrope effect is the predominant, if not the only, clinical manifestation. Leptospirosis, listeriosis, infectious bovine rhinotracheitis (IBR), bovine viral diarrhea (BVD), parainfluenza-3 (PI-3) and blue tongue are characteristic examples.

Historically, discoveries of specific infections have stimulated search for immunizing procedures. Infectious diseases affecting bovine reproduction are no exceptions, and immunizing methods have been developed for several, but not all, of them.

Application of all available biologicals in any given herd is seldom, if ever, indicated. Therefore, immunization programs must be selective, and a decision to vaccinate or not and which diseases to include in the vaccination program must be made in each individual case. Final decision rests with the owner of the particular herd. This decision is made on the basis of professional advice from a consultant or resident veterinarian. This veterinarian bears responsibility for the design of immunization program if such is indicated.

REQUIREMENTS

A program to be successful must meet certain requirements. First, in order to be incorporated in the program of a given herd, a

TABLE 1. *Immunization Guide*

Disease	Vaccine	Recommended Application	Comments
Brucellosis[a]	S–19	Calfhood, 2–6 months	60 to 70 per cent protected residual titers, danger of self-inoculation
	S–45/20	Any time	Not approved for use in United States
Leptospirosis	Bacterins[b]	Calfhood, not < 6 months; adults, any time; revaccination in enzootic areas[c]	Protection for 6–12 months
Campylo-bacteriosis (Vibriosis)	Bacterin	30–120 days before breeding, annual revaccination	Vaccinated females exposed to infected bull(s) may transmit to other
IBR	MLV Intramuscular	Calfhood, 4–6 months;[d] nonpregnant replacements < 30 days before breeding	Life-long protection, Do not vaccinate (1) if animal pregnant, (2) during outbreak, (3) during stress
	MLV Intranasal	Calfhood, 4–6 months;[d] any adults	Life-long protection
	IBR Inactivated	Any age or stage of pregnancy	Two injections initially, annual revaccination
BVD	MLV Intramuscular	Calfhood, 6–8 months;[d] nonpregnant replacements < 30 days before breeding	All precautions listed for IBR intramuscular MLV vaccine valid also for BVD MLV vaccine.
PI-3	MLV Intranasal	Calfhood, 4–6 months;[d] adults any time	Life-long protection

[a]Some authorities suggest vaccination.
[b]Leptospira serotype of the bacterin must match that of the etiological agent.
[c]Follow manufacturer's directions for revaccination.
[d]Can be administered simultaneously to normal calves.

disease must actually be responsible for reduced reproductive efficiency. Second, there must be adequate epidemiological indication that such a disease poses a definite threat to maximum reproductive performance. Third, a beneficial effect on reproduction must be one of documented advantages of immunization. Finally the efficiency of immunization must justify its cost to the owner.

These requirements are not easy to meet. Most programmed immunizations are initiated after an outbreak of abortions or other forms of infertility. Unfortunately, the etiological diagnosis required for justification of proposed immunization is made in only 25 to 30 per cent of cases. The lack of a definite diagnosis compounds the dilemma of a veterinarian who is expected to establish programs.

Similar problems are encountered when the potential danger of an infection is assessed prior to designing and implementing preventive programs. Extra- and intraherd carriers and sources of infection and managerial practices facilitating introduction, as well as spread, of infection must be considered before vaccination is recommended.

The third requirement is the most difficult to meet. With the exception of brucellosis and campylobacteriosis (vibriosis), reproductive parameters are not generally used for efficiency testing of biologicals. Clinical comparisons of reproductive performance between years of immunization and years without are highly misleading. Economic justification of immunization depends almost entirely on epidemiological indications and the efficiency of the program.

These requirements, although of principal concern to veterinarians, must also be understood by herd owners. Likewise, herd owners must have a clear understanding of the following general facts about vaccination: (1) it does not always provide complete protection, (2) immunization is not always and completely safe, (3) immunization is a control rather than an eradication measure and (4) immunization supplements but does not substitute for sanitation and other prophylactic measures.

Every infection affecting reproduction is different etiologically and epidemiologically. Immunological properties and other characteristics of particular biologicals vary among diseases and among manufacturers. Likewise, there is great variation in managerial and breeding practices among herds. Therefore, immunization programs must be custom designed for individual herds.

IMPLEMENTATION

Once it is decided that immunization for a certain disease or diseases is indicated, plans must be made for implementation of the program. Selection of the proper antigen from the commercially available products is the first step. The product selected for leptospirosis vaccination must match the variant or serotype of the etiological agent. *Leptospira pomona* bacterin cannot be expected to prevent leptospirosis caused by the serotype *hardjo*. Immunological properties of the selected product, such as the time required to produce a protective level of anti-

bodies and the duration of induced immunity, are also important for planning.

There are modified live vaccines capable of inducing mild disease and causing maternal and fetal stress.

Safe and effective vaccination depends on the proper selection of animals to be immunized. Age, stage in the reproductive cycle (particularly pregnancy) and stress such as concurrent other disease, high production, transportation and so forth are important factors to consider.

A rational approach requires that each infection known to affect reproduction be considered individually by taking into account all the aforementioned factors and considerations before a complete program is prepared for a particular herd.

A summary of pertinent highlights regarding immunization for maximum reproductive performance is present in Table 1. This should be useful as a guide for designing vaccination programs. Review articles served as source materials.[1, 2]

REFERENCES

1. Kahrs, R.F.: Rational basis for an immunization program against the common diseases of the bovine respiratory tract. Can. Vet. J., *15*:252, 1974.
2. Zemjanis, R.: Vaccination for reproductive efficiency in cattle. JAVMA, *165*:689, 1974.

Use of Clinical Chemistry Techniques in the Investigation of Bovine Infertility

ELDEN G. LAMPRECHT
3M Center, St. Paul, Minnesota

The use of clinical chemistry techniques for the dairy cow is not new. Clinical chemistry test procedures have been run on serum for decades in the bovine species. The history of their use follows the development of individual metabolite tests for human medicine. Traditionally, a limited number of tests have been used in dairy cattle showing specific clinical signs of disease. An example is the measurement of serum calcium and

phosphorus levels in the downer cow syndrome.

In 1970 a multiple test profile concept was introduced to monitor the metabolic state of the dairy herd and, in particular, to assess the adequacy of dietary intake for production.[3] A flurry of investigative activity was stimulated throughout the world as a result of this. The literature suddenly contained recommendations concerning which chemistry tests to run, numbers of cows to sample, methods of reporting results and disease problems to investigate. Proponents of the concept soon produced numerous sets of blood chemistry test averages for cattle populations, which were represented as being industrial normal values.

Beneath the enthusiasm for this new concept was a general absence of coherent guidelines and indications for the use of the metabolic profile test in cattle. Normal sources of physiological variation were frequently not considered when reporting test results. Also absent was a universally recognized system of handling samples from the time of collection until laboratory results were returned. Some test results are affected by the anatomical site of sampling because of selective nutrient removal by vital organs that are drained by the respective blood vessels. Other serum metabolites exist in a dynamic state of equilibrium with blood cells. This makes proper sample handling critical. Often the laboratory performing the analysis is not the same one that published standard values. The choice of laboratory is another potential source of error if standardization procedures are not identical. The investigator must have a clearcut objective in mind and a rational means of interpreting the data generated before performing a multiple serum chemistry test.

PHYSIOLOGICAL SOURCES OF VARIATION

Much information has been accumulated on the effect of physiological and environmental factors on clinical chemistry and hematology test results in cattle. This is a confusing area to summarize because either the reasons for the changes in results are not understood or these changes cannot be consistently reproduced.

Increasing age of cattle is associated with changes in more test values than any other physical or environmental factor. Serum cholesterol concentrations increase with increasing age, with most of this change taking place by 3 years of age. Also, the albumin/globulin ratio decreases because of increasing globulin concentrations. The following tests show the opposite pattern of decreasing concentrations with increasing age: inorganic phosphorus, calcium, serum glutamic-pyruvic transaminase (SGPT) and alkaline phosphatase determinations. Many of these patterns of changes hold true for increasing lactation number as well as age.

The stage of lactation follows increasing age of the cow as a factor influencing chem-

istry values. Serum glutamic-oxaloacetic transaminase (SGOT) activity rises at parturition. This increase probably results from enzyme release following tissue damage at parturition. SGOT values remain high during the first stage of lactation and decrease to their lowest activity in the dry cow. Albumin concentrations follow the opposite pattern. They fall at calving and rise slowly during the first 120 days of lactation. Serum inorganic phosphorus and magnesium concentrations start to decrease 7 to 14 days before parturition. Calcium levels, on the other hand, decrease 12 per cent from dry period levels at 2 days' postpartum. This appears to be independent of dietary calcium intakes. Hemoglobin concentrations start to decline during late pregnancy. This trend continues during early lactation, with lowest concentrations being reached in the 30- to 100-day postpartum interval. It should be noted that most appreciable changes occur in blood metabolites during the 3 months both before and after parturition. This unfortunately is the time interval that the investigator is most interested in from a diagnostic viewpoint.

The season and environmental temperature appear to influence very few chemistry test results. Notable exceptions are SGOT and SGPT values, which are highest in the summer, and hematocrit values, which are depressed in hot weather possibly because of hemodilution.

One of the earlier objectives of the multiple chemistry profile test concept was to assess the adequacy of dietary intakes to meet production demands. Many metabolites have been investigated for their merit as indexes of micromineral, macromineral, protein and energy intake in production situations. However, only the serum urea nitrogen test has been shown to be of value, providing a rough estimation of nitrogen intake with respect to nitrogen utilization. Even this nutrient can be more easily and economically evaluated by calculating protein demand for production versus protein intake. Under conditions of experimental starvation or massive nutrient overage, deviations in the respective metabolite tests have been reported. These are not consistently reproducible and often apply to the specific set of circumstances under which the investigation was carried out.

The ability to identify individual cows that possess great potential for annual milk production at or before maturity has been an objective of biochemistry investigations. Reports occasionally appear in the scientific literature regarding association of biochemical values with high levels of milk production. Quite often the basis for these observations has been previously discussed sources of variation including age, lactation number and stage of lactation in which the cow was sampled. Notwithstanding serious attempts, it is presently not possible to predict individuals with superior milk production ability on the basis of a battery of chemistry test results.

SITE-OF-SAMPLING VARIATION

The composition of venous blood is in part dependent on the physiological demands of the anatomical region being drained. The jugular vein, the mammary vein and the coccygeal artery and vein have all been used as blood collection sites in establishing standard clinical values in cattle. Figure 1 summarizes the magnitude of the blood chemistry differences observed in a population of 10 dairy cows simultaneously sampled at each of the three anatomical sites. In light of the reported dairy cow population averages (Table 1), the differences in values among sample sites is great for albumin,

calcium, glucose, inorganic phosphorus, SGPT and total protein.

The mammary vein site is undesirable for obtaining blood samples for serum glucose and calcium because their concentrations are appreciably lower (approximately 45 per cent and 5 per cent, respectively) than at both the jugular vein and coccygeal vessel sites. Lower mammary vein glucose concentrations are a reflection of the high maintenance requirement of the mammary gland for glucose. The lower jugular vein levels of inorganic phosphorus and the large amount of dispersion among the inter-site ratios result in an average of 10 per cent (range of 5 to 15 per cent) lower concentration at the jugular vein site than at the coccygeal vein site. It is not unusual for jugular vein concentrations of inorganic phosphorus to be 0.7 mg/dl lower than the coccygeal vessel values within the same animal. These differences result from the removal of inorganic phosphorus from circulating blood while concentrating it in saliva.

SGPT enzyme shares a wide distribution within bovine tissues. The principal location and function of the enzyme are within the cell. Its presence in moderate activity levels in serum is a consequence of normal tissue destruction and subsequent enzyme release. Increased levels measured in serum are evidence of cellular injury. Jugular vein activities average 27 per cent higher (range to 52

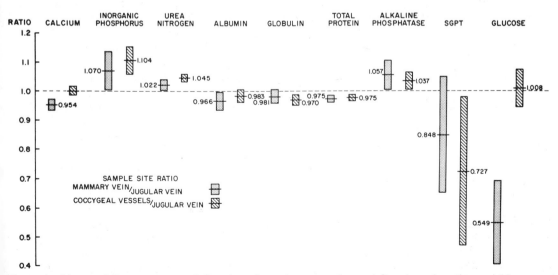

Figure 1. Means of the mammary vein/jugular vein and coccygeal vessels/jugular vein ratios and 95 per cent confidence limits of blood components in 10 dairy cows sampled simultaneously from the three anatomical sites. (All 95 per cent confidence limits of interlaboratory ratios including the ratio of 1.0 are considered to yield the same results. The intersite mean ratios × 100 equal the per cent results of the sites compared are of jugular vein reference values.)

TABLE 1. *Chemistry Test Means and Standard Limits from Blood and Serum of Four Dairy Cow Populations Reported by Separate Laboratories*

	California, USA[a]		Compton, England[b]		Minnesota, USA[c]		Pennsylvania, USA[d]	
	MEAN	1SD*	MEAN	2SD	MEAN	1SD	MEAN	1SD
Albumin gm/dl	3.7	0.3	3.2	0.5	3.1–3.7	0.6	2.74	0.30
Calcium mg/dl	9.3	0.6	9.5	0.8	9.01	0.58	9.31	0.69
Globulin gm/dl	4.8	0.7	4.4	1.2	–	–	4.82	0.76
Glucose mg/dl	–	–	45.0	8.5	74.0	11.0	–	–
Magnesium mg/dl	2.6	0.3	2.5	0.5	2.13	0.28	2.20	0.23
Phosphorus, inorganic mg/dl	5.4	0.9	6.0	1.7	5.74	1.13	6.03	1.07
Potassium mEq/L	5.1	0.6	5.0	0.7	4.60	0.39	5.12	0.50
Urea nitrogen mg/dl	18.0	6.0	14.5	5.0	15.0	3.0	–	–
Hematocrit %	33.0	3.0	32.5	5.5	31.4–34.8	3.5	32.27	3.10
Hemoglobin gm/dl	–	–	12.0	2.2	10.5–11.6	1.0	10.81	1.20

[a]Lamprecht, E.G.: PhD thesis, University of California, Davis, California, 1978.
[b]Rowlands, G.J. and Pocock, R.M.: Vet. Rec., *98*:333, 1976.
[c]Stevens, J.B.: An. Nut. Health, *30*(6):14, 1975.
[d]Stout, W.L., Kradel, D.C. and Jung, G.A. Pennsylvania State University Progress Report 358, 1976.
*SD = standard deviation.

per cent higher) than coccygeal vessel levels (Fig. 1). This increase in activity could be associated with tissue trauma resulting from nose-lead restraint. The large range of inter-site ratios probably indicates differing degrees of trauma experienced by individual restrained cows. Saliva production and the resulting hemoconcentration lead to higher jugular vein protein concentrations than at the other two sites. This difference is small but very important when compared with published population averages and ranges.

The results of samples from the coccygeal vessels give a better overall representation of most chemistry tests. This is especially true for serum calcium, glucose and inorganic phosphorus determinations. The coccygeal vessels are preferred because blood that either supplies or drains the tail is not affected by nutrient demands of organ systems involved with secretory processes.

SAMPLE HANDLING VARIATION

The chemical and enzymatic composition of blood represents a dynamic state of equilibrium between its cellular and fluid components. Once removed from an animal, the blood sample is subject to alterations in this equilibrium. The understanding of proper sample handling is important to obtaining interpretable laboratory results. There are two intervals of time that influence chemistry test results. The first is the sample handling time between the collection of blood and the separation of serum or plasma from

blood cells. The second is the storage time between separation of blood cells and analysis of the serum.

Hemolysis should be avoided initially during collection and processing of blood samples. Higher concentrations of magnesium, iron and potassium occur in red blood cells than in plasma. The opposite is true for calcium. Almost all serum enzymes are present in much higher concentrations in erythrocytes than in plasma. Any visible amount of hemolysis can produce elevated serum levels. Serum should be rapidly separated from the clot to prevent exchange of electrolytes from cells. This is especially critical for potassium because potassium ions are passively concentrated within red blood cells as a result of an active enzymatic extrusion of sodium ions. A much greater exchange of potassium ions occurs in clotted specimens stored at 4° C than at 25° C. This phenomenon results from a slowing down of the active enzymatic process responsible for maintaining a high extracellular sodium concentration at the cooler temperatures. Potassium then is not allowed to remain passively concentrated within the red blood cells. Leakage of potassium results in artificially higher serum concentrations. The clotted blood should be kept at room temperature if separation of red blood cells from serum must be delayed during transportation or storage.

Serum is an inappropriate specimen for glucose analysis. Initially glucose concentrations are higher in serum than in whole blood. Glycolysis by red blood cells rapidly depletes serum glucose in the sample. The process is slowed by refrigeration and can be stopped for 8 to 12 hours at room temperature or for 48 hours of refrigeration by using an enzyme inhibitor such as sodium fluoride anticoagulant.

The red blood cell maintains a higher level of calcium in plasma than in blood cells.When adenosine triphosphate (ATP) is depleted, the cell can no longer maintain this gradient and calcium moves passively toward equilibrium into the cell. This phenomenon does not happen until after 12 hours storage at 37° C.

Following separation of serum from blood cells, enzyme activities of serum and plasma are still subject to change over the storage time period. SGOT, SGPT, lactic dehydrogenase (LDH) and alkaline phosphatase are stable at room temperature for at least 8 hours, for at least 8 days at 4° C and for 1 month or longer when frozen. Either plasma or serum may be used for enzyme determinations. The suitability of plasma depends on the type of anticoagulant used. Anticoagulants containing enzyme inhibitors, such as sodium fluoride, or metal chelates, such as EDTA, must be avoided. LDH loses activity in oxylated plasma. Serum sodium, phosphorus, calcium, magnesium and iron are not affected by storage at room temperature for at least 8 hours, refrigerated for 1 day or frozen for 1 year. If the sample is left refrigerated or at room temperature for several days, the precipitation of protein or growth of microbiological contaminants may interfere with precise measurements.

CHOICE-OF-LABORATORY VARIATION

The mean values of a sampled cow population are compared with average values of a much larger cow population in the proposed clinical application of the metabolic profile test. Table 1 lists four reports of chemistry test means and standard deviations derived from four dairy cow populations analyzed by four laboratories. The marked differences in mean values raise the possibility of the following sources of variation among the four locations: Actual differences in serum metabolite levels in the population of cows, standardization differences among the investigating laboratories or some combination of these.

The control of accuracy and precision in clinical chemistry technology is the most pressing problem in providing useful clinical laboratory results for the clinician. Precision is defined as a closeness of agreement between repeated assays of the same specimen; accuracy is the closeness with which the results of a given test on a known specimen agree with the true value. Precision is established within the laboratory by repeated analysis of known laboratory standards followed by equipment calibration. Accuracy is checked among laboratories by running replicate samples or standard reagent blanks. Automation has had a positive influence on precision within the clinical chemistry laboratory. It has eliminated much of the tedium of repetitive procedures while making many tests more affordable. Figure 2 illustrates that evidence of high precision obtained for test results from three different laboratories was a very narrow 95 per cent confidence limit of interlaboratory ratios. Data were based on 10 tests on replicate serum samples from 180 dairy cows (five herds) submitted to the laboratories. This clue of high precision was seen more often for the two fully automated laboratories (A and B) than for the conventional laboratory (C).

The standardization among clinical chemistry laboratories has been a longstanding problem. A result of this problem is a lack of agreement, or low accuracy among laboratories. None of the ten chemistry tests met the requirements of accuracy defined by capturing 1.0 within the 95 per cent confidence limits of the ratios for both interlaboratory comparisons. Two laboratories gave comparable results on only three tests (SGOT, globulin and total protein). Six of the 20 test ratio means differed from the reference laboratory by at least 10 per cent.

The choice of laboratory to which the field investigator sends serum samples will have a definite effect on the results received. For results to be meaningful and interpretable among laboratories, each lab offering a profile service should consider one of the following: (1) establishing a data bank by using intralaboratory population averages and standard limits, (2) recognizing a reference laboratory and establishing a bias factor adjustment for each metabolite in the blood chemistry profile or (3) using a universally recognized control substance to achieve standardization among laboratories.

The choice of laboratory subjects test results to another related source of variation

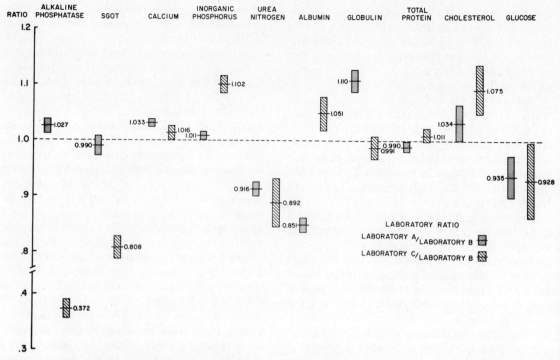

Figure 2. Means of interlaboratory ratios and 95 per cent confidence limits of blood components for 180 cows from five dairy herds analyzed by three laboratories. (All 95 per cent confidence limits of interlaboratory ratios including the ratio of 1.0 are considered to yield the same results. The interlaboratory mean ratios × 100 equal the per cent results of the laboratory compared are of laboratory B reference values.)

called herd by laboratory interaction. Both dairy herds and laboratories influence test results of metabolite concentrations in serum because of physiological variation and accuracy, respectively. The metabolite concentration levels maintained by dairy herds are, however, not consistently reflected by laboratory test sample means (Fig. 3). From the time of sample collection until results are reported, many steps can contribute to herd by laboratory interaction.

RELATIONSHIPS BETWEEN BLOOD COMPOSITION AND FERTILITY

A limited number of published field investigations have linked specific nutritional deficiencies to decreased reproductive efficiency by use of their respective serum metabolite levels. One example of this was the increased number of services per conception in heifers that had low levels of blood phosphorus along with a deficiency of dietary phosphorus. Similar reports describe infertility problems linked to overages and deficiencies in protein intake as reflected by

serum urea nitrogen and serum protein concentrations. Improperly balanced dry cow rations have been demonstrated to cause secondary effects on serum enzyme and cholesterol levels. SGOT and cholesterol tests have been used to predict increased risk of postpartum disease.

Somewhat less optimistic results have been obtained following the use of the multiple chemistry test concept in evaluating the nutritional etiology of infertility problems. Blood chemistry, nutrition, milk production and fertility were monitored and their relationships examined in groups of cows from 15 commercial dairy herds.[2] Plasma urea nitrogen, albumin, glucose, nonesterified fatty acids, acetone, calcium, magnesium inorganic phosphorus, blood copper, hemoglobin and packed cell volume were examined in relation to dietary intakes. Within the dietary ranges examined, the dietary calcium-to-phosphorus ratio appeared to have no effect on fertility. No significant differences were found in the other blood components for results of first and second services. For the ranges of blood components and nutrient intake levels recorded, there was little apparent correlation with fertility, and little

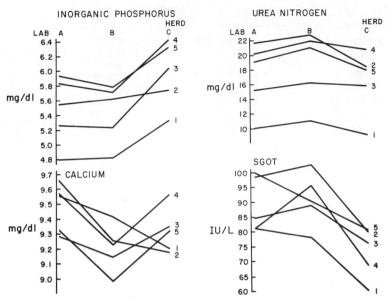

Figure 3. Examples of herd by laboratory interaction for four chemistry tests run of 36 cows from each of five dairy herds by three laboratories.

indication could be found for optimum blood component concentrations near service for maximum fertility. Abnormal blood component values may sometimes draw attention to a possible nutritional defect that can be confirmed by conventional methods, but abnormal values are not necessarily undesirable nor are normal values always consistent with an optimum situation. An oversimplified interpretation of blood analytical data in isolation may lead to erroneous conclusions.

The incidence of metabolic disturbances in dairy cows is highest during the period commencing with parturition and continues until peak lactation. This is the time period in which predictive tests have their greatest potential for recognizing imminent problems while still allowing time for ration changes and other relevant corrective measures.

The predictive value of the metabolic profile test concept for fertility complications was clinically evaluated in 10 high-producing California dairy herds.[1] A total of 800 cows were sampled and the following tests run: hematocrit, serum albumin, alkaline phosphatase, calcium, cholesterol, inorganic phosphorus, magnesium, potassium, SGOT, SGPT, total bilirubin, total protein and urea nitrogen. The laboratory results from cows with normal reproductive histories were compared with results from those

experiencing the specific reproductive abnormalities of retained placenta, abnormal vaginal discharge and repeat breeding. The mean values for the individual clinical chemistry tests for cows experiencing reproductive diseases were not appreciably different to discriminate them from the population of normal cows. The multiple chemistry profile test concept offered no advantage in detecting cows subject to reproductive diseases. Low predictive values were due primarily to the lack of sensitivity, that is, the lack of the ability to identify cows later affected by reproductive diseases. Neither the individual chemistry tests nor the series of tests were able to characterize cows subject to retained placenta, abnormal vaginal discharge or repeat breeding.

Reports in the scientific literature have and will continue to link high or low levels of blood components with susceptibility to metabolic diseases. This is not surprising because it is not difficult to find test values for either individual cows or herd means that are outside standard limits regardless of the metabolic disease status of the herd. Herds tend to have characteristic values for certain blood constituents. This effect is most pronounced in samples taken during the winter and tends to recur in successive winters.

At present, the multiple chemistry test concept is not a good substitute for a complete clinical investigation of herds experiencing infertility. The future of the metabolic profile test hinges on the development of new chemistry tests that have the ability to describe the cow's environment more inexpensively than traditional means. Ration analysis and balancing remain the investigative procedures of choice if nutritional influences are suspected to affect reproductive efficiency.

REFERENCES

1. Lamprecht, E. G.: An evaluation of the metabolic profile test predictive value for post partum disease and sources of error in field applications of clinical chemistry and hematology tests in dairy cows. PhD thesis, University of California, Davis, California, 1978.
2. Parker, B. N. and Blowey, R. W.: Investigations into the relationship of selected blood components to nutrition and fertility of the dairy cow under commercial farm conditions. Vet. Rec., *98*:394, 1976.
3. Payne, J. M., Dew, S. M., Manston, R. and Faulks, M.: The use of a metabolic profile test in dairy cows. Vet. Rec., *87*:150, 1970.

Estrous Detection in Cattle

HOWARD L. WHITMORE
University of Minnesota, St. Paul, Minnesota

DEFINITION

Estrous detection is a major problem for all dairymen using artificial insemination (AI). Most dairymen have cows that calve each month and cows to inseminate each month, and so estrous detection is a year-round task. Because the length of gestation is fixed, the calving interval depends on how soon cows are inseminated and become pregnant following calving. Recent studies show that the calving to first-service interval is 85 to 90 days. In order for cows to maintain a 12-month calving interval, this interval should be 70 days or less. Many dairymen apparently understand that most cows are cycling and that the primary problem is failure to observe estrus. Veterinarians who have personally spent time (by the clock) checking cows for estrus by visual observation know how boring and unrewarding the task is and can readily sympathize with dairymen. It is surprising how many days it rains, snows or is very hot, cold or windy, resulting in reduced mounting activity. However, the role of the practitioner is to explain to dairymen the extreme economic importance of the rather dull task of estrous detection to an artificial insemination program. If dairymen elect to use AI, they should understand that they must be willing to commit some of their time to estrous detection.

CLINICAL SIGNS OF ESTRUS

The signs of estrus can be divided into primary and secondary behavioral traits. The primary and most important signs of true estrus is the cow's *standing firm* (all four legs braced) while being mounted by another cow. This is the only sign that indicates true estrus and occurs only during the period of true estrus. Secondary signs of estrus include mounting of other cows, swollen vulva, mucous discharge, hyperactivity and bellowing. These secondary signs of estrus can be present before, during and after the period of standing heat. Diarymen should be advised that at least 90 per cent of their cows should be inseminated on the basis of standing heat. A few cows may have to be inseminated on the basis of secondary estrous signs if standing heat cannot be detected. Cattle inseminated on the basis of primary heat signs (standing firm) usually have high pregnancy rates, whereas those inseminated on the basis of secondary heat signs usually have lower pregnancy rates and frequently result in repeat breeder problems. Some dairymen who are experiencing poor breeding results with AI state that estrous detection is a minor problem and that repeat breeders are their major problem. Many times in this situation, dairymen are inseminating cows on the basis of secondary heat signs so that in reality the main problem is faulty heat detection. When veterinarians are searching for causes of repeat breeders, they should always determine whether primary or secondary heat signs are being used as the basis for AI.

METHODS OF ESTROUS DETECTION

Visual Observation

The best and most common method of estrous detection may be direct visual observation of a cow standing firm while being mounted by another cow. Studies show that twice-daily visual observation of herds detects 90 per cent of the cows that are cycling. However, there is much variation among dairymen. A few dairymen can achieve a 1-year calving interval with only once-a-day heat checks, whereas many dairymen detect only 60 per cent of their cows in estrus with two or three daily heat checks. Veterinarians should be aware of this great difference among dairymen and should try to give repeated individualized advice to those having problems with the visual method of heat detection.

Many dairymen using stanchion barns are not willing to let their cows out of the stanchion for estrous detection. Therefore, cows are checked for heat and inseminated on the basis of secondary signs of estrus observed while the animals are in stanchions. Some dairymen using this method achieve fairly satisfactory reproductive performance, whereas others have moderate to severe problems with missed heats and low conception rates. Veterinarians should be acutely aware of this type of problem and should try to determine what individualized type of advice might be followed. Grouping cows by reproductive status, turning out selected cows once or twice daily, predicting estrus by rectal palpation and placing breeding dates above the stalls may be helpful.

Several studies have been performed in which cows in loose housing were observed continuously (24 hours per day) for estrous behavior. These studies showed that 70 per cent of mounting interactions between cows occurred between 6:00 PM and 6:00 AM, whereas only 30 per cent occurred during the daytime hours. This emphasizes the importance of the time of day during which heat checks should be performed.

Visual observation for estrus may be a boring task for dairymen, but it is vital to the success of any AI program. Veterinarians should probably urge herd owners to offer monetary incentives to employees responsible for estrous detection and for cows gotten pregnant by AI. In problem herds, this may be the most effective method of achieving satisfactory reproductive efficiency.

Heat Detection Aids

There are several types of heat detector aids that can be used to augment direct visual observation, particularly in dairies using loose housing. One of the more common heat detection aids is the heat mount detector patch. These patches, containing a small plastic capsule of red dye, are glued to the rump of each cow. When the cow is in heat and stands to be mounted, pressure from the mounting animal ruptures the capsule of red dye and changes the color of the detector patch to bright red.

Australian researchers compared four different methods of heat detection in a large group of cows during a 21-day period. The methods were: (1) heat mount detector patches, (2) team watching 24 hours per day, (3) herdsmen checking twice daily and (4) two dairymen checking at milking. The proportion of cows detected in heat by each method was 98, 89, 56 and 56 per cent, respectively. When heat mount detector patches are properly used, they are very helpful, particularly in catching the cows that may have short estrous periods during the night. These patches are not a substitute for good management but are useful in helping to detect normal and problem cows. Patches may be applied to all cows ready for breeding, and following breeding a new patch may be applied to help detect cows that do not become pregnant.

Another heat detection aid is the use of "marker bulls." These bulls have been surgically prepared to prevent mating and possible spread of disease. The bulls are fitted with a halter that contains a marking device under the chin. When the bull mounts a cow that is in standing heat, marks are applied over the cow's back and shoulders. A study was performed comparing use of dairymen watching for signs of heat 30 minutes twice daily with use of a marker bull for 1 hour twice daily. The dairymen detected 72 per cent of the cows in heat, and the marker bull found 87 per cent in heat. When marker bulls are properly prepared and carefully managed, they are a valuable heat detection aid for certain dairymen. Steers and cows that have been treated with testosterone to induce mounting behavior (discussed in an earlier article) compare favorably with marker bulls for detection of estrus.

Another heat detection aid that appears to be gaining popularity is the practice of putting a fresh yellow chalk mark on each cow's tailhead each morning. This is done while cows are at the feed bunk or locked in stanchions for feeding. Cows whose chalk marks have been rubbed off are assumed to have been in standing heat during the previous 24 hours. Selection of a chalk that rubs off easily appears to work better than paint sticks or crayon-like marking chalks.

HORMONAL INDUCTION OF ESTRUS

Prostaglandin (presently available in some countries) appears to be the drug of choice to induce estrus in cattle. It can effectively cause regression of the mature corpus luteum and induce estrus in 48 to 96 hours. Fertility of cows with induced estrus compares favorably with fertility of control cows. Although estrogens have been widely utilized for induction of estrus, their use for this purpose has been questioned. Recent reports indicate that estrogen is of no, or questionable, value and may actually reduce the conception rate compared with rates for uninjected controls. Estrogen has been shown to cause partial luteal regression during the first 10 days of the estrous cycle and to produce cystic ovaries when injected in cows during the last half of the cycle. Because of the risk of producing cystic ovaries and lowering conception rates, estrogens should no longer be used for induction of estrus.

Numerous hormonal and miscellaneous treatments have been used for anestrus. However, because most cows are cycling normally, better methods of estrous detection are usually the treatment of choice.

IMPROVING ESTROUS DETECTION

It may be helpful to review the following list of management factors with all new dairymen and with those having problems detecting estrus.

1. Identify all cows by using visible neck chains, ear tags or brands. Accurate identification of cows is a very important and sometimes difficult procedure in large herds. It is essential that all cows can be easily identified from a distance so that all heat dates can be recorded.

2. Enter all cows on a barn breeding chart at the time of calving instead of at the time of breeding. If cows are entered in chronological order at calving, with heat and breeding dates recorded as they occur, problem cows can be readily detected by looking at the chart. Such cows should receive a veterinary examination, diagnosis and treatment, if indicated, to gain conception by 85 to 100 days after calving.

3. Make one person responsible for heat detection. This employee should be a very responsible and conscientious individual, such as the herdsman. It may be advisable to offer a bonus for every cow that is pregnant by 100 days after calving. Many dairymen having herds with heat detection problems have failed to delegate this responsibility to one individual. This is a very common mistake in herds with infertility problems. On many large farms, all employees are expected to watch cows for heat, with each one assuming that the other one is doing it.

4. Recognize the signs of heat. The final criterion of heat is the cow that stands to be mounted by another animal. Standing heat usually last for 8 to 18 hours. The highest conception rate occurs when cows are bred in the middle of or late in standing heat.

5. Spend 20 to 30 minutes observing cows for heat early in the morning and late in the evening. This can be the most profitable time spent during the entire day. Cows are more likely to show heat at these times than during the day, especially during hot weather.

6. Observe cows for heat when they are moving. There is greater tendency for cows to show heat when they are going to or from the milking parlor or the feeding and loafing area. Pastured animals are more likely to show heat when being moved to or from the pasture.

7. Observe cows for heat before feeding. An ideal time is while they are waiting to be fed after leaving the parlor. It is a waste of time to observe cows just after hay or silage has been placed in the bunk. If the feed bunks are routinely filled while the cows are being milked, they should be observed for heat before milking. It may be advisable to postpone feeding for 20 minutes after milking to observe cows for heat while they are

waiting to be fed. A busy person watching cows while they are busy eating will not be very successful in detecting heat.

8. Record *all* heat and breeding dates on a heat expectancy chart. This chart should be located at the entrance to the barn or in another readily available place to remind employees to observe cows for heat. The chart serves as a reminder of animals that are close to heat and need careful observation. Many dairymen do not record early heats; however, these dates may be beneficial at a later time.

9. Heat detection is just as important after breeding as before breeding. Approximately 40 per cent of the cows will fail to conceive following first service; however, cows are frequently not observed as carefully for heat after breeding as they were before breeding. All cows should receive a veterinary examination to confirm pregnancy as soon as possible after breeding. If pregnancy diagnosis is performed early after breeeding, it will still be economical to treat and rebreed those cows detected open.

CONCLUSIONS

Estrous detection is a continuous task for dairymen using AI. Dairymen must recognize that good estrous detection is the key to reproductive efficiency in an AI program. Direct visual observation of a cow *standing firm* while being mounted by another cow should probably be the primary method used for estrous detection. Heat detector patches, marker bulls and chalk marks applied to tailheads appear to be satisfactory methods of assisting management in detection of estrus. Cows inseminated on the basis of primary heat signs (standing firm) have high pregnancy rates, whereas those inseminated on the basis of secondary heat signs have lower pregnancy rates that may result in a repeat breeder problem.

REFERENCES

1. Barr, H. L.: Influence of estrus detection on days open to dairy herds. J. Dairy Sci., *58*:246, 1975.
2. King, G. J., Hurnik, J. F. and Robertson, H. A.: Ovarian function and estrus in dairy cows during early lactation. J. Anim. Sci., *42*:688, 1976.
3. Williamson, N. B., Morris, R. S., Blood, D. C. and Cannon, C. M.: A study of estrous behavior and estrus detection methods in a large commercial dairy herd. Vet. Rec., *91*:50, 1972.

Early Postpartum Breeding

HOWARD L. WHITMORE

University of Minnesota, St. Paul, Minnesota

Breeding cows at less than 60 days following calving is a subject of much concern for dairymen, artificial insemination (AI) organizations and veterinarians. Early postpartum breeding has been reported to actually lengthen the calving interval rather than shorten it and to be detrimental to the later reproductive life of cows. Close examination of the very limited studies concerning the dangers of early breeding revealed that these studies were not planned experiments but were primarily opinions expressed on the basis of retrospective interpretation of herd breeding records. It was also possible that some of these herds could have been experiencing venereal disease. Other studies have clearly shown that first service pregnancy rates are higher if breeding is delayed 60 to 90 days following calving. Based on these reports and the fact that some AI organizations offered repeat inseminations at no charge, it was logical for the AI industry to strongly recommend that breeding of dairy cattle should not begin for at least 60 days following calving. These recommendations were followed for many years.

During the 1960's, investigators and dairymen began to question whether or not the advantages of early postpartum breeding might outweigh the disadvantages. The availability of detailed breeding records from a large number of herds made it possible to evaluate total reproductive performance of cows bred at various intervals after calving.

EVALUATIONS OF HERD BREEDING RECORDS

A study in Kentucky on more than 36,000 cows evaluated the effect of breeding at consecutive 10-day intervals after calving on fertility and calving interval. The number of services per conception declined from 1.69 to 1.36 as the interval from calving to breeding increased from 21 to 30 days after calving to 121 to 130 days postpartum. The length of the calving interval increased from 343 days to 423 days as the interval from calving to breeding increased from 21 to 30 days after calving to 121 to 130 days postpartum. This study indicated that breeding cows at 40 instead of 60 days after calving would increase the mean number of services only about 0.08 per cow and would shorten the calving interval by 15 days. It was not clear from this study whether early postpartum breeding influenced the incidence of nonbreeders.

A study in Israel on more than 39,000 cows showed that earlier postpartum breeding resulted in shorter calving intervals. The average interval to first insemination decreased from 78 days during the first year of the study to 61 days during the fourth year. This reduced the interval between calvings from 385 to 376 days. Thus, for each day sooner after calving that cows were inseminated, the calving interval was shortened by 0.54 day. Although the cows were bred approximately 6 days earlier each year of this 4-year study, the percentage of cows not pregnant by day 150 after calving did not change. Thus, there did not appear to be a detrimental effect from early breeding based on the percentage cows pregnant at 150 days.

EXPERIMENTAL EVALUATION OF EARLY POSTPARTUM BREEDING

Studies in Wisconsin were specifically designed to evaluate the long-term effects of early postpartum breeding on reproductive characteristics in consecutive calving intervals. A herd of approximately 75 dairy cows was randomized into two groups. Group 1 cows were inseminated at the first observed estrus following calving (early breeding), and group 2 cows were inseminated at the first observed estrus after 74 days postpartum (late breeding). The study was performed over 7 consecutive years (1965 to 1972). The herd was on a weekly schedule of palpation of the reproductive organs *per rectum* to closely monitor their reproductive performance.

The results of this experiment are presented in Table 1. The fertility at first insemination for the early breeding group was 37 per cent, whereas it was 67 per cent for the late breeding group. The number of inseminations per pregnancy was higher for the early breeding group compared with the late bred group (2.2 versus 1.6 inseminations). However, the number of open days was much less for the early breeding group compared with the late bred group (64 versus 101 days). Statistical evaluation of these three endpoints showed highly significant differences between breeding groups. Significant differences were not found for the incidence of lost pregnancies, retained placenta, acute metritis, dystocia, twins, abortions and nonbreeders between the two groups.

The conclusions from this experiment were that early postpartum breeding could

TABLE 1. *Average Values of Different Reproductive Endpoints for Two Different Intervals of Postpartum Breeding*

Reproductive Endpoints	Bred at First Observed Estrus Following Calving	Bred at First Observed Estrus After 74 Days Postpartum
No. of calving intervals	184	180
Fertility at first insemination (%)	37	67*
Inseminations per pregnancy	2.2	1.6*
No. of open days	64	101*
Lost pregnancies (%)	2	5
Retained placenta (%)	15	9
Acute metritis (%)	6	3
Dystocia (%)	4	3
Twins (%)	5	1
Abortions (%)	3	3
Nonbreeders (%)	4	4

*Statistically significant, P < 0.005

definitely be used to shorten the calving interval and that repeated early breedings over consecutive calving intervals did not have a detrimental effect on the later reproductive life of cows. Breeding cows sooner after calving does require more services per conception because fertility is lower. Thus dairymen can compare the economics of a shorter calving interval with the cost of semen to assist in making their management decision of when to start breeding following calving.

CALVING INTERVAL AND MILK PRODUCTION

It is quite clear that shorter calving intervals result in higher average milk production per day of the calving interval. Studies on nearly 5000 completed lactations in North Carolina herds show that there was an average decrease of 2.4 kg of milk for each additional day open. Days open did not affect first calf heifers in the same manner as older cows. This study showed an actual increase of 1.16 kg of milk for each additional day open for first lactations and a decrease of 3.58 and 3.68 kg of milk for each additional day open for second and third lactations, respectively. This differential response for first calf heifers was attributed to their higher persistency and needs for growth. Based on these results, the authors suggested that a calving interval of 13 months for first calvers and 12 months for second and later calvers may be the optimum length for attaining maximum milk production. Other studies indicate that milk production per day of calving interval will

increase for each day that the calving interval is shortened, at least to 11 months. Additional studies would help to clarify if 11-month calving intervals give greater daily milk yields compared with 12-month calving intervals, especially in high-producing herds.

The optimum length of the dry period has been reported to be 40 to 45 days. Dry periods of less than 40 days result in a decrease in the next lactation milk yields, whereas dry periods longer than 45 days reduce daily milk yields.

CONCLUSIONS

Breeding cows sooner after calving has been shown to shorten the calving interval and thereby increase milk production. The only detrimental effect observed was a slight increase in services per conception when cows were bred at 40 days instead of 60 days following calving. Veterinarians can recommend to clients that cows found to be normal on the 30-day postpartum examination be bred after 45 days postpartum.

REFERENCES

1. Britt, J. H.: Early postpartum breeding in dairy cows. A review. J. Dairy Sci., *58*:266, 1975.
2. Louca, A. and Legates, J. E.: Production losses in dairy cattle due to days open. J. Dairy Sci., *51*:573, 1968.
3. Olds, D. and Cooper, T.: Effect of postpartum rest period in dairy cattle on the occurrence of breeding abnormalities and on calving intervals. JAVMA, *157*:92, 1970.
4. Whitmore, H. L., Tyler, W. J. and Casida, L. E.: Effects of early postpartum breeding in dairy cattle. J. Anim. Sci., *38*:339, 1974.

Reproductive Management of Large Dairy Herds

JOHN M. WOODS
Mesa, Arizona

T. H. HOWARD
Colorado State University,
Fort Collins, Colorado

OBJECTIVES

All objectives are subordinate to the economic success of the dairyman. Animal health exists for and is justified by the maximization of profit. Accordingly, the medical soundness of any therapeutic or management procedure must be subordinate to its economic soundness.

Management and medical techniques should provide the normal cow with the greatest possible opportunity to achieve a short calving interval. Reproductive health programs are designed for the benefit of dairymen, not cows. By exerting management pressure on natural reproductive phenomena, the animals are forced to perform efficiently. The cow is reliable; she can be depended upon to cycle and conceive with acceptable efficiency if management can identify and control the human errors that are responsible for her prolonged calving intervals. This means that fertile semen must be delivered to a healthy uterus at the right time.

The cow with a reproductive disorder should be given ample opportunity to achieve an acceptable calving interval within time limits necessary for profitability. Her disorder should be detected early and timely therapy instituted. Therapeutic heroics for chronically infertile cows constitute an unsound practice. A pregnancy initiated late in lactation contributes nothing to the dairyman other than a few extra pounds of gross weight at slaughter.

Maximum utilization of available labor is necessary to multiply the theriogenologist's efforts. The owner or manager and labor force must be systematically trained and retrained in the techniques necessary to perform their jobs. This performance should be regularly and objectively evaluated.

We have assumed for purposes of this article that the following conditions necessary for success of the program have been met: There is adequate nutrition for cycling and conception, housing or drylot facilities have been provided and the cows are free from infectious disease. The philosophy and techniques described have evolved under the conditions of drylot management systems typical of southern California, Arizona and New Mexico.

METHODS

Adequate facilities must exist to restrain large numbers of cattle in a short time with little manpower. Under drylot conditions, lockable stanchions at the manger are most successful (Fig. 1). Cows are locked in the stanchions each morning for insemination, application of heat detection aids or genital examination.

Cow identification by ear tag and record-keeping by individual cow cards are the systems most compatible with the lockable stanchion facility. Cards are kept in a vehicle in the alley in front of the manger, and card entries are made at the time that each procedure is carried out (Figs. 2 and 3).

Records have no value unless they are used to understand and control herd performance. Cows should be segregated by their reproductive status for most efficient heat detection. For management purposes, the important parameters are calving interval, average days in milk at first service, first service conception rate and culling percentage for reproductive inefficiency. These data can be obtained from electronic data processing (EDP) records of herds following official tests. The exhaustive herd summary and individual records provided by the EDP centers make this system indispensable to large herds.

After each herd check, the veterinarian should compute the 24-day heat detection percentage and percentage of cows presented for pregnancy diagnosis and found to be open. He should also satisfy himself that EDP entries are properly made, particularly if there is absentee ownership. The goals

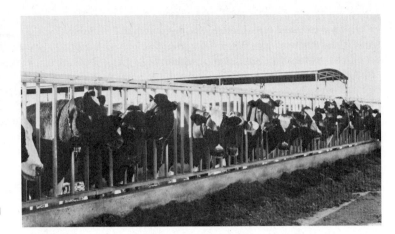

Figure 1. Cows are restrained daily in lockable stanchions.

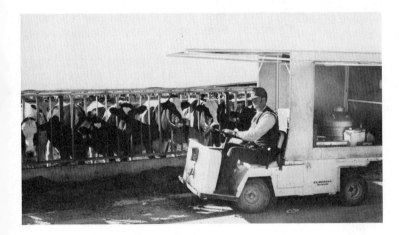

Figure 2. A vehicle equipped with all records, breeding equipment and supplies.

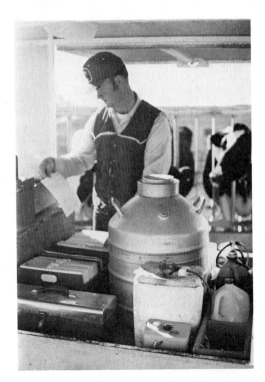

Figure 3. All events and treatments are immediately recorded on the cow cards.

for these parameters are listed in Figure 4.

The most important records for evaluation of herdsman performance are the 24-day heat detection checklist, percentage of cows diagnosed open and the monthly conception rate of each inseminator. The manager and veterinarian should review these records each month.

THE ROLES OF PHYSICAL DIAGNOSIS AND THERAPY

We will not repeat the appropriate therapies for reproductive dysfunction described elsewhere in this volume. In large herds it is crucial that early, accurate diagnoses be made, since the opportunity for observation of individual cows is not as great as in smaller units. Wholesale intrauterine antibacterial treatment is not the basis for efficient reproduction. Under conditions found in the southwestern United States, the authors have *never* observed a herd problem when nonvenereal uterine infection or hormonal dysfunction was the principal cause of loss. Wholesale treatment is a waste of herdsman and veterinarian time.

Early detection and treatment of metritis by competent herdsmen should be encouraged. At each visit, the veterinarian should examine all postpartum cows regardless of interval, in order to achieve the earliest possible detection of metritis. Nonirritating broad-spectrum antibiotic preparations should be administered to infected cows, using clean equipment. Problem cows should be re-examined as frequently as economic considerations and herd visitations permit.

All cows inseminated 30 days or more previously should be examined for pregnancy. Pregnancy should be reconfirmed at 60 to 90 days of gestation and again just before the cow is dried off.

QUALITY CONTROL OF HUMAN FACTORS

The ability of good heat detection procedures to achieve efficient reproduction can be illustrated by the following example: Assume two herds have 100 open cows each. Each herd has 60 per cent conception at first service, but dairymen detect 90 per cent of the cows in heat in Herd A and only 70 per cent in Herd B. The numbers of cows expected to become pregnant in each herd during one 21-day interval are as follows:

Herd A: 90 detected × 60 per cent conception = 54 cows pregnant
Herd B: 70 detected × 60 per cent conception = 42 cows pregnant

To achieve optimum detection and conception rates, visual observation of standing heat is necessary. This not only identifies the cow but establishes more precisely the best time for insemination. The adequacy of the amount of time spent in observing the cows is determined by the results obtained.

Heat detection aids are useful if excessive dependence on them is avoided. The most successful method in drylots with lockable stanchions is daily application of marking paint (All-Weather Paint Stik) to the tailhead (Fig. 5). Kamar patches can also be used. Remember however, that smeared pigment or a red Kamar can indicate three potential states: proestrus (as high as 15 to 20 per cent), estrus or metestrus, particularly if the aids are poorly monitored. The Kamar patches can be lost during estrus, especially if applied when the hair is wet or has been clipped.

Teaser animals are another heat detection aid. If the cow:teaser ratio exceeds 40:1, some cows will not be marked. Chin

CALVING INTERVAL:
13 months maximum

24-DAY HEAT DETECTION:
90% of eligible cows

DAYS OPEN AT FIRST SERVICE:
Desired interval + 11 days
For example, a herd starting rebreeding at
50 days postpartum has a goal of 61 days

FIRST SERVICE CONCEPTION RATE:
55% minimum

COWS EXAMINED FOR PREGNANCY
AND FOUND OPEN:
15% maximum

CULLING % FOR REPRODUCTIVE INEFFICIENCY:
6% maximum

% OF HERD PREGNANT WITH
THREE OR FEWER SERVICES:
88%
Figure 4. Herd reproductive performance goals.

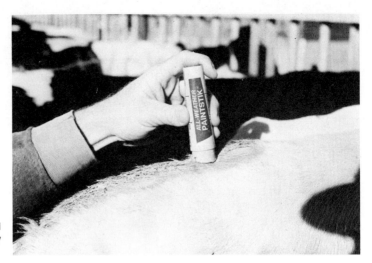

Figure 5. Marking paint is applied to the tailhead of each cow every morning.

ball marks require interpretation. The long stripes on the withers and loin are most significant and the short ones on the rump least significant. Techniques for preparation of teaser bulls that leave any possibility of intromission are unacceptable.

Heat detection is a duty that cannot be totally automated nor left to incompetent personnel. The *only* assurance of consistency is regular use of a 24-day heat detection checklist. This checklist should not be used merely to summarize past success or failure. Rather, it should be used to assess heat detection efficiency on a current basis. For example, if there are 100 eligible cows at least 45 days postpartum and one assumes that 5 per cent are not cycling and 5 per cent of heats go undetected, the remaining 90 cows should all be detected in 24 days, an average of 3.7 cows per day, or 30 cows by day 8, 59 cows by day 16 and 90 cows by day 24. If the herdsmen are lagging behind the minimum at day 8 or 16, something can still be done to improve their future performance.

Most large dairies in the southwest United States inseminate cows once daily when the cows are locked in the stanchions. Usually all cows observed in standing heat in the previous 24 hours are inseminated each morning. Far too many dairymen agonize over precise timing of insemination, rather than trying to breed only the cows that are truly in heat. If the records indicate 7 per cent or more of estrous cycle lengths are short and 7 per cent or more are long, this usually

means that many nonestrous cows are being inseminated.

All cows in heat that have reached the desired postpartum interval should be inseminated regardless of their medical history. Certainly cows with a history of recent metritis or other problems may not conceive at a high rate, but an additional 21 days of being open is a certainty if they are not inseminated: better a 90 per cent chance for a 40-dollar loss than a 100 per cent chance. Semen costs are much lower than days open. Postbreeding infusion with appropriate antibiotics may enhance the conception rate of cows with recent metritis.

Managers of herds using artificial insemination should test the semen placement proficiency of each inseminator by utilizing the dye test in extirpated genital tracts at least twice yearly. Retraining in sanitation and semen handling techniques should also be done at this time. Not everyone can successfully inseminate cows. Each inseminator's monthly conception rate should be computed and those whose performance is consistently low should be replaced.

Dairymen should demand responsible, consistent semen quality control. Nonreturn rates are a useful guide to rank the fertility of bulls, but they should not be considered pregnancy rate goals. Some dairymen in large herds regularly summarize first service conception rates within the herd by the performance of the bull and use the results as a guide to future semen purchases. Remember, not every bull nor every ejaculate is suitable for artificial insemination use.

Labor should be devoted to recently postpartum normal cows. A maximum heat detection and insemination effort should be made for this group. Chronically infertile cows should be grouped with a cleanup bull. It is a misapplication of labor resources to expend time on such animals. We recommend use of young (less than 2 years old) semen-tested bulls from within the herd. Herd owners or managers using natural service or those that purchase replacements should have all cows vaccinated for vibriosis postpartum.

CONCLUSION

Good reproductive efficiency in large herds can be achieved by the execution of certain fundamentals. First, the burden of achieving good reproductive performance should be shifted from the cow to the dairyman — recognize human error as the principal cause of losses and control it. Second, maintain good records and use them to group cows by reproductive status. Finally, expend time and labor resources on those animals that will return the most, i.e., the recently parturient normal cows. If the dairyman or veterinarian fails to master these fundamentals, sophistication in secondary skills is useless.

Computer Programs for Evaluating Reproductive Performance in Dairy Herds

LAWRENCE E. HEIDER
Ohio State University, Columbus, Ohio

At least one commercial business, Herd Reproductive Services, Inc. (HRS), and the Dairy Herd Improvement (DHI) programs offer computerized systems for evaluating reproductive efficiency in a herd.

HRS utilizes a computer in the dairy farm office. It provides direct access to reproductive information, as well as to accounting, payroll and least-cost ration programs, and is undoubtedly a forerunner of agribusiness practices of the near future. The HRS reproduction program provides a numerical index (HRS = n) that is indicative of the current status of the herd.[2] The index is based on the following formula:

$$\text{HRS} = 100 - \left(\frac{\text{DO}}{\text{TC}} \times 1.75 \right)$$

In this formula, DO equals the total number of days open for cows open more than 100 days, and TC equals the number of animals in the herd, with 1.75 as a constant value. An HRS value of 100 would be a perfect score achieved by having all animals pregnant or open less than 100 days.

There are six major computer centers in the United States that process most DHI records. The analysis and options available at each of these centers are essentially the same. However, the printout or data summaries are not in identical form. There is a trend in many of our important dairy areas to administer the business of DHI through dairymen-controlled corporations; however, the responsibility for education in DHI continues to be a responsibility of extension services. In any state, there will be at least one state extension person who can provide additional information on utilizing the DHI printouts regardless of their format.

Veterinarians who work with dairymen need to be capable of interpreting and utilizing the information provided on these printouts, which are called Monthly Herd Summaries. Correct interpretation of computer printouts can help to evaluate the reproductive program in a herd. If the parameters are less than optimal, a correct interpretation and comparison of parameters can help determine if the problem is one of disease or management error.

MEASURING REPRODUCTIVE EFFICIENCY

In working with management in reproductive health programs, one of the important parameters to check on a computer printout is "days of milk to first breeding." This number is influenced by the manager's option concerning how long to wait after calving before breeding the cows. Too often this waiting period will be 60 days, with 40 days being desirable in many herds. Days in milk to first breeding is also influenced by the ability of management to detect heats, assuming that artificial insemination is being used. Surveys of reproductive data indicate that dairymen observe about 50 per cent of all heats. Practically, with the use of planned observation and heat detection aids, this can be improved to above 75 per cent. "Services per conception" (S/C) is another heading listed on computer printouts to use in evaluating reproductive performance. This figure will range between 1.5 SC and 2.5 SC, with an average of 1.7 SC. Herds with average S/C figures above 2.5 should be examined critically for causes of infertility.

"Days open" is the most valuable current index of reproductive efficiency. If yearly calving intervals are to be achieved, this number should not exceed 85 days. A practical goal for days open is 100 days. In problem herds in which this parameter is prolonged, a comparison of days open to days in milk at first breeding and S/C will help determine if the problem is more likely related to disease or management error.

Tables 1 and 2 are guides to help evaluate reproductive efficiency.[1] Remember that the average time required to observe heats in a herd after a waiting period will be equal to about one-half the days in an estrous cycle. All animals will not be in heat on day 61.

Other measurements are available on computer printouts. One in particular deserves comment because of the interest it sometimes receives. "Average calving interval" is sometimes used to measure reproductive efficiency. The average calving interval in DHI herds is 13.4 months. This is an historical figure and tells us what happened in the herd last year. Although it is valuable for comparison and for determining progress, it is not a current index of reproductive efficiency.

Printouts also list figures for "culling rates" and "average age at last calving." Averages for these figures in dairy herds are 30 per cent and 4.5 years, respectively. Excessively high culling rates are undesirable and may be a sign of a disease problem. Low culling percentages, although possibly desirable, can raise the average age of the herd. If excessive, this could exert a negative influence on reproductive measurements since cows 4 years and older in DHI herds require more services/conception and have slightly longer open intervals.

Another advantage of computer programs in reproductive management is the availability of prelists. A variety of options are available for these prelists. As an example, one prelist useful to veterinarians and managers is a prelisting of cows due for pregnancy examination. One reason that these lists are not used frequently may possibly be that their availability is not widely known.

In summary, decision-making and problem-solving in business-oriented dairies can be facilitated by computer systems that analyze reproductive data and provide the analysis in a form that can be readily interpreted. A first glance at a printout is likely to be discouraging, but brief study will reveal information vital to helping maintain reproductive efficiency by use of reproductive health management programs.

TABLE 1. *Partition of Days Open in Average Midwestern DHI Herd**

Calving 0 days	1st Service 85 days		Conception 127 days		Calving 408 days (13.4 months)
60 DAYS	10 DAYS	15 DAYS	14 DAYS	28 DAYS	281 DAYS
Voluntary waiting	Average days to next heat	Missed heats prior to first service	Days lost owing to conception failure, 0.7 additional services	Missed heats between services	Gestation

*From Barr, H. L.: Observer, 9(2):5, 1977.

TABLE 2. A Model for Reproductive Performance*

Calving 40 DAYS	1st Service 55 days		Conception 85 days		Calving 366 days (12.0 months)
	10 DAYS	5 days	24 DAYS	6 DAYS	281 DAYS
Voluntary waiting	Average days to next heat	Missed heats prior to first service	Days lost owing to conception failure, 1.2 additional services	Missed heats between services	Gestation

*From Barr, H. L.: Observer, 9(2):5, 1977.

REFERENCES

1. Barr, H. L.: Evaluation and use of DHI reproduction information. Ohio herd improvement. Observer, 9(2):5, 1977.

2. Johnson, A. D., Myers, R. M. and Ulberg, L. C.: A method of evaluating the current reproductive status of a dairy herd. JAVMA, 144:994, 1964.

What Are Cow Indexes and How to Use Them

RON BUFFINGTON

Select Sires, Inc., Plain City, Ohio

Cow indexes are estimates of genetic transmitting ability for milk and fat as well as estimates for per cent test and dollars for gross income. Such indexes are based on lactation records made for official Dairy Herd Improvement (DHI) and Dairy Herd Improvement Registry (DHIR) dairy record-keeping programs. Cow indexes are calculated on all registered cows on test by the United States Department of Agriculture (USDA) and the top (best) 2 per cent are published three times a year—the same as sires' proofs.

Indexes are calculated from information on the cow's own production as determined by (1) the average deviation from her herdmates, (2) an adjustment for the herd genetic level and (3) the proof of the cow's sire. This index procedure produces the most accurate possible assessment of genetic merit by taking appropriate account of the degree of genetic influence on milk yield, the number of lactations of the cow and the number of paternal half-sisters. The index is expressed in terms of a plus or minus difference from zero.

An important contribution can be made to the genetic improvement of milk production and to the income from a herd if effective selection of cows is continually made. Cow index values should always be considered if they are available, since they give a more accurate estimate of genetic transmitting ability than a cow's lactation yield or even her herdmate deviation.

TABLE 1. Cow Index Record for an Ex-97 All American Aged Cow

Age (years–months)	Days	Milk (pounds)	Fat (%)	Fat (pounds)
6–4	365	27,690	3.5	982
7–8	365	35,276	3.7	1319
9–8	302	23,280	3.5	815

Cow's sire: Reg. No. 1080108
Sire's Predicted Difference (PD) = − 1400 pounds of milk
Cow's USDA Cow Index = − 506 pounds of milk

Table 2. *Cow Index Record for an Ex-94-4E Cow*

Age (years–months)	Days	Milk (pounds)	Fat (%)	Fat (pounds)
6–6	305	19,620	3.8	754
7–8	351	25,870	3.9	1013
9–0	365	26,126	4.1	1082

Cow's sire: Reg. No. 1189870
Sire's Predicted Difference (PD) = +630 pounds of milk
Cow's USDA Cow Index = +1005 pounds of milk

Some dairymen believe that if a cow has a top record, she must be genetically superior. This is illustrated by records of an Ex-97 All-American aged cow (Table 1) and an Ex-94-4E cow (Table 2).

Many dairymen would select the first cow as the superior animal because she produced 35,276 pounds of milk. However, the important factors are the herd average in both herds and the first three or four records of each of the two cows. The first cow did very poorly as a young cow, whereas the second cow had three records that averaged 20,000 pounds of milk and 900 pounds of fat prior to the 6-year-old record. Also, the sire of each cow is important in evaluating the genetic ability of the cow. There is a great difference between a sire that is minus 1400 pounds of milk and a sire that is plus 630 pounds of milk.

Dairymen interested in breeding genetically superior cattle should be concerned about cow index values for all cows on test and should know the index value of any cow before purchasing at a farm dispersal or state sale. In addition, dairymen interested in breeding better cattle should encourage all pedigree organizations to include cow indexes in all sale categories. The Ayrshire, Brown Swiss, Guernsey and Jersey Breed Associations are actively involving cow indexes in all breed literature.

Dairymen can really benefit from evaluating cow indexes. All dairymen with registered Holstein cows can receive a complete ranking of their cows by sending their registration numbers of each cow to the Holstein-Friesian Assn. of America (HFAA), Box 808, Brattleboro, Vermont, 05301 and requesting the cow inquiry. The cost is $3.00 for the first cow and 15 cents for each additional cow (registration number).

As shown in Table 3, the cows ranked genetically should be *C-B-D-A*, with *C* being the most genetically superior cow and *A* the least. One will note that cows A and B are classified higher at Excellent (93-3E) and Excellent (93-4E), respectively. However, classification scores indicate only a cow's physical conformation and do not have any-

TABLE 3. *Ranking Cows for Genetic Superiority**

A. N-Del-Cee Lodestar Duchess 5514944
Excellent (93-3E)

2–3	364d	18969M	3.6%	685F
3–5	347	10751	3.5	377
4–7	289	16550	3.7	606
5–7	352	22420	3.6	804
7–4	305	20480	3.5	718
9–4	365	24038	3.8	906
11–5	305	13490	4.5	606
Lifetime:		110148M	3.7%	4096F
Cow Index:		+584M		+16F

B. Pearl Ivanhoe Comet 5372146
Excellent (93-4E)

2–4	312d	14065M	3.8%	531F
3–5	350	27006	4.4	1179
4–7	305	25049	4.5	1116
5–8	300	28600	3.9	1115
6–7	330	31188	3.8	1173
7–8	305	22460	3.8	860
10–3	305	17240	3.9	676
Lifetime:		17460BN	3.9%	6650F
Cow Index:		+1203M		+57F

C. Maplewood Lane Dora Mega 4448454
Excellent (90) Gold Medal Dam

7–4	365d	32504M	3.6%	1180F
8–10	305	24210	3.2	772
10–5	309	23450	3.3	780
11–6	357	23650	3.5	829
12–8	305	23060	3.5	805
13–11	305	24260	3.3	793
15–2	338	25200	3.5	882
16–4	365	28730	3.0	855
Lifetime:		311330M	3.4%	10653F
Cow Index:		+2047M		+60F

D. Wapa Excellency Bridget 5924244
Very Good (85)

2–4	305d	15760M	3.3%	516F
4–2	305	23130	3.6	822
5–9	342	21720	3.3	709
Cow Index:		+882M		+24F

*Taken from pedigrees listed in Select Sires Holstein Sire Directory.

thing to do directly with her genetic transmitting ability for production.

In summary, cow indexes are another tool for dairymen to use in purchasing or culling cows. Top dairymen with registered herds know the index values of their cows.

What Is a Pedigree Index and How to Use It

RON BUFFINGTON

Select Sires, Inc., Plain City, Ohio

Pedigree indexing is the best tool yet available for figuring the probable breeding worth of a bull too young to have milking daughters or of a heifer too young to be in milk.

A Pedigree Index (PI) combines information on paternal half-sisters, the dam and the paternal half-sister of the dam into a pedigree summary of the young animal's potential for production. A Pedigree Index is computed by averaging the Predicted Difference (PD) of the sire and the Cow Index (CI) of the dam:

Pedigree Index = 1/2 PD of sire + 1/2 CI of dam

For example, if a sire had a PD of +1200 pounds of milk and the dam had a United States Department of Agriculture (USDA) Cow Index of +800 pounds of milk, the son's or the daughter's Pedigree Index would be + 1000 pounds of milk.

In several studies of the pedigrees of young sires, it was found that, on the average, the eventual PD was related to the Pedigree Index in the following manner:

PD = −200 + 60% (Pedigree Index)

The −200 represents the genetic trend in cattle, that is, the progress in milk production that dairy cows make from the time a bull is born and from the time his daughters complete records. The 60 per cent represents the proportion of the index that future daughters are expected to produce. Assuming that this relationship holds for future progeny test sires, Pedigree Index relates to PD as is shown in Table 1.

Pedigree indexing works best when applied to a number of animals. Remember that pedigree indexes are highly unreliable for individual animals but are quite accurate for large groups of animals.

Butcher and Legates[1] at North Carolina State University studied 340 Holstein sons that entered artificial insemination (AI) at less than 3 years of age and for which complete pedigree information was available. They compared the pedigree index of the animals with their PD. The 340 sons were divided into four equal groups based on their pedigree indexes. The top 25 per cent ranged from a pedigree index of +763 to +1515 pounds of milk, with an average of +891 pounds of milk. On the other hand, the bottom 25 per cent of the sons ranged in pedigree indexes from −595 to +331 pounds of milk, with an average of +117 pounds of milk. The progeny test results of the four groups are listed in Table 2.

Taken as a group, there was a strong relationship between the sons' pedigree indexes and the PD. The top 85 sons, as determined by their pedigree indexes, had an average PD of +305 pounds of milk compared with −253 pounds of milk for the 85 sons in the bottom 25 per cent. A study of Ayrshire, Brown Swiss, Guernsey and Jersey bulls showed similar results. Obviously, much time, effort and expense were wasted in sampling the 85 bulls in the bottom group.

Since pedigree indexing was developed, several studs and the USDA have designed a new AI pedigree index formula for young bulls. This index is not popular with dairy-

TABLE 1. *Relationship of Pedigree Index to Predicted Difference (PD)*

Factor	Value (pounds of milk)					
Pedigree Index	0	+500	+800	+1000	+1200	+1500
PD	−200	+100	+280	+400	+520	+700

TABLE 2. *Progeny Test Results of 340 Holstein Sons Divided into Four Groups*

Group Based on Index	Son's Average Index*	PD of Sons		
		AVERAGE*	PLUS SONS	PLUS 500 SONS
Top 25%	+891	+305	71%	35%
Second 25%	+671	+159	61%	18%
Third 25%	+453	−9	47%	7%
Bottom 25%	+117	−253	27%	4%

*Expressed in pounds of milk.

men because it eliminates the cow from the index. However, it has been proved to be very accurate in predicting the final information on groups of proven bulls.

AI Pedigree Index = 1/2 PD of sire + 1/4 PD of maternal grandsire

For example, if a sire had a PD of +1200 pounds of milk and the grandsire had a PD of +1000 pounds of milk, the young sire's pedigree index would be +850.

$$\text{AI Pedigree Index} = 1/2 \times 1200 + 1/4 \times 1000$$

or

$$\text{AI Pedigree Index} = 600 + 250$$

or

$$\text{AI Pedigree Index} = 850$$

One AI organization summarized 116 young sires. Their average AI pedigree index was +283 pounds of milk. These 116 bulls, when proven, had an average PD of +290 pounds of milk.

Pedigree indexing or AI pedigree indexing is a valuable tool to help evaluate a group of bulls. However, any bull can greatly deviate from his pedigree index, as is shown in Table 3.

In conclusion, pedigree indexing has been very helpful in evaluating young bulls prior to having milking daughters. Dairymen owning a young bull should make sure that the animal's pedigree index is +1000 or more to be certain that the genetic contribution to his herd will be constantly improving. The AI studs are sampling very few young sires with pedigree indexes below +1000 or AI pedigree indexes below +750. Both indexes include 1/2 of the sire's predicted difference. The pedigree index includes 1/2 of the dam's cow index. The AI pedigree index includes 1/4 of the maternal grandsire's predicted difference, with no contribution from the dam. Both indexes are good tools, but there is a variation that must be noted to interpret the results.

REFERENCE

1. Butcher, K. R. and Legates, J. E.: Estimating son's progeny test from his pedigree information. J. Dairy Sci., *59*:137, 1976.

TABLE 3. *Deviations in Pedigree Index*

Bull	Pedigree Index*	AI Pedigree Index*	Final Predicted Difference*
Astronaut	+366	−596	+827
Bootmaker	+324	−68	+1132
Elevation	+831	+426	+1256
Conductor	+1180	+776	+1303
Amos	+1051	+890	+630
Standfast	+967	+720	−64

*Expressed in pounds of milk.

Reproductive Health Management in Beef Cows

LAWRENCE RICE
Oklahoma State University, Stillwater,
Oklahoma

REPRODUCTIVE EFFICIENCY

Criteria such as interval to first estrus, interval to first breeding, days open, first service conception rate, services per conception, calving interval and others are often used as measures of reproductive efficiency by dairymen and veterinarians involved in dairy herd health programs. Such measures are important for proper control of the reproductive cycle and milk production of dairy cattle. These criteria are easy to evaluate from the good records avilable in many dairies.

Beef cattle are not as intensively managed, and there is neither the economic importance nor the management opportunities required to maintain the necessary records. Many beef operations with low input-low output management use only the number of calves weaned or sold as their measure of reproduction and production.

The objectives of this article are to discuss a philosophy that production is reproduction and to present a plan whereby production is increased by improved reproduction. Items discussed include production and reproduction goals, production losses and a total reproductive program.

PRODUCTION AND REPRODUCTION GOALS

Production Goals

Average weaning weight and number of calves weaned are the most commonly used measures of production. These are often inaccurate, however, because young calves born late in the calving season are often weaned too late to be included in the calculation. The best measure of production efficiency available today is pounds of calf weaned per animal unit. This evaluates

breeding, survival and growth efficiency. An animal unit (AU) is the production unit used and is a measure that best relates production efficiency to expenses. An animal unit based on production and maintenance costs is approximately 0.1 AU per 100 pounds of body weight.

Mature cow	– 1.0 AU
Bull	– 1.5 AU
Yearling replacements	– 0.6 AU
Horses	– 1.2 AU
Cow-calf pairs	– 1.2 AU

Average weaning weight should and will continue to be utilized as an important measure of beef production. This measure becomes more meaningful if it is compared with pounds of calf weaned per animal unit. With today's increased production costs, the following goals are necessary to make beef production profitable:

1. Average weaning weight (WW) =
$\dfrac{\text{Total weight}}{\text{Number of calves}}$ (Goal = 500 pounds)

2. Pounds of calf per AU =
$\dfrac{\text{Total weight}}{\text{Number AU}}$ (Goal = 75% of average WW)

A 500-pound average weaning weight is highly desirable but also exceptional. Therefore, the goal (expressed in pounds of calf per AU) of 75 per cent of that weaning weight represents maximum reproductive efficiency. For example, to maintain a herd size of 100 cows, which necessitates adding 15 per cent replacements each year, plus adequate bull power, the herd must have a minimum of 121 animal units as follows:

100 cows	–	100 AU
22 yearling replacements	–	13 AU
5 bulls	–	8 AU
127		121 AU

These animal units should produce 90 weaned calves at 500 pounds each if all reproduction and production goals are met. This represents 374 pounds of calf per animal unit or 75 per cent of the weaning weight.

Reproduction Goals

High reproduction goals must be set to achieve these production goals. Every phase of breeding, calving and nursing must be managed at maximum efficiency to avoid loss of beef production.

The most common causes of loss of beef production are: (1) too few cows in estrus the first 21 days of the breeding season, (2) low first service conception rates and (3) excessive calf losses at or near birth.[16] Low input-low output management contributes to these losses of production. Increased reproductive efficiency by use of more intensive management is necessary to increase pounds of calf weaned.

The following criteria and their respective goals are suggested as measures of reproduction and production for intensive beef reproductive management.

Adult Cow Breeding Efficiency

1. Per cent cows cycling during first 21 days breeding =
$$\frac{\text{Number cows in estrus first 21 days}}{\text{Total cows}} = \times\ 100$$
(Goal = 90%)

This criterion is important and easy to measure in beef artificial insemination (AI) herds. It is of equal economic importance in herds using natural service, but observations of estrus are less accurate and therefore unreliable in measuring estrus activity.

2. First service conception rate =
$$\frac{\text{Number cows pregnant first service}}{\text{Number bred first service}} \times 100$$
(Goal = 70%)

This criterion is especially important for all beef herds. The combination of high conception rates and high cycling rates insures a high percentage of calves born early in the calving season (90 per cent cycling first 21 days × 70 per cent conception = 63 per cent pregnant first 21 days).

3. Percent cows pregnant =
$$\frac{\text{Number cows pregnant}}{\text{Total cows}} \times 100$$
(Goal = 95%)

This value is the one most commonly used to measure reproductive performance in beef cows. The goal of 95 per cent has greater significance when the breeding season is short. The goal should be a breeding season of 63 days (three cycles) to insure ideal weaning weights. Each rancher must set his own goals, but his veterinarian can provide much help in shortening the breeding season to 63 days.

Replacement Heifer Breeding Efficiency

Heifers that calve late the first year always tend to calve late in subsequent years or have a greater tendency not to get pregnant. Replacement heifers must cycle early and be bred during a 42-day breeding season to prevent late calving the first and subsequent years. High reproductive performance must be demanded from replacement heifers:

1. Per cent cycling first 21 days. (Goal = 85%)
2. Per cent pregnant after 42 days. (Goal = 85%).

Reproductive performance is lowest in heifers suckling their first calves.[8] However, goals need to be kept at the same high standards as for the adult cows. Management must be planned and adopted to achieve these goals for first calf heifers, as described later.

Calf Survival at Birth

The best measure of calf survival is expressed as the per cent of pregnant cows that have live calves 24 hours after birth. This percentage reflects losses due to abortions and perinatal calf mortality. The accumulative measure of efficiency is defined as the percentage of total cows exposed to breeding that had live calves 24 hours after birth. This reflects both breeding efficiency and calf survival.

Calf Survival:
$$\frac{\text{Live calves at 24 hours}}{\text{Number pregnant cows retained}} \times 100$$
(Goal = 95%)

Accumulative Reproductive Efficiency:
$$\frac{\text{Live calves at 24 hours}}{\text{Total cows exposed to breeding}} \times 100$$
(Goal = 90%)

If the accumulative goal is achieved, it means that the previous breeding efficiency goals were met and that calf survival at birth was equal to expectations (95 per cent pregnancy rate × 95 per cent survival = 91 per cent live calves at 24 hours).

Calf Survival at Weaning

The percentage of calves weaned from the total cows exposed to breeding during the previous breeding season measures (1) breeding efficiency, (2) calf survival at birth and (3) nursing survival. This figure can be no greater than the lowest of the three exponents involved. Therefore nursing survival must have a high goal:

1. Nursing survival =
$$\frac{\text{Calves weaned}}{\text{Calves alive at 24 hours}}$$
(Goal = 85%)

2. Per cent calf crop weaned =
$$\frac{\text{Calves weaned}}{\substack{\text{Total cows exposed to} \\ \text{breeding previous season}}}$$
(Goal = 85%)

(95% breeding efficiency × 95% survival at birth × 95% nursing survival = 86% calf crop)

Achieving each of these reproductive efficiency goals is difficult; however, herd records prove it is possible. High goals must be set as the first step toward making progress.

LOSS OF PRODUCTION

Genetic Management

Loss of production can be due to poor genetic management. Careless selection of both cows and bulls will result in low weaning and yearling weights, especially if replacements are selected for factors other than growth. Cattlemen have too often selected bulls that have "eye appeal," popular blood lines and impressive pedigrees. Physical soundness should always guide bull selection, but visual appraisal has little objective value beyond utilizing soundness and size for age comparison.

An evaluation including three criteria — pedigree, performance test and progeny test — would meet the ultimate goal in sire selection. A pedigree will tell how a bull is expected to perform on the basis of the performance of his ancestors. A performance test will tell how the bull actually did perform. A progeny test will tell how a bull's offspring perform and is therefore the most important of the three factors. Unfortunate-

ly, very few bulls are selected on the basis of all three values. Some bulls in AI studs have accurate progeny information, but bulls in natural service are primarily selected by visual appraisal with perhaps either pedigree or performance test evaluation.

Cattlemen participating in production testing programs are those making the most genetic progress in producing replacements with better growth rates. Performance tests identify bulls that have the ability to achieve rapid growth rates during the first year of life. Yearling weight is a highly heritable trait; therefore, a bull with a heavy yearling weight and one that grew better than his herdmates should be expected to produce better growing calves. Production records are useful in (1) identifying the top producing individuals and blood lines within a herd, (2) helping the producer evaluate the genetic progress of his herd and (3) identifying cattlemen who are producing superior quality cattle. Veterinarians can and should encourage their clients to select bulls on the basis of performance and production records.

The Beef Improvement Federation (BIF) is a national organization of producers, extension personnel and scientists devoted to improving beef production by use of performance and production records. There is currently a move by this organization to encourage its members to incorporate reproductive performance in the selection of replacements. The following is quoted from the 1976 BIF Guidelines.[3]

Reproduction or fertility is the most important trait in beef cattle. Breeders are urged to record reproductive performance in both the female and the male and to build this data into their herd records. They are urged to use this data in culling and selection, even though heritabilities may be low. Recommendations for this section are based on experience and limited research information. Research workers are urged to further study reproductive traits and measures for future refinement and improvements.

The accepted BIF Gudielines for male reproductive performance are those adopted by the Society for Theriogenology. The guidelines for female reproductive performance give high scores to cows that calve early and wean a live calf every 12 months.

Artificial insemination has long been recognized as being responsible for increased milk production in dairy cattle. Beef cattle breeders who utilize AI have demonstrated similar genetic progress. However, less than 5 per cent of all beef cows are bred by AI so increased production as a result of genetic progress has been much slower in the beef industry. Breeders having herds with good reproductive performance find AI to be a useful management tool. Such breeders usually depend on more veterinary assistance with their herd health programs.

The significant point is that progressive producers recognize the importance of good reproductive performance. Veterinarians can and should provide leadership by promoting and evaluating beef cattle reproductive and genetic performance for their clients.

Reproductive Management

Causes of decreased pounds of calf weaned per animal unit can be classified into three categories: (1) increased calf mortality, (2) reduced weaning weights and (3) reduced pregnancy rates.

Increased Calf Mortality

High calf mortality means there have been excessive deaths at or near birth or from birth to weaning, or both. Although control of losses from birth to weaning is crucial in a herd health program, this topic will not be discussed as part of reproductive health management.

Perinatal calf deaths from dystocia have been reported to range from 4 to 16 per cent.[2] Reports indicate that cows experiencing dystocia have subsequent conception rates reduced by as much as 15 per cent.[6, 10] Calf losses and breeding problems following dystocia are most commonly seen in replacement heifers. Dystocia and obstetrical procedures are discussed elsewhere in this book, as the present article only discusses a management program designed to minimize losses due to dystocia in replacement heifers.

Studies have been conducted to attribute various maternal and fetal traits as causes of dystocia. In all studies, calf birth weight was determined to be the single most important trait related to dystocia.[5, 13] Data from the United States Meat Animal Research Center show that as birth weight increases the dystocia rate and the perinatal calf mortality rate also increase.[2] Dystocia and calf mortality increase markedly in the common

English beef heifers when birth weights exceed 70 pounds.[11] Recently imported large European breeds have considerably heavier birth weights and higher dystocia rates than do the English breeds.

A review of calving data from the Simmental Association indicated that for every pound increase in birth weight the number of 2-year-old cows requiring assistance increased by 2 per cent.[7] The effect on older cows was not as dramatic until calf birth weights exceeded 90 to 95 pounds. Calving difficulties increased rapidly from less than 10 per cent to 40 per cent when calves weighed 115 pounds or more at birth.

Breed association and artificial insemination organization progeny test records have demonstrated large differences in birth weights and dystocia rates among different sire progeny groups. These records indicate that bulls can be selected to sire calves that cause relatively fewer dystocias.

Dam size has been shown to affect birth weights and dystocia. Restricted prepartum nutrition will reduce calf birth weights but will not reduce the dystocia rate in heifers. This is because maternal growth is stopped early in poorly grown heifers, and they will subsequently have smaller pelves.

Properly grown replacement heifers with roomy pelves will have lower dystocia rates, and losses will be minimized when these heifers are bred to bulls known to be "easy calvers." Replacements produced under very intensive management may be selected even more critically by performing pelvic area measurements at breeding time or when pregnancy testing.[11] Heifers must be properly grown and should be bred to an "easy calving" bull. The very best replacements will be selected when the bottom 20 to 30 per cent of heifers with the smallest pelvic measurements are culled.

Reduced Weaning Weights and Pregnancy Rates

Low weaning weights and reduced pregnancy rates can be directly attributed to poor reproductive efficiency. Too few cows are in estrus during the first 21 days of the breeding season, and low first service conception rates directly affect weaning weights and pregnancy rates. Assuming that a calf will gain from 1.5 to 2 pounds per day from birth to weaning, one can calculate that a weaned calf will weigh from 30 to 40 pounds less for every 21-day cycle that the dam missed during the breeding season. Table 1 shows the effects of per cent calf crop and age of the calf on pounds of calf weaned per cow bred.

Note that a 20-day reduction in age at weaning is nearly as devastating to pounds of calf weaned as a 10 per cent reduction in calf crop.

These weights were calculated on the assumption that growth rate throughout the suckling period was similar for all calves; however, this is not true since calves born late in the calving season do not have as high average daily gain as calves born early in the calving season. This means that late calves will always be lighter at weaning regardless of when they are weaned. This phenomenon is not fully understood or completely accepted. An explanation is that most ranchers tend to select the calving season that results in the best weaning weights for their particular area. Late calves will be out of phase with maximum growth for that environment and will have lower weaning weights regardless of age at weaning.

Maximum weaning weights are obtained when the calving season is short with the majority of the calves born early in the calving season. A survey of 8742 calves in Wyoming showed that (1) 70 per cent of the calves in the top third of weaning weights were born during the first 20 days of the calving season and (2) calves in the top third of weaning weight gained more than those in the bottom third (1.68 versus 1.28 pounds per day). This reduction in average daily gain for calves in the bottom third of weaning weights can be due to (1) late calving cows not milking as well when they are out of phase with the most productive forage and (2) calves not being old enough to get maximum utilization of the most productive forage.[14]

A cow must have a calf every 12 months to be an efficient production unit. The very nature of a beef cow's reproductive physiology is a major obstacle to that 12-month goal. The gestation period averages 283 days, with ranges from 275 to 290 days. Therefore, a cow must become pregnant from 75 to 90 days after calving to produce a calf every 12 months. The onset of estrus following calving is delayed in beef cows that are suckling calves. The interval from calving to first estrus has been reported to be from 35 to 54 days longer in cows suckling calves than in dry or milked cows.[9]

Inadequate nutrition before calving delays the onset of estrus in beef cows that are suckling calves. The effect of nutrition is discussed elsewhere in this section, but the combination of suckling and reduced prepartum nutrition has a marked effect on the percentage of cows cycling before 90 days postpartum. Tables 2 to 5 have been calculated from research conducted at the United States Department of Agriculture (USDA) Beef Research Station, Fort Robinson, Nebraska. They represent the percentage of lactating beef cows expected to be in estrus at different postpartum intervals.[17]

The important point is that we expect cows to become pregnant by 90 days or less after calving, but 60 to 80 days of postpartum rest is necessary for 80 per cent of beef cows to start cycling (Table 4). Cows that calve late have two distinct disadvantages. First, they have fewer chances to cycle and therefore make up the greater number of open cows. Second, even when cows show estrus at less than 50 days postpartum, con-

TABLE 1. *Pounds of Calf Weaned per Cow Bred*

Age of Calf (days)	Calf Crop (pounds)			
	90%	80%	70%	60%
220	454	404	353	303
200	418	372	325	275
180	382	340	298	255
160	346	308	270	231
140	310	276	242	207

TABLE 2. *Availability Projection Tables for First-Calf Heifers — Per Cent Cycling — Prepartum Nutrition Level (Last Trimester)**

Days' Rest	Low (5 lb) TDN†	Moderate (7 lb) TDN	High (9 lb) TDN
110	85%	92%	95%
100	80%	90%	95%
90	70%	85%	92%
80	47%	80%	90%
70	25%	62%	77%
60	25%	45%	65%
50	10%	29%	40%
40	10%	12%	15%
30	7%	8%	10%

*From *The Cowpedia,* Syntex Agribusiness, Inc. (IBB), 1975.

†TDN = total digestible nutrients.

TABLE 3. *Availability Projection Tables for First-Calf Heifers—Per Cent Conception—Postpartum Nutrition Level (Before Breeding)**

Days' Rest	Low (8 lb) TDN†	Moderate (12 lb) TDN	High (16 lb) TDN
110	52%	64%	67%
100	47%	60%	67%
90	42%	55%	67%
80	40%	51%	62%
70	37%	48%	58%
60	28%	37%	45%
50	20%	27%	33%
40	15%	17%	20%
30	10%	15%	20%

*From *The Cowpedia*, Syntex Agribusiness, Inc. (IBB), 1975.
†TDN = total digestible nutrients.

TABLE 4. *Availability Projection Tables for Mature Cows—Per Cent Cycling—Prepartum Nutrition Level (Last Trimester)**

Days' Rest	Low (5 lb) TDN†	Moderate (7 lb) TDN	High (9 lb) TDN
90	85%	92%	95%
80	80%	90%	95%
70	70%	85%	92%
60	47%	80%	90%
50	25%	62%	77%
40	25%	45%	65%
30	10%	29%	40%
20	10%	12%	15%

*From *The Cowpedia*, Syntex Agribusiness, Inc. (IBB), 1975.
†TDN = total digestible nutrients.

ception rates are below 50 per cent (Table 5). This is illustrated in Table 6.

After 80 or 90 days of breeding, the total conception rate exceeds 90 per cent, but cows that calved in the third and fourth 21-day-period of the calving season are the poorest producers. Eighty per cent of the cows that calved in the first 21-day-period are pregnant at the end of 42 days breeding, whereas only 20 per cent of those calving in the fourth 21-day-period are pregnant at the same time. Many of these cows will be open or will continue to calve late and wean lighter calves in successive years.

The following conclusions are valid: (1) cows tend to calve at the same time every year if conditions are favorable, (2) unfavorable conditions tend to extend calving intervals or cause pregnancy failures and (3) the probability of early calving increases when replacement heifers calve early and when the calving season is short. A short calving season can be attained over a 4- or 5-year period if all replacements calve early in the first two calving seasons.

Three-Year Heifer Control Program

The first-calf heifer has more difficulties cycling and conceiving than all other cows. At calving she still has high growth requirements and is then suddenly subjected to two new stresses, calving and nursing. These three stresses require the first-calf heifer to have 20 more days of postpartum rest before breeding than older cows to insure comparable cycling rates. Therefore, the breeding of the replacement heifer must be controlled throughout the first 3 years of her life. Control thereafter is much easier since the calving pattern of adult cows is established in the first 2 reproductive years and rarely changes unless adverse conditions cause her to calve later.

What is the controlled 3-year heifer program?[12] The goals are:

1. Breed 13- to 15-month-old virgin heifers for 42 days, starting 21 days before the regular breeding season. Eighty-five per cent of the heifers should be cycling and bred during the first 21 days and 95 per cent by the end of 42 days. Eight-five per cent of the heifers bred should be pregnant.

2. Two-year-old heifers nursing their first calves should be cycling at a rate of 85 to 95 per cent during the first 42 days of the regular breeding season and 85 per cent or more should be pregnant at the end of 63 days' breeding.

To accomplish these breeding goals, three growth requirements should be achieved during specific times:

1. First year (from birth to puberty). Heifers should reach 65 per cent of their mature weight at 13- to 15-months of age.

2. Second year (from first breeding to first calving). Heifers should reach 85 per cent of their mature weight at 2 years of age.

3. Third year (from second breeding to second calving). Heifers should reach 95 per cent of their mature weight at 3 years of age.

Figure 1 illustrates the required growth curve of either replacement heifers for 1000-

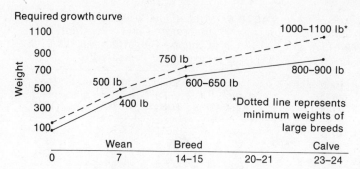

Figure 1. Growing replacement heifers. (See text for explanation.)

pound adult English cows or replacements for 1200-pound mature, large, exotic half-blood cows. The solid line represents the growth curve for the English heifers and the dotted line the growth curves for the large breed heifers. Although puberty is affected by both age and body weight, the latter is more important.

How to Establish a Heifer Program. The following steps are required to establish a 3-year controlled heifer program:

1. Select approximately 1.5 times as many heifers as will actually be needed for replacements and start breeding 21 days before the regular breeding season. These heifers should be selected on the basis that they will be between 12 and 15 months of age at the beginning of the heifer breeding season. Younger heifers will not be old enough or have sufficient weight by the start of breeding. Less than 30 per cent of properly fed heifers will be cycling at 12 months of age, whereas 85 to 90 per cent of the same heifers will be cycling at 15 months of age.[16]

TABLE 5. *Availability Projection Tables for Mature Cows—Per Cent Conception—Postpartum Nutrition Level (Before Breeding)**

Days' Rest	Low (8 lb) TDN†	Moderate (12 lb) TDN	High (16 lb) TDN
90	52%	64%	67%
80	47%	60%	67%
70	42%	55%	67%
60	40%	51%	62%
50	37%	48%	58%
40	28%	37%	45%
30	20%	27%	33%
20	15%	17%	20%

*From *The Cowpedia*, Syntex Agribusiness, Inc. (IBB), 1975.

†TDN = total digestible nutrients.

2. Weigh all heifers as a group and determine average weights. If there are wide ranges between the smaller and the larger heifers, they should be divided into two groups for feeding in order to reach 65 per cent of their mature weight by breeding time. Achieving this goal is very important. Less than 50 per cent of heifers that reach 50 per cent of their mature weight at 15 months of age will be cycling.[16]

3. Calculate the days between initial weighing and beginning of the breeding season. Determine the average daily gain necessary to reach the growth goal of 65 per cent of the mature weight, and feed to attain that average daily gain. Table 7 shows the minimun daily nutritional requirements for heifers prior to breeding and throughout the period of calving.

4. Weigh a random sample of the heifers every 30 days to check growth rates. Poorer gaining heifers should be sorted and fed more to make necessary gains.

5. At 1 year of age, it may be necessary to remove approximately 10 per cent of heifers as undesirable for replacement breeding. These heifers should be fattened for slaughter or sold to reduce carrying costs.

6. A final check weight should be obtained on a random sample of heifers shortly before breeding.

7. Breed for 42 days, starting 21 days before breeding the cows. Preferably, all breeding should be by artificial insemination, using semen from a progeny tested bull proved to be an "easy calving" bull. Such a bull should also have the genetic ability to transmit above average growth rates to his offspring. A bull should not be used for replacement heifers simply because he is an "easy calving" bull.

8. The heifers may be pregnancy tested any time after 35 days following the end of the 42-day breeding season. The sooner the

TABLE 6. *Percentage of Cows Cycling and Conceiving at Different Postpartum Intervals*

Calving Season	Per Cent in Heat 1st 21 Days of Breeding*		Per Cent 1st Service Conception		Per Cent Pregnant after Breeding		
					21 DAYS	42 DAYS	84 DAYS
1st 21 days	90	×	60	=	54	81	96
2nd 21 days	80	×	57	=	46	73	94
3rd 21 days	45	×	37	=	17	53	90
4th 21 days	12	×	17	=	2	18	76

*Cycling and conception rates based on 7 lb of total digestible nutrients (TDN) prepartum and 12 lb of TDN postpartum.

heifers are pregnancy tested, the sooner one will be able to sell all open heifers. Pelvic measurements may be taken at this time, and the bottom 20 to 30 per cent of heifers may be removed from the replacement group to decrease calving problems. Pelvic measurements, however, are of no value unless the heifers are properly grown by breeding and calving time. Culling the bottom 20 to 30 per cent from a group of small heifers will not significantly reduce calving difficulties. Second, selecting replacement heifers with large pelvic areas is not helpful if they are bred to "hard calving" bulls. The use of the pelvimeter is recommended only in herds that are under intensive management and in instances when it will provide the additional selection pressure necessary to select the very best replacement heifers.

9. Once the pregnancy replacement heifers have been selected, maintain their growth rate to reach 85 per cent of mature cow size at calving. This will help insure proper cycling rates for the second breeding and will decrease the incidence of calving problems.

10. Maintain growth through 3 years of age (95 per cent of mature body weight).

The culling rates in an intensive management program may seem severe, but cull heifers make cull cows if not eliminated. Intensive culling at early stages permits sales of cows at peak value, not at 3 to 4 years of age when the inferior cows will be sold for lower prices. The practice of early severe culling will produce maximum performance in the herd and avoid carrying costs for poor-producing females.

Maintaining control of replacement heifers through the first 3 years of life results in a herd of early calving, high-producing mother cows. After having been on a controlled heifer replacement program for approximately 5 years, calves from first-calf heifers will have weaning weights equal to the herd average. This is possible because the heifers' calves will be weaned at an average age of approximately 20 days older than the rest of the calves. Also, if artificial insemination has been used, the genetic merit of replacement heifers will exceed the average genetic merit of the cow herd.

Unfortunately, less than 5 per cent of beef females are bred artificially; consequently, genetic improvement in beef cattle is very slow. This should not detract from the utilization of the 3-year controlled heifer progrm with natural service. The growth requirements and length of breeding season will be the same. An attempt should be made to

TABLE 7. *Nutritional Requirements for Replacement Heifers**

Body Weight	Average Daily Gain (lb)	Total Digestible Dry Matter (lb)	Nutrients† (lb)	Total Protein† (lb)
400	1.10	11.0	7.1	1.25
660	1.10	18.0	10.4	1.85
660	1.65	19.0	12.0	2.00
800–900 (last 3 months gestation)	0.75	17.0	8.5	1.40
800–900 (suckling calf)	0.5	23.0	13.0	2.10

*From Nutrient Requirements of Beef Cattle. National Academy of Sciences, Washington, D.C., 1971.
†Per cent represented on dry matter basis.

select "easy calving" bulls, but this is very difficult without accurate progeny information. Genetic progress will not be as rapid with natural service, but all reproductive goals can be achieved.

TOTAL REPRODUCTIVE MANAGEMENT PLAN

An overall reproductive management plan should be decided upon by a producer and his consulting veterinarian. The plan should have enough flexibility to allow for year-to-year economic variations and differences in management abilities of producers. For example, some ranchers may find feeding of replacement heifers to calve at 2 years of age totally unfeasible. It may be necessary for replacements to calve first at 3 years of age, but all replacements should be bred to calve in a short time interval early in the calving season. The following requirements must be adopted if the plan is to yield increased pounds of weaned calves.

1. Plan 15 per cent replacements each year.
2. Maintain the same number of animal units in the herd, but reduce the number of late calving cows to permit adding more early calving replacements each year.
3. Feed and manage replacement heifers to start breeding 21 days before older cows. Select herd replacements from those becoming pregnant in a 42-day breeding season. This applies to heifers that calve first at 3 years of age as well as to those that calve first at 2 years of age.
4. Maintain first-calf heifers separately from older cows and on a higher level of nutrition through their second breeding season while nursing their first calves.
5. Maintain older cows on moderate levels of nutrition during the last trimester of pregnancy, calving and the early postpartum period. Moderate levels of nutrition during the postpartum period are nearly double moderate prepartum nutritional levels.

A 5-year projection of reproduction should be calculated initially and then updated each year. The projection will not always be accurate each year but will be helpful in establishing and evaluating both short- and long-range goals. Goals may change with economic changes in the beef cattle business and, in turn, alter projections.

A 5-year reproductive projection simply involves determining the number of cows eligible to breed during any 21-day segment of the breeding season. This is done by analyzing the postpartum interval and levels of prepartum and postpartum nutrition and evaluating body condition to estimate cycling rates.

The following data are required:
1. Calving dates. When calving dates are not recorded, the veterinarian and the rancher can estimate the number of calves born during each 20 or 30 days of the calving season. This is often necessary for the first year in the initial 5-year projection, but calving dates should be available after that for yearly updates.
2. Nutritional levels before and after calving. These are often estimates during the first year, but subsequent years records should be readily available to determine feed consumed.
3. Estimation of body condition before and after calving. This is a subjective but very important aid in the evaluation of the nutritional status. Cows may be fed according to the best recommendations of nutrition authorities but may not be in the desirable body condition for suitable reproductive performance. Data show that cows most likely to cycle and become pregnant early are those in good condition at calving, regardless of nutrition level.[15]

Given the herd information shown in Table 8, the availability tables can be used to project a 5-year reproductive plan.

The calving pattern has been similar for many years. The cows have been on low nutrition levels before calving and in relatively poor condition at calving. Nutrition has improved to moderate levels following calving, especially as summer pasture improved. Ten per cent replacements have been added annually and have been bred at the same time as the cows.

Projections for the 5-year reproductive plan should include the following changes:
1. Add 15 per cent replacements annually. Breed heifers for no more than 42 days, starting 21 days before the cows.
2. Increase prepartum feed to insure that cows are in good condition at calving, and postpartum nutrition must be increased to maintain good body condition.
3. Maintain young cows separately from older cows and separate prepartum cows from postpartum cows to insure that all receive adequate nutrition.

TABLE 8. *Calving Pattern**

Calving group	1	2	3	4	5	6	Total calves	Total open
Days of calving season	21	42	63	84	105	126		
First-calf heifers	3	4	1	1			9	1
Adult cows	14	27	27	13	4	2	87	3
Total	17	31	28	14	4	2	96	4

*Number of pregnant adult cows—90.
Number of pregnant heifers—10.

The form in Figure 2 can be used to calculate the number of cows expected to be cycling and become pregnant during each 21 days of the first controlled breeding season.[1] The calculations in the form are based on the recommended changes just listed and the information in Tables 4 and 5. This form can be used for each of the 5 years, and progress can be projected in summary, as shown in Table 9.

Three-year control of replacement heifers is the key to the program. Twenty-two heifers will be exposed to breeding to acquire 15 pregnant replacements. Ten heifers would be expected to become pregnant 21 days before the cows. Approximately seven more heifers would become pregnant in the second 21 days of the heifer breeding. Five of these would be selected to complete the 15 replacements. The combination of controlled replacement breeding and improved nutrition for the adult cows would increase the number of calves born in the first 21 days from the current 17 animals to a projected 42 calves next year.

The projection calls for shortening the cow breeding season to 63 days during the third breeding season. However, this cannot be accomplished unless at least 50 per cent of the calves are born within the first 21 days of calving (actually 42 days — 21 days of heifers only and 21 days of heifers and cows). Little change will occur in the calving season once it has been reduced to 63 days. Management failures will lengthen the breeding and calving season and will cause return to previous unsatisfactory patterns of performance.

REFERENCES

1. Anonymous: The Cow Availability Study. *The Cowpedia*, Syntex Agribusiness Inc., 1975, p. 53.
2. Anonymous: Germ plasm evaluation program. Progress Report No. 2. USMARC ARS-NC-22, 1975.
3. Anonymous: Guidelines for uniform beef improvement programs. Beef Improvement Federation USDA Program Aid, 1020, 1976.
4. Bellows, R. A., Short, R. E., Anderson, D. C., Knapp, B. W. and Pahnish, O. F.: Cause and effect relationships associated with calving difficulty and birth weight. J. Anim. Sci., *33*:407, 1971.
5. Brinks, J. S., Olson, J. E. and Carroll, E. J.: Calving difficulty and its association with subsequent productivity. J. Anim. Sci., *36*:11, 1973.
6. Burfening, P. J.: Possible effects on growth with selection for lighter birth weights. National Sire Summary of American Simmental Association, 1976, A.12, 1976.
7. Dunn, T. G., Ingalls, J. E., Zimmerman, D. R. and Wiltbank, J. N.: Reproductive performance of 2-year-old Hereford and Angus heifers as in-

TABLE 9. *Five-Year Reproductive Plan*

	First-calf Heifers	21-Day Calving Groups						Total Calves	Total Open
		1	2	3	4	5	6		
		21 DAYS	42 DAYS	63 DAYS	84 DAYS	105 DAYS	126 DAYS		
This year	0	17	31	28	14	4	2	96	4
Next year	10	32	26	22	5			95	5
2	10	39	27	16	3			95	5
3	10	44	27	14				95	5
4	10	46	27	12				95	5
5	10	46	28	11				95	5

AVAILABILITY FORM

TYPE OF CATTLE: _____

PLANNED Starting Dates: Calving _____ Breeding _____

Nutritional Levels:
(Mark with X)   Low _____   Moderate _X_   High _____

BEFORE CALVING

AFTER CALVING   Low _____   Moderate _X_   High _____

FIRST 21 DAYS' BREEDING

Calving Group	Total Head	Days Rest	% Cycling	No. Cycling	% Conception	No. Pregnant	AI or Bulls	No. Open
1	17	80	90	15	60	9	8	
2	31	60	80	25	51	13	18	
3	28	40	45	13	37	5	23	
4	14	20	12	2	17	0	14	
5	4	0	0	0	0	0	4	
6	2	-20	0	0	0	0	2	
7								
Totals	96		57	55	49	27	69	

SECOND 21 DAYS' BREEDING

Days Rest	% Cycling	No. Cycling	% Conception	No. Pregnant	AI or Bulls	No. Open
100	95	8	64	5	3	
80	90	16	60	10	8	
60	80	18	51	9	14	
40	45	6	37	2	12	
20	12	0	17	0	4	
0	0	0	0	0	2	
	0					
(Totals)	70	48	54	26	43	

THIRD 21 DAYS' BREEDING

Days Rest	% Cycling	No. Cycling	% Conception	No. Pregnant	AI or Bulls	No. Open
120	95	3	60	2	1	
100	95	8	64	5	3	
80	90	13	60	8	6	
60	80	10	51	5	7	
40	45	2	37	1	3	
20	12	0	17	0	2	
(Totals)	84	36	58	21	22	

FOURTH 21 DAYS' BREEDING

Days Rest	% Cycling	No. Cycling	% Conception	No. Pregnant	AI or Bulls	No. Open
140	95	1	50	0	1	
120	95	3	60	2	1	
100	95	6	64	4	2	
80	90	6	60	4	3	
60	80	2	51	1	2	
40	45	1	37	0	2	
(Totals)	86	19	58	11	11	

Total pregnant after 84 days = 85/96 = 89%

Summary No. 1: All Groups _____
Conception Rate _____

Summary No. 2: Selected AI Groups _____
Conception Rate _____

Projected Pregnant × 100 / Rejected Services = _____ % Projected Conception Rate

Figure 2. Availability form to calculate the number of cows expected to be cycling and become pregnant during each 21 days for the first controlled breeding season.

fluenced by pre- and post-calving energy intake. J. Anim. Sci., *29*:719, 1969.

8. Dunn, T. G., Wiltbank, J. N., Ingalls, J. E. and Zimmerman, D. R.: Dam's energy intake on milk production and calf gains. Proc. West. Sect. An. Soc. An. Sci., *16*:VI, 1965.

9. Graves, W. E., Lauderdale, J. W., Hauser, E. R. and Casida, L. E.: Relation of postpartum interval to pituitary gonadotrophins, ovarian follicular development and fertility in beef cows. *In* Studies on the Postpartum Cow. University of Wisconsin Research Bulletin 270, 1968, p. 23.

10. Lasater, D. B., Glimp, H. A., Cundiff, L. V. and Gregory, K. E.: Factors affecting dystocia and the effects of dystocia on subsequent reproduction in beef cattle. J. Anim. Sci., *36*:695, 1973.

11. Rice, L. E.: Coping with calving difficulties. Proceedings 2nd Annual O-K Cattle Conference, Oklahoma State University, 1976, pp. 11–12.

12. Rice, L. E.: Heat detection is key to successful beef AI. AI Digest, *24*:8, 1976.

13. Rice, L. E. and Wiltbank, J. N.: Factors affecting dystocia in beef heifers. JAVMA, *161*:348, 1972.

14. Schoonover, C. O.: Factors that affect weaning weight in Wyoming calves. Proceedings University of Wyoming Extension Service, 15th Annual Beef Cattle Short Course, Worland, Wyo., 1974, pp. 15–20.

15. Whitman, R. W., Remmega, E. E. and Wiltbank, J. N.: Weight change, condition and beef cow production. J. Anim. Sci. (abstr), *41*:387, 1975.

16. Wiltbank, J. N. and Faukner, L. C.: The management of beef breeding programs. Proceedings of Conference on Reproductive Problems in Animals. ASSBS and University of Georgia Center for Continuing Education, 1969, pp. 1–15.

17. Wiltbank, J. N., Rowden, W. W., Ingalls, J. E., Gregory, K. E. and Koch, R. M.: Effect of energy level on reproductive phenomena of mature Hereford cows. J. Anim. Sci., *21*:219, 1962.

Reproductive Health Program for Beef Cattle

LAWRENCE RICE

Oklahoma State University, Stillwater, Oklahoma

The preceding article discussed reproductive management of beef cows, including causes of production losses and methods for improving reproductive efficiency. A reproductive health program must also include control of other causes of production losses. Factors affecting male and female reproductive efficiency are thoroughly discussed elsewhere in this text. The purpose of this article is to outline a reproductive herd health calendar for beef cattle. Specific details are presented elsewhere in appropriate sections.

There is no single program that can be utilized for all herds. The consulting veterinarian should have a basic plan that is flexible enough to be applicable for any herd. One rancher may ask only for pregnancy diagnosis and culling assistance. Another may expect a complete program to include reproductive examination, vaccinations, therapeutic procedures and nutritional and selection consultations. The program will therefore depend upon the objectives and goals of the individual rancher.

The veterinarian should be prepared to:

1. Determine possible health problems and evaluate the impact upon the rancher's income. For example, if an immunization or therapeutic procedure fails to increase profitability or decrease loss, the procedure should be eliminated.

2. Recommend an adequate vaccination and therapeutic program.

3. Perform diagnostic procedures including necropsy and submission of samples to diagnostic laboratories. The diagnostic laboratory is invaluable for determining causes of health problems.

4. Train the rancher/herdsman to properly perform procedures that do not require the services of a veterinarian. This is particularly important for vaccination and simple obstetrical procedures. The veterinarian should train every herdsman to use proper sanitation and examination procedures for every animal he examines for dystocia. The herdsman must learn his limitations. He should be trained to make a decision after 15 minutes of examining and manipulating a dystocia if a veterinarian's assistance is required.

A herd health program should consist of a calendar of events that take place during specific times of the reproductive year (Fig. 1). A good starting point is weaning time. No specific dates are given in this calendar. The program is designed for approximately 60 to

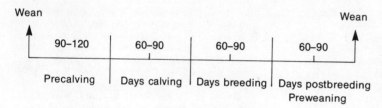

Figure 1. Calendar of events for herd health program.

90 days of calving and breeding, but it can be applied to any herd, even a herd with two calving periods in a year.

CYCLE OF BEEF HERD HEALTH AND REPRODUCTIVE CALENDAR

Weaning Period

1. Identify and weigh calves if on production testing program.
2. Complete necessary immunizations of calves. This should include vaccinations for blackleg and malignant edema bacterins, necessary respiratory disease vaccinations and other immunizations applicable to the particular area if not already completed before weaning.
3. Use pour-on product for warble control if applicable at that time of year. Follow manufacturer's directions.
4. Control internal parasites.
5. Pregnancy test all cows and examine for general health.
6. Cull open cows, old and nonproductive cows (i.e., those with cancer eye, chronic lameness, poor teeth, previous vaginal prolapse, nonproductive udders).
7. Remove operable squamous cell carcinoma lesions.
8. Immunize against leptospirosis and vibriosis if necessary. Be aware of all the *Leptospira* serotypes for which it is necessary to immunize in your area.

Weaning to Calving Interval — 90 to 120 Days

1. Monitor herd nutrition. Separate herd by age and body condition into three groups: (a) replacement heifers, (b) pregnant first-calf heifers and thin cows and (c) pregnant mature cows in good condition. Each has different nutritional requirements and should be fed accordingly.

2. Control external and internal parasites.
3. Vaccinate pregnant cows when appropriate to aid in building maximum immunoglobulin levels in the colostrum for the prevention of neonatal calf diseases. An example is the use of *Clostridium perfringens* type C and D toxoid for the prevention of enterotoxemia or hemorrhagic enteritis of baby calves.

Calving Period — 90 Days (Fig. 2)

The events listed here are applicable to any length calving season. The implementation of preventive medicine and therapeutic procedures during this time greatly influences the per cent calf crop weaned.

The following questions form a check list in preparing for the calving season.

1. Is there adequate shelter? Is there a plan to provide 24-hour surveillance for first-calf heifers, while at the same time using minimum confinement. Experience and research have shown that minimum confinement reduces neonatal disease. Likewise, inadequate confinement may result in inadequate surveillance of calving heifers.

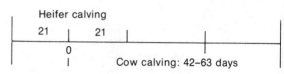

1. IDEAL: Heifers start 21 days before cows and calve for 42 days.

   COWS: 42 days   TOTAL: 63 days

2. PRACTICAL: Heifers start 21 days before cows and calve for 42 days.

   COWS: 63 days   TOTAL: 84 days

Figure 2. Diagram of 90-day calving period.

2. Has the herdsman been trained to use good judgment when assisting heifers and to call for veterinary service? The goal is a live calf to be delivered from a functional heifer. This will not be achieved unless the herdsman or owner knows his limitations and calls the veterinarian at the proper time.

3. Is there a plan to insure that all calves receive colostrum during the first 2 to 6 hours of life? Most healthy, vigorous calves will nurse during that time, but weaker calves will not and must be helped or hand fed to insure adequate colostrum consumption. Each calf should receive 5 to 6 per cent of body weight in colostrum during the first 24 hours of life. Maximum immunoglobulin absorption occurs during the first 6 hours of life, and these large molecules will not be absorbed from the intestine after 24 hours. Some heifers do not have adequate colostrum or will not allow the calf to nurse; therefore, these calves must be given special attention. Pints or quarts of stored frozen colostrum provide good insurance for such cases. Frozen colostrum can be thawed quickly and administered with a nursing bottle or stomach tube.

4. Is there a plan to separate cows with newborn calves from the rest of the herd? These cows require nearly twice as much feed as the prepartum cows. Maximum feed economy is attained by this separation.

5. Are calves identified and records kept of obstetrical and disease problems? These are important for production and reproduction analysis.

6. Is there a plan to prevent enteric diseases and to provide appropriate treatment when scours occurs?

During the calving season, cow health and nutrition need monitoring.

1. Is nutrition adequate for a nursing cow?

2. Are there adequate preparations to treat calving injuries such as vaginal lacerations, uterine prolapses and obturator paralysis? Most of these can be prevented by proper care at calving time, but some will occur and will need supportive treatment.

3. What are the plans for handling retained placenta? A small percentage of the cows will have retained placenta. The recommended treatments are intrauterine infusions and parenteral antibiotics. The membranes should not be manually removed unless they are already detached from the uterine caruncles and can therefore be easily removed. Records should be kept of treated cows so that follow-up treatments can be administered if necessary.

Replacement heifers must not be neglected during the busy calving season. They are approximately 1 year old and at the proper age to obtain yearling weights, and their growth should be monitored to insure proper breeding size by 14 to 15 months of age. Will these heifers achieve 65 per cent of their mature weight at 14 to 15 months of age? Cull heifers should be removed and should go to a feedlot or be placed on a cheaper ration. This is the proper time to give replacement heifers booster infectious bovine rhinotracheitis (IBR) and bovine viral diarrhea (BVD) immunizations, which should impart lifetime immunity. It is also time to start vibriosis vaccination where necessary.

Prebreeding Period — 30-day period

Herds that have desirable 60-day calving periods will have approximately 20 to 30 days between calving and breeding to prepare for the breeding season. When herds have longer calving seasons the following must be accomplished, approximately 30 days before breeding:

1. Brand, vaccinate and, if applicable, castrate the bull calves.
2. Control internal and external parasites if necessary.
3. Prepare the cow herd for breeding:
   a. Perform breeding soundness evaluations of bulls.
   b. Have all artificial insemination (AI) facilities ready and cows properly identified. If the owner/herdsman is doing the breeding, he should refresh his technique.
   c. Separate cull cows that are not intended to be bred. This is particularly important if there are many cows that will not be kept in the herd. They require additional feed and bulls if left in the breeding herd and are usually an economic liability.

Breeding Season — 60 to 90 days
(Fig. 3)

Regardless of the length of the breeding season the herd must be watched closely for

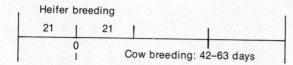

1. IDEAL: Heifers start 21 days before cows and breed for 42 days

   COWS: 42 days   TOTAL: 63 days

2. PRACTICAL: Heifers start 21 days before cows and breed for 42 days

   COWS: 42 days   TOTAL: 84 days

Figure 3. Diagram of 60- to 90-day breeding season.

disease problems and treated appropriately. In some areas internal and external parasites may need constant surveillance and control. In other areas toxic plant problems or pulmonary emphysema (cow asthma) may become herd problems, depending on pasture conditions. Many ranchers will spray periodically for flies during this time, which is also a good time for brucellosis immunization of heifer calves. Heifers should be within the recommended 2 to 6 months immunization age range at this time.

Ranchers who use AI must maintain superior estrous detection programs and excellent records for satisfactory results. Veterinarians serving such herds must be totally familiar with all new heat detection and breeding procedures.

Postbreeding-Preweaning Period

In this calendar there are approximately 90 days between the end of the breeding season and weaning. This period is shorter if the breeding season is longer. Few problems occur, but there may be specific pregnancy palpation or vaccination programs that some owners wish to implement during the 90 days before weaning.

1. Early pregnancy diagnosis (30 to 45 days after breeding) is primarily done to identify those cows that became pregnant to AI breeding. In such herds it is an important tool for identifying and selecting replacement heifers and for separating AI pregnancies from natural service pregnancies by clean-up bulls. Make an appointment to palpate for pregnancy 35 days after the last cow was bred by artificial insemination. Instruct the owner *not* to put any bulls with the cows for a 5-day period following the last AI breeding. This means that the youngest AI conceptus is 35 days old, which is palpable by the experienced veterinarian, and the oldest natural service conceptus is 30 days old, which is not palpable. All pregnant cows are identified as AI pregnancies. All open cows must be palpated again at weaning to determine their pregnancy status. At this time an owner may apply some parasite control measures.

2. Ranchers who retain ownership of their calves beyond weaning should consider some preweaning immunizations. Such programs are quite diverse in different sections of the United States. The goal is to reduce death and weight loss from postweaning diseases, especially respiratory diseases. This should be done approximately 3 to 4 weeks before weaning. The plan should be thoughtfully developed by the veterinarian and owner to satisfy individual herd needs. Starting calves on creep feed is recommended as an aid in adjusting to weaning. Ranchers who market calves at weaning have not thought that they have benefited from preconditioning programs. Purchasers of calves do not usually offer adequate premiums to cover preconditioning expenses. Even though data indicate that preconditioning reduces death loss and postweaning weight loss, it is difficult to recommend to clients who have found it unprofitable.

CONCLUSION

This completes one cycle of the beef herd health and reproductive calendar. This discussion does not provide all procedures for all beef herds. Rather, the purpose is to present a philosophy of planning a herd health program on an annual basis.

Examination Schedule for a Dairy Reproductive Health Program

DAVID A. MORROW

Michigan State University, East Lansing, Michigan

The objective of a reproductive health examination schedule is to prevent and control reproductive problems in cattle in order to maintain a profitable 12- to 13-month calving interval. This examination schedule is designed to include animals in certain reproductive categories at specific times. The frequency of farm visits will vary from weekly to monthly, depending on herd size and location.

Due to the low heritability and repeatability of reproductive disorders, the following examination schedule should be adhered to for best results and maximum return from veterinary service.

GROUP I

Cows with retained fetal membranes at 24 to 72 hours postpartum should be examined in a sanitary manner and treated conservatively if indicated with local or parenteral antibiotics. A broad-spectrum antibiotic such as 1 to 2 gm of oxytetracycline should be inserted into the uterus daily for several days for localized infection indicated by a fetid discharge. A therapeutic dose of the same drug should be administered locally or parenterally daily for several days for systemic infection. The administration of an estrogenic hormone may be helpful to increase uterine blood supply, to increase resistance to infection and to stimulate uterine contractions.

Drugs placed in the uterus are capable of causing milk and meat residues. Please follow directions on the label carefully for drugs used in food-producing animals.

Fetal membranes should not be forcibly removed by manual manipulation. The cotyledonary-caruncular attachment will become necrotic and separate at 5 to 10 days postpartum. Separation will permit the fetal membranes to be discharged intact. The removal of these detached membranes may be inhibited by a partially closed cervix. Mild tension should be applied to the exposed portion of the membranes daily to determine if detachment has occurred with passage of membranes restricted by the partially closed cervix.

The cervix, uterus and both ovaries will be located primarily in the abdominal cavity at 7 to 14 days postpartum. The normal involuting uterus should be firm with longitudinal grooves sometimes detectable. The detection of uterine fluid or lochia is normal. A thin-walled uterus containing an excessive amount of fluid is an indication of postpartum metritis. Manipulation of this type of reproductive tract should be minimized to help prevent development of perimetritis and salpingitis.

GROUP II

Cows with fetid or purulent vulvar discharge following dystocia, retention of the placenta or other postpartum complications should be examined in a sanitary manner to determine the source of the infection and treated conservatively. Once therapy is initiated with broad-spectrum antibiotics or other antibacterial agents, it should be continued daily for several days.

The reproductive tract is partially located in the pelvic canal at 14 days postpartum and can frequently be retracted by manipulation *per rectum*. The cervix is approximately 6 cm in diameter but is significantly larger in pluriparous than primiparous cows and in cows with periparturient diseases compared with cows with normal parturitions. Both uterine horns are palpable in primiparas and many pluriparas by the fourteenth day. The diameter of the uterine horns just craniad to the bifurcation is approximately 7 to 10 cm for the previously gravid horn but is larger in pluriparas than primiparas and in cows with periparturient diseases than cows with normal parturitions. Both ovaries are palpable. The regressing corpus luteum of pregnancy is frequently palpable until 14 days postpartum. It is a small, firm, slightly elevated mass on the surface of the ovary. Frequently one to three follicles ranging from 1.0 to 2.5 cm in

549

diameter are present in cows with normal parturitions. First ovulation frequently occurs by 15 days postpartum in normal cows. Ovaries are often small and inactive in cows with debilitating diseases or in high producing cows with a negative nutrient intake. The ovaries frequently remain inactive until recovery from disease occurs, production declines or the nutrient intake increases.

GROUP III

Cows should be examined at 20 to 40 days postpartum prior to breeding to determine if any detectable infection is present and if follicular or corpus luteum development has begun. The reproductive tract is located in the pelvic canal in all primiparas and most pluriparas 30 days postpartum.

The cervix is firm with a uniform diameter of approximately 3.5 to 4.0 cm 30 days postpartum. An enlarged external cervical os indicates prolapsed cervical rings or cervicitis, which is frequently secondary to metritis. Successful treatment of metritis usually corrects the cervicitis. The cervix is slightly larger in pluriparous than primiparous cows at this stage and slightly larger in cows with periparturient disease than normal cows at 30 days postpartum. The cervix is slightly larger than either uterine horn.

The diameter of uterine horns just craniad to the bifurcation is approximately 3.5 cm for the previously gravid horn and 3.0 cm for the nongravid horn 30 days postpartum. A uterine horn diameter greater than 4.0 cm after 20 days postpartum is an indicator of delayed uterine involution and reduced fertility.

Major differences in uterine horn diameter between age groups and between cows with or without periparturient disease do not usually exist 30 days postpartum. The lumina of both uterine horns should not be palpable. A palpable lumen is an indicator of delayed uterine involution most likely due to endometritis.

The vaginal discharge should be examined following rectal massage. Visual inspection of the vagina and cervix with the aid of a speculum will frequently be beneficial to confirm the diagnosis.

Gross abnormalities, such as pyometra, can be detected by palpation *per rectum* at 20 to 40 days postpartum; however, subtle involutionary changes and chronic endometritis may not be palpable. When an abnormal discharge is present, the site of infection, i.e., uterus, cervix, vagina, should be determined by vaginal examination. An infected cervix frequently indicates endometritis. If speculum examination reveals a clear cervical mucus, the vagina should be considered as the site of infection. Vaginitis is generally easily recognized on speculum examination. Cows that had a retained placenta or have reproductive infection indicated by purulent or fetid discharge or cloudy mucus during estrus should be treated by intrauterine infusion with antibiotics or other antibacterial agents during postpartum examination. Clinical evidence indicates that treatment of infected cows is helpful in reducing days open and services per conception. Controlled clinical research is needed to evaluate various postpartum treatment procedures and to determine the drug of choice, dosage and optimum time for administration of intrauterine infusion. Routine uterine infusion of normal cows is contraindicated.

At 30 days postpartum many cows have several developing follicles and a regressing normal or cystic corpus luteum that formed after estrus about 15 days postpartum. Large, thin-walled, cystic follicles greater than 2.5 cm in diameter are present on some ovaries. The average interval from parturition to first estrus is approximately 35 days in cows with periparturient disease postpartum. Many of these cows have small, inactive follicles, and a few have developing corpora lutea.

Since silent estrus and ovulation are most commonly observed during the early postpartum period, standing estrus may have been observed by the dairyman in only 20 to 30 per cent of cows with corpora lutea at the time of the postpartum examination. Silent or unobserved estrus may also be more common in high producing cows.

Normal corpora lutea will usually be present in 70 to 75 per cent of cows with functional ovaries, cystic corpora lutea in 10 to 15 per cent and cystic follicles in 15 to 20 per cent. Cows with cystic corpora lutea have estrous cycles of normal duration and often conceive when bred; therefore, treatment is not indicated.

Cystic follicles appear to be more common from 15 to 45 days postpartum than at any other time and are usually associated with anestrus. They are present more often in cows with periparturient disease than in cows following normal parturitions. Treatment is not recommended until later in the postpartum period unless signs of nymphomania are present because nearly one-half of early cases of cystic follicles recover spontaneously.

The reproductive tract frequently feels normal, from 20 to 40 days postpartum as determined by examination *per rectum;* therefore, the periparturient history, length of postpartum interval and absence of gross abnormalities on clinical examination are the main criteria for establishing the diagnosis, prognosis and treatment and for evaluating breeding soundness.

GROUP IV

Cows not showing estrus and those with abnormal estrous cycles 45 to 60 days postpartum should be re-examined. The diameters of the uterine horns are approximately the same size and the diameter of the cervix is slightly greater in the completely involuted reproductive tract. The most frequent causes of anestrus at this time are:

1. Pyometra with a retained corpus luteum of estrus. This condition develops in cows with postpartum metritis and is frequently prevented in herds on reproductive health programs. It responds well to intramuscular prostaglandin therapy (prostaglandin $F_{2\alpha}$ [25 mg Lutalyse]), with the expulsion of uterine contents at estrus in 3 to 5 days. The uterus should then be infused with broad-spectrum antibiotics following estrus.

2. Small inactive ovaries due to disease, high production, insufficient energy intake or a combination of these factors. After the predisposing cause is remedied, several weeks may be required before follicular development and estrus occur. Hormonal therapy to induce estrus is not usually indicated or necessary.

3. A functional corpus luteum in the absence of pathogenic uterine abnormalities, such as fetal mummification or pyometra, is not a retained corpus luteum, but indicates silent or unobserved estrus and ovulation. It is not necessary to manually remove a corpus luteum or to make frequent use of hormones. The stage of the estrous cycle should be estimated by palpating the size and consistency of the corpus luteum. Then the herdsman should be alerted to the time period for observing the animal to detect estrus. Animals with functional corpora lutea between days 6 and 16 of the estrous cycle also respond to intramuscular prostaglandin-$F_{2\alpha}$ (25 mg Lutalyse) therapy by coming into estrus 3 to 5 days after treatment. They should be bred at that time. Individual animals bred with expensive semen should be inseminated near the end of standing estrus, whereas groups of animals can be inseminated at approximately 80 hours after prostaglandin-$F_{2\alpha}$ therapy. Improved estrous detection is also indicated in herds with large numbers of animals in this category.

4. Cystic follicles are a common cause of anestrus and the most common cause of irregular cycles in the postpartum cow. Cows with anestrus should be treated 3 weeks prior to anticipated breeding time and bred at time of first estrus to prevent recurrence of cystic follicles. Cows with nymphomania or irregular estrous periods should be treated with luteinizing or gonadotropin-releasing hormone (GnRH) when diagnosed. These hormones produce luteinization of the cystic follicles and estrus in approximately 21 days in responsive cases. This treatment should not be repeated for 30 days unless signs of nymphomania persist in order to permit sufficient time for recovery.

GROUP V

Cows bred three or more times should be examined the day following estrus and breeding to detect possible causes of repeat breeding such as delayed ovulation, salpingitis, endometritis and pneumovagina. Consideration must also be given to egg and sperm quality as well as timing of insemination. If an intrauterine infusion is indicated, it must be administered no later than 2 days after estrus to avoid altering the estrous cycle.

GROUP VI

Cows should be examined for pregnancy 30 to 45 days after breeding to detect open cows. Abortions can occur from 30 days after breeding to term in 5 to 10 per cent of the cows. Since many early abortions will be undetected, individual cows with a history of infertility should be re-examined later in the gestation period.

REFERENCE

1. Morrow, D. A.: Postpartum ovarian activity and involution of the uterus and cervix in dairy cattle. Scope, *XIV*:2, 1969.

Records Essential for Reproductive Herd Health Programs in Cattle

DAVID A. MORROW

Michigan State University, East Lansing, Michigan

An effective reproductive record system must provide the livestock owner and veterinarian with the key information required to make reproductive management decisions. The system must be able to readily identify the animal and indicate reproductive status and action required by herdsman, management and veterinarian.

The record system must be flexible to accommodate different herd sizes. A loose-leaf notebook may be adequate for a small herd, whereas a computer is desirable for a large herd. The information must be recorded, summarized and utilized on a regular basis for best results.

The ideal goal for reproductive efficiency in cattle is a 365-day calving interval, which requires conception by 85 days after calving.

Records that can help veterinarians and herdsman achieve these goals will be discussed.

BARN BREEDING CHART

All cows should be listed on the Barn Breeding Chart in the order of calving (Fig. 1). Then estrus and breeding dates can be entered as they occur. This chronological listing of cows makes it easy to detect problem cows by observing the blank spaces under the heat and breeding columns and helps to maintain a 12-month calving interval. For example, cow 565 has not been bred, and cows 601 and 618 have not been observed in estrus. One essential criterion that all types of records must possess is the ability to identify cows for the herdsman that require his attention at a particular time. A chronological listing of cows in the order of calving on the Barn Breeding Chart fulfills this criterion; however, the conventional way of listing cows at the time of first service does not.

Barn Breeding Chart

Name or Ear Tag of Animal	Date Fresh	Heat Dates 1st	Heat Dates 2nd	Date Bred	Bull	Date Rebred	Bull	Date Rebred	Bull	Due Date
709	1-18	2-21	3-14	4-4	H 90	6-9	H 90	8-12	H90	5-22
677	3-14	4-11		6-17	H 90					3-29
700	3-18	5-14		8-10	H 90					5-20
676	3-20	4-30	5-20	6-10	H 99	6-30	H 99	7-17	H 99	4-27
693	6-4			8-2	H 99	9-16	H 99	10-8	H 99	7-20
673	6-7	7-20	8-14	9-4	H 90	10-16	H 90			7-26
660	6-23	7-21	8-20	9-10	H 95	10-24	H 95			8-4
565	9-22	10-30	11-20							
680	10-14	11-18	12-8	12-29	H 90	1-19	H 90			11-9
689	10-15	11-10	12-1	12-19	H 90	1-29	H 90			11-15
601	10-18									
618	10-20									
670	10-23	11-8	11-26							
690	11-27	12-13	1-1							
704	12-25	1-16								

Figure 1. Barn Breeding Chart. All cows should be listed on this record in order of calving. Estrous and breeding dates are added periodically.

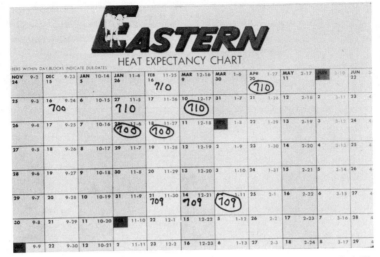

Figure 2. Estrous Expectancy Chart. All estrous periods are recorded. The cow's name is circled at the time of breeding. This chart should be displayed in a prominent place in the barn.

ESTROUS EXPECTANCY CHART

All estrous dates should be recorded on the Estrous Expectancy Chart (Fig. 2). This record, which should be located at the entrance to the barn, indicates when certain cows can be anticipated to be in estrus and should thus be observed more closely. Estrus can be more readily detected when the time of breeding approaches by referring to previously recorded dates. Irregular estrous cycles can also be readily detected by this chart. All estrous periods accompanied by breeding should be circled. Cows should be observed closely for estrus at approximately 21- and 42-day intervals after breeding. This observation should continue until pregnancy is confirmed by veterinary examination. The information on the Estrous Expectancy Chart should be transferred to the Barn Breeding Chart at weekly intervals.

DAIRY HERD MONITOR (BREEDING WHEEL)

This device combines the function of the Barn Breeding Chart and the Estrous Expectancy Chart and is a valuable management tool (Fig. 3). A color-coded key identifies individual cows by reproductive status, and the location of the wheel indicates the action required (Fig. 4). The value of the Breeding Wheel increases with the size of the herd and is essential for good fertility management in herds or groups of up to 200 cows.

The cow is entered on the Breeding Wheel by adding a tag or tape containing the proper identification in the area corresponding to the current date. The color used corresponds with the reproductive status such as calving, estrus or breeding. As the wheel is rotated clockwise on a daily basis, the cow's tag or

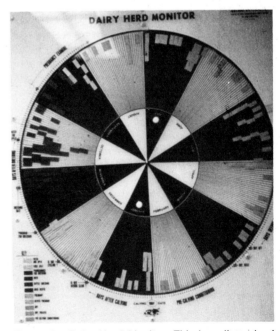

Figure 3. Dairy Herd Monitor. This breeding wheel helps the dairyman monitor the reproductive status of all cows in the herd.

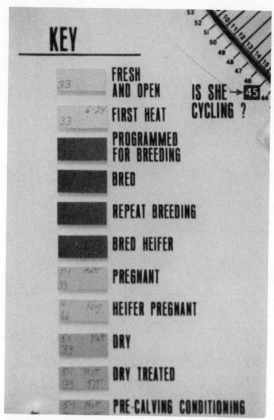

Figure 4. Dairy Herd Monitor Key. The color-coded key indicates to the herdsman the type of action required at a specific time.

Wheel. The information on the individual cow is recorded with a colored pencil that corresponds with the reproductive activity. This system has 12 sections that correspond to the 12 months in the year. Each month a new section is added for the current month, and the oldest section, which corresponds to the thirteenth month prior to the present date, is removed and can be filed for a permanent record. This system usually accommodates less than 100 cows and is less flexible than the Breeding Wheel.

COMPUTERS

Computerized systems provide the most efficient method of recording and summarizing data on individual cows and groups of cows. Dairy herd improvement (DHI) centers provide monthly lists of cows with a common reproductive status requiring the same management action; however, current information is frequently needed on a daily or weekly basis.

Recent advances in computer technology have led to the development of minicomputers located on farms and timesharing systems connected by telephone to a large, centrally located computer (Fig. 5). Although both computer systems are still in the developmental stages, they are currently being used on large farms on a limited basis. It is anticipated that computers will receive extensive future use for record keeping in large herds. These systems will electronically identify cows as they enter the parlor, determine the amount of grain to be received by each cow, record the milk weights and identify potentially sick cows. Computers will collect, sort and summarize large amounts of current information that will be used by management to make intelligent decisions in the areas of reproduction, general health, feeding and culling.

tape passes areas that indicate the need for action such as a postpartum reproductive examination, breeding or pregnancy examination. Since the color of the tag or tape changes with a change in the reproductive status, a color-coded profile is available of the reproductive status of all cows in the herd. Cows with reproductive problems can be readily identified by a color that does not match those in the same area of the wheel. The major disadvantage of the wheel system is that it does not provide a permanent record for each cow. For example, each time the status changes, the old tag or tape is discarded and a new one is added for the current date. The tag of a repeat breeder may be moved to date of breeding several times without realizing that a problem exists.

COW CALCULATOR

This device operates like a slide rule on a chronological basis, similar to the Breeding

HEALTH RECORD SYSTEMS

The system described here consists of a temporary Barn Sheet and a permanent Individual Cow Lifetime Health Record. Although intended to supplement each other, they are quite flexible and may be used either separately or together to fit the needs of an individual herdsman.

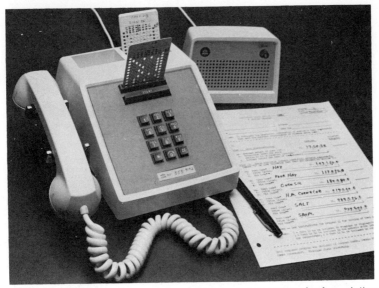

Figure 5. A telephone is used to contact a central computer for formulating least-cost balanced rations and obtaining reproductive health management information.

Individual Cow Lifetime Health Record

This record should be kept on each cow, starting at birth (Fig. 6). An 8½ × 11-inch card that fits into a three-ring notebook is illustrated. At the top of the card are the numbers 1 through 12, indicating the month of the year. Blue, white and red signal tabs are placed over the corresponding number of the months when a cow is examined and found ready to breed — the month of service and the month due to freshen, respectively. The location of these tabs enables the herdsman to determine at a glance the cows that are due to be dried off in a given month. He is also able to decide quickly which one should be observed closely for estrus. Located beneath the numbers is a space to identify the individual cow and to record all the necessary information to complete a health chart at the time of show or sale. The top half of the front page is for recording the prebreeding examination, estrus, breeding date, sire used, date examined pregnant, date due to calve and date of calving. The bottom half of the page contains space to record the results of the examination and treatment of the genital tract. Columns are provided for entering the information found on examining the vulva and vagina, cervix, uterus, right ovary and left ovary. There are additional columns for recording treatments and remarks.

The general health information is recorded on the back of the card (Fig. 7). Here conditions such as indigestion, mastitis, pneumonia and traumatic gastritis are recorded with appropriate information under columns for diagnosis, symptoms and treatment. There is also a space to include the vaccination dates for diseases such as leptospirosis, infectious bovine rhinotracheitis (IBR) and bovine virus diarrhea (BVD). This record is copied in ink by the herdsman from the barn sheet following the veterinarian's visit.

Barn Sheet

Before the veterinarian's regular visit, the herdsman organizes the work on the Barn Sheet (Fig. 8). The records of cows due for reproductive tract examinations are placed on the front of the work sheet in numerical order or in the order in which they stand in the barn. The cows to be examined can be rapidly determined by the color and location of the signal tabs on the Lifetime Health Records. The dates of parturition, time of estrus and pregnancy examination information are recorded under the appropriate column from the front of the Lifetime Health Records. At the time of examination, the herdsman accompanies the veterinarian and records the findings. It is very important that the herdsman be present at the time of

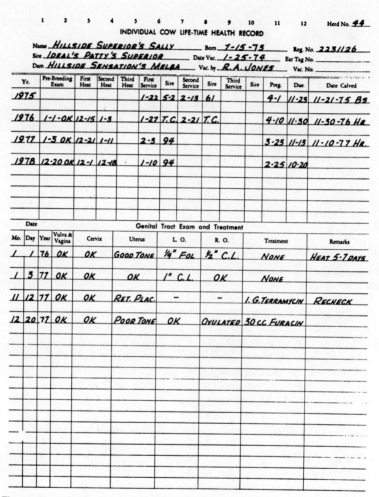

Figure 6. Individual Cow Lifetime Health Record. The front of the card is used to identify the cow and record her complete breeding history (top). Notes from reproductive tract examinations and treatment are recorded (bottom).

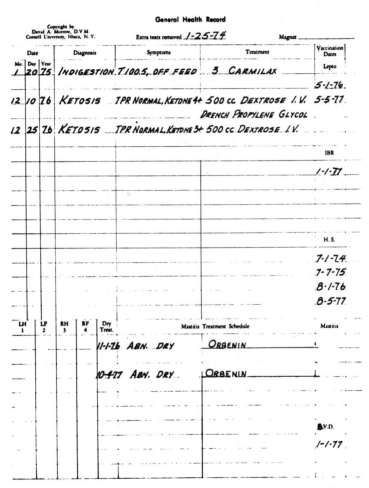

Figure 7. General Health Record. The back of the Individual Cow Lifetime Health Record card is used to record general disease conditions (top), mastitis (bottom) and immunizations (right).

Record of Cows for Monthly Reproductive Examination

Name _HILLSIDE_   Date _8-8-79_   Barn Sheet

	Cow	Fresh	Pre-Breeding	Estrum	Bred	Pregnant	Remarks
1							
2	SONJA	6-29	8-8 OK	7-10, 7-28			O.K. TO BREED
3							
4	GRACE	6-10	7-15 OK	6-27			CYSTIC L.O. 10,000 CHORIONIC
5							WATCH HEAT 2-3 WEEKS
6	SUE	1-9	2-15	1-20	4-7		
7					5-14		
8					6-23	PRH	
9							
10	POLLY	2-16	3-20	3-21, 4-15	5-5		
11					6-1	PLH	
12							
13	LADY	4-7	5-12	4-20, 5-10	6-21	PRH	RECHECK
14							
15							
16							
17							
18							
19							
20							
21							
22							
23							
24							
25							
26							
27							
28							
29							
30							

Figure 8. Barn Sheet (front). The dairyman records the reproductive history of each cow from the Barn Breeding Chart (Fig. 1) and the Individual Cow Lifetime Health Record (Fig. 6) prior to the veterinarian's arrival for the monthly reproductive examination.

Record of Animals

Cow	Fresh	Estrum	Bred and Pregnant (P)	Symptoms Noticed	Watch(?)	Instructions to Owner
						ACUTE MASTITIS
NOVA	2-25	3-9		OFF FEED HARD QUARTER	✓	TREAT QUARTER P.M. 17900
MARY	3-1			OFF FEED DRY MANURE		KETOSIS DRENCH PROP. GLYCOL
PATTY	6-10	7-12 7-30	8-19 (P)	LAME REAR LEG		FOOT ROT - KEEP IN BARN
LUCY	8-4	8-24 9-12	8-5 (P)	DROP IN MILK		INDIGESTION - GIVE TONIC

Copyright by
David A. Morrow, D.V.M
Cornell University, Ithaca, N.Y.

Figure 9. Barn Sheet (back). General health problems are recorded by the herdsman. The veterinarian may enter instructions for aftercare. This record should be located on a clipboard near the entrance to the barn.

the veterinarian's regular visit for communication purposes.

On the back of the Barn Sheet (Fig. 9) are recorded the sick animals and their location in the barn, along with the pertinent history and symptoms observed. There is also a space for the veterinarian to record his findings, leave instructions to the owner and indicate if milk is to be withheld on account of antibiotic therapy. The Barn Sheet is usually kept on a clipboard beside the barn desk so that the veterinarian can quickly locate sick animals on emergency or routine calls.

The veterinarian and herdsman must select the record system that is best for the herd size and goals of a particular operation. These systems are designed to provide rapid information for decision-making purposes that will help to obtain the goal of a 12-month calving interval.

Analysis of Records for Reproductive Herd Health Programs

DAVID A. MORROW

Michigan State University, East Lansing, Michigan

The reproductive health records must be summarized and evaluated periodically in both healthy and problem herds to compare results with desired goals. A plan of action then must be developed and implemented for the high priority areas indicated by the analysis for an effective reproductive health program.

The criteria for evaluation and the procedures for making the calculations are outlined in Table 1. Recommendations for achieving these goals are listed. The criteria for evaluation will vary with the objectives of the operation.

REPLACEMENTS (Table 1)

Mortality. Losses can be classified by periods, as follows:

1. *Birth.* Recent field surveys indicate that more than 5 per cent of calves are born dead.[3] The goal of keeping losses below 5 per cent at birth can be achieved by proper conditioning of the dam during the dry period, good herdsmanship and veterinary care at calving.

2. *Zero to 30 days.* Recent field surveys indicate that calf mortality during the first month of life may be as high as 10 to 15 per cent of all calves born alive.[3] A majority of these calf losses are due to colibacillosis. The goal of keeping losses below 5 per cent can be achieved by hand feeding colostrum immediately after calving, with 10 to 12 pounds being fed during the first 24 hours; feeding fresh or frozen colostrum for the next 3 to 4 days; and then feeding fermented colostrum, whole milk or milk replacer at the rate of 8 per cent of body weight daily until the calf is consuming 1.5 pounds of starter at 4 to 6 weeks of age. A dry, draft-free environment is also helpful in reducing mortality. Calf hutches have proved to be beneficial in reducing mortality in many situations.

3. *One to 24 months.* The primary cause of mortality during this period is both acute and chronic pneumonia. This disease can frequently be prevented by proper ventilation, which is essential to achieve the goal of keeping mortality below 2 per cent during this period.

4. *Total mortality.* Losses at birth and during the first 2 years of life due primarily to colibacillosis and pneumonia should be kept below 10 per cent. This goal can be achieved by good herdsmanship, feeding, management and veterinary care. The diagnostic laboratory can frequently aid the practitioner in arriving at a diagnosis and in instituting therapy based on the results of bacterial cultures and sensitivity testing.

Breeding Age and Weight. Holstein replacement heifers should be pregnant at approximately 15 months of age and at 800 pounds tape weight. This goal can be achieved by feeding heifers to gain approximately 1.5 pounds daily for 450 days (15 months) and by starting to breed these heifers at 14 months of age when they weigh

TABLE 1. *Reproductive Herd Health Management Program Goals*

Herd _____ Evaluator _____ Date _____			
	NO.	%	GOAL
I. Replacements			
A. Mortality			
1. Birth $= \dfrac{\text{calves dead at birth}}{\text{calves born}}$	=	=	< 5%
2. 0–30 days $= \dfrac{\text{calves died 0–30 days}}{\text{calves born}}$	=	=	< 5%
3. 1–24 months $= \dfrac{\text{calves died 1–24 months}}{\text{calves born}}$	=	=	< 2%
4. Total $= \dfrac{\text{calves died birth to 24 mo.}}{\text{calves born}}$	=	=	< 10%
B. Breeding			
1. Age $= \dfrac{\text{interval birth to first service}}{\text{total heifers}}$	=	=	< 15 mo.
2. Weight $= \dfrac{\text{total weight at first service}}{\text{total helfers}}$	=	=	> 750 lb.
C. Calving			
1. Age $= \dfrac{\text{interval birth to parturition}}{\text{total heifers}}$	=	=	> 24 mo.
2. Weight $= \dfrac{\text{total weight at parturition}}{\text{total heifers}}$	=	=	> 1200 lb.
II. Reproductive Efficiency			
A. Interval to first estrus $= \dfrac{\text{calving to first estrus}}{\text{total cows}}$	=	=	< 45 days
B. Interval to first service $= \dfrac{\text{calving to first service}}{\text{total cows}}$	=	=	< 60 days
C. Days open $= \dfrac{\text{days calving to conception}}{\text{total cows}}$	=	=	< 100 days
D. Calving interval $= \dfrac{\text{days calving to calving}}{\text{total cows}}$	=	=	< 380 days
E. Services per conception $= \dfrac{\text{no. services in all cows}}{\text{total conceptions}} =$	=	=	< 2.0
III. Periparturient Conditions			
A. Milk fever $= \dfrac{\text{cows with milk fever}}{\text{total parturitions}}$	=	=	< 3%
B. Ketosis $= \dfrac{\text{cows with ketosis}}{\text{total parturitions}}$	=	=	< 3%
C. Displaced abomasum $= \dfrac{\text{cows with displacements}}{\text{total parturitions}} =$	=	=	< 3%
D. Mastitis $= \dfrac{\text{cows with mastitis}}{\text{total cows}}$	=	=	< 10%
IV. Culling Rate			
A. Involuntary $= \dfrac{\text{number culled}}{\text{total cows}}$	=	=	< 15%
B. Voluntary $= \dfrac{\text{number culled}}{\text{total cows}}$	=	=	< 10%
C. Total $= \dfrac{\text{total culled}}{\text{total cows}}$	=	=	< 25%

approximately 750 pounds. Heifers should be bred by artificial insemination (AI) to proven bulls that sire smaller than average calves. These bulls should have a predicted difference dollar value greater than $125 with the repeatability greater than 60 per cent.

Calving Age and Weight. Holstein heifers pregnant at 15 months and 800 pounds will calve at 24 months and at 1200 pounds providing they are fed to gain 1.5 pounds daily for the 280-day gestation period. Calving difficulty will be minimized providing all the above criteria for breeding and calving are met; however, failure to meet one or more of these criteria for age, weight and calf size can be disastrous.

REPRODUCTIVE EFFICIENCY
(Table 1)

These criteria are usually calculated separately for cows and heifers. The intervals for first estrus and first service are applicable only for cows.

Interval to First Estrus. This criterion is a good indicator of the estrous detection and recording procedures in the herd. There is a tendency for the herdsman not be concerned about estrus until the cow is ready to breed. A recorded estrus soon after calving can be beneficial in helping to detect a subsequent estrus for breeding. Healthy cows fed to meet approximate nutrient requirements will frequently have their first estrus by 20 days after calving; however, the signs of this early estrus are frequently not as strong as those of later estrous periods. A herdsman doing a good job of estrous detection should observe a majority of cows in estrus by 30 to 40 days postpartum. A realistic goal for all cows should be a maximum interval of 45 days from calving to first observed estrus.

Interval to First Service. In order to maintain a 12-month calving interval, the average interval to first service must be less than 70 days. Research indicates that the calving interval can be reduced by early breeding after calving; however, there is a slight reduction in fertility.[2] As a result, the herdsman should wait at least 60 days after calving for the first service when expensive semen is being used.

Cows that are examined by a veterinarian at approximately 30 days after calving and found satisfactory to breed can be serviced at the first estrus after 45 days. Since the estrous cycle is 21 days long, the average interval to first service should be approximately 10 days longer than the minimum interval required for breeding. The interval to first service should not be greater than 60 days in herds starting to breed at 45 days. It averaged 87 days in 125 New York dairy herd improvement (DHI) Holstein herds.[4] The interval to first service frequently exceeds 100 days in herds with reproductive problems due to poor estrous detection.

Days Open. This factor measures the interval from calving to conception. It is an excellent measure of reproductive efficiency because days open can be calculated as soon as the cow is examined by the veterinarian and found pregnant, permitting the early detection of infertility. If the first service occurs at 60 days postpartum, it is possible to have one or two additional services to obtain conception and still maintain a days open interval of less than 100 days.

Days open is the most important measure of reproductive efficiency because it combines the ability to detect estrus and fertility of both male and female. An excessive number of days open may be due to delayed breeding and failure of cows to come into estrus after calving due to disease, high production, low energy intake, cystic follicles, poor estrous detection, repeat breeding or infertile semen. In 76,610 cows in Ohio DHI herds, dairymen lost 14.7 days due to conception failure and 40.3 days due to missed estrous periods.[1] Approximately one-half of the estrous periods were being missed in these herds. The Ohio results are supported by a New York field study with 125 herds and 9750 cows, which found the average interval between two services to be approximately 50 days or the equivalent of two estrous periods.[4] The most efficient method of reducing the days open is to increase the accuracy of estrus detection.

Calving Interval. This factor measures the interval from calving to calving. The approximate interval can be determined by adding the length of the gestation period in cattle (280 days) to the days open. As a result, the length of the calving interval is determined by the same factors that affect days open. A realistic goal is 380 days or less, which is equivalent to a 12.5 month or less calving interval.

Since days open and calving interval provide the same information, there is no need to calculate both. Days open should be used when possible because it permits earlier detection of potential infertility problems.

PERIPARTURIENT CONDITIONS
(Table 1)

Milk Fever. This metabolic disease occurs about the time of parturition owing to hypocalcemia. Since a majority of milk fever cases can be prevented by regulating the calcium and phosphorus intake during the dry period, the occurrence of this disease should be kept below the goal of 3 per cent. Feeding a calcium-deficient diet for 10 to 14 days prepartum is also helpful in decreasing the incidence of milk fever in problem herds.

Ketosis. This metabolic disease occurs during the first 6 to 8 weeks postpartum because of hypoglycemia. Cows that are overconditioned at parturition or underfed during early lactation are predisposed to ketosis. The feeding program during late lactation, the dry period and early lactation will help to prevent many ketosis cases and keep the occurrence below the goal of 3 per cent.

Displaced Abomasum. This condition usually occurs during early lactation. It is frequently associated with milk fever and retained fetal membranes. Two nutritional factors that have been incriminated in causing displaced abomasum are high concentrate feeding and low fiber diets during the periparturient period. This condition can be prevented by (1) challenge feeding concentrate postpartum rather than lead feeding prepartum, (2) maintaining a high fiber level in the balanced ration and (3) making a minimum number of gradual changes in the ration of periparturient cows. These recommendations should be helpful in keeping the occurrence of displaced abomasum below the goal of 3 per cent.

Mastitis. Acute cases of mastitis frequently occur during early lactation, whereas chronic cases can occur throughout the lactation period. The occurrence of both types should be kept below the goal of 10 per cent by teat dipping, dry cow treating, good sanitation, proper milking practices and a milking machine that is functioning properly.

CULLING RATE (Table 1)

Involuntary. Forced culling for infertility, mastitis, other disease conditions and injuries should be kept to a minimum and below the goal of 10 per cent. The losses due to injury in large herds in free stall housing are important. A low involuntary cull rate permits cows to have more profitable lactations in the herd, herd expansion and selective culling for herd improvement.

Voluntary. Selective culling for functional type traits such as udder conformation, feet, legs and milking speed, low production and dairy purposes will be possible only in herds with good herd health management. A reasonable goal for voluntary culling and herd improvement is approximately 15 per cent.

Total Culling Rate. The total culling rate is a good indication of the quality of herd health management. A low culling rate is generally desirable because it provides the cows with a greater number of lactations to make a profit. A culling rate of 20 per cent means the average cow will have five lactations in the herd. The culling rate increases with the size of the herd and is more than 30 per cent in some large herds, requiring the purchase of herd replacements. A reasonable goal for total culling is less than 25 per cent.

Equally important to the culling rate are the reasons for culling. If the number of cows culled for disease can be minimized, the herd can be expanded or improved by culling for poor type and low production. Added income can also be gained by selling cows for dairy purposes.

SUMMARY

Criteria were established to evaluate the reproductive health status of a herd. Goals that can be successfully achieved were developed in the areas of raising replacements, breeding efficiency, periparturient conditions and culling rate. Suggestions for achieving these goals were oulined as a means of conducting an effective herd health management program.

REFERENCES

1. Barr, H. L.: Influence of estrous detection on days open in dairy herds. J. Dairy Sci., *58*:246, 1975.
2. Olds, D. and Cooper, T.: Effects of postpartum rest period in dairy cattle on the occurrence of breeding abnormalities and on calving interval. J.A.V.M.A., *157*:93, 1970.
3. Oxender, W. D., Newman, L. D. and Morrow, D. A.: Factors influencing dairy calf mortality in Michigan. J.A.V.M.A., *162*:458, 1973.
4. Spaulding, R. W., Everett, R. W. and Foote, R. H.: Fertility in New York artificially inseminated Holstein herds in dairy herd improvement. J. Dairy Sci., *48*:718, 1975.

Effects of a Reproductive Health Program on Reproductive Performance

LAWRENCE E. HEIDER
Ohio State University, Columbus, Ohio

As dairy farms become larger, there is an increased desire and need to utilize economically sound programs as part of management. Reproductive health programs must also be based on cost benefit analysis. If they are not, they will be discarded.

Britt[2] has reported the loss of income per cow per day of delayed conception beyond 85 days after calving at four production levels (Table 1). This shows the economic advantage of optimal reproductive performance. The loss was lower in group 4 than in group 3 because the highest production group had a shorter dry period with a higher percentage of days in milk during the calving interval.

Several investigators have sought answers to questions concerning the influence of reproductive health programs on reproductive efficiency, costs and returns. In 1971, Barfoot *et al.*[1] reported their evaluation of a total herd health program, at different levels of acceptance and expense, on five health parameters including average days open, culling rate and milk production. This economic appraisal demonstrated a positive influence on reproductive health and net income.

More recently, Galton[3] has evaluated the effects of a reproductive health program in a well-controlled study on reproductive and economic performance. In this study, 144 cows within one herd were divided into two groups on the basis of parity. The cows were observed through 184 parturitions, 94 in the reproductive health group and 90 in the control group. The reproductive health group received postpartum, pregnancy and anestrous examinations on a regular basis as well as infertility examinations following fourth services. The control group was examined, and the information was recorded for comparison and analysis only. This information was not used as an indication for therapy or management decisions. Both groups were housed, fed and managed as one unit, and only the evaluator knew the group identity of cows. Several reproductive parameters were measured to determine differences between the two groups (Table 2).

Accounts of actual receipts and expenses were maintained during the trial. The herd health group had slightly increased income from more total milk and calves produced. There was slightly more income from culling in the control group because of increased turnover of cows. Expenses for semen and replacements were greater in the control group. Veterinary costs were greater in the reproductive health group. The differences in income were not significant; however, there were significant differences (P < 0.05) in the total reproductive expenses. Net difference was about 16 cents per cow per day or $58.40 per year in favor of the herd health group (Table 3).

This kind of information should encourage cattlemen and veterinarians to work co-

TABLE 1. *Loss in Income per Cow per Day of Delayed Conception beyond 85 Days after Calving**

| Calving Interval (days) | Production less than 5455 kg | Ability of Cows (5455–6363 kg) | Kg/305 Days | |
			6363–7272 kg	OVER 7272 kg
Less than 365	0	0	0	0
366–395	$1.11	$0.44	$2.18	$0.44
396–425	$1.05	$1.64	$2.48	$1.37
Greater than 426	$1.13	$1.74	$2.08	$1.49

*From Britt, J. H.: J. Dairy Sci., *58*:266, 1975.

TABLE 2. *Comparison of Reproduction Performance Variables*

Group	No. Service/Conception[a]		Days to First Service[b]	Days Open[c]
Control group	90	2.37	86.8	140.0
Reproductive health group	94	1.73	73.1	99.2

[a](P < 0.05).
[b](P < 0.01).
[c](P <0.001).

TABLE 3. *Reproductive Cost Factors per Cow per Experimental Day**

Receipts	Herd Health			Control		
Milk value[a]	$4.08			$4.03		
Calves[b]	0.14			0.12		
Primary culls[c]	0.06			0.10		
Primary and secondary culls[c]		0.14			0.21	
All culls[c]			0.23			0.34
	$4.28	4.36	4.45	$4.25	4.36	4.49
Expenses:						
Semen costs[d]	0.049			0.075		
Veterinary costs[e]	0.046			0.042		
Replacements costs[f]						
Primary	0.17			0.29		
Primary and secondary		0.38			0.59	
All culls			0.66			0.91
	$0.28	0.49	0.77	$0.41	0.71	1.03[g]
Income–Expenses	$4.00	3.87	3.68	3.84	3.65	3.46

*From Galton, D. M.: Dissertation, Ohio State University, 1976.
[a]Milk value—$9.00 per 45.45 kg.
[b]Calves (males—50% of total calves—average 38.64 kg body weight).
[c]Per cull—$0.484 per kg—average 545.45 kg.
[d]Total services—$10.00 per service.
[e]Actual costs of the program (reproduction).
[f]Replacement value of $750.00 per animal culled.
[g](P < 0.05).

operatively in health management programs to achieve economic success.

REFERENCES

1. Barfoot, L. W., Cote, J. F., Stone, J. B. and Wright, P. A.: An economic appraisal of a preventive medi-cine program for dairy herd health management. Can. Vet., *12*:2, 1971.
2. Britt, J. H.: Early post partum breeding in dairy cows: A review. J. Dairy Sci., *58*:266, 1975.
3. Galton, D. M.: Effects of a herd health program on reproductive performance of dairy cows. Dissertation, Ohio State University, 1976.

CANINE

Consulting Editor

VICTOR M. SHILLE

Sexual Behavior and Problems with Sociosexual Behavior

JAN LADEWIG
and BENJAMIN L. HART
University of California, Davis, California

The concept of sexual dimorphism is critical in understanding sexual behavior. Anatomical differences in the brain between males and females have been noted particularly in the medial preoptic hypothalamus. These structural differences may be accompanied by physiological and biochemical differences and relate to differences in behavior between males and females.

Sexually dimorphic behavior in dogs is evident in several respects. With few exceptions, males are more aggressive than females. Male dogs display mounting and pelvic thrusting toward estrous females much more readily than will normal females, whereas the female receptive posture is only rarely seen in males. Male dogs have a urination posture that is only infrequently displayed by female dogs. This behavior is more sexually dimorphic in canids than in most other mammals. Males show the leg-lift posture during urination as opposed to the squat posture in females, and the frequency of urination is much higher in males than in females. Urination in males serves, presumably, a double purpose of emptying the urinary bladder and of scent marking territorial objects, whereas in females the primary purpose of urination is to empty the bladder, although an increase in urinations may be seen around the time of the estrous period. The latter is presumably not related to territorial marking but is used to advertise her reproductive state.

The existence of sexually dimorphic differences in behavior does not mean that males and females are not able to display the behavioral patterns typical of the opposite sex. Females certainly are capable of being fiercely aggressive and on occasion may display male-like urine marking. The difference between the sexes therefore is one of frequency or probability rather than of qualitative difference.

In males, sexual behavior, as well as urine marking and fighting, is often reduced by castration. Sexual receptivity of females is permanently eliminated by ovariectomy. However, gonadectomy does not bring the sexes to some neutral plane, and it is apparent that animals remain basically true to their behavior even following gonadectomy.

For the most part, the administration of the hormone of one sex to animals of the opposite sex does not change behavioral characteristics, although some aspects of behavior may be enhanced such as the occurrence of mounting in testosterone-treated spayed females or sexual attractiveness to males in estrogen-treated males. Sex-typical behavioral patterns are fundamentally a function of neonatal gonadal androgen secretion and the influence of androgen secretion upon certain brain areas.

ONTOGENY OF SEXUAL BEHAVIOR

Sexual dimorphism reflects the differentiation of the fetal or neonatal brain into a masculine or a feminine direction. In the male fetus and neonate a surge in gonadal androgen presumably acts on the central nervous system to promote a masculine differentiation of certain parts of the brain including the preoptic area. In the female there is no significant secretion of any fetal or neonatal sex hormone. Thus, the development of a "female nervous system" reflects the absence of testosterone.

Early deprivation of androgen in the male by neonatal castration will cause a permanent reduction of masculine sexual behavior even if exogenous testosterone is given in adulthood. The administration of testosterone to the fetal and/or neonatal female, on the other hand, will cause varying degrees of behavioral and genital masculinization and behavioral defeminization depending upon the time of treatment.

After the perinatal surge testosterone levels do not rise again until the time of puberty. The prepubertal sexual activity often seen in male dogs therefore occurs prior to postpubertal androgen secretion. This behavior consists of sexual mounting, pelvic thrusting and various degrees of penile erection and is most commonly seen in connection with play. This so-called "play sex" undoubtedly facilitates the development of normal sexual behavior and copulatory efficiency in adulthood. Male dogs raised in a semi-isolated condition with little physical contact with other animals showed sexual excitement as adults in the presence of receptive females but displayed a high frequency of incorrectly oriented mounting.[1]

During the prepubertal period there is sexual dimorphism in the urination posture of males and females. Females display the squat posture and, in fact, retain this posture into adulthood. Males, for the most part, develop a stand-lean posture soon after they are able to walk easily. Thus, this sexually dimorphic behavior is also somewhat independent of concurrent androgen secretion. At about the time of puberty, urination posture changes in males from the stand-lean to the adult leg-lift posture. Also, sexual behavior characteristic of the adult male is seen shortly thereafter. It was earlier assumed that these changes were the result of the pubertal rise in testosterone secretions, but recent observations on male dogs castrated on the first day of life have shown that these castrates will eventually display the adult leg-lift posture on at least some occasions.[3] It appears that testosterone exerts its primary influence on urination posture during the fetal and neonatal period, and the later change in urination posture is more a function of maturation of the nervous system. Males castrated before puberty tend to have delayed display of the male leg-lift posture, and they frequently revert to the juvenile posture.

NORMAL SEXUAL BEHAVIOR

In order to describe sexual activity it is convenient to categorize it into appetitive and consummatory responses. The appetitive or precopulatory responses vary considerably among individual animals and are readily influenced by learning and environmental factors. The consummatory or copulatory responses are rather stereotyped in both the male and female. Ejaculation and, to some degree, erection are basically spinal reflexes. The receptive posture of the female, especially the lateral curvature of the hindquarters, is also apparently largely reflexive.

Appetitive Sexual Behavior

In free-ranging dogs and in canids related to the dog, long distance communication may play a role in bringing sexual partners together. In canids, as in most other mammalian species, this type of communication is accomplished by the use of sex pheromones. In the female, estrogens, metabolites thereof or secretory products resulting from estrogen secretion are apparently excreted or secreted into the urine. The urine that is deposited by the estrous female has an excitatory effect upon the male and plays some role in attracting him to the female's vicinity. During estrus, females show an increased tendency to urinate and may occasionally assume the leg-lift posture and therefore deposit urine on prominent vertical objects. Available evidence indicates that anal sac secretions do not play a role as a sexual attractant or pheromone.

Once a sexually active male dog and a receptive female dog are together, some elements of what may be referred to as sexual foreplay occur. The male will investigate the anogenital region of the female and may mount soon thereafter. The duration of this foreplay varies among individual males. Often an experienced stud may achieve intromission after only a brief anogenital investigation. Less experienced males may spend a considerable amount of time not only investigating the female but also urine marking the surrounding territory and playing with the female. Play-inviting behavior is sometimes observed in which the male, facing the female, may crouch on his elbows and spring at the female. Some females respond to this by dashing a short distance, as if inviting the male to chase them.

During anogenital investigation and mounting, the female will usually remain in a position of sexual presentation. This consists of the rear quarters being curved to one side or the other (usually toward the male) and the tail looped over to one side. Tactile stimulation of the vulvar region evokes contraction of the constrictor vestibuli muscle, which tends to elevate or move the vulvar orifice toward the side that the male is on. If the male dismounts without intromission, begins playing or seems to lose interest in the female, she can become excited and may mount the male and engage in pelvic thrusting. This, in turn, seems to stimulate the male to further sexual activity.

The experienced male dog will mount the female from the posterior, clasp her flank region with his front legs and start pelvic thrusting. At this time the fibrous erectile body of the penis (corpus cavernosum) becomes erect, causing a protrusion of the penis by a few centimeters out of the prepuce. Penetration seems to be achieved by trial and error pelvic thrusting. Once partial insertion has occurred, the intensity and frequency of thrusting increase until there is complete intromission.

Less experienced male dogs spend considerably more time mounting and thrusting. It is not uncommon to see such males mount from the front or side before finally orienting from the posterior position. This lack of orientation is especially evident in males that have not had a chance to interact sociosexually with other dogs during prepubertal development.

Occasionally, in a very excited male erection of the glans penis may progress to the point at which intromission is not possible. Usually a period of rest or manual palpation of the coronal part of the erect glans will induce detumescence.

Consummatory Sexual Responses

Once there is complete intromission, the intensity and frequency of pelvic thrusting by the male are increased. The clasp with the front legs is tightened, and the front legs are pulled posteriorly. The tail is deflected downward, and there is the onset of alternate leg stepping of the hind legs, which accompanies intense pelvic thrusting. This reaction, called the intense ejaculatory reaction lasts about 15 to 30 seconds and is terminated by the male dismounting or the female throwing the male. During this reaction the bulbus glandis of the penis becomes completely erect and is too large to be pulled from the vulvar orifice. Thus, the sexual partners become locked together.

The sperm-dense fraction of seminal fluid is expelled during the intense ejaculatory reaction. Seminal ejaculation occurs as a result of peristaltic contractions of smooth muscle in the urethra together with rhythmic contraction of the bulbospongiosus muscle that surrounds the urethra after it leaves the pelvic cavity.

Occasionally during mating attempts the male dog may act as though intromission has occurred and will go through a complete intense ejaculatory reaction as a result of the penis being wedged between the perineum of the female and the pelvic region of the male.

The female remains relatively inactive in the receptive position during the major part of the intense ejaculatory reaction. She will usually begin twisting and turning vigorously at about the time the bulbus glandis of the penis would reach its maximal size. Females that have been bred only a few times may show evidence of pain by reacting more excitedly or even yelping. If the male has not already dismounted, as most experienced males do before the onset of the twisting and turning, this behavior is likely to throw him off. Inexperienced male dogs are often reluctant to dismount and may even appear a bit puzzled.

The genital lock, which continues immediately after the intense ejaculatory reaction, has a duration of usually 10 to 30 minutes. However, it may be as brief as 5 minutes or as long as 1 hour. The dogs remain locked together because the swollen bulbus glandis is too large to be withdrawn from the vaginal orifice. There is no direct evidence suggesting that contraction of the constrictor vestibuli muscles by the female plays a significant role in retaining the penis within the vagina or in occluding the venous return and thus prolonging erection.

Since the glans penis cannot rotate within the vagina, the body of the penis is twisted 180° as it is reflected posteriorly. During the lock, males tend to remain rather passive, but sometimes the females move about and may drag the males behind them.

The adaptive value or function of the genital lock is not understood. It has been suggested that with the engorgement of the penis within the vagina during the lock, deposition of sperm into the uterus rather than the vagina is assured.

When detumescence of the penis allows the bulb to pass through the vaginal orifice, the lock is terminated and the two dogs separate. The penis may still be somewhat erect just after the lock, and frequently the male dog will sit or lie down and lick the genital area. Sometimes he will also investigate the female genitalia immediately after copulation but will usually not attempt to mount again.

COLLECTION OF SEMEN FOR ARTIFICIAL INSEMINATION

Copulatory responses appear to be mediated at a spinal level, and the central nervous system seems to exert an inhibitory influence on the sexual reflexes. This central inhibition must be diminished before ejaculation can occur. A calm and familiar environment and presentation of an estrous female will help to decrease the central inhibition and thereby help ejaculation.

During the intense ejaculatory reaction, the area of the corpus of the penis, just posterior to the bulbus glandis, and the urethral process receive maximal tactile stimulation, causing expulsion of seminal fluid. Stimulation of corpus penis with one hand and stimulation of the urethral process either with a finger of the other hand or with the edge of the collecting tube will most closely resemble the natural situation and facilitate ejaculation.

PROBLEMS WITH SEXUAL AND RELATED BEHAVIORS

Aggression, roaming and urine marking in inconvenient places are problems frequently presented to the practitioner. Sexual mounting of animals other than estrous bitches, inanimate objects or people is probably not as common, but is not rare and was found to occur in about one-third of the dogs in a survey of 234 dog owners.[6]

Socialization occurs during the period from the third to the twelfth week of life. Contact with the mother, littermates and people at that time is of paramount importance for the development of normal social responses later in life. Isolation from conspecifics (e.g., in the case of bottle feeding a puppy) may make a dog unable to interact socially with other dogs. Severe aggression or profound timidity may be seen, rather than more subtle threat display and submission. On the other hand, lack of human contact during this sensitive period (e.g., in the case of puppies raised in animal shelters), will often result in dogs being unable to interact with people.

Causes of sexual behavior directed toward inappropriate objects are unknown and are not likely to be due to "hormonal imbalance"

or the occurrence of testicular or adrenal tumors.

BEHAVIORAL EFFECTS OF GONADECTOMY

The most widely used correctional procedure for sexual behavior problems is castration. A prognosis about the success of this operation is difficult. In some dogs sexual behavior is abolished almost immediately, whereas others will continue to mate apparently unaffected for many years. Recent work in other species suggests that the continuation of sexual activity cannot be explained by residual amounts of gonadal androgens. Also, since adrenalectomy does not affect sexual activity of castrated male dogs, adrenal androgens cannot be the reason for persistence of the behavior.[2]

Experiments on the effect of castration in dogs showed that elements of sexual behavior can survive for years after castration of mature dogs regardless of whether they were sexually experienced or not. Dogs castrated as juveniles had difficulty with intromission as adults and were unable to achieve lock. This deficiency was attributed to the small size of the penis and the reduced diameter of the erect bulbus glandis. The decline of sexual behavior, when apparent, occurred within 6 months after castration. Frequency of mating declined, and there was increase in the latency to the first mount and decrease in the duration of the genital lock.

In order to compare these experimental results with a more practical situation, Hopkins et al.[5] analyzed the effect of castration of 42 dogs with behavioral problems. Interviews with the dog owners about 2 years after the operation revealed that roaming was most affected by castration, with 44 per cent of the dogs showing a rapid decline in this behavior (i.e., within 14 days), 50 per cent showing a gradual decline (i.e., within 6 months) and only 6 per cent showing no decline. Intermale aggression was affected in a total of 63 per cent of the dogs, urine marking in the house in 50 per cent and mounting of people or animals other than estrous bitches in 67 per cent. The effect of the castration did not seem to be correlated with the age at which the operation was done, thereby indicating that sexual experience did not play a role.

EFFECTS OF LONG–ACTING PROGESTINS

Administration of a long-acting progestin such as medroxyprogesterone at the rate of about 5 mg per pound of body weight may show effects similar to castration.[4] Since this treatment, at least in some cases, will extend the effect of castration, the two methods may be combined so that if castration has proved unsuccessful in some respects, progestin treatment should be attempted for possible additional effect.

REFERENCES

1. Beach, F. A.: Coital behavior in dogs. III. Effects of early isolation on mating in males. Behaviour, *30*:217, 1968.
2. Beach, F. A.: Coital behavior in dogs. VI. Long-term effects of castration upon mating in the male. J. Comp. Physiol. Psychol., *70*:1, 1970.
3. Beach, F. A.: Effects of gonadal hormones on urinary behavior in dogs. Physiol. Behav., *12*:1005, 1974.
4. Hart, B. L.: Behavioral effects of castration. Canine Practice, June, pp. 10–21, 1976.
5. Hopkins, S. G., Schubert, T. A., and Hart, B. L.: Castration of adult male dogs: Effects on roaming, aggression, urine marking and mounting. J.A.V.M.A., *168*:1108, 1976.
6. Ladewig, J.: Unpublished data.

Clinical Reproductive Physiology in Dogs

VICTOR M. SHILLE AND GEORGE H. STABENFELDT
University of Florida, Gainesville, Florida

THE FEMALE

The onset of puberty usually occurs between 6 and 12 months of age. Smaller dogs appear to enter puberty sooner than larger ones.[11] Once cyclic activity has begun, estrous cycles occur at about 7-month intervals.[1, 2] It is important to recognize, however, that the range of intervals in clinically normal fertile cycles has been found to be as varied as 16 to 56 weeks.[2] Although breed differences are not the rule, the 26-week mean cycle interval for the Alsatian dog is significantly shorter than the 33.5-week average found for the standard dachshund.[7] The basenji dog is different in that only one estrous cycle occurs each year, mainly in the fall.[7]

It is usually wise to recommend waiting without treatment if an animal that has been cycling normally has not come in estrus at the expected time, since cyclic intervals can also vary within an individual. Estrous cycle intervals appear to increase in the older dog, although there is no evidence to suggest that there is a decrease in fertility. Smaller litter size and increased problems associated with parturition may complicate breeding of the older bitch.

Proestrus

Clinically, it is convenient to designate proestrus as the beginning of the reproductive cycle in the dog. The duration of proestrus is about 9 days, although it is important to emphasize that the range is great (3 to 16 days). Inaccurate knowledge of the duration of proestrus is most likely due to missing the start of proestrus and the natural variability of its length. The clinical changes observed during proestrus are an increased interest in the male, although without acceptance, and swelling of the external genitalia accompanied by a blood-tinged discharge. These changes are due to the increase in circulating estrogens produced by the developing follicles (Fig. 1).

In addition to the external changes, estrogens cause growth of the squamous epithelium of the vagina as well as the endometrium of the uterus. Growth of the vaginal epithelium results in progressive changes that can be seen by examination of exfoliative cells in the vaginal smear. Noncornified (parabasal) epithelial cells disappear, and there is a gradual increase of fully cornified (anuclear) cells that eventually predominate at the end of proestrus. Epithelial cells may be classified into four types according to the degree of cornification. For accurate determination of progressive changes in the vaginal smear, differential counts of these cells may be made in smears taken daily or less often during the sexually active period (Fig.

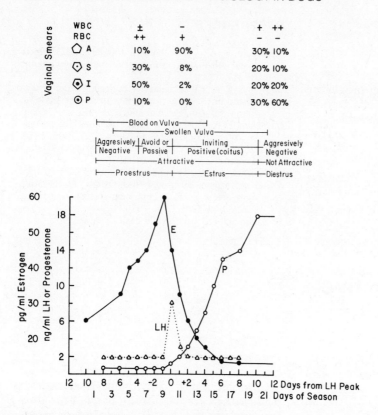

Figure 1. Schematic relationship of events occurring during pro-estrus, estrus and the luteal phase of the bitch. First day of season is the first day the bitch shows a blood-tinged vaginal discharge and becomes attractive to the male. Day 0 indicates the coincidence of the luteinizing hormone peak (LH △·△·△·) and the onset of sexual receptivity. The preovulatory surge of follicular estrogen (E ●—●) and postovulatory luteal progesterone (P ○—○) is also shown. Ovulation should occur within 24 hours after the LH peak (see text). Clinical appearance of external genitalia and behavior of the bitch toward the male are related to levels of circulating hormones (lower section of figure) and to representative differential counts of exfoliative vaginal epithelial cells (upper section of figure). The appearance of the four types of epithelial cells is shown schematically; also noted is the relative abundance of WBC's and RBC's in the vaginal smear (see text). (Adapted from Concannon, P. W., Hansel, W. and Visek, W. J.: Biol. Reprod., 13:112, 1975, with permission of authors.)

1). The increased thickness of the vaginal epithelium progressively inhibits the passage of white blood cells (WBC's) into the vaginal lumen. The presence of WBC's in the vaginal smear at the end of proestrus usually indicates the presence of a uterine infection, since WBC's can no longer penetrate the vaginal epithelium at this time.

Red blood cells (RBC's) are also observed microscopically during proestrus in the vaginal smear and macroscopically because of the red color of the discharge. They escape from the endometrium by diapedesis or hemorrhage from proliferating capillaries developing under the influence of estrogens. The RBC's tend to diminish in number at the onset of estrus when the endometrium begins to reach its mature state.

Estrus

The beginning of estrus is defined strictly as the first time that the female will accept the male. The exact time is often determined imprecisely because of various behavioral factors related to the degree of experience of the bitch and the male, her preference as to mates and the observer's knowledge of ca-

nine reproductive behavior. The onset of estrus in sexually experienced normal bitches is clearly marked by behavioral changes that include lateral deviation of the tail and presentation of the vulva to the male.

An important endocrine change takes place at the start of estrus, namely a surge release of ovulating hormone (luteinizing hormone, LH) (Fig. 1). This initiates ovulation, which usually occurs within 24 hours of the LH release or within the first day or two after the onset of estrus. It is most likely that all follicles are ovulated within a few hours. The driving force for the LH release is the rise of circulating estrogens produced by the preovulatory follicles.[9, 13, 15]

The capability of determining the onset of estrus is important because of the fact that ovulation follows shortly thereafter. In the absence of a teaser male, the time at which full cornification of the vaginal epithelium is reached, as shown by examination of exfoliated vaginal cells, often coincides fairly closely with the time of ovulation. This is because peak cornification usually occurs on the first or second day of estrus. If sequential vaginal smears can be obtained, it is possible to predict the approximate time of ovulation with some accuracy. The authors have found the examination of sequential vaginal smears useful in animals with fertility problems that were due to mistimed matings. Bitches presented by owners as just coming into proestrus (heat) were found to be in late proestrus or even in estrus, as detected by examination of the vaginal smear. The vaginal smear has also been useful in delineating cases of prolonged proestrus that were followed by normal sexual receptivity and ovulation. Analysis of blood for progesterone levels can be used for verification of the time of ovulation.

The period of sexual receptivity (estrus) lasts 9 to 10 days (range 4 to 12 days). This is in spite of the fact that estrogen levels are actually declining at the start of estrus (Fig. 1). It is obvious that once sexual receptivity is initiated, little estrogen is required to maintain it. Although ovulation occurs near the beginning of estrus, the prolonged period of sexual receptivity may be needed to allow the ovum to mature after ovulation. The canine ovum is thought to be ovulated as a primary oocyte and requires 2 to 3 days to complete the first stage of meiosis and become fertilizable.[14] If this is the case, it would appear that the actual timing of insemination may not be important and that conception can occur at any time following a breeding during the first 3 to 4 days of estrus. This seems to be borne out by experience in practice and in research colonies.[8]

Oviductal transport has been reported to range from 4 to 10 days.[5] Because of the time required for maturation of ova before they can be fertilized, actual transport of zygotes is probably closer to 4 days. The contraceptive effect of estrogen given following an unwanted mating has been shown to be due to action on zygote transport and development.[10] The earlier the exposure to estrogen, the more effective the results. Thus, early treatment for mismating is recommended.

Luteal Phase of the Estrous Cycle

One of the reasons for the long interval between estrus in the dog is the prolonged luteal phase. Luteal activity lasts for at least 75 days following ovulation in the non-pregnant animal.[3, 15] The response of the uterus to progesterone during the early part of the luteal phase involves proliferation of glandular elements and results in the production of a corkscrew-type appearance.[16] The exaggerated response of the uterus to progesterone is one of the main causes for the long involuntionary period that follows the regression of corpora lutea. Uterine involution is not complete in the nonpregnant dog until 120 to 150 days postovulation. A similar interval is required in the pregnant dog, so that involution is often not completed until 90 days postpartum.[16] Some uterine discharge thus may be present for a month or longer following parturition without being cause for concern. It is likely that the repeated, prolonged exposure of the uterus to progesterone of each ensuing cycle is the cause for the development of hyperplastic and cystic changes within the endometrium, which eventually result in the production of an environment conducive to the uterine infections that are so prevalent in the older bitch.

The term pseudopregnancy is frequently applied to dogs following the occurrence of estrus in conjunction with the normally prolonged luteal phase of the estrous cycle. There is considerable variability in the clinical manifestations of the signs of pseudopregnancy, with only minor changes occurring in most dogs. The authors feel that the term should be confined to those animals that have obvious clinical signs. The reason for the development of pseudopregnant signs is not known. It has been shown that there is no difference in the level of progesterone or the duration of the corpus luteum lifespan in dogs with or without clinical signs of pseudopregnancy.[15] The importance of prolactin in this syndrome awaits study.

THE MALE

The male dog reaches puberty several weeks later than the female, usually soon after attaining his adult body weight. The male domestic dog has not been shown to have seasonal cyclicity and thus is capable of producing sperm and breeding the entire year. A complete spermatogenic cycle has been found to take 13 to 14 days in the beagle.[6] Based on information derived from other animal studies, it is likely that 4 to 5 cycles are necessary for the completion of spermatogenesis, or 55 to 70 days.[12]

Endocrine control of spermatogenesis has not been studied in the dog *per se* to any great extent, but evidence from other species indicates that interstitial cell-stimulating hormone (ICSH), which appears to be identical to LH in the female, is active in causing production of testosterone from interstitial cells of the testicle. This hormone, or its metabolite dihydrotestosterone, is probably the main driving factor in spermatogenesis. Repeated doses of testosterone administered, for example, to stimulate libido, have been known to suppress the release of ICSH and thus depress spermatogenesis.

Semen is ejaculated in three visually distinguishable fractions. The first portion is clear and is ejaculated before or just after intromission. After the penis is intromitted, full erection follows, accompanied by intense pelvic thrusting. The second, or sperm-bearing fraction, is ejaculated at this time. The male then will usually dismount and, locked to the female by the engorged bulbus glandis, will continue to ejaculate the third fraction consisting of clear prostatic fluid for the duration of the "tie" or genital lock.

The number and quality of spermatozoa, as well as their fertility, remain stable for an indefinite period of time when the male is bred or sperm is collected every other day. Libido and morphological quality of sperm were not affected by twice daily ejaculations, although sperm motility was reduced. Canine spermatozoa survive in the genital tract up to 6 to 11 days after breeding.[4]

The prostate is the only accessory gland in the dog. It normally lies entirely within the pelvic cavity and surrounds the proximal urethra. Prostatic secretion forms the major vehicle for spermatozoa during ejaculation. It is slightly acidic (pH 6.8) and is rich in sodium and chloride. Normal prostatic function is dependent on circulating testicular androgens.

REFERENCES

1. Andersen, A. C. and Wooten, E. *In* Cole, H. H. and Cupps, P. T.(eds.): Reproduction in Domestic Animals. 1st Ed. New York Academic Press, 1959, p. 359.
2. Christie, D. W. and Bell, E. T.: Some observations on the seasonal incidence and frequency of oestrus in breeding bitches in Britain. J. Sm. Anim. Pract., *12*:159, 1971.
3. Concannon, P. W., Hansel, W. and Visek, W. J.: The ovarian cycle of the bitch: plasma estrogen, LH and progesterone. Biol. Reprod., *13*:112, 1975.
4. Doak, R. L., Hall, A. and Dale, H. E.: Longevity of spermatozoa in the reproductive tract of bitch. J. Reprod. Fertil., *13*:51, 1967.
5. Evans, H. E.: 24th Gaines Veterinary Symposium, 1974, p. 18.
6. Foote, R. H., Swierstra, E. E., and Hunt, W. L.: Spermatogenesis in the dog. Anat. Rec. *173*:341, 1972.
7. Fuller, J. L.: Photoperiodic control of estrus in the Basenji. J. Hered., *47*:179, 1956.
8. Holst, P. A. and Phemister, R. D.: Temporal sequence of events in the estrous cycle of the bitch. Am. J. Vet. Res., *35*:401, 1974.
9. Jones, G. E., Boyns, A. R., Cameron, E. H. D., Bell, E. T., Christie, D. W. and Parkes, M. F.: Plasma oestradiol, luteinizing hormones and progesterone during pregnancy and following gonadotrophin administration in beagle bitches. J. Endocrinol., *57*:331, 1973.
10. Kennelly, J. J.: The effect of mestranol on canine reproduction. Biol. Reprod., *1*:282, 1969.
11. McDonald, L. E.: Veterinary Endocrinology and Reproduction. Philadelphia, Lea & Febiger, 1975.
12. Monesi, V.: Spermatogenesis and spermatozoa. *In* Austin, C. R. and Short, R. V. (eds.): Germ Cells and Fertilization. Vol. 1. Cambridge, University Press, 1972, p. 18.
13. Nett, T. M., Akbar, A. M., Phemister, R. D., Holst, P. A., Reichert, L. E., Jr. and Niswender, G. D.: Levels of luteinizing hormone, estradiol and progesterone in serum during the estrous cycle and pregnancy in the beagle bitch. Proc. Soc. Exp. Biol. Med., *148*:134, 1975.
14. Phemister, R. D., Holst, P. A., Spano, J. S. and Hopwood, M. L.: Time of ovulation in the beagle bitch. Biol. Reprod., *8*:74, 1973.
15. Smith, M. S. and McDonald, L. E.: Serum levels of luteinizing hormone and progesterone during the estrous cycle, pseudopregnancy and pregnancy in the dog. Endocrinology, *94*:404, 1974.
16. Sokolowski, J. H., Zimbelman, R. G. and Goings, L. S.: Canine reproduction: reproductive organs and related structures of the nonparous, parous and postpartum bitch. Am. J. Vet. Res., *34*:1001, 1973.

Genetic Counseling in Small Animal Practice

D. R. JOHNSON

University of Leeds, Leeds, England

Inherited diseases and malformations are on the whole infrequently seen in dogs, but the inbreeding necessarily practiced in striving for or maintaining a breed standard may result in a problem within a particular bloodline or kennel.

Suspicions that an abnormality is genetic in origin should arise if the incidence of that abnormality is high in one breed and low in others. If data can be obtained for a particular anomaly within a breed, the incidence is often seen to be especially high in that line. Sometimes, the abnormality may be traceable to a particular group of ancestors, or even to a single dog. Pedigrees are constructed, working backward from the affected individual to its ancestors to trace its affected and nonaffected forebears. Often, the mode of inheritance can be suggested and a test mating arranged to verify it.

MODES OF INHERITANCE

In nearly all cases, genes will be inherited in different forms from the sire and dam of the individual. If a hypothetical gene *A* is considered, which can also exist as a defective form *a*, the combinations shown in Table 1 can occur.

The phenotypic expression of these genes depends on the way in which *A* and *a* interact in the heterozygote. If *A* makes an enzyme that *a* is incapable of inducing, and, in the heterozygote *Aa*, one dose of *A* is sufficient to induce enough enzyme for the needs

of the cell, *a* is recessive to *A* and its effects are not noticeable in the heterozygous animal. Another possibility is that *A* may not induce sufficient enzyme for the normal function of the cell, and in that case *AA* would be normal, *Aa* would be affected in some degree and *aa* would be abnormal. The *A* gene would then be considered semidominant.

Dominant Inheritance

Patterson and Medway[4] reported a series of cases of congenital lymphedema in the dog. This was first seen in a 10-week-old poodle × labrador bitch, which had a pitting, nonpainful edema of the hind legs. The cardiovascular system, renal functions and serum protein determinations were normal. The bitch was raised to maturity and mated to a normal poodle (Fig. 1). One of her five progeny had lymphedema. He was also raised, mated to a keeshond bitch and produced four abnormal and two normal offspring. If it is assumed that the original bitch carried a dominant mutation from *l* to *L*, which caused the lymphedema, mating her to a normal *(ll)* dog should give a ratio of one *Ll* abnormal: one *ll* normal. In fact, the

TABLE 1. *Possible Combinations of a Hypothetical Gene*

Sire (Sperm)	Dam (Egg)	Offspring
A	*A*	*AA* (homozygote)
A	*a*	*Aa* (heterozygote)
a	*A*	*Aa* (heterozygote)
a	*a*	*aa* (homozygote)

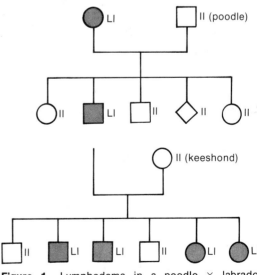

Figure 1. Lymphedema in a poodle × labrador cross. ○, female; □, male; ◇, sex unknown. Solid shading indicates affected animals. (After Patterson, D. F. and Medway, W.: J.A.V.M.A., *149*:1741, 1966.)

TABLE 2. *The Inheritance of Merle**

Mating	Breed†	Progeny		
		EXTREME DAPPLE (*MM*)	DAPPLE/MERLE (*Mm*)	FULL COLOR (*mm*)
Merle × full color	D	–	97	102
	C	–	21	24
	MC	–	12	16
			130	142
Merle × merle	D	10	11	5
	C	3	5	2
	MC	0	7	7
		13	23	14

*After Sorsby, A. and Davey, J. B.: J. Genet., *52*:425, 1954.
†*Code:* D, dachshund; C, collie; MC, miniature collie.

numbers are small, but if the second mating is added, which was also *Ll* × *ll*, the result is five abnormal: six normal progeny. It can be presumed that a mating between two abnormals would give the ratio of three abnormal: one normal, but this was not done.

Semidominant Inheritance

This form of inheritance supposes that two genes will have more effect than one. Sorsby and Davey[6] looked at merle (or dapple) in dachshunds and collies. Dapple dachshunds are a special breed, the normal black and tan, red, chocolate or cream coat being streaked with silver. The coloration is maintained by dapple × full color mating. Occasional dapple × dapple matings have occurred, which give full color, dapple and extreme dapple offspring. The latter have much white hair, are often blind or deaf and possibly have congenital heart disease. In the collie, the situation is essentially the same.

The data in Table 2 shows that merle × full color mating is similar to a lymphedema × normal situation, resulting in a 1:1 ratio. In the merle × merle matings, the expected ratio of three merle:one full color is modified to one extreme merle (*MM*), two merle (*Mm*) and one full color (*mm*). The merle class has been divided, two doses of the gene having more effect than one.

Recessive Inheritance

A condition with overshot jaw in dachshunds has been described.[2] Affected animals are viable and vigorous, but are not useful for breeding. This gene is recessive, and ab-

normal offspring can be obtained by mating two normal-appearing parents (a 1:3 ratio), or, a 1:1 ratio can be seen by crossing a heterozygote with an abnormal (Table 3).

X-Linkage

This is a special situation that arises when a gene is carried on the sex (X) chromosome. As the Y chromosome carries few genes, a male (XY) will have only one copy of the gene, whereas the female (XX) will have two. A gene that is recessive will not show its effects in the female because it is masked by its normal partner but will be noticeable in the male even though it is present in only one dose. Hemophilia in a kennel was described,[3] progeny were examined from four female carriers (heterozygotes mated to normal males). Half the male offspring were hemophiliac and half were normal, whereas all females appeared normal. If the hemophiliac male could be raised and mated to a normal female, no hemophiliacs would appear in his progeny, but all females would be heterozygous carriers.

TABLE 3. *Inherited Jaw Anomaly in Long-Haired Dachshunds**

Mating	Progeny	
	NORMAL	AFFECTED
Heterozygote (carrier) × heterozygote (carrier)	8	2
Homozygote (affected) × heterozygote (carrier)	4	3

*After Grüneberg, H. and Lea, A. J.: J. Genet., *39*: 285, 1940.

Multifactorial Inheritance

The relationship between one gene and one characteristic has been discussed; however, often the situation is more complex, with one characteristic being influenced by more than one gene pair. Assuming that two pairs of genes, *b,c,* control the fit of a hip in some way and that can mutate to *b'c'* to result in poor joints, it can be seen that animals can be *bbcc* or *b'b'c'c'* or any combination thereof. An animal with three prime genes may show a clinical abnormality and one with four, advanced form of the abnormality. If affected animals are mated, mostly affected offspring will result. If two clinically normal dogs are mated, abnormal offspring can also result. This is the simplest possible case of polygenic inheritance. This picture becomes more complicated by adding more gene pairs and introducing the effects of dominance.

Expressivity and Penetrance

Genes cannot act in isolation; their effects are modified by the sum total of all other genes present. For example, white spotting in dogs is inherited as a simple recessive *s.* If two spotted dogs are mated, both of which must be *ss,* all progeny must also be *ss.* But the amount of spotting will vary from dog to dog; some will have a larger area of white than others. The amount of white depends on the sum total of all other genes present and is a measure of the *expressivity* of *s.*

On some occasions, one or more of the progeny will not be spotted, although their progeny may be spotted. This is *penetrance;* a gene has good penetrance when all individuals appear true to the expected genotype. Poor penetrance is often concomitant with variable expressivity and will often account for abnormal progeny born to a clinically normal parent.

PRACTICAL CONSIDERATIONS

When an owner or a breeder who is worried by an abnormality that may be genetic in origin approaches a practitioner, as much information as possible should be obtained from the breeder. It is necessary to know if the abnormality has occurred before in the kennel, in the bloodline of the sire or dam or in the offspring of any stud dog in the kennel. Breeders are usually reticent about such matters, and it will be important to fully explain the need for complete information, as well as assure the individual that the information will be handled with utmost confidentiality.

After compilation of a pedigree, dominant or semi-dominant inheritance will be not difficult to discern, since one of the parents and at least one of the offspring will be affected. The remedy will simply be to avoid breeding the affected animals. If the affected animal must be used in the breeding program, abnormal offspring can be discarded. The remaining, unaffected progeny will not have the defect.

If dominance and semi-dominance can be ruled out and if it is assumed that the abnormality is recessive, it can be accepted that two-thirds of the siblings of the affected dog will be carriers, both parents of the affected dog will be carriers and one of each pair of the grandparents will be carriers. This will apply to each affected individual; often bloodlines will cross and implicate a single bloodline or mating. If data can be collected on litters containing an abnormal individual, an approximate 1:3 ratio will be seen to emerge, provided there has been no suppression of abnormals from the record, no unrecorded stillbirths, no reduced viability and no variable expressivity of penetrance. These conditions would reduce the ratio; if the ratio is more than 1:3, a recessive inheritance is highly probable.

Whether a particular dog is a carrier or whether it can be used for breeding is best determined by test mating. Test mating is time-consuming and expensive, so that the breeder should be advised of this and should be given an estimated number of normal progeny required to clear the suspected animal. If the disease in affected animals becomes evident late in life, useless puppies will have to be housed for long periods. It should be considered, however, that puppies certified free from an abnormality prevalent in a breed are sure to command a good price.

Test matings should be designed for speed and economy. It is best to test a stud dog rather than a brood bitch. The best approach is to breed the dog to an abnormal bitch. If one abnormal is produced, the stud is a carrier and the test can be discontinued. If no abnormals are produced, further test mating will be expected to result in a 1:1 ratio, and each pup will have a 50 per cent chance of being normal if the stud is not a carrier. The

TABLE 4. *Percentage Chance that a Tested Dog is a Carrier in Three Types of Test Mating for a Single Recessive Gene*

No. of Normal Offspring	Mated against Abnormal Bitch	Mated against Carrier Bitch	Mated against a Daughter
1	50.0	75.0	88
2	25.0	56.0	78
3	12.5	42.5	71
4	6.3	32.0	66
5	3.1	24.0	62
6	1.5	18.0	59
7	0.8	13.0	57
8	–	10.0	55
9	–	7.5	54
10	–	5.6	53
15	–	1.3	51
20	–	0.3	50

chance of getting two normal pups is ½ × ½ = ¼ or 25 per cent (Table 4, column 2). If seven normal pups are born, the chance of the test animal being a carrier is 1 in 100.

Another form of test mating should be considered if the abnormal animal is infertile or nonviable or if it is considered unnecessarily cruel to prolong its life. The suspected individual should be bred to a known carrier, such as its dam. The probability computation is similar to that just listed, and the chance of the first pup being normal is 75 per cent, so that 16 normal pups would be required to reduce the chance of the test animal being a carrier to 1 in 100 (Table 4, column 3).

A third type of test mating is sometimes suggested, in which the suspected dog is mated to its daughters. This is a most inefficient procedure, since the probability of the test animal being a carrier is found to be 50 per cent only after a considerable number of normal progeny has been born (Table 4, column 4).

If a polygenic mode of inheritance is involved, the veterinarian and, indeed, the geneticist will be of little practical help to the breeder. Although polygenic modes can eventually be defined, the number of test matings and progeny necessary is more suitable for use with fruit flies or mice and is not practical for dogs. If a defect seems to be inheritable but no clear pattern emerges from the pedigrees, the breeder should be advised to to breed only from least affected animals to the best animals available, expecting that the offspring quality will eventually improve.

REFERENCES

1. Burns, M. and Fraser, M. N.: Genetics of the Dog. Edinburgh, Oliver & Boyd, 1966.
2. Grüneberg, H. and Lea, A. J.: An inherited jaw anomaly in long-haired dachshunds. J. Genet., *39*:285, 1940.
3. Hutt, F. B., Rickard, C. G. and Field, R.: Sex-linked hemophilia in dogs. J. Hered., *39*:2, 1948.
4. Patterson, D. F. and Medway, W.: Hereditary diseases of the dog. J.A.V.M.A., *149*:1741, 1966.
5. Robinson, R.: Catalogue and Bibliography of Canine Genetic Anomalies. 2nd Ed. West Wickham, England, C.H.A.R.T., 1972.
6. Sorsby, A. and Davey, J. B.: Ocular association of dappling (or merling) in coat colour of dogs. J. Genet., *52*:425, 1954.

Clinical Examination for Reproductive Disorders in the Dog

VICTOR M. SHILLE
University of Florida, Gainesville, Florida

Examination of reproductive organs demands gentleness and the use of sterile, lubricated instruments or gloved hands. It is helpful to follow a routine in the examination procedures to assure thoroughness and efficiency.

HISTORY

A careful, preferably written, record kept by the owner is a great help in anamnesis. It should ideally include information about the age of the bitch at first heat, her past cyclic intervals and the clinical appearance during estrus. If the animal has been bred, timing of the breeding relative to the days of the estrous cycle should be recorded. The number of puppies delivered and their health is also of interest. In the male, information about his past breeding performance and fertility is needed. In young dogs with an apparent lack of libido, one should inquire about the environment in which they were raised during the ages of 4 to 12 weeks. During this time, peer interaction is very important for the development of normal sexual behavior.[1]

Pedigree charts can be very useful if a genetic disorder is suspected. However, they often require cooperation from more than one breeder and may be difficult to compile.

It is important to ascertain if the animal has been treated before for a similar condition or if it has had any recent treatment. If this is the case, one should inquire about the details of the treatment from the previous veterinarian. The general physical condition of the animal should also be carefully evaluated, since disorders not related to the genital organs frequently interfere with reproductive performance.

EXAMINATION OF THE FEMALE

Mammary glands should always be palpated and nipples visually inspected. At this time it is also convenient to palpate axillary and inguinal lymph nodes. The perineal region and vulva are examined, and the perivulvar skin folds are stretched to inspect for skin disorders. Before proceeding to the examination of the vestibule, it may be necessary to clip matted hair and clean the vulva. Clipping should be kept to a minimum to avoid disfiguring the haircoat of the animal. If soap or any other chemical is used for cleaning, thorough rinsing is essential to avoid subsequent skin irritation.

Entry into the vestibule and the vagina should be planned in a way that prevents contamination of the tract by instruments and lubricants before microbiological or cytological samples are taken. The insertion of a dry sterile swab to obtain a vaginal smear for cytological examination may be made easier by the use of a short nonlubricated speculum (otoscope speculum). This assures sampling from the vagina rather than from the vestibular epithelium. A sample for bacteriological culture should be obtained through a sterile long speculum (Fig. 1) using a sterile swab held with alligator forceps or a sterile pipette. A guarded culture system may also be used (see article on canine vaginitis, page 630). This assures uncontaminated samples from the anterior vagina. Vaginal infections are frequently associated with urinary tract infections, particularly cystitis. Urinalysis and urine cultures are of help in the differential diagnosis. However, catheterization of the urinary bladder in a female with vaginitis is not

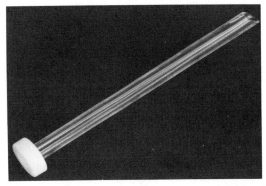

Figure 1. A Plexiglas vaginal speculum may be used in large and medium-sized breeds. It may be attached to a standard otoscope handle.

advisable. Infant and pediatric proctoscopes have been used successfully by the author and also custom-made Plexiglas tubes of 1 to 1.5 cm outside diameter and 15 to 20 cm in length. These tubes may be fitted into a standard otoscope handle and are convenient to use in most of the medium and large breeds (Fig. 1). Small breeds present a problem, since it is very difficult to see adequately through tubes of the small diameter needed for these breeds. The scope should be lubricated and sterile and should not cause undue discomfort in the mature bitch. Prepuberal bitches are more sensitive because of the small size of the vulvar opening and the tightness of the vestibular sphincter. They may require sedation prior to examination. The hyperemia caused by the passage of the scope and other instruments must be differentiated from vaginitis.

It is likely that the cervix will not be observed adequately in all except the parturient bitch. During other times in the reproductive cycle, the tendency of the vagina to stretch longitudinally with the advancing scope and the presence of the dorsal vaginal fold (pseudocervix)[6] preclude adequate exposure of the cervix. Ballooning of the vagina by a positive air pressure attachment available on some proctoscopes or by elevation of the hindquarters during passage of the scope has limited usefulness in seeing the cervix.

In addition to visual examination of the entire vagina, the condition of the posterior vagina and vestibule can be further determined by digital palpation. Placement of one or two gloved fingers into the vagina while the opposite hand manipulates the abdomen is an effective way to examine the pelvis and structures in the posterior vagina. For additional information about the dorsal wall of the vestibule and posterior vagina, one finger can be used in the vestibule while one finger of the opposite hand is inserted into the rectum.

The uterus may be palpated through the abdominal wall in females that are not unduly nervous or in pain. Visual examination of the uterus and ovaries, as well as obtaining uterine biopsy specimens, is accomplished through a laparotomy incision. This may be the only way that a definitive diagnosis can be made in some cases.

It is difficult to see the uterus on a radiogram unless the organ is grossly enlarged, as in closed pyometra, or contains radiopaque material, as in normal pregnancy or in the presence of a mummified fetus. Contrast radiography of the uterus and oviducts (hysterography) has been reported.[3] However, it remains a rather difficult procedure, since catheterization of the canine cervix cannot be accomplished easily.

Endocrine Evaluation

Animals presented with a history of unexplained infertility in the presence of apparently normal cycles or those with estrous interval abnormalities may be investigated by hormone determination. The simplest approach is to take vaginal smears either daily or at least three times a week, beginning on the first day of proestrous vaginal discharge and vulvar swelling. Progressive cornification of the exfoliative vaginal epithelium may be monitored by a differential count of the four types of epithelial cells seen in the smears (Fig. 2). The appearance of full cornification (80 per cent or more of superficial and anuclear cells) correlates well with maximal estrogen levels in the circulation and coincides with the beginning of estrus. It is important to recognize that full cornification precedes ovulation by 1 to 3 days. The occurrence of ovulation *per se* is best ascertained by measurement of plasma progesterone levels. Serial blood samples taken in conjunction with the vaginal smears throughout proestrus and estrus can be analyzed for progesterone. Occurrence of ovulation and luteinization can be timed with a good degree of accuracy in this manner.

Miscellaneous Laboratory Procedures

Routine prebreeding testing for the presence of a serum titer against *Brucella canis* may be easily done with a fast screening method (slide agglutination test). Positive results obtained by this method should be verified by the following procedure: paired serum samples should be taken 30 days apart and submitted to a laboratory for the tube agglutination test, utilizing the antigen provided by the Diagnostic Reagent Laboratory of the Veterinary Services Laboratories, APHIS, Ames, Iowa. Titers greater than 1:200 should be considered indicative of an active infection. In these cases, blood cultures confirm the presence of the organism.[4]

Infantile genitalia, failure to initiate sexual cycles (delayed puberty) and an enlarged clitoris may be due to an intersex condition caused by a chromosomal disorder. Evalua-

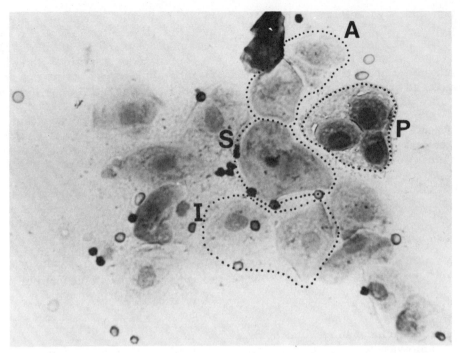

Figure 2. Differentiation of four cell types seen in vaginal smears (Wright's stain, 100×). *A,* Anuclear cell; irregular folded cytoplasm, nucleus absent. *S,* Superficial cell; angular cell outline, degenerating nucleus. *I,* Intermediate cell; angular cell outline, large normally-staining nucleus. *P,* Parabasal cell; round cell outline, small cytoplasmic volume, large, normal-appearing nucleus.

tion of this type of patient should include a cytogenetic study. Samples of buccal mucosa can be stained for the determination of Barr bodies (intracellular manifestation of X chromosomes). Also, aseptically collected blood can be used for a lymphocyte culture to determine the karyotype of the animal. More extensive tests would include a fibroblast culture and serological typing. A detailed description of these procedures is included in the article on canine cytogenetics, pages 119 to 155.

EXAMINATION OF THE MALE

The examination of the male external genitalia should include palpation and inspection of the mammary glands and nipples. The prepuce is examined, and the penis is extruded manually to allow inspection of the pars longa glandis while the amount of preputial exudate is also noted. The penis should be freely movable within the prepuce and not restricted by the narrow preputial opening (phimosis) or by adhesions of the penile retractor muscles, which may occur postcastration. In most dogs it is necessary

to use a mild sedative to examine the posterior portion of the prepuce. An otoscope may be used to search this area for foreign bodies.

Scrotal skin is inspected for the presence of inflammation and other lesions. The testes should be well into the scrotal fundus in most breeds by the time decidual dentition is complete. Unilateral or bilateral cryptorchidism or ectopic testes are undesirable in show and breeding animals. In young dogs, temporary retraction of the testes may occur from nervousness or excitement and should not be considered significant. The left testis is usually slightly more dorsal and further caudad than the right. The great differences in the breed sizes of the domestic dog preclude any statement about normal testicular size. Comparing the two testes of the male in question with those of a male of the same breed and body weight may become necessary. The testis should be smooth with a regular outline and of firm consistency.

The epididymides may be palpated starting from the dorsoanterior surface and continuing along the lateral curvature of the testis. Apparent enlargement of the epididymis may be caused by a relative decrease of the size of the testis. Epididymitis is not common in the dog.

Digital examination of the prostate is made with a gloved finger *per rectum*, while the opposite hand brings the prostate within reach by judicious pressure on the abdomen anterior to the pubis. This is successful in all but the largest breeds and should not elicit pain. The prostate is bilobate, smooth and regular in outline.

Radiography of the prostate is useful in the differential diagnosis of pelvic masses and prostatic diseases.

Semen Evaluation

A semen sample should be collected from any male with suspected infertility that has a history of testicular disease and/or a generalized febrile disease.

Collection can be accomplished by allowing the male to mount a bitch in heat or by digital manipulation. Artificial vaginas have been used successfully, although spermatozoal motility may be adversely affected by the warm latex lining.[2] Electroejaculation requires general anesthesia and is not commonly used in clinical practice. In longhaired breeds, a stockinette placed over the trunk and hindquarters will keep hair under control during semen collection. Widemouth test tubes, beakers or test tubes with a funnel, as well as casings for 6- or 12-ml-disposable syringes, are suitable for collection of semen. The collection vessel should be dry, not contaminated by soaps or detergents and sterile. It should be warmed to slightly above body temperature before collection and can then be kept sufficiently warm in the hand during collection.

In the canine, the ejaculate consists of three fractions. The second fraction of the ejaculate is characterized by a milky gray color and a thicker consistency than the first and last fractions. The second fraction contains the spermatozoa and is the only portion that needs to be collected. One should guard against missing this portion during collection from an excitable dog and, after seeing only the clear prostatic fluid of the third fraction, declaring the dog infertile.

A pipette may be used to transfer a drop of semen onto a prewarmed slide, where it is mixed with a drop of 2.9 per cent sodium citrate and examined for motility and concentration. More than 70 per cent of pro-

gressively motile spermatozoa are usually found in fertile males.

Stained smears of the undiluted ejaculate are examined for structural abnormalities. Wright's and Giemsa stains are adequate, but the eosin-nigrosin stain or India ink give excellent contrast for evaluation of morphological characteristics. The eosin-nigrosin stain may be used as follows: one drop each of 10 per cent nigrosin, 5 per cent eosin and undiluted semen are placed on a slide. The three drops are mixed gently and thoroughly for no longer than 30 seconds. A drop of this mixture is transferred onto a fresh slide and streaked across it to make a thin film. After air drying, the spermatozoa are examined under oil immersion. This stain has also been referred to as a vital or live/dead stain. However, it is not reliable for differentiating live from dead spermatozoa.

Bacterial Examination of Semen

In cases in which clinical findings indicate the presence of an infection of the male genital tract, identification of bacteria and antibiotic sensitivity testing should be done on prostatic fluid and semen. The prepuce and surrounding area should be cleaned without using any soap or detergents and, if necessary, clipped. The esthetic appearance of the dog should be preserved as much as possible. The penis is partly exposed by retracting the prepuce, and the tip of the penis is rinsed well with sterile saline. The urethra is then irrigated through a sterile disposable catheter with 2 to 5 ml of warmed sterile saline. The tip of the penis is again rinsed with sterile saline. To culture only prostatic fluid, the prostate is massaged *per rectum*, and the fluid is collected by gentle suction into the previously introduced sterile catheter. The volume of fluid collected in this manner is rather small, but it serves to differentiate testicular involvement from prostatic disease. Semen culture can be done easily by collecting semen after the preliminary cleansing, as just described. In long-haired breeds, a stockinette can be used to cover the trunk, as mentioned previously.

Testicular Biopsy

In case of acquired azoospermia, palpable testicular degeneration or suspected neoplasia, a definitive diagnosis may be aided by a testicular biopsy. It is strongly recommended that an incisional biopsy be done as described by Fahning.[5] The use of Silverman biopsy needles is to be discouraged. Not only are the specimens obtained in this manner unsatisfactory because of crushing and disarrangement of the delicate seminiferous tubules, but there is an increased possibility of causing sperm granulomas. Undue tension on the spermatic cord should be avoided during this procedure.

Miscellaneous Laboratory Procedures

Although it is possible to assay for sex steroids and interstitial cell-stimulating hormone, normal data for these hormones have not been established in the male dog. The diurnal fluctuations seen in other species presage additional difficulty in evaluating measured values in the male dog.

Serological tests for canine brucellosis and toxoplasmosis may be performed, as well as various cytogenetic procedures as described previously for the female.

REFERENCES

1. Antonov, V. V. and Hananashvili, M. M.: Significance of early individual experience in the development of sexual behavior of male dogs. Zh. Vyssh. Nerv. Deyat. *23*:68, 1973.
2. Boucher, J. H., Foote, R. H. and Kirk, R. W.: The evaluation of semen quality in the dog and the effects of frequency of ejaculation upon semen quality, libido and depletion of sperm reserves. Cornell Vet., *48*:67, 1958.
3. Cobb, L. M.: The radiographic outline of the genital system of the bitch. Vet. Rec. *71*:66, 1959.
4. Council discusses canine brucellosis as a public health problem. J.A.V.M.A., *168*:987, 1976.
5. Fahning, M. L.: Breeding soundness examination of the dog. *In* Kirk, R. W. (ed.): Current Veterinary Therapy, V. Philadelphia, W. B. Saunders Co., 1974.
6. Pineda, M. H., Kainer, R. A. and Faulkner, L. C.: Dorsal median postcervical fold in the canine vagina. Am. J. Vet. Res., *34*:1487, 1973.

Developmental Anomalies, Including Cryptorchidism

C. J. G. WENSING

State University, Utrecht, The Netherlands

NORMAL PATTERN OF SEXUAL DIFFERENTIATION

The components of individual mammalian sexual make-up are usually of one gender and conform to the chromosomal pattern established at the time of fertilization.

In the male the direction of genital duct development, differentiation of the urogenital sinus and migration of the gonad are determined by the presence or absence of hormones secreted by the fetal testis. If functional testes are present, the Müllerian structures involute, the Wolffian ducts develop, growth of the vesicovaginal septum is inhibited, outgrowth of male accessory sexual glands occurs, the genital tubercle and fusion of the genital swelling is stimulated and the testes descend.

In the female (either with or without an ovary) the Müllerian structures mature, the Wolffian ducts are resorbed, the vesicovaginal septum outgrowth separates the vagina from the urogenital sinus and fusion of the genital swellings is prevented. The ovary (if present) does not descend to a great extent. It seems quite clear that the development of the genital tract in the female direction does not need a particular stimulus — only the absence of testes is required.

The various hormone-dependent developments in the male have been subject to detailed research. It has been determined that at least two and probably three different hormones are involved in the male differentiation process (Fig. 1). The first hormone clearly established as a stimulator of male sexual development was testosterone (or, in more general terms, androgens). From experiments with castrated male fetuses subjected to androgens, experiments with male fetuses subjected to antiandrogens and experiments with female fetuses subjected to androgens, it has become clear that androgens are essential in the maintenance and differentiation of the Wolffian duct (epididymis, vas deferens and seminal vesicle). Androgens are also necessary for the male type of development of the urogenital sinus and penis. There are also a number of "experiments of nature" that substantiate these experimental findings.

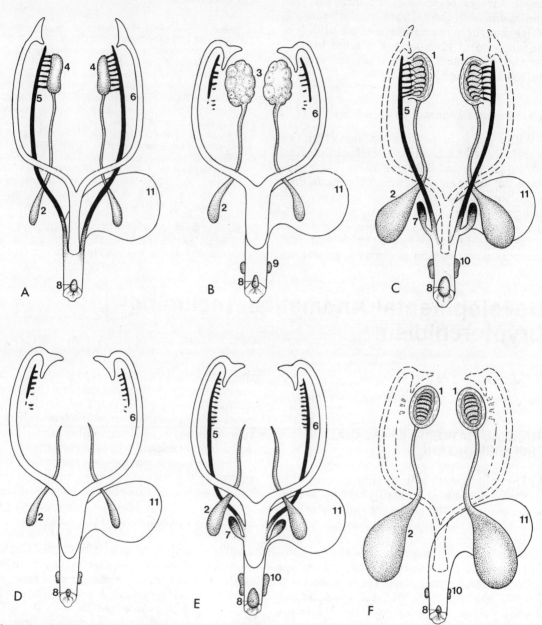

Figure 1. Schematic drawings of normal and some forms of abnormal sexual differentiation. *A,* Indifferent stage of sexual development. *B,* Normal development along the female line. *C,* Normal development along the male line. *D,* Castrate (male or female), development of the tract along the female line. *E,* Castrate treated with androgen. *F,* Male treated with antiandrogen. *(1)* Testis, *(2)* gubernaculum, *(3)* ovary, *(4)* indifferent gonad, *(5)* Wolffian duct, *(6)* Müllerian duct, *(7)* seminal vesicle, *(8)* genital tubercle, *(9)* female accessory sex glands, *(10)* male accessory sex glands (urogenital sinus), and *(11)* urinary bladder.

The regression of the Müllerian ducts in the male is brought about by a second hormone produced by the testis, named the Müllerian inhibiting factor (MIF). The first indications that Müllerian inhibition is caused by a substance other than the androgens came from androgen injection experiments. It appears to be impossible to cause the Müllerian duct to regress by the use of exogenous androgens in a castrated male fetus. It has recently been established that MIF is a nonsteroid macromolecular factor produced by fetal Sertoli cells. In calf and pig fetal testes the factor is produced during a substantial period of fetal life and seems to be present long after the regression of the Müllerian ducts.

The gonads in male and female fetuses are connected to the inguinal region by a structure called the gubernaculum. This mesenchymal structure extends from its attachment at the caudal pole of the gonad into the inguinal canal. Shortly after the differentiation of the genital ducts, an outgrowth of the gubernaculum begins in male fetuses. This outgrowth is confined to the distal part of the gubernaculum. It increases enormously in length and volume, expanding beyond the external inguinal opening into the scrotal sac. The vaginal process and the cremaster muscle are shaped by the enlargement of the gubernaculum (Fig. 2). The intra-abdominal part of the gubernaculum becomes incorporated into the enlarging extra-abdominal part because of traction. During the process, traction is also exerted on the testis, which is drawn into the inguinal canal. The outgrowth reaction can be considered the causal factor for the first phase of the descent process. Once the outgrowth reaction has occurred, the core of the gubernaculum regresses and is converted into the proper

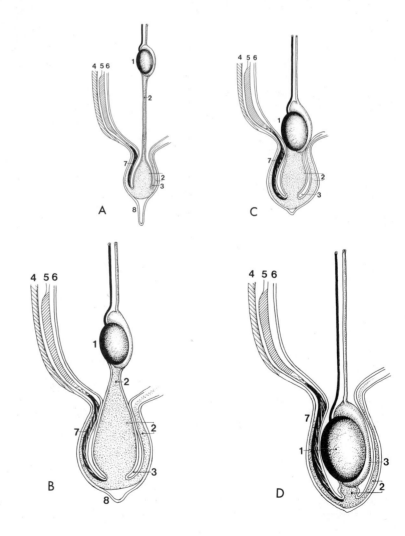

Figure 2. Schematic drawings of four successive stages in the normal descent of the testis. *(1)* Testis, *(2)* gubernaculum, *(3)* vaginal process, *(4)* external oblique abdominal muscle, *(5)* internal oblique abdominal muscle, *(6)* peritoneum, *(7)* cremaster muscle, and *(8)* external spermatic fascia.

ligament of the testis and the ligament of the tail of the epididymis. This regression enables the testis and the ligament of the tail of the epididymis. This regression enables the testis to descend further to its scrotal position. Therefore, gubernacular regression can be considered the causal factor for the second phase of the descent process. Testicular descent is the final phase of the initial events in sexual differentiation. In most domestic mammals it is completed during fetal life, but it is not completed in the dog until 2 or 3 weeks after birth.

The gubernacular outgrowth responsible for the primary phase of the descent of the testis does not depend on androgenic hormones and/or on gonadotropins but seems to be caused by a hormone of unknown chemical structure produced by the fetal testis (or neonatal testis in the dog).

ABNORMAL DEVELOPMENT

Gonads

Abnormal development of gonads either in a direction not corresponding to the apparent chromosomal sex or in an ambiguous direction (true hermaphrodism) is usually caused by minor or sometimes more profound chromosomal aberrations. The phenotype of these animals is rather variable. In swine and goats true hermaphrodism appears relatively frequently, but it is rare in other domestic mammals. Only a small number of true hermaphroditic dogs have been described.

Genital Ducts and Urogenital Sinus (Pseudohermaphrodism)

The causes of abnormal development may be endogenous or brought about by subjecting a fetus or neonate to an environment of androgens, estrogens, progestogens or anti-androgens.

In female pseudohermaphrodism the ovaries and Müllerian derivatives are normally developed, and ambisexuality is limited to Wolffian ducts and urogenital sinus derivatives. Since in the absence of testes there is an inherent tendency to feminize, a female fetus will be masculinized only if subjected to an environment of androgens. The degree of fetal masculinization is determined by the stage of differentiation at the time of androgen exposure. In the human an endogenous source of androgens is the adrenal, which accounts for most cases of female pseudohermaphrodism in those with congenital virilizing adrenal hyperplasia caused by various forms of impaired cortisol synthesis. So far these anomalies have not been encountered in domestic mammals.

Exposure of female fetuses to exogenous androgens may also result in female pseudohermaphrodism. In the dog, if exposure occurs between the fourth and seventh weeks of gestation, the genital ducts and urogenital sinus become virilized. The earlier the exposure, the more profound the masculinization will be. Early exposure may eventually lead to an almost complete formation of an epididymis, vas deferens, male urethra, prostate and penis. Exposure after the fiftieth day of gestation or after birth will result in clitoric enlargement only. It should be kept in mind that these animals have normally developed ovaries, Fallopian tubes and uterus and may be fertile.

Exposure of female fetuses to estrogens can result in an incomplete fusion of the caudal part of the Müllerian ducts, incomplete division of the urogenital sinus, incomplete formation of the vagina and occasional induction of prostate development. The connection between the Müllerian ducts and the urogenital sinus may be incomplete or entirely absent. These effects are encountered only if exposure occurs during the sensitive period of sexual differentiation. Exposure after sexual differentiation results only in hypertrophy of the uterus.

Subjecting the female fetus to progestogens may result in limited masculinization. Progesterone itself is only slightly active; various synthetic progestogens, however, are intrinsically androgenic and can produce virilization of female fetuses. In female puppies born to bitches treated with these substances, the first sign of virilization is the inhibition of vaginal development. Occasionally there may be a displacement of the orifice of the urogenital sinus, placing the vulva in a ventrocranial direction. These deviations occur only when exposure takes place during the sensitive period, which in the dog is between 30 and 50 days of gestation.

In male pseudohermaphrodism the gonads are exclusively testes, but the genital ducts and/or the external genitalia lack full masculinization and display some phenotypically female characteristics. Defective male development in such cases can be ascribed to a specific failure of the fetal testes to overcome the inherent tendency of the genital tract to feminize. Failure of the testes to secrete the necessary androgens during the critical period of sex differentiation can be due to (1) impaired synthesis of steroids, thus affecting the steroid production of both the testes and adrenals, or to (2) a specific impairment of testosterone synthesis in the testes.

In the human, several disorders belonging to the first category have been described; so far they have not been detected in domestic mammals. Patients belonging to the second category can easily go unnoticed. There are several descriptions in the veterinary literature that fit into one of these patterns, but again these anomalies have not been clearly distinguished.

Target organ insensitivity to androgenic hormones also leads to a phenotypically female development. The external genitalia are female, but the vagina is shallow and ends blindly. Since the inhibition of the Müllerian ducts is quite normal in these cases, only traces of genital ducts will be found. This hereditary disorder is usually called the "testicular feminization syndrome." Incomplete forms of this syndrome that are probably due to a lesser degree of insensitivity to androgens have also been encountered. The syndrome has been described in detail in the human, the mouse and the rat. In recent years a few cases in domestic mammals have also been described.

Exposure of male fetuses to exogenous estrogens can have variable results. If high dosages of estrogens are administered to a pregnant bitch, extensive feminization of the genital tract of the male fetuses can occur. In these cases general inhibition of the testicular function may result in partial regression of the Müllerian ducts and insufficient gubernacular outgrowth. More commonly, because of lower dosage, the effect will be limited to the external genitalia, and hypospadias is the most common finding.

Exposure to progestogens, especially the synthetic progestogens, may also result in hypospadias.

Exposure of the male fetus to antiandrogens (cryproterone acetate, chlormadinone acetate, megestrol acetate) can interfere seriously with normal sex differentiation. The outcome depends on the stage of sex differentiation at the time of exposure. Furthermore, the sensitivity of the different structures appears to be highly variable.

Hypospadias is the phenomenon that occurs most frequently and is probably due to inadequate androgenic stimulation. If a high enough dosage is administered at the proper time (30 to 44 days in the dog), complete inhibition of the Wolffian ducts and a female type of development of the urogenital sinus will result. In these cases no genital duct systems will be found, since regression of the Müllerian ducts proceeds quite normally.

Abnormalities of Testicular Descent (Cryptorchidism)

Absolute or relative failure of the gubernaculum to enlarge or aberrant growth causing the gubernaculum to extend into an unusual position (Fig. 3) can affect testicular descent.

Complete absence of the outgrowth reaction has not been observed, but substantial underdevelopment does occur in low frequency. In these cases there is a partial migration of the testis from its original position just caudal to the kidney to the vicinity of the internal inguinal opening. The final result in such cases is either permanent low abdominal cryptorchidism or delayed testicular descent.

Abnormal location of the gubernaculum can take three forms:

1. The extra-abdominal part of the gubernaculum does not expand beyond the inguinal canal but, instead, thrusts back into the abdominal cavity (reversed outgrowth). The traction normally developed by the outgrowth is absent, and the testis fails to leave its original position caudal to the kidney. This results in high abdominal cryptorchidism. Even after regression of the gubernaculum, the genesis of this anomaly can be traced owing to the topography of the cremaster muscle.

2. The outgrowth takes place partly in the inguinal canal and is partly intra-abdominal. Only slight displacement of the testis in the direction of the internal inguinal opening will then occur.

3. The reaction is partly extra-abdominal. If this occurs, descent will progress further, and the testis may even reach the internal inguinal opening.

The final outcome following these aberrations is difficult to predict, but low abdominal or inguinal cryptorchidism, often combined with inguinal hernia, is the most likely result. In some instances the gubernaculum fails to pass through the external

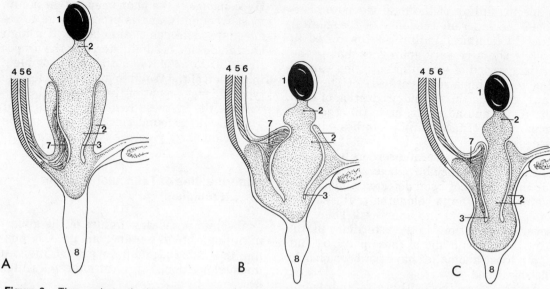

Figure 3. Three schematic drawings of abnormal gubernacular outgrowth. *A,* Reversed swelling reaction. The entrance to the vaginal process is lifted away from the internal inguinal ring, and the cremaster muscle extends intra-abdominally. *B,* Gubernacular outgrowth mainly within the inguinal canal. The anatomical relations in this area are gravely disturbed. *C,* Gubernacular outgrowth partly within the inguinal canal.

inguinal ring but instead extends between the aponeurosis of the external oblique muscle and the fleshy part of the internal oblique muscle of the abdomen. The testis is moved from the abdomen in the normal way, but, after the regression of the gubernaculum, a final ectopic extra-abdominal position of the testis is the most likely outcome.

In the female neonatal dog some gubernacular reaction occurs normally. However, due to unknown causes, this reaction can be a bit more substantial, resulting in a roomy vaginal process. This may lead to an indirect inguinal hernia in the bitch later in life.

DIAGNOSIS AND THERAPY

After birth, phenotypic sex determination may be difficult because of anatomical abnormalities of the external genitalia. Testes, if descended, are usually not palpable during the first few neonatal weeks. At about 3 months of age a more detailed examination can be carried out. The degree of penile hypoplasia and possible hypospadias or clitoric enlargement and possible fusion of genital folds can be determined. Palpation of the inguinal and the scrotal region should be carried out for presence of gonads or an inguinal hernia. Rectal palpation may yield

information about the presence of a prostate or uterus. A complete history regarding treatment of the bitch with steroids and the physical condition of the other pups in the litter may provide important aid in making a clinical diagnosis. At times a laparoscopic examination may be necessary to determine the extent of the anatomical abnormalities. It may be necessary to determine the genetic sex of the animal, and this can be done by examining cell nuclei in a buccal smear for detection of Barr bodies. If a mosaic is suspected, karyotyping of several tissues may be necessary.

Suspicion of abnormal sexual development can arise after puberty, even though the external genitalia appear normal, because the bitch does not exhibit signs of estrus.

Specific therapy for the various forms of true and pseudohermaphrodism is usually not possible; only symptomatic relief can be offered. Irritation due to hypospadias or clitoric enlargement can be abolished by a surgical correction to restore normal male or female anatomy. Removal of abdominal testes or ovotestes is recommended because of the increased risk of malignant transformation in these gonads. If the gonads are surgically removed, it is advisable also to remove the uterus whenever present.

Management of Cryptorchidism

The primary outgrowth of the gubernaculum in the dog takes place during the first 2 weeks after birth; following that period, regression starts. It is therefore not possible to diagnose maldescent of the testis until the dog is at least 1 month old. Probably it is best to wait until the third month before a final diagnosis is made. The examination must be performed very carefully because a spasm of the cremaster muscle will retract the testis toward the inguinal canal (retractile testis) and can be mistaken for cryptorchidism. Generally the testis can be manually pulled into the scrotum if the animal is calm during the examination. Until puberty, the testis can move between the external inguinal opening and the scrotum; eventually the testis will remain in the scrotum, and no treatment will be necessary. True cryptorchidism means that the testis is located either intra-abdominally or inguinally. Usually this condition is unilateral. In most of these cases it seems that testicular function is normal initially; however, destruction of the germinal epithelium develops gradually owing to the higher abdominal temperature.

Intra-abdominal cryptorchidism cannot be treated effectively, and castration is recommended. Surgical correction is possible in some cases by orchidopexy, but the risk of impairing the vascularization is extremely high. Perhaps more importantly, since there are clear indications that the condition is in some way heritable, it is questionable if therapy should be considered at all. Diagnosis of inguinal cryptorchidism is possible with careful palpation of an animal with the abdominal muscles well relaxed. Such cases have been treated with gonadotropin such as human chorionic gonadotropin (HCG). Some results have been reported with four injections of HCG (25 to 100 IU) divided over a 2-week period. If no displacement occurs following treatment, the prognosis is unfavorable. The rationale for gonadotropin treatment of cryptorchidism is questionable, since there is good reason to believe that if testicular descent occurs during treatment, the testis would have eventually come down without treatment. In any case, prolonged treatment with HCG for several weeks or more is not recommended and is probably not effective because of antibody formation and subsequent neutralization effect. Recently it has become possible to replace the HCG treatment by luteinizing hormone–releasing hormone (LHRH), which even with prolonged usage does not lead to the formation of antibodies. However, this treatment is also questionable and has not been used in the dog.*

REFERENCES

1. Curtis, E. M. and Pury-Grant, R.: Masculinization of female pups by progestogens. J.A.V.M.A., *144*:395, 1964.
2. Dain, A. R.: Intersexuality in a cocker spaniel dog. J. Reprod. Fertil., *39*:365, 1974.
3. Gier, H. T. and Marion, G. B.: Development of mammalian testes and genital ducts. Biol. Reprod., *1*:1, 1969.
4. Kelly, D. F., Long, S. E. and Strohmenger, G. D.: Testicular neoplasia in an intersex dog. J. Small Anim. Pract., *17*:247, 1976.
5. Kiesewetter, W. B., Kalayogln, M. and Sachs, B.: The effect of abnormal position, scrotal repositioning, and human gonadotropic hormone on the developing puppy testis. J. Ped. Surg., *8*:739, 1973.
6. Pendergrass, T. W. and Hayes, H. M., Jr.: Cryptorchidism and related defects in dogs: epidemiologic comparisons with man. Teratology, *12*:51, 1975.
7. Reif, J. S. and Brodey, R. S.: The relationship between cryptorchidism and canine testicular neoplasia. J.A.V.M.A., *115*:2005, 1969.
8. Schörner, J.: Gestörter descensus beim Rüden und therapeutische Massnahmen. Wien. Tierärztl. Mschr., *62*:426, 1975.
9. Shane, B. S., Dunn, H. O., Kenny, R. M., Hansel, W. and Visek, W. J.: Methyl testosterone-induced female pseudohermaphroditism in dogs. Biol. Reprod., *1*:41, 1969.
10. Weissbach, L., Heinemann, I. and Goslar, H. G.: Histochemische Untersuchungen beim experimentellen unilateralen Kryptochismus des Hundes nach HCG-Behandlung. Acta Histochem., *52*:62, 1975.

Acknowledgments: I want to express my gratitude to Mr. H. Schifferstein for preparing the drawings.

Normal Events of Gestation in the Bitch and Methods of Pregnancy Diagnosis

JAMES H. SOKOLOWSKI

The Upjohn Company, Kalamazoo, Michigan

Hypothalamic, then pituitary and then ovarian cycles produce the mediators by which all other changes in the animal organism related to reproduction occur. These cyclic events result in the period of sexual receptivity in the bitch that, if she is exposed to a stud, can result in pregnancy.

BREEDING AND CONCEPTION

It has been demonstrated that spermatozoa occur in large numbers in the lumen of the oviduct within 25 seconds after ejaculation. Because of the rapidity of spermatozoan transport, vaginal douching after coitus has little obvious value in preventing pregnancy following an unwanted mating.

Spermatozoa that are motile, but with unknown fertilization capability, can exist for up to 11 days in the lumen of the canine uterus but are absent in vaginal fluids within 24 hours after coitus. Vaginal swabs have little diagnostic value in identifying a breeding unless those swabs are taken within a few hours after coitus (Fig. 1).

Once ovulation has occurred and the bitch is in metestrus, the spermatozoa rapidly disappear so that by approximately 9 days after ovulation the uterine glands no longer contain sperm.

Ovulation in the bitch is spontaneous and is thought to occur within 24 hours after the day of first acceptance of the male. All ovulatory follicles rupture at almost the same time. Follicles that do not ovulate undergo atresia. The vaginal smear can be used to approximate the time of ovulation and therefore, presumably, the best time for breeding for maximum fertility.

Even though spermatozoa and ova can survive for several days, fertilization generally occurs in the oviducts a short time after copulation is completed. Fertility generally decreases as the interval from breeding to ovulation increases; however, fertile breedings have occurred as long as 6 to 8 days after first acceptance.

The young bitch has about 700,000 ova on her ovary. These numbers then decline rapidly — to estimates of 250,000 ova at puberty, 30,000 at 5 years of age and but a few hundred by 10 years of age. Although fertili-

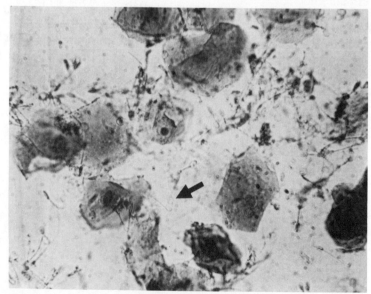

Figure 1. Vaginal smear of bitch in estrus. Cornified epithelial cells, leukocytes, debris, red blood cells and spermatozoa. (From Sokolowski, J. H.: Reproductive features and patterns in the bitch. JAAHA, *9*:71, 1973. Reprinted with permission of the editors of the Journal of the American Animal Hospital Association.)

ty wanes with advancing age, a corollary to menopause is not evident in most bitches.

FETAL DEVELOPMENT

Fertilization occurs in the oviduct, with the embryos entering the uterine horn between the 16-cell stage and the youngest blastocyst. Free-floating blastocysts then exist in the uterine horn for about 7 days. Implantation occurs over a period of time, with endometrial edema being the first indication that the blastocyst has taken up a definite position along the horn. Zonary placentation begins about day 17 to 21. By day 23 after breeding there is a structural attachment of the endometrium and trophoblast.

The earliest time that pregnancy can be accurately diagnosed is about day 17 after breeding or at the time that the blastocyst has positioned itself and the enlargement of the horn has occurred.

Embryos position along the horns without regard to the number of corpora lutea on the ipsilateral ovary and apparently migrate from one horn to the other to partially equalize the number of embryos between horns. After implantation has been completed (day 21 to 24 after breeding), embryotomy of consecutive embryos at periods from day 21 on does not result in either repositioning of embryos or abortion of the remaining embryos. Ovariectomy in the bitch at day 30 to 56

postbreeding does result in pregnancy termination, generally within 72 hours after ovariectomy. This demonstrates that the ovary (and circumstantially the production of progesterone) is required to maintain pregnancy and that the fetoplacental unit is a minor contributor to maintenance of a full-term pregnancy.

Fetal development progresses to a grossly visible stage by about day 20, when embryos of 4- to 7-mm crown-rump (C-R) length can be recovered (Fig. 2). Extreme variations can occur in embryo size (both C-R measurement and weight) within and between litters at a given time after breeding (Table 1). In the beagle bitch it has been reported that increases in fetal C-R length are linear from midgestation to about the fifty-eighth day and progress at about 6 mm per day.

Fetuses are generally larger at a given stage of development for larger bitches. Part of the between-litter variation at a given fetal age can be accounted for by size of the dam.

A blastocyst at day 17 to 18 after breeding may measure 1 to 3 mm in length but results in a segmented enlargement of the uterus of approximately 10 to 15 mm diameter (Fig. 3). It is this enlargement in the uterus that is the basis for pregnancy diagnosis by palpation.

Organogenesis advances rapidly in the embryo, so that by day 20 to 23 after breeding the aorta and mesonephric tubule are observable. By day 26 to 28 the major

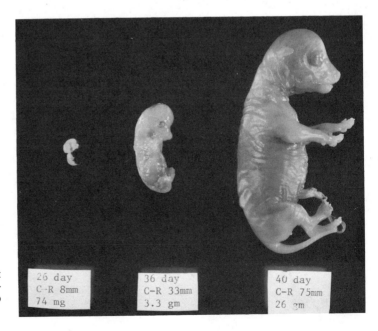

Figure 2. Canine fetal development showing the rapid change in the embryo from shortly after implantation to recognition of the fetus.

26 day
C-R 8mm
74 mg

36 day
C-R 33mm
3.3 gm

40 day
C-R 75mm
26 gm

TABLE 1. Embryo-Fetus Size and Weight at Different Stages of Gestation*

Day-Post-breeding	Number	Crown-Rump Length (mm)		Weight (gm)	
		AVERAGE	RANGE	AVERAGE	RANGE
20	1	7.0	–	–	–
26	1	8.0	–	0.074	–
28	2	12.0	(11–13)	0.244	(.191–.258)
30	2	15.5	(15–16)	0.426	(.420–.432)
32	1	19.0	–	0.794	–
33	9	32.2	(29–38)	3.50	(2.5–4.5)
35	5	42.2	(36–45)	6.10	(5.5–7.0)
36	1	33.0	–	3.3	–
37	1	46.0	–	7.0	–
38	8	54.5	(50–58)	10.6	(9–13)
40	13	71.6	(63.0–78.1)	23.9	(20.0–28.0)
52	5	114.0	(110.0–119.0)	114.0	(100.0–138.0)
54	5	138.0	(131.0–143.0)	202.4	(176.0–222.0)
57	11	132.1	(120.0–150.0)	218.0	(190.0–260.0)
Term		160.3	(147.0–170.0)	273.6	(207.0–327.0)

*Bitches of similar prebreeding size.

organs, including the undifferentiated gonad, can be observed. Microscopic identification of gonadal differentiation can be accomplished about day 30 to 34, while sex determination by the appearance of the external genitalia is not possible until after 35 days of gestation.

PHYSIOLOGIC CHANGES DURING GESTATION

The Ovary

Gross ovarian weight is greatest at approximately the time of ovulation, presumably due to size of the follicles and the luteinization that is occurring. Follicles are largest and most numerous during proestrus. The change of ovarian weight from the time of proestrus to estrus is related to the luteinizing of follicles, with corpora lutea being fully developed and most numerous about 10 days after ovulation has occurred.

The size and number of corpora lutea present on ovaries at 10 days postovulation do not differ in pregnant versus nonpregnant bitches. By 20 days after ovulation in both pregnant and nonpregnant bitches, degenerative changes are occurring in the corpora lutea. By 50 days after ovulation, changes in the corpora lutea are quite advanced, with vacuolar degeneration evident on histological examination.

Corpora lutea are a bright salmon pink color from the time of ovulation until 10 days after ovulation. They then change to yellow and finally at about 60 days after ovulation are of light tan coloration. No corpora albicantia (the whitish cicatricial remnants of a corpus luteum) are observed in

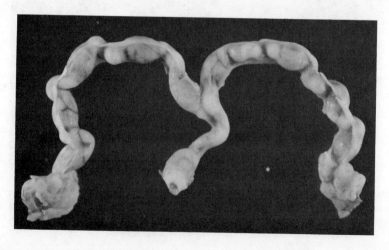

Figure 3. Pregnant canine uterus approximately 17 days after breeding (bitch weight aproximately 10 kg).

the ovaries either during or immediatly after the first heat period. They are, however, observed frequently on the ovaries of bitches after the third estrus.

It is difficult to count the total number of corpora lutea on an ovary, in that as many as one-third occur deep in the stoma and therefore are only evident after careful dissection of the ovary. It is not known if these "central" corpora lutea contribute ova available for potential fertilization. It is assumed that since these centralized corpora lutea appear functional, they contributed actively to the production of peripheral progesterone levels. Counting surface corpora lutea may lead to erroneous accounts of the precise fertility of the bitch.

The Uterus

The uterus attains maximum nonpregnant size (weight and dimension) at about 20 to 30 days after proestrus, whereas the pregnant uterus attains maximum size immediately prior to parturition. The morphological differences between a pregnant and nonpregnant uterus are insignificant until approximately day 17 to 18 after breeding, at which time spherical enlargements become evident.

The vasculature changes quite remarkably during the various stages of the estrous cycle and as fetal development progresses to term.

The Vagina

The vagina responds to estrogen influence by developing a prominent layer of cornified squamous epithelial cells. The mucous membrane becomes quite thickened and develops longitudinal folding. During proestrus and estrus the epithelium changes from cornified squamous epithelium through varying degrees of cornification and finally becomes noncornified after peripheral progesterone levels become elevated following ovulation.

Mammary Glands

As the follicles develop on the ovaries and endogenous estrogen levels increase, the epithelium of the ducts develops and the ducts proliferate. Lobuloalveolar development results from stimulation by increasing levels of endogenous progesterone. It can be speculated that prolactin or luteotrophic hormone (LTH) levels probably elevate during this period and that these changes would result in overt lactation toward the end of pregnancy. I would also speculate that prolactin is probably the mediator of the pseudopregnancy response that occurs in varying degrees in the nonpregnant bitch.

The changes in the mammary glands of the bitch are grossly imperceptible until shortly after ovulation has occurred. After that time, a bluish plaque can be observed at the base of each nipple in light-skinned bitches. As pregnancy progresses, duct development continues, and toward the end of pregnancy lobuloalveolar development reaches the peak of overt lactation.

Gestation Length

Average length of gestation for the bitch is approximately 62 days. Viable fetuses can, however, be whelped following a gestation of 58 to 66 days (duration from breeding to parturition).

PREGNANCY DIAGNOSIS

Palpation

Pregnancy diagnosis in the bitch can be determined by abdominal palpation. With the bitch in a standing position, grasp the abdomen gently as if holding a football. By applying steady pressure up toward to lumbar spine and then gently bringing the fingers together, allowing the abdominal viscera to "slip" through the fingers, you can, with practice, locate the pregnant uterus and estimate the stage of pregnancy.

During the first 18 days of pregnancy (Fig. 3) only minor gross changes occur in the uterus. About the nineteenth day, however, ovoid enlargements occur in the uterine horns in which the developing embryo is sisuated. Palpation of the abdomen between day 20 and 28 after breeding provides a method of diagnosing pregnancy. About day 20 the developing uterus will have spherical swellings approximately 10 to 15 mm in diameter. By day 28 these uterine enlargements change to an ovoid shape and increase in size to 15 to 30 mm in diameter (Figs. 4 and 5), depending on the size of the bitch.

After day 28 of pregnancy it is extremely difficult to palpate the pregnant uterus. The

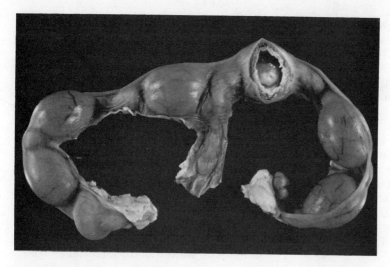

Figure 4. Pregnant canine uterus approximately 28 days after breeding (bitch weight approximately 10 kg).

embryos have enlarged to about 15 mm (crown-rump length), resulting in uterine enlargements that are more confluent and more pliable.

Digital palpation of the pregnant uterus can, of course, be complicated by a tense, fat or large bitch and by a full gastrointestinal tract or bladder. Another complication to positive pregnancy diagnosis is the presence of segmentation of the uterus in pseudopregnancy.

Radiology

Radiography can be used to obtain a positive diagnosis of pregnancy on day 42 of pregnancy or later. With careful air contrast radiographic technique, the segmented en-

largements of the uterus may be visualized prior to day 42. Radiography is probably most valuable in identifying pregnancy in large or fat animals with one or two fetuses, in identifying the number or presentation of fetuses in a dystocia or in cases of ectopic fetuses.

Ultrasonic Techniques

Ultrasonography has been used to diagnose pregnancy as early as the twenty-ninth day. The technique relies on transmission of ultrasonic waves into the medium and reflection of those waves by tissues and conversion of the reflected waves into audible signals. A similar transmitter with a visible read-out also has been developed. The major problems of ultrasound techniques used for small animal pregnancy diagnosis have been the cost of the equipment and the development of the expertise necessary for competent use of the equipment.

Other Methods

No suitable biological or chemical tests have yet been developed for use in pregnancy diagnosis in the bitch.

REFERENCES

1. Andersen, A. C. and Simpson, M. E.: The Ovary and Reproductive Cycle of the Dog (Beagle). Los Altos, Ca., Geron-X, Inc., 1973.
2. Concannon, P. W., Hansel, W. and Visek, W. J.: The

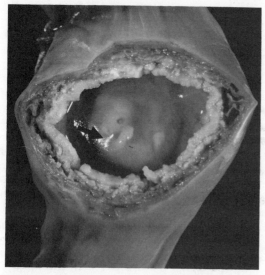

Figure 5. Twenty-eight day fetus *in situ* (also see Figure 4).

The author would like to acknowledge the technical assistance of F. VanRavenswaay.

ovarian cycle of the bitch: Plasma estrogen, LH and progesterone. Biol. Reprod., *13*:112, 1975.

3. Holst, P. A. and Phemister, R. D.: The prenatal development of the dog: Preimplantation events. Biol. Reprod., *5*:194, 1971.
4. Phemister, R. D., Holst, P. A., Spano, J. S. and Hopwood, M. L.: Time of ovulation in the beagle bitch. Biol. Reprod., *8*:74, 1973.
5. Sokolowski, J. H., Zimbelman, R. G. and Goyings, L.

S.: Canine reproduction: Reproductive organs and related structures of the non-parous, parous and postpartum bitch. Am. J. Vet. Res., *34*:1001, 1973.
6. Sokolowski, J. H.: Reproductive features and patterns in the bitch. J.A.A.H.A., *9*:71, 1973.
7. Sokolowski, J. H.: Reproductive patterns in the bitch. Vet. Clin North Am., *7*:653, 1977.

Normal and Abnormal Parturition

DAVID BENNETT
University of Glasgow, Glasgow, Scotland

NORMAL PARTURITION (EUTOCIA)

Physiology of Parturition

A knowledge of the mechanisms responsible for parturition is useful in order to appreciate the possible etiological factors responsible for abnormal parturition and how these might be managed. Unforutnately, however, the exact mechanisms of parturition in any species are still unknown. This is especially true of the canine species, principally because most research studies have been applied to the farm animals. The following account of the possible mechanisms of parturition is based on information that is available for the dog, together with reasonable extrapolations from research in other species. Until detailed studies are done specifically for the canine, a more accurate description is not possible. Physiological changes that are important for normal parturition occur within the fetus as well as within the dam, and both are closely interrelated.

Fetal Factors (Fig. I)

Recent research in man and animals has strongly implicated the importance of the fetus in determining its own time of delivery, an interesting concept in that this was also suggested by Hippocrates in 400 B.C.

It is thought that an unknown "stress" stimulus acts on the fetus through the nervous system to release corticotropin-releasing factor (CRF) from the hypothalamus, which passes to the anterior pituitary gland to cause the release of adrenocorti-

cotropic hormone (ACTH). The latter acts on the fetal adrenal glands to produce a hyperfunction, possibly accompanied by hyperplasia, with the release of adrenocorticosteroid hormones.These adrenal hormones are believed to release prostaglandins from the placenta; estrogens acting on the placenta may also assist in this release. The prostaglandins may have a local stimulatory effect on the uterine muscle that enhances contractility and may also pass into the maternal blood circulation and act on the pituitary gland of the dam to help in the release of oxytocin. A further role of prostaglandins could be a luteolytic effect, and they may also inhibit the production of the small amounts of progesterone found in the placenta of the bitch.

The "stress" factor acting on the fetal pituitary gland is unknown but could be the inability of the placenta to continue to supply sufficient nutrients to the fetus. Most of this evidence for fetal participation in determining the time of parturition is from research in other species, but some factors in the bitch could support the existence of a similar mechanism. For example, the gestation period is often increased in bitches with a single fetus and decreased in those carrying many fetuses. This could be explained by insufficient fetal steroid production in the former case and an "oversufficient" production in the latter. Puppies born with head defects have also been associated with prolonged gestation periods, and this could be explained by an abnormal pituitary/adrenal physiological relationship that interferes with normal fetal steroid production.

Maternal Factors (Fig. 2)

An alteration in the progesterone:estrogen ratio at the myometrium is generally accepted as being important for normal par-

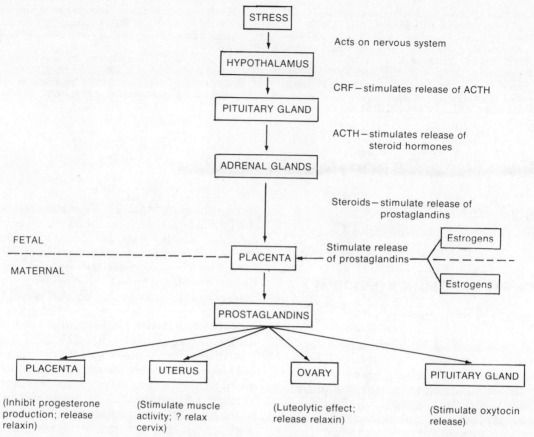

Figure 1. A summary diagram showing the main fetal factors involved in regulating parturition. CRF = corticotropin releasing factor; ACTH = Adrenocorticotropin hormone.

turition in all species. This is achieved in different ways, according to whether or not the animal secretes significant quantities of progesterone from the placenta. In placental progesterone species, e.g., the sheep, alteration of the balance is brought about by a marked increase in estrogen production in the immediate prepartum period. However, in nonplacental progesterone species, e.g., the cow, progesterone production sharply declines just before birth, and in these animals estrogens have been secreted in significant amounts for a prolonged period prior to birth. In both groups, the net effect is to alter the progesterone:estrogen ratio at the myometrium in favor of estrogen secretion.

The canine poses special problems in that it does not fit exactly into either of these two groups. Following ovulation in the bitch, the levels of circulating progesterone rise to reach peak concentrations early in pregnancy, following which a gradual decline occurs during the rest of gestation. Peripheral plasma progesterone levels are low in the imme-

diate prepartum period. However, a similar peaking occurs during metestrus in the nonpregnant animal. Although ovarian venous plasma studies have suggested an increased secretion of progesterone in pregnant animals, the majority of reported evidence indicates no apparent difference at any time in peripheral plasma progesterone levels in pregnant and nonpregnant animals.

Progesterone is certainly required to maintain pregnancy in the canine, as it is in other species. Ovariectomy of the bitch prior to day 56 of gestation causes abortion, suggesting that the corpora lutea are the major source of progesterone. However, low levels of progesterone have been detected in the placenta, and these may be an important contribution to a "progesterone blockage" of the myometrium. Hypophysectomy experiments have suggested the necessity of the pituitary gland in supporting luteal function, luteinizing hormone probably being involved.

Conflicting reports have been presented

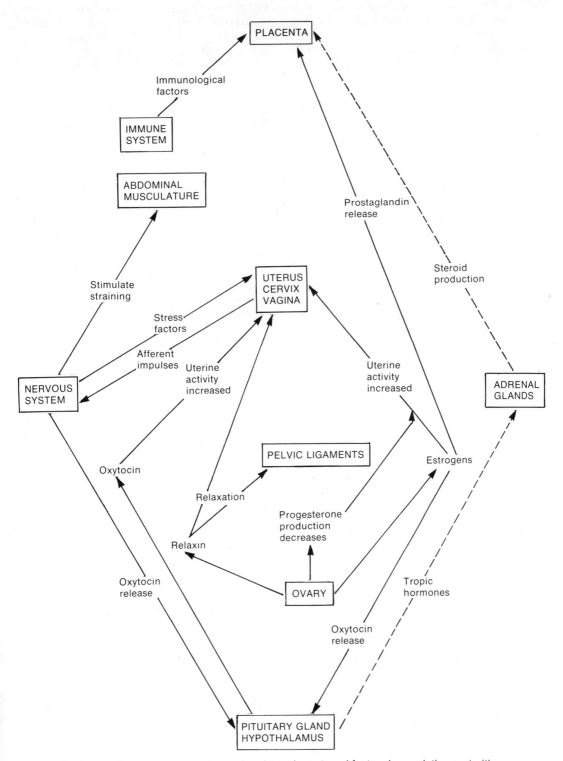

Figure 2. A summary diagram showing the main maternal factors in regulating parturition.

regarding the actual amounts and patterns of alteration of estrogens in the plasma of both pregnant and nonpregnant bitches, but no marked variation between the two has been described.

From this discussion, the bitch appears to be principally a nonplacental progesterone species and should exhibit a decrease of progesterone secretion in the presence of elevated estrogen levels at parturition. But in contrast to the polyestrous species of this group, in the bitch luteal function during pregnancy declines over a considerable part of gestation. The similarity in the pattern of secretion of progesterone in pregnant and nonpregnant bitches suggests that this pattern reflects the natural life cycle of the luteal tissue, which is unaffected by the presence of embryos *in utero*. The occurrence of low plasma progesterone levels for an appreciable period prior to fetal expulsion is difficult to explain, but some tentative evidence suggests that in spite of the large quantities of progesterone secreted in the first third of pregnancy, only very low concentrations of this hormone are actually required to ensure myometrial quiescence. In addition, some studies have demonstrated a sharp decline of the already low levels of progesterone during late gestation at the time of birth.

It is difficult to accept a simple "dying off" process of the corpora lutea as being responsible for the relatively constant duration of gestation in the bitch. It may be that a "dying off" process produces a decline in progesterone over the last two-thirds of gestation, but superimposed on this is an active mechanism that operates only in pregnant animals, producing a further sharp reduction in the secretion of progesterone immediately before birth. The absence of any marked increase in estrogen levels during late gestation suggests that the alteration in the progesterone:estrogen ratio in the bitch is caused by a decrease in the progesterone level. The removal of this so-called "progesterone block" on the uterus results in an increase in the spontaneous excitability and conductivity of the myometrium.

Oxytocin is important in initiating and coordinating strong contractions of the estrogen-dominated progesterone-free uterine muscle. In some species estrogens are believed to stimulate the release of oxytocin from the posterior pituitary gland, but of more importance is Ferguson's neurohumoral reflex, which involves stimulation of mechanoreceptors in the cervix, uterus and vagina by mechanical distension from the fetus and fetal membranes. Impulses pass via the peripheral and central nervous systems to the hypothalamus to cause oxytocin release into the bloodstream.

The nervous system is also involved in stimulating abdominal straining in the later stages of delivery. In this case distention of the cervix and vagina stimulates sensory fibers, which form the afferent input of a spinal reflex arc, the efferent output causing the abdominal muscle contractions. It is also well known that the bitch can apparently delay parturition if at all stressed (as for example when placed in unfamiliar surroundings to whelp), and this presumably involves the nervous system.

The hormone relaxin produced by the ovary or placenta, or both, may be important in the bitch by causing relaxation of the pelvic ligaments and reproductive tract, enabling a widening of the birth canal for the passage of the fetuses. Estrogens may assist in this.

The role of the maternal adrenal glands is unclear, but in some species parturition can be induced by injections of corticosteroids. It would therefore appear sensible not to administer these drugs to the bitch for any reason during late gestation. Immunological factors have been studied in relation to the dam's tolerance of the developing fetus during gestation, and such factors may possibly have a role in the eventual "rejection" of the fetus by the dam at parturition.

Clinical Stages of Parturition

The bitch shows the three recognizable stages of labor:

First Stage. During this stage the bitch usually prepares for whelping by seeking seclusion, although some prefer to have companionship from the owner. Some bitches will engage in "nest" making. Anorexia, restlessness, apprehension, trembling and occasional vomiting may be seen. The pelvic ligaments and the lower reproductive tract relax. Uterine contractions commence and increase progressively in frequency and vigor, resulting in an increase of intrauterine pressure The contraction wave commences just proximal to the most distal fetus in the uterine horn. This stage usually lasts

6 to 12 hours but may persist for as long as 36 hours in the maiden bitch.

Second Stage. Expulsion of the fetuses occurs during this stage. Tenesmus is apparent and coincides with uterine contractions. This further increases intrauterine pressure to such a degree that the fetus is propelled through the pelvis to the exterior, which is a region of lower pressure.

In describing the disposition of the fetus at the time of birth the following three terms are used — presentation, position and posture.

Presentation is described as either anterior or posterior, depending on whether the head or the hindquarters, respectively, of the fetus are delivered first. In most species anterior presentation is the norm, but in the bitch approximately 40 per cent of all fetuses are delivered in posterior presentation. Obstruction of a posteriorly presented fetus can be a problem since the umbilical cord becomes compressed against the maternal pelvis, which results in the fetus attempting to breathe and consequently inhaling fetal fluids.

Position refers to the orientation of the longitudinal axis of the pup with respect to the maternal birth canal and can be dorsal, ventral or lateral. Dorsal position with the spine of the fetus opposing the dorsal wall of the maternal birth canal is the norm.

The *posture* of the fetus is a description of the orientation of the limbs and head. Generally the head and forelegs will be extended in front of the fetus and the hindlegs extended behind.

Third Stage. This is a period of uterine contractions leading to expulsion of fetal membranes, which normally occurs within 15 minutes of the delivery of the pup. Generally fetuses are delivered from each uterine horn alternately, and thus two puppies may be born before the placentae are passed. A greenish discharge always accompanies placental separation. This color is due to the pigment uteroverdin, which is produced by the breakdown of red blood cells in the canine placenta. There is repetition of the second and third stages of labor for the delivery of each fetus in the litter, and the average period between the delivery of successive puppies is approximately 30 minutes, although this can vary greatly.

Each fetus is covered by the amnion at birth, the allantois having ruptured by the expulsive effort or having been opened by the dam's teeth at the vulva. The bitch thoroughly licks the fetus on delivery to remove the amnion, to clean the pup and to stimulate cardiovascular and respiratory function. Normally the dam will eat the fetal membranes after expulsion, and occasionally this can produce vomiting.

Signs of Imminent Parturition

Recognition of imminent parturition in the bitch can be based on a rapidly increasing body weight, abdominal enlargement, increased size of the mammary glands, enlargement of the vulva, slight vaginal mucous discharge, relaxation of the pelvic ligaments and behavioral changes. In the primigravida lactation generally occurs within 24 hours of whelping, but in the multigravida milk may be present up to 7 days prior to parturition. A sudden drop of body temperature by at least 1.1°C usually occurs within 24 hours of parturition, but as this is only transient it is difficult to detect.

ABNORMAL PARTURITION (DYSTOCIA)

Etiology

The classical division of the possible causes of dystocia is given in Figure 3, although this is slightly erroneous in that many factors overlap or are interrelated. The two principal etiological factors in the canine are primary uterine inertia and fetal obstructions of the birth canal.

Primary Uterine Inertia

This occurs when the uterine muscle fails to contract and expel the fetuses from the womb. The fetuses are of normal size, and the birth canal is generally dilated, although sometimes the cervix fails to relax completely. Primary uterine inertia may be complete, in which case the dam is unable to expel any of the pups, or incomplete, which occurs when parturition starts normally but there is insufficient activity to expel all the fetuses. This latter type is not to be confused with secondary uterine inertia, in which case the uterine muscle becomes exhausted after prolonged contraction against an obstructed fetus. There are numerous possible

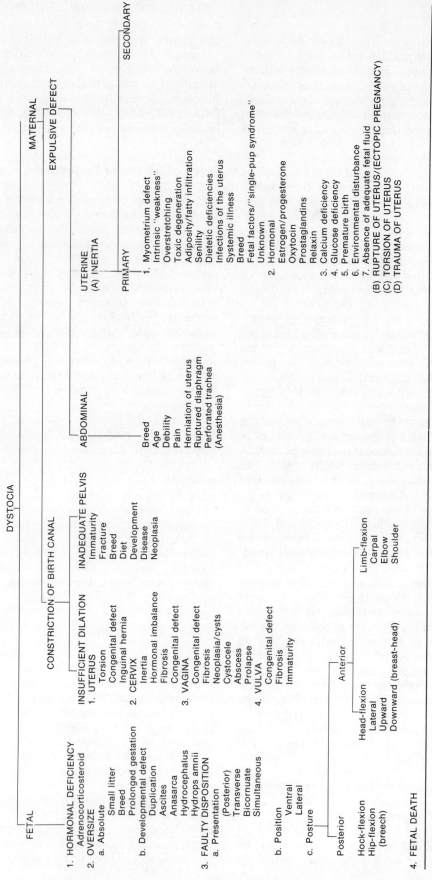

Figure 3. Causes of canine dystocia.

600

causes of primary uterine inertia, and most of these are difficult to assess and possibly somewhat academic. The "single-pup syndrome" is one important aspect of primary uterine inertia, and with maiden bitches especially, the pup often will not be delivered without assistance.

Fetal Obstruction

A fetus that is too large to pass along a maternal birth canal of normal dimensions will cause an obstruction due to absolute fetal oversize. A small litter or a prolonged gestation, or both, can be associated with fetal oversize. The term relative fetal oversize is used when a fetus of normal size is unable to pass along a maternal birth canal of abnormally small dimensions. Relative fetal oversize is thus equivalent to a maternal obstructive dystocia and can be the result of an inadequate pelvic diameter or of insufficient dilation of the birth canal. Abnormal dispositions of a fetus at birth can also produce an obstructive dystocia. Abnormal dispositions commonly occur in pups that have died *in utero* prior to delivery.

The reader is referred to Bennett[2] for further information on the causes of canine dystocia.

Breed Incidence. The brachycephalic breeds in particular are prone to an obstructive dystocia because the fetuses have comparatively large heads and the dams have narrow pelvic diameters. In addition bulldogs occasionally show slack abdominal musculature, making it impossible for uterine contractions and abdominal straining to lift the fetus into the pelvic cavity. Many terrier breeds show a high incidence of primary uterine inertia, and many of the miniature breeds show extreme variation in the size of pups and absolute fetal oversize can be a problem. Greyhounds tend to show a relatively high incidence of arrested fetal development and fetal death causing dystocia.

Placental Retention

This can be regarded as a form of dystocia and is usually associated with uterine inertia. Diagnosis is based on the presence of a copious purulent discharge at the vulva that occurs several hours after parturition. Putrefaction and septic metritis with systemic illness commonly occur and can be fatal. Sometimes the placentae can be detected on digital examination *per vaginam*.

Diagnosis of Dystocia

History

A detailed history is important for correct evaluation of any dystocic bitch. Previous whelping difficulties are relevant. Breeding dates and details of the male used at service are also important. The veterinarian should also consider the exact onset of whelping, the frequency and intensity of expulsive efforts, the number of puppies already born and the number of placentae produced, the time interval between births and the time of delivery of the last pup, maternal behavior and details of any assistance given by the owner.

Clinical Examination

The general observation of the patient and its environment can be of great assistance; for example, observing the character and frequency of straining, examining the bedding for any discharge and assessing the state of the pups already born. A general clinical examination should always be performed, as well as a more pertinent examination of the genital system.

Abdominal palpation may indicate the size and tone of the uterus, the presence of any fetuses and whether or not there is a fetus presented at the pelvis ready for delivery. Auscultation of the bitch's abdomen may identify the rapid fetal heartbeat, although this can be difficult during actual parturition because of the abdominal and uterine contractions.

The vulva must be examined for swelling, discharge and evidence of trauma. The perineum can be palpated for the presence of any fetuses within the vagina. Digital examination of the birth canal should be performed under clean conditions. The bitch is normally placed on a table and the forequarters raised. Palpating the abdomen with the other hand during the examination can assist in the digital exploration of the vagina. This examination can be used to assess the degree of dilation of the birth canal and to detect any congenital or acquired abnormalities. It should be realized that the cervix is situated cranial to the pelvis in the bitch, and thus in most animals palpation of this structure is not possible. The force of any uterine contractions can be assessed by digital pressure on the dorsal vaginal wall. If a fetus is felt, attempts should be made to assess its disposition. This is merely a matter of recognition of the fetal anatomy, and it is of great help to the veterinarian to practice feeling all the relevant parts of a neonate puppy with the tip of the finger and with the eyes closed. Palpation of a pup within the birth canal may stimulate fetal movement, and the insertion of a digit into the pup's mouth may initiate a sucking reflex; both these responses indicate fetal viability. Fetal membranes may be felt and can be difficult to distinguish from the folds of the vagina. However, such membranes tend to be thinner, and a finger can be inserted between them and the vaginal wall. It may be necessary to rupture the amnion over a presented puppy in order to determine its disposition.

Abdominal radiography of the bitch can be useful to demonstrate pregnancy, the number of fetuses remaining and the disposition of a fetus in the pelvis. The fetal skeleton usually becomes radiopaque within the last 2 weeks of gestation.

Criteria to Consider for Diagnosing Dystocia

1. Strong and persistent expulsive efforts failing to deliver a puppy within 20 to 30 minutes. When this occurs it is possible that although the pup is not delivered, placental separation occurs, in which case the pup cannot be expected to survive for any length of time inside the reproductive tract. Placental separation is indicated by the presence of a green discharge from the vagina. The most common cause of dystocia with this presentation is the obstructive type.

2. Weak and infrequent expulsive efforts failing to produce a pup within 2 to 3 hours. This most often indicates a primary uterine inertia.

3. More than 4 hours having elapsed since the birth of a puppy with no evidence of labor. This can indicate uterine inertia, although in some cases parturition may have naturally terminated.

4. Signs of systemic illness.

5. Prolongation of gestation. Duration of pregnancy is normally 63 to 65 days in the bitch. Normal whelping is unlikely to occur after 70 days of gestation, although the fetuses can remain viable for this length of time. Thus overdue bitches can be left for a few days in most instances.

However, there is little advantage in leaving maiden bitches with single pups for more than 24 hours, since natural delivery after this time is very unlikely. Once the bitch is overdue and treatment is to be delayed, frequent checks should be made and fetal heartbeats auscultated. A drop in the normally very rapid fetal heart rate indicates impending fetal death.

6. The presence of an abnormal discharge at the vulva.

7. An obvious cause of dystocia is apparent.

Treatment

The aim of treatment is the successful delivery of live and undamaged pups without harm to the dam.

Medicinal

Ecbolics are the most common drugs used in treating canine dystocia. Their main indication is for certain cases of primary uterine inertia, provided the birth canal is open and the uterine muscles are not under tension, although success with these drugs is limited. They also promote uterine involution, aid in the control of postpartum hemorrhage and help prevent placental retention. Ecbolics are contraindicated in cases of obstructive dystocia since uterine rupture can result. The most commonly used drug is posterior pituitary extract or synthetic oxytocin. Oxytocin has a short duration of action, tends to cause premature separation of the placentae and fetal death *in utero* and has been associated with uterine friability. The latter causes difficulty in suturing when uterine surgery has been necessary following the use of oxytocin. The ergot drugs are powerful stimulants of uterine muscle and have a much longer duration of action than oxytocin but are more likely to cause uterine rupture and are best used only after birth for controlling hemorrhage. Estrogen compounds (principally stilbestrol) can be used in conjunction with oxytocin since these cause cervical relaxation and sensitize the uterus to oxytocin.

Intravenous glucose solution is indicated in cases of primary uterine inertia due to hypoglycemia. Similarly, a calcium deficiency can cause uterine inertia, and treatment is with intravenous calcium borogluconate solution supplemented by oral administration of calcium. Calcium also helps to promote uterine involution and control postpartum hemorrhage.

Sedatives (tranquilizers) can be administered to bitches found savaging their puppies and to nervous bitches inhibiting parturition and also to uncooperative patients to facilitate vaginal examinations, although these drugs do cross the placenta and depress the fetal nervous system.

Antibiotic therapy may be indicated in certain instances such as septic metritis, and various types of supportive therapy may occasionally be indicated in treating the dystocic patient.

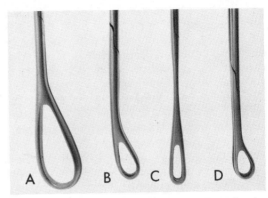

Figure 5. Obstetrical forceps as in Figure 4, showing the different types of jaws. *A* and *B*, Hobday-type (dog); *C*, Rampley-type; and *D*, Hobday-type (cat).

Surgical

Delivery *per Vaginam* by Digital and Forceps Manipulation. The bitch is best restrained on a table in the standing position, and the veterinarian must observe sterility and use adequate lubrication. Simple digital manipulation should always be tried first and in most cases will be sufficient. If instruments are used, they should be discarded as soon as possible and delivery completed by digital manipulation. Delivery with instruments should never be attempted when the fetus is totally out of digital reach. Sterile towels or gauze sponges can be used to get a good grip on the fetus with the fingers. The two main types of whelping forceps are Rampley's forceps, which engage the snout of

the anteriorly presented fetus and Hobday's forceps, which have the disadvantage of having to grip the skull of the fetus, thus increasing its effective width. An obstetrical vectis is sometimes useful (Figs. 4 and 5). With all digital and forceps manipulations it is useful to hold and anchor the fetus by abdominal palpation with the other hand, when the hand is not actively involved in the vaginal manipulation and when the bitch is sufficiently relaxed to allow useful abdominal palpation. The indications for assisted delivery *per vaginam* are:

1. To manage cases of abnormal fetal disposition that are amenable to correction *per vaginam*.

2. To manage cases of slight fetal oversize in which removal of the obstructed puppy can be expected to result in normal progression of parturition, i.e., when secondary uterine inertia has not yet developed.

3. To deliver a dead obstructed fetus if it is the last remaining puppy and when crushing of the fetus by forceps can be employed.

4. To deliver the last remaining fetus in cases of uterine inertia.

Whenever forceps are used, it is essential to check by digital palpation that the vaginal mucosa has not been included in the jaws of the forceps. Traction is applied downwards and backwards when attempting to pull a fetus from the birth canal, as dictated by the anatomy of the bitch's vagina. With maldispositions it is important to identify the abnormality and then to correct this *per vaginam*, using instruments only if necessary.

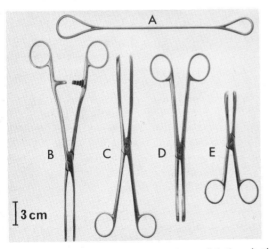

Figure 4. Obstetrical instruments for assisted vaginal delivery of puppies. *A*, Vectis; *B*, Rampley-type forceps with ratchet; *C* and *D*, Hobday-type forceps (dog); and *E*, Hobday-type forceps (cat).

It is possible to remove some retained fetal membranes during the first postpartum day by inserting a pair of sterile whelping forceps padded with sterile gauze into the uterus and rotating them in order to "wind up" the membranes, so that these are removed when the forceps are withdrawn.

Episiotomy. The indications for episiotomy are both relative and absolute constriction of the vulva, but the operation has never been found necessary by the author. The first fetus of a litter, especially in the primigravida, often becomes lodged at the vulva, but manipulation of the vulval lips over the fetus is generally sufficient to deliver the pup.

Cesarean Section (Hysterotomy) and Hysterectomy. Indications include:

1. Prolongation of gestation, complete primary uterine inertia.

2. Incomplete primary uterine inertia. Ecbolics may be successful here and can be attempted first but are less likely to be effective the greater the number of pups still remaining.

3. Secondary uterine inertia.

4. Relative and absolute fetal oversize. A cesarean section is preferable to vaginal delivery if the oversize is considerable and likely to be repeated in other fetuses, even if secondary uterine inertia has not supervened.

5. Fetal monstrosities.

6. Maldisposition of fetuses not amenable to delivery *per vaginam.*

7. Bitches with a past history of dystocia.

8. Gross abnormality of the maternal pelvis or soft tissues.

9. Fetal death following which putrefaction has supervened. This usually occurs in cases of neglected dystocia. The bitch may show systemic illness, and there is generally a malodorous greenish or blood-stained purulent discharge from the vagina; hysterectomy is often necessary.

10. Miscellaneous factors.

ANESTHESIA. Three basic anesthetic techniques have been described for the cesarean patient — local infiltration of an anesthetic agent, usually in conjunction with a parenterally administered narcotic and/or sedative agent; epidural local anesthesia, with or without sedation; and general anesthesia. The use of muscle relaxants and forced ventilation techniques that maintain the patient in a very light plane of anesthesia consistent with effective analgesia, is regularly used in human obstetrics and is now being applied to dogs by some specialist veterinary anesthetists.

Anesthetic considerations particular to the cesarean operation include the passage of sedative, narcotic and anesthetic agents across the placenta to depress the fetal nervous system, alterations in cardiovascular and respiratory function of the bitch caused by pregnancy and the effects of anesthetic agents on uterine contractility, which can influence the ease of surgery and the control of postpartum hemorrhage.

The author always uses general anesthesia for cesarean sections. Premedication with atropine is usual to help reduce respiratory secretions and to block any vagal stimulation of the heart caused by traction on the uterus or intestines, or both. Induction is generally achieved with a minimal dose of a short-acting barbiturate (methohexitone sodium) sufficient only to allow intubation, after which full anesthesia can be achieved and then maintained with a halothane and oxygen mixture. Occasionally, especially if the bitch is systemically ill, induction may be achieved with halothane and oxygen given by mask, after which intubation is performed. Vomiting is occasionally seen at induction, although this is rarely a major problem and requires only lowering the head of the patient and cleansing the mouth and pharynx of vomit before continuing with intubation. The anesthetic circuit used varies according to the size of the animal — an Ayre's T-piece is used for small breeds, a "to and fro" soda lime canister with rebreathing bag for middle-sized dogs and a soda lime circle absorber with rebreathing bag for the larger bitches. Small animals are placed on a heating pad to help prevent hypothermia. The plane of anesthesia is kept light, and the bitch is allowed to recover consciousness as soon as possible after surgery has finished so that she is able to immediately nurse and suckle the offspring.

Premedication with sedative agents will reduce the dose of barbiturates necessary for induction of anesthesia, but they too cross the placenta and tend to produce a longer-lasting depression of the fetus.

OPERATIVE TECHNIQUE. Either a flank

or midline laparotomy can be performed to exteriorize the uterus; the author prefers the midline approach.

For a cesarean section, the uterus is exteriorized and the surrounding viscera packed off with large gauze sponges to prevent fetal fluids from contaminating the peritoneal cavity. A longitudinal midline incision is made through the uterine body, and the fetuses are removed one by one from the uterus, the amnion is opened and the umbilical cord is clamped with forceps and severed about 2 cm from the fetal abdominal wall. The management of the newly delivered puppy is then taken over by a trained assistant who removes any secretions from the puppy's nose and mouth and dries the pup by vigorous rubbing with a clean towel, which also stimulates breathing. The assistant also removes the forceps from the umbilical stump and checks for hemorrhage. A source of heating, preferably an electric heating pad, is necessary to keep the pups warm while the operation is being completed. The placentae are removed at the time of surgery, but if there is any difficulty, they are best left in place because of the risk of postoperative uterine hemorrhage. If they are left, a uterine discharge will normally develop, but the placentae are usually expelled without any serious problem resulting. The uterus is closed by a double continuous inversion suture using chromic catgut. Oxytocin can be applied directly to the uterine wall or given by routine intramuscular injection to help promote postoperative involution of the uterus and control hemorrhage. Local or systemic antibiotics, or both, can be used according to the surgeon's discretion. Routine closure of the abdominal and skin wounds is performed.

The bitch and pups should be kept in a warm environment, and movement of the bitch should be restricted. Intravenous fluid therapy may be required before, during or after surgery to decrease surgical risk, counteract shock and aid recovery.

With a hysterectomy, the basic technique is similar to routine spaying. Supportive intravenous fluid therapy is important, since removal of the uterus takes away a substantial blood volume. Occasionally a fetus may be present in the lower reproductive tract, and this needs to be "milked" back into the uterine body or horn prior to removing the uterus. If this is not possible, an opening into the uterus is required to remove the offending fetus, and care has to be taken, as with the cesarean section, to prevent spillage of uterine contents. The uterine wound is closed, and removal of the uterus is then carried out.

COMPLICATIONS. Any of the usual complications associated with abdominal surgery can occur. A uterine scar caused by a previous cesarean operation can cause a defect in future placentation and produce abnormal fetal development. This can be avoided by always incising the uterine body rather than the horn. Repeated cesarean sections can be performed on the same bitch, but peritoneal adhesions may make later surgery difficult.

Prophylaxis

It is advisable to encourage owners of potential breeding bitches to have their dogs examined before mating to check their general health and assess them for any potential breeding problems, e.g., an inguinal hernia or congenital anomalies of the reproductive tract. Consideration of the dog's past medical history is also important, e.g., possible pelvic deformity resulting from a road traffic accident. A further check at 24 to 32 days of gestation for pregnancy diagnosis is useful, as is a final examination during the last days of pregnancy to assess the number of fetuses present, fetal viability and the health and well-being of the bitch. More frequent examinations may be necessary with certain patients or clients. At each examination advice to and discussion with the owner regarding management at mating, feeding during pregnancy and lactation and management of the whelping bitch should be encouraged. Frequent bodyweight recording of the pregnant bitch by the owner is useful.

Both the pregnant and lactating bitch should always be provided with a well-balanced, high-protein diet, which for the pregnant bitch will be 1.5 to 2 times its normal maintenance requirement and for the lactating bitch 3 to 4 times. Mineral and vitamin supplements are useful. The dam should not be allowed to become overweight and should receive regular exercise.

General good health must be maintained, and the bitch should be allowed to whelp in familiar, comfortable surroundings with minimal but efficient supervision. Whelping boxes should be introduced to the bitch well before the expected date of parturition.

Certain breeds have definite dystocia problems, e.g., the brachycephalic dog, and there is an obvious argument for altering breeding programs to help obviate these breed-related problems.

REFERENCES

1. Arthur, G. H.: Veterinary Reproduction and Obstetrics. 5th Ed. London, Baillière Tindall, 1975.
2. Bennett, D.: Canine dystocia — a review of the literature. J. Small Anim. Pract., *15*:101, 1974.
3. Freak, M. J.: Abnormal conditions associated with pregnancy and parturition in the bitch. Vet. Rec., *74*:1323, 1962.
4. Freak, M. J.: Practitioners'-breeders' approach to canine parturition. Vet. Rec., *96*:303, 1975.

Spontaneous Abortion

SHIRLEY D. JOHNSTON
University of Minnesota, St. Paul, Minnesota

The incidence of spontaneous abortion in the bitch is unknown. Fetal death, resorption and/or infection with vaginal discharge may be difficult to distinguish from open cervix pyometra. And bitches that do abort may eat the fetuses before they can be observed by the owner.

SIGNS

Abdominal contractions, expulsion of live or dead fetuses and vaginal discharge are consistent signs. Signs of other systemic disease, such as canine distemper, hypothyroidism, toxemia or septicemia, may also be present. Some or all of the fetuses may be aborted, and the remaining live fetuses may be born normally at term.

CAUSE

Fetal Defects

In women early abortion is usually preceded by fetal death most commonly caused by developmental abnormalities that are incompatible with life. Abnormal ova, defective germ plasm and chromosomal abnormalities (polyploidy, autosomal trisomy and aberrations of the sex chromosomes) have been incriminated. Aging of human ova and spermatozoa prior to fertilization is significantly associated with an increased inci-

dence of abortion. It is not unlikely that fetal abnormality in the dog plays a similarly important role. Chromosome analysis can be performed in the dog, but it is not commonly available. Studies in canine cytogenetics and fetal pathology may one day permit diagnosis of this cause of abortion. It is of some importance, however, for the clinician and owner to recognize the value of spontaneous abortion if a fetal defect is present.

Abnormal Maternal Environment

Hypothyroidism, a condition frequently diagnosed in dogs and a cause of infertility in the bitch, is associated with increased danger of spontaneous abortion in women. In normal pregnancy, levels of circulating thyroxine and thyroid-binding proteins are elevated. We have seen hypothyroid bitches with histories of abortions but have not established a cause and effect relationship between these two problems.

Deficient progesterone, or hypoluteoidism, was incriminated as a cause of abortion in the dog even before methods of measuring this steroid were developed. Because dogs that are ovariectomized as late as day 56 spontaneously abort, low progesterone levels must be considered a theoretical cause of abortion. This should not, however, be considered the most likely cause until rigorous endocrinological surveys are accomplished.

Caloric deprivation and vitamin deficiency of the dam can be associated with abortion, as can presence of anatomical uterine defects. Dogs with endocrinological disease (diabetes mellitus, adrenocortical dysfunction, and so forth) have not been reported to suffer an increased incidence of abortion but should probably not be used as breeding stock.

Infectious Agents

Brucella canis abortions occur most commonly between days 45 and 55 of pregnancy; early embryonic death may also be a part of *B. canis* infertility. Prolonged vaginal discharge follows abortion. Infected males and females are usually apparently healthy. The disease is most prevalent in kennel situations or in bitches bred to sexually active stud dogs (venereal transmission). *Brucella abortus* has also caused spontaneous abortion in bitches fed infected material.

Escherichia coli and other enteric bacteria are frequently cultured from the vaginal discharge or from fetal tissues after abortion. Their role in causing abortion is unknown; they may function as secondary pathogens.

Streptococcus β-hemolyticus, type L, was reported in 1961 to have been isolated from vaginal discharges or lymph node aspirates, or both, from four collies and a Doberman pinscher with histories of chronic abortion.[4] The bacteria isolated were either inoculated intravenously or given orally to six mongrel bitches in various stages of pregnancy. Four of these aborted. Two, which were infected near the end of gestation, whelped live puppies that died within several days of birth; β-hemolytic streptococci could be cultured from all of their organs.

Canine herpesvirus (CHV) is usually associated with respiratory disease and death in puppies and with mild vaginitis in the bitch. In 1971, however, CHV abortion of nearly full-term puppies was reported in several bitches from England.[6]

Canine distemper virus infection in a pregnant bitch may be associated with an increased incidence of spontaneous abortion; other debilitating diseases of bacterial, viral or neoplastic origin may also increase incidence of abortion.

Toxoplasma gondii infection can cause experimental abortion in dogs. An Italian report from 1969 documents high serological toxoplasma titers in ten bitches presented for spontaneous abortion; organisms were cultured from the uterus of six of them.[5] In our practice, active infection with this organism is uncommon, despite routine serological screening.

Trauma

In women, laparotomy will occasionally provoke abortion, especially when surgery is near the pelvic organs. Human obstetrics textbooks state that traumatic abortion is sometimes overemphasized and stress the importance of demonstrating a normal conceptus and placenta to establish this diagnosis.

DIAGNOSIS

The physical examination of a bitch with spontaneous abortion of unknown etiology must evaluate general health, nutrition, the possibility of endocrine or other disease and the magnitude of complications. Careful abdominal palpation will help determine whether other fetuses are present in the uterus. Sterile digital examination of the vagina should be done, and vaginoscopy may permit visualization of the cervix.

Laboratory evaluation should include a complete blood count, *Brucella canis* and *Toxoplasma gondii* serology determinations (paired samples are preferred) and serum thyroid hormone determination. Urine is collected for urinalysis, and a culture is taken from the anterior vagina or from the vaginal discharge. Histopathologic studies and stomach culture should be performed on the aborted fetus if possible.

TREATMENT

The bitch should be hospitalized to permit close observation and diagnostic evaluation and to enforce rest. Blood, urine and culture samples are taken immediately. If the bitch is toxic or is in shock, appropriate supportive therapy is instituted. Prophylactic antibiotics are indicated if the hemogram or rectal temperature, or both, are consistent with infection. Oxytocic agents (oxytocin, ergonovine, prostaglandin-$F_{2\alpha}$) are given to aid uterine evacuation if all of the fetuses have been aborted and if membranes are retained or if there is bleeding from the uterus. Progesterone therapy should not be given; this hormone promotes uterine quiescence, which is undesirable if either a dead fetus or infection is present.

In general, diagnosis of the cause of the abortion is more important in deciding about future breedings than as a guide for immediate therapy. Correction of caloric-, vitamin- and thyroid-deficient states is possible, and most bacterial infections can be treated specifically. To date, no permanent cure for *B. canis* infection in the dog is known; infected females must not be bred again. Canine abortions due to herpesvirus have been associated with chronic infertility and at present cannot be effectively treated. Abortion due to *Toxoplasma* does not generally occur during parasitemia caused by the tachyzoite (the one stage that is susceptible to therapy), so the bitch is not treated specifically. Bitches with a previous toxoplasma-induced abortion can probably be bred safely during subsequent cycles.

PREVENTION

Prevention of abortion in the bitch is empirical until the causes of this problem are better understood. Optimum general health, good vaccination history, negative *B. canis* titer and normal thyroid function are desirable prebreeding characteristics. Prevention of recurrent abortion in valuable bitches when infection has been ruled out may be attempted with progesterone therapy (2 mg/kg IM on days 35, 45 and 55). Serum progesterone levels can now be measured by radioimmunoassay at several veterinary schools; serial measurements during pregnancies of bitches that recurrently abort might provide a rationale for therapy. Masculinization of the external genitalia of female pups has been observed as a result of administration of progestational drugs during pregnancy.

REFERENCES

1. Carmichael, L. E. and Kenney, R. M.: Canine abortion caused by *Brucella canis*. J.A.V.M.A., *152*:605, 1968.
2. Chamberlain, D. M., Docton, F. L. and Cole, C.: Toxoplasmosis. II. Intra-uterine infection in dogs, premature birth and presence of organisms in milk. Proc. Soc. Exp. Biol. Med., *82*:198, 1953.
3. Curtis, E. M. and Grant, R. P.: Masculinization of female pups by progestogens. J.A.V.M.A., *144*:395, 1964.
4. Montovani, A., Restani, R., Schiarra, D., and Simonella, P.: *Streptococcus* L infection in the dog. J. Small Anim. Pract., *2*:185, 1961.
5. Nava, G. A.: Cases of abortion due to brucella, leptospira and toxoplasma in bitches. Atti. Soc. Ital. Sci. Vet., *23*:376, 1969.
6. Poste, G. and King, N.: Isolation of a herpesvirus from the canine genital tract: Association with infertility, abortion and stillbirths. Vet. Rec., *88*:229, 1971.
7. Sokolowski, J. H.: The effects of ovariectomy on pregnancy maintenance in the bitch. Lab. Anim. Sci., *21*:696, 1971.

Disorders in the Postparturient Bitch

J. E. MOSIER
Kansas State University,
Manhattan, Kansas

POSTPARTUM UTERINE DISEASES

The healthy uterus undergoes predictable involution and emptying following parturition. A period of 4 to 6 weeks is usually required for complete involution to occur. Palpation through the abdominal wall will reveal uterine horns that are uniform in size and consistency. Visible uterine discharge progresses from red to opaque to clear mucus.

Postpartum uterine disease rarely occurs in healthy, properly nourished bitches managed by experienced breeders. The occurrence of postpartum disease suggests the need for a thorough review of genetic background, nutritional programs and management. The more common postpartum uterine diseases include retained placenta, subinvolution, metritis and postpartum hemorrhage.

Retained Placenta

The third stage of normal parturition consists of contraction of the segment of the uterus from which the puppy came and expulsion of the fetal membranes. In many cases the puppy is accompanied by its placenta. When delivery of the placenta is delayed, it should pass within 15 minutes.

Retained placenta is suspected when the postpartum discharge is copious and dark green to black in color. Normally one should expect the green discharge to disappear within a few hours of delivery. Arthur[2] suggests that persistence of the green or black discharge 12 hours or more after delivery is indicative of a retained placenta. Palpation of the abdomen may reveal segmental enlargement of the uterus. Retained placentae are most commonly seen in bitches following prolonged whelping and in the toy breeds.

Prolonged retention of a placenta may result in necrosis of the uterine wall in the region of the placental attachment.[6] Failure to remove retained placentas will result in progressive toxemia, uterine distention and possible metritis. Death may occur in 4 to 5 days.

Early recognition of a retained placenta is best accomplished by counting placentae during the delivery. When the count reveals retention of a placenta, the administration of oxytocin (Pitocin) or ergonovine maleate (Ergotrate) followed in 5 to 10 minutes by gentle massage of the uterus through the abdominal wall may help to move the retained placenta through the cervix.

A sponge forceps holding a small pledget of gauze, inserted into the uterus and then rotated, may engage the placental membrane sufficiently to permit teasing of a portion of the placenta into the posterior vagina. Digital manipulation via the vagina may suffice to deliver a fragment of the membrane into a position where it can be grasped between the thumb and forefinger. The most difficult aspect is to avoid tearing the vaginal fragment from the undelivered placenta. Working slowly and gently teasing the placenta through the body of the uterus will result in successful delivery.

When the placenta has been retained for 12 or more hours, intrauterine injection of nitrofurazone (Utonex) is indicated for the control of early metritis. An elevation of body temperature will suggest the need for systemic antibody therapy.

If attempts to deliver a placenta through the vagina fail, laparotomy and surgical removal should be considered. When evidence of uterine wall necrosis is noted, a hysterectomy should be performed.

Subinvolution of the Uterus

Involution of the canine uterus following parturition proceeds as a gradual process of reconstruction of the endometrial layer. Failure of the uterus to undergo normal reduction in size and a delay in the regression of the endometrium are inherent in subinvolution.

Subinvolution of the uterus occurs when postparturient uterine contraction is incomplete and placental fluids and debris are retained in the uterine cavity. The cause is unknown; however, a degree of uterine inertia or muscle fatigue must be considered as etiological factors. Subinvolution usually involves both horns, but unilateral or segmented subinvolution, or both, have been observed.

Uterine subinvolution is unlikely to be a serious hazard to the bitch. Rather, it is the puppies who suffer as a result of absorption of products resulting from protein breakdown. A current hypothesis is that serum, blood, placental fluids and placental debris are retained in the uterus and as a consequence are subjected to temperatures consistent with the normal rectal temperature of the bitch. Incubation of such material at temperatures of 38.3°C for extended periods, i.e., greater than 72 hours, will result in protein breakdown and the formation of materials that, when absorbed through the exposed placental attachment sites and ultimately excreted via the milk, will create characteristic disease in nursing puppies.

Nursing puppies having a history of restlessness, crying and bloating and sometimes showing edematous red rectums suggest the presence of subinvolution of the uterus or metritis in the bitch. In the event of subinvolution, the physical examination of the bitch will reveal an active, alert, anxious female with normal rectal temperature, good appetite and a normal red discharge from the vulva. Abnormal involution is detected by abdominal palpation of the uterus. The attending clinician may note generalized failure of the uterus to involute completely or may find one horn or a segment of a horn with a larger diameter than is anticipated for normal involution. The consistency of the enlarged segment is dependent on the quantity of fluids in the affected portion.

Subinvolution of placental sites is described by Glenn.[4] He suggested that persistence of trophoblastic cells in the placental sites precludes normal involution. Rupture of the uterine wall may result in fatal peritonitis. Experience would suggest this to be a rare event. Clinicians should distinguish between subinvolution of placental sites (to be discussed) and subinvolution of the uterus.

Treatment is directed toward emptying the uterine cavity, restoring uterine tone and preventing potential metritis. Puppies are removed from the bitch for a 24-hour period. Treatment consists of instilling 5 to 10 ml of Utonex into the uterus via an insemination tube inserted through the vagina and cervix. Oral medication with 0.1 to 0.2 mg of ergonovine and appropriate doses of systemic antibiotics is recommended. Medication is continued for 7 to 10 days. Twenty-four hours after initiation of therapy the puppies can return to nursing.

Subsequent fertility is not affected and with appropriate adjustment in nutrition and management, i.e., high quality, balanced nutritional programs and adequate exercise, one can anticipate uneventful postparturient involution in subsequent breedings.

Metritis

Acute metritis, or uterine infection, is most likely to occur within the first week following parturition or abortion. A variety of organisms have been incriminated; i.e., hemolytic staphylococci, *Streptococcus, Proteus, Escherichia coli, Hemophilus* spp. and *Corynebacterium.* A retained fetus or placenta, introduction of infection by contaminated instruments or manipulation, unsanitary surroundings, traumatized tissue and a degree of uterine inertia all contribute to the development of metritis.

Infection is accompanied by depression, anorexia and toxemia. Affected bitches show elevated temperatures ranging from 39.4 to 40.5°C and rapid pulse rates. Milk flow is diminished and the bitch has little interest in her puppies. Puppies are frequently restless and cry intermittently. Growth rates decrease markedly and the puppies may develop red edematous rectums. The vaginal discharge is thin, sometimes fetid and red in color (except when retention of the placenta has occurred, in which case the discharge is green to black in color). The mucous membranes are congested and suggestive of toxemia. The bitch may strain and, unless severely depressed, will repeatedly lick the vulva. Laboratory examination variously demonstrates leukopenia or leukocytosis. Elevated leukocyte counts will be accompanied by a shift to the left.

The combination of early recognition and prompt treatment is usually effective. Patients in which signs of toxemia are well advanced are difficult to treat. The danger of uterine rupture and peritonitis must be kept in mind. The attending veterinarian should evaluate uterine tone. A flaccid uterus may respond to estrogen, calcium and either oxytocin (Pitocin) or ergonovine. Oxytocin (10 to 20 units) may be effective in ridding the uterus of fluid and debris, especially in those bitches affected shortly after parturition. Ergonovine, 0.2 mg t.i.d. for 2 or 3 days is a more consistent and prolonged ecbolic than is oxytocin. Intrauterine instillation of antibacterial/estrogen combinations (5 to 20 ml Utonex) will be useful. Appropriate systemic antibiotic therapy should be instituted to control current or potential septicemia as well as the localized infection. Antibiotic therapy should be extended a minimum of 3 days after the temperature returns to normal to assure greatest potential for subsequent breeding. Antihistamines may be used to reduce the impact of histamine release from the site of infection. Fluid therapy is indicated to combat or to prevent dehydration and to maintain effective renal function. Five per cent glucose, combined with the electrolytes, helps prevent serious damage to the liver, as the body strives to detoxify the variety of toxins generated by the bacteria and by the incubation process involving the protein components of uterine fluid and debris.

The course of the disease is usually short, ranging from 3 to 5 days. Improvement is indicated by reduction in elevated temperature, return of appetite, changing character of the discharge, drop in pulse rate and general improvement in attitude and appearance.

The potential for subsequent breeding will correlate with early recognition, prompt treatment and rapid response.

Postparturient Hemorrhage

Subinvolution of the placental sites is characterized by prolonged spotting of the bedding or kennel floor with blood following parturition. Certain kennels and certain families of dogs seem to be at higher than average risk. One might speculate that continued trophoblastic activity or failure of the healing process at the placental attachment site constitutes the basic lesion. Kirk *et al.*[5] have suggested a hormonal cause. Schall *et al.*[7] describe the lesion as large eosinophilic tissue masses protruding from the endometrium into the uterine lumen, accompanied by foci of hemorrhage. Enlarged vacuolated superficial endometrial cells, accumulation of lymphocytes and plasma cells were noted on microscopic examination. Arbeiter[1] noted uterine hyperemia, dilatation of blood vessels, cellular infiltration between myometrium and endometrium and necrosis of vessel walls with hyalinization and destruction of muscle fibers.

The vulva appears normal for the postparturient time period. Examination of the vaginal mucosa reveals healthy, normal consistency and appearance of the epithelium. A serosanguineous discharge with blood clots may be noted. Affected bitches appear unconcerned and puppies remain in good health. Palpation may reveal multiple, discrete, firm, spheroid enlargements spaced along the length of the uterus.

Periodic spotting will occur for 12 to 15 weeks postpartum.

When presented with a bitch with characteristic history and physical findings owned by a concerned breeder, the attending veterinarian should suggest continual monitoring of appetite and activity. As long as the patient continues to eat well and act normally, the owner can assume eventual recovery, and the veterinarian can reasonably reassure the owner that complete recovery is anticipated prior to subsequent seasons. The mild postparturient hemorrhage is usually noted when the bitch has been lying in one place for a period of time. As a general rule, treatment with ergonovine, calcium and intrauterine antibacterial agents is of little value. Arbeiter[1] has reported good results using medroxyprogesterone acetate, 2 mg/kg of body weight. There was rapid improvement, with the hemorrhage subsiding in 24 to 48 hours.

Postparturient hemorrhage may also occur following trauma of the uterine mucosa during parturition or when a cesarean section is performed prematurely and the placentae are forcibly removed. In such events, the administration of oxytocin or ergonovine to contract the uterus will effectively control hemorrhage. Continued hemorrhage, despite such treatment, should lead to consideration of deficits of calcium or of the clotting mechanism and to the need for possible hysterectomy.

PROBLEMS OF LACTATION

The quality of lactation of any bitch is based on genetic potential, current health and the nutritional program, both past and present. Lactation is a stress period, which should be considered during nutritional counseling.

When selecting a brood bitch, one should consider the reproductive history of the immediate ancestors. Milk quality and quantity can be enhanced by careful selection of brood stock.

The preparation for lactation begins prior to breeding. The overall health status and condition of the bitch must be considered, together with a well-managed breeding program. Appropriate energy intake, protein quality and vitamin B complex are important for adequate milk production.

A high-protein, high-caloric diet is recommended for bitches during pregnancy and lactation. The total caloric intake should be increased slowly, starting with the beginning of the last third of pregnancy. A 20 to 30 per cent increase in food intake over maintenance requirements during the last 3 weeks of gestation is followed by another 25 per cent increase per week during the first few weeks of lactation. The percentage increase will vary, depending on litter size and the activity of the lactating female.

A lack of caloric density will adversely affect milk production, puppy health and maintenance of optimum health and/or condition of the bitch.

Among the more common problems of lactation that adversely affect the bitch are agalactia, mammary congestion and mastitis.

Agalactia

Proper selection of breeding animals, a program of balanced nutrition and good health in the bitch all preclude the development of agalactia. The most common occurrence involves a poorly nourished bitch, stressed by gestation and compromised by infection. When infection exists, treatment must be promptly instituted using appropriate antibiotics, fluids and supportive therapy.

Agalactia, or failure of milk flow following parturition, can result from either the lack of milk production in the mammary gland or the failure of milk letdown. The failure of mammary development prior to whelping is generally conceded as the first indication of agalactia. The cause involves hormonal deficiency or defective secretory tissue in the mammary glands.

While estrogen activates the development of the ducts and progesterone affects development of the alveoli, their effect in the bitch is less significant than in the ruminant.

Prolactin and the growth hormone are more important and are responsible for initiation of lactation and maintenance of secretory levels, respectively. Inhibition of prolactin secretion results in a demonstrable reduction of milk production. Estrogen levels associated with parturition activate the lactogenic activity of the anterior pituitary gland. Integrity of the pituitary gland is essential for normal milk secretion. Certain proteins are more potent in supporting milk production. The protein in liver is more effective than that in egg or round steak. The act of nursing stimulates sensory nerve endings in the teat and serves as a stimulant to milk letdown and milk production. Anesthetics and tranquilizers may alter the normal response and result in temporary agalactia. If mammary gland development exists and milk letdown has not occurred, the administration of oxytocin will evoke contraction of the myoepithelial cells and forcible expression of milk into the larger ducts and teat canals.

If mammary gland development is lacking, treatment is generally not effective. Certain bitches are extremely nervous and refuse to settle down sufficiently to care for their puppies. The administration of progesterone, 0.1 mg/lb of body weight, may have a quieting effect, and subsequent nursing by the puppies will enhance milk flow.

For bitches in which milk production is marginal, the puppies should be allowed to nurse, the diet should be reviewed and the physiological parameters of good health monitored. Treatment is limited to specific therapy for demonstrated abnormalities, adequate diet and allowance of time.

Mammary Congestion (Galactostasis)

Edema and swelling of the mammary glands are sometimes noted prior to parturition; however, these usually occur a few hours to 3 days following parturition.

Galactostasis is most common in heavy milking bitches on a high level of nutrition. Affected bitches are uncomfortable and sometimes anorectic. Palpation reveals grossly enlarged, firm mammary glands, with teats that are difficult to grasp. The glandular tissue appears engorged and the mammae are warm to the touch. Milk may drop from some of the glands.

Treatment consists of withholding food and the systemic administration of diuretics. Milking those glands that are grossly distended will give temporary relief. The judicious application of hot packs or whirlpool treatment can be combined with massage to reduce the more severe congestion. Failure to relieve galactostasis may result in subsequent lactation failure of the affected glands. Careful monitoring is indicated to avoid delayed detection of infection.

Mastitis

Mastitis is an inflammation of one or more of the mammary glands. Its course may be either acute or chronic, depending on the previous history and the status of the glands at the time of infection. Acute mastitis is most frequently noted in bitches housed in questionable sanitary surroundings during hot humid weather that have recently whelped and have considerable congestion of the glands.

A variety of organisms have been incriminated, the most common being *Staphylococcus, Streptococcus* and *E. coli.*[9] The contributions of trauma and mammary congestion are a matter of conjecture, but these too are generally thought to be involved. Metritis may serve as a source or as a coincidental infection. Early signs are swelling and erythema of the affected gland. The gland becomes hot, painful and discolored. Anorexia, listlessness, elevated temperature and considerable pain or discomfort are usually noted. Affected bitches loose interest in their puppies. Puppies are restless, cry frequently and appear bloated.

The consistency of the milk gradually becomes thicker, and the color changes to yellow, pink or brown, depending on the amount of blood and the degree of purulence present. Cytological examination will reveal many leukocytes and red blood cells. Aseptically collected milk samples should be cultured and antibiotic sensitivity tests performed.

Treatment is directed toward overcoming the infection. Systemic antibacterial agents are effective in treating early mastitis. If the infection becomes localized, the resulting abscess should be lanced and drainage established. Local infiltration of the mammary gland with penicillin or penicillin and streptomycin is sometimes useful in preventing abscessation. Puppies should be prevented from nursing from affected glands by the use of bandages and tape. When the milk is not frankly purulent, the puppies may be allowed to continue to nurse. If several glands are affected or if the condition is severe, it may be appropriate to remove the puppies to an incubator and to treat them as orphans. The affected gland should be periodically milked out during the day. Penicillin at 24-hour intervals, penicillin/streptomycin at 12-hour intervals or kanamycin at 12-hour intervals for at least 5 days is usually effective.

Cold packs are useful during the early stages of congestion and infection, and hot packs are generally indicated once the inflammation is well established. Hot packs will hasten localization and give relief from swelling and pain.

There is a tendency for mastitis to recur during later lactation periods in a once-affected bitch. Recurrence in individual lines or strains within a given breed suggests a hereditary tendency toward the disease.

PUERPERAL TETANY

Puerperal tetany in the bitch is a metabolic disease characterized by hypocalcemia. While puerperal tetany may occur as either a preparturient or a postparturient episode, it is most commonly seen in heavy lactating bitches 2 to 4 weeks after parturition. Serum calcium levels are generally 8 mg per 100 ml or less and in severe cases range from 6 to 7 mg per 100 ml. Studies have indicated a relationship between the hormonal influences and hypoglycemia, acetonemia and cholesteremia in this disease.[8] Affected animals exhibit neurological signs beginning with an aura of slight disorientation, nervousness, apprehension, occasional whining and rapid breathing. Muscle tremors followed by spasms may render the animal unable to walk. The gait is stilted and sometimes erratic, and the legs are stiff. Intermittent twitching followed by short intervals of relaxation become progressively more severe until generalized convulsions of short duration are sometimes noted.

Most eclamptic bitches have temperature elevations (as high as 41.6°C) during the spastic period. The inability to rise is accompanied by labored respirations; a hard, rapid pulse; congested mucous membranes and excessive salivation. The neck and legs become extended and generalized stiffness is apparent. The patient may fall forward or to one side. Affected muscles exhibit fine fibrillary twitchings or contractions.

Treatment is generally instituted by the intravenous administration of 10 per cent calcium gluconate (5 to 15 ml). The injection should be given slowly, since emesis is likely to occur following rapid injection. Sodium pentobarbital may be used to control seizures or serious spasticity. Response to treatment is usually rapid and complete. In those animals in which the response is less than complete, one should administer glucose intravenously and should consider the use of sodium bicarbonate. Hypoglycemia and acidosis are occasional complicating metabolic deviations. If acidosis is apparent, the oral administration of sodium bicarbonate for 3 to 5 days following initial parenteral injection is beneficial. Since systemic alkalosis associated with hyperventilation may cause a decrease in ionic calcium in the blood, one should ascertain that systemic acidosis does indeed exist prior to instituting sodium bicarbonate therapy.

It is a common practice to prescribe a calcium supplement following initial therapy. Dicalcium phosphate, 0.5 gm/7 lb of body weight and a review of the diet to assure appropriate mineral balance are indicated. A determination of the levels of calcium, phosphorus, protein and fat plus a review of the sources of food ingredients may suggest the need for nutritional counseling.

Bardens[3] has recommended the use of prednisolone to prevent recurrences. The recommended dose rate is 0.5 mg/5 pounds of body weight daily for the remainder of the lactation period. Preliminary results would indicate that dexamethasone is not an effective substitute for prednisolone in the prevention of recurring puerperal tetany. The character of the discharge and the general well-being of the bitch must be monitored to avoid overlooking metritis/or toxemia or both.

The decision to allow continued nursing is dependent on the age of the puppies, the feasibility of the owner's caring for the puppies and the initial response of the bitch to therapy. When the response appears delayed or the bitch in poor condition, the decision to cease allowing the puppies to nurse should be considered.

A history of puerperal tetany in a bitch with a previous litter should command careful examination of the diet. Adequate calcium, vitamin D, trace minerals and a balanced diet should be recommended. Bitches with a history of puerperal tetany are best scheduled on a diet of high caloric density during lactation.

REFERENCES

1. Arbeiter, K.: The use of progestins in the treatment of persistent uterine hemorrhage in the post partum bitch and cow: A clinical report. Theriogenology, 4:11, 1975.
2. Arthur, G. H.: Wrights Veterinary Obstetrics. Baltimore, The Williams & Wilkins Co. 1964, p. 345.
3. Bardens, J.: Sterility in the bitch. In Kirk, R. W. (ed.): Current Veterinary Therapy II. Philadelphia, W. B. Saunders Co., 1966, pp. 681–682.
4. Glenn, B. L.: Subinvolution of placental sites in the bitch. Guelph, Ontario, Gaines Vet. Symp., October 9, 1968.
5. Kirk, R. W., McEntee, K. and Bentinck-Smith, J.: Disease of the urogenital system. In Catcott, E. J. (ed.): Canine Medicine. Wheaton, Ill., Am. Vet. Publications, 1968, p. 404.
6. Roberts, S. J.: Veterinary Obstetrics and Genital Diseases. Published by the author, Ithaca, N.Y., 1954, p. 234. Distributed by Edwards Bio. Inc., Ann Arbor, Mi.
7. Schall, W. D., Duncan, J. R., Finco, D. R. et al.: Spontaneous recovery after subinvolution of placental sites in a bitch. J.A.V.M.A., 159:1780, 1971.
8. Toivola, B. E. and Mather, G. W.: Puerperal Tetany of the Bitch. Norden News, Winter, 1968.
9. Trainor, E.: Mastitis. In Kirk, R. W. (eds.): Current Therapy II. Philadelphia, W. B. Saunders Co., 1966, pp. 673–674.

Genital Emergencies

THOMAS P. GREINER AND GREGORY M. ZOLTON

Animal Medical Center, New York, New York

Diseases of the genital tract included in this article are emergency conditions and thus require immediate care to insure best results.

MALE GENITAL SYSTEM

Paraphimosis

Paraphimosis is a condition that occurs when the penis protrudes from the preputial cavity and cannot be replaced in its normal position. A moderate degree of phimosis may be associated with or may be an inciting factor in its occurrence. Paraphimosis is most frequently observed after coitus, although there are other causes. It is assumed that the penis is protruded in the semi-erect state and remains engorged because of constriction by the prepuce behind the bulbus glandis. The inability to retract the penis leads to further congestion and engorgement, complicated by the dog's licking of the penis, thereby creating more trauma. If the condition is left untreated, urethral obstruction, necrosis and gangrene may occur. Other causes that have been observed are strangulation from rubber bands or string wound around the penis, chronic balanoposthitis with resultant engorgement from trauma due to excessive licking, trauma to the penis, fracture of the os penis, lacerations of the penis and chronic priapism. A careful examination should always be conducted to establish the cause of the condition.

Treatment

Emergency treatment should be directed toward restoring the penis to the preputial cavity. The penis may be damaged in varying degrees, ranging from mild swelling and edema to gangrene and self mutilation. The extent of injury will also vary according to the length of time that the penis has remained outside of the sheath.

The animal should first be placed under a general anesthetic and the penis and prepuce cleansed gently with surgical soap. When swelling and edema are only moderate, a more conservative approach to treatment may be utilized. Application of a cold hyperosmolar solution of glucose (or table sugar) or a solution of urea may help to reduce swelling and edema. The penis should be well lubricated with an obstetrical lubricant and replaced in the preputial cavity by manipulating the prepuce over the penis.

If the penis cannot be replaced or has been severely traumatized, an incision in the prepuce may be necessary to replace the penis. An attempt should first be made to cleanse and debride any necrotic or gangrenous tissue. If lacerations are present, they should be sutured with 3–0 or 4–0 chromic catgut to control hemorrhage. Cleansing and removal of necrotic tissue may be facilitated by the use of a solution of boric acid and ammonium alum (Massengill powder). We prefer to make the incision on the prepuce on its ventral aspect. The incision should be just long enough to allow replacement of the penis. It should then be closed with two layers of sutures, one reuniting the mucosa and the other reuniting the skin. The anterior 0.5 to 1 cm of the incision may be closed by suturing the mucosa to skin on their respective sides, thereby creating a larger opening that may help to prevent recurrence of the condition.

If the penis appears unhealthy or if swelling does not disappear after a reasonable period of time, it is preferable to pass a large indwelling male urethral catheter into the bladder for 24 to 48 hours. The catheter can be held in place by suturing it to the prepuce. A loose purse-string suture may be placed around the preputial orifice to help prevent the penis from prolapsing until such time as the inflammation has subsided. Antibiotic-steroid ointments infused around the penis are of value in controlling inflammation and infection once the penis is replaced. Adhesions between the penis and prepuce may occur in severely traumatized cases. These can best be prevented by fully extruding the penis from the prepuce daily for 10 to 12 days after formation of the adhesions. Amputation of the penis may be required in the most severely traumatized cases.

Trauma to the Penis and Prepuce

Traumatic injuries of the penis and prepuce, such as contusions and lacerations, will often also require emergency treatment. Contusions may occur in the form of blunt trauma, as in an automobile accident, or from bite wounds, creating a crushing type of injury. Lacerations can result from many causes but most commonly occur as a result of bite wounds or of the dog jumping a fence. Lacerations of the penis will usually bleed profusely and will require some means of controlling hemorrhage.

Rupture of the penile urethra, although uncommon, may also occur. The principal clinical sign of a ruptured penile urethra is the result of extravasation of urine into the surrounding subcutaneous tissues. The area at which leakage occurs shows signs of a developing abscess or cellulitis, with progressive edema developing on the ventral abdominal wall. Severe trauma to the penis may also produce obstruction of the urinary passage as a result of swelling.

Treatment

Contusions of the penis and prepuce are best treated by gentle cleansing of the tissue, infusion of a topical antibiotic-steroid ointment into the prepuce and parenteral administration of antibiotics and steroids.

Lacerations of the penis will usually require suturing to control hemorrhage. Small puncture wounds need not be sutured if they are not hemorrhaging. Gentle cleansing, infusion of an antibiotic-steroid ointment into the prepuce and tranquilization are usually all that is required. Tranquilization will be of value in preventing excitement and erection, both of which may result in hemorrhage of the wound. The ointment will help prevent the formation of adhesions between the penis and prepuce, as well as help control infection. Larger lacerations will usually require sutures to control bleeding. If the wound is excessively large, an attempt should be made to isolate and ligate the bleeding vessels while the dog is under anesthesia. The cut edges of the tunica albuginea and mucosa should be debrided and sutured with 3–0 or 4–0 chromic catgut. The prepuce should be infused with an antibiotic-steroid ointment for 10 days to 2 weeks post-operatively to prevent formation of adhesions.

Puncture wounds of the prepuce should be drained by using a Penrose drain. The local application of hot compresses in addition to systemic antibiotic therapy should be used to help control infection. Larger lacerations of the prepuce can be sutured. One must take care not to interfere with the preputial orifice.

Rupture of the penile urethra is best managed by inserting a large urethral catheter into the bladder, preferably a Foley catheter if this can be inserted. If the trauma to the urethra is extensive, a urethrostomy posterior to the site of trauma may be indicated. It is also important to drain the subcutaneous tissue where urine has collected.

Trauma of the Scrotum and Testis

Scrotal skin is extremely sensitive to a myriad of chemical irritants. Any irritated or lacerated scrotal integument will cause excessive licking by the patient. This in turn will lead to further inflammation and infection. If not treated promptly, the patient will invariably mutilate the organ, necessitating castration or complete scrotal ablation. For minor chemical irritations or abrasions, a topical antibiotic–anti-inflammatory ointment should be applied three or four times daily. The use of tranquilizers and an Elizabethan collar of sufficient size will prevent further self-mutilation. Minor lacerations can be debrided and closed with fine (3–0 or 4–0) monofilament nonabsorbable sutures. If drainage of a traumatized scrotum must be established, it is best accomplished anterior to the scrotum with small (¼ inch) Penrose drains. Drainage through the scrotal integument may result in excessive inflammatory tissue and granulation. Severe injuries to the testis may require either unilateral or bilateral castration with subsequent drainage of the scrotum or complete scrotal ablation.

Testicular Torsions

Torsion of a retained testicle is a rare entity but does require immediate surgery. The vast majority of torsed testicles are abdominal rather than inguinal. Patients with this disorder will most commonly present with severe abdominal discomfort, the absence of one or both testicles in the scrotum and extreme pain upon abdominal palpation of the involved testicle. A diagnosis is made by physical examination and confirmation of a posterior abdominal mass on radiographs. In some cases a final diagnosis must await an exploratory laparotomy. Upon entering the abdominal cavity, the torsed testicle will appear swollen and very congested or hemorrhagic. Surgical extirpation of such a testicle will alleviate all symptoms. These testicles should always be biopsied because a small percentage may be neoplastic.

Trauma of the Prostate Gland

Prostatic trauma may occur as a result of any blunt trauma to the posterior abdomen or pelvis. Although such trauma is rare, a prostatic abscess or suppurative prostatitis may present as an acute problem if ruptured. Such animals present with an acute abdomen and clinical signs of peritonitis and sepsis, including collapse, dehydration, anuria and possibly coma. The most commonly cultured organisms from prostatic abscesses are *Escherichia coli, Proteus* spp., *Pseudomonas* spp. and occasionally streptococci and staphylococci. These extremely virulent organisms can easily cause an acute abdomen, sepsis, shock and subsequent death if they enter the abdomen through a ruptured abscess. This requires immediate surgical intervention. Since these patients would seldom survive a prolonged procedure such as a prostatectomy, surgical drainage must be performed rapidly and efficiently.

Treatment

Immediate steps should be undertaken to rehydrate the patient, replacing fluid and electrolyte deficits and assuring adequate urine output at surgery. Correct choice of anesthesia is very important in these situations. We prefer to premedicate our patients with atropine sulfate (0.01 mg/lb) and acetylpromazine (1 mg/20 lb) given intravenously or intramuscularly. Anesthesia is induced via a short-acting barbiturate (sodium thiamylal, 4 to 9 mg/lb to effect) and maintained after intubation with nitrous oxide, oxygen and minimal flow of fluothane.

Upon entering the abdominal cavity a sample of fluid for culture and sensitivity should be obtained. A thorough lavage is begun with a warm physiological solution to rid the peritoneal cavity of gross contamination. The prostate gland should now be isolated. If a large abscessed cyst is ruptured, it may be resected if pedunculated or marsupialized if broad-based. If diffuse prostatic suppuration is encountered, local drainage techniques must be applied. This is best accomplished by isolating and packing off the gland with laparotomy towels. A digit should be introduced into the prostate through the rupture site to break down all fibrous cavities, producing one large cavitated prostate. This is now copiously flushed with a warm, sterile saline-antibiotic solution (such as saline/Biosol or a saline and 10 per cent Betadine solution). A second prostatic incision is made opposite the rupture site to provide a "through and through" pathway for drainage. Three ½-inch Penrose drains are placed through the prostate gland. One tip of all three drains is sutured with a single suture of 4–0 chromic catgut to the prostatic parenchyma. This prevents internal movement of drains. The drains are now exteriorized lateral to the laparotomy incision and sutured to the skin. A thorough lavage of the abdominal cavity is repeated, and a second set of ½-inch Penrose drains (three to six in number) is used to drain the periprostatic area as well as the rest of the abdominal cavity. This second set of drains should be exteriorized through the abdominal wall via a third incision and opposite the incision for the prostatic drains. This technique facilitates pulling the prostatic drains 24 to 72 hours before the abdominal drains. Castration should always be performed at this time.

Drains are removed in 5 to 10 days postoperatively. The patient's hydration, electrolytes and urinary output must be monitored closely. Maximum doses of a broad-spectrum antibiotic (such as chloramphenicol [Chloromycetin] 20/mg/lb q.i.d.) must be maintained throughout the hospitalization and the recuperative periods of 2 to 3 weeks postsurgery.

A septic insult such as a ruptured prostatic abscess will usually cause coma and death within 6 to 12 hours. If the patient survives the first 24 to 36 hours postsurgically, a favorable prognosis may be expected.

FEMALE GENITAL SYSTEM

Uterine Prolapse

This is a rare condition seen primarily in the postpartum female. At that time, the cervix is dilated and with sufficient straining, a uterine prolapse may occur. The uterus may prolapse to any degree from a mild cervical prolapse to protrusion of one or even both uterine horns.

Mild, early prolapses with healthy viable tissues may be reduced with minimal manipulation and sedation. If edema and venous congestion are present, a 50 per cent dextrose solution or a 20 per cent mannitol solution may be applied to decrease swellings and precipitate reduction.

Prolapses must always be examined closely for necrosis, self-mutilation, ruptures of uterine vessels or neoplasia. If such conditions are present or reduction even under a general anesthetic cannot be achieved, a laparotomy should be performed. If the uterus cannot be salvaged, an ovariohysterectomy is recommended. If reduction is attained and the uterus is viable and breeding is desired, the uterus should be instilled with crystalline penicillin and posterior pituitary extract should be injected intramuscularly to aid in uterine involution.

Vaginal Hyperplasia and Prolapse

Estrual hypertrophy and/or congestion of vaginal mucosa occurs in all females during estrus to one degree or another. If, however, it becomes excessive and prolonged, a vaginal prolapse may occur. Since such mucosal changes occur more so in the vagina than in the vulva, an eversion of the vaginal vault can be seen. These prolapses are usually minimal, and the majority will regress by metestrus if kept moist and clean and viable with an ointment such as a topical antibiotic-steroid preparation.

If the prolapse is nonviable, dry or necrotic or has undergone mutilation, surgical intervention is necessary. A thorough examination and cleansing should be performed to identify the extent of the prolapse as well as to rule out a prolapsed vaginal leiomyosarcoma. We routinely recommend an ovariohysterectomy if breeding is not to be considered.

If the animal is to be used for future breeding and a resection is undertaken, the owners should be made aware of the fact that even after resection, future prolapses may occur.

The most common complication with resection of vaginal prolapses is the surgeon's failure to identify, via catheterization, the urethra. Episiotomies are useful in exposing the base of the prolapse where resection will take place as well as identifying the urethral orifice. Bleeding is controlled via suturing and electrocautery.

COITAL INJURIES (MALE AND FEMALE)

Injuries sustained to the genital mucosa of the male or female during intercourse should be considered emergencies. Such injuries should be well cleansed, hemostasis attained (either by sutures or ligatures) and the wound primarily closed with fine absorbable suture material (such as 3–0 or 4–0 chromic gut). Appropriate topical and/or systemic antibiotics should be instituted.

REFERENCES

1. DeHoff, W. D., Greene, R. W., and Greiner, T. P.: Surgical management of abdominal emergencies. Vet. Clin. N. Am., *2*:141, 1972.
2. Goodger, W. J. and Levy, W.: Anesthetic management of the cesarean section. Vet. Clin. N. Am., *3*:85, 1973.
3. Johnston, D. E.: Male genital system. *In* Archibald, J. (ed.): Canine Surgery. 1st Archibald Ed. Wheaton, Ill., Am. Vet. Publications, 1965, pp. 611–640.
4. Osborne, C. A., Low, D. G., and Finco, D. R.: Canine and Feline Urology. Philadelphia, W. B. Saunders Co., 1972, pp. 249–253.
5. Smith, K. W.: Female Genital Tract. *In* Archibald, J. (ed.): Canine Surgery. 1st Archibald Ed. Wheaton, Ill., Am. Vet. Publications, 1965, pp. 641–676.

Induction of Estrus in the Bitch

LAWRENCE E. EVANS
Iowa State University, Ames, Iowa

Induction of estrus in the bitch may be utilized in several ways. In the research laboratory it is often desirable to breed a number of bitches to whelp at the same time. This is also an effective tool for teaching canine reproduction. With induced estrus, a particular mating or pregnancy may be timed for the convenience of the private owner. Induction may be used in the treatment of prolonged anestrus or incomplete estrus in the bitch. Because of the variable causes of anestrus, including heritable factors, it is desirable to investigate such cases fully before reproduction is encouraged.

The pituitary and placental gonadotropins have been used in various combinations to induce estrus in the bitch. Placental gonadotropins have a considerably longer half-life and are therefore more desirable; however, they have become increasingly more difficult to obtain commercially in the United States. The following treatment schedules have been shown to be relatively effective for estrus induction.

Treatment I. Pregnant mare serum gonadotropin (PMSG) and human chorionic gonadotropin (HCG) are given as separate subcutaneous injections on the same day (Table 1).

TABLE 1. *Treatment I. Administration of Pregnant Mare Serum Gonadotropin (PMSG) and Human Chorionic Gonadotropin (HCG)*

	Weight of Dog (kg)		
	5–10	10–25	≥25
PMSG	200–300 IU	300–500 IU	600 IU
HCG	100–150 IU	150–250 IU	300 IU

TABLE 2. *Treatment II: Administration of Sheep Pituitary Gonadotropin*

	Weight of Dog (kg)		
	5–10	10–25	≥25
Day 1	1 ml	1–2 ml	2 ml
Day 4	1 ml	2 ml	2 ml

Treatment II. Sheep pituitary gonadotropin, Vetrophin, which contains the equivalent of 1 mg of follicle-stimulating hormone (FSH) and 1 mg of luteinizing hormone (LH) per ml, may be administered subcutaneously or intramuscularly. Cattle or swine pituitary preparations are similar to sheep preparations in gonadotropin content (Table 2).

Treatment III. Equine pituitary gonadotropin, Pitropin, contains 25 Fevold-Hisaw rat units per ml. It may be administered subcutaneously or intramuscularly. Equine pituitary extracts have lower LH content than sheep or swine extracts and should be supplemented with HCG (Table 3).

Vulvar swelling and a hemorrhagic discharge usually will occur in 4 to 5 days after treatment. A second treatment may be repeated at 5 to 7 days if proestrus has not occurred. Once initiated the estrous cycle should proceed normally. However, the proestrous period is often shortened, with acceptance of the male beginning about 10 days after treatment.

Estrus can be induced during any phase of the estrous cycle, but fertility should be expected only if induction and matings occur approximately 4 months or more after the previous estrus. Animals treated during early diestrus often develop cystic follicles, presumably because existing progesterone levels block LH release from the pituitary. Approximately 85 per cent of the normal dogs induced at the proper time and 65 per cent of the animals with prolonged anestrus will show a good standing estrus after treatment. Normal conception rates and litter sizes can be expected in the mated bitches.

Animals in deeper stages of anestrus (prolonged anestrus or during hot summer months) require increased dosages or longer periods of therapy for induction. Primer doses of PMSG or pituitary gonadotropins at the recommended levels just listed may be given 3 to 4 days prior to treatment. Previous studies have indicated that excessive dosage levels of therapy may produce multiple follicular development in some dogs or a refractory stage in others, in which the ovaries fail to develop follicles. Care should be taken not to overtreat individual animals.

Repeated therapy with gonadotropins, particularly those of placental origin, should not be extended beyond 2 weeks because of the possibility of immune response to the drug. Immune response will render the drugs less effective and will enhance the possibility of anaphylactic reaction. Studies in the bitch have not been done to indicate when a second regimen of therapy would be effective and safe, but gonadotropin immune studies in the male dog suggest that 6 months would be a safe interval. The animal's owner should be advised of the dangers of anaphylactic reaction with these drugs.

TABLE 3. *Treatment III: Administration of Equine Pituitary Gonadotropin*

	Weight of Dog (kg)		
	5–10	10–25	≥25
Day 1	0.5–1 ml	1 ml	2 ml
Day 4	1 ml + 100 IU HCG	2 ml + 200 IU HCG	2 ml + 200 IU HCG

REFERENCES

1. Faulkner, L. C.: An immunological approach to population control in dogs. J.A.V.M.A., *166*:479, 1973.
2. Nett, T. M., Akbar, A. M., Phemister, R. D., Holst, P. A., Reichert, L. E., Jr. and Niswender, G. D.: Levels of luteinizing hormone, estradiol and progesterone in serum during the estrous cycle and pregnancy in the beagle bitch. Proc. Soc. Exp. Biol. Med., *148*:134, 1975.
3. Wright, P. J.: Studies of the response of the ovaries of bitches to PMS and HCG. Proceedings VII International Congress Animal Reproduction AI. Munich, 1972.

Abnormal Estrous Activity

ROBERT D. PHEMISTER

Colorado State University,
Fort Collins, Colorado

PUBERTY

Normal Puberty

Puberty in the bitch is defined by the first estrous period. Ovulation occurs at this time and the bitch is fertile, although generally not capable of producing as many young as later in life when full sexual maturity is reached. Puberty in the female represents the onset of cyclic reproductive function and is preceded by months of follicular growth and atresia. It has been estimated that in the bitch half of the follicles present at birth have been lost by the time of puberty. As puberty is reached, some follicles, presumably responding to increasing follicle-stimulating hormone (FSH) secretion, become enlarged and the associated estrogen secretion leads to signs of proestrus and estrus and to ovulation.

The age of puberty varies greatly within and among breeds. Most summary-type articles give a range of 6 to 12 months of age, but the relatively few published reports of original data suggest that the normal range extends to about 24 months in most breeds. Free-roaming bitches reportedly experience their first estrus earlier than confined animals, but this conclusion does not seem to be based on any systematic study. Puberty tends to appear earlier in small breeds compared with larger breeds of dogs. This is consistent with the relationship between growth, attainment of adult size and the onset of puberty in other species. When puberty occurs early, before a bitch is fully grown, breeding is followed by a greater likelihood of difficulty at parturition. Accordingly, it seems wisest to avoid breeding bitches during their first estrus unless this occurs after growth is complete.

Some bitches approaching puberty may exhibit episodes of false proestrus. These episodes are characterized by slight palpable enlargement and increased turgidity of the vulva and a slight sanguineous vulvar discharge. The bitch may attract but will not accept the male at this time. These signs usually subside after a few days but can recur sporadically over several weeks and are eventually followed by normal proestrus and estrus.

Delayed Puberty

Puberty and the establishment of a cyclic pattern of reproductive function are primarily endocrine-controlled phenomena but can be modified by the external environment and by genetic factors. Nutrition may be a factor influencing the onset of puberty in the bitch. In some species a high plane of nutrition hastens and a low plane or specific nutritional deficiency delays puberty. Specific studies apparently have not been reported for the bitch. It is known, however, that age at first estrus is genetically controlled and can be modified by inbreeding.

Occasionally a healthy young bitch in good physical condition will reach 2 years of age without having been observed in estrus. The ovaries in such animals typically are smaller than normal and lack evidence of follicular development. The incidence of this condition is not known but is probably quite low. In a group of 758 beagle bitches that we observed from birth to 30 months of age, all but two experienced at least one estrus during this period. Hormonal treatment has usually proved unsuccessful.

ABBREVIATED OR PROLONGED ESTRUS

When considering abnormalities of the estrous period, it is important to know the range of normality and to understand the relationship between endocrine and behavioral events and ovulation. Most bitches are in proestrus for 7 to 10 days and in estrus for 7 to 10 days, a combined time of 2 to 3 weeks. At the extremes, an individual bitch may complete both proestrus and estrus in less than 1 week or extend as long as 5 to 6 weeks.

Much of the variability can probably be explained by the fact that the physical and behavioral signs that characterize proestrus and estrus are imprecise indicators of hormonal and ovarian function. Follicular development prior to ovulation in the bitch normally requires about 2 weeks. It is accompanied by estrogen secretion, which produces marked changes in the genital tract and alters the bitch's behavior. The interval between hormone secretion and observable effect, the rate at which these changes occur and their intensity and duration are all variable and subject to misinterpretation.

From a breeding standpoint, what is important is the time of ovulation. Estrus can be defined as the first day that the female accepts the male. The vast majority of bitches ovulate early in estrus, usually by the fourth day. However, exceptional animals have been reported to ovulate as early as 2 days before the estimated onset of estrus or as late as 7 days after the onset.

Successful breedings of bitches with widely differing estrous periods can be achieved by considering the following: (1) ovulation is normally completed within a few hours, (2) the ova require about 3 days after ovulation to mature in the oviduct before they are capable of being fertilized, (3) once mature, canine ova have a fertilizable life of about 24 hours and (4) canine spermatozoa can normally survive and function for at least 7 days in the female genital tract. Thus, a single mating at any time during the first week of a normal 7 to 10 day estrus is likely to be successful. It seems prudent to plan a mating at the first opportunity, since some bitches evidently ovulate prior to acceptance of the male and some allow breeding for only a few (1 to 3) days. A second mating should be planned about 4 or 5 days later to provide for bitches that ovulate late. A single, properly timed breeding achieves as high a conception rate and litter size as multiple breedings. The principal reason for breeding more than once is to assure proper timing between ova and spermatozoa.

Reproductive failure occasionally occurs because the clinical signs of proestrus and estrus are misinterpreted by the dog handler. A sanguineous genital discharge, interpreted as proestrus, may continue well into estrus, causing the owner to unduly delay having the bitch bred. Conversely, proestrus may be prolonged and followed eventually by a normal estrous period with ovulation. The cytological study of the vaginal smear usually provides a more accurate indication of the progression of hormonal and ovarian events than do outward clinical signs. In many bitches with unusually short or unusually long estrous periods, vaginal cytological and hormonal analysis reveals that the cycle is progressing normally, i.e., it is only the bitch's estrual behavior that is aberrant.

Some bitches display what has been termed a "split estrus." Typically in this condition estrus follows a normal period of proestrus but is interrupted by a few days during which the bitch will not accept the male. The initial period of acceptance is brief (1 to 2 days) and, based on vaginal cytology, is premature. Although the condition has not been studied extensively, follicular growth and ovulation apparently proceed normally. The condition does not appear to affect fertility.

Polyestrus has also been described in the bitch; however, it is rare. It is characterized by recurrent estrous periods separated by short intervals. The condition may persist for years. Matings during this time are usually infertile. A bitch after experiencing extended polyestrus will occasionally conceive, have a normal pregnancy and resume a normal estrous cycle. This suggests that gonadotropin therapy might be of benefit, but documented studies are not available.

Prolonged or continuous estrus is usually attributed to the presumed presence of multiple, bilateral, estrogen-secreting follicular cysts. Such cysts are common in older bitches, but their pathogenesis is not known. Affected bitches are sterile and because their behavior is considered objectionable, they are usually treated by ovariohysterectomy. If the cysts are limited to one ovary, unilateral ovariectomy may be curative and allow for subsequent pregnancy. Surgical rupture of the cysts following laparotomy usually fails to correct the condition. The daily intramuscular injection of chorionic gonadotropin in doses of 100 to 500 IU or more has been recommended but reportedly has not been particularly successful.

Luteinizing hormone (LH) is not invariably deficient in bitches that display protracted estrus. A bitch that was part of a study to determine hormone levels during the normal estrous cycle remained in estrus for 4 weeks. During this time her plasma levels of LH remained at values comparable with the normal ovulatory surge. The levels subsequently dropped and she went out of estrus, apparently without ovulating (progesterone levels did not become elevated). Constant estrual behavior is also occasionally seen in ovariohysterectomized bitches in which not all the ovarian tissue was removed and in bitches with metritis, vaginitis or vulvitis.

PROLONGED ANESTRUS

Since proestrus, estrus, metestrus and diestrus or pregnancy normally differ in total duration by less than about 3 weeks, it is the variable length of anestrus that accounts for the major differences observed in cycle length. The mean interestrous interval in young, healthy bitches is 7 to 8 months, but the range is considerable — from 3 to 14 months. The idea that small breeds have short cycles and large breeds have long cycles appears to be invalid. Two of the larger breeds studied, Labrador retrievers and German shepherd dogs, have among the shortest average interestrous intervals, 4.6 and 6.1 months, respectively. In general, breed differences are not significant. The interestrous interval observed for any given bitch is also variable. Some bitches cycle at a relatively constant interval while others may vary by 5 months or more in the lengths of their cycles.

Little information is available concerning the effect of advancing age on the estrous cycle. There is little change until about 8 years, at which time the cycles become progressively longer, regularly exceeding 12 or more months in length. While the bitch may continue to experience estrus and be fertile beyond 8 years, there is evidence that reproductive efficiency is greatest between 3 and 5 years and declines thereafter.

Prolongation of the anestrous period beyond about 15 months in a bitch that has cycled normally suggests a hormonal problem. Physical examination should be complete. Obese bitches sometimes remain in anestrus for extended periods. Correction of the obesity may lead to a resumption of normal cycling. Similarly, in cachectic bitches if the cause of the cachexia can be corrected and the normal condition restored, a return to estrus may occur. Anestrus has also been associated with hypothyroidism and with hyperadrenocorticism. If nutritional and other metabolic or systemic disease can be ruled out, the condition is likely to be the result of absent or insufficient pituitary gonadotropic stimulus.

Specific hormone therapy for inducing fertile estrus consists of giving FSH and LH in proper sequence. A number of preparations, dosages and schedules have been used, but it is difficult to determine how successful they have been. Most studies have failed to include mating or have failed to report the results of mating. A variety of FSH preparations given at least twice at intervals of 3 to 9 days have successfully stimulated follicular development and produced clinical signs of proestrus or estrus. Estrogen may be administered to enhance breeding receptivity when proestrus is fully established, but the dose should be small and the action brief, so as not to interfere with fertility. Administering LH-containing preparations to produce ovulation of the exogenously stimulated follicles has not been uniformly successful.

A modification of a previously described regimen[2] has proved successful in limited testing on *normal* anestrous bitches in our laboratory. Two or three injections of FSH (15 to 25 mg subcutaneously or intramuscularly) are given at weekly intervals. Signs of proestrus usually follow the second or third injection. One week after the onset of proestrus, estrogen may be administered intramuscularly (0.5 mg of estradiol) to enhance the bitch's estrual behavior. Two days later LH is injected (1 to 2 mg intravenously), and the bitch is bred after 24 hours and again 48 hours after the initial breeding. Bitches that fail to respond with signs of proestrus within 3 months are given LH (5 mg intravenously) and after 10 days the entire regimen is repeated.

REFERENCES

1. Andersen, A. C. and Simpson, M. E.: The ovary and reproductive cycle of the dog (beagle). Los Altos, Ca., Geron-X, 1973.
2. Bardens, J. W.: Hormonal therapy for ovarian and testicular dysfunction in the dog. J.A.V.M.A., *159*:1405, 1971.
3. Phemister, R. D.: Nonneurogenic reproductive failure in the bitch. Vet. Clin. N. Am., *4*:573, 1974.

False Pregnancy

SHIRLEY D. JOHNSTON
University of Minnesota, St. Paul, Minnesota

False pregnancy (also called pseudopregnancy or pseudocyesis) in the bitch is a physical and behavioral syndrome that may occur 2 to 3 months after estrus. At one time, false pregnancy was thought to be caused by a functional (i.e., progesterone-secreting) corpus luteum. It is now known that all bitches that ovulate produce functional corpora lutea and remain under progesterone influence for a variable 60 to 100 days. Serum concentrations of progesterone are similar in bitches that manifest signs of false pregnancy and in those that do not. Except for a sharp decline 1 to 2 days before parturition in pregnant bitches, progesterone levels are approximately the same in pregnant, nonpregnant, asymptomatic and false pregnant animals. The terms overt and covert pseudopregnancy have been used to describe nonpregnant bitches in the luteal phase, with and without clinical signs of false pregnancy. Future studies of pituitary hormones and of the magnitude of progesterone drop at the onset of false pregnancy may help clarify the pathogenesis of this condition.

The incidence of overt pseudopregnancy in the bitch is unknown. Reports in the literature place it as high as 50 to 75 per cent. Because many pet dogs are ovariohysterectomized, the true incidence in a susceptible population is not reflected by the number of clinical cases. Also, many breeders recognize the syndrome as a physiological event and do not present their animals for veterinary care.

In 59 cases of false pregnancy evaluated at the University of Minnesota Companion Animal Hospital (primarily a referral practice), no breed predisposition was observed; 28 breeds were represented. There was no age predilection; of the 59 cases, 6 were presented after their first estrus (at 7 to 11 months) and 14 bitches were over 7 years of age. Overt pseudopregnancy has also been observed 3 to 4 days after surgery in several bitches ovariohysterectomized during diestrus, in the luteal phase. This is not surprising, since lactation and nesting behavior occur when luteolysis and sharp progesterone decline occur in the pregnant bitch. The occurrence of false pregnancy is not influenced by previous pregnancies.

SIGNS

Mammary gland development, lactation and personality changes are the most commonly noticed signs. Lactation may persist for 2 weeks or longer and is encouraged by self-nursing or by the adoption of unrelated neonates. Personality changes include nesting, mothering activity, restlessness and irritability. A mucoid vaginal discharge is often present. Abdominal distention is common; the uterus may be palpably increased in length and diameter and shows endometrial hyperplasia on histological examination. Abdominal contractions that mimic those of parturition are observed in occasional bitches. Vomiting, diarrhea, polyuria, polydipsia, anorexia and polyphagia have all been reported.

DIAGNOSIS

The diagnosis is made on the basis of breeding history and physical examination. If the abdomen is difficult to palpate and the breeding history is uncertain, abdominal radiographs will rule out normal pregnancy after 42 days' gestation. If depression and abdominal distention are observed 2 to 3 months following estrus, closed cervix pyometra should be considered as a differential diagnosis; abdominal radiography and a complete blood count help distinguish these two conditions.

TREATMENT

In the absence of extreme discomfort, the pseudopregnant bitch should be treated supportively (i.e., care of mammary glands, light sedation if necessary) until she proceeds into anestrus. Hormonal therapy is usually unnecessary, although treatment with any of the sex steroids will cause remission of signs, mediated by a negative feedback inhibition effect on the hypothalamic-pituitary axis. Male steroids are preferred; testosterone at a dose of 1 to 2 mg/kg given once intramuscularly is effective. Mibo-lerone, an androgenic steroid, may soon be available as an oral preparation for treatment of false pregnancy. Megestrol acetate (2 mg/kg orally, once daily for 8 days) is also effective, although some bitches at our clinic have relapsed after megestrol acetate thera-py.

PREVENTION

Although there is evidence that this con-dition does not predispose to other reproduc-tive tract diseases, false pregnancy may recur with subsequent heats. Later fertility, however, is not affected. Ovariohysterec-tomy is the only known preventative meas-ure.

REFERENCES

1. Concannon, P. W., Hansel, W. and Visek, W. J.: The ovarian cycle of the bitch: Plasma estrogen, LH and progesterone. Biol. Reprod., *13*:112, 1975.
2. Fidler, I. J., Brodey, R. S. Howson, A. E. and Cohen, D.: Relationship of estrous irregularity, pseudo-pregnancy, and pregnancy to canine pyometra. J.A.V.M.A., *149*:1043, 1966.
3. Hadley, J. C.: Unconjugated oestrogen and proges-terone concentrations in the blood of bitches with false pregnancy and pyometra. Vet. Rec., *96*:545, 1975.
4. Nett, T. M., Akbar, A. M., Phemister, R. D., Holst, P. A., Reichert, L. E. Jr. and Niswender, G.: Levels of luteinizing hormone, estradiol and progesterone in serum during the estrous cycle and pregnancy in the beagle bitch. Proc. Soc. Exp. Biol. Med., *148*:134, 1975.

Cystic Endometrial Hyperplasia–Pyometra Complex

ROBERT M. HARDY
University of Minnesota, St. Paul, Minnesota

INTRODUCTION

Canine pyometra is a complex polysys-temic metestrual disease of the mature bitch. It is often associated with diverse clin-ical and pathological manifestations related to both genital and extragenital lesions. Other synonymous terms include pyometra complex, pyometritis, catarrhal endometri-tis, purulent metritis and chronic cystic en-dometritis.

ETIOPATHOGENESIS OF GENITAL LESIONS

There is general agreement that genital lesions seen in canine pyometra result from hormonal and bacterial interaction. Hor-monal dysfunction is considered a predispos-ing and perpetuating factor in all cases.

The metestrual timing of this disease led most investigators to suspect progesterone as a causative or contributing substance. Plasma progesterone concentrations are highest during this stage of the estrous cycle, and corpora lutea are usually found when the ovaries from dogs with pyometra are examined. All of the clinical signs and pathological lesions can be experimentally produced following the administration of progesterone alone. Furthermore, numerous iatrogenic cases were documented in the mid-1960's. These developed subsequent to therapeutic injections of progestational com-pounds used to delay or suppress estrus. Such data supported the concept that increased plasma progesterone activity was the initiat-ing factor in the disease.

With the advent of newer technology, measurement of plasma progesterone and estrogen levels became possible, and no dif-ferences in plasma progesterone or estrogen concentrations were detected between the normal and the diseased animals. It has been suggested that a defect in the metabolism of progesterone and estrogen by the target organ (uterus), rather than excessive proges-terone production, may be the primary ab-normality in this disease. A change in the number or affinity of endometrial receptor sites could lead to abnormal accumulations of hormones within the uterus and result in the observed histological changes.

The uterus undergoes a number of mor-phological changes under the influence of progesterone and estrogen. The most fre-quently observed hormonally induced patho-logical change in the uterus is cystic en-dometrial hyperplasia (CEH). CEH is an exaggerated response of the uterus to progestational stimulation during the luteal phase of the estrous cycle. It is considered to be the initial phase in the development of pyometra. Estrogen stimulation accelerates the rate of development of these progesterone-induced lesions but is not necessary for their development. Prolonged or repeated progesterone stimulation produces an acute inflammatory reaction that may be aggravated by bacterial infection. When regression of the corpus luteum occurs, progesterone levels decrease. The acute inflammatory reaction undergoes resolution, and the uterine wall becomes infiltrated with plasma cells. Repeated cycles in dogs with functionally closed crevices result in the development of chronic endometritis. The degree of cervical patency is variable. Closure of the cervix is usually associated with more severe clinical signs.

Secondary bacterial contamination of the uterus is a frequent complication of pyometra. The type of bacteria most frequently isolated in canine pyometra is *Escherichia coli*. Sixty to 74 per cent of clinical cases yield this organism. Other less frequently isolated bacteria include staphylococci, streptococci, *Proteus* spp., *Klebsiella* spp. and *Salmonella* spp. Data collected from clinical patients at the University of Minnesota are similar to other reported surveys.

The source of the uterine bacteria is probably the urinary tract or anogenital region. Bacteria are thought to gain entry to the uterus during estrus and proliferate in metestrus. In a recent study, the same strain of *E. coli* was isolated from the urine and uterus of 23 bitches with pyometra. Specific endometrial and myometrial receptors for *E. coli* antigens were present in the infected uteri, theoretically enhancing the colonization of bacteria in the uterus.

Spontaneous recovery may occur following regression of the corpus luteum, relaxation of the cervix and discharge of the uterine contents. However, such dogs are prone to recurrent attacks at subsequent estrous cycles.

ETIOPATHOGENESIS OF RENAL MANIFESTATIONS

Although many dogs with pyometra develop renal disease, few have lesions severe enough to produce renal failure. The types of renal disease observed with pyometra may be classified as follows: (1) prerenal uremia; (2) primary glomerular disease; (3) reduced tubular concentrating capacity; (4) concomitant renal disease, the etiology of which is unrelated to pyometra and (5) combinations of these.

Prerenal azotemia may develop in pyometra patients secondary to dehydration or shock, or both. If decreased renal perfusion persists, ischemic tubular disease may develop.

A mixed membranoproliferative glomerulonephropathy has been observed in dogs with pyometra. This lesion is probably caused by immune-complex deposition in the glomerular capillary walls. Although glomerular injury is a frequent finding in canine pyometra, the severity of such lesions has not been observed to result in primary renal failure. From a prognostic standpoint, the glomerulonephropathy is apparently reversible following removal of the diseased uterus.

Impaired tubular ability to concentrate urine is a common finding in canine pyometra. The urine specific gravity in such dogs is usually below that of glomerular filtrate (<1.008). Such hyposthenuria occurs in spite of adequate circulating levels of antidiuretic hormone. This is one of the few examples in veterinary medicine of "renal diabetes insipidus." The exact mechanism (or mechanisms) responsible for this impaired concentrating ability is poorly understood. A decrease in renal medullary solute concentration is known to be present. Recent evidence also indicates that the epithelial surfaces of Bowman's capsule and the renal tubular epithelium have an affinity for *E. coli.* antigen, suggesting that the tubular defect may have an immunological basis.

Both the frequency with which renal failure and pyometra occur concomitantly and the instances in which the renal failure is unrelated to pyometra are unknown. Renal calculi, pyelonephritis and chronic generalized nephritis have been observed in dogs with pyometra at the University of Minnesota.

PATHOPHYSIOLOGY OF DISEASE IN OTHER SYSTEMS

In addition to the genital and renal lesions previously considered, the bone marrow, liver, spleen and adrenals may be altered in canine pyometra. The bone marrow alteration is one of a marked increase in the myeloid: erythroid ratio due to hyperplasia of the myeloid elements. The tremendous chemotactic influence of the inflamed endometrium causes a massive outpouring of neutrophils into the peripheral blood. A marked immature neutrophilia commonly occurs (Table 1). In severely toxic animals, bone marrow depression results in decreased white blood cell (WBC) counts associated with immaturity and in mild to severe anemias. The liver, spleen and adrenal glands often exhibit evidence of extramedullary myelopoiesis. This reflects an inability of the bone marrow to keep pace with peripheral demands for neutrophils. Acute adrenal cortical collapse may occasionally develop as a complication of pyometra.

CLINICAL FINDINGS

History. Pyometra occurs most often in dogs over 6 years of age. The mean age of 134 dogs with pyometra evaluated at the University of Minnesota was 6.9 years. However, dogs less than 1 year of age have been seen with this problem. No breed predilection is known to exist.

The severity of clinical illness is dependent upon cervical patency, stage of the estrous cycle, the presence of bacterial infection of the uterus, the duration of illness and the severity of uterine and extragenital lesions.

The most common clinical signs are depression, anorexia, vaginal discharge, vomiting, polydipsia, polyuria, nocturia and diarrhea. Signs less commonly observed by owners are abdominal enlargement and vulvar swelling. The volume of vaginal discharge is highly variable and depends in part

on the degree of cervical patency. The discharge is usually yellow-grey or reddish-brown and has a fetid odor. Nondraining pyometra cases tend to be more "toxic" because of the accumulation of large volumes of pus within the uterus. Polyuria and polydipsia are frequently observed clinical signs. Although not pathognomonic for canine pyometria, such signs in middle-aged, non-spayed bitches are highly suggestive of this disease.

The duration of clinical illness is variable. Of 92 cases evaluated at the University of Minnesota in which the duration of illness was known, the mean length of illness was 14 days. An association of clinical illness with recent estrous cycles is often present. Of 105 cases evaluated by the author, the mean time from the last observed estrus to clinical presentation was 5.7 weeks.

Contrary to popular belief, there is no substantial evidence that pseudopregnancy, irregular heat cycles and/or lack of previous pregnancies predisposes dogs to this condition.

Physical Examination. Physical examination of dogs with pyometra often detects a number of abnormalities. The most frequent irregularities are dehydration, depression, palpable uterine enlargement and a vaginal discharge. Rectal temperatures are usually normal. Subnormal temperatures are occasionally observed, usually in severely toxic animals.

LABORATORY FINDINGS

Hemogram. An immature neutrophilia is a consistent finding in most cases of pyometra (Table 1). Total WBC counts are variable but usually range from 20,000 to

TABLE 1. *Results of Complete Blood Counts Obtained from 127 Dogs with Canine Pyometra**

	PCV (%)	Hemo-globin (gm%)	WBC/cmm ×10³	Lymph. (%)	Neut. (%)	Juv. (%)	Stab. (%)	Seg. (%)	Eos. (%)	Mono. (%)	Total Plasma Protein (gm%)
Number Examined	119†	120†	127	127	127	127	127	127	127	127	67†
Mean	39	12.8	39.3	11.2	81.9	4.6	26.4	48.8	2.3	6.69	8.2
Mode	40	14.5	27.5	8.0	83.0	0.0	32.5	44.5	1.0	1.0	9.0
Median	40	13.5	32.5	9.0	83.0	3.0	32.5	44.5	1.0	4.0	8.4
Range	15–56	4.1–19	2.5–196.8	0–36	49–97	0–43	0–67	8–86	0–21	0–25	6.5–10.6

*Of 134 cases evaluated, hemograms were obtained in 127. All hemograms were obtained prior to initiation of medical and/or surgical therapy. (Survey conducted at the University of Minnesota.)
†Data were not obtained from some patients because the quantity of blood obtained was insufficient.

100,000/cu mm. Dogs with higher counts usually have a closed cervix and bacterial infection of the uterus. When normal WBC counts are found, a severe degenerative left shift is usually present. Occasionally, a normal WBC count and differential are detected in a dog with a very enlarged uterus. These uteri are usually noninfected and contain clear, mucoid-like material. They are classified clinically as a "mucometra" or "hydrometra."

Following removal of the uterus, many dogs exhibit a marked rise in total WBC counts, sometimes two to three times presurgical levels. This postsurgical increase reflects continued myelopoiesis from the previously stimulated bone marrow, an effect that persists for several days.

A mild to moderate normocytic, normochromic anemia occurs in many dogs with pyometra. Of 119 cases surveyed, 34 (28 per cent) had such an anemia (packed-cell volume less than 36 per cent). The anemia is thought to result from toxic bone marrow depression or loss of red cells into the uterine lumen, or both.

Serum Proteins. Moderate to marked hyperproteinemia occurs in most cases of pyometra. This is due almost entirely to an increase in gamma globulins. Fibrinogen concentrations are usually normal, while hypoalbuminemia is a frequent finding. The mean plasma protein concentration of 67 cases surveyed by the author was 8.2 gm/dl (Table 1).

Blood Urea Nitrogen or Creatinine. Because of the potential for renal failure to develop in all dogs with pyometra, it is recommended that a complete urinalysis and blood urea nitrogen (BUN) or creatinine concentration be determined presurgically. Serum BUN concentrations were evaluated in 93 of 134 patients with pyometra surveyed at the University of Minnesota; 15 (16.1 per cent) were abnormally elevated (Table 2).

Urinalysis. Because all dogs with pyometra have the potential to develop prerenal or primary renal failure, or both, a complete urinalysis should be performed in conjunction with a BUN determination in all patients. Data from presurgical urinalyses on 57 dogs are tabulated in Table 2. Hyposthenuria and proteinuria were present in a significant number of cases.

To prevent contamination of the urine with genital tract inflammatory cells, the vulva should be cleansed thoroughly prior to collecting a midstream urine sample. Samples collected via catheterization or cystocentesis will eliminate introduction of inflammatory cells from the genital tract, which tends to confuse urine sediment interpretation.

Cytology. Vaginal cytological studies can be useful in cases with either an open or closed cervix. By the tenth to twentieth days of metestrus in normal dogs, vaginal smears contain primarily small, noncornified or large, flat epithelial cells with vacuolated cytoplasm. In contrast, vaginal smears from dogs with pyometra contain excessively large numbers or masses of neutrophils and bacteria that persist into late metestrus and anestrus.

RADIOGRAPHY

Abdominal radiography is of greatest value in dogs that have no vulvar discharge or in which abdominal palpation does not detect uterine enlargement. In animals whose clinical history and physical examination are diagnostic, abdominal radiography serves to confirm the presence of an enlarged uterus and permits evaluation of the abdomen for unsuspected, concomitant abdominal disorders (abnormal kidney size, renal calculi, tumors, and so forth). All degrees of severity of pyometra should be visible on survey radiographs if the patient has been properly positioned and prepared.

Radiographically, the uterus of a dog with pyometra is characterized by the presence of a homogeneous, tubular, fluid density mass in the posterior abdomen. If interpretation is hampered by overlying intestines, abdominal compression techniques may be used to displace the intestines cranially. Contrast hysterography is contraindicated for routine use, as it subjects the patient to unnecessary risks of uterine trauma or rupture.

Normal nongravid canine uteri, as well as uteri from dogs in estrus or that are pseudopregnant, cannot be visualized on survey films. Enlarged normal uteri are radiographically evident only during the later stages of pregnancy and for a variable period of time following parturition.

DIFFERENTIAL DIAGNOSIS

The diagnosis of canine cystic endometrial hyperplasia–pyometra complex is usually

TABLE 2. *Results of Presurgical Evaluation of Urine Specific Gravity, Urine Protein and Serum BUN Concentration Obtained from Dogs with Pyometra**

	Urine Specific Gravity				
	<1.007	1.008–1.024	>1.024	**BUN > 35 mg%**	**Proteinuria†**
Number affected	10	28	19	15	15
Per cent of total	17.5	49.2	33.3	16.1	26.3

*Total numbers tested: urine specific gravity, 57; urine protein, 57; BUN concentration, 93.
†Significant numbers of RBC and/or WBC were not detected in the urine sediment.

uncomplicated. Occasionally, the clinical signs are nonspecific and/or they mimic other diseases so that pyometra is not considered. Dogs with pyometra but without physical or historical evidence of vaginal discharge present the greatest diagnostic difficulty. Other diseases associated with polydipsia, polyuria, nonspecific signs of illness or an enlarging abdomen must also be considered. Occasionally, a pregnant bitch will be presented with no history of recent breeding. The gravid uterus will be radiographically indistinguishable from that of pyometra prior to the time of fetal skeletal calcification (40 to 45 days). The uterus should be carefully palpated at surgery to eliminate the possibility of pregnancy.

Other disease syndromes characterized by a sick animal with polydipsia and polyuria include renal failure, diabetes mellitus, hepatic failure and occasional cases of hypoadrenocorticism. The rapidity with which diagnostic tests are selected to rule out these diseases depends on the clinical status of the patient and the economic constraints imposed by the client.

Conditions characterized by a vaginal discharge that may resemble pyometra are normal estrus, vaginitis and vaginal neoplasia. A specific diagnosis can usually be established on the basis of physical examination, exfoliative cytology, radiography and so forth.

DIAGNOSIS

The diagnosis of pyometra is most often made on the basis of clinical signs, laboratory data, radiography and vaginal discharge. Detecting concomitant diseases, especially renal failure, requires laboratory confirmation. It is recommended, therefore, that a urinalysis, hemogram and BUN or creatinine concentration be performed in all pyometra cases.

TREATMENT

Surgical Treatment

The most satisfactory treatment for the majority of patients with pyometra is ovariohysterectomy. The use of supportive therapy (i.e., fluids, antibiotics, blood transfusions) may be required prior to, during and after surgery. All unnecessary therapeutic delays prior to surgery should be avoided, as these are rarely associated with clinical improvement of the patient.

Any of the complications associated with routine ovariohysterectomy surgery have the potential to develop in pyometra patients. Complications related strictly to pyometra surgery include peritonitis, uterine rupture and uterine stump abscess. If peritoneal contamination occurs, the abdominal cavity should be flushed thoroughly with warm lactated Ringer's solution. Water-soluble antibiotics should be placed into the peritoneal cavity prior to closure of the abdominal incision.

The incidence of postoperative renal failure in canine pyometra as compared with other major abdominal surgery is unknown. Since the incidence of renal disease is high in dogs with pyometra, the potential for renal complications to develop may be greater in these animals. Careful presurgical, surgical and postsurgical attention to the patient's fluid and electrolyte needs should reduce the likelihood of this complication developing.

Medical Treatment

Medical therapy should be reserved primarily for valuable breeding animals or animals that are so toxic that immediate surgery carries too high a risk of mortality. A number of medical or combined medical-surgical approaches to treating canine pyometra have been proposed. Although most of the earlier medical treatments were strictly empirical, newer therapeutic approaches have been devised to reverse the pathophysiological mechanisms that initiate the disease. Preliminary results of limited clinical experience with these approaches appear encouraging. The objectives of medical therapy should include: (1) restoration of the reproductive capacity to valuable breeding animals, (2) drainage and lavage of the uterus, (3) elimination of bacterial infection from the uterus and (4) removal of the source of progesterone responsible for initiating the disease.

Estrogens, testosterone and oxytocin are hormones that have been used to treat pyometra. Estrogens alone provide a variable degree of success. They initiate cervical relaxation and increase uterine muscular tone and contractility, promoting the expulsion of exudate from the uterine lumen. Estrogens also increase the resistance of the uterus to bacterial infection. Even though clinical improvement may occur following estrogen therapy alone, severe exacerbations often develop that require surgical intervention.

Testosterone has also been used as a medical treatment of pyometra. In one study, the parenteral administration of 25 mg of testosterone twice weekly produced clinical remissions in 7 of 10 dogs within 3 weeks. One of the 7 had a relapse and required an ovariohysterectomy. Testosterone is thought to act by causing ovarian atrophy. So little documented material is available on the use of this drug in canine pyometra that meaningful conclusions are impossible to formulate.

Both oxytocin and various ergot alkaloids have been used to stimulate expulsion of uterine contents by increasing uterine motility. Since oxytocin is most effective on an estrogen-primed uterus and since pyometra is associated with high progesterone activity, a priming period with estrogen should be considered prior to the use of this drug. Ergonovine maleate, one of the ergot alkaloids, is also more effective on an estrogen-primed uterus. The recommended parenteral or oral dosage is 0.2 mg twice daily for 10 days.

Progesterone and related compounds should not be given to dogs with pyometra. Such agents only aggravate the disease. The use of progesterone to delay or prevent estrus may also occasionally result in the development of pyometra.

Several procedures are available that allow drainage of the uterus with minimal trauma to the patient. Self-retaining male Foley catheters (No. 20) can be manually passed through an open cervix. Following catheterization, instillation of mucolytic agents (Alevaire) into the uterus may allow for more effective drainage of inspissated uterine exudate. When the cervix is closed, catheters may be inserted following cervical dilatation via a hysterotomy incision. If severe systemic toxicity prevents complete surgical removal of the uterus, it may be marsupialized through a small stab incision in the abdomen. This allows for drainage while supportive presurgical care is continuing. This procedure can often be completed using only local anesthesia.

Surgical removal of corpora lutea, if present, has been advocated as part of a combined medical-surgical approach to pyometra therapy, since these structures play a significant role in the pathogenesis of the disease. The objective of this procedure is to promote regression or pathological uterine changes by removing the major source of endogenous progesterone.

A potential nonsurgical method of inducing "luteolysis" is with the use of prostaglandins. The luteolytic agent prostaglandin $F_{2\alpha}$ is being used on an experimental basis to induce regression of the corpus luteum in dogs with pyometra. Although initial results appear encouraging, too few cases have been evaluated for meaningful conclusions to be drawn.

Systemic and intrauterine antibiotics are valuable for eliminating any secondary bacterial infections associated with pyometra. Broad-spectrum antibiotics (chloramphenicol, ampicillin) should be used while awaiting the results of culture and sensitivity data on uterine exudate. Intrauterine irrigation and lavage with dilute nitrofurazone solutions may be helpful in eliminating uterine infections.

Recently, medical therapy alone, combining diethylstilbestrol and ergonovine maleate with systemic and local antibiotics has produced encouraging results. Several dogs have been returned to health and have whelped normal litters. The best success appears to occur when bitches are bred the first estrus following therapy. Diethylstilbestrol is given orally at a dosage of 1 mg twice daily for 10 days. Ergonovine maleate is also given for 10 days at a dosage of 2 mg twice daily, either orally or parenterally. Antibiotics should be continued for 4 to 6 weeks, with the choice of drug based on antibiotic sensitivity data. It should be emphasized again that medical therapy should be attempted only in valuable breeding animals in relatively good physical condition.

REFERENCES

1. Borresen, B.: Pyometra in the dog — A pathophysiological investigation. Nord. Vet. Med., 27:508, 1975.
2. Ewing, G. O., Schecter, R. D., Whitney, R. C. and Wind, A. P.: The therapy of canine pyometra. J. Am. Anim. Hosp. Assn., 6:218, 1970.
3. Gourley, I. M.: Treatment of canine pyometra without ovariohysterectomy. *In* Bojrab, M. J. (ed.): Current Techniques in Small Animal Surgery. Philadelphia, Lea and Febiger, 1975.
4. Hadley, J. C.: Unconjugated oestrogen and progesterone concentrations in the blood of bitches with false pregnancy and pyometra. Vet. Rec., 96:545, 1975.
5. Hardy, R. M. and Osborne, C. A.: Canine pyometra: pathophysiology, diagnosis and treatment of uterine and extra-uterine lesions. J. Am. Anim. Hosp. Assn., 10:245, 1974.
6. Sandholm, M., Vesenius, H. and Kivisto, A. K.: Pathogenesis of canine pyometra. J.A.V.M.A., 167:1006, 1975.

Canine Vaginitis

PATRICIA SCHULTZ OLSON
Colorado State University,
Fort Collins, Colorado

Client education has significantly increased the number of dogs being examined by the veterinarian for reproductive disorders. Vaginitis in the dog is also being recognized with increased frequency. This may be related, at least in part, to the fact that breeders have become more conscientious about the potential dissemination of infectious agents by the transportation of breeding animals throughout the country.

CLINICAL FINDINGS

Any animal presented with a vaginal discharge and congested vaginal mucosa should be suspected of having vaginitis. The discharge should not be confused with normal proestrous bleeding, the lochia immediately following parturition or abnormal uterine discharges. Proestrous bleeding is a normal occurrence in the bitch and is usually seen along with vulvar swelling. Lochia, a greenish-colored material seen following parturition, rapidly diminishes in quantity within a few days after parturition and completely subsides within a few weeks. Uterine discharges may be associated with metritis or pyometra. In these cases the animal is often febrile and has signs of systemic illness. A thorough history, radiographic studies, abdominal palpation and a complete blood count will help differentiate vaginal from uterine discharges.

Puppies often develop vaginitis prior to their first estrus. Although juvenile vaginitis is not normal, it usually subsides following the first estrus and requires no treatment. Cases of several weeks' duration, however, may require treatment.

DIAGNOSIS

A thorough vaginal examination should be performed using a sterilized vaginal endoscope, otoscopic cones for small breeds or young animals, fiberoptic equipment if available or a modified human anoscope.[4] The anterior vagina should be evaluated for inflammation or other abnormalities. A well-lubricated, gloved finger may detect tumors, foreign bodies or malformations. A urine sample should be obtained to rule out the possibility of concomitant cystitis.

Smears should be prepared by means of a direct impression of the vulvar mucosa on a microscope slide, which is then stained with new methylene blue and a coverslip applied. Deeper vaginal smears may be obtained by rubbing cotton-tipped applicators or glass rods against the vaginal mucosa and transferring cells to a glass slide for cytological examination. Large numbers of leukocytes will usually be present in smears taken from a dog with clinical signs of vaginitis. This finding must be interpreted with knowledge of the time of the animal's estrous cycle, since leukocytes are normally present in diestrous smears. Bacteria will be present in most vaginal smears, regardless of whether or not the dog suffers from clinical vaginitis.

Vaginal cultures should be taken from any animal suspected of having vaginitis. This can be done using a sterile culturette or a sterilized cotton-tipped applicator, which is passed through the otoscope cone or vaginal speculum at the time of vaginal examination. A guarded culture system can also be utilized in obtaining anterior vaginal cultures. Both aerobic and anaerobic cultures can be prepared utilizing sheep blood agar plates and thioglycollate broth. Normal female canines usually harbor bacteria in the vagina. Fewer bacterial isolates are obtained from anterior samples than from posterior samples.[2] Puppies under 6 months of age harbor significantly more coagulase-positive staphylococci than do older animals.[2] Once a potential pathogen is isolated, antibiotic sensitivity tests should be performed in order to formulate proper antimicrobial therapy.

TREATMENT

Treatment for vaginitis is variable, being dependent on the cause of the infection, the stage of the estrous cycle and the antibiotic sensitivity results obtained by vaginal culture. In animals with primary bacterial infections, antibiotics may be infused directly into the vagina. Since no information is available at present to indicate which antibiotics are spermicidal to the canine spermatozoon, those antibiotics used for vaginal infusions must be chosen discriminately. Nitrofurazone, 0.2 per cent, has been used safely 48 hours prior to natural breeding or artificial insemination in the canine.

One should always advise the owner not to breed the animal during the first estrus after a diagnosis of vaginitis has been made. Some breeders will not delay breeding, especially if the vaginitis is a recurring problem. In such cases rigorous treatment is recommended if the animal is to be freed of the infection prior to breeding. Bitches due to whelp within a few days may also be given antibiotic infusions in an attempt to reduce exposure of puppies to potentially pathogenic bacteria in the vaginal canal. Such intravaginal infusions are given during the last few days of gestation. Systemic antibiotics have been used in some dogs throughout their gestation, but the drugs should always be evaluated for possible teratogenic effects.

In the nonpregnant animal that is not being bred, intravaginal infusions of antibiotics may be performed daily in conjunction with systemic antibiotic therapy. Diethylstilbestrol may be used for control of vaginal infections, but possible deleterious side effects of the drug should be considered.[1]

When treating secondary vaginitis, the inciting cause should be eliminated (neoplasia, foreign bodies and so forth) in addition to the recommendations just described.

PREVENTION

Some measures may prevent the dissemination of a vaginal infection or its recurrence in an animal. Animals with a known history of vaginal infections should have vaginal cultures obtained prior to breeding. If a culture is taken on the first day of proestrous bleeding, results are ready in time for intravaginal infusions to be used prior to breeding. Males used for breeding should also have preputial and urethral cultures taken. Although the means for dissemination of vaginal bacteria is unknown, animals grouped together seem to harbor similar bacteria.[2]

REFERENCES

1. Jöchle, W.: Hormones in canine gynecology. A review. Theriogenology, *3*:152, 1975.
2. Olson, P. N. S.: Canine vaginal flora. M. S. thesis, University of Minnesota, St. Paul, Minn., 1976.
3. Osbaldiston, G. W., Nuri, S. and Mosier, J. E.: Vaginal cytology and microflora of infertile bitches. J. Am. Anim. Hosp. Ass., *8*:93, 1972.
4. Pineda, M. H., Kainer, R. A. and Faulkner, L. C.: Dorsal median postcervical fold in the canine vagina. Am. J. Vet. Res., *34*:1487, 1973.
5. Platt, A. M. and Simpson, R. B.: Bacterial flora of the canine vagina. Southwest Vet., *17*:76, 1974.

Canine Herpesvirus Infection

LELAND E. CARMICHAEL
Cornell University, Ithaca, New York

Canine herpesvirus (CHV) causes a fatal septicemic disease of infant puppies that are usually less than 1 month of age. Clinical features of the disease consist of the sudden death of apparently healthy puppies after a brief period of illness that usually lasts no more than 24 hours. Most commonly, pups are affected between the first and third weeks of life, with occasional fatal cases occurring after the third week. Herpesvirus infection has only rarely been found to be a cause of puppy deaths within the first 3 days of life. Generalized, nonfatal infection occurs in older pups but clinical signs are usually not apparent. Signs are virtually absent in pups infected after weaning. The incubation period varies between 3 and 8 days in newborn puppies given virus intranasally.

Signs in older dogs inoculated with virus are limited to mild rhinitis or vaginitis. British investigators have associated a canine herpesvirus with abortions, stillbirths and infertility in a kennel of Alsatians.[3] The virus recovered from the genital tracts of affected dogs was antigenically indistinguishable from canine herpesvirus strains isolated previously from neonatal pups; however, certain cultural differences were noted. Unfortunately, the genital isolate was not stored and is no longer available for study. Nevertheless, when vesicular lesions affecting the genital tract are observed, especially if recurrent infection is noted, attempts at virus isolation should be made.

The disease is transmitted principally by contact between susceptible pups and infective oral or vaginal secretions, usually from the bitch. It also may be spread from an infected dog to susceptible newborn pups by kennel owners or contaminated objects. There is only one reported case of prenatal transmission; however, it is likely that such instances occur occasionally.

The differential lesions that distinguish this disease from canine hepatitis and toxoplasmosis are the focal areas of renal and hepatic necrosis and hemorrhage. Microscopic examination may reveal intranuclear "type A" inclusions in occasional cells at the periphery of necrotic foci, especially in the kidneys and liver. Inclusions are not numerous.

Inapparent infections are common in dogs. Although such infections occur without significant clinical signs (these being limited to mild serous rhinitis or vaginitis), the epizootiological importance is apparent. Periodic shedding of the canine herpesvirus in nasal secretions, similar to that reported in humans infected with herpes simplex viruses or cattle infected with infectious bovine rhinotracheitis viruses, also has been observed in infected dogs. By use of immunosuppressant agents (corticosteroid drugs, antilymphocyte serum), viral recrudescence has been demonstrated as long as 6 months after primary intranasal infection. Despite persistent infections of the dog, bitches that had lost their pups because of the herpesvirus have not been reported to have suffered additional losses at subsequent whelpings.

Pups with maternal antibody are readily infected by CHV; however, there is no clinical illness, since the infection remains localized. Neutralizing antibodies develop after the infection and have persisted at low levels for at least 2 years.

REFERENCES

1. Carmichael, L. E.: Herpesvirus canis: aspects of pathogenesis and immune response. J.A.V.M.A., *156*:1714, 1970.
2. Carmichael, L. E., Squire, R. A. and Krook, L.: Clinical and pathologic features of a fatal viral disease of newborn pups. Am. J. Vet. Res., *26*:803, 1965.
3. Poste, G. and King, N.: Isolation of a herpesvirus from the canine genital tract: association with infertility, abortion and stillbirths. Vet. Rec., *88*:229, 1971.
4. Wright, N. G. and Cornwell, H. J. C.: Experimental herpesvirus infection in young puppies. Res. Vet. Sci., *9*:295, 1968.

Canine Brucellosis

LELAND E. CARMICHAEL
Cornell University, Ithaca, New York

Brucellosis in dogs due to *Brucella canis* (*B. canis*) has been recognized since 1966, when widespread abortions were observed in colonies of beagles. Since that time the disease has occurred in various breeds, and its presence has been recorded on several continents. Although canine brucellosis is widespread in the United States, the reported incidence rates vary from approximately 1 to 6 per cent, depending on the area sampled and the type of diagnostic test employed. The recent availability of a rapid slide test has made *presumptive* diagnosis of this disease relatively simple. However, the occasional occurrence of nonspecific agglutination when the stained antigen (Canine Brucellosis Diagnostic Test, Pitman-Moore, Inc.) is mixed with a patient's serum emphasizes that the plate (slide) test should not be the only criterion applied to the diagnosis of this disease. False-positive reactions have been observed with a small proportion of serums obtained from dogs proved noninfected by extensive bacteriological and serological studies.

Since no treatment for the disease is certain and the implications are very serious for dogs proved infected, vigorous attempts to establish a diagnosis by all available means should be sought before declaring an animal infected. Unfortunately, there have been many instances when inadequate diagnostic procedures were applied and dogs were needlessly destroyed. Each case deserves extensive study. A knowledge of the general nature of brucellosis and the protein nature of the disease in the dog, especially in the nonpregnant female and in apparently normal males, is important. The reference list includes useful articles that may be consulted to amplify the brief description presented here.

ETIOLOGY

The disease is caused by a small gram-negative cocobacillus that grows aerobically on enriched media, such as Albimi brucella broth and agar or trypticase soy tryptose media. Growth is relatively slow, requiring 48 to 72 hours for colonies to form. Unlike some *Brucella abortus* biotypes, growth is not favored by carbon dioxide. After several days' incubation, growth of translucent colonies becomes very mucoid (ropy in broth). Because of the mucoid nature of the organism, it does not possess the smooth (O) antigens of *B. abortus* or *B. melitensis;* therefore, the usual brucellosis test antigens available for diagnosis of this disease in other domestic species are useless. *B. canis* cross-reacts extensively with *B. ovis*, with rough variants of other *Brucella* species and with additional gram-negative bacterial species. Cross-reactions with as yet unidentified microorganisms may give rise to nonspecific agglutinins and confuse the serodiagnosis. Biochemically, the canine brucella is similar to *B. suis*. Especially useful diagnostic characteristics, in addition to cultural and morphological aspects, are dye inhibition reactions (no growth on basic fuchsin; growth in the presence of thionin) and the rapid production of urease by *B. canis*. The canine brucella does not produce hydrogen sulfide but is oxidase positive.

EPIDEMIOLOGY

Since the initial recognition of canine brucellosis in commercial and private breeding kennels, the disease has been found to be widespread in the dog population throughout the United States. Accurate incidence rates are not available because uniform test procedures have not been established; however, an "average incidence" appears to be about 1.5 per cent. Incidence rates of 5 to 6 per cent have been reported in certain areas of the country. The disease now has been confirmed in Japan, Mexico, Germany, Czechoslovakia and, most recently, in Brazil. Serological evidence of the disease has been reported in Peru and Tunisia. Outbreaks in Czechoslovakia and Japan occurred after importation of infected dogs from the United States.

Transmission occurs principally by way of infectious vaginal discharges or mammary secretions following an abortion and by the seminal fluids of infected males at the time of breeding. Spread via urine or other discharges is possible, but is unproved and not likely. Males may shed organisms in semen for weeks or months after apparent recovery, presenting a formidable diagnostic challenge. Dogs are the only known natural host, although foxes were proved highly susceptible by experimental inoculation. Cats are clearly susceptible, but this species has not been adequately studied. As noted later in this article, there have been human infections.

CLINICAL SIGNS

Clinical signs in bitches include abortion after the thirtieth day of gestation, most commonly between the forty-fifth and fifty-fifth day. Occasional litters may be born with some pups alive and some dead. Early embryonic deaths with termination of pregnancy may occur, suggesting to the owner that the bitch had failed to conceive. Generalized lymph node enlargement, principally due to reticular cell hyperplasia, is common in both sexes. In the male, epididymitis and orchitis, often followed by testicular atrophy, are common. *B. canis* can be isolated readily from the blood or vaginal discharges of infected animals and from the fetal and placental tissues. Prolonged bacteremia, often lasting more than 2 years, is a notable feature of the canine disease. After several months' infection, bacteremia may be intermittent.

An important aspect of the disease in males is infertility. Between postinfection weeks 2 and 5, abnormal sperm (30 to 80 per cent) are evident, with bent tails, swollen midpieces and distal protoplasmic droplets. By 20 weeks' postexposure by the oral route, more than 90 per cent of the sperm may be abnormal with severe reduction in motility. Neutrophils and monocytes are common in the ejaculate, and detached heads are evident. Clumps of spermatozoa with head-to-head agglutination are readily observed. Spermagglutinins have been found in both serum and seminal fluid samples from infected males. Brucella organisms may be isolated from ejaculated semen in abundance during the second month after infection; however, the number of organisms decreases rapidly after this time. Shedding is sporadic thereafter, although organisms have been recovered from the semen of infected dogs for as long as 60 weeks. The prostate gland is an abundant source of the organisms.

It is important to recognize that many infected animals appear normal, even though they may have bacteremia. There is no fever. Agglutinins appear in the serum approximately 3 weeks following oral infection and persist at high levels (titer value will depend on the particular test system employed) until recovery commences, typically 1 year or longer. Recovered animals are immune to reinfection; however, the duration of immunity is not known.

DIAGNOSIS

A diagnosis should not be made until adequate clinical, serological and bacterial examination are carried out. A history of abortions, infertility, testicular abnormalities (epididymitis, atrophy) and poor semen quality or of lymph node enlargement with or without these signs should lead to consideration of *B. canis* infection. A rapid slide agglutination test that produces *presumptive* diagnostic information in a few minutes is now available (Pitman-Moore, Inc.). This test has proved rapid and highly accurate in identifying infected animals, for "false-negatives" have not been observed. Occasional "false-positive" reactions have been found, however, and the slide test always should be followed by additional examinations. Several laboratories offer diagnostic assistance; however, there is no standardized procedure and interpretations of tube agglutination test results vary.* Serum samples must be clear and not contaminated. It is not possible to interpret agglutination test results on serums from dogs that have received antibiotic treatment for brucellosis unless an interval of at least 4 weeks has elapsed since cessation of treatment. One test requires incubation of serum dilutions and antigen for 48 hours at 52°C; another test uses 2-mercaptoethanol. The lat-

---

*The Diagnostic Laboratory, New York State College of Veterinary Medicine, Ithaca, New York, 14853, offers a *B. canis* diagnostic service in which positive reactions in one laboratory are confirmed by additional tests in an independent facility. Diagnostic assistance also may be obtained from the Veterinary Service Diagnostic Laboratory, U.S.D.A., Ames, Iowa, 50010. Instructions for shipping serum samples or blood for culture may be obtained from the Biologic Reagents Section, V.S.D.L., Ames, Iowa, 50010.

ter gives lower titers but reduced nonspecific reactions. Serological evidence of infection (generally indicated by tube agglutination test titers in excess of 1:200 or 2-mercaptoethanol titers in excess of 1:100) should always be followed by attempts to isolate the organism by blood cultures or by cultures of lymph node or bone marrow biopsy specimens. Because of the serious prognosis, especially as regards use of an infected dog for breeding purposes, all available diagnostic aids should be employed.

TREATMENT

There is no certain treatment; however, some success has been achieved experimentally. Evaluation of any treatment regimen must be followed by periodic bacteriological and serological tests, since early apparent success at treating the disease often has proved disappointing, even though a period of abacteremia occurred for a few weeks after cessation of a course of antibiotic therapy. The goal of treatment is to eliminate the organism from the infected animal, a difficult task for eradication of all brucella infections. Treatment may be considered for dogs when it is made clear to the owner that the procedure is expensive in both cost and time and that success cannot be assured. Follow-up blood cultures and serological tests are essential. These should be done 6 to 8 weeks after cessation of any treatment.

Several treatment schedules have been tried (most unsuccessful!); however, the following ones have been claimed successful in several instances.

1. Tetracycline hydrochloride given orally (t.i.d.) for 3 weeks at 30 mg/lb body weight. Treatment is discontinued for 3 to 4 weeks. A second course of tetracycline hydrochloride is then given, together with streptomycin (20 mg/lb, b.i.d.) with or without sulfadimethoxyine (25 mg/lb, once daily).

2. Minocycline hydrochloride given orally (b.i.d.) for 14 days at 25 mg/lb body weight. Simultaneous intramuscular administration of streptomycin (10 mg/lb, b.i.d.) is given for the first 7 days and then is discontinued. This treatment resulted in complete clearance of *B. canis* from the tissues of four of five treated female animals examined at necropsy 6 weeks after cessation of treatment. In the unsuccessful an-

imal, a few colonies of *B. canis* were isolated only from cultures of the spleen.

Only treatment schedules as intensive as those just described have proved successful. Eradication of organisms from the prostate tissue of infected males has not been reported. Infected males should not be used for breeding purposes; transmission may be interrupted by castration and antibiotic treatment.

CONTROL

Control and prophylactic measures should include the use of serum agglutination tests, blood cultures, isolation and removal of infected animals, good sanitation and common sense.

All females that have aborted or failed to conceive after successive matings or males that have genital disease should be considered as possibly being infected with *B. canis*. Such dogs should be isolated immediately and a serum sample taken and tested by the slide or tube agglutination test. Blood should be cultured. Dogs in a breeding kennel found positive by cultures of blood and serology should be destroyed. Treatment may be considered for valuable pets and working dogs; however, owners should be advised of the cost and the uncertain outcome. Control within a breeding kennel consists of serological testing and, if possible, blood cultures followed by elimination of all positive animals.

Repeated tests at monthly intervals should be performed on all dogs in a colony with infected animals. Animals found positive should be removed, and at least three negative monthly tests should be obtained on all dogs before a kennel can be considered negative. All dogs introduced into a kennel, especially if they are to be used for breeding, should be maintained in separate quarters until at least two negative tests, done at monthly intervals, are obtained. The entire kennel should be cleaned and disinfected daily. Roccal solution and Wescodyne have proved to be bactericidal. Animal handlers should wear disposable gloves. Hands should be rinsed in disinfectant between examinations of animals for heat. Animals with "suspicious" agglutinin titers should not be introduced into a kennel unless repeated tests suggest nonspecific reactions.

Bacterins are not available for prophylaxis.

PUBLIC HEALTH ASPECTS

Human infections have been observed. At the present writing, eighteen human cases have been reported. Eight were laboratory workers. All infections have been relatively mild, and infected individuals responded well to tetracycline therapy. Headache, fatigue, enlarged regional lymph nodes without splenomegaly and mild fever were the principal signs. The owners of infected dogs should be informed of the public health risk but should not be alarmed since man, like other noncanine species, appears relatively resistant.

REFERENCES

1. Carmichael, L. E. and George, L. W.: Canine brucellosis: Newer knowledge. International Symposium on Brucellosis (II), Rabat, 1975. Published in Develop. Biol. Standard., *31*:237, 1976.
2. Carmichael, L. E. and Kenney, R. M.: Canine brucellosis: The clinical disease and immune response. J.A.V.M.A., *156*:1726, 1970.
3. Fredrickson, L. E. and Barton, C. E.: A serologic survey for canine brucellosis in a metropolitan area. J.A.V.M.A., *165*:987, 1974.
4. George, L. W.: Studies on the immune response in canine brucellosis. Thesis, Cornell University, Ithaca. New York, 1974, pp. 1–124.
5. George, L. W. and Carmichael, L. E.: A plate agglutination test for the rapid diagnosis of canine brucellosis. Am. J. Vet. Res., *35*:905, 1974.
6. Lewis, G. E.: Canine brucellosis. *In* Kirk, R. W. (Ed.): Current Veterinary Therapy V. Philadelphia, W. B. Saunders Co., 1974, pp. 974–976.
7. Moore, J. A. and Gupta, B. N. Epizootiology, diagnosis and control of *Brucella canis*. J.A.V.M.A., *156*:1737, 1970.
8. Pickerill, P. A., and Carmichael, L. E.: Canine brucellosis: Control programs in commercial kennels and effects on reproduction. J.A.V.M.A. *160*:1607, 1972.

Epidemiological Aspects of Mammary and Genital Neoplasia

ROBERT SCHNEIDER

University of California, Davis, California

INTRODUCTION

Data presented here are from the collection of the population-based Animal Neoplasm Registry (ANR) covering Alameda and Contra Costa counties, California.[1] Cases are submitted by veterinarians practicing in the area, and attempts are made to register every case. A very rapid pathology service, free of charge to the practitioners, provides them and the ANR with a histopathological diagnosis for each case. More than 30,000 pet animals that have had at least one tumor are in the ANR collection. Periodic population surveys yield population-at-risk data.[2] Thus, for any demographic variable, incidence rates (or the number of new cases occurring on the average per year per 100,000 dogs in the population) can be calculated. Since cancer incidence rates vary with age, adjustment to a standard aged population is necessary. Comparisons can then be properly made between subgroups having different age distributions, such as the different sexes and breeds. The rates presented in this article, therefore, reflect tumor occurrence in a standard aged population.

Age standardized incidence rates for tumors of the major reproductive organ sites are presented in Table 1. Mammary gland tumors accounted for 32 per cent of the total malignant and benign tumors in the female; tumors of the genital system consituted 2 per cent of the total. In the male approximately 10 per cent of tumors were in the genital system and 1 per cent in the mammary glands. The principal male genital organ having tumors was the testes, contributing 89 per cent of the genital system tumors and 9 per cent of all tumors. It should be kept in mind, however, that tumor rates for the mammary glands and the genital system are related to the number of dogs neutered in a population and, with some organs, to the age at neutering as well. Thus, in other populations the proportions of tumors and the incidence rates at these sites could vary from those presented in this article.

TABLE 1. *Age Standardized Tumor Incidence Rates per 100,000 Dogs per Year by Primary Reproductive Site for Female and Male Dogs—July, 1967 to June, 1974*

Primary Site	Total		Malignant Only		Benign Only	
	FEMALE	MALE	FEMALE	MALE	FEMALE	MALE
All sites	995.2	831.6	267.5	221.1	727.7	610.5
Mammary glands	319.3	8.9	92.2	1.6	227.1	7.3
Genital system	20.0	85.7	3.4	39.4	16.6	46.3
Ovary	4.6	–	1.9	–	2.7	–
Uterus	2.3	–	0.5	–	1.8	–
Testes	–	76.3	–	31.7	–	44.6
Prostate	–	7.4	–	7.2	–	0.2
External genitalia	13.1	2.0	1.0	0.5	12.1	1.5

TUMORS OF THE MAMMARY GLAND

An overwhelming majority of mammary tumors occur in the bitch. However, unlike man and the cat in whom the ratio of neoplasms is approximately one male case to every 100 female, the dog has approximately two cases in the male to every 100 in the female.

Neutering of the bitch has a sparing effect on mammary tumor occurrence. However, neutering must occur before maturity in order to exert an influence.[3] Bitches neutered prior to any estrous cycles had 200 times less mammary cancer, those neutered after one cycle had 12 times less risk and those neutered after maturity had no reduced risk.[3] Regardless of the age at which neutering occurred, the overall reduction in risk attributable to most populations is five to seven times. This low overall rate is due to the dilution effect of females neutered after maturity. On the other hand, while neutering reduced the risk in the female, it had no effect on the male. Castrated males had standardized rates approximately equal to those for intact males.

The principal tumor type found in the mammary gland was the mixed mammary tumor. Of approximately 4000 mammary tumor specimens submitted to the ANR, 67 per cent were of the mixed mammary type. Various adenomas and adenocarcinomas constituted 32 per cent. Most of the mixed mammary tumors were benign (6.5 to 1), while most of the adeno- group were malignant (2 to 1). The probability of a mammary tumor being malignant or benign at various ages is shown in Table 2. This table can aid in prognosis when pathological services are not available. It is seen that the probability of malignancy increased with the age of the animal at veterinary diagnosis. An interesting observation in Table 2 is that neutered females over 3 years of age have a 5 to 10 per cent increased probability of having a malignancy. Since neutered females have approximately five to seven times less mammary cancer than intact animals, it would appear that early neutering has a stronger sparing effect on future benign development rather than malignant mammary tumor development.

Rates for the major breeds were examined for excess occurrence of mammary tumors in a specific breed by comparing standardized rates, after adjustment for the reduced incidence in the neutered proportion of each breed. Table 3 compares rate ratios of the nine most popular breeds in the population. Using the rate for the breed with the lowest incidence (Chihuahua) as equal to 1.00, all of the other breeds had approximately 1.75 to 4 times more mammary tumors than the

TABLE 2. *Probability (%) of Malignancy of a Mammary Tumor in a Female Dog— By Age*

Age Group (yrs)	All Females	Intact Females	Neutered Females
<2	0	0	0
2–3	10	10	0
4–5	10	10	15
6–7	15	15	20
8–9	25	20	25
10–11	35	30	40
12–13	45	40	50
14–15	45	40	50
>15	45	40	50

TABLE 3. Comparison of the Ratios* of Mammary Tumor Occurrence in Nine Major Breeds, Using Age Standardized Breed Incidence Rates Adjusted for Differential Risk in the Neutered Proportions of Each Breed

Breed	Population-at-Risk	Ratio of Adjusted Rates*
Chihuahua	2,696	1.00
Pekingese	927	1.15
Labrador retriever	1,506	1.74
Beagle	1,559	1.75
Poodle, all sizes	15,258	2.31
German shepherd dog	6,079	2.41
German shorthaired pointer	1,273	2.60
Dachshund	4,502	2.67
Cocker spaniel	1,445	4.03

*Ratio is the age standardized incidence rate adjusted for the reduced incidence in the proportion neutered in the population for that breed, divided by the same rate for the Chihuahua breed.

Chihuahua. The cocker spaniel had the highest rate among the breeds listed.

Survival data indicated that animals that had malignant mammary tumors removed had excess deaths concentrated in the first year after cancer removal. The death rate was 2.5 times the rate in a matched control population not having mammary cancer.[3] Because of treatment costs and the age of the animals, euthanasia or death is likely if additional tumors or complications develop. Over 70 per cent of dogs studied developed additional tumors.[3] The younger the dog, the longer the period before additional tumors or complications developed. In 42 months after diagnosis of the first cancer, 50 per cent of dogs 6 years or younger developed additional mammary cancer, whereas 75 per cent of dogs 10 years and over developed such cancer. As there are eight to ten mammary glands, a variable number of glands may independently express tumors. This expression, however, appears to be age-related: the older an animal, the sooner a subsequent mammary tumor may occur.

Neutering animals after cancer development did not prolong life. It appeared that younger animals were more likely to be neutered as part of the cancer treatment. In a group of 75 animals with first malignancies, 20 animals neutered before mammary

tumor diagnosis had a mean age of 11.0 years, 41 animals not neutered had a mean age of 11.1 years and 14 animals neutered as part of the cancer treatment had a mean age of only 9.0 years, at least 2 years younger than the other two groups.[3] Average ages of death for the three groups were 12.2 years, 12.5 years and 11.3 years, respectively. Thus while the group neutered as part of the cancer treatment survived on the average about 1 year longer, this can be attributed to their increased life expectancies at the time of cancer diagnosis. From life tables that I have calculated for the dog, an 11-year-old female can be expected to live 3.6 years more, while a 9-year-old female can be expected to live an additional 4.9 years.

TUMORS OF THE FEMALE GENITAL SYSTEM

The median age for female dogs having genital tumors was between 9 and 10 years. Most tumors of the ovary were adeno- types, with malignancies constituting about 33 per cent of the total. Of 44 tumors, three were dysgerminomas (the female counterpart of the seminoma in the male), suggesting that this tumor may not be as rare in the bitch as previously thought.

About 75 per cent of tumors of the uterus were smooth muscle lesions, principally benign (leiomyomas). Almost all of the tumors of the external genitalia occurred in the vagina. Since tumors of the vulva consist of skin tumor types, they were not included in this article. The vaginal tumors were overwhelmingly benign, with approximately 80 per cent being either leiomyomas or fibromas.

The effects of neutering on tumor rates for the female genitalia are shown in Table 4. The external genitalia tumor rate was approximately 12 times greater in intact females. The primary tumor of both the uterus and vagina was the leiomyoma, and possibly the expression of this tumor type at both sites is hormonally related.

TUMORS OF THE MALE GENITAL SYSTEM

The median age for male dogs having genital tumors was between 10 and 11 years. The principal site was the testes. Of approxi-

TABLE 4. *Genital Tumor Expression In Intact and Neutered Female and Male Dogs*

Site	Rates per 100,000 per year		
	BOTH	INTACT	NEUTERED
Female:			
All genital	20.0	53.2	3.0
Ovary and uterus	6.9	20.5	0.2*
External genitalia	13.1	32.7	2.8
Male:			
All genital	85.7	104.9	9.7
Testes	76.3	96.5	—
Prostate	7.4	7.2	8.4
External genitalia	2.0	1.2	1.3

*An adenocarcinoma occurred at the stump of the uterus in a neutered female.

mately 600 testicular tumors, about 50 per cent were Sertoli cell tumors and 33 per cent were seminomas. Most of the others were interstitial cell tumors. Because of the potential for malignancy, seminomas were classified as malignant and accounted for most of the malignant testicular tumor rate in Table 1. However, few testicular tumors are metastatic in the dog, even by local extension. Retained testicles have a very high rate of tumors. The prostatic tumors were practically all adenocarcinomas. Tumors of the external genitalia, primarily of the penis, were mostly transmissible venereal tumors. These were diagnosed in dogs recently imported into the area; this tumor does not appear to be able to maintain itself in the native population. Other tumors of the penis included various epithelial and connective tissue lesions. Tumors of the skin of the penis and of the scrotum were not included in this article.

Neutering males had no effect on genital tumor occurrence. The apparent eleven-fold reduction in all male genital system tumors (Table 4) was due to the absence of testicular tumors in neutered males. Prostatic and external genitalia tumor rates were the same in neutered and intact groups.

SUMMARY

In summary, mammary tumors are the most frequent tumors of the reproductive system in the bitch. Neutering before maturity reduces the risk of their development. Neutering after mammary tumor expression does not prevent additional tumors or prolong the life of a bitch. Once a mammary tumor occurs, there is a high probability that a subsequent mammary tumor, or mammary tumor complications, will occur in that animal. How soon this will happen is related to age: the older the bitch, the sooner it can be expected.

The principal tumor of the uterus and vagina was the leiomyoma. The expression of this tumor at these sites may be hormonally related, since it occurs in such high frequency in intact bitches.

The principal tumor of the male genital system was the Sertoli cell tumor in the testes. Neutering had no effect on genital tumor occurrence in the male.

REFERENCES

1. Schneider, R.: A population-based animal tumor registry. *In* Ingram, D. G., Mitchell, W. R. and Martin, S. W. (Eds.): Animal Disease Monitoring. Springfield, Ill., Charles C Thomas, Publisher, 1975.
2. Schneider, R. and Vaida, M. L.: Survey of canine and feline populations: Alameda and Contra Costa counties, California, 1970. J.A.V.M.A., *166*:481, 1975.
3. Schneider, R., Dorn, C. R. and Taylor, D. O. N.: Factors influencing canine mammary cancer development and postsurgical survival. J. Nat. Cancer Inst., *43*:1249, 1969.

Neoplasms of the Reproductive Organs and Mammary Glands of the Dog

STEVEN E. CROW

Michigan State University, East Lansing, Michigan

INTRODUCTION

While tumors of the mammary glands of dogs are frequently encountered by the small animal practitioner, neoplasms of the reproductive organs are less commonly observed. Clinical recognition, however, is not necessarily indicative of the relative incidence of these neoplasms. Although uncommonly recognized as a cause of clinical disease, tumors of the testes are exceeded in frequency only by those of the skin and connective tissue in male dogs. In contrast, the relatively rare ovarian tumors in female dogs are almost always recognized clinically. Transmissible venereal tumor is rarely encountered in much of the world; yet in certain areas of the world, it is a common neoplasm.

Treatment for tumors of the reproductive tracts and mammary glands of the dog has previously been limited to surgical excision. In animals with advanced, inoperable neoplasms, euthanasia has been recommended. However, in recent years other treatment modalities have been incorporated into the management of these neoplasms. These include radiotherapy, chemotherapy, immunotherapy and cryosurgery and may be employed as the primary treatment or as an adjuvant to surgery.

The ultimate goal of any treatment is cure. However, in advanced cancer cases in which cure is unlikely, treatment may serve other useful purposes including: (1) temporary palliation of symptoms, (2) prolonged survival and (3) improved quality of survival. Benign tumors are almost always successfully treated by surgical resection, whereas malignant neoplasms are rarely cured by surgery because they frequently metastasize to inoperable sites. Therefore, it is essential that the clinician obtain tissue for histopathological examination before proper treatment can be prescribed or a prognosis rendered. Whenever feasible, wide excisional biopsy is preferred. If general anesthesia is required, biopsy is delayed until physical status can be evaluated.

Since most of these patients are older animals, an extended data base should be obtained. After a careful physical examination and clinical history have been completed, the performance status, including liver and kidney function, should be carefully evaluated. Staging procedures should include a complete blood count, urinalysis, blood urea nitrogen (BUN), serum glutamic pyruvic transaminase (SGPT), serum alkaline phosphatase (SAP) and thoracic radiographs. Regional lymph nodes should be carefully examined. Abdominal radiographs are indicated for detection of mammary and testicular tumors or when abnormal structures are suspected by palpation or ballottement.

Following clinical staging procedures and the establishment of a histological diagnosis, a treatment program is devised and a prognosis for disease-free interval and survival is estimated. While no scheme for staging of canine reproductive tract or mammary tumors has been widely accepted, the reader is referred to a scheme for staging of solid tumors, which classifies the size of the primary neoplasm and the presence of metastases in lymph nodes and other organs.[3] An appreciation of tumor mass and tissue involvement should afford guidelines for the selection of the various modes of treatment.

Surgery remains the treatment of choice for most solid neoplasms (with a few exceptions to be discussed later in this article) and should be employed whenever possible without disrupting the function of associated structures. Subtotal resection may be of value by decreasing tumor mass and thereby reducing the cell population prior to the initiation of adjuvant therapy.

While cryotherapy is useful in several tumor types, it is unlikely that it will receive wide usage in the treatment of reproductive tract or mammary tumors. Specific advantages are that cryotherapy may be used with minimal anesthesia (local or mild sedation) and that it may stimulate recognition of tumor antigens by the immune system.

Radiation therapy may be used either as the primary therapy or as an adjunct to surgery or cryosurgery. Superficial tumors that are known to be radiosensitive are treated with 4000 to 6000 rads total dose of external beam irradiation administered in 500-rad fractions three times weekly. For deeper lesions, a cobalt teletherapy source should be used to avoid serious complications such as moist desquamation or deep ulceration of the skin. Concomitant chemotherapy should be avoided, as it may potentiate these cutaneous complications.

Chemotherapy is most often used as palliative treatment in disseminated malignancies. However, it may be used "prophylactically" as an adjunct to surgery when the development of metastatic disease is expected. The use of cytotoxic drugs must always be closely controlled and monitored. Anticancer agents are dosed on the basis of body surface area, which may be calculated from body weight using conversion factors (Table 1). Weekly examination, including packed cell volume (PCV), total white blood count (WBC) and differential and platelet quantitation, is recommended. Cytotoxic agents are discontinued temporarily if the PCV is less than 25 per cent, WBC less than 3000/μl, neutrophils less than 1000/μl and platelets less than 50,000/μl. A list of frequently used, commercially available compounds and recommended dosages and frequency of administration is also provided (Table 2). Specific indications and effective combinations will be given for individual tumors in later sections of this article.

Immunotherapy is a promising mode for treating cancer. It is best used when the tumor load has been reduced to microscopic size. Exciting data from many laboratories have prompted its application in the management of cancer at several veterinary institutions. However, since immunotherapy remains a poorly understood and experimental procedure, specific treatment recommendations would be premature.

TUMORS OF THE EPIDERMIS OF THE EXTERNAL GENITALIA

All tumors of the skin and adnexal tissues may occur on the prepuce, scrotum or vulva. Mast cell tumors and melanomas are fre-

quently seen on the scrotum. Fortunately, most melanomas in this site are benign, and surgical removal is curative. Ulcerated lesions of the male inguinal region are frequently mast cell tumors and should be approached cautiously. Diagnosis is best made by fine needle aspiration and cytological examination using new methylene blue or Wright-Giemsa stains. Unless wide surgical extirpation can be accomplished, such as by scrotal ablation, these tumors may be better treated by radiation therapy or cryosurgery. Inadequate surgical removal of associated tissues frequently results in inguinal dissemination. The inguinal lymph node should be palpated and removed if suspected of having tumor infiltration. The prepuce or scrotum may be extremely hot, swollen, bruised and painful because of histamine release from neoplastic mast cells. Significant improvement in these cases is not expected, but palliative therapy with high oral doses of

TABLE 1. *Conversion Table of Weight to Body Surface Area in Meters for the Dog**

kg	m^2	kg	m^2
0.5	0.06	23.0	0.81
1.0	0.10	24.0	0.83
1.5	0.13	25.0	0.85
2.0	0.15	26.0	0.88
2.5	0.18	27.0	0.90
3.0	0.20	28.0	0.92
3.5	0.23	29.0	0.94
4.0	0.25	30.0	0.96
4.5	0.27	31.0	0.99
5.0	0.29	32.0	1.01
6.0	0.33	33.0	1.03
7.0	0.36	34.0	1.05
8.0	0.40	35.0	1.07
9.0	0.43	36.0	1.09
10.0	0.46	37.0	1.11
11.0	0.49	38.0	1.13
12.0	0.52	39.0	1.15
13.0	0.55	40.0	1.17
14.0	0.58	41.0	1.19
15.0	0.60	42.0	1.21
16.0	0.63	43.0	1.23
17.0	0.66	44.0	1.25
18.0	0.69	45.0	1.26
19.0	0.71	46.0	1.28
20.0	0.74	47.0	1.30
21.0	0.76	48.0	1.32
22.0	0.78	49.0	1.34
		50.0	1.36

*After Theilen, G. H.: *In* Ettinger, S. F. (Ed.): Textbook of Veterinary Internal Medicine. Philadelphia, W. B. Saunders Co., 1975.

TABLE 2. *Dosage, Frequency of Administration, Route and Associated Toxicities of Certain Antineoplastic Drugs*

Drug	Dosage and Frequency	Route	Major Toxic Effects
Chlorambucil (Leukeran)	2.0 mg/m² BSA* 2 × weekly	Oral	Myelosuppression
Cyclophosphamide (Cytoxan)	50 mg/m² BSA 4 × weekly	Oral	Myelosuppression, hemorrhagic cystitis
Cytosine arabinoside (Cytosar)	100 mg/m² BSA 4 × weekly	Subcutaneous or intravenous	Myelosuppression
5-fluorouracil (Fluorouracil)	200 mg/m² BSA once weekly	Intravenous	Neurological
Methotrexate	2.5–5.0 mg/m² BSA q2d	Oral	Gastrointestinal, myelosuppression
Prednisone	20–40 mg/m² BSA b.i.d. daily × 7d; then 10–20 mg/m² BSA b.i.d. q2d	Oral	Polyuria, polydipsia, polyphagia, muscle wasting
Vinblastine (Velban)	2.0 mg/m² BSA once weekly	Intravenous	Myelosuppression
Vincristine (Oncovin)	0.5 mg/m² BSA once weekly	Intravenous	Myelosuppression

*BSA = body surface area.

prednisone and antihistamine (Benadryl, 100 mg/m² t.i.d.) may make the animal more comfortable. Partial remissions of 1 to 3 months have been seen in dogs given cytosine arabinoside, cyclophosphamide and vinblastine in combination with prednisone.

Squamous cell carcinoma of the prepuce or vulva is treated with surgery or radiation. The prognosis varies from favorable to poor, depending on the size and depth of the lesion. Metastasis to the inguinal lymph nodes may occur.

TRANSMISSIBLE VENEREAL TUMOR

Transmissible venereal tumor (TVT), now rare in the United States, is unique in several respects. First, TVT is spread by transplantation during coitus. Second, its cells contain from 57 to 62 chromosomes instead of the normal canine complement of 78 chromosomes. Dogs of any breed or age not previously exposed are susceptible, but sexually-active young adult dogs are most frequently affected. There is considerable variation in the appearance and behavior of TVT, ranging from small hyperemic papules to ulcerated, lobulated, sessile masses up to 5 cm in diameter. Tumors are located on the penis and prepuce or on the vulva or vagina of the female dog. Occasionally, TVT may metastasize to the inguinal lymph nodes and skin and less often to the liver, spleen and eyes. Many lesions may undergo spontaneous regression, but some will persist and may result in the death of the animal.

Treatment of TVT is not clearly defined. Many authors recommend surgical excision for immediate relief, but recurrence is not unusual. Response of localized lesions to radiation has been reported. Since TVT should be considered malignant until proved otherwise, chemotherapy should be used as an adjuvant to surgery or in treatment of established metastatic disease. Vincristine, methotrexate and cyclophosphamide used in combination will usually cause regression within 4 to 8 weeks. Treatment should continue for several weeks after complete regression is noted.

Dogs that have recovered from TVT are said to be immune for subsequent infection, but the mechanism is not fully understood. Transfusion of blood or serum from "immune" dogs has been recommended as a treatment for TVT.

TUMORS OF THE MALE REPRODUCTIVE TRACT

Testicular Tumors

Tumors of the testes are usually found in dogs over 7 years of age. Three main types of tumors are the Sertoli cell tumor (SCT), the interstitial cell tumor (ICT) and the seminoma. The incidence for all three types is about equal when clinical bias is eliminated. Cryptorchid testes are said to have an increased incidence of tumors, especially of Sertoli cell tumors.[2]

Sertoli cell tumors develop from the nurse cells of the seminiferous tubules. When these cells become neoplastic, a firm mass may be palpated in the testis. SCT occurs bilaterally or simultaneously with either seminoma or interstitial cell tumor. Signs of feminization occur in approximately 25 per cent of all dogs with SCT.

Most SCT's are biologically benign. However, since 10 per cent or more of these tumors are malignant, staging procedures are completed prior to bilateral orchiectomy. Metastases to the inguinal, iliac and sublumbar lymph nodes and to the lungs, liver, spleen, kidney and pancreas have been reported. Undetected metastases should be suspected when feminization signs persist for more than 4 to 6 weeks after castration. Malignant SCT may respond to cyclophosphamide or methotrexate treatment.

Seminomas arise from the spermatogenic cells of the seminiferous tubules. Because these tumors are usually less than 2 cm in diameter, only one-third of these lesions are detected clinically as an enlargement of one of the testicles. Occasionally, alopecia and feminization signs occur. Bilateral orchiectomy is again the treatment of choice and is usually curative. Whereas this neoplasm metastasizes rapidly and frequently in man, it rarely does so in the dog. Localized lesions are quite radiosensitive. Vincristine and cyclophosphamide have been recommended for disseminated seminoma, but the prognosis for these cases is grave.

The interstitial cell tumor arises from the cells of Leydig that are located between seminiferous tubules. Due to its lack of clinically detectable hormone production and relatively small size, ICT is rarely recognized clinically. Metastases are rare. Castration is almost always curative.

Prostatic Neoplasms

While benign glandular and smooth muscle tumors of the prostate have been reported, adenocarcinoma is the most frequently diagnosed neoplasm of the canine prostate. Affected dogs are usually older than 8 years of age. These malignant neoplasms tend to spread by extension and invade the urethra, urinary bladder and pelvic skeleton. Hydronephrosis and hydroureter sometimes result. Fine needle aspiration, catheterization with prostatic massage and contrast cystography help to confirm the diagnosis of prostatic adenocarcinoma.

Unfortunately, metastases to the lungs and regional lymph nodes have usually occurred prior to diagnosis. Castration followed by exogenous estrogen therapy (estradiol cypionate, ECP, 0.5 to 2 mg intramuscularly every 3 to 6 weeks) may be temporarily palliative. Invasive carcinomas that do not respond to hormonal therapy are treated with a combination of cyclophosphamide and 5-fluorouracil. The prognosis in all cases is unfavorable.

Penile Tumors

Squamous cell carcinoma and fibroma have been reported to occur on the penis. Extension of the former to the prepuce is common, and such cases should be treated by surgery and radiotherapy as previously described. In extensive lesions, penile and preputial amputation are indicated. Antepubic or perineal urethrostomy should be performed prior to amputation.

TUMORS OF THE FEMALE REPRODUCTIVE TRACT

Ovarian Tumors

Primary tumors of the canine ovary have been infrequently reported. As in the testicular-stromal tumors, ovarian neoplasms may cause endocrine abnormalities or may be an incidental finding during physical examination. No consistent clinical features are associated with these tumors, although persistent or prolonged estrus, vaginal discharge and gynecomastia are frequently noted. Cystic endometrial hyperplasia or pyometra may occur concurrently. Abdominal distention with ascites is frequently the presenting sign. The granulosa-theca cell tumor, which arises from ovarian follicular cells, is the most common. Ovariohysterectomy is the treatment of choice. The tumor is usually benign but has been reported to metastasize via lymphatic vessels or direct extension in the peritoneal cavity. Therefore, the abdominal lymph nodes and peritoneum are carefully examined during surgery for evidence of tumor spread; any abnormal tissue is resected. Adjuvant chemotherapy with 5-fluorouracil and cyclophosphamide is recommended for such cases.

Ovarian adenomas (serous cystadenoma and pseudomucinous cystadenoma) are the second most common ovarian tumors. These benign tumors originate from the coelomic epithelium of the ovary and occur most often in older nulliparous bitches. Both tumors are treated successfully by ovariohysterectomy.

Serous cystadenocarcinoma is a rare neoplasm in the dog. Ascites with no endocrine disturbance may lead the clinician to suspect the presence of peritoneal dissemination. Cytological examination of free abdominal fluid may reveal cellular rosettes or "signet ring" cells characteristic of adenocarcinoma. These neoplasms grow rapidly and metastasize readily to the liver and lungs. Therefore, therapy is merely palliative. Subtotal resection should be attempted to reduce the tumor mass. Combination chemotherapy with chlorambucil, cyclophosphamide and 5-fluorouracil plus judicious use of a diuretic (furosemide, chlorothiazide) may temporarily control the peritoneal effusion. One author has recommended intraperitoneal infusion of triethylenethiophosphoramide (Thio-TEPA) at a dose of 0.2 to 0.4 mg/lb after drainage of fluid by paracentesis. A grave prognosis must be offered.

Dysgerminomas develop from the germinal epithelium of the ovary and are the female analog to testicular seminoma in the male dog. These tumors are considered malignant and are reported to metastasize to the lymph nodes, kidneys and liver. Disseminated tumors should be treated aggressively. Chemotherapeutic agents that are recommended include vincristine and cyclophosphamide. The prognosis for metastatic dysgerminoma is unfavorable.

In addition to its primary neoplasms, the ovary may be the site of visceral metastasis of other malignancies and should always be examined during exploratory celiotomy.

Uterine and Vaginal Tumors

The most common neoplasms of the female genital tract are the fibroma and leiomyoma. They occur in older bitches and are rarely associated with clinical signs, usually presenting as a mass protruding from the vulva. Occasionally, tenesmus or constipation is noted. Surgical resection (ovariohysterectomy for uterine masses) is curative.

Their malignant counterparts, leiomyosarcoma and fibrosarcoma, are rarely seen. These tumors spread by local invasion but will sometimes metastasize via blood or lymphatic vessels. Surgery is again the treatment of choice. Radiotherapy may afford temporary control of unresectable masses.

Lipomas of the vagina are slow-growing, well-circumscribed masses occurring outside or within the vaginal lumen. Intraluminal lipomas are frequently pedunculated, while extraluminal masses cause bulges in the perineum. Fine needle aspiration will often provide the diagnosis. Surgical excision is usually effective when elected. Many animals with lipomas are obese; weight reduction may discourage recurrence or the development of new lipomas.

MAMMARY GLAND TUMORS

Neoplasms of the mammary glands are the most common tumors of the bitch. Less then half of these tumors are diagnosed histologically as malignancies. Nevertheless, mammary cancer accounts for almost 50 per cent of all malignancies of the bitch. Mammary tumors are seen in older dogs, with a mean age of 10.5 years at diagnosis. Purebred dogs appear to have an increased risk relative to mixed breed dogs. The sparing effect of early ovariohysterectomy on the development of mammary tumors has been documented.

Approximately 65 per cent of the tumors involve the fourth and fifth glands, while the first gland is least commonly affected. The reasons for this are unknown, although trauma by the hindlegs and increased hormonal influence have been suggested. Multiple tumors in one or both chains of mammary glands are a common finding.

Benign mammary lesions include adenomas, fibromas, ductal papillomas and mixed mammary tumors. Commonly encountered malignant tumors are carcinomas and mixed tumors. The latter, which contain both epithelial and mesenchymal (myoepithelial) components, may differentiate into carcinomas or sarcomas. All malignant mammary neoplasms may potentially metastasize, although fewer than 50 per cent do. The most frequent sites of metastasis are the lungs, liver, skin and bone.

Proper management of mammary tumors requires strict adherence to an established plan. All mammary enlargements should be evaluated for possible neoplasia. Mammary nodules or swellings should be biopsied. Depending on the size and characteristics of the lesion and the preference of the surgeon, a core or an excisional biopsy is submitted for histopathological examination. Presurgical evaluation should include all procedures discussed in the opening remarks of this article. While many dogs are geriatric patients, most of these animals are acceptable surgical candidates.

Benign neoplasms are treated by excision of the affected gland. While a good prognosis may be given, many of these dogs will develop new mammary tumors in the future. Each new tumor should be considered cancerous until proved otherwise. In the case of multiple mammary nodules, radical resection of the entire affected chain of glands is the preferred method of treatment. When both groups of mammae are involved, a two-step bilateral radical mastectomy is recommended. Previously unspayed bitches are ovariohysterectomized when bilateral mastectomy is performed. While spaying may have no effect on the progression of the mammary neoplasms, it will prevent unwanted pregnancy and resultant nursing problems.

Malignant mammary tumors are treated by radical mastectomy of the entire affected chain. If there is gross enlargement or cytological evidence of tumor infiltration of the axillary or superficial inguinal lymph nodes, these should be removed and sectioned by the pathologist. Apparently normal or reactive lymph nodes should be spared, as they are the body's first line of defense against metastasis. This is especially true for carcinomas.

Adjuvant chemotherapy for breast cancer in women has had only limited success in improving 5-year survival statistics. Useful agents for carcinomas in women include cyclophosphamide, methotrexate and 5-fluorouracil. These drugs used in combination have shown improved remission and survival data over single-agent chemotherapy. Sarcomas, generally less responsive to anticancer drugs than their epithelial counterparts, are treated with cyclophosphamide and vincristine.

Some mammary gland malignancies have metastasized by the time of diagnosis. Chemotherapy in such cases is sometimes palliative. In particular, progression of skin metastases may be checked for periods up to 2 to 3 months, and inflammatory tumor nodules become quiescent for similar periods. Regression of pulmonary nodules has not been witnessed by this author.

Radiotherapy, a vital modality in the management of human breast cancer, has received very little attention in treating canine mammary cancer. The extensive field of mammary tissue and the potential damage to underlying viscera are reasons for omitting this mode of therapy. However, treatment of cutaneous metastases by external beam irradiation is highly successful in women and would likely be so for dogs. Cryosurgery of cutaneous and subcutaneous nodules may be a satisfactory way to handle skin metastases as well. Immunotherapy for canine mammary cancer is presently being investigated.

Several factors have been correlated with prognosis in evaluating mammary cancer patients. In general, malignant mammary tumors are larger than benign neoplasms. However, small, ulcerated tumors suggest a poorer prognosis. Ulceration in large tumors is more a reflection of trauma or pressure necrosis than of malignancy. Breed variation in postoperative survival has been evaluated, with German shepherds having a significantly shorter length of survival than dachshunds and beagles. In addition, bitches whose tumors had been present for greater than 6 months lived longer than those with shorter preoperative courses.[1]

The single most important prognostic factor remains the histogenetic classification of the tumor. Among the malignant tumors, mixed mammary tumors carry an intermediate prognosis with a mean postoperative survival period of 10 months. Tubular and papillary carcinomas arising in mixed tumors warrant a fair prognosis (mean survival approximately 24 months), while solid and anaplastic carcinomas bear a grave prognosis (mean survival approximately 7 months). Scirrhous (fibrous) reaction in a mammary carcinoma is associated with early, frequent recurrences following surgery. In addition, the presence of lymphatic infiltration must be assessed. Histopathological evidence of lymphatic vessel invasion portends a short survival period after diagnosis (approximately 4 to 12 months).

REFERENCES

1. Bostock, D. E.: The prognosis following the surgical excision of canine mammary neoplasms. Europ. J. Cancer *11*:389, 1975.

2. Lipowitz, A. J., Schwartz, A. and Wilson, G. P.: Testicular neoplasms and concomitant clinical changes in the dog. J.A.V.M.A., *163*:1364, 1973.
3. Madewell, B. R.: Clinical diagnosis of cancer. Proceedings 42nd Annual Meeting American Animal Hospital Association, II. Cincinnati, Ohio, 1975, pp. 90–92.
4. Theilen, G. H.: Veterinary Medical Oncology. *In* Ettinger, S. J. (Ed.): Textbook of Veterinary Internal Medicine. Philadelphia, W. B. Saunders Co., 1975, pp. 127–149.

Infertility in the Male Dog

ROLF E. LARSEN

University of Florida, Gainesville, Florida

Little information concerning fertility in the male dog is available in the scientific literature. This is due partially to the limited number of females that any particular male breeds in a lifetime and, until recently, to the lack of emphasis on the use of artificial insemination.

Patients presented as infertile can be classified as never fertile (primary infertility), subfertile, or infertile with a history of previous fertility (acquired infertility). The group diagnosed as infertile but with a history of past fertility appears to be the largest. This probably reflects management and owner concern more than an actual incidence of genital lesions in the population. In one review of 200 dogs presented for fertility evaluation, 158 of the 200 had similar histories of reproductive failure and azoospermia at an average age of onset of 3 1/2 years. This may reflect purebred dog management in areas where males are used at stud once or twice at a young age before gaining a reputation in the show ring. Another common pattern is for males to be presented after three to four failures at stud with no history of any breeding attempts before 2 or 3 years of age. Degenerative changes may have appeared during this time span in many animals and have gone unrecognized.

PRIMARY INFERTILITY

Testicular hypoplasia may occur in varying degrees, although it is commonly associated with complete azoospermia. Testicles are small and may be either hard or soft in consistency. The epididymides are easily palpated. Libido in most cases is not affected. Hereditary hypoplasia has been described for other domestic animals. Whether oligospermic dogs may be placed in this category is questionable, but partial hypoplasia may explain why many dogs show oligospermia from puberty in the absence of any clinical signs or historically significant event. Histologically, testicular structure may vary from only a single layer of Sertoli cells in the tubules to the presence of all spermatogenic cell types. Leydig cells and other interstitial tissue appear normal, and tubule walls and basement membranes have a normal thickness.

Bilateral segmental aplasia of the epididymis is known to occur, resulting in azoospermia but maintaining normal ejaculatory reflexes. The defect may be detectable by careful palpation.

Epididymo-orchitis may occur prepuberally and result in permanent damage to the epididymis or testicular tissue. Historical information related to such an event is seldom available, and evidence of long-term damage must be diagnosed on physical examination or biopsy.

Defects in the hypothalamic-pituitary-gonadal axis may be suspected in an animal with a juvenile appearance or other signs of endocrine disorders. Eunuchoidism or hypogonadotropic hypogonadism has not been specifically diagnosed in the dog with laboratory confirmation. These animals, however, should respond to gonadotropic treatments; the general absence of response of infertile dogs so treated suggests either that this is not a common condition or that proper treatments are not in use. Biochemical defects in androgen synthesis are known to occur in man but have not been specifically identified in the dog.

Animals with sperm in the ejaculate may be completely sterile if there is a high percentage of sperm abnormalities. High percentages of acrosomal defects, cytoplasmic droplets, midpiece defects or reversed tails have been observed in sterile dogs that appear clinically normal. Rapid loss of sperm motility has also been associated with infertility.

SUBFERTILITY

Most males classified as subfertile are oligospermic or normospermic with poor motility of or abnormal spermatozoa. The testes of these animals are often small. The animal may have a history of siring small litters. The presence of proximal droplets, detached heads, doubled structures, tail defects or abnormal acrosomes with an incidence of over 20 per cent for any one defect results in subfertility. Inguinal hernia with omentum or intestine extending into the scrotum has been associated with poor morphology, motility and concentration of sperm. Irritation caused by movement of abdominal tissue within the vaginal tunics and insulation of the scrotum are possible explanations for poor semen quality. Although the hernia is most often unilateral, function of both testicles may be adversely affected. Varicocele, i.e., tortuosity of the testicular veins within the spermatic cord, is often associated with subfertility in man. This condition involves venous congestion and abnormal blood flow related to man's upright walking position. It is unlikely that this condition occurs in the dog.

ACQUIRED INFERTILITY

Acquired testicular and excurrent duct (includes the efferent ducts, epididymis and vas deferens) injury may be due to a variety of factors, and even infertility due to infectious diseases may be mediated by changes in the circulation and temperature of the testicle. Heat, ischemia, advanced age, sexual overuse, chemical toxicities, tumors, scrotal dermatitis, psychological and environmental stress, duct obstruction, infectious diseases, autoimmune phenomena and hormonal disturbances have all been shown to have detrimental effects on the canine testis.

Heat

Warming the testes to body temperature has been shown to cause loss of sperm motility and eventual loss of sperm production. Experiments with cryptorchid dogs have clearly shown loss of spermatogenic function in abdominal testes. In scrotal testicles, however, warming to body temperature for 10 days is not sufficient to cause irreversible damage. Dogs appear to have the capacity to recover from the degeneration caused by elevated scrotal temperatures to a greater degree than some other species. Testosterone production by the testis is not adversely affected by temperatures up to 39.7° C. Therefore, degenerative changes probably cannot be blamed directly on alteration in testosterone secretion.

Ischemia

Testicular ischemia has been investigated in a number of ways in the dog and has the potential for producing severe, permanent damage. Complete ischemia, as might be seen with torsion, produces loss of spermatogenic capability within 1 to 2 hours, although some Leydig cells may remain even after days of torsion if blockage of blood flow is not complete. It has been suggested that low arterial irrigation of the canine testis for even short periods of time may produce semipermanent damage to testosterone-producing cells.

Age

Senile atrophy of the testis is commonly seen in dogs over 10 years of age. The American Kennel Club (AKC) does not recognize litters produced by a sire of more than 12 years of age unless breeding soundness is confirmed by a veterinarian. The giant breeds seldom can be used past 8 years of age.

Sexual Overuse

Collection of semen every other day, while maintaining sperm numbers, is possible for indefinite periods in the normal dog. However, this appears not to be true in some individuals. Proper management of these individuals will help maintain acceptable fertility. In one documented case of spermatogenic "fatigue" and azoospermia, the dog responded to 3 months of sexual rest with a full recovery.

Scrotal Dermatitis

Canine scrotal skin is extremely sensitive to both traumatic and chemical irritation. In most surgical procedures, an attempt should be made to approach scrotal contents through incisions in abdominal or perineal skin proximal to the skin with the underlying tunica dartos. Surgical preparation of the scrotum should involve careful clipping, rather than shaving of the skin, with minimal abrasions or shaver burns. It is common for dogs to lick open incisions or cuts of the scrotum, causing healing to take place by granulation. Dogs forced to sit on cement floors that are cleaned and dampened with disinfectant solutions will often show a wrinkled, hyperemic scrotal skin. Dogs with a painful epididymitis or orchitis may cause scrotal dermatitis by constant licking. Insect bites and stings in the scrotal area have resulted in sterility and abnormal sperm morphology for periods up to a year. Poor motility, bent tails and loose heads have been the findings in reported cases.

Environmental Stress

Healthy dogs caged in new surroundings may develop changes in the germinal epithelium. These changes are reversible, and a return to normal may be seen after 6 months in the new environment. High environmental temperatures for extended periods may result in scrotal heating.

Duct Occlusion

Obstruction of the vas deferens or epididymis is seldom diagnosed in the dog but may be a sequela of epididymitis or spermatocele. Vasectomy in the dog results in degenerative pressure changes in the testis, but these changes are not permanent, and the testes return to normal in most males. The effects of ligation of the cauda epididymidis result in softening and reduction of size of the testis. Leydig cells remain unchanged, but the seminiferous tubules undergo degenerative changes in 1 to 3 months. It has been shown in other species that the closer the epididymal blockage to the testis, the more severe the damage. Atrophic and degenerative changes may be a result of blood stasis caused by the increase in pressure within the tubules and the resistance of the tunica albuginea to that pressure.

Autoimmune Phenomena

Spermatozoa are antigenic to the male producing them, as are certain other body tissues and products such as thyroglobulin. Diseases or trauma exposing testicular tissue or spermatozoa to the immune system may cause the formation of antibodies and the development of sensitized white blood cells, as well as causing a local reaction. A lymphocytic thyroiditis described in certain strains of beagles has been associated with a genetic predisposition to the development of lymphocytic orchitis. Pathological changes associated with this condition include reduction in size and weight of the testis and sterility or reduced fertility. Lymphocytic infiltrations are present in the epididymis and all portions of the testis. Focal degeneration, segmental atrophy and diffuse atrophy of the testis may be seen in this condition.

Inflammatory responses due to any agent may interrupt the integrity of duct walls and cause release of spermatozoa, with exposure of the body to the foreign spermatozoal antigens. Spermatozoa escaping into surrounding tissue initiate the formation of sperm granulomas. Sperm stasis caused by congenital or acquired blockage of the ducts may also result in the formation of spermatoceles, with eventual rupture or degeneration of the duct and further exposure to antigenic elements. When sperm granulomas occur at the level of the efferent ducts, the inflammatory response in severe cases will completely block the passage of sperm to the epididymis.

Chemical Toxicities

Cadmium has been shown to cause severe damage to both Leydig cells and seminiferous tubules, initiating a rapid necrosis of the testis at dosages having no known side effects on other body organs. α-Chlorohydrin, an alkylating agent experimentally used to render epididymal sperm infertile in many species, causes pathological changes in both the epididymis and the testis in the dog. Certain antibiotics such as amphotericin B cause testicular atrophy, and antineoplastic mitotic inhibitors such as cyclophosphamide and vinblastine affect cell division in the testis. Many other drugs, particularly those with estrogenic or antiandrogenic activity, may also cause testicular atrophy. Cytostatic drugs such as the alkylating agents (chlorambucil, cyclophosphamide) are capable of causing genetic damage. Adenomyosis of the epididymis, characterized by invasion of the muscular layers of the tubule by the epithelial lining, may occur as a result of estrogenic stimulation. Sperm migrate into the blind sacs formed as part of this process, and sperm granulomas develop in some cases. Normal, sterile urine, experimentally injected into the vas deferens of normal dogs and forced into the epididymis, causes inflammation of the epididymis. Retrograde flow of urine into the epididymis during violent exercise or traumatic injury could, therefore, be an explanation for occasional incidents of acute epididymitis with negative bacteriological laboratory results.

Epididymitis

Escherichia coli, Proteus spp., *Streptococcus* and *Staphylococcus* spp. are common isolates from acute suppurative epididymitis or epididymo-orchitis. *Mycoplasma* spp. has been found in the preputial cavity of a large percentage of clinically normal dogs. This organism has been isolated from a few dogs with epididymitis. Prostatic disease is frequently associated with epididymitis and may be a primary focus of infection or contribute to retrograde movement of infectious material from the urinary tract. Infectious agents can enter the epididymis by way of the vas deferens or from the seminiferous tubules. Hematogenous movement or entrance via the lymph vessels from sites of infection elsewhere in the body, entrance through the vaginal tunic from the peritoneal cavity or direct laceration of the scrotum are also possible entry routes for infectious agents. In man, gonococcal infection of the urethra is thought to cause a breakdown in the normal resistance to movement of bacteria into the posterior urethra and vas deferens. This allows urethral flora to move into the epididymis, causing infection and acute inflammation. A specific organism causing similar problems has not been identified in the dog.

Acute infections are characterized by the presence of pus in the ducts and by abscess formation. Chronic epididymitis reveals local induration that may be accompanied by evidence of chronic obstruction, distention of the ductules, fibrous scarring and obliteration or distortion of the lumen. Recurrent acute or sustained chronic infection may result in microabscesses, scrotal sinuses or sperm granulomas.

Certain general infections of bacterial, viral, fungal or parasitic etiology have been associated with painful swelling of the scrotal contents and other effects on the testis and epididymis in different species, including the dog. The epididymis is a specific target for *Brucella canis,* and the bacteria are harbored in this organ. Transmission to a susceptible bitch can occur at the time of mating. Abnormal sperm make up 30 to 80 per cent of the ejaculate within 2 to 5 weeks after acute *B. canis* infection. More than 90 per cent of the sperm cells may be abnormal 5 months after infection. Neutrophils and monocytes are seen in the ejaculate. Evidence of an immune reaction against spermatozoa has been detected with spermagglutination tests. Lesions in the epididymis have been seen following outbreaks of distemper, and it is thought that distemper virus can cause epididymitis. During an active infection with distemper, dogs will often lose the capability to produce fluid of any kind during ejaculation. Although behavioral and physical responses may appear normal in dogs strong enough to attempt mating, neither spermatozoa nor prostatic fluid is produced by the ejaculatory reflexes. In dogs affected by this condition, testosterone in the peripheral blood drops to extremely low levels. Sperm production and testosterone secretion may return after recovery.

Orchitis

Acute orchitis may follow trauma, systemic infection, prostatitis and epididymitis. Routes of infection are the same as those causing epididymitis, and the term epididymo-orchitis is often used to describe inflammation of the scrotal contents. *Brucella canis,* distemper virus and other systemic infectious diseases cause testicular changes as well as epididymal effects. This is particularly true if infections are associated with prolonged fever. A case of ehrlichiosis was acccompanied by azoospermia and infertility for a duration of 1 year. Mild trauma, as experienced during testicular biopsy, results in a drop in sperm output that may or may not be accompanied by decreased motility. Common morphological spermatozoal defects observed following testicular trauma are bent tails, other tail defects, proximal cytoplasmic droplets and damaged acrosomes. Minor traumatic injuries, such as biopsy procedures, are usually followed by complete recovery. Complications resulting in infection, hemorrhage and continued exposure to sperm antigens or other foreign bodies may result in testicular atrophy or adhesions of the common and proper vaginal tunics.

Hormonal Disturbances

Testicular degeneration and atrophy may occur because of tumors or abnormalities of the pituitary gland or hypothalamus that interfere with gonadotropin production and release. When associated with obesity and skin changes, this syndrome is called dystrophia adiposogenitalis. Hypothyroidism may be associated with decreased spermatogenesis in the male and prolonged anestrus in the bitch. Alterations in the levels of the adrenal steroids may affect pituitary and testicular function, but laboratory analysis of the effects of Cushing's or Addison's syndrome on testosterone levels or spermatogenesis has not been performed in the dog.

Tumors

Seminomas, Sertoli cell tumors and interstitial cell tumors reduce sperm cell production and fertility. Testicular degeneration is probably due to a combination of compression on adjacent tissue and steroid production, which may act at both the pituitary and the local level. Adenomyosis of the epididymis is a common sequela of the estrogenic stimulation provided by Sertoli cell tumors. The most frequent clinical sign associated with testicular neoplasia is prostatic disease, which may contribute to further inflammation and complications in the epididymis and testis.

Balanoposthitis

Inflammation of the mucous membrane surface of the penis and prepuce may be characterized as a constant dripping of greenish pus and smegma from the prepu-

tial orifice. This condition rarely affects fertility or libido in the male. Bacterial flora of the penis is changeable and unpredictable. One case of infertility and uterine infection with *Streptococcus canis* in the bitch has been related to the presence of the same organism in the urethra of the stud. Balanoposthitis may also be diagnosed when lymphoid follicles enlarge on the penis and prepuce over the bulbus glandis area. These follicles are often cyst-like and appear to be fluid-filled. Mild irritation, such as mating or semen collection, can cause hemorrhage into the follicles and sometimes frank bleeding from the surface. In dogs used for mating and semen collection, the follicles show constant changes. Hemorrhagic cysts that cover the bulbus glandis may be completely resolved a week later, leaving no evidence of scarring or infection. The enlargement of lymphoid follicles should be considered a local mechanism of response to irritation and infection and not the cause of dripping pus and smegma. Balanoposthitis is often seen concurrently with infections of the skin and surface structures such as the ear canals and anal sacs. Urinary tract infections may also predispose an animal to the condition.

DIAGNOSIS

History and Physical Examination

A complete history, thorough physical examination and semen evaluation are the basis for the diagnosis and prognosis of infertility and testicular disease. The history should include all illnesses, injuries, treatments, management environments and owner observations related to development, behavior and mating experiences. Semen evaluation should be done in a quiet, isolated area before any other handling is attempted. A bitch in standing heat is preferable as a mount animal, although many dogs will respond to collection procedures with a proestrous or anestrous bitch. Certain dogs will refuse to respond to a bitch except for a limited period of her standing heat. Judgments should not be made concerning libido and fertility until the male has had semen collected and has been observed with a standing, flagging, estrous female. During collection of semen, the total mucous membrane surface of the penis can be examined and the os penis palpated. After the ejaculate is obtained, a complete physical examination should be performed, including careful palpation and recording of measurements of the prostate, testis, epididymis and spermatic cord.

Semen Evaluation

Semen is usually ejaculated in three distinct fractions — the presperm, the sperm-rich and the prostatic fractions. Presperm and sperm-rich fractions are generally collected in the same tube. The combined volume of these two fractions in most dogs ranges from 1.5 to 3.5 ml. The approximate volume of presperm should be noted. Some dogs have no presperm fluid, while an occasional dog will produce 8 to 10 ml. of clear fluid that may be erroneously regarded as sufficient for evaluation unless the ejaculatory reflexes are closely observed. The sperm-rich fraction is milky or opalescent in color and is easily differentiated from the clear prostatic portion. The tube can be changed when the ejaculate becomes clear, and the prostatic fraction is collected separately. The penis becomes more engorged with blood throughout the first two fractions, and care must be taken with the collection device (artificial vagina, rubber cone) to relieve pressure at the tip of the penis. The penile membranes may rupture and bleed if this is not done. If blood appears in the ejaculate, it is of immediate importance to determine whether the hemorrhage is from the surface of the penis or is issuing from the urethra together with the semen.

Gross motility and wave motion or mass activity depends on semen density and motility. Owing to the large volume of prostatic fluid in the ejaculate, sperm cell concentration must be related to total numbers of spermatozoa. A count of 200 million cells has been suggested as a minimum total acceptable, but a total of 500 million cells is generally expected from mature dogs weighing over 30 pounds. Motility is evaluated by dilution of semen with isotonic saline or 2.9 per cent sodium citrate on a heated, coverslipped glass slide. Most normal fertile dogs will have at least 80 per cent progressively motile cells. Less than 70 per cent should be considered below the standard of the general population. Abnormal movement often reflects the type of structural defect seen on morphological examination of spermatozoa. Rapid loss of motility in collected semen may be an indicator of poor fertility. Normal spermatozoa, collected as a separated sperm-rich fraction, will maintain motility for several hours and are relatively resistant to cooling. Dilution of the sperm-rich fraction with prostatic fluid will cause a more rapid loss of motility on standing.

Sperm morphology may be evaluated with a live-dead stain or a wet mount of formalin-fixed cells visualized with phase microscopy. An eosin-nigrosin stain is used in this laboratory for negative staining of spermatozoa, which are easily visualized against the dark nigrosin background. Oil immersion should be used for evaluation of sperm morphology. Although specific information on the relationship between the percentage of abnormal cells and conception rate or litter size is not available, males having conception rates unacceptable to the owner often show 40 per cent or more abnormalities of the head and midpiece. Morphological deviations from normal in the acrosome, including knobbed structures and flattening of the apical portion, are associated with infertility. Bent tails may be an indication of scrotal irritation or trauma. An incidence of any abnormality of greater than 20 per cent should be considered below the population standard. Immature dogs often show high numbers of cytoplasmic droplets; however, this is not always associated with infertility in the young animal. Because semen quality may markedly improve with age, care should be taken in the evaluation of the young dog. A follow-up examination is frequently necessary in establishing the diagnosis and prognosis in reproductive tract disorders.

Testicular Biopsy

Testicular biopsy provides a better analysis of spermatogenic function than semen evaluation alone can provide. Complete azoospermia in the mature dog with no history of former sperm production carries a very negative prognosis, which in the absence of disturbances in other organ systems is unlikely to improve regardless of the biopsy findings. In dogs with acquired infertility or a history of oligospermia, the biopsy may suggest both the etiology and severity of the degeneration.

The testicular biopsy should be obtained via a skin incision in the anesthetized dog. Surgical preparation is similar to that for castration. The incision is made over a testicle moved up under the nonscrotal skin slightly lateral to the prepuce. A 1-cm incision is made in the common vaginal tunic. The testis surface is then incised, with an attempt to avoid large surface vessels. Gentle pressure on the testis causes tissue to bulge through the incision. This tissue may be removed by cutting it with a razor blade or fine scissors. Small, fibrosed or hardened testicles often will not exude tissue from the incision, and a wedge must be taken. Closure is accomplished with one layer of sutures in the common vaginal tunic and one layer in the skin. The tunica albuginea is not sutured. Fixation should be in Bouin's fixative or other solutions that have proved valuable for testicular tissue. Formalin should not be used since it distorts tubule walls.

Oligospermic dogs often have normal-appearing seminiferous tubules and interstitial tissue. Testicular histological findings in azoospermic dogs and males with acquired infertility may range from complete loss of normal testicular architecture, to tubules with a single layer of Sertoli cells and to tubules with arrested spermatogenesis at one stage of the spermatogenic cycle. Normal structure and spermatogenic activity may suggest a lesion in the excurrent duct system. The interstitial cells may be hypertrophied, but in the absence of inflammatory cell infiltration the interstitial tissue seldom appears abnormal.

Hormonal Status

Testosterone can be accurately measured by radioimmunoassay, but this hormone has a wide range of values in both normal and abnormal dogs. Values ranging from 0.5 ng/ml to 9.0 ng/ml have been observed in fertile dogs with normal semen. There is a wide range of values during a single day, with 2.5 ng/ml or more often separating the highest and lowest values. Infertile or azoospermic dogs often have testosterone concentrations within the same range observed in normal males. Dogs with signs of systemic disease, trauma or inflammation have been observed with testosterone levels ranging from nondetectable to 5.0 ng/ml. With the exception of the very low values, it is difficult to associate testosterone concentration with spermatogenic function.

The existence of other endocrine disorders must be considered. Thyroid function should be evaluated. Skin and haircoat changes,

distribution of body fat, appetite, water consumption and general condition should be noted by both client and veterinarian.

Behavior

Mating behavior and copulatory reflexes can be evaluated only by observation of the stud with an estrous bitch. Detailed descriptions of mating attempts can often be obtained from the owner and should include time involved in foreplay, mounting attempts, response to observers, receptiveness of the bitch, type of thrusting attempted by the male and presence of an erection outside or within the prepuce. The male and female should not be in contact for a period of 12 hours before the controlled observation. Males refusing to mount an estrous bitch in a free-running situation should be allowed exposure to a muzzled and secured female. When difficulty with intromission is noted, the genitalia of the bitch should also be examined for obstructions, such as a persistent hymen, vaginal hyperplasia or vaginal tumors. Males demonstrating poor libido must be evaluated relative to their rank in a kennel social hierarchy and with the bitch herself. Males with adequate libido but unable to mount or mate should be examined for physical defects causing pain or weakness. Occasionally, an inexperienced male or a male attempting to mate a difficult bitch will develop a full erection of the bulbus glandis before intromission. When this occurs, he should immediately be isolated from the female until the penis is flaccid and then should be allowed to make another attempt.

TREATMENT

Treatment of Diagnosed Lesions

Infection and Trauma. Local infection of the testis and epididymis may be treated by antibiotic therapy and establishment of drainage. When only one testicle is seriously affected, unilateral orchiectomy is a valid approach. This surgical approach may also be used as an alternative to unilateral vasectomy in cases of epididymitis caused by retrograde flow of urine in the vas deferens. A male suffering from brucellosis should not be used at stud, and the destruction of the animal must be seriously considered. Other systemic diseases should be resolved and the dog allowed 10 to 12 weeks of sexual rest before a serious fertility evaluation is repeated.

Developmental Defects. Preputial stenosis and a persistent ventral frenulum may occasionally be observed. Surgical correction is indicated, but thought must be given to a surgical technique that will not significantly shorten the mucous membrane surface of the prepuce in cases of stenosis. A rare male will not be able to extend the penis during his thrusts, although his genitalia are normal on examination. Collection of semen and artificial insemination may be possible with such dogs, but the owner should be allowed to reflect on the use of animals with abnormal reflexes in purebred breeding programs.

Tumors. Neoplasia in scrotal testes is most often seen in aging animals. Since semen quality will be affected by the presence of the tumor, fertility may be enhanced by the removal of a single testis when the neoplasm is unilateral. If attempts to breed the dog are planned for an extended period into the future, unilateral orchiectomy with a 10 to 12-week rest period is the treatment of choice.

Inguinal Hernia. A standard surgical approach with replacement or excision of herniated omentum may be used. The testis on the affected side will swell for a week or more, and semen concentration and morphological structures will degenerate significantly. In 10 to 12 weeks, the semen should return to normal.

Balanoposthitis. The treatment of penile and preputial surface irritation and infection should include treatment of any infection of the urinary tract or skin and adnexa. Infusions of antibiotic solutions into the sheath may be effective in some cases. Hair should be clipped from the urethral orifice to facilitate examination and local treatment. Preputial culture and skin culture should be done in cases of persistent drainage of pus from the prepuce, and both local and systemic treatment should be instituted with antibiotics selected by sensitivity testing. When the lymphoid follicles themselves appear to be infected and draining, chemical cautery with astringents may be warranted, but antibiotic therapy should be explored first. Copper sulfate (2 per cent solution) has been used to flush the mucous membrane surface of the prepuce in refractory cases. The lymphoid follicles may be cauterized by the direct application of copper sulfate crystals. Breeding animals should be treated at least 2 to 3 weeks prior to stud use.

Treatment of Idiopathic Infertility

Historical Therapies. Everything from apricot pits to garlic and from diethylstilbestrol (DES) to pregnant mare serum gonadotropin (PMSG) has been used to treat male sterility. All of these treatments have apparently given satisfactory results to an occasional dog owner willing to endorse the particular therapy. Unfortunately, little documentation exists relating pretreatment fertility, semen quality and testicular structure to post-treatment values of the same parameters. PMSG has been the most commonly advocated therapy for azoospermic and oligospermic dogs. Although it continues to be suggested and used, its efficacy remains in question. PMSG has a stimulatory effect on the spermatogenic cells, but no valid claim has appeared demonstrating a return to fertility or the acquisition of fertility in an infertile azoospermic stud. It has been suggested that azoospermic dogs do not respond to PMSG but that males with oligospermia may benefit from 200 to 500 IU of PMSG intravenously at 3 to 6-day intervals. Follicle-stimulating hormone (FSH) has also been used at a dosage of 25 mg subcutaneously once weekly.

Untested Therapies. Because no hormonal treatment has received adequate investigation in canine infertility, any treatment is speculative. Drugs that have been used in human medicine include mesterolone, a synthetic androgen that has positive steroidal effects at the testicular level but minimal negative feedback effects. Clomiphene is also used as a centrally active compound that has both weak estrogenic and antiestrogenic properties. Testosterone cannot be used for causing a positive effect on spermatogenesis. Prolonged elevated blood levels will prevent luteinizing hormone (LH) release and cause reduction of testicular concentrations of androgen. Administration of exogenous testosterone in quantities sufficient to raise testicular concentration to a functional level is not acceptable therapy because of the enormous dosages required. Hormones with FSH and LH activity are often used but with questionable results.

Prolonged stimulation is required for positive results, and antibody formation to these protein gonadotropins can be expected. When LH activity is desired, human chorionic gonadotropin (HCG) should be used. HCG is itself antigenic, but antibodies formed against it are less likely to cross-react with the dog's endogenous LH than are antibodies formed against pituitary LH products. It must be remembered that virtually all azoospermic dogs remain azoospermic, regardless of treatment, unless a specific cause has been identified and corrected.

Libido

Animals that show a lack of interest in some bitches but willingly service others are not uncommon. It is important to arrange early arrival of the bitch during proestrus so that daily play and determination of the onset of estrus are possible. The stud should not be kept in the same enclosure with the bitch except during supervised periods. Males that refuse to mate an estrous bitch can often be ejaculated manually and an artificial insemination performed. HCG can be used 24 hours before mating, at a dosage of 10 IU/lb, to elevate libido. Results obtained with hormonal treatments are inconsistent. Providing optimum socialization for the stud as a pup, positive sexual experiences at puberty and foresight in the management of a breeding pair can bypass many of the difficulties that are due to behavior. Libido is a trait that can be influenced by genetic selection and environment, and dog breeders must be encouraged to consider both aspects in their attempts to produce sound dogs.

REFERENCES

1. Bane, A.: Sterility in male dogs. Nord. Vet. Med., 22:561, 1970.
2. Fritz, T. E., Lombard, L. S., Tyler, S. A. and Norris, W. P.: Pathology and familial incidence of orchitis and its relation to thyroiditis in a closed beagle colony. Exp. Mol. Path., 24:142, 1976.
3. Harrop, A. E.: The infertile male dog. J. Small Anim. Pract., 7:723, 1966.
4. Mancini, R. E. and Martini, L. (Eds.): Male Fertility and Sterility. New York, Academic Press Inc., 1974.
5. Von Krause, D., II: Examination of fertility in the dog. Dtsch. Tierarztl. Wschr., 72:3, 1965.

Diseases of the Prostate Gland of the Dog

DELMAR R. FINCO
University of Georgia, Athens, Georgia

INTRODUCTION

Although prostatic fluids are a constituent of semen, such secretions are not essential for its fertility. This indicates that diseases of the prostate in which secretions are diminished would not affect fertility. However, other factors must be considered before drawing this conclusion. Some prostatic diseases decrease libido, apparently because of pain. Inflammatory components of prostatic secretion (white blood cells, red blood cells, bacteria) may affect semen quality and lead to infertility. For these reasons, evaluation of the prostate is an essential part of the examination of the reproductive tract of the male dog.

The prostate gland is often the innocent victim of human error. It is frequently incriminated as being the cause of signs that actually are due to other organ dysfunctions. On the other hand, the prostate gland is sometimes overlooked when it is actually the culprit. Even when the prostate is correctly diagnosed as being diseased, knowledge of the specific disease entity is frequently not obtained. Stamey has stated that in humans "The term prostatitis is all too often a waste basket of clinical ignorance, used to describe any condition associated with prostatic inflammation."[12] In veterinary medicine the term is often used even more loosely to include noninflammatory as well as inflammatory diseases. These deficiences in diagnosis will be overcome only by thorough, methodical evaluation of each patient and by additional research on diseases of this organ.

EVALUATION OF THE PROSTATE GLAND

Physical Examination

The location of the prostate depends on its size. It is present in the pelvic canal when of normal size, but it assumes an abdominal location as enlargement occurs. When in the pelvic canal, the prostate gland is best examined by a combination of abdominal and rectal palpation. After inserting a finger into the pelvic canal *per rectum,* the other hand is used to grasp the caudal abdomen and push its contents toward the pelvic inlet. This abdominal maneuver pushes the prostate back to the examiner's finger.

Pain or discomfort shown by the dog during rectal palpation must be interpreted with caution. Pain should be considered to be of prostatic origin only when digital pressure is applied directly to the gland. Palpation of the normal gland is not painful.

The size, shape, surface texture and position of the gland should be evaluated. Specific data are not available for normal prostate size in various breeds at various ages. Generally, the gland is palpable with difficulty in the sexually immature dog, while in the sexually mature dog its diameter is six to eight times that of the urethra. The prostate is normally symmetrical, with right and left lobes separated by a shallow dorsal sulcus. The surface is normally smooth, and the consistency of the gland is slightly spongy.

Radiography

The normal prostate gland usually cannot be distinctly visualized on survey radiographs. However, a space-occupying mass visualized between the pelvic inlet and the urinary bladder should be assumed to be prostate gland until proved otherwise. In order to differentiate the urinary bladder from a caudal abdominal mass, it is helpful to introduce contrast medium, such as air, into the urinary bladder.

The diagnosis of some less common prostate diseases (neoplasia, calcification, calculi) may be made from survey radiographs that reveal radiopaque areas in the gland or evidence of proliferative lesions of the lumbar vertebrae. However, more common diseases such as hyperplasia, squamous metaplasia, bacterial prostatitis and prostatic cysts cannot be differentiated radiologically.

On urethrograms made during retrograde injection of contrast medium into the urethra, reflux of medium into the prostate gland may sometimes be observed. While reflux does not occur in most normal dogs, it has not been studied adequately enough to determine if its presence is always associated with disease.

Examination of Prostatic Fluid

Prostatic fluid is actively secreted by the epithelial cells of the gland. There is no assurance that prostatic fluid will invariably contain abnormal elements found in an intracellular or interstitial location in the gland, but the probability of this seems to be high. Therefore, examination of prostatic fluid is valuable in evaluating the status of the gland.

Prostate massage is a common method of obtaining fluid in man, but it has limited application in the dog. This is because only small volumes of fluid can usually be expelled into the urethra. These small volumes are difficult to retrieve and to differentiate from urethral debris. Sufficient fluid is probably available for valid analysis only when palpation is followed by dripping of material from the urethral orifice or when dripping occurs spontaneously. Prior to obtaining a specimen, the dog should be allowed to urinate to clear the urethra of debris. The tip of the penis is removed from the sheath and gently washed with soap and water. While the penis is protruding, the prostate is massaged and fluid is collected in a sterile container as it drips from the urethral orifice.

Ejaculation of the dog is a more reliable method of obtaining prostatic fluid. To obtain an ejaculate, the dog should be handled under quiet, relaxed conditions. Dogs that become apprehensive when placed on a table should be handled on the floor. The dog is ejaculated by applying pulsatile pressure on the prepuce over the bulb of the penis. The tip of the penis is gently cleansed with soap and water after it protrudes from the sheath. Ejaculate is collected in a sterile container such as a 50-ml plastic syringe case. The ejaculate may be partially fractioned if desired. In the normal dog the clear fluid obtained during the latter part of ejaculation has a higher content of prostatic fluid. However, complete separation of testicular and prostatic components of the semen is not possible. Abnormalities found in semen could originate from the urethra, prostate, ductus deferens, epididymis or testicle. To localize the site of abnormality, other data (clinical examination, biopsy) should be obtained to correlate with evaluation of semen.

To assist in evaluating the prostate, two procedures are performed on the ejaculate:

Bacterial Culture, Cytologic Examination. Quantitative bacterial culture is performed by conventional techniques. Slides of ejaculate are air-dried and stained with new methylene blue or Wright's stain and are examined for evidence of inflammation. Normally only a few white blood cells (WBC) per high power field are present, and bacteria are not detected. Examination of semen for neoplastic cells of prostatic origin may also be done, but negative results do not rule out prostatic neoplasia.

Prostate Gland Biopsy. Percutaneous fine needle aspiration biopsy and needle punch biopsy can usually be performed on the enlarged prostate gland of the dog. Biopsy can also be performed during laparotomy.

Fine needle aspiration biopsy can be performed more quickly and easily than percutaneous punch biopsy but has the disadvantage of not providing a specimen adequate for tissue sections. Aspiration biopsy of the prostate gland is performed as follows:

1. The gland must be adequately immobilized for any biopsy procedure.

2. A transperineal or transabdominal approach may be made, depending on the location of the gland.

3. Transperineal biopsy:
   a. If the prostate can be palpated most easily *per rectum*, an assistant forces abdominal contents caudally by abdominal palpation while the operator performs the aspiration biopsy.
   b. The area lateral to the anus is surgically prepared, and the prostate is palpated *per rectum*.
   c. A 22-gauge spinal needle of appropriate length is inserted through the skin and parallel to the rectum.
   d. The needle is guided to the prostate gland, and the capsule is punctured.
   e. The stylus is removed, a syringe is attached and aspiration is performed as the needle is advanced.
   f. If fluid is not obtained, aspiration is continued as the needle is moved

through the tissue three or four times.
   g. The sample is processed for culture and cytological examination.

4. Transabdominal biopsy:
   a. If the prostate can be palpated most easily *per abdomen,* this approach is used.
   b. The gland is immobilized by abdominal palpation, and the same technique is used as described for transperineal biopsy.

Percutaneous punch biopsy is more elaborate than aspiration biopsy but has the advantage of providing adequate tissue for formalin fixation and standard histological evaluation. While physical restraint or mild sedation is usually sufficient for aspiration biopsy, sedation and infiltration with local anesthetic are required for punch biopsy. The Franklin-modified Silverman needle has been used successfully for punch biopsy of the prostate. Details of use of the needle are described in a publication on biopsy techniques.[2] In addition to obtaining tissue for histological examination, the needle may be swirled in liquid media for bacterial culture.

Biopsy after exposure of the gland at laparotomy has the advantage of allowing visualization of the prostate to aid in choosing the biopsy site. Excisional biopsy may be performed, allowing procurement of a large tissue specimen. The disadvantages of this approach are the greater time involvement, greater expense and increased risk to the patient.

Potential complications of biopsy include dissemination of infection, hemorrhage and urethral fistula. If fever, leukocytosis or acute inflammatory exudate in semen is present, biopsy is not indicated. If a punch biopsy is desired but there is concern regarding dissemination of infection, aspiration biopsy should be performed first, since leakage from the site of a fine needle aspiration biopsy is less likely than from the site of a punch biopsy. Hemorrhage and urethral fistula are possible complications that rarely occur.

BENIGN HYPERPLASIA

Benign hyperplasia of the prostate occurs in middle-aged and older dogs. Although it has been found that hyperplasia is associated with an altered ratio of androgen to estrogen, definitive knowledge is sparse concerning mechanisms and effects of sex steroids on prostatic metabolism.

Clinical Signs. Hyperplasia that is diagnosed by pathological criteria (i.e., increase in gland size, histological evidence of hyperplasia) does not invariably cause clinical signs of disease. This is because the hyperplastic canine prostate gland enlarges uniformly in an outward direction. Urethral obstruction does not develop, as it does in man. Signs are observed only when outward enlargement reaches a size sufficient to impinge on the colon. Constipation, straining and tenesmus are then observed, and the dog may pass a mucoid stool because of tenesmus. With uncomplicated prostatic hyperplasia, there is no discharge from the dog's penis and the patient is afebrile, alert and active.

Diagnostic Criteria. Prostatic hyperplasia must be diagnosed on the basis of several criteria. Clinical findings of constipation and an enlarged prostate may be observed with disease of the prostate other than hyperplasia. The character of the prostate gland is particularly important. With hyperplasia, no prostatic pain exists, enlargement is symmetrical and the gland retains its normal slightly spongy character. There is an absence of a soft, fluctuant feeling that would be anticipated with an accumulation of fluid in the gland. Signs of feminization are absent, and the testicles are usually normal. Fever and leukocytosis are absent. The dog is usually over 6 years of age. If the diagnosis is still in doubt based on the preceding criteria, cytological examination of an ejaculate is indicated. Lack of signs of inflammation is consistent with prostatic hyperplasia. Prostatic biopsy may be performed to confirm the diagnosis, but it is not indicated if other criteria are met. If treatment for hyperplasia fails, inaccurate diagnosis is probable and biopsy should then be considered.

Treatment. Although the exact mechanism is unknown, estrogens are an effective therapy for prostatic hyperplasia. If available, repositor diethyl stilbestrol is administered (intramuscularly) at a dose of 1.0 mg/kg, up to a maximum dose of 25 mg. Estradiol cyclopentylpropionate (estradiol cypionate, ECP) may be used if diethylstilbestrol is not available. ECP is about 10 times as potent as diethylstilbestrol when administered parenterally and should be used at a dose of 0.1 mg/kg IM with a max-

imum dose of 2.0 mg. A single dose of either drug is usually adequate. A decrease in size of the gland is usually apparent in 5 to 7 days. Repeated injections of estrogens or diethylstilbestrol or administration of single large doses may cause bone marrow depression and squamous metaplasia of the prostate of the dog. The bone marrow depression may be life-threatening because of thrombocytopenia and leukopenia. Consequently, both diethylstilbestrol and ECP must be used judiciously in the dog.

Estrogens may affect the reproductive ability of the dog by decreasing libido. Effects on spermatogenesis are also likely. The owner should be advised of these effects prior to administration of the drugs.

Castration is an effective, permanent treatment for benign hyperplasia that may be employed if the reproductive capacity of the dog is of no concern.

Effective, safe forms of therapy for benign hyperplasia that do not affect reproduction are presently not available for the dog.

CHRONIC BACTERIAL PROSTATITIS

The incidence of chronic bacterial prostatitis in the dog is unknown. Uncontrolled clinical studies indicate that it is fairly common. Usually, gram-negative organisms are responsible for the infection. In some human beings, chronic inflammatory prostatic disease may be present, but bacteria cannot be isolated. Efforts to isolate less common organisms (mycoplasma, anaerobes, fungi) from such patients have been futile. It has not been established whether abacterial chronic prostatitis exists in the dog.

Clinical Signs. Chronic bacterial prostatitis may cause few obvious signs, and the dog is often clinically normal and afebrile. The animal may be presented to the veterinarian because the owner occasionally notes drops of blood or pus on the dog, in the environment or in the first morning urine passed. With more severe infection, exudate may drip from the penis constantly. In some cases, exudate may accumulate within the prostate gland and penile discharge may be absent (see Prostatic Abscess later in this article).

With chronic bacterial prostatitis, findings on palpation of the prostate are variable. The gland is usually, but not invariably, enlarged. It may be symmetrical or asymmetrical and is usually nonpainful. The consistency of the prostate may vary from firm to soft and fluctuant, depending on whether focal accumulations of pus have occurred.

The hemogram may reveal a normal or an elevated WBC count, depending on the degree of prostatic involvement. Microscopic examination of an ejaculate reveals an inflammatory exudate.

Diagnostic Criteria. Because of the variation in physical findings associated with chronic bacterial prostatitis, diagnosis by physical signs alone is not possible. Any male dog with a history of dripping of blood or exudate from the penis should have chronic bacterial prostatitis ruled out by cytological examination and culture of the exudate or semen. A quantitative culture that yields greater numbers of organisms in semen than in midstream voided urine is evidence of primary genital infection. Confirmation of chronic bacterial prostatitis may also be made by qualitative culture of material obtained by fine needle aspiration of the gland. The skin at the site of aspiration should be scrubbed thoroughly prior to aspiration to eliminate contamination by skin micro-organisms.

If conventional cultures are negative, samples should be submitted for culture of *Brucella canis*.

Treatment. In man, empirical treatment of chronic prostatitis with antibiotics has generally been unsuccessful. As a result, studies were conducted on normal dogs to determine the relationship between blood and prostatic fluid levels of various antibacterial compounds. It was found that negligible concentrations of ampicillin, penicillin G, cephalothin, oxytetracycline, kanamycin, polymyxin B, nalidixic acid, nitrofurantoin and all sulfa drugs tested were found in the prostatic fluid of normal dogs a few hours after intravenous administration of the drug.

Some other antibacterial compounds had prostatic fluid levels that were actually several times higher than plasma levels. These included trimethoprim, oleandomycin and erythromycin.

Chloramphenicol was present in the prostatic fluid at a concentration of 56 to 65 per cent of the concentration in plasma. Lincomycin and tetracycline were present in prostatic fluid at concentrations roughly 12

to 35 per cent of plasma levels. Differences among drugs in their diffusion in prostatic fluid are apparently due to several factors, including lipid solubility, degree of ionization of the drug, plasma protein binding and the acidic or basic character of the drug. With regard to the latter, prostatic fluid in the dog normally is more acid than plasma is (pH 6.1 to 7.4), and basic antibiotics that diffuse in the fluid may be trapped therein to exceed plasma levels. Conversely, acidic drugs are excluded from prostatic fluid, depending on their degree of ionization. Weakly ionized acids (pK' > 7) may diffuse in prostatic fluid and can approach, but cannot exceed, plasma concentration. Neutral molecules, if lipid-soluble, can diffuse in prostatic fluid and equal plasma levels.

These studies, utilizing acute experiments in normal dogs, provide valuable information. One limitation of the studies may be their acute nature. Limited studies of a more prolonged type (drug administration for 7 days) suggested that some drugs that did not attain effective levels in the prostatic fluid immediately may do so after a longer interval. On the basis of the preceding data, antibacterial compounds that may be of value in treating chronic bacterial prostatitis in the dog are trimethoprim, erythromycin and chloramphenicol.

Trimethoprim interferes with folic acid function by inhibiting conversion of dihydrofolate to tetrahydrofolate. It acts against both gram-negative and gram-positive organisms and is synergistic with sulfonamides. A sulfonamide may enhance the activity of trimethoprim against a bacterium, even if the bacterium is resistant to the sulfa. Tribrissen is a combination of sulfadiazine and trimethoprim. Although no sulfas reach therapeutic levels in prostatic secretions, sulfadiazine has a higher penetration than most sulfa preparations. It is likely that the antibacterial activity of trimethoprim in prostatic fluid is enhanced by the quantity of sulfadiazine present.

Erythromycin is considered to be an antibiotic with a gram-positive spectrum. However, at high concentrations it is effective against most gram-negative organisms. Activity is also enhanced at an alkaline pH. The amount of antibiotic that enters the prostate gland can be increased by increasing the pH difference between plasma and prostatic fluid. For this reason, erythromycin and sodium bicarbonate have been advocated for simultaneous use in the treatment of chronic bacterial prostatitis in man caused by gram-negative organisms. The efficacy of this combination in the dog remains to be proved. Tentatively, a dose of 10 mg/lb of erythromycin and 0.2 to 0.3 grain/lb of sodium bicarbonate every 8 hours may be tried.

Chloramphenicol is effective against a high percentage of gram-negative organisms *in vitro*, and so this drug is a good choice for *in vivo* use in canine bacterial prostatitis. Since prostatic fluid levels of the drug are only about half of plasma levels, the upper range of the recommended dose of chloramphenicol should be used (25 mg/lb every 8 hours orally).

Tetracycline has been recommended for treatment of bacterial prostatitis in the dog on the basis of studies in human beings. Studies in man suggest that the high doses of this drug that can be attained by intravenous injection may result in adequate levels of this antibiotic in prostatic fluid despite it low degree of penetration. However, levels obtained by oral administration are not likely to be adequate, since blood levels do not reach the values attained by intravenous injection. In addition, plasma-protein binding of tetracycline is apparently greater in the dog than in man. For these reasons, tetracycline is not likely to be effective for treatment of chronic bacterial prostatitis of the dog.

In the treatment of chronic bacterial prostatitis, consideration must be given to the duration of therapy and the evaluation of the dog for persistent or recurrent infection. Antibacterial therapy should be maintained for a minimum of 2 weeks, and preferably for a period of 4 to 6 weeks. In choosing an antibiotic, sensitivity testing is essential because penetration of an antibacterial agent into prostatic fluid is meaningless if the organism is resistant to the drug. Obviously, *in vitro* sensitivity must be correlated with prostatic penetration of the drug. Negative bacterial cultures during therapy are probably meaningless, since such results in man are followed by positive cultures a few weeks after therapy is discontinued. Cultures of ejaculate should be performed after the drugs have been discontinued for a minimum of 5 days and should be repeated at monthly intervals for at least 2 months. Controlled studies have not been performed in the dog regarding the effects of castration on chronic bacterial prostatitis. However, clinical impressions seem to suggest that castration of these patients is beneficial.

ACUTE BACTERIAL PROSTATITIS

Clinical Signs. In contrast to chronic bacterial prostatitis, the acute disease results in clinical signs that make diagnosis much more obvious. Fever, depression and anorexia are usually present. Because of prostatic pain, the dog moves reluctantly with a stilted gait. Exudate may drip from the penis independent of the act of urination. On palpation, the prostate is enlarged and very painful. An ejaculate often cannot be obtained because of the pain associated with the disease.

Diagnostic Criteria. Clinical findings and examination of prostatic secretions for inflammatory cells are adequate for diagnosis. Cultures and sensitivity testing are helpful in formulating therapy.

Treatment. Factors limiting passage of drugs into the fluid of the normal prostate may not apply during acute prostatitis. It is hypothesized that membrane barriers to drug diffusion are altered by acute inflammation. Therapy with antibacterial agents having *in vitro* effectiveness against the organism is highly successful in eliciting a remission of clinical signs. Dogs should be evaluated several weeks after cessation of therapy to establish if infection has been eradicated or only suppressed.

PROSTATIC CYSTS AND ABSCESSES

The etiology of prostatic cysts is unknown. It is hypothesized that they arise as retention cysts or that remnants of the uterus masculinus secrete the cystic fluid. The cause and pathogenesis of prostatic abscesses are similar to those of bacterial prostatitis, already discussed. However, cysts and abscesses have the potential for assuming a massive size. Because clinical signs and treatment of these two abnormalities have many common features, these masses are discussed together.

Clinical Signs. A large abdominal mass is usually present that fills the caudal half or more of the abdomen. The mass is usually very firm, giving the impression of solid tissue. Although a catheter can usually be passed into the urinary bladder with ease, the dog may have dysuria, and urinary retention may be a complication. If partial urinary retention has been present for several days or weeks, mild hydronephrosis may develop. Fever and leukocytosis may exist if infection is present. Fluid may or may not drip from the penile orifice. Dogs with prostatic cysts or abscesses are usually too uncomfortable to be successfully ejaculated.

Diagnostic Criteria. The abdominal mass must be identified as being the prostate. Pneumocystography is the best tool to localize the mass and determine its relationship to the urinary bladder. If systemic signs of infection are absent, fine needle aspiration can be performed. As much of the fluid as possible should be aspirated to establish if the mass is exclusively cyst or if a significant portion is solid tissue. Aspirated fluid should be cultured, and the sediment obtained after centrifugation should be examined for neoplastic cells. Cytological examination is indicated because retention cyst formation may occasionally be secondary to neoplasia.

Treatment. Conservative medical treatment of these abnormalities is usually unsuccessful. Aspiration of prostatic contents is followed by progressive increase in the size of the mass as more fluid forms. Infection cannot be eradicated despite prolonged antibiotic therapy. Surgical drainage of the cyst or abscess is the preferred treatment. When long-term drainage is allowed to occur, treatment is usually successful. A method for surgical drainage of these masses has been developed by Gourley and Osborne, and their article can be consulted for details of treatment.[4]

In cases in which urinary retention was a problem preoperatively, renal function should be carefully evaluated. Postoperatively, urinary retention may persist for a variable period of time. During the postoperative period, the bladder should be kept empty so that detrusor tone can be reestablished. Use of parasympathomimetic drugs such as bethanechol (Urecholine) may be of value. A dosage of 2.5 to 15 mg orally t.i.d. is used.

PROSTATIC NEOPLASIA

Neoplasia of the prostate gland of the dog is uncommon. Surveys indicate that adenocarcinoma is most common and that leiomyosarcoma is next in frequency of occurrence.

Clinical Signs. Since there are several diseases causing prostatic enlargement, early diagnosis is usually not made. If the urethral lumen is invaded, dysuria and urinary retention may occur. On palpation, the gland may vary in size and shape from that of the normal prostate. If the capsule is invaded, extreme pain may be elicited. The gland may be very firm, and it may be adherent to surrounding structures. Metastasis to lumbar vertebrae may occur, and this may be detected radiologically.

Diagnostic Criteria. Diagnosis by histological identification of neoplastic cells is the only reliable method, although lumbar metastatic lesions are very strong presumptive evidence.

Treatment. Diagnosis is usually made too late for treatment by prostatectomy. Castration and treatment with estrogens are employed in man, but the efficacy of these procedures has not been adequately evaluated in the dog. Little data are available on other chemotherapeutic agents. In man cryosurgery has been advocated as a therapeutic tool, with implications that this procedure provides immunological antitumor benefits for the patient.

SQUAMOUS METAPLASIA

Squamous metaplasia of the prostate is caused by excess estrogen production. This may be due to a Sertoli cell tumor of the testicle, or it may be iatrogenically induced.

Clinical Signs. Squamous metaplasia causes signs identical to those of hyperplasia. However, generalized signs of excess estrogen production may aid in differentiating the two conditions. Biopsy will reveal metaplasia.

Treatment. Therapy involves removal of the source of excess estrogens.

REFERENCES

1. Berg, O. A.: Parenchymatous hypertrophy of the canine prostate gland. Acta Endocrinol., *27*:140, 1958.
2. Finco, D. R.: Prostate gland biopsy. Vet. Clin. North Am., *4*:367, 1974.

3. Goland, M. (Ed.): Normal and Abnormal Growth of the Prostate. Springfield, Ill., Charles C Thomas, Publisher, 1975.
4. Gourley, I. M. G. and Osborne, C. A.: Marsupialization — A treatment for prostatic abscess in the dog. J. Am. Anim. Hosp. Assoc., 2:100, 1969.
5. Hessl, J. M. and Stamey, T. A.: The passage of tetracyclines across epithelial membranes with special reference to prostatic epithelium. J. Urol., 106:253, 1971.
6. Leau, I. and Ling, G. V.: Adenocarcinoma of the canine prostate. Cancer, 22:1329, 1968.
7. Lloyd, J. W., Thomas, J. A. and Mawhinney, M. G.: Androgens and estrogens in the plasma and prostatic tissue of normal dogs and dogs with benign prostatic hypertrophy. Invest. Urol., 13:220, 1975.
8. Madsen, P. O., Wolf, H., Barquin, O. P. et al.: The nitrofurantoin concentration in prostatic fluid of humans and dogs. J. Urol., 100:54, 1968.
9. Mobley, D. F.: Erythromycin plus sodium bicarbonate in chronic bacterial prostatitis. Urology, 3:60, 1974.
10. Reeves, D. S. and Ghilchik, M.: Secretion of the antibacterial substance trimethoprim in the prostate fluid of dogs. Br. J. Urol., 42:66, 1970.
11. Reeves, D. S., Rowe, R. C. G., Snell, M. E. et al.: 23 further studies on the secretion of antibiotics in the prostatic fluid of the dog. Proceedings Second National Symposium on Urinary Tract Infection. London, 1972.
12. Stamey, T. A.: Urinary Infections. Baltimore, The Williams and Wilkins Co., 1972.

Artificial Insemination and Storage of Canine Semen

KJELL ANDERSEN
Veterinary College of Norway, Oslo, Norway

INDICATIONS FOR USE OF ARTIFICIAL INSEMINATION IN THE DOG

The first successful pregnancy following artificial insemination (AI,) was obtained in the dog as early as in 1780 by the Italian scientist Lazzaro Spallanzani. During the next 150 years relatively little progress was made within this field, but in the last few decades artificial insemination has become an important factor in modern breeding programs for several domestic species, especially cattle and swine. In the dog, however, the use of AI is still rather limited, partly because of the difficulties in establishing rational criteria and methods for the selection of animals with a high breeding value and partly because of the fact that dog breeding is, after all, of comparatively little economic importance.

Nevertheless, artificial insemination has been performed in dogs, at least on a small scale, for quite a number of years in some countries. The indications for the use of AI in this species may be systematized into three main categories:

1. *Mating problems due to the bitch.* In nonparous animals, especially when they are young, the outer part of the female genitalia may be rather narrow with more or less pronounced constrictions in the vestibulovaginal region. This condition may evidently induce a certain degree of pain in connection with the introduction of the penis, causing the bitch to interrupt the copulatory act at this stage. In some cases the bitch seems to display a tendency toward selecting her sexual partner, refusing to accept the male chosen by the owner. A nervous, sensitive or aggressive temperament can also hamper acceptance of the male dog. It is questionable, however, whether AI is justified in the latter case. Different forms of chronic vaginitis may further impair the fertility after natural mating, although these conditions are reported to have little influence on the results of artificial insemination.[10]

2. *Mating problems due to the male dog.* These problems are mainly caused by different forms of impotence. Especially in old dogs, weakness, stiffness and pain in the back and the hindquarters may impede a normal accomplishment of the copulatory act. In small dogs, and particularly in short-legged breeds such as the dachshund and Pekingese, there seems to be a general tendency toward mating difficulties that are more or less irrespective of age.

Psychological forms of impotence are also encountered in dogs. The lack of libido in some of these cases may be caused by temporary shyness and sexual inexperience. On the other hand, in some rare cases copulation is prevented by habitual premature erection, probably due to an exceptionally strong sexual drive.

3. *Difficulties in bringing the female and male together. These pertain specifically to geographical distances and other obstacles.* For several breeds such problems have constituted a definite limit to the genetic improvement of the dogs. As in other species, progress in breeding often seems to be dependent on supply of genetic material from other geographical areas, within the countries as well as across national borders. In the latter, quarantine restrictions enforced to prevent spread of contagious disease may be an additional factor that is interfering with improvement of the quality of various breeds in certain countries.

COLLECTION AND HANDLING

For Immediate Use of Undiluted Semen

In the case of mating difficulties caused either by the bitch or by the male dog, undiluted ejaculates are used immediately after collection. This procedure can be performed by use of an artificial vagina[8] or by digital manipulation of the penis. Collection of semen by means of digital manipulation is preferably carried out in the presence of an estrous bitch. The preputial skin is pushed back, permitting the bulbus glandis to be exposed, and the masturbation is started by applying a moderate pressure on the caudal part immediately behind bulbus glandis. In most cases this will initiate the erection and will also cause the subsequent thrusting movements that seem to be of importance for obtaining a representative ejaculate from the dog. These reactions are usually rather easy to provoke if the male dog shows some sexual interest in the bitch, especially if he is mounting or trying to mount her.

The ejaculate of the dog consists of three fractions that are not always easy to separate. The first fraction usually has a volume of 0.5 to 2 ml and is of a clear, watery consistency with very few spermatozoa. Normally, the deposition of this part of the ejaculate occurs during the thrusting movements. As these movements cease and the penis reaches maximal erection, the second fraction is deposited. This portion of the ejaculate is of about the same volume as the preceding one, is almost white in color with a

rather viscous consistency and contains the major number of spermatozoa. Subsequently, there is a gradual transition to a third fraction, which usually is very voluminous (3 to 25 ml) and is deposited within a period of 5 to 45 minutes. As a rule, this last portion of the ejaculate has the same clear, watery consistency as the first fraction, which was previously thought to be secreted by urethral glands, a concept probably extrapolated from the human. Such glands are, however, not present in domestic animals.[12] In the dog it is therefore likely that the prostate, being the only accessory gland in this species, has already started secreting fluid before the spermatozoa are ejaculated and that the prostatic secretion begun at the onset of the erection is continued during the entire process of ejaculation.

The ejaculate is preferably collected in a special glass tube shown in Figure 1, but an ordinary test tube provided with a glass funnel can also be used. To avoid cold shock, it is important that the equipment be warmed to 30 to 35° C and tentatively kept at that temperature in the hand of the operator, especially if the collection is taking place in a cold room. As the insemination dose should have a sperm concentration of at least 200×10^6 cells per ml., only the second portion of the ejaculate is of interest. In some cases it is, however, very difficult to obtain well-fractioned material, and in order to avoid too great a loss of spermatozoa, some of the third fraction must sometimes

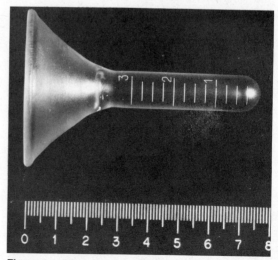

Figure 1. Glass tube used for collection of dog semen.

be included. As soon as the semen is obtained, it is tested for density, motility and morphological defects and then used for insemination as quickly as possible, preferably no more than 10 minutes elapsing from collection until deposition in the female genitalia.

For Storage of Diluted Semen, Liquid or Frozen

The conditions under which canine spermatozoa can be preserved for distribution and storage have been the object of intensified investigation during the last several years, and in several countries experiments have been conducted to solve different problems within this field. The collection of sperm is performed by the same procedure as described for undiluted semen. However, when preservation of canine spermatozoa is desired, it is important to obtain a well-fractioned ejaculate, since seminal plasma seems to have an unfavorable effect on both the survival time and the freezing tolerance of the sperm cells. This may be due to activation produced by certain factors in the plasma, one of which is believed to be a reduced stability of the cell membrane, thus rendering the spermatozoa more vulnerable to cold shock and to the special physical and chemical conditions connected with the process of deep freezing.

Prolongation of the viability of sperm cells for a limited period of time (12 to 48 hours) can be achieved by adding special diluents to the sperm-rich fraction of the ejaculate. The dilution rate usually ranges from 1:5 to 1:10. Pasteurized milk has been used for short-term storage of canine semen, and semen was found to be fertile after storage for more than 48 hours.[7] Another extender that has been tried with some success is a solution of 1.16 per cent sodium citrate dihydrate, 0.75 per cent glycine and 1 per cent glucose, to which is added 20 per cent volume for volume (v/v) egg yolk.[6] A solution of 1.46 per cent sodium citrate dihydrate, 0.93 per cent glycine and 1.25 per cent glucose mixed with 20 per cent (v/v) egg yolk is also recommended.[5] Furthermore, the Illini Variable Temperature (I.V.T.) extender[16] has been used for prolonging the viability of canine spermatozoa, and pregnancy has been obtained more than 24 hours after collection of the semen. Antibiotics, usually 500 to 1000 IU of penicillin and 1 mg of dihydrostreptomycin per ml, are added to the different extenders to obtain a bacteriostatic effect. The diluent should have a temperature of about 35° C when added to the sperm-rich fraction. The diluted semen is then placed in a water bath having the same temperature and is subsequently cooled in a refrigerator to about 4° C over a period of 2 to 3 hours.

For long-time preservation of sperm, deep freezing has to be performed. Dog semen is usually frozen in pellets or payettes (straws) by use of carbon dioxide ice or liquid N_2 respectively, after dilution with extenders containing egg yolk, glycerol and antibiotics. Precautions similar to those previously described should be taken to avoid cold shock. The first pregnancy after insemination with frozen dog semen was obtained in the United States in 1969.[13] The semen was diluted 1:3 with 11 per cent lactose containing 4 per cent (v/v) glycerol and 20 per cent (v/v) egg yolk and was frozen in pellets. Semen handled and frozen by approximately the same procedure was used the following year in the Netherlands for insemination of two bitches, which both conceived.[15] Tris-fructose-citric acid extender containing 8 per cent (v/v) glycerol and 20 per cent (v/v) egg yolk has been used with good results for freezing dog semen in payettes.[3] As a rule, the dilution rate is somewhat higher than in pellets, usually ranging from 1:3 to 1:5 depending on semen density. Both medium-sized (0.5 ml) and minimum-sized (0.25) payettes have been used. The freezing technique is the same as that used for bull semen,[9] and the material has been stored from 3 weeks to 1½ years in liquid N_2 before use. Immediately before insemination, which usually is performed twice during the period of heat, 4 to 5 medium payettes (or 8 to 10 mini-payettes) constituting a dose of 2.0 to 2.5 ml containing about 200×10^6 spermatozoa are thawed in water at 75° C (6.5 seconds for medium and 5 seconds for mini-payettes).[1]

INSEMINATION PROCEDURE AND RESULTS BY VAGINAL AND UTERINE DEPOSITION OF THE SEMEN

The method of vaginal deposition of the semen is rather easy to perform and may be used with fairly good results with undiluted sperm-dense fractions of ejaculates of good quality immediately after collection. The conception rate does seem to be somewhat lower than by natural mating.[2] However, since the indications for artificial insemination in the dog make this method applicable for only a rather select group of animals, the basis for a real comparison is rather uncertain. Vaginal insemination has also been used with some success for diluted semen stored for 12 to 48 hours. Even when using frozen semen, this insemination method has resulted in a conception rate of 46 per cent in a group including 32 bitches.[14] One type of equipment used for vaginal deposition of semen is demonstrated in Figure 2. The sperm-rich fraction of the ejaculate is drawn into the plastic catheter by means of the pump. When using diluted, more voluminous semen doses, a syringe, instead of a pump, has to be connected to the catheter. The catheter is inserted in a dorsocranial direction through the vestibule. Subsequently the rear part of the instrument is somewhat elevated, kept in a horizontal position and introduced into the cranial portion of the vagina. This part of the vagina, which is very narrow, is also called the pseudocervix[11] because when observed through a speculum, it may have the appearance of the vaginal portion of the cervix with a ventral fissure indicating the presence of an external orifice. This rather special appearance of the genital tract has led to the erroneous concept that the insemination dose is deposited in the uterus when the conventional technique is used. To prevent loss of semen, elevation of the bitch's hindquarters for some minutes is recommended.[8] Insertion of a gloved finger into the vestibulum for 5 to 10 minutes and masturbation by massage of the clitoris immediately after semen deposition seem to cause contractions of the genital tract, thereby possibly promoting the transport of spermatozoa from the vagina into the inner genitalia.

Natural mating in the dog involves an indirect form of uterine deposition of the semen, a good deal of it being transported through the cervical canal into the uterus during the copulatory act. This form of uterine deposition is the result of a mechanism involving several factors, such as retention of the penis and high ejaculate volume, as well as vaginal and uterine contractions.[17] As a result of preservation of semen, especially the process of freezing and thawing, it seems very difficult to avoid a certain reduction of the number of living spermatozoa. In addition, a dilution of the semen before freezing is necessary. The result of these factors is presumably a low number of fertile spermatozoa reaching the site of fertilization when deposited in the vagina.

In order to achieve a real intrauterine deposition of the insemination dose, thus insuring that a sufficient number of fertile spermatozoa reach the oviducts, a special technique has been developed.[3] The bitch is placed on a table of convenient height and is held by an attendant. Administration of sedatives is seldom necessary. The plastic tube is inserted into the narrow anterior part of the vagina by the same technique described for the introduction of the catheter used for vaginal insemination. By placing the tube against the posterior part of the cervix uteri, which protrudes into the vagina as a small portio, it is possible to push the organ forward and somewhat downward. This procedure will facilitate the fixation of the cervix, which normally undergoes a pronounced enlargement during proestrus and estrus, thus becoming rather easily accessible by abdominal palpation. Subsequently, the insemination catheter, which can be connected with a syringe, is passed through the tube. By careful manipulation of the cervix and the catheter, the latter is inserted via the external os and through the short cervical canal into the corpus uteri for semen deposition. To improve the semen transport from the uterus

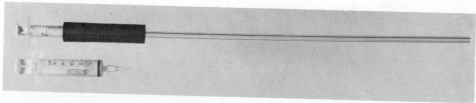

Figure 2.   Equipment used for vaginal insemination, including plastic catheter, pump and syringe provided with an adapter.

to the oviducts, uterine motility is tentatively stimulated by the same kind of masturbation described in connection with vaginal insemination.

The effect of uterine insemination has been tested by use of liquid as well as frozen semen in a small trial including 37 animals.[4] In one group, 17 bitches of various breeds were inseminated with the sperm-rich fraction of the ejaculate immediately after collection. Of these animals, 13 conceived — the litter size ranging from 2 to 12 living puppies. Another group of 20 bitches of various breeds were inseminated with semen frozen in N_2 vapor and stored for various lengths of time (ranging from 3 weeks to 18 months) in liquid N_2. In this group 16 bitches conceived, with a litter size ranging from one to nine living puppies.

SCIENTIFIC AND PRACTICAL ASPECTS

More experimental work is still required to solve the different problems connected with artificial insemination and storage of canine semen. In particular, when frozen semen is being used, very little is known about the minimum number of living spermatozoa per dose and the optimal time of insemination. Since these factors may be interrelated, inasmuch as an excess of spermatozoa seems to some degree to compensate for the unfavorable effect of an early insemination, comprehensive and systematic experiments have to be conducted within this field.

The use of frozen dog semen on a greater practical scale would probably make a valuable contribution to an improvement of the breeding program in this species. The method that permits uterine deposition of the semen seems to enhance fertility, especially following insemination with frozen semen. However, it is somewhat complicated and time-consuming unless one has some training. A simplification of the procedure resulting in some form of a modified vaginal deposition could be advantageous under practical conditions. The technique must, however, secure an effective transport of semen into the inner genitalia of the bitch, thus simulating the events of a normal copulatory act.

REFERENCES

1. Aamdal, J. and Andersen, K.: Fast thawing of semen frozen in straws. Zuchthygiene, *3*:22, 1968.
2. Andersen, K.: Kunstig sædoverføring på hund (artificial insemination in the dog). Medlemsbl. Norske Vet. Foren. *21*:482, 1969.
3. Andersen, K.: Insemination with frozen dog semen based on a new insemination technique. Zuchthygiene, *10*:1, 1975.
4. Andersen, K.: Artificial uterine insemination in dogs. Proceedings Eighth International Congress Animal Reproduction and A. I. Cracow, Poland. *IV*:960, 1976.
5. Foote, R. H.: The effects of electrolytes, sugars, glycerol and catalase on survival of dog sperm stored in buffered yolk mediums. Am. J. Vet. Res., *25*:104, 32 (1964).
6. Foote, R. H. and Leonard, E. P.: The influence of pH, osmotic pressure, glycine and glycerol on the survival of dog sperm in buffered yolk extenders. Cornell Vet., *54*:78, 1964.
7. Harrop, A. E.: Artificial insemination of a bitch with preserved semen. Br. Vet. J., *110*:424, 1954.
8. Harrop, A. E.: The physiology of reproduction in the dog and bitch. *In* Kirk, R. (Ed.): Reproduction in the Dog. London, Bailliere, Tindall & Cox., 1960.
9. Jondet, R.: Congelation rapide de sperm de taueau conditionné en paillettes. Proceedings Fifth International Congress Animal Reproduction and A. I. Trento, Italy, *IV*:463, 1964.
10. Leonard, E.: Dogs. *In* Perry, E. C. (Ed.): Artificial Insemination of farm animals. New Brunswick, N.J., Rutgers Univ. Press, 1968.
11. Pineda, M. H., Kainer, R. A. and Faulkner, L. C.: Dorsal median postcervical fold in the canine vagina. Am. J. Vet. Res., *34*: 1487, 1973.
12. Roberts, S. J.: Veterinary Obstetrics and Genital Diseases. Ithaca, N.Y., 1971.
13. Seager, S. W. J.: Successful pregnancies utilizing frozen dog semen. A.I. Digest, *17*(12):26, 1969.
14. Seager, S. W. J. and Fletcher, W. S.: Progress on the use of frozen semen in the dog. Vet. Rec., *92*:6, 1973.
15. van Gemert, W.: Puppies from deep frozen semen. Neth. J. Vet. Sci., *4*:1, 1971.
16. VanDemark, N. L. and Sharma, V. D.: A preliminary report on preservation of bovine semen at room temperature. J. Anim. Sci., *15*:1212, 1956.
17. Walton, A.: Copulation and natural insemination. *In* Parkes, A. S. (ed.): Marshall's Physiology of Reproduction. Vol. 1, Part 2. London, Longmans, 1960, pp. 130–160.

section **VII**

POPULATION CONTROL IN URBAN PETS

Consulting Editor

VICTOR M. SHILLE

Overpopulation of Dogs and Cats: Demographic Aspects

ROBERT SCHNEIDER
University of California, Davis, California

Since 1970 there has been increased concern about a possible overpopulation problem among dogs and cats. It appeared that the initial concern was brought about by a temporary imbalance in the supply-demand for puppies.[1] During the decade starting in 1960, there was increasing demand for pets. Part of this demand was due to the long period of prosperity experienced during the 1960's and part to the needs for personal protection. As an illustration, in Alameda and Contra Costa Counties, California, in 1961, there were approximately 40,000 puppies entering households. This number steadily increased, until peaking in 1967 at approximately 73,000 puppies. In the following 3 years, 1968, 1969 and 1970, 71,000, 57,000 and 43,000 puppies, respectively, entered households. It was the sudden large decrease in demand in 1969 and 1970 that triggered the increase in concern about animal population overproduction, since many of the excess puppies found their way to pounds or shelters to be euthanized. In addition, as the economy of the country slowed down in the early 1970's, owners suddenly either no longer wanted or could not keep some of their pets. These animals also found their way to pounds or shelters. A summary of reports of local animal control activities sent to the California Department of Health indicated that for all of California between 1970 and 1971 (Table 1), there was a 12.4 per cent decrease in owner redemption of their dogs from these facilities, the first redemption decrease of any size in 20 years!

The major demographic characteristics of animal populations will be presented in this paper. Much of the data were obtained from animal population surveys done as part of the needs of a population-based animal cancer registry. Specifically, data were from the 1970 survey[2] and from a follow-up survey done 1 year later on all animals alive and resident on December 31, 1970. These survey data are particularly relevant because they were done when concern about overpopulation of dogs and cats was beginning. If one better understands the demographic characteristics of dog and cat populations, one may better be able to constructively help prevent overpopulation problems.

LIFE EXPECTANCIES OF THE DOG AND CAT

Life expectancies of the average dog and cat determined for chronological ages up to 15 years are shown in Table 2. All calculations excluded causes of death that were owner-related such as "did not want," "could not keep" and so forth. For the group under 1

TABLE 1. *Number of Dogs Licensed, Reclaimed by Owners and Placed in New Homes (From Animal Control Activities in California, 1966–1975)*

Year	Number Licensed	Number Reclaimed	Number To New Homes
1966	1,079,615	66,458	86,492
1967	1,229,069	72,451	78,453
1968	1,260,414	80,641	89,548
1969	1,297,710	85,984	95,389
1970	1,534,756	98,973	93,523
1971	1,733,727	86,662	92,791
1972	1,728,266	113,701	92,734
1973	1,688,011	115,342	91,303
1974	1,859,578	120,626	93,023
1975	1,819,151	136,460	102,940

TABLE 2. *Expected Age at Death by Current Ages for Dogs and Cats**

Current Age (yrs)	Age at Death (yrs)	
	CANINE	FELINE
<1	8	5
1	10	7
2	11	9
3	11	11
4	12	12
5	12	12
6	13	13
7	13	13
8	13	14
9	14	15
10	14	15
11	15	16
12	15	16
13	16	16
14	16	17
15	17	18

*Excluding human-related reasons characterized as "unwanted."

year of age, only animals placed in households after weaning were considered.

Life expectancies are a combination of a number of factors. Purebred dogs have approximately a 1 year longer life expectancy at 2 months of age than crossbreds; however, by 2 years of age and older, crossbreds can be expected to live ¾ to 1½ years longer than purebreds. Purebred cats, on the other hand, have a consistent edge on crossbreds and domestics of approximately ¾ to 2 years throughout their lifespan. Female dogs will outlive males anywhere from 1 month to 1½ years. Female cats will outlive males anywhere from 2 months to 2½ years. The size of the dog is also related to life expectancy. The trend appears to be that the smaller the dog, the longer the life expectancy. Dividing purebred dogs into three groups on the basis of median weight for each breed (up to 25 pounds, 25 to 64 pounds and over 64 pounds) yielded life expectancies of 9.4, 8.4 and 7.2 years, respectively, at 2 months of age. This compares with a life expectancy of 8.2 years for all purebreds combined at the same age.

AGE CONSIDERATIONS

The median ages for most dog and cat populations will be between 2 and 4 years, depending on the number of puppies and kittens in the population. Cat populations tend to have a median age approximately ½ to 1 year less than dogs. Throughout a calendar year, the total number of puppies and kittens entering households will amount to 20 to 40 per cent of the total population. The actual proportion will depend on supply-demand factors. However, at any given time, animals under 1 year of age will constitute only 10 to 25 per cent of the total population.

It is of interest to compare dog and cat age distributions with those of man. This now can be done because of the availability of reasonable age conversion equivalents for dogs and cats. For the dog, the age conversion system developed by Lebeau can be used. Lebeau considered that once maturity was reached, aging occurred at a constant rate in both canine and human. He considered 2 years of age as the age of maturity in the dog and 24 years as maturity in humans. Each year of life after maturity in the dog was equivalent to 4 years in humans. For feline-to-human age conversion, we developed a similar system based on life expectancies. Animals euthanized because of human-related reasons were excluded. For the cat, maturity is reached by 1½ years of age, and 2 years was considered equivalent to 26 years of age in the human. Each year of life after 2 years was found equal to 3⅓ years in man. Table 3 shows some of the comparative age equivalents of human, dog and cat.

What is noted in dog and cat populations compared with human populations is that

TABLE 3. *Some Equivalent Ages of Humans, Dogs and Cats*

Human Age (yrs)	Equivalent Canine Age (yrs)	Equivalent Feline Age (yrs)
24	2	1.5
32–35	4	4
52–55	9	10
72–75	14	16
>91	>18	>21

death of members occurred earlier with animals. In a comparative sense, age-converted survival curves of the dog and cat resemble those of man 50 to 100 years ago when man had a shorter life expectancy and more deaths in the early years of life due to disease.

SEX DIFFERENCES

There is a general tendency to choose males as pets if possible, particularly with cats, and this is reflected in the male/female numbers of both species. In Alameda and Contra Costa Counties in 1970 there were approximately 20 per cent more males for animals under 1 year of age. However, numbers of males exceed numbers of females only in the early years of life. By approximately 4 or 5 years of age, females predominate in both species, and this predominance increases throughout the remaining lifespan of each species. Interestingly, as with women, the bitch and queen are more adaptive to survival in our environment.

BREED DISTRIBUTION

Popularity of canine breeds in different localities determines breed numbers. For Alameda and Contra Costa Counties, breed preference in 1970 is shown in Table 4. Purebred-crossbred numbers indicate almost as many purebreds as crossbreds in the population (47 per cent versus 53 per cent). The lack of correlation between distributions of purebred and crossbred animals of the same breed was probably due to the more dominant expression of certain breeds in crossbred situations and the tendency to group certain crossbred-type animals together as crossbreds of the same breed.

TABLE 4. *Proportional Distribution of the Principal Dog Breeds, Alameda and Contra Costa Counties, 1970*

Breed	Per Cent Purebred	Per Cent Crossbred
Poodle, all sizes	13.3	5.3
German shepherd dog	6.1	6.1
Dachshund	3.5	2.0
Chihuahua	2.2	2.6
Labrador retriever	1.6	2.2
Beagle	1.3	1.7
German shorthaired pointer	1.1	0.2
Cocker spaniel	1.1	5.9
Pekingese	1.0	1.2
Doberman pinscher	0.9	0.3
Fox terrier	0.9	4.3
Shetland sheepdog	0.8	0.5
Collie	0.8	1.6
Pomeranian	0.8	0.6
Brittany spaniel	0.7	0.2
Basset hound	0.6	0.1
Boston terrier	0.6	0.1
Boxer	0.6	0.3
Keeshond	0.5	0.2
Miniature schnauzer	0.4	0.1
Other breeds	8.3	6.6
Mixed	–	10.9
TOTAL	47.0	53.0

The preference for cat breeds is governed by the supply of particular breeds. Since cat breeding remains largely uncontrolled by owners, the readily available supply of kittens is predominantly crossbred, classified as domestic shorthair or domestic longhair. In the survey, only 14 per cent of the cat population were purebreds, and about 80 per cent of these were purebred Siamese. There is a tendency to discuss disease conditions in both canine and feline breeds without adequate documentation of the population-at-risk for each breed. Obviously, one cannot consider the interaction between a disease condition and a particular breed without adequate knowledge of the breed numbers of the population-at-risk. As shown in Table 4, the popularity of the various breeds can yield large differences in population-at-risk numbers. These differences will be reflected in the number of cases of a disease occurring by chance in each breed.

UNWANTED PETS

An important consideration from the pet's standpoint is not only its life expectancy but also how long it may be expected to stay in a specific household. Table 5 presents the number of additional years the typical dog or cat can be expected to stay in a given household for chronological ages up to 15 years. Table 5 differs from Table 2 in that all reasons for leaving a household were included in calculations, whereas in Table 2 only calculations of deaths attributable to disease and accidents were included.

A marked impact in the calculations for Table 5, especially in the younger ages, concerned losses due to a pet no longer being wanted. In the follow-up survey 1 year after the initial survey, it was found that, excluding animals having moved out of the area, approximately 15 per cent of the canine and 25 per cent of the feline population were no longer in their original households. Of these losses, approximately 40 per cent of dogs and 30 per cent of cats were given away by their owners.

Among dogs, those under 1 year of age suffered the greatest population losses; approximately 35 per cent were removed. More than one-half of this loss was because the animals were no longer wanted, and one-third of the loss was due to dogs being given to pounds or shelters. The median time spent in a household by an adopted puppy that left during its first year of life was 4.4 months. Assuming the typical puppy entered a household at 6 weeks to 2 months of age, the median age at which such puppies were disposed of was 7 months of age. This age agrees with the age pattern of dogs found in pounds and shelters. Most unwanted dogs turned in to those facilities are half-grown. Reasons for disposal of that large a proportion of such pets need to be clarified.

REPRODUCTIVE ACTIVITIES

Lack of understanding of the dynamics of pet population reproduction has led to gross underestimates of the proportions of female dogs and cats neutered in a population. In Alameda and Contra Costa Counties in 1970, it was found that 48 per cent of bitches and 65 per cent of queens were neutered. These proportions were initially unbelievably high since puppy and kitten production

TABLE 5. *Expected Remaining Length of Residency in a Given Household, by Current Age, for Dogs and Cats**

Current Age (yrs)	Additional Period Expected in Household (yrs)	
	CANINE	FELINE
<1	6.1	4.9
1	6.9	5.6
2	7.0	6.0
3	6.9	6.5
4	6.5	6.7
5	6.1	6.5
6	5.7	6.4
7	5.2	6.1
8	4.6	5.8
9	4.1	5.4
10	3.5	4.9
11	3.2	4.3
12	2.8	3.8
13	2.3	3.4
14	2.0	2.9
15	1.9	2.5

*All causes of leaving a household combined, including human related reasons characterized as "unwanted."

that year was 31 per cent and 76 per cent more, respectively, than households available to take them. However, generally the supply of puppies does not greatly exceed demand, and in this population, having 48 per cent of bitches neutered would normally be adequate. The 31 per cent excess puppies in 1970 were approximately 13,219 puppies more than the 42,661 adopted. The sum of these two figures, 55,880, approximated the 56,604 puppies entering households in 1969. Apparently, the 1970 reproduction rate was closely related to the 1969 demand. Had the demand in 1970 been as great as or greater than that of 1969, there would not have been any overproduction of puppies. For kittens, however, production continued in excess in 1970 as in previous years. An excess of kittens would be expected in this population (at 1970 demand levels) until 75 to 80 per cent of all queens were neutered, a difficult objective to achieve.[1]

Some of the important reproductive considerations found in the survey were that in general for each intact bitch, one offspring was weaned annually; for each intact queen, three offspring were weaned. Reproductivity was concentrated in the 1 to 3-year-old females in both species to whom 63 per cent of dog litters and 74 per cent of cat litters were born. There were 1½ puppies and 5¼ kittens weaned annually per intact female in the 1 to 3-year-old group.

Advocates of low cost neutering clinics thus would do well to concentrate on neutering females 3 years of age and under. However, it should be pointed out that owners appear to be less inclined to neuter such animals, possibly because of the large numbers that leave households during these ages. Survival data indicated that approximately only 50 per cent of bitches and 33 per cent of queens were still in households by 3 years of age. The replacement rates needed to maintain the population after losses in early life of these magnitudes make it difficult to control reproduction by neutering because of the constant large supply of females entering these prime reproductive ages.

Another reason that a major emphasis on neutering may not help control reproduction in dogs is because estimated demand appears to be a major factor affecting puppy production. Annual litter production per intact bitch was 0.2 litters in the 1970 survey. This rate appears low when considering the feline reproductive rate of 0.9 litters annually per queen found in the survey. Although canine and feline breeding activities may not be directly comparable because of differences in type and frequency of estrus, females of both species still are expected to produce only two litters per year at maximal breeding efficiency. Hence, the difference between 0.2 and 0.9 litters is quite large. A major part of this difference represents the ability of owners of bitches to better control their pets' breeding activities. Economic factors and ease of placement of puppies, both constituting a demand measurement for owners of intact bitches, are strong motivating factors in canine breeding considerations. An increase of only 0.1 litter per intact bitch (from 0.2 to 0.3 litters) per year, which is still only one-third of the reproductive rate of cats, would result in 50 per cent more puppies in the Alameda and Contra Costa area.[1]

POPULATION GROWTH OUTLOOK

Another population survey was done in Alameda and Contra Costa counties to estimate the dog and cat population changes that had occurred during 1975. In the 5-year period from 1970 to 1975, the owned dog population increased from 224,815 to 299,460 (33.2 per cent); the cat population during the same period increased from 151,176 to 193,788 (28.2 per cent). Life expectancies improved, and inroads appeared to have been made in reducing the numbers of unwanted pets. Neutered percentages in 1975 were 52, 10, 74 and 57 for female dog, male dog, female cat and male cat, respectively. The corresponding 1970 percentages were 48, 7, 65 and 52. Thus, the proportion neutered also increased. Puppy and kitten excesses were considerably reduced in 1975, but even with 74 per cent of queens neutered, there were still approximately 10 per cent excess kittens. As the early 1980's are being approached, it does not appear that the growth of pet dog and cat populations has ceased.

REFERENCES

1. Schneider, R.: Observations on overpopulation of dogs and cats. J.A.V.M.A., *167*:281, 1975.
2. Schneider, R. and Vaida, M. L.: Survey of canine and feline populations: Alameda and Contra Costa Counties, California, 1970. J.A.V.M.A., *166*:481, 1975.

Pharmacological Control of Estrus in the Bitch and Queen

THOMAS J. BURKE
University of Illinois, Urbana, Illinois

INTRODUCTION

The last decade has seen increasing pressure placed upon the veterinary profession to provide alternatives to traditional surgical methods of birth control in companion animals. Current opinion within the profession suggests that the present veterinary medical health delivery system cannot provide the level of quality low-cost surgical birth control that has frequently been demanded. Furthermore, increasing leisure time has allowed many dog and cat owners to become involved in various animal competitions that preclude surgical castration, either by written regulation or by tradition. It is equally apparent to most clinicians that a segment of the population is unalterably opposed to "desexing surgery" for a variety of reasons. The need for relatively low-cost, safe, efficacious and readily available forms of birth control has been amplified by the pet population explosion and its effects upon man and his environment. Confinement and physical control remain the least expensive means of pregnancy prevention but often are either undesirable or unattainable by the owner.

Although it can be conceded that no one drug or device will totally solve the problem and that public education and owner responsibility will be an integral part of any solution, the practitioner should be aware of current advances in the field of medical control of estrus. To be sure, other nonsurgical avenues are being explored, and the reader is referred to the appropriate articles in this text. Safe and effective methods of pregnancy termination also are needed.

Veterinarians must be willing to assist the owner in planning and providing control of reproduction, whether permanent or temporary, for his pet just as they provide disease prophylaxis, parasite control and other routine health care services.

Several drugs have been used to alter reproductive function in the dog and cat. A complete review of all of these compounds cannot be undertaken in the space provided. Only drugs widely in use or those whose future clinical use seems promising to the author will be considered.

Current physical means of estrus control, excluding contraceptive devices, are limited to the cat. Since she is an induced ovulator, vaginal-cervical stimulation of the queen has been used to terminate estrus. Glass rods and cotton-tipped swabs have been employed, as have the services of castrated or vasectomized tomcats. However, the former method is not always reliable. Although some castrated toms do not lose their libido, it is preferable to maintain a vasectomized tom in the hospital, perhaps a blood donor, to use for terminating estrus in clients' queens. This method is also safer for the clinician, as he is less likely to be scratched or bitten.

PHARMACEUTICAL AGENTS

Progestogens

The first hormone to be used to control estrus in animals was progesterone, and the first report of its use in the bitch appeared in 1952. Since then a number of compounds possessing primarily progestational activity have been used for estrous inhibition in the dog and cat. The reader is referred to relatively recent reviews[5, 6, 10] of the use of these compounds, since several have not been widely used in the United States and only one, megestrol acetate (Ovaban), is currently approved for this indication in this country. Those compounds having the widest use, past or present, by American veterinarians are progesterone, hydroxyprogesterone acetate, medroxyprogesterone acetate and megestrol acetate.

The most severe side effect of chronic progestogen administration in dogs and cats is, cystic endometrial hyperplasia, with or without subsequent infection. This is well recognized by most veterinarians[10] and need not be discussed further. Prolonged progestational therapy in cats also has been correlated with the development of mammary neoplasia, although mammary adenomas have been seen in association with the luteal phase of the cycle in untreated queens. The injection of repositol forms of progestogens for suppression of estrus continues today but the risk:benefit ratio dictates that this practice should be discontinued in both dogs and cats.

Megestrol Acetate

Megestrol acetate is a potent, orally active progestogen with a relatively short half-life (8 days) in dogs.[3] It has been used by European veterinarians for prevention and postponement of estrus in the dog and cat since the mid-1960's and has been available to veterinarians in the United States since April, 1975.

There currently are two label indications for estrus control in the dog: stopping a cycle in proestrus (prevention of estrus) and postponement of an anticipated estrus prior to the onset of proestrus. Clinical trials have demonstrated 92 per cent and 97 per cent efficacy, respectively.[3] Treatment did not affect subsequent cyclicity and fertility.[3]

For prevention of estrus, megestrol is administered daily for 8 days at a dose of 2. 2 mg/kg (1 mg/lb), beginning during the first 3 days after the onset of sanguineous discharge *and* vulvar swelling. Starting treatment too early results in an early posttreatment heat. A marked decrease in efficacy occurs if treatment is delayed beyond the third day of proestrus. Although timing of the first post-treatment heat cannot be accurately predicted, it will usually occur 4 to 6 weeks earlier than usual following administration of a correctly timed course of prevention therapy. British workers report that return to estrus can be delayed by administering megestrol at 2. 2 mg/kg for 4 days, beginning during the first 3 days of proestrus, followed by 0.55 mg/kg (0.25 mg/lb) for 16 days.[1]

If mating occurs during the first 3 days of treatment, megestrol therapy should be stopped and the bitch treated for mismating.[1] If mating occurs after 3 days of treatment, therapy should be continued since the drug will prevent pregnancy in most cases.[1]

For postponement of an anticipated heat, megestrol is given at a dose of 0.55 mg/kg (0.25 mg/lb) daily for 32 days, beginning at least a week prior to the onset of proestrus based upon the patient's history. British veterinarians have prescribed megestrol at a dose of 0.1 to 0.2 mg/kg twice weekly for up to 4 months following a postponement course of therapy for extended suppression.[1] Bitches so treated should be allowed to have a normal cycle before being retreated.

If postponement therapy is begun in late anestrus, the next heat should occur in 5 to 6 months. Treatment during early to mid-anestrus may have no effect on the occurrence of the next cycle.

Vaginal cytological examination often is useful in timing megestrol therapy. If a sample, obtained atraumatically, shows erythrocytes, postponement therapy should not be given. Rather, that cycle should be treated with properly timed prevention therapy since proestrus is imminent.

Temporary minor side effects of increased appetite, decreased activity, weight gain and, rarely, lactation may occur during treatment. Changes in hair coat and olfaction have not been observed.

Bitches with grossly abnormal cycles are not candidates for megestrol therapy, as correct timing cannot be assured.

Megestrol is not currently approved for use in cats in the United States. The author treated laboratory cats at 0, 2.5 and 5 mg/animal every 7 days for 70 days. Estrus was prevented in those animals receiving 5 mg, but not 2.5 or 0 mg, weekly. Limited clinical trials using 5 mg/cat have shown that daily administration for 3 days will stop estrus and continued therapy on a once weekly basis for 10 weeks prevents further heats during treatment. Return to cyclicity depends upon the time of year and other factors, possibly exposure to prolonged light and other estrous queens.

British recommendations for postponement of estrus in the queen are 2.5 mg/cat/day for 8 weeks or 2.5 mg/cat/week for up to 18 months.[1] Treatment is begun during diestrus or anestrus, respectively.

In summary, megestrol acetate appears to be a safe and efficacious drug for temporary estrus control in the bitch and, potentially, the queen. Care must be exercised by the clinician to insure proper timing and avoidance of gross overdosage.

Androgens

Testosterone

Testosterone propionate has been used to prevent estrus in working dogs, particularly racing greyhounds. Oral and parenteral routes have been used. Greyhound bitches given 25 mg of oral testosterone weekly have been kept out of estrus for as long as 5 years with apparent return to normal reproductive status.[7] Side effects of clitoral hypertrophy and vaginitis have been noted, with the former being prominent enough to have affected bitches referred to as "tail-lighters." Silcone tube implants containing testosterone effectively prevented estrus in beagle bitches for as long as 840 days with return to normal cyclicity and fertility.[6] The effective dose released per day was calculated to be 168.6 μg/kg. Clitoral hypertrophy and vaginitis were observed in about 20 per cent of the treated bitches. Androstenedione at approximate doses of 200 to 450 μg/kg/day failed to inhibit estrus.[6]

Doses of testosterone sufficient to inhibit estrus may produce side effects that are undesirable to some owners. In addition, premature epiphyseal closure may occur if immature bitches are treated. Inadvertent treatment of pregnant bitches may cause severe urogenital anomalies in female puppies. Thus, testosterone cannot currently be recommended for estrus control.

Mibolerone

A synthetic 19-norsteroid compound, mibolerone, was recently approved for long-term estrous inhibition. Mibolerone is an androgenic, anabolic antigonadotropic steroid that does not possess progestational or estrogenic activity.[9] In purebred and mixed breed bitches treated for periods up to 1300 days, estrus inhibition was more than 95 per cent successful.[9] Dosage ranged from 30 μg/day for dogs weighing 1 to 12 kg up to 180 μg/day for dogs more than 45 kg, and for German shepherds and German shepherd cross-breeds.[9] Mild clitoral hypertrophy has been observed. Administration of mibolerone to estrous bitches did not interfere with conception or gestation. However, female puppies were masculinized.

Daily administration of 50 μg of mibolerone to adult queens for 180 days prevented estrus, while doses of 20 μg/day or 50 μg/week did not.[4] Side effects seen clinically were mild clitoral hypertrophy and thickening of the cervical dermis. Histological examination of tissues obtained at necropsy from treated queens revealed evidence of thyroid dysfunction and clitoral hyper-

trophy with a few clitorides that contained bacula. Return to cyclicity and subsequent fertility were not impaired. Field testing of mibolerone in the queen has recently been suspended by the manufacturer, as mortality occurred at doses as low as twice the minimum effective dose. It is apparently hepatotoxic in cats.

Mibolerone will not arrest proestrus or estrus in either the bitch or queen, and therapy may need to be begun as much as 30 days prior to the onset of proestrus. Such therapy will effectively suppress estrus in dogs for long periods of time and may prove capable of being used for the lifetime of the animal.

Prostaglandins

Recently F-series prostaglandins have been employed to alter the estrous cycle of mares. Although they may not prove useful in suppressing estrus in the dog and cat, they have the potential for shortening the normal interestrous interval and for use as abortifacients as a result of their luteolytic properties.

THE ACYCLIC ANIMAL

Reproductive biologists today generally agree that the hypothalamus is responsible for sexual cyclicity or acyclicity. If exposed to androgens at the appropriate (critical) time, the hypothalamus becomes acyclic (male). A nonandrogen-sensitized hypothalamus releases appropriate gonadotropic releasing factors that result in hypophyseal elaboration of gonadotropins, thus creating estrous cycles (female). Exposure of neonatal rats or mice to testosterone creates an acyclic animal, regardless of phenotypic sex.[2] The critical time for rats and mice ends during the first few days of postnatal life.[2] The guinea pig, an animal with a gestation period approximating that of the dog and cat, has a critical time for hypothalamic sensitization that occurs totally *in utero*.[2] Exposure of dog and cat fetuses to androgens has resulted in multiple urogenital anomalies, many of which are surgically uncorrectable and are esthetically undesirable. Some androgen-treated acyclic rodents remain in anestrus while others remain in permanent behavioral estrus[2] — a distinct disadvantage for the pet owner. At this time it appears unlikely that hormonal treatment of the puppy, kitten or pregnant dam will provide a satisfactory means of estrus control.

REFERENCES

1. Anonymous: A Glaxo Guide to Ovarid. Greenford, England, Veterinary Division, Glaxo Laboratories Ltd., 1976.
2. Barraclough, C. A.: Alterations in reproductive function following prenatal and early postnatal exposure to hormones. *In* McLaren, A. (Ed.): Advances in Reproductive Physiology. Vol. 3. New York, Academic Press, 1968, pp. 81–112.
3. Burke, T. J. and Reynolds, H. A.: Megestrol acetate for estrus postponement in the bitch. J.A.V.M.A., *167*:285, 1975.
4. Burke, T. J., Reynolds, H. A. and Sokolowski, J. H.:

A 180-day-tolerance-efficacy study with mibolerone for estrus suppression in the domestic cat. Am. J. Vet. Res., *38*:469, 1977.
5. Christie, D. W. and Bell, E. T.: The use of progestogens to control reproductive function in the bitch. Anim. Breed. Abstr., *38*:1, 1970.
6. Cox, J. E.: Progestogens in bitches: A review. J. Small Anim. Pract., *11*:759, 1970.
7. Pegram, L.: Personal communication. Ralston-Purina Co., St. Louis, Mo., 1976.
8. Simmons, J. G. and Hamner, C. E.: Inhibition of estrus in the dog with testosterone implants. Am. J. Vet. Res., *34*:1409, 1973.
9. Sokolowski, J. H. L: Androgens as contraceptives for pet animals with specific reference to the use of mibolerone in the bitch. *In* Davis, L. E. and Faulkner, L. C. (Eds.): Pharmacology in the Animal Health Sector. Ft. Collins, Col., Colorado State University Press, 1976, pp. 164–175.
10. Stabenfeldt, G. H.: Physiologic, pathologic and therapeutic roles of progestins in domestic animals. J.A.V.M.A., *164*:311, 1974.

Immunological Control of Fertility in Dogs

LLOYD C. FAULKNER
University of Missouri,
Columbia, Missouri

Protection against microbial antigens is a common veterinary usage of immunology, and the neutralization of biologically active molecules is a basic property of antibodies. It has long been recognized by veterinarians that repeated injections of heterologous gonadotropins commonly become successively less effective. Present knowledge suggests that this reduced efficacy is the consequence of the formation of antibodies to the hormones. The antigenicity of protein hormones can be enhanced when appropriate adjuvants are used. In addition, small peptides or steroid hormones may be rendered antigenic by using them as haptens conjugated to an appropriate carrier protein. The specificity of antibodies to steroid hormones can be manipulated by selection of the site of conjugation.[4]

Antibodies, specifically for a hormone, have been used to study the sites of production and to identify the individual cells that produce the hormone. Levels of hormones in the blood and tissues have also been quantified in a variety of reproductive states.[5]

The use of antibodies for the neutralization of the hormones that regulate reproduction is a relatively recent field of exploration. Immunization of rats and rabbits against luteinizing hormone (LH) was associated with atrophy of the gonads and accessory sex organs.[8, 13] Active immunization of rabbits of both sexes caused genital atrophy and reproductive failure.[6, 7] Antibodies against the beta subunit of placental gonadotropin were associated with failure to establish pregnancy in ovulating primates.[12] Specific antiserum to LH decreased ovarian blood flow and circulating levels of progesterone in ewes, and anti-LH serum reduced luteal function in sows and cows.[3, 9-11] Antibodies to conjugated gonadotropin-releasing hormone (GnRH) reduced levels of gonadotropin and impaired fertility in immunized rats.[2]

Dogs have been immunized with LH and human chorionic gonadotropin.[1] Antibodies to bovine and ovine LH were associated with genital atrophy and reproductive failure in actively immunized adult dogs. Immunization delayed puberty in bitches and tended to delay puberty in males. Reproductive disturbances were attributed to cross reaction between antibodies to exogenous gonadotropins and endogenous hormone.[1]

Antibodies might be raised against a variety of molecules, including antigenic sites on gametes, which are vital to normal reproductive function. Active immunization might be utilized for long-term control of fertility, while passive transfer could be used for short-term effects. In addition to their use in the control of fertility, antibodies to reproductive hormones might be valuable in the control of cellular proliferations or excessive growth of tissues that are hormone-dependent. Thus, immunological methods might be used in cases of mammary and genital neoplasms and in cases of genital hypertrophy or hyperplasia.

Immunological techniques suggest exciting possibilities for the control of fertility in dogs, but the applicability of these methods to clinical practice remains obscure. Laboratory studies have confirmed the biological feasibility of using antibodies to control fertility in dogs, but several problems prevent the clinical application.

Active immunization is the best hope for inducing prolonged infertility as an alternative to surgical sterilization. An adjuvant that eliminates the need for repeated injections of antigen and does not stimulate an unacceptable inflammatory response is required. Single injections of gonadotropic antigen have raised levels of antibody, causing reproductive failure, but the primary response was of inadequate duration. Antibodies produced in response to second or third injections of antigen did not consistently result in reproductive failure.[1] The passive transfer of antibodies for short-term control of fertility offers the best hope for the near future. Passive transfer of immunity allows the use of a standardized quantity of a purified antibody that has been previously characterized for its ability to inhibit fertility.

Active or passive immunization against reproductive hormones provides a promising nonsurgical method for fertility control. However, in addition to the fundamental problems of immunology involved in the development of a "vaccine" for controlling fertility, several mechanisms of reproductive functions in dogs need to be elucidated before a safe and long-lasting vaccine for controlling fertility becomes available.

REFERENCES

1. Faulkner, L. C., Pineda, M. H. and Reimers, T. J.: Immunization against gonadotropins in dogs. *In* Nieschlag, E. (Ed.): Immunization with Hormones in Reproduction Research. Amsterdam, North-Holland Publishing Co., 1975, p. 199.
2. Fraser, H. M.: Effects of antibodies to luteinizing hormone releasing hormone on reproductive functions in rodents. *In* Nieschlag, E. (Ed.): Immunization with Hormones in Reproduction Research. Amsterdam, North-Holland Publishing Co., 1975, pp. 107–117.
3. Hoffman, B., Schams, D., Bopp, R., Ender, M. L., Gimenez, T. and Karg, H.: Luteotrophic factors in the cow: Evidence for LH rather than prolactin. J. Reprod. Fertil., *40*:77, 1974.
4. Niswender, G. D.: Influence of the site of conjugation on the specificity of antibodies to progesterone. Steroids, *22*:413, 1973.
5. Niswender, G. D., Nett, T. M. and Abbar, A. M.: The hormones of reproduction. *In* Hafez, E. S. E. (Ed.): Reproduction in Farm Animals. Philadelphia, Lea and Febiger, 1975, pp. 57–81.
6. Pineda, M. H., Lueker, D. C., Faulkner, L. C. and Hopwood, M. L.: Atrophy of rabbit testes associated with production of antiserum to bovine luteinizing hormone. Proc. Soc. Exp. Biol. Med., *125*:665, 1967.
7. Pineda, M. H., Faulkner, L. C., Hopwood, M. L. and Lueker, D. C.: Effects of immunizing female rabbits with bovine luteinizing hormone. Proc. Soc. Exp. Biol. Med., *128*:743, 1968.
8. Quadri, S. K., Harbers, L. H. and Spies, H. G.: Inhibition of spermatogenesis and ovulation in rabbits with anti-ovine LH rabbit serum. Proc. Soc. Exp. Biol. Med., *123*:809, 1966.
9. Reimers, T. J. and Niswender, G. D.: Effects of specific neutralization of luteinizing hormone and prolactin on ovarian blood flow and progesterone secretion. *In* Nieschlag, E. (Ed.): Immunization with Hormones in Reproduction Research. Amsterdam, North-Holland Publishing Co., 1975, p. 95.
10. Snook, R. B., Brunner, M. A., Saatman, R. R. and Hansel, W.: The effect of antisera to bovine LH in hysterectomized and intact heifers. Biol. Reprod., *1*:49, 1969.
11. Spies, H. G., Slyter, A. L. and Quadri, S. K.: Regression of corpora lutea in pregnant gilts administered antiovine LH rabbit serum. J. Anim. Sci., *26*:768, 1967.
12. Stevens, V. C.: Female contraception by immunization with HCG — Prospects and status. *In* Nieschlag, E. (Ed.): Immunization with Hormones in Reproduction Research. Amsterdam, North-Holland Publishing Co., 1975, p. 217.
13. Wakabayashi, K. and Tamaoki, B.: Influence of immunization with luteinizing hormone upon the anterior pituitary-gonadal system of rats and rabbits, with special reference to histological changes and biosynthesis of luteinizing hormone and steroids. Endocrinology, *79*:477, 1966.

section VIII

EQUINE

Consulting Editors
EDWARD MATHER
and
DOUGLAS MITCHELL

Factors Affecting Stallion Management

B. W. PICKETT

Colorado State University, Fort Collins, Colorado

INTRODUCTION

Responsible stallion management requires a potential fertility examination, including a seminal evaluation, prior to the breeding season. However, potential fertility evaluation of stallions has been neglected because of failure to identify the factors responsible for the extreme variation in seminal characteristics and the lack of information on the relationship between these factors and fertility. The season of the year influences many of the physical and chemical characteristics of stallion semen, as well as blood hormone levels, sexual behavior and fertility.[1, 9, 14, 15] Other factors affecting seminal characteristics are sexual stimulation, frequency of ejaculation, age, testicular size and method of seminal collection.[3-5, 13, 16, 18]

SEMINAL EVALUATION

In an attempt to improve reproductive efficiency, a series of experiments has been conducted with primary emphasis on factors that influence seminal characteristics and on developing a rationale for an appropriate seminal evaluation. This first study was designed to determine the effect of the season on seminal characteristics, so that collection of semen during any month of the year could be used as a measure of reproductive capacity during the breeding season.

First and second ejaculates of semen were collected from each of five aged quarter horse stallions once each week for 13 months, May through May. Attempts were made to collect the second ejaculate 1 hour after the first. Presented in Table 1 are the overall means and monthly ranges of the seminal characteristics for first and second ejaculates.

Presented in Figure 1 is a graph of the mean monthly volumes of gel-free semen for first and second ejaculates. The difference between 58 ml for first ejaculates and 50 ml for second ejaculates, although relatively small, was statistically significant ($p < 0.05$). Thus, a slightly lower volume can be expected for second ejaculates collected 1 hour after the first. Volume is measured primarily to provide an essential factor in calculating the number of spermatozoa per ejaculate. Gel-free semen was obtained by incorporating a filter into the neck of the collection bottle; thus, the gel was removed during collection and was never mixed with the sperm-rich fraction of the ejaculate.[10]

Presented in Figure 2 is the mean monthly volume of gel. Mean volume of gel was 7 ml for all first and 2 ml for all second ejaculates (Table 1). However, in the 75 first ejaculates (29 per cent) that contained gel, the mean gel volume was 27 ml, while 29 second ejaculates (11 per cent) contained an average of 19 ml. It appeared that the seminal vesicles, which secrete the gelatinous fraction, were slower to replenish their secretion than the other secondary sex glands. This may be due to an inability of certain stallions to become sexually stimulated during certain seasons or after an extended regimen of seminal collection. Although no evidence was presented, Nishikawa[9] reported that gel served as a bacteriostat. Regardless of the function of gel, semen from some stallions rarely, if ever, contains gel, and yet, their fertility appears normal. Thus, the presence or absence of gel in an ejaculate may not reflect the fertility of that ejaculate. Furthermore, when mares are bred utilizing artificial insemination (AI), the gel is a nuisance and must be removed during seminal collection.[10] Fertility of semen appeared to be normal although the gel was never mixed with the "sperm-rich" fraction.[17]

The gel must be removed during seminal collection to obtain a representative sample for estimation of spermatozoal concentration. The gel can be removed after seminal collection, but more spermatozoa are lost.[18] This is an important consideration when the maximum number of spermatozoa are needed for AI.

During an evaluation for potential fertility, measurement of gel is necessary only if one is attempting to carefully estimate daily spermatozoal output (DSO). It has been es-

TABLE 1. *Physical Characteristics of First and Second Ejaculates of Stallion Semen**

Characteristic	Ejaculate	Mean	Range LOW	Range HIGH
Volume (ml)				
Gel-free	1	58	45	81
	2	50	42	63
Gel	1	7	0	30
	2	2	0	11
Total	1	66	45	104
	2	52	42	68
Spermatozoa/ml (10^6)	1	281	224	321
	2	170	111	234
Spermatozoa/ejaculate (10^9)	1	15	10	22
	2	8	5	12
Sperm motility (%)	1	73	70	75
	2	74	70	77
pH	1	7.47	7.36	7.57
	2	7.59	7.46	7.70

*Adapted from Pickett, B. W., Faulkner, L. C. and Voss, J. L.: J. Reprod. Fertil. (Suppl.), *23*:25, 1975.

timated that there are approximately 19 million spermatozoa per ml of gel.[18] Considering the variation and the difficulty in counting the spermatozoa in gel, it is highly unlikely that the information is worth the effort for any practical purpose.

Presented in Figure 3 are the mean monthly total seminal volumes, while the mean monthly ranges are listed in Table 1. The total volume of first and second ejaculates increased 38 and 21 per cent, respectively, from winter to spring. Total seminal volume, generally including gel, is the most commonly reported seminal characteristic. However, this characteristic is probably of least importance, since excellent fertility can be obtained by AI with 1.5 ml of raw semen, and as little as 0.6 ml may be ade-

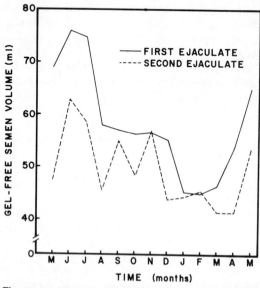

Figure 1. Mean monthly gel-free seminal volumes. (Adapted from Pickett, B. W. and Voss, J. L.: Proc. 18th Ann. Conv. A.A.E.P., pp. 501–531, 1972.)

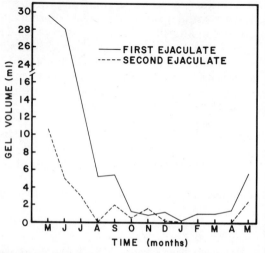

Figure 2. Mean monthly gel volumes. (Adapted from Pickett, B. W. and Voss, J. L.: Proc. 18th Ann. Conv. A.A.E.P., pp. 501–531, 1972.)

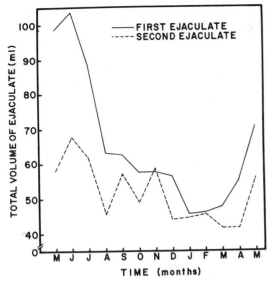

Figure 3. Mean monthly total seminal volumes. (Adapted from Pickett, B. W. and Voss, J. L.: Proc. 18th Ann. Conv. A.A.E.P., pp. 501–531, 1972.)

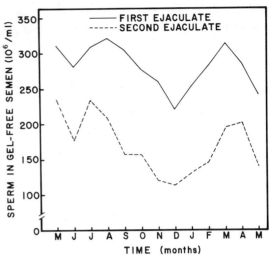

Figure 4. Mean monthly concentrations of spermatozoa per ml of gel-free semen. (Adapted from Pickett, B. W. and Voss, J. L.: Proc. 18th Ann. Conv. A.A.E.P., pp. 501–531, 1972.)

quate.[17] In addition, up to 100 ml of semen can be obtained without the occurrence of complete ejaculation.[13] Furthermore, when stallions were used as teasers, gel volume increased from an average of 8 to 23 ml, and mean gel-free seminal volume increased fom 37 to 63 ml without an increase in spermatozoal output.[12]

The relationship between seminal volumes in first and second ejaculates in this study was reasonably consistent. However, a low first ejaculate volume followed by a high second ejaculate volume is not uncommon when semen is collected from inexperienced 2- or 3-year-old stallions. The first may serve as a stimulus for the second ejaculate.

The concentration of spermatozoa per ml of gel-free semen was estimated with a Bausch and Lomb "Spectronic 20" spectrophotometer. Utilizing this method, total spermatozoa per ml can be quickly and accurately determined. This item of equipment is absolutely essential for anyone seriously intent upon determining accurate potential fertility evaluation of stallions and/or utilizing AI for *maximum reproductive efficiency*.

Average concentrations of spermatozoa per ml of gel-free semen are presented in Figure 4. Second ejaculates collected approximately 1 hour after the first contained approximately 60 to 65 per cent as many sperm as first ejaculates. This relationship was true when stallions were collected at weekly intervals or when two ejaculates were col-

lected two times per week.[16] The number of spermatozoa per ml is less important than the total number of spermatozoa per ejaculate. In fact, total spermatozoa per ejaculate (provided frequency of ejaculation is known) and motility of spermatozoa are the two most valuable measurements in a seminal evaluation.

First ejaculates contained a mean of 15 billion spermatozoa; second ejaculates contained 8 billion. First ejaculates ranged from 10 billion in January to 22 billion in July. Second ejaculates ranged from 5 billion in December to 12 billion in July (Fig. 5). The

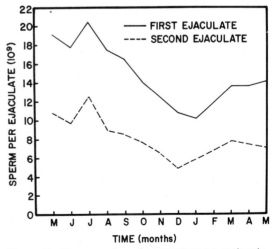

Figure 5. Mean number of spermatozoa per ejaculation (billions) by month. (Adapted from Pickett, B. W. and Voss, J. L.: Proc. 18th Ann. Conv. A.A.E.P., pp. 501–531, 1972.)

difference in mean total spermatozoa per ejaculate between first and second ejaculates was 53.7 per cent, and the difference in monthly means between the ejaculates ranged from 46.9 to 56.9 per cent.

In a previous 12-month study, the difference between the means of 170 paired first and second ejaculates was 49.8 per cent. When the ejaculation frequency was doubled to two ejaculates twice per week, the percentage of spermatozoa in second ejaculates was 45.8 per cent of the total in first ejaculates.[16] The relationship of spermatozoal numbers in first and second ejaculates was so consistent that the second ejaculate can be used to determine how representative the first ejaculate was of a normal ejaculation. If a stallion has been sexually rested for at least 4 days and the second ejaculate does not contain approximately 50 per cent of the total number of spermatozoa in the first ejaculate, one of the following must be suspected: (1) one of the ejaculates was incomplete, (2) the stallion's extragonadal spermatozoal reserves (EGR) had been depleted, (3) excessive spermatozoa had accumulated in the excurrent ducts,[13] (4) the excurrent ducts were incapable of storing large quantities of spermatozoa or (5) the stallion was sexually immature.[19] This approximately 50 per cent relationship (6 versus 12 billion) was also observed when one ejaculate per day was collected at intervals of six times per week compared with three times per week after the EGR had been stabilized.[16]

Although others[9, 21] found no difference in spermatozoal output due to season, Pickett *et al.*[15] reported a 52.0 and 46.2 per cent reduction in spermatozoal output from the highest to the lowest month in first and second ejaculates, respectively. In this study, corresponding reductions average 46.2 and 42.4 per cent (Fig. 5). This dramatic decrease in spermatozoal output probably represents a true decrease in spermatogenesis. Since season influenced spermatozoal numbers for both ejaculates (p <0.01), season must be considered when stallions are evaluated for breeding soundness.

Daily spermatozoal production (DSP) in the stallion was 8 billion and DSO accounted for 87 per cent of DSP.[3] Since DSP was 8 billion spermatozoa and mean extragonadal transit time was 7.5 to 11.0 days, the EGR should range from 60 to 88 billion. The EGR of 11 stallions 24 hours after the last ejaculation was 58.6 billion.[4] When one ejaculate of semen was collected from each of nine stallions at frequencies of one, three or six times per week, mean spermatozoal numbers were 13.5, 12.7 and 7.2 billion, respectively. Therefore, if the number of spermatozoa per ejaculate is more than the total DSP for 2 to 3 days, it is suspected that the stallion is accumulating spermatozoa in the excurrent ducts.[16]

Seminal characteristics of five successive ejaculates collected at hourly intervals from a stallion presented to our laboratory for seminal evaluation are presented in Table 2. This horse had a history of settling his mares when pasture-bred, but he did rather poorly when hand-bred. This is a classic example of accumulation of sperm in the seminal ducts. The numbers of sperm in the fourth and fifth ejaculates compared favorably with those of first and second ejaculates of normal stallions. This stallion was used rather sparingly in hand-breeding, compared with what his sexual activity probably was in the pasture. It was therefore recommended that he be used more frequently. When he was not used daily or every other day, two covers per day on the same mare were recommended.

When time is critical, two ejaculates collected 1 hour apart are minimal for a seminal evaluation. Ideally, DSP should be determined, which can be predicted from DSO.[5] To obtain DSO, semen must be collected daily for approximately 1 week, and DSO is dependent upon events initiated approximately 2 months prior to seminal collection.[22]

Testicular size determined by scrotal circumference permits a relatively accurate es-

TABLE 2. *Seminal Characteristics of Five Ejaculates from a 13-Year-Old Quarter Horse Exhibiting Sperm Accumulation**

| | Semen Volume (ml) | | | |
Ejaculate	GEL	GEL-FREE	Total Sperm (billions)	pH
1	29	75	60.8	7.40
2	16	57	47.6	7.49
3	19	89	25.3	7.64
4	0	56	16.5	7.67
5	0	48	8.4	7.77

*Adapted from Pickett, B. W. and Voss, J. L.: Proceedings 18th Annual Convention, A.A.E.P., 1972, pp. 501–531.

TABLE 3. *Stallion Semen Extender for Motility Estimations**

Ingredients	Per Cent
Dried skim milk	5.0
Glucose	5.0
Antibiotics/ml of extender: 500 IU polymyxin B sulfate 500 U penicillin	

*Adapted from Pickett, B. W. and Voss, J. L.: Proceedings 18th Annual Convention, A.A.E.P., 1972, pp. 501–531.

timation of spermatozoal output in bulls.[6] Stallion testicular weight was significantly correlated with DSP and DSO (0.77); this was expected, as 21 million spermatozoa were produced per gram of testicular parenchyma.[4, 5] However, *in vivo* testicular measurements accounted for only 32 per cent of the variation in DSO.[5] In spite of the relatively poor correlation, the testes should be palpated and measured during a routine breeding soundness examination because a stallion with small testes is a potentially poor producer of spermatozoa. The number of mares that can be bred utilizing AI or natural service is dependent upon the number of spermatozoa available for ejaculation.

Freshly ejaculated stallion spermatozoa tend to clump or agglutinate.[15] To reduce the influence of clumping on motility, semen must be extended in a diluent that prevents clumping. The formula for such an extender is presented in Table 3. Prepare a relatively

large quantity of this extender, and pipette 4.75 ml into glass vials for storage in a deep freezer. Prior to seminal evaluation, an appropriate number of the vials are thawed in a water bath maintained at 38°C (100°F). When the extender is warmed to 38°C (100°F), 0.25 ml of raw semen is added. Motility is then estimated at 200× magnification under phase-contrast microscopy. *A word of caution*: This extender has not been fertility tested.

Mean motility of spermatozoa from first ejaculates was 73 per cent with a range from 70 to 75 per cent; mean motility in second ejaculates was 74 per cent and ranged from 70 to 77 per cent (Fig. 6). No influence of season on motility was observed for first or second ejaculates. Motility of spermatozoa from first ejaculates is occasionally lower than motility of spermatozoa in second ejaculates. This difference generally disappears when the frequency of ejaculation is sufficient to prevent spermatozoal accumulation.[13]

Illustrated in Figure 7 are the monthly changes in pH. The mean pH of gel-free semen from first ejaculates was 7.47 compared with 7.59 for second ejaculates. The range for first ejaculates was 7.36 to 7.57, while the range for second ejaculates was 7.46 to 7.70. The pH is a useful diagnostic tool for seminal evaluations because in a "normal situation" the pH of second ejaculates is always higher than that of corresponding first ejaculates regardless of season.[15] When the pH of a second ejaculate is lower than that of the corresponding first

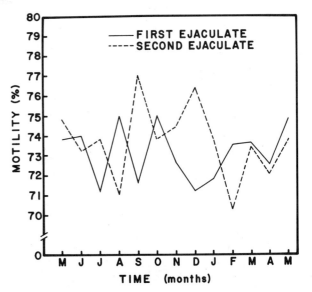

Figure 6. Mean monthly motility of spermatozoa. Adapted from Pickett, B. W. and Voss, J. L.: Proc. 18th Ann. Conv. A.A.E.P., pp. 501–531, 1972.)

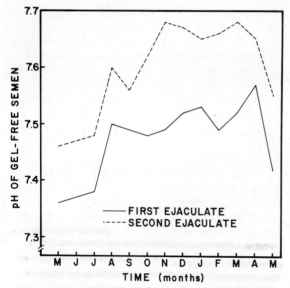

Figure 7. Monthly variation in pH of gel-free semen. (Adapted from Pickett, B. W. and Voss, J. L.: Proc. 18th Ann. Conv. A.A.E.P., pp. 501–531, 1972.)

ejaculate, the first ejaculate must be considered incomplete or abnormal.

The pH of accessory sex gland fluid, devoid of epididymal contributions, will be approximately 8.0. Kirton et al.[7] collected four consecutive ejaculates of semen from bulls within 1 hour and found that pH increased from 6.26 to 6.92. These investigators postulated that the contributions of the seminal vesicles to the ejaculate were relatively constant but that the contributions of the epididymides decreased with repetitive ejaculations. This is an extremely important observation in relation to potential fertility evaluation of stallions, since it is possible to obtain relatively large quantities of seminal fluid and some spermatozoa without the occurrence of ejaculation, or at least without a contribution from the epididymides.[13] This postulation is in excellent agreement with Seidel and Foote,[20] who calculated that the bull epididymides contributed 31 to 36 per cent to the seminal volume of first ejaculates compared with 19 per cent to the volume of second ejaculates. Therefore, when the pH of the first ejaculate is higher or equal to the pH from a corresponding second ejaculate, particularly if the normal relationship in spermatozoal output is altered, the first ejaculate must be considered incomplete or abnormal.

We believe that the percentage contribution to volume of the stallion is higher from the accessory sex glands and less from the

epididymides in second ejaculates than the percentage contribution of the bull, primarily because the volume of the second ejaculate does not change, in relation to first ejaculates, as dramatically as spermatozoal output. Second ejaculates from bulls usually contain 56.2 to 91.6 per cent of the number of spermatozoa found in first ejaculates.[7, 8, 11] After the stallion has had 3 days of sexual rest, the stallion ejaculate normally contains more total spermatozoa than the bull ejaculate. Furthermore, the ductus deferentes and ampullae contain sufficient spermatozoa for a complete ejaculate,[4] whereas the corresponding structures in the bull contain too few spermatozoa for a complete ejaculate.[2]

The seminal vesicles contribute significantly to the bovine ejaculate, which must correspond to the bulbourethral glands in the stallion, because the seminal vesicles in the stallion secrete gel. The gel has a higher pH than gel-free semen but probably contributes very little to the seminal pH since it is removed during collection. For pH to be of diagnostic value, the gel must be separated from the "sperm-rich" fraction because (1) the pH of gel-free semen in the first ejaculate is lower than that of second ejaculates, (2) the pH of gel is higher than that of gel-free semen, (3) there is a greater quantity of gel secreted in first than in second ejaculates and (4) if the gel and "sperm-rich" fractions mix during collection, the difference in seminal pH between first and second ejaculates would be greatly reduced.

FREQUENCY OF EJACULATION

From routine examination of semen for breeding potential, it was concluded that one of the most common causes of infertility and sterility among popular stallions is overuse. Horses are seasonal breeders, and spermatozoal output early in the breeding season is only 50 to 75 per cent of the output at the peak of the season. Mares are in heat longer and have fewer fertile ovulations early in the breeding season. These factors cause the breeder to use the stallion more frequently, which further contributes to the infertility problem.

To study the effects of frequency of ejaculation on some characteristics of equine semen, nine Quarter Horse and Thoroughbred stallions were randomly assigned to three groups.[16] The groups were assigned to a

TABLE 4. *Effect of Frequency of Ejaculation on Mean Stallion Seminal Characteristics over Last 2 Weeks of 4-Week Collection Period**

Characteristic	Frequency of Ejaculation per Week		
	1×	3×	6×
Volume/ejaculate (ml):			
Semen, gel-free	47	56	51
Gel	18	8	6
Total	65	64	57
Spermatozoa:			
Concentration/ml (10^6)	288	248	142
Total/ejaculate (10^9)	11.4	11.7	5.9
Total/wk (10^9)	11.4	35.2	35.3
Motility (%)	54	52	56

*Adapted from Pickett, B. W., Sullivan, J. J. and Seidel, G. E., Jr.: J. Anim. Sci., *40*:917, 1975.

seminal collection frequency of one time (1×), three times (3×) or six times (6×) per week for 4 weeks (one collection period). At the end of each collection period, the animals were sexually rested for one week, and groups were reassigned to a different collection frequency for the next collection period. This protocol was continued until each stallion had been collected at each frequency for 4 weeks. The results are presented in Table 4.

There were no differences in seminal volume due to frequency of seminal collection; thus, it is possible for a stallion to produce large volumes of semen containing very few sperm. Spermatozoal concentration per ml of gel-free semen remained essentially the same whether a stallion was collected once per week or every other day (Table 4). However, when semen was collected 6× per week, the number of sperm per ml dropped abruptly.

When the total number of sperm per ejaculate was calculated, the 1× averaged 11.4 billion, compared with 11.7 at 3× and 5.9 at 6×. There was no difference between the 1× and 3× (11.4 versus 11.7 billion) in total sperm per ejaculate. From a practical point of view, this was interpreted to mean that a stallion being used every other day still ejaculates as many sperm per cover as if he were being used once per week.

The total spermatozoal output per week averaged 11.4, 35.2 and 35.3 billion per week at frequencies of 1×, 3× and 6×, respectively. Total spermatozoal output per week was identical at 3× and 6× frequencies. With an every-other-day collection schedule, all the sperm that are available for ejaculation are being collected. For maximum efficiency, we recommend artifical insemination. Stallions should be collected every other day, and all mares in heat that have been in standing heat for 2 days or longer should be inseminated.

CONCLUSIONS AND RECOMMENDATIONS

1. Semen from each stallion should be evaluated prior to the breeding season and before sale if the animal is to be used for breeding.

2. The stallion should have at least 4 days and preferably 1 week of sexual rest prior to seminal evaluation.

3. At least two ejaculates should be collected an hour apart for the evaluation. Ideally, two ejaculates should be collected followed by daily collections for 1 week.

4. The volume of gel-free semen is relatively unimportant.

5. Second ejaculates normally contain about one-half the number of spermatozoa found in first ejaculates.

6. Total spermatozoal output per ejaculate from normal stallions will vary from one billion to 30 billion spermatozoa, depending upon testicular size, frequency of ejaculation, season and age.

7. For reliable estimations of motility, equine semen should be extended (1:20) in an extender that prevents clumping of the spermatozoa.

8. The pH of normal first ejaculates is always lower than the pH of corresponding second ejaculates unless the stallion is very young.

9. A sample of stallion semen and a swab from the urethra and prepuce should be cultured during a breeding soundness examination and periodically during the breeding season.

10. The variation in stallion seminal characteristics is extremely large because of season, and this must be considered during seminal evaluation.

11. Testes should be measured for a complete breeding soundness examination.

REFERENCES

1. Berndtson, W. E., Pickett, B. W. and Nett, T. M.: Reproductive physiology of the stallion. IV. Seasonal changes in the testosterone concentration of peripheral plasma. J. Reprod. Fertil., *39*:115, 1974.
2. Bialy, G. and Smith, V. R.: Number of spermatozoa in the different parts of the reproductive tract of the bull. J. Dairy Sci., *41*:1781, 1958.
3. Gebauer, M. R., Pickett, B. W. and Swierstra, E. E.: Reproductive physiology of the stallion. II. Daily production and output of sperm. J. Anim. Sci., *39*:732, 1974.
4. Gebauer, M. R., Pickett, B. W. and Swierstra, E. E.: Reproductive physiology of the stallion. III. Extra-gonadal transit time and sperm reserves. J. Anim. Sci., *39*:737, 1974.
5. Gebauer, M. R., Pickett, B. W., Voss, J. L. and Swierstra, E. E.: Reproductive physiology of the stallion: Daily sperm output and testicular measurements. J.A.V.M.A., *165*:711, 1974.
6. Hahn, J., Foote, R. H. and Seidel, G. E., Jr.: Testicular growth and related sperm output in dairy bulls. J. Anim. Sci., *29*:41, 1969.
7. Kirton, K. T., Hafs, H. D. and Hunter, A. G.: Levels of some normal constituents of bull semen during repetitive ejaculation. J. Reprod. Fertil., *8*:157, 1964.
8. Macmillan, K. L., Desjardins, C., Kirton, K. T. and Hafs, H. D.: Relationship of glycerylphosphorylcholine to other constituents of bull semen. J. Dairy Sci., *50*:1310, 1967.
9. Nishikawa, Y.: Studies on reproduction in horses. Japan Racing Association, Shiba Tamuracho Minatoku, Tokyo, Japan, pp. 1–340.
10. Pickett, B. W. and Back, D. G.: Procedures for preparation, collection, evaluation, and insemination of stallion semen. Colorado State Univ. Exp. Sta., Anim. Reprod. Lab. Gen. Series 935. 1973, pp. 1–26.
11. Pickett, B. W. and Komarek, R. J.: Lipid and dry weight of bovine seminal plasma and spermatozoa from first and second ejaculates. J. Dairy Sci., *50*:742, 1967.
12. Pickett, B. W. and Voss, J. L.: Reproductive management of the stallion. Proceedings Eighteenth Annual Convention A.A.E.P., 1972, pp. 501–531. Published by The A.A.E.P., Golden, Col., 80401.
13. Pickett, B. W. and Voss, J. L.: Abnormalities of mating behaviour in domestic stallions. J. Reprod. Fertil. (Suppl.), *23*:129, 1975.
14. Pickett, B. W., Faulkner, L. C. and Voss, J. L.: Effect of season on some characteristics of stallion semen. J. Reprod. Fertil. (Suppl.), *23*:25, 1975.
15. Pickett, B. W., Faulkner, L. C. and Sutherland, T. M.: Effect of month and stallion on seminal characteristics and sexual behavior. J. Anim. Sci., *31*:713, 1970.
16. Pickett, B. W., Sullivan, J. J. and Seidel, G. E., Jr.: Reproductive physiology of the stallion. V. Effect of frequency of ejaculation on seminal characteristics and spermatozoal output. J. Anim. Sci., *40*:917, 1975.
17. Pickett, B. W., Back, D. G., Burwash, L. D. and Voss, J. L.: The effect of extenders, spermatozoal numbers and rectal palpation on equine fertility. Proceedings Fifth N.A.A.B. Technical Conference on A. I. Reproduction, 1974, pp. 47–58. Published by N.A.A.B., Columbia, Mo., 65201.
18. Pickett, B. W., Gebauer, M. R., Seidel, G. E., Jr. and Voss, J. L.: Reproductive physiology of the stallion: Spermatozoal losses in the collection equipment and gel. J.A.V.M.A., *165*:708, 1974.
19. Pickett, B. W., Faulkner, L. C., Seidel, G. E., Jr., Berndtson, W. E. and Voss, J. L.: Reproductive physiology of the stallion. VI. Seminal and behavioral characteristics. J. Anim. Sci., *43*:617, 1976.
20. Seidel, G. E., Jr. and Foote, R. H.: Compartmental analysis of sources of the bovine ejaculate. Biol. Reprod., *2*:189, 1970.
21. Skinner, J. D. and Bowen, J.: Puberty in the Welsh stallion. J. Reprod. Fertil., *16*:133, 1968.
22. Swierstra, E. E., Gebauer, M. R. and Pickett, B. W.: Reproductive physiology of the stallion. I. Spermatogenesis and testis composition. J. Reprod. Fertil., *40*:113, 1974.

Use of Artificial Insemination in Stallion Management

B. W. PICKETT

Colorado State University, Fort Collins, Colorado

INTRODUCTION

The primary objective during the breeding season is to settle the maximum number of mares in the minimum amount of time. This will reduce labor and other expenses and provide earlier foals, thus shortening the foaling season and, again, reducing labor and so forth. Artificial insemination (AI) can aid in accomplishing these goals. The following is a list of the advantages of AI and a brief discussion of these advantages.

1. The procedure permits disease control. AI is effectively used in the cattle industry to control certain venereal diseases. This is accomplished in two ways: (a) the semen is diluted sufficiently so that the number of organisms is reduced below the number necessary to cause the disease and (b) the diluent or extender used to dilute the semen

contains antibiotics that either kill the organisms or destroy their pathogenic properties. It is suspected that these same factors would be useful in the control of reproductive diseases in horses.

2. AI reduces the possibility of injury to the mare and/or stallion. The reason why a stallion will occasionally object violently to a particular mare is unknown, but this has resulted in many mares and an occasional handler being severely injured. When AI is practiced, a gentle mare acceptable to the stallion can be used for collection so that injury to the mare, stallion or personnel is greatly reduced. The use of a gentle mare during seminal collection is extremely important in getting maximum use from a stallion that is extremely shy or is being retrained after a poor breeding experience. In addition, many stallions can be trained to mount a phantom and ejaculate. Furthermore, AI eliminates the problem associated with mating animals of different size.

3. Stallions that have developed poor breeding habits or have been injured may be used in an AI program when natural service may not be possible. Stallions have been trained to ejaculate into an artificial vagina without mounting a mare. A stallion that has been injured or has developed chronic lameness or other problems and then is trained to ejaculate in this manner could be used in an AI program. In at least one instance in which a stallion was unable to get an erection but showed excellent sex drive, training to an artificial vagina was accomplished. Stallions that have been mismanaged, kicked or otherwise injured during the breeding process generally develop poor breeding habits. It is quite common for these horses to dismount quickly while in the process of ejaculating. Under these circumstances, much of the ejaculate is lost on the ground. This can sometimes be circumvented by catching the dismount sample and reinforcing the natural cover with AI. However, the exposure of semen to these conditions results in loss of quality and is a very poor management practice. When semen is collected with an artificial vagina, the ejaculate is collected in its entirety. Furthermore, collection of semen with an artificial vagina generally aids in correcting this habit.

4. Semen can be evaluated at each collection; thus, minor changes in seminal quality are observed immediately. Formation and maturation of sperm require about 60 to 70 days in the horse. Thus, periodic seminal evaluation, as is done in AI, in conjunction with an effective herd health program, will aid in identification of causes of reproductive failure that would otherwise go undetected.

5. AI aids in identification of reproductive problems. Many times use of AI is criticized for being responsible for low fertility when it only aided in pointing out the problems.

6. The procedure prevents overuse of a stallion, particularly early in the breeding season. One of the most common causes of infertility or sterility is overuse. Some stallions can be used daily and occasionally twice or even three times per day without reducing spermatozoal output below the number needed for maximum fertility, while other stallions become infertile or even sterile after daily use. Stallions in the latter category should never be used more than three times per week.

7. More mares can be bred on a given day to the same stallion. When two or more mares need to be bred on a given day, AI is beneficial in preventing overuse of the stallion but still getting the mares bred at the proper time. Cattle semen can be collected, extended and used to breed cows for at least 3 days without an appreciable loss of fertility. However, too little information is available to follow this procedure with stallion semen. Although there are several extenders that have been used for stallion spermatozoa, our current recommendation is to collect the semen and use it immediately without dilution.

8. AI permits more effective use of older, more valuable stallions. As stallions age, degenerative changes occur that reduce the total number of sperm produced, and in many cases those that are produced have a greater number of abnormalities, which further reduce fertility. A properly spaced collection schedule and reliable seminal evaluation program, plus insemination of the proper number of sperm into the uterus at the proper time, will result in more conceptions than by natural service. In fact, in many cases this may be the only method to obtain foals from an old, valuable stallion.

9. Mares can be bred at the most opportune time for the maximum chance of conception. When 40 to 50 mares are booked, AI is the only realistic solution to breeding these mares for *maximum reproductive efficiency.* Our current recommendation is to collect the stallion every other day and breed all mares that have been in heat 2 days and longer.

Before entering into an AI program, the moral obligations, mechanics of collection, handling of semen, insemination techniques and costs must be thoroughly understood by all parties involved. Artificial insemination offers no complete solution to breeding problems. In fact, it can compound the problem if incorrectly practiced. Artificial insemination has been criticized or labeled as a means of reducing the accuracy of sire identification. Quite the contrary is true. Accurate records and keen observation are absolutely necessary in any successful AI program.

Inherent fertility, nutrition, age, disease, sexual behavior and season are factors affecting fertility. Equine fertility can be improved by the use of artificial insemination. However, certain factors such as extender composition, manipulation of the reproductive tract, methods of handling semen, insemination techniques and the number of spermatozoa per insemination can affect fertility in an AI program.

Artificial insemination allows utilization of the minimal number of spermatozoa for *maximum reproductive efficiency*. Small inseminate volumes, containing adequate numbers of spermatozoa for maximum fertility, are less likely to cause a reaction or induce infection than are larger volumes. In a controlled experiment, a mean volume of only 1.5 ml of raw semen was used to inseminate 24 mares.[3] A pregnancy rate of 75.0 per cent was obtained during cycle 1 and 91.7 per cent after two cycles. It is obvious that good pregnancy rates can be obtained with small volumes of semen, but care must be used during insemination of small volumes to insure that the calculated amount of semen, containing the appropriate number of spermatozoa, is placed in the body of the uterus. Appropriate techniques for handling semen and sanitary procedures should always be followed.

SEMINAL EXTENDERS

Artificial insemination permits one to utilize a seminal extender. This is especially beneficial with stallions shedding pathogenic bacteria. The extended semen can be treated with appropriate antibacterials, thus reducing the danger of contamination of the mare's uterus. The equine industry very much needs an extender that will promote fertility and prolong survival of sper-

matozoa. Semen in some extenders appears to offer good fertility when used with certain extenders such as skim milk, skim milk-gelatin or cream-gelatin. However, insemination with raw semen is easier and simpler than preparing the extender and so forth. Therefore, raw semen is still recommended except when it is necessary to:

1. Permit effective antibiotic or antibacterial treatment of semen containing pathogenic organisms.

2. Enhance viability of spermatozoa from stallions with low fertility.

3. Prolong the survival of equine spermatozoa.

4. Protect the spermatozoa from unfavorable environmental conditions.

5. Extend the volume of inseminate for stallions that produce exceedingly low volumes of semen containing large numbers of spermatozoa per milliliter of raw semen.

6. Aid in proper evaluation of sperm motility.

In 1973, 72 mares were randomly assigned to a factorial experiment that included three seminal treatments.[3] Insemination was initiated on May 1 and continued for three estrous periods or until pregnancy was diagnosed. Semen was collected from three stallions every other day, and all mares in estrus for 2 days or longer were inseminated.

The three seminal treatments, which utilized 500 million motile spermatozoa per insemination, were as follows:

1. Semen plus 10 ml of a 2.4 per cent Tris extender.

2. Semen plus 10 ml of a cream-gelatin extender.

3. Raw semen.

Presented in Table 1 are the results of that study.

Only 37.5 per cent of the mares settled when bred with spermatozoa in the 2.4 per cent Tris extender during cycle 1, compared with 75.0 per cent in cream-gel and 75.0 per cent bred with raw semen. After three cycles the pregnancy rates were 75.0, 95.8 and 91.7 per cent for the Tris, cream-gel and raw semen treatments, respectively. Spermatozoa in the cream-gel treatment settled 23 of 24 mares. Fertility was depressed (p <0.01) by extension of semen in the Tris extender, probably caused by the presence of glycerol.

Pregnancy rates of 75.0 per cent during a single cycle are much higher than normally reported for dry mares and would be consid-

TABLE 1.   *The Effect of Seminal Treatments on Pregnancy Rates of Mares**

| | Extended[a] | | | | Raw[b] | |
| | Tris | | Cream-Gel | | | |
Cycle	NO. OF MARES	PREGNANT (%)	NO. OF MARES	PREGNANT (%)	NO. OF MARES	PREGNANT (%)
1	24 (9)[c]	37.5	24 (18)	75.0	24 (18)	75.0
2	13 (5)	38.5	5 (4)	80.0	6 (4)	66.7
3	7 (4)	57.1	1 (1)	100.0	1 (0)	0.0
Total	24 (18)	75.0[d]	24 (23)	95.8[e]	24 (22)	91.7[e]

*Adapted from Voss, J. L. and Pickett, B. W.: Colorado State Univ. Exp. Sta., Anim. Reprod. Lab. Gen. Series 961, 1976, pp. 1–29.

[a] 500×10^6 motile spermatozoa extended in 10 ml of extender.

[b] 500×10^6 motile spermatozoa.

[c] Numbers in parentheses are the number of mares that became pregnant.

[d,e] Percentages within rows with different superscripts are significantly different at the 1 per cent level of probability (analysis of variance).

ered excellent for other classes of livestock, including cattle. It has been assumed that fertility is much lower in the equine species than in other species of livestock. Obviously, this is not true when AI is used under proper management conditions.

Because of the excellent results obtained with the cream-gel extender, the method of preparation is included here.

Preparation of 100 ml of cream-gelatin extender: Needed are 1.3 gm of Knox gelatin, 10 ml of deionized water and 90 ml of half and half cream.

1. Weigh out 1.3 gm of Knox gelatin.

2. Add Knox gelatin to 10 ml of deionized water.

3. Autoclave Knox gelatin and deionized water for 20 minutes.

4. Heat half and half cream in a double boiler for 10 minutes at 92°C (198°F), being sure that it does not boil or exceed 95°C (203°F).

5. Remove any scum from the half and half cream after heating.

6. Add the half and half cream to the Knox gelatin solution to make a total volume of 100 ml.

7. Freeze in 10-ml doses and store in the deep freezer until used.

Note: Be sure that the extender is warmed to body temperature, i.e., 38°C (100°F), before the raw semen is added.

During 1975, an experiment was conducted utilizing 48 normally cycling, nonlactating mares to determine the effect on fertility of three extenders, skim milk-gelatin, skim milk alone and cream-gelatin.[3] All mares were teased daily with one or two stallions and inseminated every other day beginning on day 2 or 3 of their first normal estrus following May 1.

The results by extender are presented in Table 2. Pregnancy rates for the skim milk-gel and skim-milk alone were both 62.5 per

TABLE 2.   *Effect of Extenders on Fertility of Equine Spermatozoa**

| | Extender | | | | | |
| | Skim Milk | | Skim Milk-Gel | | Cream-Gel | |
Cycle	NO. OF MARES	PREGNANT (%)	NO. OF MARES	PREGNANT (%)	NO. OF MARES	PREGNANT (%)
1	16 (3)†	18.8	16 (3)	18.8	16 (3)	18.8
2	13 (6)	46.2	13 (5)	38.5	13 (3)	23.1
3	7 (1)	14.3	8 (2)	25.0	10 (1)	10.0
Total	16 (10)	62.5	16 (10)	62.5	16 (7)	43.8

*Adapted from Voss, J. L. and Pickett, B. W.: Colorado State Univ. Exp. Sta., Anim. Reprod. Lab. Gen. Series 961, 1976, pp. 1–29.

†Numbers in parentheses are the number of mares that became pregnant.

cent, while 43.8 per cent of the mares bred with spermatozoa in the cream-gel became pregnant. Although there were no significant differences among the pregnancy rates, because of the small number of mares involved, it appeared that spermatozoa extended in the skim-milk extenders will provide as good or better fertility than the spermatozoa in the cream-gel extender.

The skim milk extenders provide an advantage over cream-gel in that motility of the spermatozoa can be observed microscopically, whereas in cream-gel, movement of the spermatozoa is obscured by fat globules. However, it must be pointed out that the skim milk extenders have never been compared with raw semen in a controlled experiment. The methods of preparation of both skim milk extenders are as follows:

1. *Skim milk:* 100 ml of skim milk (nonfortified) is required.
   a. Heat the skim milk in a double boiler for 10 minutes at 92°C (198°F). The temperature should never fall below this point or exceed 95°C (203°F).
   b. Freeze in 10-ml doses and store in the deep freezer until used.
2. *Skim milk-gelatin:* 1.3 gm of Knox gelatin and 100 ml of skim milk (nonfortified) are required.
   a. Weigh 1.3 gm of Knox gelatin.
   b. Add to 100 ml of skim milk and agitate for 1 minute.
   c. Heat mixture in a double boiler for 10 minutes at 92°C (198°F). The temperature should never fall below this point or exceed 95°C (203°F). Swirl the mixture periodically during the heating process.
   d. Freeze in 10-ml doses and store in the deep freezer until used.

SPERMATOZOAL NUMBERS

The number of mares that can be bred per ejaculation is dependent upon the number of spermatozoa obtained and the number of spermatozoa required per insemination for *maximum reproductive efficiency.* The number of spermatozoa obtained per ejaculation is dependent upon libido, testicular size, age, season and frequency of ejaculation.

Presented in Table 3 are the results of 100 million versus 500 million spermatozoa per insemination unit. There were only 14 mares per group in this study, and the fertility was

TABLE 3. *Effect of Number of Motile Spermatozoa on Pregnancy Rates in Mares[*]*

	Spermatozoa			
	500 Million		**100 Million**	
Cycle	NO. OF MARES	PREGNANT (%)	NO. OF MARES	PREGNANT (%)
3	9 (4)†	44.4	9 (3)	33.3
4	5 (2)	40.0	5 (2)	40.0
Total	14 (6)	42.9	14 (5)	35.7

[*]Adapted from Pickett, B. W., Back, D. G., Burwash, L. D. and Voss, J. L.: Proceedings Fifth N.A.A.B. Technical Conference on A.I. Reproduction, 1974, pp. 47–58.

†Numbers in parentheses are the number of mares that became pregnant.

low, probably because the mares had not settled in a previous experiment and were undoubtedly subfertile. The difference between the 42.9 and 35.7 per cent was not significant. As a matter of fact, there was only a difference of one mare in favor of the treatment with 500 million sperm. These mares were bred with raw semen, and the average volume per inseminate for the mares in the 100 million group was only 0.6 ml of semen.

Presented in Table 4 are the results of a study utilizing 72 mares, comparing 100 million versus 500 million spermatozoa in a cream-gelatin extender. The overall difference in fertility of 63.9 versus 75 per cent for the 100 million and 500 million sperm, respectively, was not statistically significant.

TABLE 4. *Effect of Spermatozoal Number on Pregnancy Rate in Mares[*]*

	Spermatozoa			
	500 Million		**100 Million**	
Cycle	NO. OF MARES	PREGNANT (%)	NO. OF MARES	PREGNANT (%)
1	36 (14)†	38.9	36 (9)	25.0
2	22 (10)	45.4	27 (9)	33.3
3	12 (3)	25.0	18 (5)	27.8
Total	36 (27)	75.0	36 (23)	63.9

[*]Adapted from Demick, D. S., Voss, J. L. and Pickett, B. W.: J. Anim. Sci., 43:633, 1976.

†Numbers in parentheses are the number of mares that became pregnant.

TABLE 5. *Effect of Spermatozoal Number by Seminal Treatments on Pregnancy Rates in Mares**

| | Spermatozoa | | | |
| | 500 Million | | 100 Million | |
Seminal Treatments	NO. OF MARES	PREGNANT (%)	NO. OF MARES	PREGNANT (%)
Fresh	9 (9)†	100.0	9 (8)	88.9
Cooled (2 hr)	9 (7)	77.8	9 (8)	88.9
Cooled (2 hr) + glycerol	9 (5)	55.6	9 (3)	33.3
Cooled (24 hr)	9 (6)	66.7	9 (4)	44.4
Total	36 (27)	75.0	36 (23)	63.9

*Adapted from Demick, D. S., Voss, J. L. and Pickett, B. W.: J. Anim. Sci., *43*:633, 1976.
†Numbers in parentheses are the number of mares that became pregnant.

Presented in Table 5 are the results, using the same data in Table 4, of the effect of number of sperm by seminal treatments. Please note, in the first two seminal treatments, i.e., fresh and cooled 2 hours, 16 of 18 mares, or exactly the same number, settled to treatment with both the 100 million and 500 million spermatozoa. However, when semen was cooled 2 hours and 7 per cent glycerol was added or semen was stored for 24 hours, fertility was depressed by using 100 million spermatozoa per insemination unit. *Therefore,* it must be concluded that when severe stress, such as the addition of glycerol or storage for 24 hours, was placed on equine spermatozoa, 100 million spermatozoa per insemination was not sufficient to maintain *maximum reproductive efficiency,* but if the stallion and mare are fertile and the methods of collection and insemination are satisfactory, 100 million spermatozoa will provide *maximum reproductive efficiency.*

It is obvious from these studies that not enough information is available concerning the physiological requirements of equine spermatozoa to prepare an extender that will protect the spermatozoa to the same degree that bovine spermatozoa can be protected.

REFERENCES

1. Demick, D. S., Voss, J. L., and Pickett, B. W.: Effect of cooling, storage, glycerolization and spermatozoal numbers on equine fertility. J. Anim. Sci., *43*:633, 1976.
2. Pickett, B. W., Back, D. G., Burwash, L. D. and Voss, J. L.: The effect of extenders, spermatozoal numbers and rectal palpation on equine fertility. Proceedings Fifth N.A.A.B. Technical Conference on A.I. on Reproduction, 1974, pp. 47–58. Published by the N.A.A.B., Columbus, Mo. 65201.
3. Voss, J. L. and Pickett, B. W.: Reproductive management of the broodmare. Colorado State Univ. Exp. Sta., Anim. Reprod. Lab. Gen. Series 961, 1976, pp. 1–29.

Physical Examination and Genital Diseases of the Stallion

DEAN P. NEELY

Maryland Equine Center, Inc.,
Cockeysville, Maryland

INTRODUCTION AND BASIC PHYSIOLOGY

In addition to the semen examination for evaluating the stallion's breeding soundness, one should consider the psychological and physical ability of the stallion to deliver semen to the mare. Along with examination of the reproductive organs, a complete physical examination should be performed with attention directed toward the functions of the musculoskeletal, neurological, optic and olfactory systems. Evaluation of these systems can be aided by observing the stallion's approach to the mare — his ability to achieve and maintain an erection; to mount the mare; to complete intromission, copulation and ejaculation and to dismount quietly from the mare.

To properly interpret parameters being evaluated, a basic knowledge of the physiological events necessary to produce and ejaculate semen is needed. Briefly, it takes the stallion's testis approximately 49 days to produce spermatozoa. The spermatozoa then leave the testis and traverse approximately 80 yards of the single epididymal tubule in which they achieve maturation and develop motility. This transit takes approximately 5 to 11 days, or combined with spermatozoal production by the testis, approximately 60 days are required to produce mature, motile spermatozoa. On ejaculation the spermatozoa pass up the ductus deferens into the urethra and are rhythmically ejected in a series of jets from the end of the penis. Of the approximate eight successive jets of semen expelled, the first three jets contain nearly 80 per cent of the spermatozoa in the ejaculate. The remainder of the ejaculate consists primarily of accessory gland secretions. The bulbourethral (Cowper's) glands secrete shortly before ejaculation, with the suggested purpose of neutralizing the urethral pH. This is referred to as the pre-sperm fraction of the ejaculate. The second or sperm-rich fraction of the ejaculate follows and contains the spermatozoa being ejected from the ductus deferens, plus the secretions of the prostrate gland and the glands of the ampullae. Lastly, the third or gel fraction of the ejaculate appears and contains the gelatinous secretion of the seminal vesicles and relatively few spermatozoa.

PROCURING THE HISTORY

As with any clinical examination, one must consider three important factors: The history of the animal, the environment in which the animal is maintained and the animal itself. The history should establish proper identification, including breed, color, markings, brands, tattoos and the age of the animal. Drawings or photographs of the markings are desirable to avoid errors and legal complications.

Pertinent information should also be obtained about any past illnesses, present and/or past treatments, behavioral difficulties, past conception rates and any problems related to breeding ability or performance. As always, care should be taken to construct proper questions so that the answers convey a valid history.

GENERAL PHYSICAL EXAMINATION AND ASSOCIATED PROBLEMS

A complete soundness examination should be performed and all parameters evaluated toward determining the ability of the stallion to maintain and withstand a vigorous breeding regimen. Prior to direct physical examination, the condition of the stallion should be noted. A stallion in poor flesh may reflect improper nutrition and/or management or chronic disease. Chronic disease is likely to be a problem specific to the individual stallion, but improper nutrition or poor management may encompass the entire breeding farm operation. Correction of these underlying problems should be done prior to evaluating the breeding soundness of the stallion. Once a satisfactory condition is established, it is desirable to delay semen evaluation for 60 days so that spermatogenesis and epididymal transit time reflect the improved condition of the stallion.

On direct physical examination, the conformation of the stallion should be assessed. Although most stallions that are retired to stud have excelled in competitive events and should therefore have good conformation, certain conformational defects may be observed. For a breeding animal, it would be useful to know what conformational defects are inherited. In the horse, suspected inherited defects include overshot jaws, undershot jaws, sickle hocks, umbilical hernias, inguinal hernias, cryptorchidism and testicular hypoplasia, to name a few. Because of their probable polygenic nature, the inheritance of these traits in the horse has not been documented by genetic studies. Therefore, it is difficult to deny a satisfactory breeding soundness opinion based on the possibility of transmitting these defects. Fortunately, most breed associations disallow registering cryptorchid stallions. Testicular hypoplasia may cause a stallion to be rejected on the basis of a poor semen evaluation.

Of prime concern in evaluating conformation are abnormalities involving the back and rear legs. This is because most of the physical stress of breeding is oriented to these areas. Old back injuries and spondylosis may cause pain and delay or prevent proper mounting and copulation. The presence of neurological defects, exhibited by incoordination, nerve paralysis or spasmotic conditions of the rear legs, may also prevent natural breeding. Bursitis, osteoarthritic conditions and associated muscle atrophy in the rear legs, especially those disorders involving the hock and stifle joints, may inhibit or prevent natural breeding attempts and reduce libido because of pain. Disturbed libido associated with pain may be reflected by lack of interest in mares, failure to achieve an erection, repeated attempts prior to mounting or dismounting prior to ejaculation.

Decreased libido may be related to psychological problems and should be differentiated from that associated with arthritic pain. Stallions that are continually mistreated by their handlers may exhibit disinterest in breeding. Careful observation while the stallion attempts to breed a mare, along with the physical examination, will help distinguish the origin of the problem.

Arthritic, pain-related conditions may respond to anti-inflammatory drug therapy, such as phenylbutazone, aspirin or steroids. When artificial insemination is permitted, the use of small mares or the training of the stallion to a "phantom" or "dummy" constructed low to the ground may be employed for semen collection. This helps reduce pain by preventing the excessive stress on the back and rear legs.

All pain-related conditions, and their response to treatment, should be evaluated as to the ultimate effect on the duration of the stallion's breeding ability. Such interpretations should be included in the stallion's report and considered in the overall breeding soundness evaluation.

An ophthalmological examination, rectal examination and olfactory evaluation should be included as part of the physical examination. A stallion with developing blindness may have difficulty in approaching and mounting mares. A rectal examination should include a thorough abdominal exploration, rather than just evaluation of the internal genitalia. Aneurysms, abscesses or abdominal adhesions may be detected and reflect on past or present illnesses that could influence the final soundness evaluation. Olfaction is difficult to evaluate, but the presence of a normal "flehmen" reaction, or curling up of the upper lip after smelling the mare, is an indication that normal olfactory perceptibility is present.

EXTERNAL GENITALIA

The stallion's external genital organs are usually examined prior to or while washing the stallion's penis and sheath for breeding or semen collection purposes. Some prefer to examine these organs after semen collection, when the horse is more tractable.

Penis and Prepuce

Examination Procedure

To examine the stallion's penis and prepuce, the animal is exposed to a mare long enough to stimulate "let-down" or the extension of the penis from the preputial sheath. Stallions may resent examination of their external genitalia and will kick straight out to the rear or sometimes "cow-kick" toward the examiner. Thus, the stallion should be examined in an open area where the examiner has freedom of movement and where the stallion will not kick solid objects, which could cause leg injuries. The individual examining the stallion should protect himself by standing with his body beside the front quarters of the stallion and should gently slide his hand with a slow but steady movement down the chest wall and under the abdomen and then grasp the penile shaft.

The penis and prepuce are examined by palpation and visual evaluation. The glans penis is examined with special attention to the urethral process, along which vesicular and/or space-occupying lesions may be noted. The urethral diverticulum is carefully evaluated for abnormalities and collections of smegma, often referred to as the "bean." The examination is continued back over the shaft of the penis, observing closely for injuries and scars. While the penis remains extended, both the internal and external folds of the prepuce will be visible and are evaluated for scars and vesicular or space-occupying lesions. Normally, a dense, brown-black, greasy smegma is present near the base of the penis but may be a deep violet color on lightly pigmented preputial skin.

Diseases and Abnormalities

In a review of 119 stallions with diseases of the penis and prepuce, Vaughan[11] noted the following incidence: 31 per cent had lesions associated with trauma, 24 per cent had neoplasia, 15 per cent had penile paralysis, 12 per cent had parasitic lesions, 5 per cent had urinary calculi and 3 per cent had penile and preputial anomalies. The remaining 10 per cent had conditions of nonspecific preputial edema, venereal pox, hemospermia, diverticulitis, urethritis, pendulous sheaths and deviated penises.

Trauma and Hematoma of the Penis. Trauma to the stallion's penis and prepuce may occur as the result of the stallion's getting entangled in fencing, the mare's kicking the stallion's erect penis, sudden movements of either the mare or stallion during intromission, improperly positioned breeding stitches in mares or tight-fitting or dirty "stallion rings." Deep lacerations of the penis require complete sexual rest to limit erection stimuli, since the high blood pressures within the erect penis can result in continued hemorrhaging. Surgical repair of glans penis lacerations should be considered if it appears that these may heal in a manner that will obstruct the urethral orifice at ejaculation. For example, a laceration extending into the urethral diverticulum may heal as a flap of tissue deflected over the urethral process and may act to divert the course of semen that is normally ejaculated directly into the mare's cervical os.

"Stallion rings" fit over the shaft of the penis, proximal to the glans penis, and are designed to prevent masturbation by causing pain when erection occurs. These rings are available in various sizes and should be properly fitted to each individual stallion. Stallion rings that are too small or that are not cleaned at weekly intervals may cause irritation, scarring and eventual constrictive fibrosis to the shaft of the penis. Such conditions, if allowed to persist for a long time, can interfere with normal erection and may cause ischemic necrosis.

Hematomas of the penis (so-called "fractures of the penis") are often the result of blunt trauma associated with breeding attempts in which the stallion was kicked. Severe bending of the penile shaft during intromission or improper handling of artificial vaginas during semen collection can also produce penile hematomas. Following trauma or severe bending of the penile shaft, vessels that lie subcutaneously and outside the dense tunica albuginea will hemorrhage. This differs from hematoma of the bull's penis in which hemorrhage occurs from the corpus cavernosum penis because of rupture of the tunica albuginea that encloses it.

The traumatized penis of the stallion rapidly becomes enlarged because of acute inflammatory edema that increases the size of the penis to 10 to 13 cm in diameter and 30 to 35 cm in length. The penis hangs ventrally and is usually curved, with the glans penis pointing posteriorly. The penis cannot be retracted into the prepuce because of its increase in size and weight. Medically, this represents an acute traumatic balanoposthitis with paraphimosis. Use of tranquilizers is contraindicated in the stallion with a hematoma of the penis, since they cause the penis to drop even further ventrally and to become more edematous.

Treatment of the hematoma of the penis should be instituted rapidly to prevent the occurrence of secondary thrombosis of veins and lymphatics. Since the great increase in size is primarily related to edema, treatment is directed toward reducing the edema and preventing its recurrence. Cold water hydrotherapy and compression therapy via massage, pneumatic bandages or wrapping the penis tightly with a towel will aid in decreasing the edema. Glycerin, sulfaurea or other nonirritating hydrophilic agents may be applied under the compression bandage to further reduce the edema.

Excoriation of the superficial epithelium of the penis leaves a raw, reddened, exposed surface and is commonly encountered with or without compression-type therapy. Protectants in the form of ointments can be applied to prevent further excoriation. Anti-inflammatory drugs, such as phenylbutazone or aspirin, may be administered.

Once the edema and penile size have been reduced, the penis should be suspended to prevent the recurrence of edema. This can be accomplished with the use of a "stallion supporter" or a large bed sheet wrapped around the horse's abdomen and tied over his back in the form of a "many-ties" bandage. Once the edema is sufficiently reduced, the stallion may be anesthetized and the penis forced back into the prepuce and retained there by a heavy purse-string suture placed in the preputial orifice. An opening, approximately the size of two fingers, should be maintained to allow for urination. The sutures can be removed in 4 to 7 days.

Finally, and of utmost importance, it is necessary to provide freedom from sexual stimuli, which could encourage an erection and cause additional hemorrhage. If the stallion is not being considered as a breeding animal, castration should be recommended to help prevent any recurrence of this problem.

Rupture of the corpus spongiosum has, on rare occasions, also been reported in the stallion as the result of trauma. The corpus spongiosum penis is that portion of the erectile tissue that surrounds the urethra and is associated with the pulsatile ejaculation events; it should not be confused with the corpus cavernosum penis, which is responsible for penile erection. One recently reported case of rupture of the corpus spongiosum penis occurred at the level of the ischial arch and was thought to be the result of a kick to this site. Urethral stricture resulting in rupture of the bladder caused the death of this stallion.

Neoplasms of the Penis and Prepuce. Squamous cell carcinoma is the most common neoplasm of the horse's penis and prepuce (accounting for 20 to 21 per cent of the neoplasia reported in the horse). When classified by anatomical region involved, squamous cell carcinomas occur on the penis and prepuce approximately 45 per cent of the time, with only the head and ocular regions sharing a similar incidence. The lesion initially may appear as a small, heavily keratinized plaque on the penis and prepuce, but being infiltrative, it soon forms a shallow, crusted, fungating, ulcerative neoplasia. Malignancy is considered low for squamous cell carcinomas of the penis and prepuce since the disease spreads primarily by local infiltration within the epithelial tissues. Cryosurgery is recommended for early lesions, but radical surgical removal in the form of penile amputation or the preputial reefing operation is considered necessary for extensive neoplasia involving these organs.

Melanotic tumors of older gray-colored horses occasionally occur on the prepuce. Treatment is usually not attempted since the disease is often also present in the perineal areas, develops slowly, is nonulcerative and does not impede breeding.

Squamous papillomas, sarcoids and hemangiomas may also occur on the penis and prepuce. The squamous papilloma is considered of viral origin and usually is self-limiting and requires no treatment. Sarcoids of the prepuce, also considered of viral etiology, may require repeated cryosurgery or deep excision surgery followed by electrocautery, since recurrences are common. Persistent treatment of the associated exuberant granulation tissue should also be instituted.

Paralysis of the Penis. Penile paralysis in the stallion is characterized by the penis remaining extended from the prepuce in a flaccid state. Causes of this disease are varied, but most cases are thought to be associated with damage to the third and/or fourth sacral nerves or their branches that innervate the penis. Infectious diseases such as equine herpesvirus I, rabies and streptococcal-associated purpura hemorrhagica have been associated with penile paralysis and neurological disease. Phenothiazine-base tranquilizers, notably propionylpromazine and rarely acepromazine maleate, have been implicated in causing stallion penile paralysis. In addition, spinal disease, direct trauma to the penis and unattended cases of hematomas of the penis have been related to causing penile paralysis. Exhaustion and starvation, for unexplained reasons, have also been associated with the disease. On one farm, penile paralysis occurred in five stallions because of prolonged neglect and starvation. More commonly, individual cases occur when the stallion has been turned out on inadequate pasture without any supplemental feed.

The paralyzed penis initially develops a pendulant edema with excoriation and hyperkeratosis of the epithelial surfaces. Fissures and ulcerations in the thickened penile epithelium frequently follow. The majority of these stallions retain their libido and will mount mares in estrus but fail to acquire an erection of the penis. These stallions rarely regain their ability to retract the penis. Thus, treatment is often by penile amputation or the use of a penis retraction operation (reefing operation or Bolz's technique), which obviously halts the stallion's reproductive ability. In one case, when continued breeding use was desired, it was possible to train a stallion with a penile paralysis of 1 year's duration to an artificial vagina, resulting in 18 out of 18 mares conceiving via the use of artificial insemination. All 18 mares foaled the following year, and 15 out of 16 mares later rebred to the same stallion via artificial insemination also conceived. The thickened, keratinized, paralyzed penis is often insensitive over the majority of its surface and does not achieve an erection; therefore, modifications of available artificial vaginas are needed. Increasing the temperature of the water in the artificial vagina and adjusting its size should be considered. Persistence is the key to the training of the stallion to an artificial vagina.

Parasitic Lesions of the Penis and Prepuce. The larval forms of *Habronema muscae* (a horse stomach parasite) and *Callitroga hominivorax* (the screw-worm fly) are the most commonly reported parasitic lesions of the equine penis and prepuce. The screw-worm eradication program in the southern states has controlled this larval disease within the United States, but in countries in which the disease persists, infestations of the horse's prepuce and glans penis can occur. The fly's eggs are deposited on the edge of moist wounds and hatch out their larvae within 6 to 21 hours. The larvae invade the exposed tissue and cause a necrotic, granulomatous, ulcerative lesion. Treatment for the screw-worm lesions consists of cleaning the wounds, applying topical larvicides and insect repellent and protecting the wound from further exposure.

H. muscae larval lesions (summer sores, genital bursatti, cutaneous habronemiasis) most frequently occur near the preputial ring or on the urethral process of the glans penis. The fly (commonly the house fly, *Musca domestica*), serving as an intermediate host for *Habronema,* deposits the larvae while feeding on the moist areas of the preputial ring and urethral process. The larval invasion stimulates the rapid formation of a granulomatous lesion that contains numerous small yellow caseous granules, characteristic of the disease. The necrotic foci are composed primarily of the larvae, their remnants and a heavy infiltration of eosinophils.

Lesions on the urethral process of the glans penis can enlarge and cause difficult urination because of constriction of the urethra. Large lesions may leave severe scars on the prepuce, which interfere with the normal extension and retraction of the penis which may require surgical corrective measures. *Habronema* granulomas frequently have an associated intense pruritus, which subjects the area to continued trauma, bleeding and delayed healing.

In northern climates the lesions may disappear spontaneously during the winter months with complete healing. In warmer climates therapy should be instituted, but success is often variable. Most veterinarians agree that the lesions should be surgically exised and that steroid therapy is beneficial. The organic phosphates are the most commonly used larvicidal drugs. They may be used systemically, topically or via both routes simultaneously. One suggested therapeutic regimen is an anthelmintic dose of organophosphate via stomach tube, plus 300 mg/day of prednisone orally for 14 days. At 2 weeks the lesions are re-evaluated; if they persist, the same drug combinations are repeated. At 4 weeks, if the lesions still persist, the horse is given 300 mg/day of prednisone orally for another 14 days. The organic phosphate therapy is not repeated because of the possibility of toxicity. Since the granulomatous lesion is primarily associated with dead larvae, many feel that the steroids contribute to the major regression of the lesions.

Infectious Diseases Involving the Penis and Prepuce

EQUINE COITAL EXANTHEMA. Equine coital exanthema (genital horsepox, equine venereal vulvitis or balanitis) is caused by equine herpesvirus III, which was first isolated in 1968. The disease is transmitted during coitus and has an incubation period of about 6 to 10 days before lesions appear. Initial lesions, which appear primarily on the prepuce and shaft of the penis, are small, raised, reddened, vesicular blisters measuring 1 to 2 mm. These watery blisters rapidly progress to form pustular papules, with the number of the lesions increasing over a 2- to 5-day period. By the sixth day, most of the primary pustules appear as encrusted, scab-like lesions. The scab is easily rubbed off, revealing purulent ulcers. The encrusted ulcers may coalesce into an area approximately 2 cm in diameter, with the ulcers demarcated by a narrow erythematous border. The disease usually causes mild pain, but the temperature, pulse, respiration and appetite remain normal. Rarely, secondary bacterial infections may complicate the disease, causing an elevated temperature with marked edema of the prepuce and a thick, mucopurulent exudate over the involved area. Uncomplicated lesions usually heal in 7 to 9 days, leaving depigmented white scars on the dark-skinned areas.

Other than the presence of the lesions, the stallion appears to be little affected, except for a possible decrease in libido associated with pain caused by the lesions. The virus itself does not appear to affect the fertility of the stallion or of the mare. The virus has been inoculated directly into the pregnant uterus without causing abortion.

The antibody titer to coital exanthema is short-lived, probably about 1 year in duration. With exposure to the disease, the titer usually remains low for 7 to 9 days and then develops rapidly, reaching a maximum in 13 to 21 days, which correlates with the healing of the lesions. Equine coital exanthema may be spread by asymptomatic carriers, as the disease often appears sporadically without any other mares or stallions on the farm exhibiting lesions.

The disease is self-limiting, so treatment is aimed at preventing secondary bacterial infections. This is done with the use of antibiotic ointments applied to the prepuce and penile shaft. Sexual rest while the lesions are present helps prevent the spread of the disease.

DOURINE. Dourine is caused by *Trypanosoma equiperdum* and is a venereally transmitted disease in the equine. It has been eradicated in the United States but still exists in other countries, notably Asia and Africa. The incubation period is recorded as being from 1 to 12 weeks, with early signs of fever, inappetence and edematous swelling of the stallion's prepuce and scrotum. Exudate may be observed passing from the urethral orifice. Urticarial plaques 2 to 5 cm in diameter may appear on the sides of the body or elsewhere in the skin. Such plaques are considered pathognomonic of the disease. Dourine may eventually result in the development of muscle paralysis and atrophy, starting in the cranial regions and progressing to the rear limbs. Penile paralysis may also occur. Eventually, severe emaciation occurs, and a 60 to 75 per cent mortality rate is reported. The diagnosis is best made by a complement fixation test. Treatment is reported as being impractical because of the poor results and the expense involved. If eradication is the goal, all diseased and reactor animals should be destroyed.

HEMOSPERMIA. Hemospermia refers to the presence of blood in the semen. It may render such ejaculates infertile. Most frequently the presence of blood in the stallion's semen is transient in nature, is of unknown etiology and only affects the ejaculates involved. On occasion, chronic hemospermia may be noted. Voss[12] has correlated chronic cases of hemospermia with bacterial urethritis, *Pseudomonas* often being the organism involved. Affected stallions often had heavy breeding use and exhibited some reluctance to cover mares, requiring several mounts to complete the act. This is believed to be associated with pain that accompanies the urethritis and increases in intensity during ejaculation.

The bleeding appears to occur from ulcers and prolapsed subepithelial vessels that protrude into the urethral lumen. Endoscopic examination of the urethra can aid in diagnosing such lesions, but a subischial urethrotomy may be needed to view lesions present in the most proximal portions of the urethra.

Treatment consists primarily of sexual rest, which is often the only therapy needed, although occasionally systemic and local antibiotic therapy may be used. It should be noted that even with prolonged usage and high dosages of antibiotics, infections of the stallion's genital system usually fail to respond to systemic therapy. Local therapy in the form of urethral suppository inserts at the sites of the urethritis has been used by Voss.[12] These are usually placed through a subischial urethrotomy for lesions in the proximal urethra.

Blood in the semen may also occur from

small lacerations or puncture wounds in the stallion's glans penis that bleed only at the peak of erection. Close inspection of the penis and urethra will reveal which site is involved.

During natural breeding, if blood is noticed on the stallion's penis, the mare should be checked as a possible source, since rupture of the mare's anterior vagina by a stallion with a long penis does occur. This is especially prominent in maiden and small mares bred to such stallions. The use of "breeding-rolls," or a roll of cotton placed above the stallion's penis and against the buttocks of the mare, can help prevent deep penetration and tears of the vagina. Blood may also occur from torn hymens or ruptured varicose veins in the area of the mare's hymen.

URETHRAL CULTURES. Urethral cultures are frequently used as part of the stallion's breeding soundness examination. Extreme care is needed in interpreting the results of such cultures, since the distal portion of the stallion's urethra usually harbors a wide range of microbial flora that do not cause an active disease of the stallion's genital system. An active infection of the stallion's genital system would be characterized by the presence of high numbers of inflammatory cells in the semen.

Urethral swab cultures are taken both prior to and after semen collection to provide evidence of the type of bacteria present and to determine if a decrease in the quantity of these organisms occurs after the semen has flushed through the urethra. Hughes[4] reported that 73 per cent of the urethral cultures from 70 stallions revealed bacterial growth, but none of these stallions exhibited disease of their genital system. Thirty-five per cent of these stallions had *Pseudomonas* cultured, and without any therapy these animals achieved conception rates ranging from 71 to 82 per cent. A similar study by Merkt *et al.*[9] involving 74 stallions showed that 40 per cent of the stallions had *Klebsiella* cultured from the pre-ejaculatory secretion and/or prepuce. They also reported that of 607 mares covered by stallions having *Klebsiella*-positive cultures, 77 per cent conceived.

Even though *Klebsiella* is considered very pathogenic in the genital system of the equine, studies of *Klebsiella aerogenes* show that some 230 different capsule types of this organism exist. Only *Klebsiella* capsule types 1 and 5 have definitely been associated with infections of the equine genital system. The remainder apparently exist as surface contaminants without causing an active disease.

Most treatments of stallions with active genital infections are unsuccessful using present methods. High levels of antibiotics administered over periods of 10 to 14 days to achieve necessary systemic levels have failed to rid stallions of the bacteria despite the great expense involved. Infection soon recurs with the resumption of breeding activity. Most likely, events are similar to that observed in the mare, in whom resistance to certain infections is diminished because of a defective local defense mechanism in the mucosal lining of the genital tract. If the spermatozoa remain viable in stallions harboring bacteria in their genital tract, special management procedures can be instituted when they are bred to mares susceptible to such infections. The preferred technique utilizes artificial insemination, and the semen is first treated by placing it in a semen diluent containing antibiotics to control the bacteria. Burns *et al.*,[2] using a semen extender containing an antibiotic, showed a 93 per cent reduction in the bacterial count of the semen after 15 minutes. Similarly, Kenney[7] found semen with a high bacterial count practically free of bacterial growth after only 5 minutes in a semen extender containing an antibiotic. The two most commonly used antibiotics in semen extenders are potassium penicillin or sodium penicillin at the level of 1000 IU/ml and gentamicin sulfate at the level of 1 mg/ml. These appear to effectively control any bacterial contamination within the semen without causing significant spermicidal effects. When breeding regulations prevent the use of artificial insemination, approximately 100 to 300 ml of the antibiotic-containing semen extender may be infused into the uterus of the mare immediately prior to service to help control bacteria and prevent possible infections.

In summary, most stallions simply harbor bacterial organisms on their genital organs and are not diseased. No stallion should be condemned for breeding soundness solely on the basis of a positive bacterial culture from his urethra or semen.

Anomalies of the Penis and Prepuce

MALE PSEUDOHERMAPHRODITISM. Male pseudohermaphroditism is the most common form of equine intersex reported. These animals have hypoplastic, retained testicles, either abdominal or inguinal, and usually exhibit a stallion-like behavior. The genitalia are ambiguous and vary from appearing quite female, with only a slightly enlarged penile clitoris, to appearing more stallion-like. In the latter, the penis and prepuce are positioned further caudal than normal. Many animals lack complete preputial development. Often the penis is pointed ventrally or posteriorly and positioned near the perineal area. These animals can achieve an erection when sexually stimulated.

The karyotype of the equine male pseudohermaphrodite also varies widely from the normal 64,XX of a female (these animals frequently have a hypoplastic uterus), to the XXY,XXXY Klinefelter-type karyotypes and to a wide variety of mosaics and mixoploidy, such as XX/XY, XX/XXY or XO/XX/XXY. These animals are sterile and usually cannot copulate with the mare. Some have been utilized as teasers and are run with the mares on pasture. Marking harnesses, similar to those used in sheep, may be placed under the pectoral regions of the hermaphrodite. The mares that have been mounted will have a chalk or crayon mark left on their posterior quarters by the harness.

VARICOSITIES OF PREPUTIAL VEINS. Large, distended veins in the prepuce of the stallion occur on occasion but usually do not interfere with breeding. When the colt is young, these veins are noted as a soft, fluctuant, swollen area, often on one side of the prepuce. The swelling lacks the heat and edema associated with trauma or abscess formation.

Scrotum

Examination and Function

The scrotum is best evaluated while palpating the testicles. The scrotal skin is normally thin and pliable and may be slightly oily to touch because of the numerous sweat glands present within it. Little or no subcutaneous fat should be present in the scrotum, since it shares a testicular thermoregulatory function along with the cremaster muscle and the pampiniform plexus of the spermatic cord. This function is mandatory, for if the temperature around the testicle increases for any period of time, it can disturb the ability of the testes to produce spermatozoa. It has been shown in the bull that the sperm output decreases markedly by 14 days after the scrotum has been artificially insulted. With persistent high testicular temperatures, permanent testicular atrophy may eventually occur.

Diseases and Abnormalities

Scrotal Trauma. Trauma causes most scrotal problems in the stallion, usually occurring in the form of lacerations or blunt trauma with associated hematomas. Trauma-derived inflammation in the scrotum causes an increase in temperature and therefore should be carefully evaluated as to severity and duration. Superficial lacerations may require only cold water hydrotherapy and protective ointments; deep lacerations may require surgical debridement, extensive cooling, antibiotic therapy and even unilateral castration if a single testis is involved or if suppurative infections have occurred between the parietal and vaginal tunics.

Hematoceles are usually the result of blunt trauma, such as occurs when the stallion is kicked during attempted breedings. The hematocele is characterized by the collection of blood between the testicular tunics. Initially, this is a warm, fluctuant, somewhat painful swelling of the scrotum. As the hemorrhage organizes, it is palpable as a firm area; however, the majority of the scrotal pouch consists of a fluctuant, painless swelling because of the seroma formation. Extensive adhesions often form within the tunics and can be detected by the failure of the testicles to slide easily within the scrotum. Unilateral castration of the affected testis is recommended if a decrease in sperm production occurs and lasts longer than 60 to 90 days, since any initial detrimental and temporary effect on spermatogenesis should have been reversed by this time.

Scrotal Edema and Dermatitis. Scrotal edema in the stallion may be associated with systemic diseases such as equine infectious anemia or be the result of venous abnormalities. We have noted stallions with pendulous, edematous scrotums that become apparent during the summer months when the scrotal and cremaster muscles are relaxed. Often the edema will disappear with exercise or with diuretic therapy. Associated with scrotal edema, we have observed distended veins near the scrotal attachment and/or in the spermatic cord and thus suspect varicosities of such veins as one cause of this problem. Persistent scrotal edema may eventually result in atrophied testicles and sterility.

Edema may also result from scrotal dermatitis, although scrotal dermatitis in the stallion is rare when compared with the other domestic species with more exposed scrotums. The thin, delicate scrotal skin of the stallion is easily irritated by various chemicals, soaps or ointments. Chronic irritation by strong soaps during the washing procedure in stallions may cause thick, edematous plaques to form on the ventral scrotum. In the few cases that we have observed, fertility did not appear impaired, possibility because the edema was only on the ventral portions of the scrotum.

Scrotal Neoplasms. Neoplasms of the stallion's scrotum are rare. We have observed one case of squamous cell carcinoma originating as a small nodule in the scrotum of a 3-year-old Morgan stallion and spreading rapidly over the scrotum and posteriorly onto the perineum. Melanotic tumors of the scrotum may also occur.

Testicles and Epididymides

Examination and Structure

Normally the stallion has two scrotal testes positioned with their longitudinal axes in an anterior-posterior orientation. The testicles and epididymides are palpated through the scrotal wall to determine size, shape, symmetry and consistency. Testicular size is estimated either by determining each testicle's three-dimensional measurement or by ascertaining the scrotal width of both testicles. The normal testis varies from 8 to 12 cm long, 5 to 7 cm high and 4.5 to 6 cm wide. Normal scrotal width ranges from 9 to 13 cm. The thumb and forefinger can be used as calipers to estimate individual testicular measurements, while mechanical calipers can be used to determine scrotal testicular widths. Scrotal testicular widths should be determined while the penis is in a nonerect state, since erection of the penile shaft causes the testes to move further apart. It is best to palpate both testicles simultaneously, using one hand on each testicle. By utilizing deep palpation and moving the hand slowly along each testicle, minor degrees of variations in shape and consistency can be noted. Normal testicles are of a uniform size and shape and have a semi-firm or turgid consistency throughout, except for the shallow, fluctuant feel of the veins present in the vaginal tunics.

The epididymides are palpated to determine size, shape, consistency and location. The head of the epididymis is positioned on the anterior-dorsal aspect of the testis. The epididymal head is frequently difficult to palpate because the cremaster muscle and spermatic vessels attach in this area and obscure demarcation of this structure. The body of the epididymis passes over the dorsal-lateral aspect of the testicle as a long, narrow structure measuring 5 to 10 mm in diameter. In younger stallions both the body and tail of the epididymis are loosely attached, making them more easily evaluated than in older stallions. The tail of the epididymis is prominently displayed and easily palpated in most stallions. It measures 2.0 to 2.5 cm in diameter and has a slightly soft, uniform consistency. The ligament of the tail of the epididymis, or scrotal ligament, which is a remnant of the gubernaculum, attaches the tail of the epididymis to the scrotum. It forms a firm, nodular area at the posterior-dorsal aspects of the epididymis, approximately 5 to 10 mm in size. This serves as a landmark for identifying the proper location of the tail of the epididymis and should not be misinterpreted as an abnormality, such as a spermatocele.

Diseases and Abnormalities

Orchitis. Acute orchitis is rarely reported in the stallion but can result from trauma or hematogenous spread of infectious organisms. Affected testes will be quite warm, sensitive and very tense because of the swelling within the unyielding vaginal tunics. Frequently an epididymitis accompanies the condition. A larger number of polymorphonuclear leukocytes will be present in the semen, and the spermatozoa concentration will be greatly reduced.

Beta-hemolytic streptococci are the most common organisms involved, although *Streptococcus equi* has also been noted to spread hematogenously to the testes. The organism causing glanders and *Salmonella abortus equi* organisms were previously reported to cause equine orchitis.

Treatment of acute orchitis consists of cold water hydrotherapy and high systemic levels of the appropriate antibiotics. If the condition affects only one testis, unilateral castration of the involved gland should be considered since the swelling and increased temperature within the unyielding vaginal tunic may affect both testes and, in addition, result in testicular degeneration.

Lymphocytic inflammatory foci, often perivascular in location, are a frequent occurrence within the equine testes and are indicative of various forms of chronic, undetected orchitis. The seminiferous epithelium surrounding these lesions is frequently degenerated. The perivascular location of the foci suggests a relationship to vascular lesions. Viral diseases such as equine viral arteritis and equine infectious anemia have been suggested as one cause of such vascular lesions. The migrating larvae of *Strongylus edentatus* have also been suggested as a cause of these lymphocytic foci. One report indicates the investigators were unable to find *Strongylus* larvae in the normal scrotal testes, even though these could be recovered from cryptorchid testes. The focal areas of seminiferous tubule degeneration in the testicular parenchyma appear to be related to the presence of immature spermatozoa in the semen.

Testicular Hypoplasia and Degenerative Atrophy. Testicular hypoplasia and degenerative atrophy result in decreased-to-zero sperm production. Testicular hypoplasia refers to small testes of soft consistency that have failed to develop properly. This is usually the result of congenital factors or failure to develop at puberty due to even more obscure etiologies.

The degenerative, atrophied testis is one that had once achieved normal size and function and then regressed in size and productive ability following insults such as disturbances in the thermoregulatory function or orchitis. Nutritional deficiencies (vitamin A), autoimmune factors and anabolic steroids have also been suggested as causing testicular degeneration. Bullard and Kerr[1] administered low therapeutic levels of an anabolic steroid to approximately 16-month-old stallions at 4-week intervals for a period of 6 months. They suggested that spermatogenesis was not adversely affected following such administration. It should be noted that two of the five stallions treated had moderate-to-heavy desquamation of germ cells into the seminiferous tubule lumina. These immature forms of spermatozoa were not observed in four of the five control stallions.

Studies on the use of routine x-ray therapy in the horse have been unable to show any correlation between such therapy and significant testicular degeneration. A wide variety of uncommon substances, such as lead salts, thallium, cadmium, nitrofurans and griseofulvin, have also been associated with testicular degenerative changes in other species and may be suspected in the horse.

Atrophic testes are small and frequently firm on palpation because of the fibrosis that has replaced much of the seminiferous epithelial tissue. Occasionally, focal testicular atrophy may be noted as the result of focal intratesticular hemorrhage. Such areas may calcify, forming localized nodules in the testicular parenchyma.

If both testicles are hypoplastic or atrophic, no known therapy, including hormonal treatments, is effective. These stallions are considered unsatisfactory for breeding soundness. Also, if only one testicle is atrophic, the sperm output may be insufficient for classification as a sound breeding animal.

Testicular Neoplasms. Seminomas, teratomas, lipomas and interstitial cell tumors have been reported in the stallion's testicles. Sertoli cell tumors are apparently very rare in the stallion.

The seminoma appears to be the most common neoplasm, with rough calculations suggesting a maximum of approximately a 0.5 per cent incidence in the intact-male equine population. Usually only one testicle is involved, and a history of sudden enlargement of the testicle is frequently reported. The affected testicle may be 15 to 18 cm in diameter and have a soft-to-fluctuant consistency. Seminomas are subject to hemorrhage, which may account for the fluctuant, fluid consistency felt on palpation.

On cross section, the tumor resembles neoplastic lymphoid tissue, appearing somewhat lobulated, with a glistening pale gray surface in the nonhemorrhagic areas. Normal testicular parenchyma will be crowded off to one edge of the enlarged testicle and be the usual brownish-tan color. The equine seminoma often metastasizes to an inguinal lymph node and then throughout the posterior abdomen and pelvic areas.

Testicular biopsy may be used to aid in diagnosis if the history and clinical evidence suggests other possible causes. Nevertheless, castration is usually recommended for any testicle that becomes 15 cm or more in diameter. Castration should include as much of the spermatic cord as possible, and sections of the spermatic cord should undergo histopathological examination to determine the possibility of metastasis having already occurred. Rectal exploration of the inguinal lymph nodes may also be used to evaluate such metastasis.

Testicular Torsion. True torsion of the stallion's testicle is rare. When it does occur, testicular torsion is a very acute, painful condition, causing the stallion to exhibit signs of severe colic. Examination usually indicates that the testicle has rotated at least 360° within the scrotum, causing an occlusion of the spermatic vessels. Castration of the affected testicle is required if the vascular supply has been occluded sufficiently to cause tissue devitalization.

More common in the stallion is partial testicular rotation within the scrotum. The testicle may be situated in a complete 180° rotation with the tail of the epididymis pointing anteriorly. Most frequently, this is a developmental abnormality associated with the descent of the testicle into the scrotum, as indicated by such rotations being noted in young stallions and by the testicle subsequently remaining in this position. Rotation of the testicle through approximately 90° as it is retracted up close to the abdomen is another form of partial testicular rotation. This rotation appears to be related to the improper attachment of the cremaster muscle to the vaginal tunic of the testis. Partial testicular rotations usually are observed in only one testicle, and any detrimental effect on semen quality is rare.

Epididymal Disease. Diseases of the epididymis are rare in the stallion. Anomalies of the epididymis, such as the segmental aplasia common in bulls, rams and dogs, have not been reported in stallions. Epididymitis due to infectious organisms can be associated with concurrent orchitis, as previously discussed. Spermatic granulomas, which result from blind epididymal tubules being impacted with sperm, have occasionally been reported in the equine.

Epididymal stagnation, sperm stasis or sperm accumulation in the seminal ducts has been observed within the past 5 to 6 years and is being diagnosed with increasing frequency in low fertility stallions. The disease appears to be related to a disturbance in sperm transport, resulting in spermatozoa accumulating in the tail of the epididymis and probably in the ductus deferens and accessory glands as well. The stagnated spermatozoa are usually dead, lack motility and may have a high percentage of head-tail separations. Initial semen collections may reveal unusually high concentrations (900 to 1300 × 10⁶/ml), and the dense semen may appear similar to rich cream in color and consistency. In most of these stallions, repeated hourly ejaculates will begin to yield intact motile spermatozoa of normal concentration (100 to 200 × 10⁶/ml) after about the fourth or fifth ejaculate. A fair percentage of these motile spermatozoa have cytoplasmic droplets attached, indicating that they have just recently traversed the epididymis and achieved maturation.

One stallion observed with this syndrome required ejaculation two to three times daily for 6 days before normal motile spermatozoa were recovered. The initial ejaculates were of such high concentration that clumps of spermatozoa resembling mastitic milk were caught in the filters used to separate off the gel fraction of the ejaculate. Smooth, elongated, blunt-ended pellets or casts of solid, dense spermatozoa were observed to be floating freely in the gel fraction of the ejaculate, indicating that probably sperm stasis had also occurred in the seminal vesicles.

Stallions with the sperm stasis or sperm accumulation syndrome require frequent ejaculation, usually at least once daily, if maintenance of normal motile spermatozoa is desired. These stallions also required repeated monitoring of semen collections for concentration, as well as motility, to insure that the stallion is maintaining a sufficiently high concentration of spermatozoa in the ejaculate to provide satisfactory conception. A more exact control over the management of these stallions would utilize artificial insemination with adequate numbers of normal spermatozoa being inseminated (500 × 10⁶ progressively motile spermatozoa).

Spermatic Cords

The spermatic cords of the stallion should be palpated for determination of size, shape and consistency. Normally they are about 2.5 to 3.0 cm in diameter with a uniform, soft consistency. The more tubular ductus deferens usually cannot be delineated since it is surrounded by the cremaster muscle and spermatic vessels. Varicoceles, or dilatations of the spermatic veins, may occur, especially near the tortuosities of the pampiniform plexus. These can occasionally be observed during routine castrations. As previously discussed, large varicosities are suspected of being one cause of some forms of scrotal edema. Verminous granulomas have been reported in the spermatic cord of the stallion, although these are more commonly noted in the cords of cryptorchid testes.

INTERNAL GENITALIA

Evaluation and Diseases of the Accessory Glands

Some of the accessory glands of the stallion's genital tract may be evaluated via rectal examination. The ampullae that form the upper ends of the ductus deferens are readily distinguished because they lie outside the genital fold and have a slightly turgid, tubular form. They are approximately 12 to 20 cm long and have a 1.5 to 2.5 cm diameter. The ampullae are located near the pelvic brim and branch out over the urinary bladder in a Y-shaped fashion.

The seminal vesicles, which are hollow, elongated, sac-like glands lying dorsal-lateral to the ampullae, average about 8 to 10 cm in length and 3 to 5 cm in diameter. Normally they are quite flaccid and lie partially within the genital fold, which makes them difficult to palpate. To delineate the seminal vesicles it is best to do a rectal examination prior to the semen collection while the glands still contain a full supply of their gelatinous secretion, thus giving them a more distended outline. Seminal vesicles often cannot be delineated in those stallions that secrete very little gel in their semen.

The prostate gland, which is situated within the pelvic canal, consists of two nodular lobes on either side of the pelvic urethra connected by an isthmus overlying this structure. Both the prostrate gland, which is buried within retroperitoneal tissue, and the bulbourethral glands, which are deep within the bulbourethral muscles, elude rectal palpation.

Diseases of the stallion's accessory glands are rare. Seminal vesiculitis has been associated with streptococcal and pseudomonal infections. The seminal vesicles, when inflamed, become enlarged and may feel lobulated. Pus in the semen accompanies seminal vesiculitis, and rectal massage of the seminal vesicles will often cause an increase in the inflammatory cell content of the semen. As previously noted, systemic antibi-

otic therapy is usually unsuccessful for stallion genital infections. Surgical removal as performed in bulls with seminal vesiculitis has been suggested. If the prostate becomes palpable, enlarged and firm, infection of this organ may be suspected.

A case of apparent unilateral hypoplasia of the left ampullar gland has been observed, although acquired atrophy of this organ cannot be ruled out since the animal was an 18-year-old standardbred stallion. The affected ampulla was only 7 mm in diameter and lacked the normal turgid, tubular nature of the unaffected 15-mm-diameter ampulla on the right side. This stallion also exhibited the sperm accumulation syndrome previously described.

Evaluation and Problems of the Internal Inguinal Canals

The internal inguinal canals are an easily detected landmark for evaluating the stallion's genital system. Their slit-like openings, which are approximately 4.0 to 4.5 cm long, can be examined rectally by sliding the fingers down the internal abdominal wall from the pelvic brim. The internal inguinal rings are located approximately 10 to 12 cm ventral to the pelvic brim and anywhere from 6 to 10 cm lateral of midline. The slit-like openings are positioned in a diagonal dorsal-medial to ventral-lateral fashion. By inserting two or three fingers into the opening, one can palpate the spermatic artery and ductus deferens.

Abnormalities to check for in the internal inguinal canal include adhesions and inguinal hernias. Abnormally enlarged internal inguinal rings may be prone to inguinal hernias, and owners must be alerted to the possibility that such hernias may occur during the stress of breeding, with a rapid onset of severe colic following.

REFERENCES

1. Bullard, T. L. and Kerr, K. M.: The effect of a new anabolic steroid on spermatogenesis in young stallions. The Southwestern Vet. 26:39, Fall, 1972.
2. Burns, S. J., Simpson, R. B. and Snell, J. R.: Control of microflora in the stallion semen with a semen extender. J. Reprod. Fertil. (Suppl.), 23:139, 1975.
3. Evans, L. H.: The soundness examination and soundness examination form. A.A.E.P., 1968, pp. 57–79.

4. Hughes, J. P., Asbury, A. C., Loy, R. G. and Burd, H. E.: The occurrence of *Pseudomonas* in the genital tract of stallions and its effect on fertility. The Cornell Vet. *57*:53, 1967.

5. Hughes, J. P. and Loy, R. G.: The relation of infection to infertility in the mare and stallion. Eq. Vet. J., 7:155, 1975.

6. Jubb, K. V. F. and Kennedy, P. C. (Eds.): Pathology of Domestic Animals. Vol. 1, 2nd Ed., New York, Academic Press, 1970, pp. 443–481.

7. Kenney, R. M.: Clinical fertility evaluation of the stallion. A.A.E.P., 1975, pp. 336–355.

8. Kenney, R. M., Bergman, R. V., Cooper, W. L. and Morse, G. W.: Minimal contamination techniques

for breeding mares: Technique and preliminary findings. A.A.E.P., 1975, pp. 327–336.

9. Merkt, H., Klug, E., Bohm, K. H., and Weiss, R.: Recent observations concerning *Klebsiella* infections in stallions. J. Reprod. Fertil., (Suppl.), *23*:143, 1975.

10. Roberts, S. J. (Ed.): Veterinary Obstetrics and Genital Diseases. 2nd Ed. Ithaca, New York, 1971, pp. 604–697. Distributed by Edwards Brothers Inc., Ann Arbor, Mi.

11. Vaughan, J. T.: Surgery of the penis and prepuce. A.A.E.P., 1972, pp. 19–40.

12. Voss, J. L. and Wotowey, J. L.: Hemospermia. A.A.E.P., 1972, pp. 103–112.

Clinical Examination and Abnormalities in the Mare

JOHN P. HUGHES

University of California, Davis, California

REPRODUCTIVE CYCLE OF THE MARE

Although mares will breed in any month of the year, they must be classified as seasonal breeders. The length of the estrous cycle, the length of estrus and ovarian activity in the nonpregnant mare should not be characterized without indicating what season of the year is being used to make these definitions. One of the major problems in equine reproduction is that the physiological breeding season does not necessarily coincide with the breeding season imposed on horses by many breed associations. In the Northern Hemisphere the universal birthday of January 1 means that breeding commences during mid-February, which is outside the physiological breeding season for mares. Studies at the University of California have indicated that 75 to 85 per cent of mares develop signs of estrus and then ovulate from April through October, but only 20 to 25 per cent of mares come into heat and ovulate in January and February. Irregularities in the estrous cycle of the mare are strongly tied to season, which is related primarily to length of daylight, nutrition and climatic factors.

Estrous Cycle

The length of the estrous cycle is defined as the period from one ovulation to another when accompanied by estrus and/or a low plasma progestin level (1 ng/ml). Using a figure of 1 ng/ml of plasma progestin eliminates those ovulations that occur during the luteal phase of the cycle. During California's physiological breeding season from April through October, estrous cycle length averages 21 to 22 days, estrus lasts 5 to 6 days and ovulation occurs 24 to 48 hours before the end of estrus.

Osborne's study of Australian slaughter specimens indicated that a low of 18 per cent of mares ovulated in the winter, with a highest mean of 91 per cent observed in the summer. In South Africa, during winter and early spring 85 per cent of mares had either little follicle development with long estrous periods or follicle growth with failure of ovulation. During the summer months, at least 96 per cent of the estrous periods ended in ovulation.

There are areas of the world in which a large proportion of mares cycle the year around. Periods of ovarian inactivity in the mare can last from 2 months to 4 or 6 months, depending on the latitude and possibly the climate of the area in which the animal is located. The further north or south of the equatorial line, the more pronounced the occurrence of a period of ovarian inactivity during the winter.

Light affects the mare's estrous cycle significantly. She responds to decreasing light by slowly terminating cyclic ovarian activity over a period of 4 or 5 months following the summer solstice (June 22) and then responds slowly to increasing light with the establishment of cyclic ovarian activity in the spring, usually about 3 or 4 months after the winter solstice (December 22). The influence of light on the cyclic activity of the mare has been used in many parts of the world to renew ovarian activity and initiate ovulation early in the spring, so that more mares may be covered by the stallion.

Variations in patterns of cyclic behavior may include erratic cycle length, erratic estrous behavior, failure of ovulation, failure of follicle development and spontaneous prolongation of the corpus luteum. These behavioral patterns fall into three general groups; however, there is considerable overlapping of the responses of the mares in these three groups:

1. *Polyestrous mares.* A few mares cycle fairly regularly throughout the year. While there may be some variations in the length of the estrous cycle (i.e., estrus and diestrus), particularly in the winter, these variations are within normal limits. The cervix may fail to relax or secretions may remain scant or sticky, particularly as the mares come out of the winter period. This is another indication of seasonal cyclicity.

2. *Seasonally polyestrous mares.* Mares in this group have a definite cyclic period and a rather definite noncyclic or anestrous period. The noncyclic period varies greatly both in length (from 40 days to as long as 8 months) and in time of occurrence in individual mares. In general, the anestrous period occurs during winter and early spring. The response of mares when teased during anestrus may vary considerably. Anestrous mares with little, if any, follicular activity detectable on palpation often respond passively to the stallion, neither rejecting nor accepting his advances. The cervix and the uterus may become completely flaccid and difficult to delineate. On vaginoscopic examination, the cervix will appear pale and free of mucus and in some instances will be partly to fully dilated. Other mares have considerable ovarian activity during winter anestrus, with follicles growing to moderate size and then regressing, to be replaced by others. These mares actively resist the advances of the stallion, and the cervix is pale, dry, tight and sticky.

Mares may start cycling abruptly when they begin to come out of the winter anestrous period. More commonly, however, there is a prolonged period during which the degree of sexual receptivity varies until intense standing estrus is evident. Mares will stand to be covered by a stallion for periods of 15 to 60 days or more during this phase. During these periods of prolonged heat, the ovaries may have little, if any, detectable follicular development, or they may have many small follicles, a few larger ones and finally one or two follicles that progress to ovulation.

3. *Seasonally polyestrous mares with erratic reproductive patterns.* This group includes mares that show heat without ovulation and ovulation without heat, as well as variations in the length of the estrous cycle and heat, in intensity of heat and in responses to the stallion when teased. These patterns of variability more often occur in the winter and early spring. Of the patterns observed, ovulation without estrus and prolonged anestrus leading to a persistent corpus luteum are the most common.

It is important to remember that mares in anestrus, in prolonged estrus and in the transitional phase of erratic reproductive behavior from winter anestrus to regular cyclic ovarian activity or mares with a prolonged corpus luteum are poor prospects for a fertile mating. Given time, these mares will resume regular patterns of estrous cyclic activity.

Estrus

The reproductive cycle of the mare is more easily understood if it is divided into the follicular (or estrous) phase and the luteal (or diestrous) phase. The follicular phase is characterized by the growth of follicles in the ovary, secretion of estrogen and signs of sexual receptivity in the mare. The length of time that a mare is in heat decreases from February through June, with shortening of the interval from onset of estrus to ovulation. One study showed that the length of estrus averaged 7.6 days from February through April (with a range of 2 to 60+ days) and 4.8 days from May to October. Another study revealed that by June two-thirds of the estrous periods are 4 days or less, and all are less than 9 days, and that by July three-quarters of the periods are short.

Estrous Behavior. Determination of estrous behavior in the mare by using a teaser stallion is one of the most important functions in the management of brood mares for maximum fertility. This should be carried out daily or every other day, using a stallion that has good libido and will tease the last mare of the day as vigorously as he did the first mare of the day. There are a number of different methods used for teasing mares. They can be teased in a stock, at a teasing bar or even in some instances in the pasture. Whatever the method, each mare must be teased as an individual unless she breaks down with the usual signs of estrus at sight or sound of the stallion. A few broodmare farms employ a stallion that has had the penis everted posteriorly by a surgical procedure. A marking harness is placed on the stallion, and he is turned loose with the mares. Those mares in estrus can be noted by the mark left by the stallion. This has been useful under certain specialized management conditions in which mares are particularly difficult to find in heat when hand-teased. Another common practice is to put a stallion in a pen or stall in one corner of the paddock where the mares can come up to him and show signs of estrus voluntarily.

The usual response of the mare in heat is one of interest in and acceptance of the stallion. Although there may be initial rejection of the teaser, most mares accept his advances without agitation. A typical mare in estrus does not kick, the tail is elevated without switching, the legs are spread apart, the pelvis is flexed and contraction and relaxation of the labia of the vulva with urination and eversion of the clitoris occur. Behavioral changes of less intensity are often observed just before and after true heat.

During diestrus, follicles grow and regress, and those destined to ovulate begin to increase in size and become prominent before the mare comes into heat. Usually, only one follicle continues to grow to ovulatory size of 35 to 60+ mm (average being 45 mm), but on occasion two or more follicles may grow at a similar rate and double ovulations occur. Occasionally, a follicle will rupture when a second smaller follicle (20 to 30 mm) is present on one of the ovaries. The second follicle will then grow rapidly and ovulate 24 to 48 hours or more later. On occasion, an ovulatory follicle that develops to a diameter of 10 cm or more persists for a variable period of time (up to 60+ days) and then regresses without disrupting normal estrous cycle length or subsequent ovulations.

In a group of mares studied at the University of California, multiple ovulations occurred 25 per cent of the time, with a higher incidence in March than in other months. Some mares have a much greater tendency for multiple ovulation than others. The interval between multiple ovulations averages 1 day, but 2 or 3 days is not uncommon. Multiple ovulations are not significantly different whether on the same or opposite ovaries, and there is no reason to believe that multiple ovulations appearing on the same ovary are not just as apt to result in twins as are multiple ovulations occurring on opposite ovaries. In slightly more than half of the estrous periods, two or more follicles over 25 mm in diameter were palpable. In our study, 78 per cent of the mares ovulated within 48 hours prior to the end of heat, 10 per cent of the mares were out of heat before ovulation occurred and 76 per cent of the ovulations occurred between 4 P.M. and 8 A.M.

Failure of ovulation during the physiological breeding season is rare. Only one case of ovulatory failure was recorded in a series of 300 estrous periods studied. A perceptible softening of the follicle usually occurs just prior to ovulation, but based on twice daily palpation, this may not be detected. Pain is usually associated with ovulation, but there is considerable variation among mares and some do not show discomfort.

Estrogens that are secreted by the follicle cause sexual receptivity or heat, are responsible for changes in the reproductive tract that permit passage and transport of the sperm and have a role in initiating luteinizing hormone (LH) release, which leads to ovulation. These events must occur in a definite time sequence if mating is to occur and sperm are to be available when the egg reaches the oviduct. Failure of any one or a combination of these events, or of the timing, may result in infertility, the rate of failure being greatly influenced by seasonal changes.

Visual Changes within the Reproductive Tract. Visual changes are noted during estrus that are usually characterized by alterations in color, amount of edema, degree of relaxation and amount and consistency of secretions detectable on vaginoscopic examination. Although considerable variation in these characteristics occurs among mares, changes in individual mares are fairly consistent. Usually, just prior to or at the onset of estrus, the cervix begins a progressive softening and relaxation, changes in color from pale to shades of pink or red and becomes edematous, and the secretions become more abundant and fluid in consistency.

Although the greatest degree of cervical change (color, edema, relaxation and consistency of secretions) usually occurs near ovulation, such changes are sometimes present earlier or later in the cycle. Therefore, these changes alone are not an accurate indication of the time of ovulation. The best judgment of when to breed the mare is derived from the psychological behavior of the mare when teased by the stallion, the condition of the cervix when palpated and viewed with a speculum and the follicular development of the ovary as determined by palpation. It should be remembered that some mares in anestrus that have little, if any, follicular activity will have a flaccid cervix, which on visual examination is fully dilated, allowing one to see into the uterus.

Diestrus

The diestrous phase of the estrous cycle, initiated by ovulation, the formation of the corpus luteum and the secretion of progesterone, averages 15 days in length during the physiological breeding season.

Diestrus is characterized by active resistance of the mare to the teaser stallion. The mare will lay her ears back, switch her tail, squeal, bite and kick at the stallion. Some mares, however, may be only slightly agitated and then only when aggressively teased.

When ovulation occurs, the collapsed follicle begins to fill with blood and within 8 to 10 hours is very soft and fluctuant on palpation; by 24 hours a corpus luteum is usually palpable. The corpus luteum has a functional life span of about 14 days. Progesterone secreted by the corpus luteum takes the mare out of heat and is responsible for sealing off the uterus from the exterior and preparing its tissues for the support of pregnancy, if this occurs. During diestrus, the cervix is tightly constricted and white in color, with no edema and only a scanty amount of viscous mucus present. Mares will ovulate during the diestrous phase of the estrous cycle. These ovulations occur between days 2

and 15 of the luteal phase and are unaccompanied by signs of estrus. The cervix remains pale, dry, tight and sticky. Diestrous ovulations are a diagnostic problem to the veterinarian unable to follow ovarian activity in the mare on a regular basis. The problem becomes even more confusing in trying to determine which follicle to breed to when dealing with a mare known to have a period of cyclic ovulation without showing estrus to the teaser. There can be no doubt that each subsequent palpation of the ovaries becomes more valuable in accumulating information when managing this type of mare.

On occasion, the follicular cavity continues to fill with blood after ovulation and forms a hematoma that may reach 10 to 12 cm in length and persists beyond the next ovulation without affecting the length of the cycle. One case has been recorded of a hematoma measuring 27.5 cm in diameter and weighing 7.5 kg that did not affect normal cyclic activity on the opposite ovary. Care must be taken not to confuse these hematomas, which occur following ovulation and which occasionally persist for several months, with ovarian tumors. From a differential diagnostic standpoint, mares with hematomas of the ovary continue to cycle normally, whereas mares with granulosa cell tumors of any duration do not cycle normally.

BARREN MARES

There are a number of reasons why mares fail to conceive or remain in foal during any particular breeding season. The more important factors contributing to a mare's failure to produce a live foal after breeding are as follows:

1. Failure to select broodmares based on reproductive performance.
2. Short breeding season.
3. Failure of the imposed breeding season to coincide with the physiological breeding season.
4. Improper teasing of the mare (failure to detect heat).
5. Endocrine factors.
6. Uterine infections.
7. Physical abnormalities of the mare that contribute to infertility.
8. Pathological developments affecting the reproductive tract.
9. Chromosomal abnormalities.
10. Nutrition.

11. Age.
12. Immunological factors.
13. Foal heat breeding.
14. Abortion.
15. Stallions of marginal fertility.

Failure to Select Broodmares Based on Reproductive Performance

The basic fertility of horses is not any less than that of other species, such as cattle. Mares have a heat period of several days compared with a heat period of 1 day or less in cattle. Thus, mares have a greater opportunity to be covered several times during any one heat period.

A problem in equine reproduction is that little selection for reproductive performance has been practiced among mares that have demonstrated a high level of excellence on the race track or in the show ring. Thus, we may be presented with a mare that is barren season after season, with a poor reproductive history, uterine infection or adhesions and fibrosis in the cervix or uterus.

Short Breeding Season

In areas where foals become 1 year of age on January 1, the breeding season starts on February 15 but often does not continue beyond June. Mares that fail to start normal cyclic activity until late April or May may be bred over one or two estrous cycles and then passed over for the season. Mares that foal in late May or June will often be bred only at the foal heat or will be skipped entirely for that year.

Failure of the Imposed Breeding Season to Coincide with the Physiological Breeding Season

The major problem related to the short breeding season of breeds using the January 1 birthday is that the imposed breeding season ends before the peak of the physiological breeding season is reached. The normal breeding season for mares in California, or areas of a similar latitude, is April to October, when most mares develop signs of heat and ovulate. During the early part of the imposed breeding season from February to March, only 20 to 40 per cent of the mares are cycling and ovulating normally. Irregularities of estrous cycle length and ovulation are mostly confined to the early part of the breeding season in barren and maiden mares. Regular estrous cycle lengths, in general, are established as soon as the first ovulation of the new season has occurred. During the early part of the breeding season, it is not unusual for mares to stay in heat 40 to 60 days or longer without ovulating or even showing significant follicular activity. The stallion and the mare respond to increasing daylight, and fertility reaches a maximum during the summer. As the daylight increases, the estrous period decreases in length and the ovulation rate increases.

Increasing the photoperiod with artificial lighting beginning December 1 can be used to establish ovarian activity earlier in the spring. Artificial lighting will not increase inherent fertility.

Improper Teasing of the Mare (Failure to Detect Heat)

When mares are hand bred, detection of heat using a proper teaser stallion is extremely important. Inadequate teasing or failure to detect heat will severely reduce reproductive efficiency. Teasing is dependent upon presenting the mare to a vigorous stallion and evaluating her reactions. The teasing program must be carried out by a careful observer of animal behavior who must record observations for each individual mare.

Endocrine Factors

Failure to show heat is an important cause of infertility in mares. It should not be forgotten, of course, that pregnancy causes mares to stop showing heat, and mares already in foal are occasionally presented for breeding or as a breeding problem.

It is now apparent that a number of mares have spontaneous prolongation of the corpus luteum. This spontaneous prolongation occurs in mares that appear to be normal except for failure of the corpus luteum to regress. Persistence of the corpus luteum may occur at any time during the breeding season and averages 60 to 70 days in duration. Persistence of the corpus luteum is an important cause of infertility in the breeding of mares because the affected mare fails to show normal cyclic ovarian activity and heat as long as the corpus luteum is retained. These mares may grow follicles that occasionally ovulate, but these animals do not show heat in conjunction with this follicular development and ovulation. Mares in deep winter anestrus will respond to 1 to 10 mg of estradiol and show anovulatory estrus in 3 to 6 hours. Mares with active corpora lutea will not respond to estrogen in this manner. Prolonged corpora lutea can also occur following embryonic loss.

Mares that lose embryos before the thirty-sixth day of gestation and mares with spontaneously prolonged corpora lutea respond consistently to prostaglandin treatment. If loss of the conceptus occurs after the thirty-eighth to fortieth day, when the "endometrial cups" are formed that secrete pregnant mare serum gonadotropin, mares will not return to heat until approximately 120 days from the estrus at which they conceived. The response of these mares to prostaglandin treatment to bring them back into heat is inconsistent.

A few mares will fail to show heat even though normal cyclic ovarian activity is occurring. These mares will have normal ovulatory intervals and corpora lutea of normal life span. Why these mares are behaviorally anestrus is unknown. It may be related in some way to failure of the sex center in the hypothalamus to respond or to inhibiting factors such as anxiety or trauma. Improper teasing is one of the most common reasons why mares fail to show estrus. These mares can be managed successfully by observing physiological changes in the genitalia, either by speculum examination or by rectal palpation.

As previously pointed out, many mares during the winter months have spontaneous cessation of cyclic ovarian activity. Mares are obviously infertile during this period. Treatment for winter anestrus is to wait until seasonal ovarian cyclicity begins or to use artificial light. Gonadotropin-releasing hormone given on days 1 and 2, days 11 and 12 and days 21, 22 and 23 of treatment, along with parenteral injections of progesterone on days 5 through 16, has recently been shown to induce follicle formation and ovulation in "winter-anestrus" mares.

Multiple ovulations occurred 25 per cent of the time in a group of mares under our observation. One mare in this group had multiple ovulations 75 per cent of the time. Despite this level of multiple ovulations, the incidence of twins is only 1 to 2 per cent (range 0.5 to 5 per cent). Most twins are aborted or die soon after delivery. One study reported 266 twins from 8252 mares, only 13 of which had a foal that could be reared. In another report on 62 pairs of twins, one foal

was born alive in 21 per cent of cases and both foals were born alive in 14.5 per cent of cases, but 42 per cent of all foals born alive died by 2 weeks of age. There appears to be a much higher survival rate in twins born to the draft breeds.

Uterine Infections

Bacterial infections of the genital tract have been recognized for many years as an important cause of infertility in the mare. Kentucky workers in 1928 recovered bacteria from 36.6 per cent of all barren mares examined, and 24 per cent of the bacteria recovered were *Streptococcus zooepidemicus*. Surveys of mares in Ireland and England have suggested a similar incidence of infected mares. In 1966, Bain found 12 per cent infected mares in his area of practice in Australia. In 1971, workers in New Zealand indicated a highly significant relationship between culture results and subsequent breeding performance; 43 to 45 per cent of mares with a positive culture before breeding produced a live foal, compared with 64 to 71 per cent that had negative culture results. Scott and co-workers found that obtaining routine cultures of mares can result in the isolation of many organisms that are not associated with any pathological process.

These surveys do not necessarily demonstrate that sterility was directly attributable to disease of the genital tract that was due to infection by the organisms recovered. A variety of species of bacteria may be recovered during a single estrous period in one animal. A number of workers have pointed out the importance of differences in the susceptibility of mares to infection and that recovery of bacteria from the cervix or uterus does not necessarily mean a diseased mare. There are also strain differences in pathogenicity of bacteria that infect the uterus of mares, particularly *Klebsiella* and *Pseudomonas* organisms. It has been suggested that uterine infections are more easily incurred during the luteal phase of the cycle when the uterus is under the influence of progesterone and that the uterus is more resistant to infection during the follicular phase when it is under the influence of estrogens.

Although we do not know what percentage of barrenness is due to uterine infection, there can be no doubt that bacteria are a causative factor and that properly selected and administered antibiotics are effective in eliminating bacterial endometritis. It is well recognized that stallions harbor bacteria in their genital tracts and on their external genitalia. The semen from the stallion contains numerous types of bacteria and is ejaculated into the uterus during cover of the mare. *Proteus* sp. *Streptococcus, Escherichia coli, Pseudomonas, Staphylococcus, Aerobacter* sp. and *Corynebacterium* sp. are commonly isolated from the semen or urethra of stallions with no visible or palpable lesions of the genital tract and no significant pus cells in their semen. These organisms are usually normal surface contaminants. Multiple pure cultures or an increase in bacterial numbers in a second ejaculate of semen, taken 1 hour after the first, would warrant investigation.

It is apparent, therefore, that the act of breeding introduces organisms into the reproductive tract of the mare in a high percentage of cases. Bryans reported on a group of 97 mares whose cervices were examined by bacteriological culture 24 hours after being bred. Ninety per cent of foaling mares, 87 per cent of barren mares and 81 per cent of maiden mares had positive culture results. None of the group became infected despite the fact that six species of bacteria and fungi found in these mares were known to produce genital infections. Breeding hygiene practiced on most equine breeding farms has been used to reduce contamination when the mare is bred by the stallion, but it is impossible to sterilize either the stallion's penis or the mare's vulva and vagina. Texas workers found that washing the stallion's penis before and after cover of the mare lowered the bacteria count only by a factor of 10. With this in mind, the following experiments were performed to determine if young, clinically normal mares would develop genital disease and fail to conceive if repeatedly inoculated with pathogenic bacteria into the uterus:

In the first experiment, three virgin mares were inoculated with a rapidly growing culture of *Streptococcus zooepidemicus* at each estrus over a period of approximately 1 year. Prior to each inoculation, bacterial cultures were obtained from the cervix and uterus. At the first estrus following the last inoculation, the mares were bred by a stallion of established fertility. In all, 37 intrauterine inoculations of the organism were made in these three animals. Two became pregnant during the first heat, and one became preg-

nant during the third heat. All three delivered normal, healthy foals at term with no abnormal or retained fetal membranes.

In the second experiment, five virgin mares were inoculated with a rapidly growing culture of *S. zooepidemicus* at specific stages of the estrous cycle. Within 5 hours of inoculation the uterus became distended and turgid. The cervix enlarged to as much as six times the preinoculation size and relaxed, allowing the inoculated broth now containing large amounts of pus to flow out of the uterus. This occurred both in mares inoculated when not in heat and in those inoculated during heat. The reaction began to subside by 12 hours' postinoculation in all mares, and within 96 hours the reproductive tract had regained its normal appearance and condition. It was possible to recover *S. zooepidemicus* at the subsequent estrus in only one of eleven examinations. None of the inoculations performed during heat, including the day of ovulation, altered cycle length. Between heats (luteal phase), however, five of seven inoculations resulted in a reduction of the interval between ovulations. These results suggest that mares with short cycles and a poor breeding record may be suspected of having established uterine infections.

In another experiment, two mares, one young, clinically normal mare and one chronically infected mare, received intrauterine inoculations of *S. zooepidemicus* and were examined 5 hours later. The reaction to inoculation differed markedly between these two mares. The maiden mare showed distention of the uterus and relaxation of the cervix, allowing pus to escape. The mare with the long-standing infection exhibited little, if any, cervical or uterine reaction to the inoculation. The results of this study demonstrate clearly the ability of the healthy uterus of the young mare to eliminate infectious organisms. This is markedly different from the situation in many older mares and in some mares following a number of pregnancies, in which the ability to respond defensively to organisms has been lost or diminished.

These studies suggest that mares that become susceptible to infection have had their normal defense mechanisms disrupted, which may be related to immunological and cellular mechanisms of resistance.

The following points should be kept in mind concerning uterine infection in the mare:

1. The normal stallion will harbor bacteria in the urethra or semen but will not be diseased.

2. The majority of the stallions that harbor bacteria in their genital tracts are of normal fertility.

3. A stallion should not be considered unfit for breeding based only on the recovery of bacteria from the urethra or semen.

4. The normal stallion contributes significantly to exposure of the mare's uterus to pathogenic organisms.

5. Mares in good reproductive health are highly resistant to infection introduced into the uterus at breeding.

6. Mares whose defense mechanisms have been altered, by whatever cause, may develop uterine disease when exposed to infectious organisms during breeding.

7. Certain strains of bacteria may have a greater effect than others on survival of the sperm or establishment of infection. Whether a mare becomes infected appears to be related to the pathogenicity of the bacteria causing uterine infection and the susceptibility of the mare.

8. With repeat-breeding mares, it is impossible to say whether a bacterial disease of the uterus will respond readily to treatment and whether the mare will continue to be fertile. There is a good chance that she has lost some degree of ability to resist infection and will become readily reinfected, even if the original infection is eliminated.

A number of management procedures can be used to reduce exposure of the mare to bacteria at breeding. Artificial insemination of the mare with diluted semen that has been treated with antibiotics to control bacteria is the most logical method, but horse breed organization rules may restrict or prohibit its use. Mares easily reinfected or those with mild uterine infections may be treated during estrus, prior to and after cover of the mare by the stallion. In those breeds that do not permit artificial breeding, the instillation into the uterus of a semen diluent containing antibiotics, administered just prior to cover by the stallion, is a useful procedure.

Pyometra. Pyometra is marked by the presence of abnormal fluid in the uterine cavity. This fluid may accumulate because of interference with natural drainage but may also be present when the cervix is patent. Mares with pyometra may show normal cyclic ovarian activity with associated signs of heat, whereas others may have prolonged periods of anestrus.

Studies have shown that noncycling mares with pyometra have a prolonged corpus luteum (CL). Based on histological examination and hormone analysis, it appears that mares with pyometra and with a prolonged CL have pathological changes in the endometrium that inhibit release of the factor (prostaglandin) that causes CL regression. The mare with pyometra that maintains cyclic ovarian activity still has enough normal endometrium present to control regression.

Physical Abnormalities of the Mare that Contribute to Infertility

Pneumovagina (wind-sucking) is one of the important predisposing causes of uterine infection. It is more often seen in old or debilitated mares with a flat croup and thin, poorly developed vulvar lips. Mares that tend to become swaybacked with age also are more prone to the condition, as are angular mares with prominent pin bones.

The suspensory ligament of the anus originates from the second and third coccygeal vertebrae and runs ventrally and around the ventral portion of the anus, acting as a sling. It then crosses below the anus and proceeds down the side of the vulva to form the suspensory ligament of the vulva. Some of these fibers blend with the retractor ani muscle. Therefore, when the anus recedes anteriorly, these fibers exert a pulling effect on the vulva, with a consequent tilting forward of the vulva and opening of the vulvar lips. Pneumovagina is most often noted during estrus or when the mare is in motion. The treatment for pneumovagina is suturing of the vulvar lips (Caslick's operation).

Mares with the type of conformation that predisposes to wind-sucking will, on occasion, pool urine in the vagina, particularly if the tissues of the vagina have lost their tone and the ligament supporting the uterus stretches and allows the uterus to hang down in the abdominal cavity over the brim of the pelvis. In severe cases the accumulation of urine in the anterior vagina will flow through the cervix into the uterus when the mare comes into heat. The urine may result in chronic irritation and, of course, is spermicidal. Less severe cases of urine pooling may be treated by merely wiping the urine out of the vagina prior to cover by a stallion.

More severe cases require an operation to extend the urethra back to the vulvar lip so that the pooling of urine cannot occur.

A persistent hymen is not unusual in maiden mares. Rather than allowing a stallion to rupture the hymen at the time of service, it is preferable to gently break it down with the sterile-gloved hand and dilate the area with the three-pronged or Caslick speculum before cover by the stallion. Rarely, mucous epithelial debris will collect behind a persistent hymen and is released at the time the hymen is incised.

Pathological Developments Affecting the Reproductive Tract

Cervical and uterine adhesions may occur following a difficult birth, particularly if fetotomy was performed. These may also occur following intrauterine irrigation with irritating solutions, such as iodine. While mild adhesions of the external os of the cervix may be broken down and mares with such lesions may conceive, more severe adhesions extending anteriorly or involving the uterus are associated with poor fertility.

Endometrial cysts are not commonly encountered in the uterus of the mare. They can range from microscopic in size to a few millimeters in diameter, particularly when there is cystic distention of uterine glands, or they can be several millimeters to several centimeters in diameter, as a result of collections of lymphatic fluid in the endometrium. On occasion, an endometrial cyst will extend into the lumen of the uterus in a bladder-like fashion and can be easily mistaken for an early pregnancy. The effect of endometrial cysts on fertility is not completely understood, but such cysts may interfere with a mare's fertility if they are large or occur in sufficient numbers. According to Kenney, lymphatic lacunae resulting from collections of lymphatic fluid are seen in mares only over 10 years of age.

Ventral uterine enlargements occur on occasion. The endometrium in the region of these enlargements undergoes atrophy, and the number of endometrial glands is reduced. It is considered that these areas may contribute to infertility in mares.

Studies of mares with granulosa cell tumors involving one ovary indicate that there is complete suppression of activity in the other ovary as far as follicle growth and ovulation are concerned. Thus, the granulosa cell tumor is able to exert a powerful negative feedback effect on the hypothalamus, which prevents cyclic growth of follicles. Three types of sexual behavior have been noted in these mares: (1) anestrus, or failure to show heat, was the most common finding, (2) aggressive stallion-like behavior in the presence of other mares also occurred or (3) male-type behavior was noted following a period in which no signs of heat were shown or in which continuous estrus was exhibited when teased by a stallion. Mares that have granulosa cell tumors and that are in continuous estrus are in a state of ovarian inactivity similar to mares coming out of the winter anestrous period that exhibit like behavior. Following surgical removal of the infected gonad, recovery of activity in the remaining ovary varied among mares and was significantly affected by the season of the year when surgery was performed. In some mares, up to 8 months or more were required for resumption of cyclic ovarian activity, and some mares, it appears, may never recover. Two mares that failed to resume cyclic ovarian activity in the 18 months after removal of a granulosa cell tumor had the remaining ovary removed. These ovaries were found to be completely inactive on histological examination. Chromosome analysis of these mares revealed a normal 64,XX female constitution.

Chromosomal Abnormalities

Cytogenetic studies of horses that are phenotypically female but that are infertile because of chromosomal abnormalities have recently appeared in the literature.

Affected mares are usually presented as fertility problems. They tend to be smaller in height and weight than the average for their breeds. All breeds appear to be involved, as chromosomal abnormalities have been reported in the Appaloosa, Quarter Horse, Arabian, Thoroughbred and Pony. The reaction when teased by a stallion varies from rejecting his advances to allowing him to mount. There is no cyclic pattern to estrous behavior, as such mares may show estrus for days and then become passive or resistant to teasing by the stallion.

External genitalia appear normal to slightly small. The uteri and cervices are small and flaccid on rectal palpation. The ovaries are extremely small, smooth and firm and contain no palpable follicles in most cases. When removed and examined, the ovaries lack germ cells and consist of undifferentiated ovarian stroma. On speculum examination, the cervical os is frequently dilated.

Mares with chromosomal abnormalities of this type are sterile. Although the number of cases of sterility caused by chromosomal abnormalities is small, it is important to realize that the condition does occur and is being found with increasing frequency.

For a further discussion of chromosomal abnormalities, see Section IV, Cytogenetics.

Nutrition

The effect of nutrition on fertility in the mare needs a great deal of study before useful judgments can be made. It has been shown that mares on a higher plane of nutrition started ovarian activity earlier in the breeding season than mares fed maintenance rations. Van Niekerk in South Africa reported that embryos of mares on a low plane of nutrition usually died at 25 to 30 days of gestation. The mares with resorbed fetuses failed to return to heat for many weeks.

Aging

Although there are great individual variations among mares, it is generally accepted that fertility gradually declines after 12 to 14 years of age.

Immunological Factors

In man, much interest and study have gone into the concept that immune phenomena may be involved in unexplained infertility. Sperm are antigenic, and antispermatozoal antibody may be formed. What role this phenomenon may play in horses is unknown. Sexually active women are exposed continually to semen and therefore have a much greater opportunity to form antispermatozoal antibody. It is difficult to interpret the significance of spermatozoal agglutinating antibodies found in serum of women because such antibodies occur in women and men proved to be fertile at the time of their detection. Autoagglutination of sperm has also been shown to occur, owing to antibodies in the semen and serum of men. It is considered that in these cases agglutination of the sperm occurs rapidly after ejaculation and, therefore, ovum penetration cannot occur. Complicating this finding is the fact that some men with antibodies are fertile. Further study needs to be done in this area of antispermatozoal antibody before any sound judgments as to its effect on infertility in the equine species can be made.

Foal Heat Breeding

Most studies have indicated that breeding mares at the first postpartum estrus (foal heat) results in a greater rate of infertility and early embryonic loss than breeding at subsequent heat periods. The problem has been considered to be due to uterine defense mechanisms not having recovered fully and uterine epithelium not being completely involuted and prepared for conception by the time of foal heat. Recent studies have shown that there seems to be greater repair of uterine structures by day 15, but the difference is minimal compared with the repair shown at days 5 and 10. Reports on conception rates following mating at foal heat have ranged from 28 per cent to 62 per cent. Lieux, in California, indicated that 40 per cent of mares bred at foal heat were found to be pregnant and 33 per cent foaled, as compared with a conception rate of 51 per cent of mares bred at the second heat postfoaling, of whom 43 per cent foaled. An interesting point brought out in this study was that foal heat breeding did not appear to interfere with the overall conception rate for the season when compared with the overall seasonal conception rate for mares bred at an estrus subsequent to the second heat postfoaling. Tolksdorff, in Germany, reported that 36 of 60 mares (60 per cent) conceived when bred at the foal heat, as compared with 25 of 41 mares (61 per cent) that conceived at the second heat postfoaling. Of the 36 mares that conceived during foal heat, 6 (16.6 per cent) resorbed their fetuses, while only one (4 per cent) of the 25 mares bred at the second postfoaling resorbed her fetus. As can be seen, controversy still exists over whether or not to breed at the first postpartum. If mares are to be bred at foal heat, they should meet several criteria to qualify: (1) the foal should be delivered without significant difficulty; (2) the placenta should be passed within 3 hours postpartum; (3) the foal should be live, strong and healthy; (4) when examined at 7 days postpartum, the cervix should be free from bruises and no abnormal discharges should be noted and (5) the uterus, on rectal palpation, should be involuting normally.

Bacteria can usually be cultured from cervical swabs taken during the foal heat, so that a positive culture result is probably significant only if the mare is clinically infected. Two management procedures have been suggested to allow more time for uterine involution and endometrial repair to occur following foaling, without waiting until the second heat postpartum. One procedure has been to delay the onset of postpartum estrus, using progesterone to inhibit the release of gonadotropins by the pituitary. The second procedure has been to allow the mare to ovulate at the foal heat, wait 5 days and then administer prostaglandins. These mares would usually return to heat within 2 to 5 days and ovulate about 4 days after coming into heat.

Abortion

Abortion contributes in a very important way to the overall problem of reproductive failure in the mare. Studies show that from 8 to 19 per cent of mares diagnosed in foal at approximately 40 days of gestation subsequently fail to foal. Osborne, in Australia, indicated a difference of approximately 9 per cent between diagnosis of pregnancy made by the Aschheim-Zondek test and the final findings. South African workers reported a fetal loss from 35 days onward of 14 per cent, and Platt, in a study at an English breeding farm, reported an overall abortion rate of 12.8 per cent. He noted an increased number of abortions in mares that conceived within 21 days of foaling, as compared with longer intervals. He also noted a greater liability to abortion in mares over 18 years of age. The abortion rate was also higher in barren mares, as compared with foaling mares. Early embryonic and fetal loss occurring before 100 days has had little study. The aborted embryos or fetuses are seldom seen, and this makes study difficult. Between 4 and 6 months of gestation, abortions tend to be autolyzed and, again, are often of undetermined etiology. Bacteria are responsible for a number of abortions during this stage of gestation. From 6 months of gestation to term, aborted fetuses tend to be fresh, with specific lesions present to aid in the diagnosis. Studies in humans indicate that as high as one third of early abortions are due to chromosomal abnormalities. As was pointed out previously, twinning is one of the most important causes of abortion in mares. Placental disease may be a cause of abortion, but its exact role is not really understood. Some examples of placental disease of a noninfectious nature leading to abortion might be premature placental separation, a body pregnancy, torsion of the umbilical cord and hypoplasia of the chorionic villi. Bacteria, viruses and fungi are all important causes of abortion in the mare. In the United States, herpesvirus is the most important infectious agent causing abortion, and most of these abortions occur from the seventh to the ninth month to term.

Stallions of Marginal Fertility

Stallions should have a fertility examination prior to the start of the breeding season and periodically during the breeding season. This subject has been covered in previous articles in this section.

The broodmare farm that must use a marginally fertile stallion to cover mares requires a very carefully controlled breeding program. Management procedures to be considered for the stallion might include the following:

1. A determination of his semen quality.
2. A determination of his sperm output.
3. The effect of frequency of ejaculation on sperm concentration. This would be important in determining how many mares the stallion could cover and how frequently.
4. Longevity of the ejaculated spermatozoa. This could give a clue as to how closely cover of the mare by the stallion should be correlated with ovulation. Careful observation will sometimes reveal that if a mare is to conceive she must be bred much closer to ovulation by some stallions than by others.
5. Bacteria should be cultured from the semen and urethra (on occasion, bacteria may be recovered that are detrimental to the longevity of the spermatozoa). This may require injecting semen extender containing antibiotics into the uterus immediately prior to cover of the mare by the stallion or collection of the stallion and dilution of the semen extender, depending on the rules of the breed association.
6. Centrifugation of the semen sample to separate the spermatozoa from the seminal plasma. It has occasionally been noted that the seminal plasma is detrimental to the spermatozoa, and resuspension of the spermatozoa in a semen diluter will greatly enhance their longevity.
7. It will be noted that stallions have an increase in the number of live, motile sper-

matozoa in ejaculates collected at short intervals after the first ejaculate. This indicates that the environment within the epididymis is detrimental to the spermatozoa. Management in this case would require more frequent ejaculations to achieve maximum fertility.

PHYSICAL EXAMINATION

This should follow a definite set of guidelines that will determine to the best of our ability the mare's potential fertility. Whether all parameters outlined are used would depend on the particular animal being examined and the judgment of the veterinarian. A maiden mare, for example, would not usually require a fiberscopic examination or uterine biopsy, and even culture of the uterus is often unnecessary.

Interpretation of the findings of the veterinary examination must be done carefully. Judgment must be exercised to avoid interpretations that falsely condemn an animal for breeding purposes. For example, the growth of three or four colonies of bacteria on a blood agar plate from a swab of the cervix or uterus of a clinically normal mare with no history of infertility is unlikely to indicate disease of the uterus. At the same time, obtaining a negative culture result from the uterus does not necessarily mean a reproductively normal animal.

I. Identification. The mare should be identified by owner, breed and age. Color, markings and brands or tattoos should also be recorded. This could be done on an outline of the horse similar to those filled out on registration forms. A Polaroid picture might be useful.

II. History. It is often difficult, if not impossible, to obtain an accurate history with pertinent details. The following information is appropriate:

1. Maiden, barren, foaling.
2. Previous foals and dates.
3. Date of last foal, gestation length and survival to 2 weeks.
4. Problems associated with foaling.
5. Fetal membranes:
   a. Abnormalities.
   b. Retained.
6. Repeat breeding:
   a. Years bred.
   b. Times bred per estrus.
   c. Cycles bred.
   d. Cycles bred per conception.
7. Previous treatment for reproductive, medical or surgical problems.
8. Hormone injections.
9. Sexual behavior:
   a. Anestrus.
   b. Prolonged heat.
   c. Silent heat.
   d. Agitated heat.
10. Feeding program.
11. Use:
   a. Racing.
   b. Performance.

III. Clinical External Examination. The external examination should include:

1. Physical condition and general health: The mare must be capable of carrying a fetus to term. A general examination of the cardiovascular, respiratory, locomotor and nervous systems, including the eyes, should be done.
2. Vulva:
   a. Configuration, size and degree of closure.
   b. Scars or other lesions.
   c. Discharges.
3. Sexual behavior during estrus and diestrus: It may be necessary to determine to your own satisfaction the response of the mare when teased during the follicular and luteal phases of the estrous cycle. Any situation that inhibits the response of the mare should be avoided.

IV. Clinical Internal Examination. The speculum examination should include:

1. Vagina:
   a. Color.
   b. Discharges, urine and/or exudate.
   c. Size and normality, including position, adhesions or rectovaginal fistulae.
2. Cervix:
   a. Color.
   b. Edema.
   c. Degree of relaxation.
   d. Character of the secretions, i.e., sticky, stringy or fluid.
   e. Discharges and their nature.
   f. Normality: tears, scars or adhesions should be noted.

One must not confuse physiological variations with pathological conditions of the vagina and cervix.

Palpation should include the following:

1. The vagina and cervix should be palpated for any abnormalities such as adhesions or, more rarely, strictures. On occa-

sion, during estrus, one may pass the hand through the cervix and palpate the internal surface of the uterus.

2. The cervix, uterus and ovaries should be palpated *per rectum*. These structures are carefully examined for any abnormalities in *size, consistency, tone, symmetry* and *content*. Abnormalities most often noted in the uterus are endometrial cysts (lymphatic lacunae), pyometra, mucometra and tumors. Ovarian abnormalities most commonly observed are hematomas, tumors and the extremely small ovaries associated with Turner's syndrome. One must be very careful before assuming that small, non-functioning ovaries are pathological, however, as they may become active. A chromosome analysis would be required to make a positive diagnosis of gonadal dysgenesis.

After carefully evaluating the information obtained from the examination to this point, the veterinarian must decide whether to utilize cervical and/or uterine culture, uterine cytological studies, fiberscopic examination, chromosome analysis and hormone analysis as further aids.

V. Culture of the Cervix and/or Uterus. Although cultures are routinely taken from the uterus, there is considerable controversy about whether this is necessary. One study that we conducted indicated that if there was clinical evidence of disease, the results of cervical cultures correlated with uterine cultures in more than 96 per cent of cases caused by beta-hemolytic streptococci and *Pseudomonas* and 87 per cent of cases caused by *Escherichia coli*. Correlation was only about 80 per cent with a clinically normal cervix and vagina.

Uterine cultures are taken during estrus, but again the definitive work has not been done to prove that this is the only reliable time to culture. If the mare is in heat, one is less likely to introduce infection, as her resistance should be at its greatest. The fluid mucus during estrus makes a culture from one area more representative of the entire uterus. With an instrument such as the Knudsen culture and sampling apparatus, reliable cultures can be obtained from the diestrous uterus if as much of the uterus as possible is swabbed.

Culture of the reproductive tract is a useful diagnostic aid, but is not an end in itself. The requirement of a negative culture result is inappropriate in some circumstances. The normal, healthy mare can, on occasion, have bacteria cultured from her reproductive tract. The culture medium used will influence the results. One or two organisms growing in broth may appear to be significant. A few scattered colonies on a blood agar plate cultured from the uterus of a barren mare may be much more significant than the same finding in a maiden mare. Responsibility for interpretation of results must be exercised by the veterinarian and not by the diagnostic laboratory.

VI. Cytological Examination of the Uterus. A swab should be obtained from the uterus of the mare and a smear made on a slide for cytological examination. The smear can be stained with new methylene blue or orcein stains.

Mucus from the uterus of normal mares shows some epithelial cells with few, if any, lymphocytes or neutrophils. The leukocytes increase if endometritis is present. An increase in neutrophils suggests an acute process, whereas lymphocytes are more often noted in chronic disease. Bacteria may be noted in some smears.

An alternative technique is to put on a sterile, disposable surgical glove and insert the finger into the cervix of the mare in estrus. A smear from the finger is made on a clean slide and stained as previously indicated.

Cytological examination is an important procedure in deciding whether a mare is diseased. If bacteria are causing disease in the uterus, there should be some cytological evidence that this is true.

VII. Fiberscopic Examination. This technique is of limited value in relation to the cost of the instrument. The procedures just described will provide a diagnosis in most instances. This instrument can be useful to visualize endometrial cysts, uterine adhesions, tumors and small areas of exudate.

VIII. Uterine Biopsy. This is a very useful aid in making a prognosis when examining barren, repeat-breeding mares. Not every mare requires a biopsy, but it is very helpful in determining the breeding potential of the problem mare. Uterine biopsy (technique, indications and evaluation) is covered elsewhere in this section.

IX. Chromosome Analysis. Cytogenetic studies of phenotypical female but infertile mares with small, inactive ovaries and no cyclic pattern to their estrous behavior are justified to obtain a complete evaluation of their fertility (see Section IV, Cytogenetics).

X. Hormone Analysis. Progesterone analysis to determine the presence of a prolonged corpus luteum (CL) is the most common procedure utilized by clinicians at present. Estrogen, luteinizing hormone, follicle-stimulating hormone and prostaglandin are also being assayed. These new assay techniques will allow a better understanding of irregularities in the estrous cycle of the mare and a more rational approach to the use of hormones in broodmare practice. Several workers (Irvine, Loy, Hughes) have reported that most mares in "deep" winter anestrus will come into estrus within 3 to 6 hours when injected with 1 to 10 mg of estradiol. Mares with a prolonged CL or those in the luteal phase of the estrous cycle will not come into heat. This may be a useful approach to the diagnosis of a prolonged CL.

REFERENCES

1. Allen, W. R.: The immunological measurement of pregnant mare serum gonadotrophin. J. Endocrinol, 43:593, 1969.
2. Allen, W. R.: Endocrinology of early pregnancy in the mare. Equine Vet. J., 2:64, 1970.
3. Allen, W. R. and Moor, R. M.: The origin of the equine endometrial cups. I. Production of PMSG by foetal trophoblast cells. J. Reprod. Fertil., 29:313, 1972.
4. Allen, W. R. and Rossdale, P. D.: A preliminary study upon the use of prostaglandins for inducing oestrus in non-cycling Thoroughbred mares. Equine Vet. J., 5:137, 1973.
5. Allen, W. R. and Rowson, L. E. A.: Control of the mare's oestrous cycle by prostaglandins. J. Reprod. Fertil., 33:539, 1973.
6. Alm, C. C., Sullivan, J. J. and First, N. L.: Induction of premature parturition by parenteral administration of dexamethasone in the mare. J.A.V.M.A., 165:721, 1974.
7. Andrews, F. N. and McKenzie, F. F.: Estrus, ovulation and related phenomena in the mare. University of Missouri Research Bull., p. 329, 1941.
8. Barty, K. J.: Observations and procedures at foaling on a Thoroughbred stud. Aust. Vet. J., 50:553, 1974.
9. Bengtsson, G. and Knudsen, O.: Feed and ovarian activity of trotting mares in training. Cornell Vet., 53:404, 1963.
10. Berliner, V. R.: The estrous cycle in the mare. In Cole, H. H. and Cupps, P. T. (eds.): Reproduction in Domestic Animals. 1st Ed., New York and London, Academic Press, 1959, pp. 267–289.
11. Berthelon, M. and Rampin, D.: Infection utérine et fonctionement des ovaires chez la jument. Revue Méd. Vét., 119:653, 1968.
12. Betteridge, K. J. and Mitchell, D.: Direct evidence of retention of unfertilized ova in the oviduct of the mare. J. Reprod. Fertil, 39:145, 1974.
13. Bhavnani, B. R., Short, R. V. and Solomon, S.: Formation of estrogens by the pregnant mare. I. Metabolism of 7-³ H-dehydroisoandrosterone and 4-¹⁴ C-androstenedione injected into the umbilical vein. Endocrinology, 85:1172, 1969.
14. Bielanski, W., Tischner, M. and Zapletal, Z.: Effects of intrauterine injection of stallion semen in mares not showing oestrus. Bull. Acad. Pol. Sci., 22:519, 1974.
15. Britton, J. W.: Breeding farm practices. In Catcott, E. J. and Smithcors, J. F. (eds.): Equine Medicine and Surgery. Wheaton, Ill. American Veterinary Publications, 1973, p. 649.
16. Clegg, M. T., Cole, H. H., Howard, C. B. and Pigon, H.: The influence of foetal genotype on equine gonadotrophin secretion. J. Endocrinol, 25:245, 1962.
17. Cole, H. H.: High gonadotropic hormone concentration in pregnant ponies. Proc. Soc. Exp. Biol. & Med., 38:193, 1938.
18. Cole, H. H. and Hart, G. H.: The potency of blood serum of mares in progressive stages of pregnancy in effecting the sexual maturation of the immature rat. Am. J. Physiol., 93:57, 1930.
19. Cole, H. H., Howell, C. E. and Hart, G. H.: The changes occurring in the ovary of the mare during pregnancy. Anat. Rec., 49:199, 1931.
20. Cole, H. H., Hart, G. H., Lyons, W. R. and Catchpole, H. R.: The development and hormonal content of fetal horse gonads. Anat. Rec., 56:275, 1933.
21. Day, F. T.: Sterility in the mare associated with irregularities of the estrous cycle. Vet. Rec., 51:1113, 1939.
22. Dunn, H. O., Vaughan, J. T. and McEntee, K.: Bilaterally cryptorchid stallion with female karyotype. Cornell Vet., 64:265, 1974.
23. Evans, J. W., Faris, D. A., Hughes, J. P., Stabenfeldt, G. H. and Cupps, P. T.: Relationship between luteal function and metabolic clearance and production rates of progesterone in the mare. J. Reprod. Fertil. (Suppl.), 23:177, 1975.
24. Evans, M. J. and Irvine, C. H. G.: Serum concentrations of FSH, LH and progesterone during the oestrus cycle and early pregnancy in the mare. J. Reprod. Fertil. (Suppl.), 23:193, 1975.
25. Gerneke, W. H. and Coubrough, R. I.: Intersexuality in the horse. Onderstepoort J. Vet. Res., 37:211, 1970.
26. Geschwind, I. I., Dewey, R., Hughes, J. P., Evans, J. W. and Stabenfeldt, G. H.: Plasma LH levels in the mare during the oestrous cycle. J. Reprod. Fertil. (Suppl.), 23:207, 1975.
27. Ginther, O. J.: Occurrence of anestrus, estrus, diestrus, and ovulation over a 12-month period in mares. Am. J. Vet. Res., 35:1173, 1974.
28. Ginther, O. J. and First, N. L.: Maintenance of the corpus luteum in hysterectomized mares. Am. J. Vet. Res., 32:1687, 1971.
29. Ginther, O. J., Pineda, M. H., Wentworth, B. C. and Nuti, L.: Rate of disappearance of exogenous LH from the blood of mares. J. Anim. Sci., 39:397, 1974.
30. Girard, A., Sandulesco, G., Fridenson, A. and Rutgers, J. T.: Sur une novelle hormone sexuelle cristallisée retireé de l'urine des juments gravides. C. R. Acad. Sci. (Paris), 194:909, 1932.
31. Gonzalez-Angulo, A., Hernandez-Jauregui, P. and Marquez-Monter, H.: Fine structure of gonads of the fetus of the horse. Am. J. Vet. Res., 32:1665, 1676, 1971.

32. Hart, G. H. and Cole, H. H.: The source of oestrin in the pregnant mare. Am. J. Physiol., *109*:320, 1934.

33. Holtan, D. W., Nett, T. M. and Estergreen, V. L.: Plasma progestins in pregnant, postpartum and cycling mares. J. Anim. Sci., *40*:251, 1975.

34. Hughes, J. P. and Loy, R. G.: Artificial insemination in the equine: A comparison of natural breeding and artificial insemination of mares using semen from six stallions. Cornell Vet., *60*:463, 1970.

35. Hughes, J. P. and Loy, R. G.: The relation of infection to infertility in the mare and stallion. Equine Vet. J., 7:155, 1975.

36. Hughes, J. P., Benirschke, K., Kennedy, P. C. and Trommershausen-Smith, A.: Gonadal dysgenesis in the mare (a report of 5 cases). J. Reprod. Fertil. (Suppl.), *23*:385, 1975.

37. Hughes, J. P., Kennedy, P. C. and Benirschke, K.: XO-gonadal dysgenesis in the mare (report of two cases). Equine Vet. J., 7:109, 1975.

38. Hughes, J. P., Stabenfeldt, G. H. and Evans, J. W.: Estrous cycle and ovulation in the mare. J.A.V.M.A., *161*:1367, 1972.

39. Hughes, J. P., Stabenfeldt, G. H. and Evans, J. W.: Clinical and endocrine aspects of the estrous cycle of the mare. Proc. 18th Ann. Conv. Am. Assoc. Eq. Pract., 1973, pp. 119–151.

40. Hughes, J. P., Stabenfeldt, G. H. and Evans, J. W.: The oestrous cycle of the mare. J. Reprod. Fertil. (Suppl.), *23*:161, 1975.

41. Kenney, R. M., Ganjam, V. K. and Vergman, R. V.: Non-infectious breeding problems in mares. Vet. Scope, *19*:16, 1975.

42. Lovell, J. D., Stabenfeldt, G. H., Hughes, J. P. and Evans, J. W.: Endocrine patterns of the mare at term. J. Reprod. Fertil. (Suppl.), *23*:449, 1975.

43. Loy, R. G.: Effects of artificial lighting regimes on reproductive patterns in mares. Proc. 14th Ann. Conv. Am. Assoc. Eq. Pract. 1968. 1969, pp. 159–169.

44. Merkt, Von H.: Artificial insemination and horse breeding. VI Int. Cong. Anim. Reprod. & Art. Insem., Paris, Vol. II, 1968, pp. 1581–1583.

45. Mitchell, D. and Betteridge, K. J.: Persistence of endometrial cups and serum gonadotrophin following abortion in the mare. VII Int. Cong. Anim. Reprod. & Art. Insem., Munich, I, 1972, pp. 567–570.

46. Mossman, H. W. and Duke, K. L.: Comparative Morphology of the Mammalian Ovary. Madison, Wis., University of Wisconsin Press, 1973.

47. Neely, D. P., Hughes, J. P., Stabenfeldt, G. H. and Evans, J. W.: The influence of intrauterine saline infusion on luteal function and cyclic ovarian activity in the mare. Equine Vet. J., 6:150, 1974.

48. Nett, T. M., Holtan, D. W. and Estergreen, V. L.: Plasma estrogens in pregnant and postpartum mares. J. Anim. Sci., *37*:962, 1973.

49. Noden, P. A., Oxender, W. D. and Hafs, H. D.: Estrus, ovulation, progesterone and luteinizing hormone after prostaglandin F$_{2\alpha}$ in mares. Proc. Soc. Exp. Biol. Med., *145*:145, 1974.

50. Noden, P. A., Oxender, W. D. and Hafs, H. D.: The cycle of oestrus, ovulation and plasma levels of hormones in the mare. J. Reprod. Fertil. (Suppl.) 23:189, 1975.

51. Osborne, V. E.: Analysis of the pattern of ovulation as it occurs in the annual reproductive cycle of the mare in Australia. Aust. Vet. J., *42*:149, 1966.

52. Pattison, M. L., Chen, C. L., Kelley, S. T. and Brandt, G. W.: Luteinizing hormone and estradiol in peripheral blood of mares during estrous cycle. Biol. Reprod., *11*:245, 1974.

53. Pineda, M. H., Garcia, M. C. and Ginther, O. J.: Effect of antiserum against an equine pituitary fraction on corpus luteum and follicles in mares during dioestrus. Am. J. Vet. Res., *34*:181, 1973.

54. Purvis, A. D.: Elective induction of labor and parturition in the mare. Proc. 18th Ann. Conv. Am. Assoc. Eq. Pract. 1972. 1973, pp. 113–116.

55. Rossdale, P. D. and Mahaffey, L. W.: Parturition in the Thoroughbred mare with particular reference to blood deprivation in the newborn. Vet. Rec., *70*:142, 152, 1958.

56. Rowlands, I. W.: Levels of gonadotropins in tissues and fluids, with emphasis on domestic animals. *In* Cole, H. H. (ed.): Gonadotropins. San Francisco, Freeman, 1963.

57. Short, R. V.: Progesterone in blood. IV. Progesterone in the blood of mares. J. Endocrinol., *19*:207, 1959.

58. Solomon, W. J.: Rectal examination of the cervix and its significance in early pregnancy evaluation of the mare. Proc. 17th Ann. Conv. Am. Assoc. Eq. Pract. 1971. 1972, pp. 73–79.

59. Squires, E. L. and Ginther, O. J.: Collection technique and progesterone concentrations of ovarian and uterine venous blood in mares. J. Anim. Sci., *40*:275, 1975.

60. Squires, E. L., Douglas, R. H., Steffenhagen, W. P. and Ginther, O. J.: Ovarian changes during the estrous cycle and pregnancy in mares. J. Anim. Sci., *38*:330, 1974.

61. Stabenfeldt, G. H., Hughes, J. P. and Evans, J. W.: Ovarian activity during the estrous cycle of the mare. Endocrinology, *90*:1379, 1972.

62. Stabenfeldt, G. H., Hughes, J. P., Evans, J. W. and Geschwind, I. I.: Unique aspects of reproductive cycle of the mare. J. Reprod. Fertil. (Suppl.), *23*:155, 1975.

63. Stabenfeldt, G. H., Hughes, J. P., Evans, J. W. and Neely, D. P.: Spontaneous prolongation of luteal activity in the mare. Equine Vet. J., 6:158, 1974.

64. Stabenfeldt, G. H., Hughes, J. P., Wheat, J. D., Evans, J. W., Kennedy, P. C. and Cupps, P. T.: The role of the uterus in ovarian control in the mare. J. Reprod. Fertil., *37*:343, 1974.

65. Steffenhagen, W. P., Pineda, M. H. and Ginther, O. J.: Retention of unfertilized ova in uterine tubes of mares. Am. J. Vet. Res., *33*:2391, 1972.

66. Stickle, R. L., Erb, R. E., Fessler, J. F. and Runnels, L. J.: Equine granulosa cell tumors. J.A.V.M.A., *167*:148, 1975.

67. Trum, B. F.: The oestrous cycle of the mare. Cornell Vet., *40*:17, 1950.

68. van Niekerk, C. H.: Early clinical diagnosis of pregnancy in mares. J. S. Afr. Vet. Med. Ass., *36*:53, 1965.

69. van Niekerk, C. H. and Gerneke, W. H.: Persistence and parthenogenetic cleavage of tubal ova in the mare. Onderstepoort J. Vet. Res., *31*:195, 1966.

70. van Niekerk, C. H. and van Heerden, J. S. Nutrition and ovarian activity of mares early in the breeding season, J. S. Afr. Vet. Med. Ass., *43*:351, 1972.

71. van Rensburg, S. W. J. and van Niekerk, C. H.: Ovarian function, follicular oestradiol-17β, and luteal progesterone and 20α-hydroxypregn-4-en-3-one in cycling and pregnant equines. Onderstepoort J. Vet. Res., *35*:301, 1968.

72. Von Lepel, J. F.: Maintenance of fertility in the horse including artificial insemination. Equine Vet. J., 7:97, 1975.
73. Warszawsky, L. F., Parker, W. G., First, N. L. and Ginther, O. J.: Gross changes of internal genitalia during the estrous cycle in the mare. Am. J. Vet. Res., 33:19, 1972.
74. Whitmore, H. L., Wentworth, B. C. and Ginther, O. J.: Circulating concentrations of luteinizing hormone during estrous cycle of mares as determined by radioimmunoassay. Am. J. Vet. Res., 34:631, 1973.

Systematic Approach to the Diagnosis of the Infertile or Subfertile Mare

C. B. BAKER
Lana Lobell Farms, Montgomery, New York

R. M. KENNEY
University of Pennsylvania, Kennett Square, Pennsylvania

INTRODUCTION

The evaluation of the fertility of a mare is often requested to determine if a mare has a satisfactory potential for breeding or to determine why a mare, after repeated breeding attempts, has failed to conceive or produce a foal. A variety of techniques have been developed to aid in the evaluation and prediction of a mare's fertility. Utilizing the techniques in a logical manner enables systematic identification of known causes of infertility. A systematic approach should preclude the necessity of performing *all* diagnostic tests on *all* mares of reduced fertility.

The approach described in this article is based upon behavioral and physical findings as well as the utilization of a model of endocrine interactions in the mare. As our understanding of endocrinological events is refined and expanded, the model can be expanded or corrected and the systematic approach modified to accommodate new knowledge.

MANAGEMENT OF MARES FOR BREEDING

The most important factor in achieving maximum reproductive efficiency is proper management. This includes good nutrition, proper parasite control, immunization programs, regular teasing and breeding to a fertile stallion in concert with ovulation. The utilization of a systematic approach to evaluation of the mare assumes that management factors are optimal. If that is an unsafe assumption, the examiner must investigate all facets of the mare's breeding management. Such investigation should not be underestimated since infertility problems in many mares associated with poorer breeding operations are usually due to some aspect of breeding mismanagement.

Estrous Behavior and Ovarian Size versus Season

Understanding the normal seasonal pattern of reproductive activity in the mare is essential before one can correct problems of infertility. Often we are examining animals that exhibit periods of "physiological" infertility not associated with pathological conditions. It is necessary, therefore, to consider these natural phenomena as a differential diagnosis in the systematic approach to infertility in the mare. In as much as the mare is a seasonally polyestrous animal, 70 to 80 per cent of the population is anestrous during the winter season and truly polyestrous during the physiological breeding season (April 15 to August 15). Between these two seasons, mares go through a period of transition that can commence at any time from February to June and can vary in duration from days to weeks or even months. A few exceptions to the pattern are those mares that cycle throughout the year.[5]

Behaviorally, mares in winter anestrus

are either passive or resistant to the teaser, yet they can be in either "shallow" or "deep" anestrus depending upon the type of ovarian activity. In deep anestrus the ovaries are very small (approximately 4.0 cm × 3.0 cm × 2.5 cm) and very firm. The occasional mare with small, hard ovaries will exhibit behavioral signs of estrus, just as will the occasional ovariectomized mare. In shallow anestrus the ovaries are larger, with an occasional small follicle (usually 10 mm or less) definable on palpation. Ovulations rarely, if ever, take place during this period, and full behavioral estrus will seldom be displayed. The small ovaries are caused by the seasonal lack of gonadotropic stimulation to the ovarian follicles.[14]

The transition period is marked by the appearance of large, irregularly lobulated ovaries (8.5 mm × 5.0 cm × 4.5 cm). These "transitional" ovaries are characterized by clusters of many small (10 to 25 mm), viable, and atretic follicles. The estrous behavior during this period is often erratic, and mares may be in constant estrus or may continually act as if they were coming into estrus. Prolonged estrous periods of receptivity without ovulation or with delayed ovulation are common during the transitional period.

During the summer months the ovaries are larger (7.0 cm × 4.0 cm × 3.5 cm) and lobulated because of the presence of follicles and corpora lutea. Estrus will be exhibited on a regular, recurrent basis. The large follicles that develop on these ovaries usually ovulate at regular intervals.

Toward the end of April and certainly after May 1, most mares are in the physiological breeding season in the United States. Mares will come into estrus, ovulate promptly and promptly go out of estrus in a span of 3 to 5 days. This is termed the season of ovulatory receptivity.[5]

The ovaries will usually have several palpable follicles during estrus, with one follicle assuming "dominance" in that it will be larger and will mature to ovulation before the others. Mature follicles vary in size but tend to be 2.5 cm or more in diameter, average 4.5 cm in diameter and can be up to 10 cm immediately prior to ovulation. As a follicle matures, it protrudes increasingly above the surface of the ovary. At maturity, it will protrude several centimeters, thereby creating a steep angle with the ovarian surface (Fig. 1). The follic-

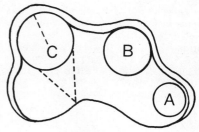

Figure 1. Ovary.

ular wall feels thinner as maturation progresses and sometimes becomes softer. The rate of softening (if it occurs) is correlated to an estrous period of 3 to 5 days.

Fertile breeding with natural service is highest when follicular maturation is accompanied by synchronous changes in the uterus and cervix, which explains the decreased fertility seen in early transition cycles when cervical relaxation does not consistently take place. Cervical edema and relaxation are a result of estrogens that are produced by the maturing follicle.

To evaluate what effect the follicular estrogen is having on its target tissues, the amount of edema and relaxation of the cervix should be estimated. This is done by first palpating and evaluating the cervix and attempting to predict what will be found on the ovaries and then ascertaining the maturation of the most advanced follicle. If the prediction was correct, the mare's reproductive system is highly correlated; if the prediction was incorrect, the system is poorly correlated and fertility will be subnormal. These classifications will be covered in the section concerned with the examination of the tubular system later in this article.

MODEL OF ENDOCRINE CONTROL OF FOLLICULAR GROWTH, OVULATION AND LUTEINIZATION

The sequence of hormone interaction is discussed in detail in Section I and will not be repeated here except to elucidate some important hormonal characteristics of the mare.

Gonadotropin-releasing hormone (GnRH) produced in the hypothalamus travels to the anterior pituitary and initiates the release of follicle-stimulating hormone (FSH) and luteinizing hormone (LH), the levels of which remain high for several days following ovulation. There is some evidence that at least LH is luteotropic in the mare. It appears that the FSH levels peak twice during each cycle at approximately 10-day intervals.[4] One rise starts shortly before estrus and reaches a peak after ovulation. This rise is associated with a concurrent rise in LH levels, follicular maturation and ovulation. A second FSH surge, without a concomitant rise in LH levels, occurs between ovulations. This surge produces a palpable increase in size of the ovaries because of an increased number of small follicles during and after the onset of estrus. In contrast to FSH, there is only one LH surge per cycle. It commences with the onset of estrus, is still climbing at ovulation and reaches a peak in early diestrus.[4]

With the formation of the corpus luteum after ovulation, progesterone levels climb rapidly and remain elevated until 3 to 6 days prior to the onset of the next estrus, at which time they exhibit a rapid decline. The elevated diestrous levels of progesterone do not appear to interfere with the release of FSH but may inhibit release of LH. Alternatively, the pre-estrous rise of estradiol release may be involved in LH release, as it is in other species. Circulating estradiol levels start to rise 2 days before the onset of estrus. They reach a peak 1 or 2 days before ovulation, after which they rapidly decline and remain at low levels until the next cycle.

Normal midcycle levels of progesterone do not appear to suppress the midcycle surge of FSH in the mare, and, in fact, fertile ovulation has been shown to occur in face of high progesterone levels.[6] The mechanism of these fertile diestrous ovulations also remains obscure (Fig. 2).

The scheme described here and in previous articles applies to the operation of the endocrine system of the mare during the long photoperiods (summer) but not during the short photoperiods (winter), when most mares do not cycle. The seasonal (photoperiodic) effect in other species that are seasonal breeders seems to be mediated via the pineal body. There have been no published studies on the role of the pineal body in regulation of seasonal estrus in the mare. However, by extrapolating from the data available for other polyestrous mammals, it is possible to speculate that the pineal body plays a similar role in the mare.

Antigonadotropic substances have been

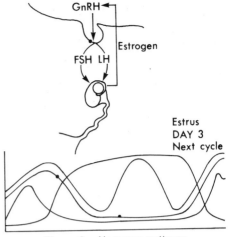

Figure 2. Hormone patterns.

shown to be produced by the pineal body in response to darkness. During periods of short days (long nights), these antigonadotropic substances appear to inhibit the synthesis or release of GnRH. This, in turn, inhibits the synthesis or release of FSH and LH from the pituitary. Without gonadotropin (FSH and LH) stimulation, the ovaries become small and hard because of the regression of any follicles and corpora lutea that are present. The condition of the genital tract in the mare reflects changes consistent with this model. The ovaries of mares in deep winter anestrus are small and hard. Because corpora lutea are not present, they do not respond to prostaglandin-$F_{2\alpha}$ ($PGF_{2\alpha}$) or its analogs or to intrauterine saline infusions during these periods. The uterus is flaccid because of the lack of gonadal steroids (i.e., estrogen and progesterone which are produced in response to the gonadotropins).

With increasing length of day, the amounts of antigonadal activity gradually decrease. Gonadotropin release will increase proportionately. These gradual changes result in the "transitional" manifestations characterized by the formation of multiple small follicles and the occurrence of erratic or prolonged cycles. Ovulation may occur, but fertility during these cycles is lower. This lowered fertility can be explained by the condition of the uterus. Endometrial biopsies taken during this period show that the uterus is still in the atrophy of winter anestrus. In essence, changes in the uterus are one step behind those of the ovaries. These mares commonly have a flaccid uterus during early transition. Later in the transition, the uterus gains some tubular-ity. The cervix frequently remains tight throughout this cycle. Normal fertility will be achieved when the hypothalamus, pituitary, ovaries, uterus and cervix are all operating in synchrony.

This preceding description of the endocrine system, even if simplified, is very complex. Nonetheless, the astute clinician will benefit from recent knowledge so that he knows how and when to intervene.

SYSTEMATIC APPROACH TO DIAGNOSIS

Figure 3 is a schematic representation of the steps to follow in diagnosing fertility problems in the mare.

The first and foremost step in evaluating fertility problems in a mare is to determine whether or not she is pregnant.

If not, the next step is to determine whether the problem lies in the endocrine or the tubular system. If a mare exhibits estrous behavioral response to a stallion, ovulates, forms a corpus luteum and returns to estrus in approximately 14 days, it can be assumed for diagnostic purposes that the hypothalamus, pituitary, ovarian follicles, corpora lutea and uterine luteolytic mechanism are operating normally. In this case the tubular system (i.e., oviducts, uterus, cervix, vagina and vulva) should be examined for the cause of infertility. If the mare is not cycling normally, e.g., either shows no estrus or abnormal estrous cycles, one must consider endocrine dysfunction. Behavior findings should be observed by knowledgeable personnel over two or more estrous periods before being considered significant.

Examination of the Ovaries

The first step in determining the cause of such abnormal behavioral findings is the evaluation of the ovaries. Examination of the ovaries *per rectum* allows classification into four basic groups:

1. Small, hard ovaries much like those found in a mare during deep winter anestrus.

2. Transitional ovaries, much like those found in mares during February, March and April in the Northern Hemisphere, which can become larger than normal. Some vet-

erinarians compare them to a "cluster of grapes."

3. A large disparity in ovarian size. One ovary is small and firm like a winter anestrous ovary, and the other ovary is much larger than normal, being 3 to 6 inches or greater in diameter.

4. Normal ovaries of cyclic mares during the period of ovulatory receptivity. These are basically 2.5 to 3 inches in length and contain a variable number and size of follicles and corpora lutea, depending upon the stage of the cycle. The normal ovary possesses a readily detectable ovulation fossa ventrally.

Small, Hard Ovaries

The small, hard ovary is found in normal mares during winter, in mares with certain types of chromosomal abnormalities, severe malnutrition, severe stress, and probably in mares with endocrinopathies involving the hypothalamus, pituitary and ovary. The winter anestrous ovary is by far the most common. Therefore, it is important to consider the time of the year in which the mare is examined. During November, December, January and February, it will be safe to conclude that in the majority of cases these findings are probably due to winter anestrus. Several options are available for "treating" these cases:

1. Wait for the physiological breeding season.

2. Use artificial light 8 to 10 weeks prior to desired breeding date.

3. Administer exogenous GnRH.

Finding small, hard ovaries during the remainder of the year should lead the clinician to consider malnutrition, intersexuality or an endocrine disorder of the hypothalamus, pituitary or ovary.

The first step in making a firm diagnosis of small, inactive, nonseasonally related ovaries is a chromosomal analysis. The vast majority of mares with abnormal karyotypes found thus far have been sterile. If the karyotype is normal, endocrinopathies of the hypothalamus or pituitary or nonresponsive ovaries should be considered.

The next consideration is the mare's behavior. True nymphomaniacs have small, hard ovaries; show some signs of estrus for prolonged periods and are frequently dangerous to be around. Reportedly, ovariectomy does not eliminate these signs and such mares are infertile if breeding can be accomplished.

A potential method of differentiation would be the use of GnRH, according to the method of Evans and Irvine.[4] The occurrence of estrus and ovulation subsequent to injection of GnRH would indicate that the problems primarily pertained to the hypothalamus. This procedure should

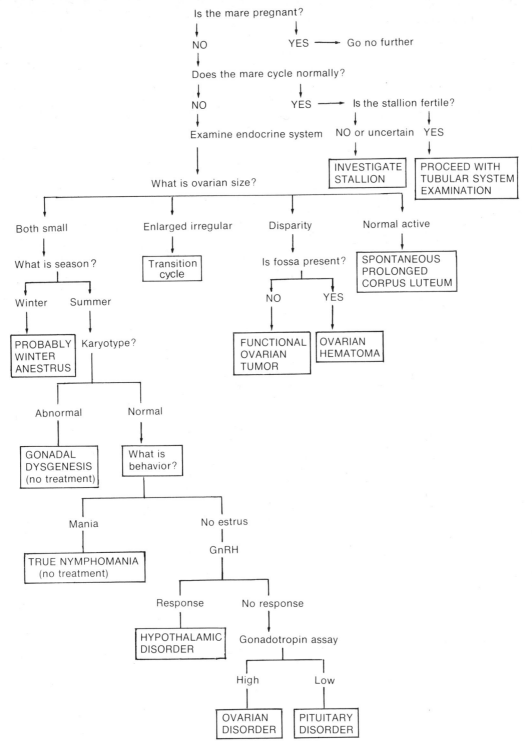

Figure 3. Flow chart for diagnosis of fertility problems in the mare.

also be therapeutic. Lack of response would indicate either a pituitary or an ovarian dysfunction. Laboratory assays of FSH and LH levels may be of potential benefit in differentiating between these conditions. One could speculate that abnormally high levels of gonadotropins might be found in cases of nonresponsive ovaries, similar to that demonstrated in women. Subnormal FSH and LH levels would be consistent with a pituitary disorder. Assays for equine FSH and LH levels are only available at a few veterinary colleges in the world at present. A purified equine pituitary extract that does not induce refractoriness may prove to be effective in treating mares with pituitary dysfunction.

Transitional Ovaries

The second classification includes ovaries with multiple small follicles. During this period, follicles develop but fail to mature. Again, this is part of the natural seasonal progression of ovarian development. It is best handled by waiting until the endocrine system becomes fully operational, usually in late April or early May at 41° North. The later stages of transition will be recognized by the progression of one follicle, which will develop, ovulate and undergo luteal formation. However, endometrial biopsies during the transitional period usually reveal endometrial atrophy consistent with winter anestrus. These findings help explain the reduced fertility of transition cycles. The time required for transition varies, on an individual basis, from 1 or 2 weeks to 1 or 2 months. GnRH has the potential to be used to hasten transition. Injection of 200 mg of repositol progesterone daily for 7 to 10 days is useful in suppression of estrus during this period and appears to hasten the first ovulation.[17]

Disparity in Ovarian Size

The third ovarian type is that in which there is a great disparity in ovarian size. In this case, one ovary will vary from the size of a winter anestrous ovary to a normal ovary, while the other will be larger than normal. Such enlarged ovaries usually contain either a functional granulosa cell tumor (GCT) or an ovarian hematoma. These conditions can usually be differentiated by the presence or absence of an ovula-

tion fossa, behavior or persistence of findings. Open mares with ovarian hematomas continue cycling. Hematomas appear rapidly and regress to normal ovarian size, whereas GCTs do not regress. If the enlarged ovary lacks an ovulation fossa, a granulosa cell tumor is probably present. Granulosa cell tumors are usually steroidogenetically active. Estrogens, progestins and testosterone produced by the tumor inhibit the hypothalamic-pituitary axis. Therefore, gonadotropic stimulation to the contralateral ovary is lacking. The behavioral signs seen in a mare with a granulosa cell tumor may vary. These include lack of estrous signs, persistent proestrus, persistent estrus or stallion-like behavior. These signs are probably dependent on the relative amounts of each gonadal steroid produced. Endometrial biopsy has not yet revealed a consistent diagnostic feature correlated with these tumors. The treatment is surgical removal of the enlarged ovary, provided the mare is normal in other respects, including having a normal endometrial biopsy. The inactive ovary can be expected to resume spontaneous activity from within a few days to a few months after surgery, depending upon the season and other incompletely understood intrinsic factors.

The presence of an ovulation fossa supports a diagnosis of ovarian hematoma. These hematomas usually regress within a few days but may persist for up to 6 months and generally do not affect the function of the contralateral ovary. Examination of the ovary at 15- to 30-day intervals for signs of regression would also support this diagnosis. If the mare fails to cycle or shows manic behavior, surgical removal of the ovary would be indicated.

Mares exhibiting estrous mania are sometimes diagnosed as having "cystic follicles." However, "true" cystic follicular degeneration has not been shown to exist in the horse. The structures that do meet most of the criteria of authorities in this area are the atretic or avascular follicles found most often in transitional periods (anovulatory receptivity).[9]

Normal Ovaries

The fourth classification of ovaries of mares that do not display the normal estrous patterns is that in which two apparently normal ovaries are present. These mares will frequently develop large follicles, occasionally ovulate and yet fail to exhibit behavioral estrus. This combination of normal ovaries and lack of estrus is most common in the late spring and summer period of ovulatory receptivity. Such mares usually have a persistent corpus luteum, probably as a result of the failure of the uterine luteolytic mechanism.[6] The administration of $PGF_{2\alpha}$ or its analogs or of intrauterine saline infusions will cause luteolysis of these persistent corpora lutea. Endometrial biopsy and cervical manipulation[8] have been reported to be very effective in inducing luteolysis with a return to normal estrus. Mares with pyometra may also have decreased $PGF_{2\alpha}$ release and usually will not cycle normally.[15] These mares may be considered to have both a tubular system lesion and an endocrine lesion.

Examination of the Tubular System

Let us consider next the mare that cycles and ovulates normally but fails to become detectably pregnant after repeated breedings or fails to carry a foal to term. Because of repeated normal cycles, it is safe to assume that her endocrine system is operating normally. Provided the mare has been bred to a fertile stallion, we should next examine her tubular system for the cause of her infertility.

The simplest way to determine the stallion's fertility is to determine pregnancy rates in mares already bred by him. If the rate is acceptable, the stallion need not be examined further. If pregnancy rates are not acceptable or are unavailable, the stallion should be investigated. Stallion examinations were covered earlier in this section, and for purposes of this discussion we will assume that the stallion is fertile.

The tubular system is examined by several procedures that closely follow each other and overlap in findings; these will be presented in the order in which they are done.

Visual Examination and Vaginal Air Test

This evaluation begins with a careful visual examination of the tail, perineal region and vulva for evidence of exudate or other vaginal discharge and is followed by visual appraisal of the vulvar lips for size, shape and defects. The vulvar lips should close over the orifice and be no more than 10° from vertical. The adequacy of closure is tested by placing the palm of the hand on each vulvar lip gently pulling the lips apart while listening for the aspiration of air into the vagina (air test). Aspiration of air indicates the potential for pneumovagina, which can usually be corrected by suturing the lips of the vagina. The Caslick procedure should not be carried out until the entire tubular system examination is completed. The degree of vulva that extends above the floor of the vestibule should be determined. The dorsal commissure should extend no more than 4 cm above the floor of the pelvis in the average normal thoroughbred or standardbred. This distance will increase as the vulva tilts or is pulled forward, which further increases the incidence of pneumovagina. These mares also frequently have a "downhill vagina" (anterior vagina lower than the floor of the vestibule) that can interfere with normal drainage of the tubular system and pull the urethral opening forward and upright. Endometritis and urine pooling are often a problem in these mares and will be covered more fully later in this article.

Rectal Palpation

The internal genitalia are evaluated by palpation *per rectum*. The cervix is first evaluated for location, diameter, length, degree of edema and relaxation. These determinations should allow the examiner to classify the cervix into one of six categories: P, X, OX, A, B or C (Fig. 4). With these classifications, one should be able to predict which structures one would expect to find on the ovaries and the expected condition of the uterus. Ovarian palpation usually follows cervical palpation. A highly desirable feature is a positive correlation between dominant features of the ovaries and the uterus and the state of the cervix.

The cervix of the pregnant mare (P) usually undergoes characteristic changes. It will feel longer (10 cm) and firmer than the cervix of the nonpregnant mare and will often feel so distinct that it feels separated from the uterus. The length and firmness are the primary findings that should alert the examiner to the possibility of pregnancy. Another frequent finding with a P cervix is that it does not lie longi-

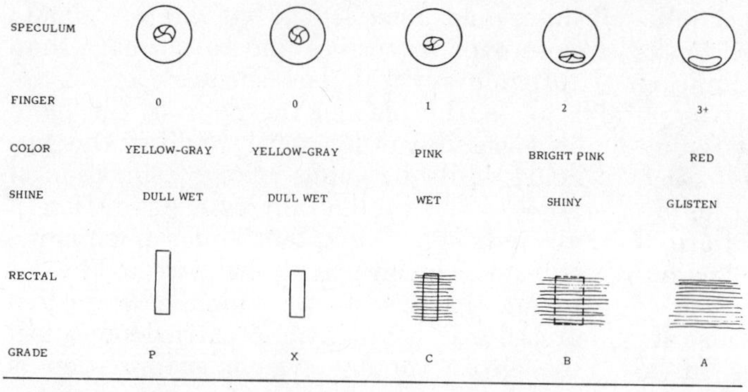

SPECULUM	⊘	⊘	◉	◒	◯
FINGER	0	0	1	2	3+
COLOR	YELLOW-GRAY	YELLOW-GRAY	PINK	BRIGHT PINK	RED
SHINE	DULL WET	DULL WET	WET	SHINY	GLISTEN
RECTAL	▯	▯			
GRADE	P	X	C	B	A

Figure 4. Cervix—speculum—palpation.

tudinal to the axis of the mare's body but instead lies at an angle to the axis (skewed). These features appear as early as day 16 to 18 of pregnancy and last up to day 90, after which they become less reliable. Uterine findings that correlate with a P cervix are tense uterine tone, an amniotic vesicle and frequently a kink in the non-pregnant horn. The kink is most commonly found in primiparous (maiden) mares. The characteristic P cervix is slower to evolve in rebred, recent postpartum mares, and the uterus usually does not develop the kink. If pregnancy is found, further examination of the tubular system is not required.

An X cervix is characteristically about 8 cm long, 2 cm in diameter and firm, and its outlines are readily definable. It will feel much like a good-sized thumb. An X cervix is most commonly found in mares during winter anestrus and transition phases. If a significant degree of cervical relaxation is present, the structure is designated an OX cervix for "open X." One would expect to find a flaccid uterus with an X or OX cervix.

The C cervix reflects the early effect of estrogen. A circumferential edema can be palpated (as indicated by the shading in Figure 4).

The B cervix reflects the continued effects of estrogen. It will have doubled in width compared with the X cervix, has more uniform relaxation and is much flatter and shorter and more edematous. The B cervix will be found in mares coming in or going out of heat.

The A cervix reflects maximum estrogenic influence. It is very wide and uniformly relaxed with abundant edema. The borders are difficult to palpate. This type of cervix will be found in mares during estrus only at the time of the physiological breeding season and indicates synchrony of the entire genital tract. If no other abnormalities are found in the tubular examination, these mares are ready to breed.

The ovaries should be evaluated for size, texture and the presence of ovulation fossa, as well as for specific palpable structures such as follicles and corpora lutea. Again, cervical findings should be used to predict the ovarian structures present (Table 1). With an X cervix, there usually will be no palpable follicles, corpora lutea or corpora hemorrhagica. If a follicle or follicles are present, they will be less than 20 mm in diameter. With a C cervix, one would expect to find at least one follicle $\geq$ 20 mm in diameter or in corpus hemorrhagicum (CH) or corpus luteum.

The mare with a B cervix will usually have at least one follicle 30 mm or larger that is protruding prominently and often softening (mare "coming in") or a CH (mare "going out"). The mare with an A cervix should contain a major large follicle that may be undergoing preovulatory softening.

The ovulation fossa normally faces ventrally in a mare but can face in any direction when being palpated, depending on technique used. The fossa can normally be either a large or a small depression. Absence or filling in of the fossa is highly suggestive of a neoplasm, usually a granulosa cell tumor.

The next step in the internal genital examination is palpation of the uterus. It is important to first rule out the possibility of pregnancy, since further examination would be contraindicated. The reader is referred to other sources for methods of pregnancy diagnosis based on rectal palpation. It is occasionally difficult to differentiate large pyometras that are not draining from 90-day pregnancies by rectal palpation alone. The mare immunological pregnancy

TABLE 1. *Findings on Rectal Examination in Mare with Synchronous Tract*

Findings	Classification of Cervix				
	P	A	B	C	X or OX
Behavior	Cold	Hot	Coming in or going out	Cold	Indifferent to cold
Uterine tone	Turgid, to turgid with bulge	Edematous	Edematous to tubular	Tubular	Flaccid
Size of follicle	25–50 mm, if present	25–50 mm	15–30 mm, if present	± follicles	Usually none, small if present
Corpus luteum (CL) or corpus hemorrhagicum (CH)	Present but not characteristic	No	CH if going out	CL early	No
Palpable endometrial folds	Don't palpate for folds	Palpable and prominent	Going or coming	Palpable but not prominent	Usually not palpable
Overall ovarian size	Normal	Normal	Normal	Normal	Small and hard, to transition ovaries
Cyclic endometrial changes	Don't biopsy	Tall, columnar	Medium, columnar	Low, columnar	Cuboidal, atrophy

(MIP) test is of value in differentiating these conditions.

Once pregnancy is ruled out, the uterus should be palpated for the degree of tone due to edema or turgidity and the presence or absence of endometrial folds. The uterus is very commonly flaccid during winter anestrus and early transition because of the lack of gonadal steroid influence that prepares the uterus to receive a conceptus. A flaccid uterus should be correlated with an X or OX cervix; small, hard ovaries and indifferent or cold behavior when the mare is teased. Occasionally, mares with these rectal findings will show estrous behavior for extended periods of time. The mechanisms causing these behavioral changes are obscure at present.

Normally, as the season progresses the uterus will begin to gain some tone and become more readily palpable. These changes are correlated with the development of larger ovaries with multiple small follicles (often very firm). The cervix may be classified as X during the early stages and as C later. Behavior is quite variable during this period, and may range from the mare's acting cool and indignant to the teaser, to indifferent, to behavior associated with periods of prolonged estrus.

During the physiological breeding season, the entire uterus should reflect edematous changes comparable to those observed in the cervix. Edema increases the tone of the uterus. The desirable correlation during estrus is an A cervix; a large, fluctuant follicle on the ovaries and an edematous uterus (edematous but flaccid). These ovarian, cervical, behavioral and uterine findings detected simultaneously will indicate that synchrony of the tract has been achieved and that normal fertility is expected if no other abnormalities of the mare's tract exist.

Edema of the endometrial folds makes them readily palpable. The endometrial folds are palpated by holding the four fingers together and under the uterus and placing the thumb dorsal to the uterus. By traversing the uterus from end to end, the endometrial folds can be felt to slip between the fingers and the thumb. Absence or atrophy of the folds should be noted.

After the mare ovulates, the cervix closes rapidly and will go from A to C in 1 to 2 days and the follicle will fill with blood (forming the corpus hemorrhagicum, CH). Rectally, a CH and an early corpus luteum (CL) will feel like a water balloon filled with clotted blood. The uterus becomes less edematous and more tubular (rounded). The endometrial folds become less prominent, and no effort should be made to palpate the folds at this time if the possibility exists that a conceptus is present in the uterus, i.e., if the mare had been bred. The endometrial folds should be palpated in the mare not bred on or before day 5. Prominent isolated endometrial folds are probably abnormal (endometrial cyst or edematous endometrial fold).

A great aid in palpating uterine abnormalities and in defining endometrial folds is the remarkable relaxation of the rectum produced by intravenous injection of 15 to 30 mg of propantheline bromide (Pro-Banthine).

Uterine Swab

Uterine swabs are far more reliable as an indicator of disease than are cervical swabs. It has been shown that the numbers of organisms are reduced drastically from those found in the vagina to the external cervical os to the cervical canal to the uterus, respectively. Data indicate that bacteria are isolated from the external cervical os three times as often as they are from the uterus. Thus, cultures obtained from areas other than the uterus itself probably result in "false positive" cultures in a significant number of cases.

A culture of a properly acquired swabbing of the endometrium should be accomplished in a dust-free, draft-free area. The examiner's hand and arm are first covered by a plastic sleeve; the hand, in turn, is covered by a sterile surgical glove. The sheath of the swab is capped by the middle finger and carried to the cervix, where the index finger is inserted into the lumen and used to guide the apparatus into the uterus. Once in the endometrial lumen, the swab is unsheathed, rotated, resheathed and then withdrawn to the external cervical os. The sheath is recapped with a finger and withdrawn from the vagina. The swab is reinserted into its sterile plastic bag. The swab should be plated promptly or kept moist with transfer media

at 4°C (refrigerated) until plated. It is always wise to remember that the *routine* of culturing the endometrium will only detect many aerobic bacteria and fungi. Special culturing techniques are required for detecting microaerophilic and anaerobic bacteria, *Mycoplasma* and viruses. (See Contagious Equine Metritis, page 779.)

If growth occurs on the plate, the clinician should determine if there is an infection occurring in the uterus or if the organism is, in fact, a contaminant. If no growth occurs on the plate, the clinician should determine if the mare is clean or if an organism was missed for some reason. Inflammatory cell changes found in endometrial biopsies therefore add support to interpretation of uterine cultures.

Because of the potential for significant numbers of both "false positive" and "false negative" cultures, it is desirable to correlate culture results with the presence or absence of inflammatory changes in the endometrial biopsy (Table 2). In this way it is often possible either to rule out an organism as a contaminant or to suspect the presence of an organism that was not cultured.

Speculum Examination

Speculum examination is an important and integral step in the process of fertility evaluation; however, it is a potentially dangerous procedure if the instrument is not sterile. Chemical disinfection of the speculum is insufficient to guard the genital health of the mare. For ease of handling, we prefer the black, plastic cylinder; a sterile, disposable speculum or a Caslick's speculum and a pocket flashlight. The mare's tail is first wrapped. Then, after thorough cleansing of the vulva and perineum with soap and water, the specu-

TABLE 2. *Correlation of Results from Endometrial Swab and Inflammatory Changes Found on Endometrial Biopsy*

Uterine Swab	Endometrial Biopsy	Interpretation of Conclusion
Positive	Positive	Mare is infected, treat with appropriate antibiotics based on sensitivity tests
Positive	Negative	Swab probably contaminated
Negative	Positive	Infected, organism not recovered
Negative	Negative	Mare is clean, not infected

lum is inserted into the vagina. If it does not pass beyond 20 cm, withdraw it and examine the vagina manually for a persistent hymen.

After inserting the speculum, the vaginal walls and floor are examined for the presence of foam and fecal debris, both indicators of pneumovagina. The vaginal walls are examined for evidence of scars, lacerations and transluminal adhesions or vaginal septae. The floor is examined for pools of mucus, pus or urine. These materials accumulate not only when they are produced in abundance but also when there is loss of tone in the vaginal tissues, particularly in the older multiparous mares and in mares with a predisposing conformation (downhill vagina). The source of excess mucus is usually from the anterior vagina or cervix and less often from the uterus. Pus can occur from any or all of these organs.

The appearance of the cervix is frequently used by clinicians to index the stage of the estrous cycle and pregnancy. During winter anestrus the X cervix will be small, tight and yellowish-pink to gray and will lie in the center of the vaginal vault. It will not readily admit one finger. However, at times during winter anestrus the cervix will be open and will enable the examiner to see inside the uterus (an OX cervix). The cervix will be pale and lack evidence of edema and mucus. A P cervix will be in the center of the vagina. It will have a long portio, and a characteristic blue-gray tenacious mucus will be found on the speculum when the instrument is removed from the vagina. This mucus makes insertion of the speculum more difficult during pregnancy. A C cervix will be pink, slightly flattened and slightly swollen on speculum examination. The orifice may be slightly open. The C cervix is still in the center of the field or has dropped slightly.

The B cervix is deep pink, the orifice is larger and some mucous secretion is apparent. This type of cervix will have dropped below the center of the field, and its folds will be limp and edematous. The membranes will be deep pink and shiny because of abundant mucus. The lumen readily admits two fingers.

The A cervix is also deep pink with abundant secretion, making it appear shiny. The orifice is larger still. The A cervix usually lies on the vaginal floor and will readily admit three fingers.

The portio vaginalis of the cervix is given particular attention. It should be observed for possible adhesions to the vaginal wall and can also be used to index involution of the uterus in the postpartum mare.

Oviduct Evaluation

It is not possible at present to evaluate the oviduct reliably with clinically applicable techniques. Only occasionally is it possible to palpate the oviduct.

Vandeplassche and Henry[16] found evidence of chronic, nonocclusive salpingitis in slaughtered mares in the Netherlands—88 per cent of these mares were 11 years old or older. The incidence of infundibulitis, ampullitis and isthmitis occurred up to 37 per cent, 21 per cent and 9 per cent, respectively. Similar studies have not been done in the United States, and it is not known what effect these changes have on the foaling rate.

Internal Cervical Palpation

While inserting the culture swab and biopsy punch, the cervix should be carefully evaluated for adhesions, cervical defects and lacerations, as well as for transluminal adhesions and cysts.

Endometrial Biopsies

The endometrium is a critical component of mare fertility because it alone is in contact with fetal tissue after day 5 of pregnancy. Traditional uterine palpation and swabbing are not capable of revealing all endometrial changes that may depress the mare's ability to carry a foal to term. Proper palpation of endometrial folds and endometrial biopsy, when added to the physical examination, greatly increase the clinician's ability to evaluate and establish a prognosis for mare fertility.

The endometrial biopsy is obtained immediately after obtaining the uterine swab for culture. Aseptic precautions similar to those used to obtain the culture sample are taken. The biopsy punch is carried through the vagina to the cervix and passed into the uterine lumen. The gloved hand used to guide the punch is then removed from the vagina and inserted into the rectum, where it is used to guide the biopsy punch to the appropriate site, or sites, in the uterus. When a site has been chosen, the biopsy punch is laid with the handle parallel to the floor. The entire punch is withdrawn about 1 inch so that it does not cut the anterior side of the uterine lumen.

The floor of the lumen is gently pushed up by the index or middle finger of the gloved hand in the rectum. The biopsy punch is then open and closed and the punch retracted. A properly sharpened biopsy punch will cut the tissue much like a Metzenbaum scissors will, but a dull punch will cause some resistance to be encountered on removal of the closed punch. If this happens, pull the punch until the resistance is encountered. At this point a quick, short tug will separate the specimen from the rest of the endometrium. This tearing of the specimen from the rest of the endometrium is undesirable, and the punch should be returned to the manufacturer for resharpening.

If no abnormalities were noted on palpation of the uterus, one biopsy specimen is taken at the junction between the body and either of the uterine horns. Additional samples may be collected from any abnormal areas noted on previous portions of the examination. The biopsy sample should be carefully removed from the punch with a needle (to minimize artifacts) and immediately placed in Bouin's fluid. The tissue should be left in Bouin's fluid for 2 to 24 hours and then switched to a solution of 70 per cent ethanol or 10 per cent formalin for submission to the laboratory.

It is recommended that two slides be made, one for the clinician to examine and the other for interpretation by a pathologist who is familiar with reading equine endometrial biopsies. A collection of slides and reports can thus be obtained for future reference and training. For interpretation of endometrial biopsies the reader is referred to a recent article by Kenney.[9]

Interpretation of samples is most reliable when 2 linear cm or more are examined. Reliability is lost with samples 1 cm long or less. In mares with dilated, thin or flaccid uteri, the difficulty of obtaining sufficient tissue with one sampling is increased. Additional samples should be obtained until 2 cm of tissue is recovered.

On the basis of the extensiveness and severity of histological changes, the endometrium can be divided into three categories of decreasing ability to carry a foal to term:

Category I. The endometrium will not interfere with the ability of the mare to conceive and carry a foal to term. Such an endometrium will have:

1. Either no detectable pathological changes or only slight, widely scattered foci of inflammation, fibrosis or lacunae.

2. No evidence of hypoplasia.

3. No evidence of atrophy.

Category II. In this category the endometrium will interfere with the ability of the mare to carry to term, but the condition is considered correctable or not severe. The endometrial tissue can possess each of the following changes or a wide variety of combinations of these changes:

1. Slight to moderate, diffuse cellular infiltrations of upper lamina propria.

2. Scattered, frequent inflammatory or fibrotic foci throughout the lamina propria.

3. Frequent but scattered periglandular fibrosis of individual gland branches of any degree of severity.

4. "Nests" of gland branches — up to an average of three per 5.5 linear mm in at least four fields.

5. Widespread lymphatic lacunae that do not produce palpable changes.

Category III. The endometrium will interfere with the ability to carry a foal to term, and the condition is not correctable or else will be extremely difficult to correct. Such an endometrium will have one or more of the following changes:

1. Widespread periglandular fibrosis of any degree of severity. This means five or more "nests" of branches in at least four fields of 5.5 mm each.

2. Widespread, diffuse cellular infiltration of the upper lamina propria.

3. A high percentage of plasmacytes compared with lymphocytes (the higher the percentage of plasmacytes, the graver and prognosis).

4. Lymphatic lacunae so extensive as to produce a "jelly-like" or fluid-like feel to the uterine wall.

5. Endometrial and gonadal hypoplasia accompanying chromosomal abnormalities.

6. Pyometra with cellular changes similar to item 2.

These changes seriously interfere with the ability of such endometria to carry a foal to term. Mares with endometria in Category III frequently become pregnant but infrequently carry the fetus to term.

The foaling rate within each category

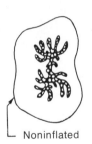 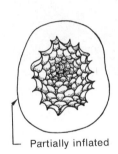 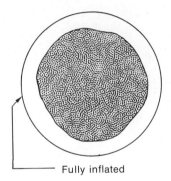

Noninflated   Partially inflated   Fully inflated

Figure 5. Normal fiberoptic examination.

varies significantly — Category I being 70 to 90 per cent; Category II, 50 to 67 per cent and Category III, 4 to 10 per cent.

In general, the high foaling rates in Categories I and II were associated with very good farm management and only fair veterinary care. The foaling rate in Category II is often improved with more extensive veterinary supervision. The lower foaling rates in Categories I and II were associated with less careful management and veterinary attention. Neither management nor medical care effectively alters the outcome in Category III.

As might be anticipated, there is a direct correlation of category with age. In most cases, Category I is dominated by young and maiden mares, with an average age of 9 years, whereas the average age in Category II is 12 years and in Category III 15 years. Whether this is due to the aging effect in itself or to repeated endometritis remains to be determined.

Interuterine Palpation

For internal palpation of the uterus an existing A cervix or a cervix made an A cervix by use of exogenous estrogens is generally required. The examiner and the mare are prepared as for taking an endometrial swab. The hand, covered with a sleeve and sterile glove, is passed into the uterine lumen, while the other sleeved arm is passed into the rectum. In this manner the uterine wall can be grasped and evaluated between two sets of fingers.

It is questionable if veterinarians with large hands can safely perform an internal uterine palpation. If one cannot pass a hand through the cervix, an instrument such as a Chambers catheter or a biopsy punch can be passed into the uterus, which is palpated between the instrument and the hand in the rectum.

Fiberscopic Examination of the Uterus

If abnormalities of the uterus were noted on prior examinations or if the mare has long-term unexplained infertility, a fiberscopic examination of the uterus can be carried out. The equipment used must have a device for inflating the uterus, a mechanism for cleaning the lens and preferably a mechanism for manipulating the viewing field while the instrument is in the uterus. Also some method of stiffening the fiberscope is desirable. The cross section of the normal noninflated mare's uterus contains very little space (having a large potential space but a very small real space); thus, the normal equine uterus must be inflated to be viewed (Fig. 5).

The fiberscope is passed through the cervix in a manner identical to passage of the swab or biopsy punch. The gloved hand is used to hold the external os of the cervix closed when the uterus is inflated with air. As the uterus is inflated (it will usually take 2 to 3 minutes), the normal nonestrous uterus will appear as a hollow pipe.

(Partially inflated)

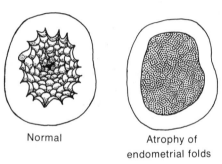

Normal   Atrophy of endometrial folds

Figure 6. Endometrial fold atrophy.

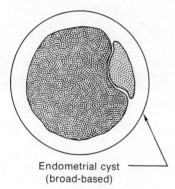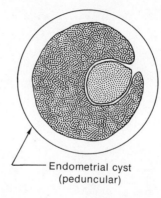

Endometrial cyst
(broad-based)

Endometrial cyst
(peduncular)

Figure 7. Endometrial cyst.

The examiner will see the endometrial folds begin to flatten. The folds are similar to pink cherries attached to the uterine wall. At times the lumen becomes readily apparent on first viewing, before the 2- to 3-minute inflation time takes place, which should alert the examiner to consider atrophy of endometrial folds (Fig. 6). This will be seen in focal myometrial atrophy, segmental endometrial fold atrophy and in seasonally anestrous mares.

The fully inflated uterus should have an even inside curvature. A segmental reverse curvature is suggestive of an edematous endometrial fold or an endometrial cyst. Endometrial cysts are of two types:

1. Lymphatic—a collection of fluid in the lymphatic channel(s) up to 10 cm.

2. Glandular—a collection of secretions within a gland, usually less than 2 mm in diameter.

Lymphatic cysts can often be palpated *per rectum* and can be either turgid or flaccid. The folds filled with lymphatic lacunae can also be detected if one is used to palpating endometrial folds. At times these cysts can be removed or ruptured with a biopsy punch. Glandular cysts are usually very small, are not usually felt rectally, and are seen only with the fiberscope. The so-called edematous folds are usually the result of collections of lymphatic fluid within lymphatic channels and are in fact lymphatic lacunae.

Transluminal adhesions may be detected with the aid of a fiberscope or by direct intraluminal palpation. These adhesions may be classified into two types: longitudinal and transverse. The majority of these adhesions have been found in mares with a Category III uterus by biopsy. Transluminal adhesions appear to be adherent endometrial folds. Atrophy of adjacent endometrial folds is also common in these mares.

There is a normal structure present in all mares that appears somewhat like a transluminal adhesion and is called the internal intracornual frenulum (or septum). Care should be taken not to interpret this as a transluminal adhesion (Fig. 8).

At times the adjacent endometrial folds are adherent and will cause short adhesions or blind pockets. Transluminal adhesions and all their variations are commonly seen in biopsy Category III mares with atrophy of endometrial folds. The reproductive prognosis for these mares is poor.

Diagnosis of complete transverse transluminal adhesions with the fiberscope will be

(Fully inflated)

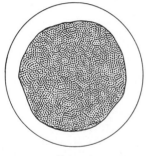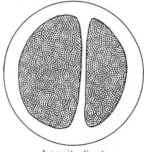

Normal

Longitudinal
transluminal adhesion

Figure 8. Luminal adhesion.

(Fully inflated)

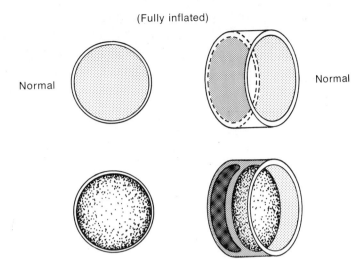

Normal   Normal

Figure 9. Luminal adhesion.

Transverse transluminal adhesion

potentially difficult. These adhesions may appear identical to other portions of the endometrial wall (Fig. 9).

Multiple transluminal adhesions have been observed that appear like bands of cellophane. Repeated biopsies revealed that the endometrium was lacking. The history revealed a *Pseudomonas* metritis and reported intrauterine infusion with 7 per cent tincture of iodine.

When performing a fiberscopic examination, the air used for inflation may form bubbles, which should suggest possible mucometra.

Endometritis does not consistently show a pattern, but acute *Pseudomonas* endometritis will reveal angry red walls (other organisms may also, but extensive work in this area has not been done).

Pyometras should be definitively diagnosed prior to fiberscopic examination, but if a fiberscope is inserted in a mare with pyometra, the fluid will appear as a yellowish to greenish accumulation of fluid. Insertion of the fiberscope too far into the uterus will cause it to be submerged in exudate and a clear viewing field will be lost.

Segmental lesions that appear as pustules or plaques have also been seen.

Few reports concerning intrauterine fiberscopic examinations are available and more information is needed.

CONCLUSION

The utilization of this systematic approach will yield a diagnosis in the large majority of mares. As more causes of infertility are demonstrated, this systematic approach can be refined and expanded to accommodate this new knowledge.

REFERENCES

1. Allen, W. R. and Cooper, M. J.: The use of synthetic analogues of prostaglandins for inducing luteolysis in mares. Ann. Biol. Bioch. Biophys., *15*:461, 1975.
2. Arthur, G. H.: The induction of oestrus in mares by uterine infusion of saline. Vet. Rec., *86*:584, 1970.
3. Caslick, E. A.: The vulva and vulvovaginal orifice and its relation to genital health of the Thoroughbred mare. Cornell Vet., *27*:178, 1937.
4. Evans, M. J. and Irvine, C. H. G.: Induction of estrus and ovulation in the anestrous mare with exogenous gonadotrophin releasing hormone. Cracow, VIII International Congress on Animal Reproduction and A.I., 1976, p. 79.
5. Greenhoff, G. R. and Kenney, R. M.: Evaluation of reproductive status of non-pregnant mares. J.A.V.M.A., *167*:449, 1975.
6. Hughes, J. P. and Stabenfeldt, G. H.: Conception in a mare with an active corpus luteum. J.A.V.M.A., *170*:733, 1977.
7. Hughes, J. P., Benirschke, K., Kennedy, P. C. and Trommershansensmith, A.: Gonadal dysgenesis in the mare. J. Reprod. Fertil. (Suppl.), *23*:385, 1975.
8. Hurtgen, J. P.: Alterations of the equine estrous cycle following uterine and/or cervical manipulations. Proceedings of the 21st Annual Convention of American Association of Equine Practice, 1975, pp. 368–377.
9. Kenney, R. M.: Cyclic and pathological changes of the mare endometrium as detected by biopsy with a note on early embryonic death. J.A.V.M.A., *172*:241, 1978.

10. Kenney, R. M. and Ganjam, V. K.: Selected pathological changes of the mare uterus and ovary. J. Reprod. Fertil., (Suppl.), *23*:335, 1975.
11. Kenney, R. M., Ganjam, V. K., Cooper, W. L. and Lauderdale, J. W.: The use of prostaglandin $F_{2\alpha}$-Tham salt in mares in clinical anestrus. J. Reprod. Fertil. (Suppl.), *23*:247, 1975.
12. Loy, R. G. and Swan, S. M.: Effects of exogenous progestogens on reproductive phenomena in mares. J. Anim. Sci., *25*:821, 1966.
13. Moore, R. Y., Heller, A., Bhatnager, R. K., Wurtman, R. J. and Axelrod, J.: Central control of the pineal gland: visual pathways. Arch. Neurol., *18*:208, 1968.
14. Oxender, W. D., Noden, P. A. and Hafs, H. D.: Estrus, ovulation and serum progesterone, estradiol and LH concentration in mares after an increased photoperiod during winter. Am. J. Vet. Res., *38*:203, 1977.
15. Stabenfeldt, G. H., Hughes, J. P., Kindahl, H., Neely, D. P. and Granstrom, E.: The influence of chronic uterine infection on luteal activity in the mare. VIII International Congress on Animal Reproduction and A.I. Krakow, 1976, pp. 645–648.
16. Vanderplasse, M. and Henry, M.: Salpingitis in the mare. Proceedings of the 23rd Annual Convention of the American Association of Equine Practitioners, 1977, pp. 123–131.
17. Van Niekerk, C. H., Coubrough, R. I. and Dans, H. W. H.: Progesterone treatment of mares with abnormal oestrous cycles early in the breeding season. J. S. Afr. Vet. Med. Assoc., *44*:37, 1973.

Gestation and Pregnancy Diagnosis in the Mare

S. J. ROBERTS
Woodstock, Vermont

Equine theriogenology has rapidly advanced in the past 20 years, with many significant reports being published on ovulation, fertilization, embryology, fetal and placental physiology and disease, endocrine studies, methods of pregnancy diagnosis, abortion and other diseases associated with pregnancy.

OVULATION, FERTILIZATION, EMBRYOLOGY, FETAL AND PLACENTAL DEVELOPMENT

Ovulation in mares requires a healthy, well-nourished mare and occurs naturally during seasons with increasing or long periods of daylight, such as late spring through early fall, or by artificial lighting in late fall through the early spring months. The transition period between anestrus and the normal breeding season in the early spring and late fall is characterized by irregular estrous cycles, abnormal estrous behavior and failure of ovulation. Maturing graafian or ovarian follicles grow rapidly during estrus and reach 1 to 3 or more inches (2.5 to 7.5 cm) in diameter before ovulation. Just prior to ovulation, which occurs in the ovulation fossa or concave aspect of the ovary, the follicle wall becomes softer and less tense. Once estrous cycles in mares have commenced in the breeding season, ovulation usually can be induced within 24 to 48 hours during estrus by the intramuscular or subcutaneous injection of 2500 to 10,000 IU of human chorionic gonadotropin (HCG). Repeated injections at subsequent estrous periods during the same breeding season have not been effective in inducing early ovulations, probably because of the production of antihormones to HCG.

Most ovulations in the mare occur toward the end of estrus or within 24 to 48 hours before signs of estrus cease. Only occasionally do ovulations occur prior to 48 hours before the end of estrus or after estrus terminates. Following ovulation, the follicle fills with a large, soft blood clot, the corpus hemorrhagicum, that on rectal palpation may be mistaken for a follicle just prior to ovulation. The corpus luteum develops rapidly in the ovarian substance but is seldom palpable because of the thick ovarian tunic. Various studies have reported that 15 to 30 per cent of equine estrous periods are characterized by twin or double ovulations.

Since sperm capacitation time is short and normal spermatozoa survive from 2 to 4 or more days during estrus in the mare's genital tract, most mares are bred and fertile sperm are present in the oviduct at the time of ovulation.

Equine ova are probably ovulated as primary oocytes that mature and are capable of being fertilized within a few hours after entering the oviduct. Fertilization occurs soon afterward, with the first cell cleavage within 24 hours after ovulation. The fertilized, dividing ovum enters the uterus about 4 to 5 days after ovulation. Unfertilized ova ovulated during estrus or pregnancy frequently remain in the oviducts for weeks or months. Recently ovulated ova die or lose their ability to be fertilized within a short period after ovulation, probably within 2 to 12 hours.

The gestation period, or pregnancy, extends from fertilization to parturition and has been divided into three periods:

The period of the ovum in the mare is the first 12 to 15 days of pregnancy during which time the fertilized ovum, usually in the morula stage, enters the uterus from the oviduct. The zona pellucida fragments, and the blastula, or blastocyst, develops and inhibits the release of the luteolytic substance, probably prostaglandin, from the endometrium. This prevents the normal involution of the corpus luteum, which is secreting progesterone necessary for endometrial development and release of uterine glandular secretions to nourish the blastocyst and early embryo.

The period of the embryo extends from 12 to 15 days to about 55 to 60 days of gestation. During this period major tissues, organs and body systems are formed; most of them in the first half of this period of rapid growth and differentiation of tissues and organs. By 38 days of gestation the embryo is recognizable as a horse. The embryonic (chorionic) vesicle, which is round in shape until about 25 to 30 days of gestation, increases in size from 6 cm at day 18 to 11 cm at day 38 of gestation. After day 30 the embryonic vesicle becomes more oval in shape. The chorionic girdle of the embryonic vesicle develops rapidly between days 25 and 36, when it is about 5 mm in width. Between days 36 and 38, the girdle separates from the fetal membranes, and its cells invade the endometrium to form the endometrial cups that by 40 days of gestation are producing large amounts of equine gonadotropin. By day 45 of gestation, the chorioallantois has extended beneath and replaced the entire surface of the chorioallantoic vesicle. It is probable that firm attachment of the placental villi to the endometrial sulci occurs between 50 and 70 days of gestation. Before 70 days of gestation there is definite evidence of transuterine migration of the conceptus between the right and left uterine horns,

which occurs in about 20 per cent of pregnant mares.

The period of the fetus extends from 55 to 60 days of gestation to parturition. During this period minor details in the differentiation of tissues, organs and systems occur, along with the growth and maturation of the fetus (Table 1). The increase in the size of the fetus during gestation is a geometric-like curve, with the weight increasing very rapidly during the last 2 to 3 months of pregnancy. For this reason special attention to the level and quality of nutritive intake should be considered during the latter third of gestation. The equine fetal gonads reach a total weight of 50 grams or more at about 250 days of gestation because of a marked increase in the interstitial cells. By 300 days the fetal gonads have begun their regression in size, with degenerative changes being apparent. The cause of this great increase in size of the equine fetal gonads between 180 to 280 days of gestation is not known.

Prior to the development of the chorioallantois, the nutritive needs of the developing ovum and embryo are absorbed from endometrial secretions through the blastodermic vesicle, the yolk sac and the amniotic chorion, respectively. At 20 to 30 days the yolk sac has largely regressed and the chorioallantois is nearly completely formed. By 90 days the chorioallantoic villi attached in the endometrial crypts provide for nutrients to and waste removal from the fetus via their respective circulatory vessels in the diffuse placenta characteristic of Equidae. Toward the end of gestation the amount of amniotic fluid surrounding the equine fetus is 3000 to 7000 ml, and the amount of allantoic fluid is 8000 to 18,000 ml. Amorphous, semisolid, amber-colored, soft, pliable, rubber-like, irregular-shaped, flattened masses or bodies with thin edges, 2.5 to 15 cm in diameter and 0.3 to 3.8 cm in thickness, are commonly found floating in fluids in the allantoic cavity. These are called hippomanes or "colts' tongues." In mares, the fetus is surrounded by the viscous amniotic fluid derived from the skin, amniotic epithelium, fetal urine, saliva and secretions of the nasopharynx of the fetus. The volume of amniotic fluid is probably regulated by swallowing by the fetus. The fetus and the amniotic membranes in the mare float freely in the allantoic cavity, which is filled with watery allantoic fluid primarily from the excretion of the fetal kidneys. The equine fetus is attached to the amniotic and chorioallantoic membranes only

TABLE 1. Size and Characteristics of the Equine Fetus and Uterus During Pregnancy*

Day of Gestation	Size and Shape of Chorionic Vesicle	Amount of Fetal Fluids (ml)	Diameter of Horn Containing Fetus	Weight of Fetus	Length of Fetus (Crown-Rump)	Fetal and Placental Characteristics
16	5.2 cm Pigeon's egg (round)				0.32 cm	
20	6.0 cm Bantam's egg (round)				0.66 cm	
25	6.8 cm Pullet's egg (slightly oval)	30–40			0.6–0.85 cm	
30	7.5 cm Small hen's egg (oval)	40–50	4.5–5 cm	0.2 gm	0.9–1.0 cm	Eyes, mouth and limb buds visible, chorionic vesicle present only in the uterine horn
35	8.5 cm Large hen's egg (oval)	60–90	4.5–6.5 cm		1.5 cm	
40	10.0 cm Turkey's egg (oval)	100–150	7–8.5 cm		1.8–2.2 cm	Eyelids and pinnae have appeared
45	10.5 cm Goose's egg	150–200	7.5–9 cm		2.0–3.0 cm	
50	11.5 cm Orange (oval)	200–350	8.3–9.5 cm		3.0–3.5 cm	
60	13.3 × 8.9 cm Small melon (oval)	300–500	8.9–10 cm	10–20 gm	4–7.5 cm	Lips, nostrils and development of feet observed; eyelids partially closed; placenta not attached but beginning to go into the body of uterus
90	23 × 14 cm Small football (oval)	1200–3000	12.5–15 cm	100–180 gm	10–14 cm	Villi of placenta present but without firm attachment, mammary nipples and hooves visible, body and horn of uterus both involved and enlarged
120		3000–4000		700–1000 gm	15–20 cm	External genitalia formed but scrotum is empty, placenta attached, ergots and orbital areas prominent
150		5000–8000		1500–3000 gms	25–37 cm	May or may not have fine hair on orbital arch and tip of tail, prepuce not yet developed
180		6000–10,000		3–5 kg	35–60 cm	Hair on lips, orbital arch, nose and eyelashes and fine hair on mane
210		6000–10,000		7–10 kg	55–70 cm	Hair on lips, nose, eyelids, edge of ears, tip of tail, back and mane
240		6000–12,000		12–18 kg	60–80 cm	Hair on mane and tail, back and distal portion of extremities
270		8000–12,000		20–27 kg	80–90 cm	Short fine hair over entire body
300		10,000–20,000		25–40 kg	70–130 cm	Body completely covered with short hair, prepuce developed, hair on mane and tail increased
330		10,000–20,000		30–50 kg	100–150 cm	Complete hair coat and hair coat gets its final color, testes descend

by the long, 40- to 80-cm umbilical cord, which is usually moderately twisted.

The fetal membranes and fetus develop mainly in the body and one horn of the uterus with a small extension of the membranes into the nongravid horn. Villi are present on the entire surface of the chorioallantois except in the region of the internal os of the cervix, the cervical "star" region. During the first half of gestation the equine fetus, which is small, can lie in any direction, but after the seventh month the fetus is longer than the diameter of the gravid uterine horn and body and is located longitudinally in these structures. Very rarely, 1 in 1000 gestations, single equine fetuses may develop in both horns as bicornual or transverse pregnancies. These usually result in severe dystocia at the time of parturition. During late equine pregnancy it is generally agreed that the fetus rests with its back on the ventrolateral abdominal wall in the dorsoilial or dorsopubic position. More than 99 per cent of equine fetuses are in anterior presentation with the fetal head toward the cervix by the eighth or ninth month of gestation.

TWINNING IN THE MARE

Twin births occur rarely, about 0.5 per cent, in the equine species. If observed abortions of twins are included, this figure increases to about 1.5 per cent. Double ovulations occur in 15 to 30 per cent of equine estrous periods and especially in certain "twin-prone" mares. There is presently a lack of published data to link twinning in mares with heredity, as occurs in other species. Most double ovulations occur within 48 hours of each other. Nearly all equine twin pregnancies are of the fraternal or dizygotic type. Monozygotic twin pregnancies are rare. The incidence of triplets in mares is extremely rare, possibly 1 in 300,000 births. Evidence would indicate that in 95 per cent of mares with twin ovulations one or both ova or embryos are lost early in the gestation period. This could be a common cause of equine infertility. The surviving twin embryos are usually bicornual in location. Between 6 and 9 months of gestation, one or both fetuses may die and abortion of both fetuses is common. Even in twin pregnancies proceeding to term, both twins are seldom born in a viable state. Usually one is expelled dead or as a mummified fetus, together with a live but frequently small or weak twin. This high death rate, greater than 90 per cent, in twin pregnancies is apparently due to a competition between twin fetuses for placental area. Although the chorions may fuse, anastomosis of blood vessels between the two placentae does not occur. One chorion invaginates into the other, and the smaller, debilitated fetus with the smaller placental area dies because of a lack of nutrients and is expelled prematurely along with the larger fetus. Alternatively, it may mummify and remain in the uterus to be expelled at parturition with the live fetus that had the larger placental area.

Various procedures have been tried in mares to avoid or prevent twin pregnancies. These have included:

1. Following ovulations by repeated rectal examinations of the "twin-prone" mare's ovaries and breeding only when one follicle matures.

2. If two large, mature follicles are found on rectal palpation, either:
    a. Don't breed the mare until possibly the next estrus (see previous discussion).
    b. Tap one follicle *per vaginam* with an ovarian needle.
    c. Wait until one follicle ovulates and then breed 12 to 18 hours later, after the first unfertilized ovum has died.

3. Diagnose twin pregnancy very early in gestation by rectal palpation of two chorionic or embryonic vesicles and:
    a. Attempt to manually crush one embryonic vesicle or
    b. Destroy one embryo by inserting a needle or trocar into the embryonic vesicle after a laparotomy operation.
    c. Dilate the cervix and douche the uterus to cause abortion and then rebreed at the next estrus.
    d. Inject the mare intramuscularly with prostaglandin-$F_{2\alpha}$ ($PGF_{2\alpha}$) at 12-hour intervals in doses of 5 to 10 mg to produce abortion and then rebreed at the next estrus.
    e. Allow the twin pregnancy to proceed to term with the hope that twin abortion will not occur and that one or both fetuses will be born alive.

None of these procedures used to prevent or "treat" equine twin pregnancies is highly satisfactory in the control of this common condition.

HORMONAL CONTROL OF EQUINE GESTATION

After ovulation the corpus luteum develops in the ruptured follicle and produces progesterone, which reaches a significant blood plasma concentration of 6 to 10 ng/ml or more by day 5. This production rate continues in the pregnant mare until days 35 to 40 of gestation, when pregnant mare serum gonadotropin (PMSG) is produced by the endometrial cups. The endometrial cups originating from the chorionic girdle of the embryonic vesicle produce PMSG levels detectable as early as 32 to 36 days of gestation. However, high or diagnostic levels of 40 to 80 IU/ml are not reached until 40 days of gestation and then persist at a high level until 90 days, after which the serum levels of PMSG usually decline rapidly. Mares carrying mule conceptuses have greatly reduced (one-tenth) production of PMSG, while donkeys carrying hinny conceptuses show greatly increased PMSG levels. It is generally considered that from 50 to 70 days of gestation, the high levels of PMSG, together with the pituitary gonadotropins, maintain the primary corpus luteum and increase its activity and stimulate the formation of secondary corpora lutea from anovulatory and ovulated follicles. Thus, after 40 days of gestation the level of progestogens in the blood plasma of pregnant mares rises to about 10 to 20 ng/ml, depending on assay methods. The secondary corpora lutea, as well as the primary corpus luteum, persist in the ovaries and continue to secrete progestogens until days 140 to 160 of gestation, when they begin to regress. They become completely regressed by days 210 to 220 of gestation. Placental progesterone production probably begins at approximately day 50 to 70 of gestation and supplements the progesterone produced by the primary and secondary corpora lutea until about midpregnancy, when the corpora lutea regress and even ovariectomy can be performed in the mare without terminating pregnancy. Progestogen plasma levels gradually rise in the latter months of pregnancy to 20 to 50 ng/ml, depending on assay methods, after which they decline precipitously to very low levels of 3 ng/ml or less. Estrogen levels in the plasma of pregnant mares rise from the fourth month (120 days) of gestation to a peak at about 9 months (180 to 270 days),

decline gradually until late gestation and then fall rapidly after foaling. Apparently, the estrogens and progestogens are produced by the fetoplacental unit in the latter two-thirds of gestation.

Follicular development in ovaries of pregnant mares increases from 10 to 20 days of gestation to a peak in size and number at 50 to 60 days of pregnancy, probably under the influence of PMSG and pituitary gonadotropin. Then follicular activity decreases, and by day 220 the ovaries contain no large follicles.

The initiation of parturition or the termination of gestation in the mare is probably brought about by the presence of relatively high levels of estrogens, a modest increase in fetal glucocorticoids, an increase in prostaglandins and, terminally, an increase in levels of oxytocin. Other hormones such as relaxin may also play a role. Mares apparently can control the actual onset of labor by a number of hours, since 80 to 85 per cent of parturitions occur at night, with most occurring within 2 hours of midnight.

DURATION OF THE EQUINE GESTATION PERIOD

The duration of the gestation period of the mare varies from 327 to 357 days, with an average duration of 340 to 342 days. Draft mares may foal after a slightly shorter gestation period of 330 to 340 days. Ass-horse hybrids have a longer gestation of 350 to 355 days, approaching that of asses (356 to 375 days). Male fetuses usually have a gestation period 1 to 2 days longer than female fetuses. In the Northern Hemisphere, foals born from January through April have gestation periods about 10 days longer than foals born from May through September. Short gestation periods in conjunction with abortions or premature births may be associated with twinning. Prolonged equine gestation periods of up to 375 days and even longer, with the delivery of a live foal, have rarely been reported. The duration of gestation in the mare may be shortened slightly by injections of prostaglandins, glucocorticoids, estrogens, progesterone or oxytocin given late in gestation. The practical induction of parturition will be discussed in a subsequent article.

EQUINE TERATOLOGY OR INHERITED DEVELOPMENTAL ANOMALIES

Inherited or genetic lethal or semilethal defects reported in horses include atresia coli in Percherons, hemophilia, sterility (Fredricksborg lethal) in white horses, epitheliogenesis imperfecta of the lower limbs (sex-linked lethal), hereditary ataxia in the Oldenburg breed, "wobbles" or incoordination seen in all breeds, especially Thoroughbreds, Standardbreds and the American saddle horse. The latter is most common in male animals and is due to compression of the spinal cord in the cervical region caused by defective development of the cervical vertebrae. (In recent years four or five other causes for incoordination or symptoms of "wobbles" have been described in horses.) Other lethal defects include cerebellar hypoplasia in Arabian horses, absence of a retina, "combined immunodeficiency in Arabian foals" and hydrocephalus. Inherited nonlethal defects in horses include congenital blindness, aniridia with cataracts in Belgium horses, umbilical hernia, cryptorchidism, brachygnathia, subluxation of the patella (especially in ponies), multiple exostoses in Quarterhorses and Thoroughbreds, heaves or pulmonary emphysema, laryngeal hemiplegia (roaring) and hip dysplasia in Dole horses. Other possible nonlethal inherited defects include scrotal hernia, side bone, hypotrichosis congenita and sterility in mules and hinnies (horse × ass hybrids).

Congenital defects or anomalies of a nonhereditary nature are not uncommon in horses and may arise from ingested teratogens (including drugs or chemicals), radiation, endocrine disturbances, possibly nutritional deficiencies, possibly viral infections during the first third or half of gestation and chromosomal anomalies due to aging of the gametes in the oviduct before fertilization, which is quite possible in horses. These congenital developmental errors include cyclopia, polydactyly, polydontia, teratomas, hermaphrodites or intersexes, cardiac anomalies, cleft palate, ectopic urethra, persistent urachus, anomalies or failure in development of the gonads or genital tract, entropion, cataracts, optic nerve hypoplasia, ectopia of the patella, dentigerous cysts, dermoid cysts and others. Conjoined twin fetuses are extremely rare in horses.

PREGNANCY DIAGNOSIS IN THE MARE

Indicative or subjective history and signs of pregnancy in a mare include:
1. Services by a stallion.
2. Cessation of estrous periods as determined by regular teasing at 1- to 2-day intervals through the forty-fifth day after service.
3. Increased gentleness and docility by the third month of gestation.
4. Enlargement of the abdomen, especially the ventral portion (pear-shaped abdomen), by the fifth month.
5. Observation of fetal movements, especially after drinking cold water, by the seventh to eighth month of gestation.
6. Enlargement of the udder.
7. Relaxation of the pelvic ligaments by the tenth month.

"Spurious" conception may follow a normal service in a healthy cycling mare, in which further estrous cycles apparently cease and rectal examinations at a later date reveal that the mare is not pregnant. However, these signs, especially the early ones, may be misleading. The breeding history of the mare in previous years is helpful. Some mares may fail to conceive after breeding and have a failure of estrus due to a persistent corpus luteum. Others may conceive but abort or absorb an early embryo prior to 90 days of gestation and not exhibit estrus. Furthermore, some mares (up to 10 per cent) may show signs of estrus for a short period or be indifferent to a teaser stallion and yet be pregnant. Thus, a broodmare may exhibit widely contradictory behavior in respect to her true state of pregnancy. Ballottement of the fetus during late gestation in the mare is difficult because of the thick abdominal wall and the tensing of the abdominal muscles by the mare during this maneuver.

Internal Examination for Detecting Pregnancy in the Mare

Before the internal examination for detection of pregnancy in the mare is performed, a good clinical breeding history should be obtained, if possible. The foaling and breeding dates, dates of estrus, frequency and efficiency of teasing before and after breeding and knowledge of the regularity of the mare in her estrous cycles and past foalings are helpful.

The rectal diagnosis of pregnancy in the mare by an experienced veterinarian is the earliest and most accurate method available. In performing a rectal examination in a mare, the same equipment, dress and mode of procedure are used as for examination of the cow, with the following exceptions: Restraint is more essential in mares. Many mares require the application of a nose twitch to control and make them stand quietly and prevent them from kicking the operator. Some veterinarians have the mare's tail forced firmly dorsally and cranially over the sacrum as a form of restraint. Certain excitable mares that object to restraint must be handled gently and quietly if a rectal examination is to be performed. Often these mares may be examined only by having a foreleg elevated. In rare cases tranquilization or even sedation with acepromazine or xylazine (Rompun) in addition to using a twitch may be required. If breeding hobbles are used to restrain a mare, kicking is prevented but the hocks may be raised suddenly and injure the operator if he is standing too close to the rear quarters. A mare can be examined in stocks, over or around a stall partition or by being backed up to a manger or to several bales of hay or straw. If a mare is in stocks, the rear rope or board should be low so that if the mare drops her hindquarters suddenly the examiner's arm will not be injured. It is best to bandage the mare's tail or have it held upward and to one side by an assistant so that the long tail hair does not irritate the anus and rectum at the time the examiner's arm is inserted and the tail does not become soiled.

A bland, nonirritating lubricant should be used on the arm. The rectum of the mare is drier than that of the cow, and the operator's arm requires frequent, liberal lubrication. The author favors a bucket of soapy water made with a bland soap and applied to the arm with a sponge. Dial liquid soap (Armour, Inc.) can be applied frequently to the arm and anus during the rectal examination without causing irritation of the rectum. Commercial lubricants such as K-Y jelly are also helpful. The peristaltic waves in the mare are stronger than in the cow. The hand and arm should be withdrawn from the rectum when a peristaltic contraction occurs. Trauma to the rectum of the mare is more easily produced than in the cow and has more serious and sometimes fatal results because of the mare's increased susceptibility to peritonitis. Rectal examinations should therefore be made with quiet restraint, care and gentleness. Withholding feed, especially roughage, for 12 to 24 hours aids the examination.

After entering the rectum of the mare and locating the bony pelvis, it is easier to first locate one of the ovaries until, with more experience, the uterus can be readily found. The distinct, fibrous, bean-shaped ovary, 4 to 8 cm long by 3 to 5 cm thick, is located about 10 to 20 cm cranial to the shaft of the ilium and about 5 to 10 cm below the lumbar vertebrae in the nonpregnant mare or the mare in early pregnancy. The operator who uses his right hand can more readily locate the left ovary of the mare and vice versa. After locating one ovary, the hand is passed down the utero-ovarian ligament to the uterus. The uterus is cupped in the hand between the fingers and thumb, and palpation of the cranial border and ventral and dorsal portions of the nonpregnant or early pregnant uterine horns, the opposite ligament and the opposite ovary is performed. The nonpregnant, completely involuted uterus is pliable, soft, flat and rather flaccid and measures 4 to 7 cm wide and 2 to 5 cm thick. In the maiden or young mare the nonpregnant uterus is suspended above the floor of the pelvis and abdomen. In older mares, especially the first month after foaling, the uterus may be located more ventrally and may be hanging cranial to the floor of the pelvis in the abdominal cavity. Dimock advised operators that in circumstances in which the uterus was located well forward and downward in the abdominal cavity, traction on the broad ligament or bimanual examination, with the other hand in the vagina grasping and exerting traction on the cervix, could be helpful.

Uterine Changes during Pregnancy

In most mares, rectal palpation of the uterus to diagnose pregnancy can be performed by an experienced operator with great accuracy from 30 to 40 days of gestation. Diagnosis usually is easier for the less experienced veterinarian from 40 to 50 days of pregnancy. Pregnancy diagnosis is easier in maiden mares or primigravidae and in barren, nonfoaling mares than in mares conceiving during foal estrus when the uterus has not completely involuted. Zemjanis and others have described their apparently skilled, careful techniques for diagnosing equine pregnancy manually from 17 to 30 days of gestation. Great care must be used not to injure the embryo or the chorionic or embryonic vesicle. It is often desirable to re-examine the mare once to twice at bimonthly intervals to make certain that embryonic or fetal death and resorption or abortion has not occurred. In the mare, as in the cow, early embryonic deaths are not uncommon, with an incidence of 2 to 10 per cent or greater between early pregnancy diagnosis and 110 days of gestation.

The thickness of the uterine wall increases slightly in both pregnant and non-pregnant mares from days 10 to 16 after the onset of estrus. From day 16 to 21 there is a three-fold increase in thickness in the uterine wall in pregnant mares, while in nonpregnant mares the thickness of the uterine wall declines to a low point at the onset of the next estrus. The tone of the uterine wall follows the same pattern, showing a definite increase in the tone of the uterine wall of both pregnant and nonpregnant mares to day 16 followed by a decline in tone in nonpregnant mares to a soft, flaccid state about 1 day before the next estrus. In pregnant mares the uterine tone continues to increase after day 16, with the uterine horn becoming round and tubular about 5 days later.

Palpation of the Chorionic or Embryonic Vesicle

During pregnancy the uterine horns enlarge (see Table 1). The earliest that this can ordinarily be detected is 20 to 30 days. This enlargement is characterized by a circumscribed ventral bulge or distention of the uterine horn, usually just to the right or left of the center or bifurcation of the horns. A dorsal bulging of the horn is not observed until after 40 days of gestation and then is not marked. Rarely, the embryo and its membranes may develop more laterally in either horn or in the body of the uterus. The spherical bulge or swelling is caused by the chorionic or embryonic vesicle during early gestation and later by the oval chorioallantoic vesicle containing the enclosed amniotic sac and embryo, the vitelline or yolk sac and the allantoic fluid. From 3 to 6 weeks the vitelline or yolk sac is large and the amniotic cavity around the embryo is small. The

allantoic cavity grows rapidly from 5 to 7 weeks of gestation, during which time it contains much fluid. This embryonic vesicle at first is round or slightly oval and then, as it enlarges, assumes a more ovoid, tubular or sausage-shaped outline and extends into the body of the uterus about 60 to 90 days of gestation. The uterine wall during this early stage of pregnancy is more tubular in shape, has a more tonic feel, and is thinner over the ventral bulge. As in the cow, these changes are primarily due to filling of the uterine horn and body with fetal membranes and fluid, imparting the feel of a heavy, water-filled rubber balloon.

By 60 to 70 days the chorioallantoic vesicle is so large that it is difficult to delineate its extent, and the early tonus is less evident. Manual slipping of fetal membranes, as in the cow, is not done in the mare because the discrete, localized oval area of the uterus occupied by the conceptus in early pregnancy readily differentiates pregnancy from pyometra or mucometra. In addition, the thicker, more tonic equine rectal wall makes this technique hazardous. Furthermore, such vigorous handling of the vesicle in very early pregnancy might cause embryonic death.

Palpation of the changes in the size of the horn and body containing the fetus has been outlined in Table 1. Since the size of the round and, later, of the oval chorionic and chorioallantoic vesicle is closely correlated with the size of the uterine horn, the diagnosis and duration of early pregnancy may be ascertained.

The pregnant uterus in the mare is usually suspended above or on the level of the floor of the pelvis until the third to fourth month of gestation, when it drops enough to rest on the abdominal floor, at which time the ventral surface of the uterus cannot be palpated. In older mares the uterus may rest on the abdominal floor by the third month. When the uterus lies deep in the abdominal cavity, it can be drawn caudally by retraction on the cranial border of the broad ligament. If the mare is more than 3 months' pregnant, it will be difficult or impossible to pull the uterus back, owing to its weight; whereas if the mare is not pregnant, the uterus can be drawn back and palpated. By the fifth to sixth month of pregnancy the uterus is well forward in the abdominal cavity, and the broad ligament is under definite tension. The ovary may be 20 to 25 cm below the lumbar vertebrae and is moved with difficulty because of the stretching of the mesovarium.

Palpation of the fetus through the rectal wall can usually be performed by 90 to 120 days of gestation, at which time the fetus feels like a small, heavy, submerged but floating object as the hand contacts it. In most mares it is usually possible to palpate the fetus *per rectum* from the third month throughout the rest of the gestation period. The size and weight of the equine fetus during the various stages of pregnancy are noted in Table 1. In a few deep-bodied mares, palpation of the fetus may be difficult from the fifth to seventh months of gestation. In these mares the location of the uterus, the position of the ovaries and the palpation of the enlarged, "whirring" uterine artery will aid or confirm a diagnosis of pregnancy.

Unlike the cow, palpation of the ovaries of the mare during early pregnancy is of no value in determining which uterine horn contains the fetus. A portion of the corpus luteum is palpable for only a few days after ovulation in the region of the ovulation fossa before it is covered by the dense, fibrous ovarian tunic. Furthermore, although ovulation occurs more commonly (52 to 63 per cent) in the left ovary, about 60 per cent or more of the fetuses develop in the right horn. The fertilized embryo can undergo intrauterine migration in both directions; thus, the percentage of pregnancies in each horn is about equal or is a few percentage points more in the right horn.

Investigators have reported some interesting findings concerning the ovaries of mares during pregnancy. They divided the gestation period into four periods in relation to the changes that occur in the ovaries. The first period, from ovulation to 40 days, was characterized by the presence of a single corpus luteum of pregnancy. A number of various-sized follicles up to 5 cm in diameter were usually present in pregnant mares from 10 to 40 days of gestation on both ovaries. The second period, from 40 to 150 days, was characerized by marked ovarian activity with as many as 10 to 15 follicles over 1 cm in diameter and the formation of corpora lutea. Ovulation may occur during this period. Usually three to five or more accessory corpora lutea are present in each ovary. The diameters of the largest follicles were greatest about 50 to 60 days of gestation. This ovarian activity, with follicle and corpora lutea formation, is probably produced by the high level of gonadotropic hormones secreted by the endometrial cups in the uterine endometrium from 40 to 120 days of gestation, together with gonadotropin secreted by the anterior pituitary gland. The third period, from 150 to 210 days, was characterized by a regression of the corpora lutea, and large follicles were absent. During the fourth period, from 210 days to foaling, no corpora lutea or follicles were present. Throughout these latter two periods, gestation is maintained by steroid hormones produced in the placenta.

The vaginal examination as an aid to pregnancy diagnosis may be helpful, but it is not as accurate as the rectal examination of the uterus. By 30 days of pregnancy the normal equine vagina and cervix are very white and pale on examination with a speculum. In fact, they are more white and pale than at any time during the estrous cycle and resemble a mare's vagina in anestrus during the winter months. By 60 to 90 days of pregnancy the mucous membrane is usually very dry, sticky and gummy. There is less tendency for the vagina to balloon when the speculum is inserted than there is during the estrous cycle. More of this gummy mucus is present on the mucous membrane of the vagina during pregnancy than during the anestrous period. About 75 per cent of pregnant mares show these characteristic vaginal changes. The other pregnant mares may show a more hyperemic or congested mucous membrane with less mucus. In rare cases a vaginitis with a mucopurulent exudate may be seen. The cervix in pregnant mares is usually tightly closed and small with a puckered external os. It is usually pulled downward and to one side. The external os of the cervix usually becomes covered with gummy, sticky mucus. In advanced pregnancy it may be easier to palpate the fetus through the vagina than through the rectum, as the mare objects less to the vaginal examination.

Differential Diagnosis

Differential diagnosis as part of pregnancy examinations should be considered by the inexperienced examiner. From 70 to 110 days a distended bladder may be confused with pregnancy. Pneumovagina, or a uterus filled with air, might be mistaken for pregnancy. From 90 to 120 days an enlarged or distended right colon or pelvic flexure of the colon might rarely be confused with a pregnant uterus. Pyometra and mucometra associated with focal cystic degeneration of the endometrium are occasionally found in the mare. In this condition the uterine wall may be thick and heavy, and the fluid contents of the uterus are sluggish. Tumors, usually leiomyomas, are rare in the mare. Mummification of a single fetus has not been observed in the mare. Fetal maceration is uncommon.

Double ovulation occurs in 18 to 20 per cent of mares, and twin pregnancies are quite commonly diagnosed. But the incidence of twin births is low (0.5 per cent) because of embryonic or fetal death and abortion of possibly one or, more often, of both fetuses. Twin embryos may be detected early by the palpation of two chorioallantoic vesicles or ventral bulges, often with one vesicle in each horn. Later, twin fetuses might be palpated and both uterine arteries might be enlarged. Embryonic deaths in mares may be diagnosed at 30 to 45 days by a loss of fluid and tone in the chorioallantoic vesicle. The uterine wall, however, may remain tonic and thick for a considerable period, even though the size of the ventral bulge regresses. These mares may not return to estrus for 40 to 80 days, possibly because of the "persistence of the corpus luteum." Douching the uterus with 500 ml of warm saline, if performed before 45 or 50 days of gestation, or the injection of 10 mg of $PGF_{2\alpha}$ usually results in a return to estrus within a few days in these mares. If early embryonic death is suspected, repeated examinations *per rectum* may be needed to confirm it.

Other abnormalities of the mare's uterus that might be confused with early pregnancy include large endometrial cysts up to 5 cm or more in diameter; a doughy, flaccid myometrial lymphatic lacuna and a focal atony of the myometrium and endometrium in the region to the right and left of the uterine bifurcation that may cause ventral bulges of the uterine horn. However, careful palpation will usually reveal that these pathological structures are thicker-walled and lack the fluid feel of an embryonic vesicle and that the uterine wall lacks the characteristic marked tonicity noted in pregnant uteri. These findings are usually seen in older mares.

Biological and Other Tests for Pregnancy in the Mare

The biological tests for pregnancy in the mare are based on the presence of high levels of certain hormones at various stages of pregnancy. Some of these tests are highly accurate and useful in very nervous or vicious mares and small ponies, in which rectal examinations are dangerous or impossible, and also when the veterinarian is not experienced in the manual examination for pregnancy.

The most practical biological tests for pregnancy in the mare determine the presence of pregnant mare serum gonadotropin (PMSG) between 40 and 120 days of gestation. This hormone is produced by the endometrial cups. Tests used for detecting PMSG in mare's serum are the Aschheim-Zondek (A-Z) rat test; Friedman's modification of the A-Z test, or rabbit test; the male frog test and the mare immunological pregnancy (MIP) test. The latter test is presently the most widely used test in the United States because it can easily be performed in the field or office, is highly accurate (over 90 per cent) and results can be obtained within a few hours.

The MIP test is a hemagglutination inhibition test utilizing the principle that PMSG inhibits the agglutination of sheep erythrocytes coated with PMSG in the presence of PMSG antiserum from rabbits. Recent studies have shown that between 40 and 120 days of gestation the MIP test is more reliable than the rectal palpation method for diagnosing pregnancy unless the palpation is performed by a highly experienced diagnostician. Early embryonic or fetal death loss from 45 to 90 days of gestation is fairly common in mares. If PMSG levels become elevated before the death of the conceptus, these levels will remain high and give a false positive test. The incidence of false negative MIP tests is generally low unless blood is drawn from mares before 40 days or after 120 days of gestation, the mare is carrying a mule fetus or the serum is overheated.

Other less practical and less accurate mare biological pregnancy tests include:

1. Tests such as the Cuboni method for detecting high levels of estrogen in the urine between 120 and 290 days of gestation. This chemical test is most accurate from 150 to 250 days.

2. Tests such as radioimmunoassay (RIA) or competition protein binding for determining levels of progestogens or estrogens in blood serum can be used about 17 to 21 days after service and ovulation to determine whether conception possibly occurred or not. However, when mares are teased regularly, less than 7 per cent of the nonpregnant mares have not returned to estrus by 24 days.

3. Other biological tests in rats or mice, other chemical tests for detecting the presence of estrogens in urine and tests such as the mucin test on vaginal mucus have been described.

Other nonbiological tests for pregnancy in the mare include the use of the fetal electrocardiogram from the fifth or six month to term and the use of ultrasound or "sonar" instrumentation.

REFERENCES

1. Arthur, G. H.: Veterinary Reproduction and Obstetrics. 4th Ed. London, Baillière and Tindall, 1975.
2. Roberts, S. J.: Veterinary Obstetrics and Genital Diseases. 2nd Ed. Ann Arbor, Mich., Edwards Bros. Inc., 1971.
3. Rowlands, T. W., Allen, W. R. and Rossdale, P. D. (Eds.): Equine Reproduction, Proceedings of the 1st International Symposium on Equine Reproduction, Cambridge, England. London, Blackwell Scientific Publ., 1975.
4. Zemjanis, R.: Diagnostic and Therapeutic Techniques in Animal Reproduction. Baltimore, The Williams and Wilkins Co., 1962.

Abortion and Other Diseases of Gestation in Mares

S. J. ROBERTS
Woodstock, Vermont

Abortion is the observed expulsion of a nonviable or dead fetus. Expulsion of the embryo or fetus following death between 20 and 90 days of pregnancy is rarely noticed. Most abortions, even on a well-supervised breeding farm, are usually not observed until after 4 or 5 months of gestation.

For this reason most early embryonic and fetal deaths, which are common from 20 to 90 days of gestation, are considered to be a form of infertility. Early death of the fertilized ovum is usually associated with a regular or slightly delayed estrous cycle. The incidence of early fetal death in mares between 30 and 90 days of gestation is widely reported as 7 to 30 per cent, the average being 8 to 15 per cent. An increase in early pregnancy losses has been associated with: (1) use of certain stallions; (2) short postpartum intervals of less than 30 or 40 days before service; (3) mares over 18 years of age; (4) mares that were infertile or aborted at the previous breeding season; (5) injudicious, rough manual examination of mares in early pregnancy, i.e., before 40 days; (6) poorly managed breeding, in which excessive aging of spermatozoa or ova occurred in the oviducts prior to fertilization, resulting in chromosomal abnormalities; (7) malnourished mares between 25 and 31 days of pregnancy, (8) uterine infections; (9) an abnormal endometrium with fibrotic, atrophied endometrial glands and (10) excessive stress due to overheating, trucking, working and so forth.

The incidence of observed equine abortions after the fourth month of gestation usually constitutes only a small percentage of total pregnancy wastage (about 2 to 12 per cent of all pregnancies). Abortions may be caused by either infectious or noninfectious agents that affect the normal function and development of the fetus, fetal membranes and genital tract. Given an accurate and complete history and prompt delivery of the chilled, aborted fetus and membranes and a blood sample to a competent diagnostic laboratory, the cause of the abortion can usually be ascertained in about 50 to 60 per cent of cases submitted. Not infrequently the fetus dies in the uterus and is not expelled for 2 to 3 days, with resultant autolytic changes that make a definitive diagnosis very difficult. Autolysis of the equine fetus is characterized by opacity of the cornea; soft, mushy internal organs and gelatinous, blood-tinged subcutaneous and placental tissues.

INFECTIOUS CAUSES OF EQUINE ABORTION

Bacteria

Bacterial causes of equine abortion include *Streptococcus zooepidemicus, Salmonella abortus equi, Leptospira pomona* and possibly other *Leptospira* organisms, *Escherichia coli, Staphylococcus aureus, Corynebacterium equi, Pseudomonas aeruginosa, Brucella abortus* and other *Brucella* organisms, *Klebsiella pneumoniae* var. *genitalium, Actinobacillus, Streptococcus equi* and other streptococci and staphylococci.

Most of these organisms gain entrance to the uterus through the cervix, invade the cervical portion of the placenta and spread to the allantoic and amniotic cavities and the fetus. They are often found in the stomach or lungs of the fetus as a result of its swallowing or inhaling infected amniotic fluid. Some of these bacterial organisms, such as salmonella and leptospira, can enter the uterus from the blood stream and pass to the fetus through the placenta. Most of these organisms cause abortion during the last trimester of gestation or are present in the liveborn foal at parturition.

Streptococcus zooepidemicus, a betahemolytic streptococcus, is the most common bacterial cause of abortion at any stage of gestation. This organism is commonly found on the external genital organs of mares and stallions. It may be recovered by culture of the genital tract from more than 90 per cent of foaling mares for several days after parturition and is the most common organism associated with vaginitis, cervicitis and metritis secondary to pneumovagina. These "strep" abortions occur most commonly on poorly managed farms where proper breeding hygiene, including prebreeding examination and culture of mares, and proper washing of the external genitalia of the mare and stallion before and after breeding are not followed. In addition, such abortions are common on farms where frequent services at "foal" heat, excessive frequent breeding of older mares, unjustified vulvar suturing of mares and unsanitary foaling procedures occur.

The normal, healthy genital tract in mares not prone to infection is quite resistant to small numbers of *S. zooepidemicus* or other organisms introduced at parturition or breeding. Abortions due to this organism are sporadic because infection is limited to the genital tract and is not spread by ingestion or other means. The organism is usually readily recovered from the infected fetus, infected fetal membranes and genital discharges after abortion. Infected mares may require local antibiotic therapy of the genital tract, preferably at estrus; vulvar suturing, if the mare has pneumovagina; limited services performed in a careful, hygienic manner or artificial insemination with semen treated with antibiotics and possible douching of the uterus with antibiotics 12 to 24 hours after service. Older, chronically infected mares can be a serious problem and require a guarded prognosis.

Salmonella abortus equi as a cause of contagious equine abortion was first described in the United States in the late nineteenth century and was a common cause of outbreaks of abortion in Kentucky in the early twentieth century. Abortions due to this agent have been reported in many states, as well as worldwide. Except for two small, isolated outbreaks, salmonella abortion in mares has not been reported in the United States since 1932. The reason for the near disappearance of this previously common disease is not known.

The salmonella organism is spread by ingestion of feed and water contaminated by fecal or genital wastes. The incubation period is 10 to 28 days, and the incidence of abortion in a group of infected mares may reach 50 to 90 per cent. The fetus is usually autolyzed, and the placenta is edematous, necrotic and hemorrhagic. The organism can readily be recovered by culture, and the agglutination test performed on the mare's serum will demonstrate antibodies with a titer of 1:500 to 1:5000. The use of bacterins as a prophylactic measure has been highly effective in the past in preventing outbreaks of salmonella abortions.

Leptospira pomona and other leptospirae have occasionally been reported as a cause of abortion in mares. Abortions may occur without any history of prior disease but often occur 1 to 3 weeks after a mild illness that is characterized by moderately elevated body temperature, anorexia, slight depression and icterus. Usually the fetus shows autolysis, and demonstration of the leptospiral agent is unsuccessful by culture, staining or fluorescent antibody techniques; however, the aborting mare will frequently show a rising antibody titer.

The other bacterial agents usually cause only sporadic abortions and are associated with conditions and disease factors similar to those associated with *S. zooepidemicus*. Preventive measures and appropriate local treatment of the genital tract with antibiotics are indicated.

Viruses

Viral causes of equine abortion include rhinopneumonitis or equine herpesvirus 1, equine arteritis virus and equine infectious anemia.

Equine herpevirus 1 (rhinopneumonitis virus) is widespread in the United States, Canada, Japan and European countries. It commonly affects foals in the fall of the year at weaning time and produces a mild, febrile (102 to 104°F or 38.8 to 40.0°C) respiratory disease with coughing, nasal discharge ("snots") inappetence and depression. Occasionally ataxia, paresis, prostration and death may occur in young or older horses when the virus invades the central nervous system. The incubation period of the respiratory disease is 2 to 3 days in foals. The signs of the disease may linger in foals for 2 to 6 weeks. Spread of the disease is mainly by inhalation or droplet infection or occasionally by ingestion. The disease is highly contagious and infectious, and animals may experience several attacks at 6-month to 2-year intervals. The respiratory disease in older horses that have previously been infected is very mild, with few or no clinical signs. The incubation period for abortion in natural cases averages 20 to 30 days, but it may extend up to 90 days. This long incubation period may be due to the persistence of the virus in the leukocytes of the mare and in the chorion of the placenta before it finally invades the susceptible fetus, causing its death and expulsion.

Fetal death and abortion due to this virus rarely occur before the fifth month of gestation, and 90 per cent of cases occur from 8 months to term. Infected foals may be born at term but die within 2 to 9 hours of birth. The incidence of abortion in a group of mares varies from 1 to 90 per cent, depending on factors such as the degree of immunity, virulence of the virus, numbers of mares in advanced pregnancy and so forth. Abortions may occur over a period of 2 weeks to 3 months, with 90 per cent of abortions occurring within 60 days. Fetuses usually die and are expelled promptly in a fresh state. Some infected fetuses show no significant lesions, but many have edema and petechial hemor-

rhages in the lung or small whitish-yellow foci of necrosis in the liver. Intranuclear inclusion bodies are frequently found in the bronchial epithelium and the liver cells. Virus abortion due to equine herpesvirus 1 is probably the most common single cause of abortions in the last trimester of pregnancy. Permanent immunity, as with other herpesviruses, does not occur, and carriers of the virus are common. The prophylactic use of vaccine is discussed elsewhere.

Equine arteritis virus will produce rare outbreaks of a severe general systemic and respiratory disease, with abortion as a complication. This virus was found to cause abortion about 15 to 20 years ago soon after the occurrence of severe "shipping–fever-like" disease outbreaks, which were characterized by elevation of body temperature (103 to 106°F or 39.4 to 41.1°C), conjunctivitis, lacrimation, photophobia, palpebral edema (pink eye), severe depression, rapid respirations, weakness, stiffness, anorexia, rapid loss of weight and sometimes edema of the lungs and abdomen. Deaths occasionally occurred in old or young horses. The course of the disease was 2 to 15 days, with abortion usually occurring 1 to 14 days after the onset of illness. The incidence of abortion ranged from 1 to 50 per cent. Most abortions occurred between 5 and 10 months of gestation, and as they did not occur promptly after fetal death, the fetuses underwent autolytic changes prior to expulsion. No inclusion bodies were present, but the virus could be recovered from fetal tissues such as the liver and lung. Recovered horses had a prolonged immunity to reinfection. Although an effective vaccine has been developed, it has not been commercially produced, probably because the incidence of the disease is so low.

Equine infectious anemia in pregnant mares is occasionally characterized by early fetal death or abortion. Abortion may be due to the virus invading the fetus during the last half of pregnancy, or it may be associated with the stress produced in the mare by an acute febrile episode of the disease. Further study is needed to elucidate the mechanism of abortion in equine infectious anemia.

Fungi

Mycotic or fungal causes of equine abortion include *Aspergillus fumigatus, Mucor* spp. and *Allescheria boydii;* the first-named being by far the most common. Mycotic abortions in mares, like abortions from miscellaneous bacterial causes, are sporadic. The fungus probably invades the fetus through the cervix and placenta or possibly through the blood stream directly to the placenta. In most mycotic abortions the placenta, especially the chorioallantois, is extensively and diffusely involved. Mycosis may be responsible for 5 to 30 per cent of all infectious abortions. Most mycotic abortions occur late in gestation after the placenta has been infected for many weeks. Fetuses are usually small because of growth retardation due to chronic placental disease. Some of these infected fetuses may be expelled alive. Infection, especially with *Mucor* spp., may cause a mycotic pneumonia in the fetus. Skin lesions rarely occur. The causal organism may readily be cultured from the placenta and occasionally from the fetal organs. The chorioallantois is usually extensively diseased, edematous, thickened and necrotic.

Protozoal Causes

Protozoal causes of equine abortion include *Trypanosoma equiperdum* and *Babesia equi* or *B. caballi,* which cause dourine and piroplasmosis, respectively. Abortion due to these agents is rare in horses. It is not certain whether the fetus and placenta are invaded by *T. equiperdum.* If invasion does not occur, abortion is probably due to the stress produced by the disease in the mare. Dourine is present only in tropical countries and has been eradicated from North America. It is transmitted primarily by sexual contact.

Babesiasis or piroplasmosis may result in abortion in severely affected mares, possibly because of the stress produced by the disease. Signs of the acute disease resemble those of equine infectious anemia, except that icterus and hemoglobinuria may also be present. Presently this disease is largely limited to the state of Florida in the United States but is endemic in many tropical countries. The fluorescent antibody technique is applied to red blood cells from infected fetuses, foals or dams to demonstrate the parasite. This, together with the complement fixation test, is highly efficient for diagnosing babesiasis and for differentiating it from equine infectious anemia, leptospirosis, equine herpesvirus 1 and neonatal isoerythrolysis. Therapy for mares affected with piroplasmosis is available and is generally effective.

NONINFECTIOUS CAUSES OF EQUINE ABORTION

These may include drugs or chemicals, hormones, chromosomal abnormalities and physical causes.

Chemicals, Drugs and Poisonous Plants

Phenothiazines and thiabendazole; purgatives such as arecoline and aloes; sudan grass or sorghum pastures; sodium iodide; organophosphate anthelmintics; ergot and others have occasionally been reported as causing equine abortions. However, the evidence or scientific basis for incriminating these chemicals, drugs or agents as causes of abortion has not been adequately proved.

Hormones

Hormonal causes of equine abortion have included estrogens, glucocorticoids, oxytocin, prostaglandins and possibly a progesterone deficiency.

Estrogens in large doses induce abortion or parturition in cows and ewes. There is some reported evidence that large, repeated doses of estrogen may cause abortion in ponies. Further studies are needed to prove that estrogen can be abortifacient in the mare.

Glucocorticoids, such as dexamethasone, at doses of 100 mg/day for 4 days given during the tenth month of gestation will hasten or induce parturition. The author's experience, and that of others working with pregnant mares, has shown that the stresses of transport, close housing after pasture, sudden reduction and changes in feed and water intake, debilitating conditions or diseases, and other stresses, especially from 3 to 5 months of gestation when progesterone levels from the corpora lutea are declining, will cause abortions. Mitchell[3] reported that about 50 per cent of pregnant yearling mares aborted between 30 and 160 days of gestation, probably because of stress factors. Certain mares are definitely more easily stressed than others. Mares that conceive promptly but have a history of abortion should be managed so as to avoid stress throughout gestation, especially after 60 days.

Oxytocin, 20 to 100 IU intramuscularly, is highly effective for inducing parturition in mares in an average of 50 to 60 minutes during late gestation, near term, or during moderately prolonged gestations (see following article).

Prostaglandins in single or multiple doses, 2.5 mg of prostaglandin-$F_{2\alpha}$ ($PGF_{2\alpha}$) every 12 hours, will cause abortion in pony mares between 80 and 300 days of gestation. An average of 3.7 injections were given with a mean interval from first injection to abortion of 38.6 hours.[3]

Progesterone deficiency has been incriminated as a cause of abortion in mares and other animals. Ganjam and co-workers[3] have shown that the half-life of progesterone in the mare is extremely short. Giving 150 to 300 mg of progesterone daily maintains normal blood levels (6 to 8 ng/ml) of this hormone in ovariectomized mares or those in deep anestrus. Therapy consisting of 500 mg of repositol progesterone every 6, 10 or 30 days is presently being used as an aid in preventing equine abortion supposedly caused by progesterone deficiency. However, this is obviously a very low dose in light of the report just cited. Thus, further doubt is cast on whether abortion in mares can result from a simple progesterone deficiency.

Chromosomal Abnormalities

Chromosomal anomalies are probably seldom a cause of abortion from 3 months to term. However, as mentioned earlier, death of the fertilized ovum or early embryo or fetus, especially before 90 days, might be caused by chromosomal anomalies, as has been reported in other mammalian species.

Physical Causes

Physical causes are probably seldom responsible for abortions in mares (other than those abortions deliberately performed by man). These causes include abnormalities of the umbilical cord, trauma or severe injury to the mare or to the embryonic vesicle, natural service during pregnancy and manual dilatation and douching of the pregnant uterus.

Abnormalities of the umbilical cord that are potentially lethal to the fetus are caused by excessive length of the cord and result in:

1. Strangulation of the amniotic portion of the cord around portions of the fetus, resulting in deep grooves and local edema in the head, neck, legs, back and thorax.

2. Excessive torsion of the amniotic part of

the cord with urachal obstruction and vascular occlusion. Urachal obstruction can cause excessive distention of the fetal bladder and rupture of the bladder prior to or during birth or can even cause dystocia. Rupture of the urachus with urine passing into the amniotic cavity has also been described by Whitwell.[3] Vascular occlusion of the umbilical cord is the major cause of death and abortion of an autolyzed fetus. In these cases the amniotic portion of the umbilical cord is markedly twisted and is associated with hematomas, aneurysms, thromboses, ecchymoses and edema. Usually, a distended bladder and a dilated urachus are also present. Torsion or strangulation of the umbilical cord is responsible for about 1 per cent of fetal deaths and abortions and occurs most commonly between 5½ and 7½ months of gestation.

3. Whitwell[3] described 11 abortions in conjunction with long umbilical cords associated with ischemic necrosis of the cervical pole of the chorioallantois that was distinct from infective cervical placentitis.

Trauma or injury resulting in severe stress to a pregnant mare, such as prolonged, difficult transport; hard, sustained work; difficult, long surgical operations and vigorous struggling and trauma in a "cast" mare may cause abortion. This is probably due to stress and the production of glucocorticoids that initiate abortion, as previously described. Rough, traumatic manipulation of the embryonic vesicle during manual pregnancy diagnosis, especially from 16 to 40 days of gestation, should be avoided. Evidence would indicate that this could cause the death of the early embryo in horses as well as in cattle. Conversely, if this examination is done gently and skillfully by a highly experienced diagnostician, apparently few deaths are produced.

Natural service during the first 3 months of gestation occurs occasionally, possibly due to the increased estrogen levels associated with follicular ovarian activity during this period. Abortions following natural matings during pregnancy are rare because of the constricted cervix.

Manual dilatation of the cervix and the introduction of several hundred milliliters of physiological saline, dilute Lugol's solution or iodized oil in a clean, sanitary manner readily produces abortion within 3 to 10 days in most mares. A second treatment may occasionally be necessary. Aborting mares after 3 or 4 months of gestation is usually not recommended because complications may arise as a result of the large size of the fetus.

Induction of abortion or prevention of conception is occasionally performed when mismating has occurred or when an owner has purchased a pregnant mare with an undesired pregnancy or has decided after breeding a mare to terminate the pregnancy. If the mismated mare is still in estrus or was bred only 12 to 72 hours previously, a large, single injection of 100 to 200 mg of repositol diethylstilbestrol or several injections of 10 to 20 mg of estradiol given every 36 to 48 hours would probably prevent pregnancy, much as such therapy does in other domestic animals. If the bred mare fails to show heat signs at the next expected estrous period or if she is diagnosed pregnant then or at a subsequent examination, she may be given an intrauterine douche, as just described, or one or multiple injections of prostaglandin-$F_{2\alpha}$ or a suitable prostaglandin analog, 2.5 to 5.0 mg at 12-hour intervals, to cause abortion.[3] Insufficient information is presently available to recommend the use of large dosages of estrogens or glucocorticoids, or both, to produce abortion.

MISCELLANEOUS DISEASES AND ACCIDENTS OF THE EQUINE GESTATION PERIOD

Fetal Mummification

Fetal death in horses occurring from the third to tenth month of gestation that does not result in abortion or maceration is followed by autolytic changes in the fetus and placenta, absorption of the placental and fetal fluids and mummification of the fetus. In the horse, fetal mummification is uncommon and has only been reported as occurring in one of twin fetuses that has died during pregnancy, possibly because of placental insufficiency. In twin equine fetuses the smaller twin usually dies and both twins are aborted, but if one twin mummifies and remains in the uterus for several months, it and its fetal membranes will be expelled with the viable fetus when the latter is aborted or delivered at term. The great discrepancy in size between the mummified fetus and the viable twin may lead to an erroneous diagnosis of superfetation. The

mummified fetus and its membranes may not be observed because of its small size. Single mummified fetuses have never been reported in the mare.

Fetal Maceration

Maceration of the equine fetus is rare but may occur at any stage of gestation from 2 months to term. Fetal death may be due to any of the various causes of abortion, but if the cervix fails to dilate sufficiently and the fetus remains in the uterus, autolysis proceeds to emphysema and maceration, metritis and pyometra and in some cases to a fetid vulvar discharge. The diagnosis of fetal maceration can usually be determined from the breeding history and an evaluation, following vaginal and rectal examination, of the uterus and its contents. The cervix of the mare should be gently dilated manually with frequent lubrication and the fetus and placental remnants carefully removed. In rare cases fetal emphysema and maceration in late gestation may require a partial fetotomy or even a cesarean operation if the cervix cannot be well dilated. The uterus and cervix should then be treated as for metritis and cervicitis with broad-spectrum antibiotics in an oily base. Aftercare may also require systemic antibiotic therapy and treatment to prevent acute laminitis.

Hydrops Amnii and Hydrops Allantois, Edema of the Chorioallantois and Fetal Dropsy

These conditions are extremely rare in the equine species. Hydrops amnii has not been reported in mares. The author has observed mild-to-moderate cases of edema of the chorioallantois, no cases of fetal anasarca or dropsy or excessive fetal ascites and only one case of hydrops allantois. In the latter case rupture of the prepubic tendon and shock resulted in the mare's death.

Extensive Unilateral Ventral Hernias

Extensive unilateral ventral hernias occurring in mares during late gestation are rare. These may be associated with excessive uterine weight in cases of twinning or of hydrops allantois. Affected mares may be treated in a manner similar to that for rupture of the prepubic tendon (see following paragraph) and should be given prompt assistance at foaling to avoid the delivery of a dead foal because of the inability of the abdominal muscles to assist adequately in its expulsion. Repair of these extensive hernias is impossible, and the breeding life of the mare is usually terminated.

Rupture of the Prepubic Tendon

Rupture of the prepubic tendon (prepubic desmorrhexis) is a rare occurrence in light mares in advanced pregnancy but is more common in draft mares. Usually this condition is preceded by an area of marked, tense, painful edema, 4 to 6 inches thick on the abdominal wall, extending from the udder to the xiphoid region. Affected mares move very slowly and cautiously and refuse to lie down. In a few cases rupture of the prepubic tendon may occur suddenly because of trauma or violence without the usual development of severe edema. When rupture does occur, it is associated with severe distress, pain, sweating, rapid respiration, a fast, weak pulse and possible internal hemorrhage and shock. Collapse and death usually follow within a few minutes or hours. Even in the few animals that survive, the mare's usefulness is so severely limited that she is usually humanely destroyed. Mares that develop a severe ventral edema and a stiff, cautious gait indicative of a possible impending rupture of the prepubic tendon should be confined and have exercise limited; large, bulky feeds avoided and a light, laxative concentrate ration fed. A wide, heavy canvas girdle, with straps that can be tightened, should be placed around the mare's abdomen for support. Heavy padding should be placed over the spine to prevent pressure necrosis. Affected mares should be watched closely for the initiation of parturition so that assistance can be given promptly, since abdominal contractions are weak. Induction of parturition with oxytocin should be seriously considered.

Extrauterine Pregnancy

True extrauterine pregnancy in the mare in which the embryo or conceptus establishes nutritive relationships with tissues other than the endometrium has never been described. False or secondary uterine pregnancy in which the fetus develops normally but escapes into the abdominal cavity through a uterine wall rupture, usually late in gestation, is very rare and generally follows trauma or violence to the mare. The fetus dies promptly, often followed by the death of the dam due to abdominal complications. In the mare the uncommon rotated or compound bicornual pregnancy may be mistaken for an extrauterine fetus because the birth canal is very long and the fetus, which is located in both uterine horns, may be palpated beneath the stretched vagina and uterine body.

Torsion of the Uterus

Torsion of the uterus occurs in the later stages of gestation, possibly associated with the mare's rolling or falling or with excessive activity of the fetus. As in the cow, uterine torsion may not occur or be detected until dystocia results at the time of parturition. This condition is rare in the mare because of the dorsally attached broad ligaments, and many cases are limited to about a 180° twist. Signs of uterine torsion are restlessness, anorexia, abdominal pain or colic and frequent attempts at urination. These prolonged signs resemble those seen in the early stages of parturition, and when these are observed in advanced pregnancy, the anterior vagina should be examined for the twisting or folding of the wall indicative of torsion. A rectal examination should be performed to determine the direction of the torsion and the degree of tension on the broad ligaments. If the condition is diagnosed early and fetal death and rupture of a large blood vessel have not occurred, the prognosis is usually guarded to favorable. The torsion may be relieved by sedating or anesthetizing the mare and rolling her rapidly by means of ropes in the direction of the torsion or by using Schaffer's method that utilizes a plank placed on the abdomen to hold the fetus in place while the mare is slowly rolled in the direction of the torsion.[2] If these conservative methods fail, a laparotomy through the left flank of the standing or recumbent mare may be performed and the torsion corrected manually.

Hemorrhage of Pregnancy

Occasionally, violence or trauma, especially to an older mare in late gestation, may cause rupture of a large uterine blood vessel that results in fatal intra-abdominal hemorrhage or a large hematoma in the broad ligament. Signs of excessive hemorrhage include markedly increased respiration and heart rate, weakness, staggering, sweating, pale mucous membranes and the rapid onset of prostration, shock and death. Treatment with large quantities of blood or blood substitutes is indicated in severe cases, but this is difficult to implement within a short period.

Older mares in advanced pregnancy may rarely show occasional, slight, recurrent bleeding from the vulva. This is of concern to the owner but usually is not serious and often does not require treatment. This bleeding does not usually come from the uterine cavity but from a ruptured "varicose" or surface vein in the vaginal or hymenal region. Such lesions usually heal spontaneously after foaling, but ligation or cautery of the lesion may be indicated. Rarely, bleeding from the vulva may be due to a traumatic lesion of the vulva, hymen or vagina or to a tumor involving those structures.

REFERENCES

1. Arthur, G. H.: Veterinary Reproduction and Obstetrics. 4th Ed., London, Baillière and Tindall, 1975.
2. Roberts, S. J.: Veterinary Obstetrics and Genital Diseases. 2nd Ed. Ann Arbor, Mich., Edward Bros. Inc., 1971.
3. Rowlands, T. W., Allen, W. R. and Rossdale, P. D.: (Eds.): Equine Reproduction Proceedings of the 1st International Symposium on Equine Reproduction, Cambridge, England. London, Blackwell Scientific Publ., 1975.
4. Zemjanis, R.: Diagnostic and Therapeutic Techniques in Animal Reproduction. Baltimore, The Williams and Wilkins Co., 1962.

Induction of Parturition in the Mare

ROBERT B. HILLMAN

New York State College of Veterinary Medicine, Ithaca, New York

Elective induction of parturition has been employed for several years to insure the presence of professional assistance at the time of foaling. This technique allows a veterinarian to schedule the foaling for a time and place that are convenient for him and at the same time placates the overanxious owner.

INDICATIONS

Some of the indications for the elective induction of parturition in the mare include:

1. Delayed parturition due to uterine atony, as seen in the mare that has gone to term and appears ready to foal in every way but does not complete the act. Her udder is full of colostrum, the vulva and sacrosciatic ligaments are relaxed and, on vaginal examination, her cervix is open two to three fingers, but she doesn't foal.

2. Prolonged gestation with a pregnancy of more than 365 days duration and a foal that is getting so large that there is danger of injury to the mare or foal, or both, at parturition.

3. Leakage of colostrum.

4. Prevention of injury at foaling in mares that have suffered damage at previous foalings.

5. Impending rupture of the prepubic tendon due to excessive ventral edema or hydrops of the amnion, or both.

6. As a research technique to obtain colostrum-deprived foals.

7. As a teaching device to allow scheduling of foalings, so that a large group of students can be present to observe the foaling and the techniques employed in caring for the mare and newborn foal.

MARE SELECTION

The criteria employed to determine whether a mare is ready for induction include:

1. Length of gestation. While successful inductions have been accomplished as early as 320 days, it is best to wait at least 330 days to insure complete maturation of the fetus.

2. Udder enlargement with the presence of colostrum.

3. Relaxation of the perineal region. The vulva and the sacrosciatic ligaments should be relaxed.

4. Cervical relaxation. The cervix should be softening and allow the easy insertion of one or two fingers. If the cervix is very tight and sticky, the mare should be treated with 15 mg of diethylstilbestrol 12 hours prior to starting induction. If all other parameters are ready, the cervix will usually be soft and will dilate without treatment with estrogen.

MARE PREPARATION

1. Wrap the tail with a clean bandage.
2. Wash the perineum and udder.
3. Place the mare in a clean, well-bedded boxstall.

TREATMENT

Inject 40 to 60 IU of oxytocin intramuscularly. The degree of uneasiness, restlessness and colic shown by the mare is directly proportional to the dose of oxytocin, so high doses are avoided to eliminate severe colicky behavior. A dose of 40 to 60 IU will result in the foal's being on the ground in less than an hour in nearly every case. Therefore, higher doses are not warranted.

SIGNS

Approximately 15 to 20 minutes after the injection of oxytocin, the mare will start to sweat along the neck in front of the shoulders. About the same time, the mare will begin to pass small amounts of fecal material at frequent intervals. At 20 to 25 minutes, she will appear restless and will start circling the stall and switching her tail. Straining begins at about 25 to 30 minutes after injection, and occasionally mares given this dose of oxytocin will show a mild form of rolling at about 35 minutes. The fetal membranes should appear at the lips of the vulva at 35 to 40 minutes, and usually by 45 to 50 minutes the foaling is completed. In most instances, the placenta is passed without difficulty within a half hour of foaling when foaling is induced by using 40 to 60 IU of oxytocin.

CARE OF MARE AND FOAL

As soon as the foal's head clears the vulva, quietly break the membranes and clear the air passages. Don't disturb the mare or break the navel cord for at least 10 minutes. Once the mare gets up and breaks the cord, dip the foal's navel in iodine. Milk out 10 or more ounces of colostrum, pass a stomach tube and feed the foal to insure an adequate early supply of colostrum. Give the foal an enema to remove any firm meconium balls. If the mare has not had a tetanus toxoid booster prior to foaling, administer tetanus antitoxin to the foal. The placenta should be carefully examined for completeness and pathological lesions.

Complications

1. Premature placental separation. Occasionally, the first membrane to appear at the vulva is the dark red chorioallantois with its cervical star. This membrane should be opened to allow the amnion with the enclosed foal to be expelled first. If this is not done, the chorioallantois will separate from the uterus prematurely and the foal may be anoxic at birth.

2. Dystocia. In rare instances, the fetal membranes will not appear at the lips of the vulva at 35 to 40 minutes after the injection of oxytocin. A clean, careful vaginal examination should be done at this time to determine the position of the foal. A malpresentation is very easy to correct at this time but if left for several hours, the uterus contracts around the foal and this, combined with the forceful straining of the mare, makes the necessary corrections more difficult.

ALTERNATIVE METHODS OF INDUCTION

1. Dexamethasone. Dexamethasone administered at normal therapeutic doses will not induce parturition in pregnant mares. Parturition can be induced by daily administration of 100 mg of dexamethasone for 4 consecutive days. Foaling occurs 4 days ± 1.6 days after the last dexamethasone injection. Live, healthy foals were obtained when induction was started from 321 to 324 days of gestation.

2. Prostaglandin-$F_{2\alpha}$ has been used to induce parturition in mares near to term, but

the results have been very variable and no consistently effective dose has been found. In some trials, treatment has been associated with a very high incidence of fetal and foal death.

3. Fluprostenol. Fluprostenol (Equimate) is a synthetic prostaglandin analog. This drug has been used to successfully induce parturition in ponies (250-μg dose) and Thoroughbred mares (1000-μg dose) at from 322 to 367 days of gestation. Nine mares were used in one study, and all had viable foals within 4 hours of the first injection, although two of the foals suffered fractured ribs during foaling. The authors state it is not necessary to have colostrum in the udder or cervical relaxation prior to using fluprostenol for inducing parturition.

REFERENCES

1. Alm, C., Sullivan, J. J. and First, N. L.: Induction of premature parturition by parenteral administration of dexamethasone in the mare. J.A.V.M.A. *165*:721, 1974.
2. Alm, C., Sullivan, J. J. and First, N. L.: The effect of a corticosteroid (dexamethasone), progesterone, oestrogen and prostaglandin $F_{2\alpha}$ on gestation length in normal and ovariectomized mares. J. Reprod. Fertil. (Suppl.), *23*:637, 1975.
3. Burns, S. J.: Clinical safety of dexamethasone in mares during pregnancy. Eq. Vet. J., *5*:91, 1973.
4. Hillman, R. B.: Induction of parturition in mares. J. Reprod. Fertil. (Suppl.), *23*:641, 1975.
5. Rossdale, P. D., and Jeffcott, L. B.: Problems encountered during induced foaling in pony mares. Vet. Rec., *97*:371, 1975.
6. Rossdale, P. D., Jeffcott, L. B. and Allen, W. R.: Foaling induced by a synthetic prostaglandin analogue (fluprostenol). Vet. Rec., *99*:26, 1976.

Neonatal Problems in the Horse

PETER D. ROSSDALE

Beaufort Cottage Stables, New Market, England

INTRODUCTION

The neonatal period presents the clinician with special problems of diagnosis and therapy because it covers the transition between intra- and extrauterine existence. Physiologically, this entails a variety of adaptive responses by the newborn animal, the most immediate of which involve the pulmonary and cardiovascular systems. Clinically there are developing patterns of behavior and alterations in physical signs and levels of homeostasis. It is necessary, therefore, for the clinician to interpret the baselines of normality that reflect the adaptive processes, so that abnormal states may be recognized and interpreted. But investigatory medicine is constrained by certain limitations peculiar to the newborn period, namely:

1. The history of the individual, as far as it relates to intrauterine happenings, cannot be subjected to direct observation.

2. The physical and chemical hazards of birth impose extrinsic and indeterminate factors with effects that can be judged only in their extremity.

3. The response of the newborn mammal to any given stimulus is conditioned by the inherent needs of fetal life and may, therefore, be weaker and less effective than would normally be the case.

The newborn animal should not be regarded as a small edition of the adult but must be approached as a distinct entity in physiological and clinical terms. This peculiar status requires a working definition by which the clinician, research worker and teacher may communicate, with mutual recognition of the inter-related factors ranging over the spectrum of the disciplines of which veterinary medicine is composed.

Terminology

Neonatal period (birth to 4 days). During this period the major physiological behavioral responses are accomplished, and the signs of maladjustment and of conditions related to intrauterine existence and parturient events first appear.

Previable Period. Delivery prior to the 300th day of gestation. A foal is unlikely, even when intensive care and assistance are given, to survive for any length of time if delivered before the 300th day of gestation. Delivery before this time is therefore conveniently described as an *abortion*.

Prematurity. A foal born between 300 and 320 days of gestation. Signs include undersize and weakness, as evidenced by taking longer than normal (2 hours) to stand for the first time following birth, and having difficulty in holding the sucking position.

Dysmaturity. A dysmature foal is one that shows premature-like signs but is delivered at a gestational age of greater than 320 days.[13]

Perinatal Period. There is some difficulty in arriving at a satisfactory definition of the perinatal period. Bergin[2] described it as extending from day 30 of gestation until day 30 after birth, and Platt[7] defined it as from day 299 of gestation until day 56 after birth. Platt's definition is preferable from a clinical viewpoint because the period starts at the limit of viability. However, there is less reason to place the end of the period at day 56 postpartum, and it would be better to determine the period as day 300 of gestation until the end of the fourth day postpartum.

The purpose of clearly defined terminology is not only to facilitate communication among scientific workers but to enable data to be accumulated in such a way that useful comparisons may be made between differing geographical managerial systems on a current and historic basis. This is particularly necessary in collating information obtained in surveys. For example, Platt[7] calculated neonatal mortality as 41.1 per cent from the number of deaths occurring in the first week postpartum, but in a similar survey Merkt and Von Lepel[5] obtained a loss of 5 per cent in the first 4 weeks postpartum, whereas Rossdale and Leadon[14] reported a mortality rate of 3.6 per cent in newborns that showed signs in the first week, irrespective of the age at which death occurred.

Influences of Gestation and Birth on the Clinical Status of the Newborn Foal

The clinician, no less than the trained or untrained observer of mammalian birth, is acutely aware of the vulnerability of each newborn life. The feeling of insecurity that attends the newborn period reflects the changing physiological status of the individual from intra- to extrauterine existence, delivered by the dramatic and somewhat "explosive" event of birth. The newborn foal's well-being depends on functions that, though poorly understood, have recently been investigated by such methods as long-term catheterization of the fetal and uterine vessels.[3] These studies have thrown light on the transfer of gases and metabolites across the equine placenta,[17] and together with studies on the ultrastructural development and anatomy of the placenta[16, 18] have helped to provide a better understanding of fetal homeostasis and of maternal and fetal endocrinology in the terminal stages of gestation.[1, 6] The role of fetal kinesis in preparing the fetus for extrauterine behavior has been investigated by Fraser and co-workers,[4] using an ultrasound probe.

The physiology of parturition as it affects the fetus and its adaptive processes is also receiving the increasing attention that this subject deserves. However, the information about normal birth is, at present, confined to reports on blood gas status[8, 9, 11, 12] and blood pressure measurements in the jugular vein and carotid artery,[15] involving a protocol of study whereby the fetus was investigated during second-stage delivery. As yet there has been no report of investigations using a protocol of sequential measurements throughout first- and second-stage birth.

The effect of parturition on the fetus may vary within physiological limits related to its duration and the ease with which the fetus is propelled through the birth canal. But even within these limits the fetus is subjected to stress, as is evidenced by partial pressures of oxygen and carbon dioxide that are lower and higher, respectively, and an increased acidosis in the parturient and newly delivered period compared with values existing *in utero*.

Thus the newborn foal starts its extrauterine existence in a condition that is directly influenced by gestational and parturient events, but usually it is only when the newborn status is abnormal that the clinician becomes concerned with the phenomena of adaptation. In this situation it is necessary to be able to interpret the findings of clinical and laboratory examinations in light of the changing patterns of the period.

THE NORMAL NEONATAL FOAL: A CLINICAL APPRAISAL

The clinician requires chronologically defined criteria to interpret the changing physiological status during the neonatal period. These criteria may be selected according to the clinician's personal preference and experience, but there are certain landmarks of clinical examination that the author has found helpful and that are presented in Tables 1 to 8.

NEONATAL DISEASE

Classification

No classification of neonatal disease can be definitive because, in many cases, conditions have a multifactorial origin. For example, infection of the placenta may lead to prematurity or neonatal maladjustment, or both. Birth trauma may lead to fractured ribs that become a focus for bacterial infection and subsequent "joint ill."

Infective Conditions

Group I. Conditions characterized by fever, lethargy and reduced strength of suck. The primary sites of infection include the liver, kidney, brain, lungs, alimentary tract and synovial surfaces. Synonyms are sleepy foal disease, joint ill, diarrhea and septicemia. Causal agents include *Escherichia coli,* streptococci, staphylococci, *Actinobacillus equuli* and equine herpesvirus 1 (EVH 1).

Noninfective Conditions

Group II. Conditions characterized by gross disturbances in behavior and subdivided as follows:

1. Neonatal maladjustment syndrome (NMS) distinguished by convulsions and complete loss of suck reflex. Respiratory distress may be a feature. Synonyms are "barkers," "convulsives" and "dummies," and causal factors include asphyxia, birth trauma and other forms of fetal stress.

2. Prematurity and dysmaturity (previously discussed).

3. Meconium colic, evidenced by signs of straining, rolling and lying in awkward positions.

Group III. Developmental abnormalities that include hypo- and hyperflexion of the limbs, cleft palate, hare lip, parrot jaw, microphthalmia, umbilical urachal fistula, hernia and patent bladder.

Group IV. Immunological conditions of incompatibility between maternal and fetal tissues, e.g., hemolytic jaundice.

Differential Diagnosis

The age at which signs first appear (Table 1) provides a useful basis for differential diagnosis. Further judgment de-

TABLE 1. *Incidence of Appearance of First Signs of Equine Neonatal Disorders*

	Age (in hours)				
	0–12	12–24	24–28	48–72	72–96
Group I:					
Septicemic conditions	+†	++	+++	+++	+++
Group II:					
Neonatal maladjustment syndrome (NMS)	+++	++	+	+	
"Prematurity," "dysmaturity"	+++				
Meconium colic	+	+++	+++	+	+
Group III:					
Patent bladder				+++	++
Congenital defects	+++	+ (palate)			
Group IV:					
Hemolytic disease			+	+++	++

*From Rossdale, P. D.: Vet. Rec., *91*:581, 1972.
†Indicates maximum (+++) to minimum (+) incidence.

TABLE 2. *Normal Neonatal Findings in the Foal*

Age	Behavior	Temperature	Pulse Rate	Auscultative Findings	Respiratory Function	Excretory Function
0–1 min	At the moment of full delivery the foal is lying on its side with the hind legs to the level of the hocks remaining in the mare's vagina. The first movements are usually those of raising the head, arching the neck and thrusting forward with the forelegs.	Mean 77.6°C; range 37.1 to 38.9°C.	Range 30–90 beats/min; mean 68.8 ± 2.03 beats/min.		A respiratory rhythm is normally established with an initial predominance of the abdominal component followed by thoracic movements and thereafter by an equal contribution of both.	
1 min–2 hr	The righting reflexes appear soon after the respiratory rhythm has been established, and the foal turns onto its brisket, withdrawing its hind legs from the vagina in the process. Attempts to stand are made within the first half hour and success is achieved usually within 1 hour. The method of achieving the standing position is that of the adult, i.e., by raising the fore- and then the hindparts. Sucking movements with the tongue and lips may be present within minutes of birth, and thrusting forward of the head in the sucking position is often elicited by contact with the mare.	By 2 hrs the rectal temperature should be in the range of 37.8 to 38.3°C. Shivering occurs in the first 3 hrs postpartum.	Range 60–200 beats/min; mean 129.8 ± 6.22 beats/min.	A machinery murmur can be heard in a localized area on the left side of the chest at the level of the shoulder joint and the posterior border of the triceps muscle with the limb in the natural standing position. The murmur can be heard between age 30 min and 60 hr postpartum in most subjects.	Mean resting respiratory rate at age 3–10 min is 68.0 ± 3.9, decreasing to mean 35.1 ± 1.9 per min by age 1 hr. This rate is maintained for the remainder of the neonatal period. Tidal volume does not vary significantly, at 10 min mean values of 515.6 ± 42.9 ml have been recorded, and at age 1–48 hr, 553.2 ± 20.8 ml. Minute volume falls from 34.4 ± 2.3 to 18.7 ± 0.8 liters over the same period (Rossdale, 1969).	Meconium passed for first time at age ½ hr, and is completely voided by 2–3 days. Micturition occurs for first time at about 5 hr (colts) and 9 hrs (fillies).
2–12 hr	Thigmotaxis (udder searching) starts soon after the foal has achieved the standing position for the first time, and success at sucking is normally achieved within 1–3 hr postpartum. Patterns of following, strength of suck and the ability to get up and lie down increase with age.		Range 72–133 beats/min; mean 95.8 ± 14.8 beats/min.			

TABLE 3. *Erythrocyte Count, Hemoglobin Content, Hematocrit and Total and Differential Leukocyte Count in Jugular Venous Blood of 22 Normal Thoroughbred Foals from Birth to 96 Hours*[*]

| Age | Erythrocytes (× 10⁶/mm³) | Hemoglobin (gm/100 ml) | Hematocrit (%) | Leukocytes | | | | |
				TOTAL (/mm³)	POLYMORPHS (%)	LYMPHOCYTES (%)	MONOCYTES (%)	EOSINOPHILS (%)
Birth	10.32 ± 0.213	15.07 ± 0.238	46.7 ± 0.75	6831 ± 356	67 ± 2.34	32.5 ± 2.32	0.5	0
12 hr	9.20 ± 0.367	14.04 ± 0.567	41.7 ± 1.89	10068 ± 1022	74.4	24.2	1.4	0
24 hr	8.975 ± 0.2056	13.78 ± 0.358	40.8 ± 1.11					
36–96 hr	8.971 ± 0.3524	13.31 ± 0.20	38.7 ± 0.71		71.2	26.8	2	0

*From: Rossdale, P. D. and Ricketts, S. W.: The Practice of Equine Stud Medicine. London Baillière Tindall, 1974, p. 217.

TABLE 4. *Glucose, Cortisol, Sodium and Potassium Levels in the Jugular Venous Blood during the First 36 Hours after Birth*[*]

Age	Whole Blood Glucose (mg/100 ml)	Plasma Glucose (mg/100 ml)	Plasma Cortisol (gm/100 ml)	Serum Sodium (mEq/liter)	Serum Potassium (mEq/liter)
10 min	65 ± 2.5	95 ± 6.0	6.75 ± 0.36	—	—
1 hr	56 ± 5.5	88 ± 8.0	8.70 ± 0.63	184.4 (5 samples); range 173.9–195.6	4.38 (5 samples); range 1.4–5.7
10–12 hr	91 ± 8.7	130 ± 12.5	3.75 ± 0.53	—	—
36 hr	104 ± 5.2	133 ± 6.1	3.75 ± 1.5	—	—

*From Rossdale, P. D. and Ricketts, S. W.: The Practice of Equine Stud Medicine. London, Baillière Tindall, 1974, p. 217.

TABLE 5. *Jugular Venous Blood Protein Content Before and After Sucking for the First Time**

	Total Serum Protein (gm/100 ml)	Albumin (gm/100 ml)	Total Globulin (gm/100 ml)	α-Globulin (gm/100 ml)	β-Globulin (gm/100 ml)	γ-Globulin (gm/100 ml)
First hr before sucking	4.5	2.74 ± 0.17	1.84 ± 0.14			
	4.808 ± 0.16(12)†	3.325 ± 0.195(12)	1.483 ± 0.174(12)	0.51 ± 0.163(6)	0.523 ± 0.071(6)	0(6)
12–96 hr after sucking	6.0	2.34 ± 0.13	3.1 ± 0.26			
	4.89 ± 0.143(29)	2.824 ± 0.114(29)	2.031 ± 0.163(29)	0.659 ± 0.76(29)	0.632 ± 0.56(29)	0.81 ± 0.113(29)

*From Rossdale, P. D. and Ricketts, S. W.: The Practice of Equine Stud Medicine. London, Baillière Tindall, 1974, p. 217.
†Figures in brackets indicate number of samples.

TABLE 6. *Po_2, Pco_2, Standard Bicarbonate and Lactate Levels in Arterial and Venous Blood during the First 36 Hours after Birth**

Age	Source	Po_2 (mm Hg)	Pco_2 (mm Hg)	pH	HCO_3 (mEq/liter)	Whole Blood Lactate (mg/100 ml)
During second stage prior to delivery	Digital artery	22.6 ± 1.4	72.8 ± 2.21	7.172 ± 0.014	–	18.8 ± 2.63
0 to 60 sec, some gasping	Umbilical artery	35.4 ± 3.86	69.1 ± 3.04	7.260 ± 0.018	23.06 ± 0.86	25.5 ± 2.66
90 to 180 sec, respiration established	Umbilical artery	59.6 ± 3.24	57.6 ± 3.49	7.240 ± 0.014	–	–
12 hr	Facial and digital arteries	91.0 ± 3.3	48.4 ± 1.53	7.376 ± 0.016	27.50 ± 1.28	11.6 ± 1.11
5 min	Jugular vein	–	73.3 ± 4.29	7.277 ± 0.012	23.23 ± 0.58	29.22 ± 3.74
30 min	Jugular vein	–	72.1 ± 1.879	7.316 ± 0.019	26.90 ± 1.26	18.47 ± 2.28
1 hr	Jugular vein	–	61.4 ± 2.181	7.356 ± 0.02	26.94 ± 1.54	16.03 ± 1.47
36 hr	Jugular vein	–	57.0 ± 3.69	7.385 ± 0.0105	27.55 ± 0.914	8.160 ± 2.039
24 hr	Jugular vein	–	58.80 ± 2.29	7.392 ± 0.0065	29.30 ± 0.515	6.800 ± 0.815

*From Rossdale, P. D. and Ricketts, S. W.: The Practice of Equine Stud Medicine. London, Baillière Tindall, 1974, p. 214.

TABLE 7. *Parameters of Respiratory Function in 10 Normal Newborn Foals**

Age range (hr)	3–168
Mean ± SE† weight (kg)	32.3 ± 4.6
Mean ± SE respiration rate (per min)	30.5 ± 3.4
Mean ± SE tidal volume (ml)	429.0 ± 36.0
Mean ± SE tidal volume per kg body weight (ml/kg)	15.4 ± 0.9
Mean ± SE minute volume (1)	12.8 ± 1.8
Mean ± SE pH	7.354 ± 0.011
Mean ± SE $Paco_2$ (mm Hg) breathing air	47.5 ± 2.6
Mean ± SE Pao_2 (mm Hg)	80.1 ± 3.8
Mean ± SE Pao_2 (mm Hg) breathing oxygen	312.8 ± 37.3
Mean ± SE percentage increase in Pao_2 after breathing oxygen 3 min	310.5 ± 51.3

*From Rossdale, P. D.: Res. Vet. Sci., *11*:270, 1970.
†Standard error (SE).

pends on clinical signs (Table 2) and laboratory measurements (Tables 3 to 8).

Clinical Signs

Behavioral Disturbances

Ability to stand. Once a foal has stood for the first time, the ease with which it is subsequently able to get to its feet is a cardinal sign of its health. Difficulty in a foal that has previously been capable of standing unaided is a feature of NMS. Premature foals are weak but rapidly gain strength provided they receive adequate nursing, but foals suffering from infection progressively lose strength and become unable to get up or to stand.

Suck reflex. In Group I (infective conditions) the suck reflex gradually diminishes in strength, but it is lost suddenly in NMS. Foals suffering from meconium colic may temporarily lose the "suck reflex."

Affinity for the mare. The ability of the newborn foal to direct itself toward and locate the mammary glands of the mare is absent in NMS and reduced in cases of prematurity and Group I conditions.

Neurological signs. Spasmodic contractions (jerks or clonus), wandering and restlessness, jaw champing or chewing, sneezing, exaggerated extensor tone, motor convulsions (aimless limb movements), loss of postural tone and righting reflexes are characteristic of NMS and may be associated with cerebral hemorrhage or edema. Some foals suffering from infection and others with meconium retention may exhibit "wandering" signs.

Ophthalmological signs. Asymmetrical pupillary apertures, scleral splashing, retinal petechiae and nystagmus are indicative of cerebral hemorrhage.

Colic. Abdominal pain is commonly associated with meconium retention. Signs include frequent rolling, lying on the back, rotation of the head and lying in unusual positions. Some of these signs may be seen in patent bladder, prematurity or septicemia, especially that caused by *E. coli* and *Actinobacillus equuli.*

Rectal Temperature. The rectal temperature of foals suffering from NMS may fluctuate between 90°F (32.2°C) in coma and 105°F (40.6°C) in convulsions. Rectal

TABLE 8. *SGOT, SAP and CPK Levels in Jugular Venous Blood of 11 Normal Thoroughbred Foals between the Ages of 12 and 96 Hours**

SGOT† (IU)	SAP‡ (IU)	CPK§ (IU)
71.5 ± 4.03	566.3 ± 20.64	52.3 ± 4.25

*From Rossdale, P. D. and Ricketts, S. W.: The Practice of Equine Stud Medicine. London, Baillière Tindall, 1974, p. 216.
†Serum glutamic oxaloacetic transaminase
‡Serum alkaline phosphatase.
§Creatinine phosphokinase.

temperatures should be taken at least every 6 hours to record transient alterations. Elevated temperatures may be found in cases of septicemia, although in the terminal phase subnormal levels may be present.

Heart Rate. Bradycardia ($<$50 beats/min) immediately after birth followed by tachycardia ($>$150 beats/min) is indicative of asphyxia. Tachycardia occurs in foals suffering from convulsions, septicemia associated with high temperature and hemolytic disease following minor exertion. At rest, the heart rate during the neonatal period is normally 80 to 120 beats/min but tends to slow during coma and convalescence from NMS.

A jugular pulse in foals suffering from NMS indicates cardiac failure. Engorgement of the jugular vein may occur in Group I conditions and hemolytic disease.

Respiratory Rate. Increased respiratory rates in foals over 2 hours old may be due to (1) respiratory distress, i.e., reduced pulmonary function associated with atelectasis; (2) metabolic acidemia invoking the compensatory process of increased ventilation or (3) hyperthermia.

Differentiation of these three states requires measurement of ventilatory capacity and arterial or venous blood gas chemistry values. Tidal volume (V_T),* minute volume ($\dot{V}$)† and maximal tidal volume ($V_T$max)‡ can be measured with the aid of a Wright's respirometer attached to a latex mask.[10] A normal 50-kg foal aged 1 hour or more has a V_T of 400 to 600 ml, $\dot{V}$ of 14 to 20 liters and a $V_T$max of 900 to 1200 ml.

In respiratory distress, V_T and $V_T$max are reduced ($<$400 ml and $<$600 ml, respectively, and respiratory rates and $\dot{V}$ are increased ($>$60/min and $>$40 liters, respectively).

Expiratory sounds of "barking," grunting or high-pitched whinnying occur during convulsive episodes and are probably associated with biochemical or neurological disturbances.

Other Diagnostic Signs. The intensity of signs in Group I conditions gradually in-

creases over the course of illness, and their nature depends on the site of the infecting agent. Retraction of the eyeballs into the orbits is frequently found in cases of septicemia and diarrhea. Emaciation is seen in cases of prematurity and in dysmaturity associated with placentitis due to infection and other causes.

Patent bladder. Meconium colic must be differentiated from the much rarer condition of "ruptured" bladder. Diagnosis is based on the presence of urine in the abdomen, a sample of which should be obtained by paracentesis. The urine is distinguished from ascitic fluid by its odor, high urea content ($>$80 mg/100 ml) and absence of fibrin. Further confirmation may, if necessary, be made by introducing a dye, such as fluorescin, into the bladder and half an hour later withdrawing a sample of abdominal fluid to test for its presence.

Hemolytic disease. Clinical diagnosis of hemolytic disease rests on yellow mucous membranes, a red discoloration of urine, hemoglobin value $<$7 gm/100 ml and hematocrit $<$20 per cent, presence of "ghost" cells, bilirubin levels $>$20 mg/100 ml and an indirect van den Bergh reaction. Serological tests performed on the dam's plasma and the foal's erythrocytes complete the diagnosis.

Laboratory Measurements

Hematocrit, Hemoglobin and Erythrocytes (Fig. 1). Foals suffering from diarrhea or convulsions have increased hematocrit values ($>$44 per cent). Reduced levels ($<$35 per cent) are experienced in septicemia, inflammatory conditions of the fetal membranes and prematurity. In hemolytic disease the hematocrit level falls to $<$20 per cent.

Hemoglobin and erythrocyte counts usually follow hematocrit readings, ranging from $>$17 gm/100 ml and 9 $\times 10^6$/cu mm, respectively, in diarrhea and convulsions to $<$7 gm/100 ml and $<$4 $\times 10^6$/cu mm, respectively, in hemolytic disease.

White Blood Cell Count. A leukocytosis ($>$14,000 cells/cu mm) occurs in most septicemic conditions, although to establish a diagnosis it may be necessary to carry out serial determinations over a period of 48 hours. However, a leukopenia ($<$4,000 cells/cu mm) may be present if the infecting agent produces leukocytic substances, and low white blood cell counts are often

---

*Tidal volume (V_T) is the amount of gas passing into or out of the lungs during a respiratory movement at rest.

†Minute volume ($\dot{V}$) = V_T times respiratory rate per minute.

‡Maximal tidal volume ($V_T$max) is the amount of air employed in an inspiratory or expiratory effort when the foal has to struggle. The measurement is comparable to vital capacity in the human subject.

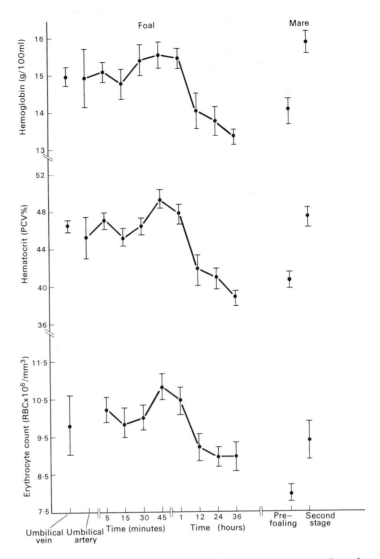

Figure 1. Hemoglobin, hematocrit and erythrocyte counts (mean ± SE) in the jugular blood of 29 newborn foals from birth to age 36 hours. (From Rossdale, P. D. and Ricketts, S. W.: The Practice of Equine Stud Medicine. London, Baillière Tindall, p. 215.)

found in premature foals and in those associated with placentitis.

Blood Glucose. Hyperglycemia (plasma levels >150 mg/100 ml) occurs during convulsions, and reduced (plasma levels <30 mg/100 ml) occur in prematurity. Hypoglycemia is usually symptomless during the neonatal period.

Blood Lactic Acid. A significant increase (>80 mg/100 ml of plasma) occurs in foals suffering from respiratory distress or convulsions.

Serum Proteins. Low levels of serum proteins occur in prematurity, and subnormal globulin levels are often present in septicemia.

Venous Blood pH. Acidemia (pH <7.10) occurs in foals that do not establish an initial respiratory rhythm and in foals suffering from convulsions. Low levels (pH <7.30) are encountered in diarrheic foals.

Arterial Blood Gas Tensions. Levels <70 mm Hg Pao_2 are a feature of NMS. Carbon dioxide tensions are raised (>70 mm Hg) in cases of respiratory distress and reduced (<30 mm Hg) in metabolic acidemia, provided pulmonary ventilation is normal.

Increments of arterial oxygen gas tensions during 100 per cent oxygen inhalation are normally 100 to 300 mm Hg, but if pulmonary ventilation is reduced by atelectasis, increments are <50 mm Hg.

Urine. Heavy deposits of protein in the urine are suggestive of nephritis, although a positive reaction may be expected in the first 36 hours of life because of the presence of low molecular weight milk proteins. Leukocytes and bacteria in smears made from centrifuged deposits or grown on culture are diagnostic of infective nephritis.

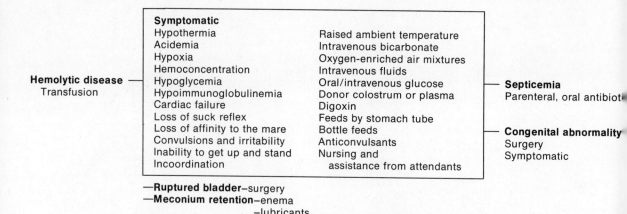

Hemolytic disease Transfusion	**Symptomatic**		Septicemia Parenteral, oral antibiot
	Hypothermia	Raised ambient temperature	
	Acidemia	Intravenous bicarbonate	
	Hypoxia	Oxygen-enriched air mixtures	
	Hemoconcentration	Intravenous fluids	
	Hypoglycemia	Oral/intravenous glucose	
	Hypoimmunoglobulinemia	Donor colostrum or plasma	Congenital abnormality
	Cardiac failure	Digoxin	Surgery
	Loss of suck reflex	Feeds by stomach tube	Symptomatic
	Loss of affinity to the mare	Bottle feeds	
	Convulsions and irritability	Anticonvulsants	
	Inability to get up and stand	Nursing and	
	Incoordination	assistance from attendants	

—**Ruptured bladder**–surgery
—**Meconium retention**–enema
　　　　　　　　–lubricants
　　　　　　　　–pain-relieving drugs

Figure 2. Summary of therapy. (From Rossdale, P. D.: Vet. Rec., *91*:581, 1972.)

Therapy

The treatment of neonatal conditions consists primarily of measures appropriate to the presenting signs. For example, if a foal cannot suck, it must be fed by artificial means; if it is hypothermic, ambient temperatures must be raised. It may be necessary to provide supportive treatment that resembles the postoperative "intensive care" situation, with the objective of stabilizing somatic function and allowing time for a rehabilitation of the adaptive process. There are, however, certain conditions in which a specific approach is required, for example, the surgical repair of patent bladder or replacement of erythrocytes in hemolytic disease.

Therapy for various neonatal conditions is outlined in Figure 2.

Group I (Infective Conditions)

Antibiotics should be administered immediately if infection is suspected because delay may make the condition less amenable to treatment. Without laboratory confirmation of the causal organism, selection of therapeutic agents is subjective. Neomycin sulfate (Biosol), ampicillin (Polyflex), cloxacillin (Orbenin, not approved for equine use in the United States) or trimethoprim-sulfadiazine (Tribrissen) may be used separately or in combination, and for broad-spectrum use chloramphenicol sodium succinate (Chloromycetin) intravenously is recommended. The total daily dosage should be subdivided into two, or preferably three, administrations and

given by parenteral or oral routes. Intra-articular administration is essential in cases of infective arthritis.

If the foal's hematocrit is less than 35 per cent, dam's plasma or whole blood should be administered intravenously after cross-matching against the foal's erythrocytes. Doses of 100 ml may be transfused by means of a syringe or transfusion apparatus at 3-hour intervals on two or three occasions. Heart and respiratory rate should be monitored during transfusion and the flow rate controlled to avoid circulatory disturbances.

Mare's blood should be collected into a sterile bottle containing 120 ml of sodium citrate per 500 ml of blood. Plasma is removed by suction after standing for 1 to 2 hours.

Ten to 20 ounces of donor colostrum should be administered within 6 hours of birth to those foals whose dams have "run milk" prior to foaling. Colostrum may be stored deep frozen in cartons for several years, and breeders should be advised to collect small quantities from mares that have ample secretions.

Group II (NMS, Prematurity, Dysmaturity, Meconium Colic)

Group II conditions, in particular, require general supportive measures.

Behavior. Incoordinated foals need constant supervision to prevent exhaustion from unavailing attempts to stand. It may be necessary for an attendant to sit with the foal and to restrain it in the recumbent position. Comatose foals should be placed on a rug to avoid bed sores, and scalding of the skin by urine may be reduced by frequent powdering of contaminated areas.

Convulsions. Convulsions and irritability can be controlled by phenytoin (Dilantin) administered intravenously (IV), intramuscularly (IM) or *per os* at the rate of 5 to 10 mg/kg of body weight, followed by maintenance doses of 1 to 5 mg/kg of body weight every 2 to 4 hours, reducing to 12-hour intervals.

Feeds. In the absence of a suck reflex, feeds should be administered through a plastic or rubber stomach tube with an outer diameter of about 1 cm and a blunt distal end. Mare's milk or reconstituted dried milk should be given at the rate of 80 ml/kg of body weight per day divided into a minimum of 10 equal feeds. Dried milk preparations should be reconstituted to provide 45 calories in 8 to 12 ml water/kg of body weight per day. For example, a 50-kg foal should receive 2250 calories in 4 to 5 liters of fluid/day. Feeds should be administered at 100°F (38°C).

Hypothermia. A normal foal maintains its body temperature against low surrounding temperatures, but those in coma or those suffering from hypoxia require special measures. Mildly affected foals may be treated by fitting a woolen pullover over the body. Severely affected foals may require surrounding temperatures of 80°F to 90°F (26.6°C to 32.2°C) before rectal temperature is restored to normal levels. Radiant heat is the most effective source of heat, although washable electric blankets or hot air blowers are useful.

Acidemia. Foals with convulsions, severe diarrhea or respiratory difficulties following birth suffer from metabolic acidemia. Five to 10 ml/kg of 5 per cent sodium bicarbonate should be administered IV through a 16GA × 1½B (blunt) hypodermic needle or a size 1 (G15) Braunula (intravenous) catheter, using a 50-ml syringe or gravity feed apparatus. Repeated administrations may be made at 2- to 3-hour intervals in the presence of continuing convulsions or diarrhea.

Hypoxia. Oxygen may be administered through a mask or by means of a rubber tube inserted into one nostril at flow rates of 10 liter/min. In either method of inhalation it is important to allow free elimination of expired carbon dioxide.

Hemoconcentration. Convulsive or diarrheic foals with hematocrit values >45 per cent should be transfused with normal saline at the rate of 10 to 20 ml/kg of body weight. If dehydration is severe, plasma should be administered IV.

Hypoglycemia. Blood glucose levels <30 mg/100 ml are rarely encountered, but supplementary energy sources are indicated when glycogen reserves are reduced, as in asphyxia or emaciation.

Cardiac Failure. Tachycardia, jugular pulse and venous engorgement may be treated by 0.5 mg of digoxin (Lanoxin) injection IM or IV, followed by maintenance doses of 0.5 mg b.i.d.

Cerebral Hemorrhage. Foals suffering from gross behavioral abnormalities, prematurity or respiratory difficulties should receive 10 mg of vitamin K (Konakion) IM b.i.d. for 2 days.

Meconium Retention. Meconium retention should be treated by the administration of 400 ml of warm liquid paraffin emulsion through a stomach tube, and pain is controlled by 200 mg of meperidine (Demerol) subcutaneously repeated at 2- to 3-hour intervals, depending on severity.

Enemas of soapy water help to break up the accumulation of meconium in the rectum, but these should be administered infrequently and with great care so as to avoid ballooning of the rectum. In the United Kingdom the condition is rarely fatal, except as a result of rupture of the rectum caused by manipulative instruments or enema tubes.

Group III (Developmental Abnormalities)

Each abnormality must be treated according to its position and severity. Hyperflexion of the limbs may be corrected successfully with splints or appliances that aid the re-establishment of normal limb positions. Surgical severance of fibers of the flexor muscle and tendons may be necessary in severe cases. Hypoflexion of the limb requires bandage support around the fetlocks and pastern joints, and general nursing is required to help affected foals to get up and suck.

Surgical intervention is indicated in cases of patent bladder and open abdominal floor. Urachal fistulae that do not respond to antibiotic and astringent applications to the umbilicus may also require surgery. Cleft palates may be repaired, depending on the extent of the abnormality, but if the soft palate is involved, the prognosis is poor.

Clinicians should carefully consider the justification for treatment in each case of developmental abnormality and carefully weigh the balance of likely future working and breeding soundness, the costs of therapy and the owner's particular interests.

Group IV (Immunological Conditions)

Replacement of erythrocytes by transfusion is necessary when the erythrocyte count falls below about 3 million/cu mm. The most satisfactory source of erythrocytes is the affected foal's dam, but it is essential that the cells are first washed free of plasma, which is heavily laden with antibody. Maternal blood is collected into flasks containing 120 ml of sterile acid citrate dextrose/500 ml of blood and centrifuged. Supernatant plasma is removed by suction and replaced by an equal volume of normal saline. The mixture is shaken, and the process is repeated two or three times before the cells are safe for administration.

A liter of erythrocytes may be administered intravenously over a period of about 1 hour, employing a 100-ml syringe and a 16GA × 1½B hypodermic needle or indwelling catheter inserted into the jugular vein. The quantity and number of subsequent administrations depend upon the cell count. When this falls below 2 million/cu mm, the prognosis is grave but should not be assumed to be hopeless.

Under ordinary conditions the disorder has a high mortality rate. Successful treatment depends upon the continued monitoring of the erythrocyte count, the transfusion of suitable erythrocytes and the application of supportive measures. It may be impractical for practitioners without adequate laboratory facilities to attempt therapy, but if the case has to be referred to an establishment that involves a long journey, it is helpful to administer a quantity of maternal cells, washed in the manner previously described, to enable the foal to survive the journey.

An alternative procedure to the administration of packed erythrocytes is an exchange transfusion in which the foal's plasma is partly replaced by suitable donor plasma.

All possible precautions should be taken to avoid exerting or exciting the foal, and during convalescence it should not be turned loose in a paddock until the erythrocyte count is above 5 million/cu mm.

Preventive Measures

The problem of preventive medicine as applied to the neonatal period is that such measures that may be available have to be applied indirectly, i.e., through the mare. This conundrum emphasizes the fact that the neonatal mammal is heir to the problems of gestation and birth, and postnatal challenges are of only relatively minor importance.

Group I Conditions

The incidence of septicemic conditions may be reduced by careful management, such as having mares foal in the environment in which they have been resident for at least 4 weeks prior to parturition. Also, the foal should be able to receive good quality colostrum within 3 hours postpartum (by bottle-feeding the dam's or donor's colostrum in circumstances in which this is necessary, e.g., "running milk" on the part of the mare or an inability of the foal to stand). Attendants should adhere to the principles of cleanliness in all procedures in which infection may be introduced through the oral or umbilical routes. Foaling boxes should be clean and, if practicable, used infrequently.

Success has been claimed for the administration of routine prophylactic antibiotic injections to the foal during the first 1 to 5 days following birth, but the efficacy of these regimens in preventing infection is rarely substantiated by the use of controls. However, on farms where neonatal diarrhea or other septicemic conditions, such as infective arthritis, exist, prophylactic antibiotic therapy is advocated.

It is important to provide protection against tetanus during the first 7 weeks postpartum, especially on farms where the disease is endemic. Prophylaxis may be based, preferably, on active immunization of the mare by administering toxoid in the last month prior to parturition or by injecting the foal with tetanus antitoxin serum during the first and fourth weeks postpartum.

Group II Conditions

No specific prophylaxis can be recommended against NMS, premature or dysmature situations or meconium colic. Advice in general terms includes avoiding measures that might interfere with the adaptive processes, such as might occur by excessive or too vigorous handling during the period in which the foal develops the behavioral bond with its dam. Strong traction or unnecessary manipulation of the foreparts should be avoided when possible during delivery. Anticonvulsant drugs, vitamin K and intravenous bicarbonate may be administered to foals that have undergone difficult birth or show evidence of behavioral disturbances in an attempt to prevent the onset of convulsions, and every effort should be made in these cases to avoid vigorous restraint. Enemas of liquid paraffin or of soap and water and liquid paraffin and castor or olive oil given orally are routine practices on many stud farms, but their efficacy in preventing meconium colic is based on a subjective assessment.

Group III Conditions

There are no known means of preventing congenital abnormalities in the horse, although attention should be given to avoiding the administration of drugs at all stages of pregnancy except when there is a reasonable and essential indication. Hereditary influences should be considered when mares have delivered a deformed foal, and subsequent selection of the stallion may be influenced accordingly. However, in the absence of objective studies for the particular deformity in question, prophylaxis in this situation is largely a matter of subjective opinion.

Group IV Conditions

Mares that have had previous foals that suffered from hemolytic disease or foals in which the disease is confirmed by pre- or immediately postparturient tests for antibody on maternal blood or colostrum should not be allowed to have their foals suck from 24 to 36 hours postpartum. In these cases the foal should be fed at least 10 ounces of donor colostrum within 3 hours of birth and subsequently should receive reconstituted milk until allowed to feed from its dam after the prescribed interval.

REFERENCES

1. Barnes, R. J., Nathanielsz, P. W., Rossdale, P. D., Comline, R. S. and Silver, M.: Plasma progestogens and oestrogens in foetus and mother in late pregnancy. J. Reprod. Fertil. (Suppl.), *23*:617, 1975.
2. Bergin, W. C.: A survey of embryonic and prenatal losses in the horse. Proceedings 15th Annual Convention American Association Equine Practitioners. 1969, pp. 121–128. Published by the A.A.E.P., Golden, Colorado.
3. Comline, R. S., Hall, L. W., Lavelle, R. and Silver, M.: The use of intravascular catheters and long-term studies on the mare and foetus. J. Reprod. Fertil. (Suppl.), *23*:583, 1975.
4. Fraser, A. F. L., Hastie, H., Callicott, R. B. and Brownlie, S.: An exploratory ultra-sonic study of quantitative fetal kinesis in the horse. Appl. Anim. Ethol., *1*:395, 1975.
5. Merkt, H. and von Lepel, J. D.: Report on the autumn 1970 examinations of West German Thoroughbreds (bloodstock). Vollblut, Zucht und Rennen, *34*:26, 1971.
6. Nathanielsz, P. W., Rossdale, P. D., Silver, M. and Comline, R. S.: Studies on foetal, neonatal and maternal cortisol metabolism in the mare. J. Reprod. Fertil. (Suppl.), *23*:625, 1975.
7. Platt, H.: Etiological aspects of perinatal mortality in the Thoroughbred. Equine Vet. J., *5*:116, 1973.
8. Rossdale, P. D.: Blood gas tensions and pH values in the normal Thoroughbred foal at birth and in the following 42 hours. Biol. Neonat., *13*:18, 1968.
9. Rossdale, P. D.: pH and pCO$_2$ of equine amniotic fluid at the time of birth. Biol. Neonat., *12*:378, 1968.
10. Rossdale, P. D.: Measurements of pulmonary ventilation in normal newborn Thoroughbred foals during the first three days of life. Br. Vet. J., *125*:137, 1969.
11. Rossdale, P. D.: Some parameters of respiratory function in normal and abnormal new-born foals with special reference to levels of p$_a$O$_2$ during air and oxygen inhalation. Res. Vet. Sci., *11*:270, 1970.
12. Rossdale, P D.: A clinical assessment of perinatal respiration in the foal. Proceedings 7th International Conference AI and Reproduction, Munich, *9*:468, 1972.
13. Rossdale, P. D.: A clinician's view of prematurity and dysmaturity in Thoroughbred foals. Proc. Roy. Soc. Med., *69*:631, 1976.
14. Rossdale, P. D. and Leadon, D.: Equine neonatal disease: A review. J. Reprod. Fertil. (Suppl.) *23*:685, 1975.
15. Rossdale, P. D., Jeffcott, L. B. and Palmer, A. C.: Raised fetal blood pressure and haemorrhage in CNS of newborn foals. Vet. Rec., *99*:111, 1976 (editorial correspondence).
16. Samuel, C. A., Allen, W. R. and Steven, D. H.: Ultrastructural development of the equine placenta. J. Reprod. Fertil. (Suppl.), *23*:575, 1975.
17. Silver, M. and Comline, R. S.: Transfer of gases and metabolites in the equine placenta: a comparison with other species. J. Reprod. Fertil. (Suppl.), *23*:589, 1975.
18. Steven, D. H. and Samuel, C. A.: Anatomy of the placental barrier in the mare. J. Reprod. Fertil. (Suppl.), *23*:579, 1975.

Nutrition and Reproduction in the Horse

H. F. SCHRYVER and H. F. HINTZ

Cornell University, Ithaca, New York

A successful breeding program requires a sound feeding program. The effects of nutrition on reproduction can be those of deficiency or excess of single nutrients or, more commonly, of many nutrients caused by rations that are imbalanced in quality and quantity. Clinicians need to know which nutrients affect reproduction, what the requirements are for these nutrients and how the requirements may be met by practical feeding programs.

NUTRIENT FUNCTIONS IN BREEDING ANIMALS

Consideration must be given to function when devising feeding programs for breeding animals. For example, the nutritional needs of the stallion during breeding season do not appear to be different from those of maintenance. A slight increase in energy intake may be necessary or beneficial during the height of the breeding season; however, it is easy to overestimate the nutrient needs of the stallion at this time. Overfed stallions are probably more common and of greater concern than are undernourished stallions.

The nutrient requirements of the mare during pregnancy depend upon the maintenance of her own body and upon the growth and metabolism of tissues formed during pregnancy. These tissues include the fetus and fetal membranes, the uterus and the mammary glands.

The fetus is completely dependent upon the dam for all nutrients. The source of the nutrients can be from stores of the mare's own body or from current dietary intake by the mare. Thus, fetal nutrition can be influenced by the mare's current dietary supply or, in the case of stored nutrients, by the recent dietary history of the mare.

Although pregnancy is customarily divided into trimesters, for purposes of discussion of nutrition, two important periods will be defined. The first occurs early in pregnancy and corresponds to the first trimester when organs differentiate and develop. During this stage, fetal growth in terms of weight gain and nutrient accretion is slight. At the end of the first trimester of pregnancy, the foal weighs only about 1 pound (Fig. 1). The nutrient requirements of the mare during this period are much the same as for maintenance of good health in any mature horse. However, restricted maternal nutrition in terms of the entire diet or of specific nutrients during this early formative and developmental period of pregnancy may result in failure of pregnancy, arrested development of the fetus or developmental abnormalities.

The second important period occurs after organ differentiation is complete and is characterized by rapidly accelerating growth and nutrient accretion. About half of the foal's

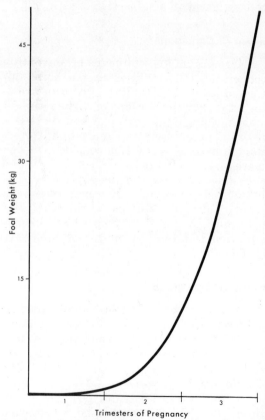

Figure 1. Weight change of the foal during gestation. A foal of one of the light breeds weighs only 1 kg at the end of the first third of gestation and 10 to 12 kg at the end of the second third. Weight gain accelerates very rapidly during the final trimester.

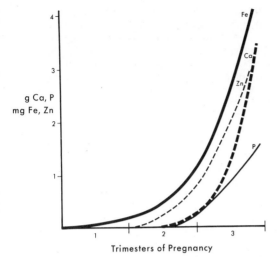

Figure 2. Accretion of minerals in the fetus is most marked during the last third of pregnancy. For example, 85 to 90 per cent of the foal's calcium is deposited in the skeleton at this time.

body protein and 85 to 90 per cent of the fetal calcium (Fig. 2) is accreted at this time when the foal begins to assume a significant part of the mare's body weight. During this period, which corresponds to the last trimester of pregnancy, the nutrient requirements of the mare accelerate very rapidly. Poor maternal nutrition during this stage of pregnancy often leads to a stunted newborn or to diminished storage of glycogen in fetal muscle and liver. Lack of stored energy sources may contribute to neonatal mortality.

From the standpoint of nutrition, lactation is another critical phase in the reproductive cycle and places far greater demands on the mare than is often recognized. An average mare may produce 500 kg of milk monthly while nursing a foal. Feed is needed not only for the secretion of protein, calcium and phosphorus in milk but also for providing energy for the process of milk secretion itself. In general, unless the requirements for lactation are met through the diet, these substances are removed from the body of the mare. Failure to provide the nutrients needed for lactation can lead to rapid malnutrition of the mare, to diminished milk production and to subsequent breeding problems.

NUTRITIONAL REQUIREMENTS OF BREEDING ANIMALS

Nutrients are required by breeding animals for their own bodily maintenance, to replace nutrients expended in reproduction and to fulfill other functions such as growth or work, which may be concurrent with reproduction.

Energy

Calories are largely supplied by carbohydrates, usually as starch, sugar and cellulose, but protein and fat are also used as energy sources. Excess energy is stored as fat. Energy is required for all bodily processes and activities. The more intense the process or activity, the greater the amount of energy that is required. Functions that consume a large amount of energy include growth, hard work, lactation and the late stage of pregnancy.

Restriction of energy intake during the growth period causes a decrease in the rate of growth and delays the onset of sexual maturity. Conversely, high intake of a balanced diet during growth increases the rate of growth within the limits of genetic potential and hastens the onset of sexual maturity. Energy restriction in mature animals may alter or stop sexual activity. Animals that have been overfed and are fat may also exhibit altered sexual activity. It is commonly accepted that excessive body fat decreases libido in the male and the efficiency of reproduction in the female. It has been noticed in many species of animals that lean females that are gaining weight at the onset of the breeding season generally have the greatest reproductive efficiency. This management tool has also been successful in horses. In some instances, overweight mares are fed a limited but balanced ration and are exercised so that they reduce to a desired weight by January. Feed intake is then increased so that the mare is gaining weight slowly as the breeding season draws near.

Pregnancy increases the need for energy to allow for storage of energy in new tissues and to replace energy expended in new tissue formation. Although the developing fetus goes through many critical phases early in pregnancy, the demands for energy above the maintenance needs of the mare are very small. However, during the last trimester, weight gains by the foal rapidly accelerate. The foal assumes a significant proportion of the body weight of the mare, and the energy needs of the foal become a significant part of the mare's energy economy. The change from a level of maintenance energy requirements to a higher level is a gradual one when needs accelerate. At the same time that energy requirements rapidly increase, the foal occupies more space in the abdominal cavity of the mare, reducing her ability and desire to consume large quantities of feeds of relatively low energy density, such as poor quality hay. Thus, her ration during the last trimester must be supplemented with high energy feeds, such as grain.

It is often recommended that mares be fed about 16 per cent more energy during the last 3 or 4 months of gestation. This is probably best distributed as an 8 per cent increase during the eighth month, 16 per cent during the ninth and tenth months and about 20 per cent during the final month. However, the safest and easiest guide is to observe the mare and adjust feed intake to achieve the desired body condition.

The energy requirements of lactation are even greater than those of pregnancy. The 1000-pound mare probably produces an average of 12 to 18 kg of milk per day at peak lactation, but some may produce as much as 24 kg. About 800 kilocalories of energy is required to produce 1 kg of milk. For many mares this translates as an increase in feed intake of about 50 per cent to meet the increased energy needs of lactation.

Protein

Protein is necessary for the synthesis of the sex hormones, for development of the gonads and maturation of the sperm and ova, for development of the embryo and fetus and for lactation. Relatively large amounts of protein are required for deposit in the fetus late in pregnancy and again during lactation, when protein is secreted in milk. A severe deficiency of protein causes many problems in breeding animals, including cessation of estrus, reduction of the amounts of circulating pituitary, ovarian and testicular hormones and, if fertilization occurs, resorption of the embryo or the birth of premature, dead or weak offspring. Even moderate protein deficiency has been shown to decrease the birth weight in foals. Protein deficiency commonly causes depressed appetite, leading to inadequate energy intake. Thus, protein deficiency and energy deficiency often occur together.

The maintenance protein requirement for mature horses is about 8.5 to 9 per cent of

TABLE 1. *Protein Requirements of Breeding Animals*

Classification	Per cent of Ration*
Mature horses	8.5–9
Pregnant mares	10–12.5
Lactating mares	11–13
In creep rations	18–20

*90 per cent dry matter basis.

the diet (Table 1). This amount should also be adequate for mares and stallions at breeding time and for the mare during the first two-thirds of pregnancy. Normal animals do not appear to benefit from greater protein intake. Mares during the last third of gestation need about 10 per cent dietary protein and during peak lactation about 12.5 per cent protein. Later in lactation, when milk production decreases, about 11 per cent dietary protein may be adequate.

During late pregnancy and peak lactation, consideration should also be given to protein quality, that is, to the balance of essential amino acids in the protein source. Examples of high quality proteins are soybean oil meal, alfalfa and the proteins of animal or fish origin (Fig. 3). Proteins of cereal grains are relatively low in lysine and some in tryptophan and methionine as well.

Calcium and Phosphorus

In phosphorus-deficient areas of the world, efficiency of reproduction is extremely low. Deficient animals exhibit irregular estrous cycles or anestrus. This is due to phosphorus deficiency itself and to loss of appetite and consequent low intake of feeds that are also deficient in protein and vitamin A.

Deficiency of calcium generally has less effect on reproduction than does phosphorus, unless the deficiency is very severe or prolonged. The dam has well-developed mechanisms for withdrawing calcium from her skeletal stores during deficiency. However, the skeleton of the severely deficient mare may become depleted of minerals during pregnancy and lactation. Unless replenished, she may be less able to support pregnancy and lactation in subsequent years.

The maintenance requirements for mature animals are about 0.3 per cent calcium and 0.2 per cent phosphorus (Table 2). It is unlikely that breeding animals other than mares in late pregnancy and lactation ben-

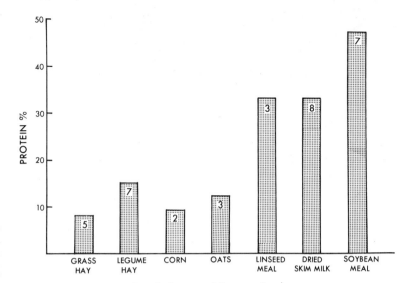

Figure 3. Protein content of some common feeds. The figures at the top of the bars give the relative lysine content of the protein and are an indication of the quality of the protein.

Protein Content of Common Feeds

efit from amounts of calcium and phosphorus above the maintenance level. However, demand for these minerals becomes great during late pregnancy and peak lactation. About 85 to 90 per cent of the foal's skeleton is mineralized during the last 90 to 100 days of pregnancy. The mare must take in 10 to 15 gm of calcium and 8 to 12 gm of phosphorus above her maintenance needs daily to provide the amounts needed by the developing foal. Mares in the last third of pregnancy should be fed diets that contain about 0.45 per cent calcium and 0.30 per cent phosphorus.

A lactating mare may secrete about 15 to 20 gm of calcium and about 7 to 10 gm of phosphorus in milk daily during peak lactation. A 1000-pound mare needs about 50 gm of calcium and 35 gm of phosphorus daily to meet these needs. Diets containing 0.45 to 0.6 per cent calcium and 0.3 to 0.4 per cent phosphorus should be adequate.

Good quality hay and pasture contain all the calcium and phosphorus needed to meet

TABLE 2. *Calcium and Phosphorous Requirements of Breeding Horses*

	Per Cent of Diet*	
Period	CALCIUM	PHOSPHORUS
Maintenance	0.3	0.2
Gestation (last third)	0.45	0.30
Lactation (peak)	0.6	0.35

*Values depend on availability of nutrient, feed intake and energy concentration of diet.

the maintenance requirements of mature horses such as stallions, open mares and mares in early pregnancy (Fig. 4). Legume hays such as alfalfa or clover are rich sources of calcium but contain no more phosphorus than the grasses. Mineral sources of calcium or phosphorus, or both, such as limestone, monocalcium phosphate, dicalcium phosphate, bone meal or monosodium phosphate are useful, effective and very inexpensive supplements for pregnant and lactating mares. The choice of supplement should be determined by the needs of the animal.

Trace Minerals

About 15 other elements are needed in trace amounts for good health and reproduction. These elements include copper, zinc, iron, manganese, iodine and selenium (Table 3).

Copper is needed for the formation and maintenance of many of the connective tissues such as bone, cartilage, ligament, tendon and blood vessels. Serum copper levels have been shown to decline in older mares, and this has been thought to be related to uterine artery rupture. *Manganese* is part of an enzyme system involved in the formation of some of the chemical constituents of cartilage. Deficiency of manganese in cattle has resulted in deformities in calves similar to contracted tendons. *Zinc* is required in many enzymes that are responsible for energy me-

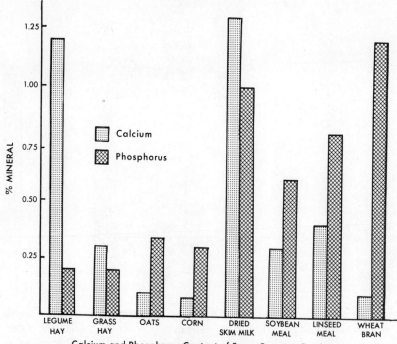

Calcium and Phosphorus Content of Some Common Feeds

Figure 4

tabolism and for new tissue formation. *Iron* is needed for the formation of hemoglobin in the fetal blood. Copper, zinc, manganese and iron are found in good quality hay and pasture plants. Free choice feeding of these trace minerals in trace-mineralized salt is a simple, safe and effective means of preventing deficiency. Increased requirements of pregnancy and lactation are likely met through increased feed intake at these times.

Iodine is also needed in reproduction and is easily supplied by trace-mineralized salt. Organic forms of iodine do not appear to be any more effective than the inorganic forms in iodized salt. Iodine deficiency occurs in distinct geographical areas. Unless preg-

nant mares in these areas are supplemented with iodine, the foals may be stillborn or weak at birth. Considerable caution must be used when supplementing pregnant mares with iodine preparations. There have been several reports of stillborn or weak foals born of mares that have been given excessive amounts of iodine during pregnancy. The enlarged thyroids of the affected foals may resemble those seen in iodine deficiency and have resulted in mistaken administration of still higher iodine supplements. Excess iodine intake has resulted from injudicious use of supplements that contain very high amounts of iodine, such as some forms of kelp.

There is increasing evidence that *selenium* is deficient in many areas of the United States. Muscle degeneration is seen in young calves, lambs, pigs and foals in these areas. In addition, there is evidence that selenium may also be involved in reproduction. In New Zealand, selenium supplementation reduced the proportion of barren ewes from about 45 per cent to about 8 per cent. Trace-mineralized salt does not contain selenium. Selenium supplements should be calculated and administered with great care because the margin of safety between the required (0.1 parts per million, ppm) and toxic amounts (greater than 3 ppm) of selenium is very small. Among the natural feeds,

TABLE 3. *Trace Element Requirements for Mature Horses*

Element	Value*
Copper	5–8
Iodine	0.1
Iron	40
Manganese	20
Selenium	0.1
Zinc	40

*The values given are estimates of the requirements for maintenance of mature horses and are ppm (mg/kg) in the diet.

linseed meal is an effective and safe supplement.

Fat-Soluble Vitamins

Vitamin A affects all epithelial tissues and thus plays an important role in reproduction. Severe vitamin A deficiency causes degeneration of the germinal epithelium of the testis, resulting in decrease or cessation of spermatogenesis. In the female, deficiency alters the epithelial lining of the reproductive tract and may result in irregular estrus and delayed breeding. In females that conceive, abortion or the birth of weak or dead young may result.

One study done in cattle more than 40 years ago should be of interest to horsemen. Continuous feeding of low quality timothy hay to cattle caused abortion or stillborn calves. Affected cows did not come into estrus until given green feed. Cattle fed high quality alfalfa in the same experiment did not develop the problem. It was later shown that deficiency of vitamin A in the timothy hay was the factor concerned with the reproductive abnormalities in this experiment.

Horses obtain vitamin A from precursors, such as carotene, that occur widely in fresh green feeds (Table 4). About 1 mg of carotene is equivalent to about 400 International Units (IU) of vitamin A. Vitamin A activity is rapidly destroyed during the sun curing and storage of hay. However, properly cured hay that has not been stored for long periods and still has some green color generally has enough vitamin A activity for most horses. Horses are able to store enough vitamin A in

TABLE 4. *Carotone Content of Feedstuffs*

Feedstuff	Carotene* (mg/kg)
Alfalfa hay (midbloom)	33
Alfalfa hay (mature)	15
Barley	0
Beet pulp	0
Bermuda grass hay	36
Bluegrass pasture	383
Clover, red	34
Corn, dent yellow	2
Oats	0
Timothy hay (midbloom)	11
Timothy hay (late bloom)	10

*Dry matter basis.

the liver to meet their requirement for 4 to 6 months after they have had access to fresh green feed for about a 4- to 6-week period. Vitamin A stored in the liver protects against reproductive problems during short periods when vitamin A deficient feeds are fed. However, horses wintered on hay that has been stored for longer than 1 year or that has been improperly cured by excessive exposure to the weather may benefit from vitamin A supplements. In most species the vitamin A content of serum is a reflection of vitamin A status.

About 25 IU/kg of body weight per day of vitamin A is adequate for the maintenance of mature horses and 50 IU/kg is adequate for pregnant and lactating mares (Table 5). This is about 22,000 IU for pregnant mares of about 1000 pounds body weight.

Vitamin E has long been known to be essential to normal reproduction in the rat, but attempts to link vitamin E to reproductive failure in many of the domestic animals have generally resulted in negative or contradictory results.

There is no clear evidence that vitamin E alone helps prevent reproductive problems in the horse. However, one study suggested that conception was improved in barren mares supplemented orally or by injection with both vitamin E and vitamin A. Barren mares given 100,000 IU of vitamin A and 100 IU of vitamin E daily for 3 months starting about 1 month before breeding had a larger number of foals than unsupplemented mares. Further studies in mares are needed before the use of vitamin A and E supplements can be recommended for widespread use.

Vitamin D is needed by the mare for the proper assimilation of calcium and phosphorus during the periods of heavy demand for these minerals in late pregnancy and lactation. It is not known whether the vitamin or its metabolites are transported across the equine placenta to the fetus. Sunlight and sun-cured forages provide all of the vitamin needed by horses. Supplements are not needed in most cases.

Water-Soluble Vitamins

Good quality hays and grains generally contain liberal amounts of all of the *B vitamins*. In addition, the micro-organisms of the horse cecum and colon synthesize large

TABLE 5. *Vitamin Requirements for Breeding Animals*

Vitamin	Requirement	Sources
Vitamin A:		
Mature horses	30 mg of carotene or 25 IU/kg of body weight	Fresh, green, leafy forage; alfalfa hay
Pregnancy and lactation	60 mg of carotene or 50 IU/kg of body weight	
Vitamin D:		
Mature horses	1.5 IU/kg	Sunshine, sun-cured forages
Vitamin E	Not known	Grains, green forage
Vitamin B₁ (thiamin)	25 mg/day	All good quality feeds, brewer's yeast
Vitamin B₂ (riboflavin)	20–40 mg/day	Green forage, alfalfa

amounts of the vitamins. Unless intestinal function is impaired and poor quality feeds are used, B vitamin supplementation is probably not necessary, even during the critical periods of pregnancy and lactation.

Under normal circumstances the horse does not appear to have a dietary requirement for *ascorbic acid* (vitamin C). Ascorbic acid supplements are used in an effort to improve stallion semen quality and reproductive efficiency of mares on some breeding farms. Controlled studies are needed to assess the value of this practice.

FEEDING SUGGESTIONS FOR BREEDING ANIMALS

The following will list examples of rations that can be used on breeding farms, but it should be remembered that these are only examples. Many feeds or combinations of feeds can be used. Selection should be based on nutrient content, cost, availability and acceptability to horses. For example, many western horsemen will substitute alfalfa for grass hay and barley for oats and corn.

The maintenance requirements of mature, nonworking horses can usually be supplied by good pasture or good quality hay plus trace-mineralized salt and clean water (Fig. 5). The amount of feed required by stallions

will depend on the individual, but about 1/2 to 3/4 pound of grain and 1 to 1 1/2 pounds of hay per 100 pounds of body weight should be adequate.

The body condition of the mare at breeding time is very important. Trim mares that are gaining weight seem to have the best chance of conception. The ration just described for the stallion should be adequate for the mare at breeding time and into the first half or two-thirds of gestation. It is important to observe the mare and adjust the feed intake according to body condition.

During the last third of pregnancy, nutrient requirements increase greatly, and the intake of bulky feeds such as hay will decrease. The mare will probably eat about 1 pound of hay per 100 pounds of body weight and will need 1/2 to 1 pound of a grain mix in addition to the hay. If grass hay is fed, the grain mix should contain 16 per cent protein, 0.5 per cent calcium and 0.4 per cent phosphorus. A typical grain ration for a pregnant mare fed grass hay could contain:

45 per cent oats.
30 per cent corn.
12 per cent soybean meal.
9 per cent wheat bran.
3 per cent molasses.
1 per cent limestone.

If legume hay is fed instead of grass hay, there is no need to use protein or calcium supplements such as soybean meal and lime-

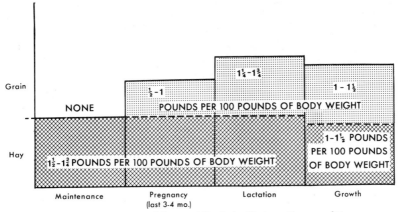

Approximate Amounts of Hay and Grain for Various Classes of Horses

Figure 5. Approximate amounts of hay and grain for horses. The pregnant mare will probably eat less roughage during the last trimester of pregnancy than is indicated in the figure. The grain ration should be increased accordingly.

stone. Many mares are fed too heavily early in pregnancy on the assumption that nutritional needs are greatly increased all through pregnancy. This is not only wasteful but the overweight mare has more difficulty foaling and may be more difficult to breed following foaling.

Lactating mares have greatly increased nutrient requirements. A mare may need as much as 1 1/4 to 1 3/4 pounds of grain per 100 pounds of body weight. Mares vary considerably in the ability to produce milk, and the best rule is to observe the mare and feed accordingly. The grain mix should contain at least 16 per cent protein, 0.7 per cent calcium and 0.5 per cent phosphorus when grass hay is fed and 12 per cent protein and 0.5 per cent phosphorus when legume hay is fed. When a grass hay is fed, the ingredients of the grain mix might consist of:

40 per cent corn.
35 per cent oats.
15 per cent soybean meal.
5 per cent wheat bran.
3 per cent molasses.
1 per cent limestone.
1 per cent dicalcium phosphate.

If legume hay is fed, the grain ration might be:

40 per cent corn.
50 per cent oats.
5 per cent soybean meal.
4 per cent wheat bran.
1 per cent dicalcium phosphate.

The mare can be helped considerably by providing a creep ration for the foal. This may be begun as early as 2 weeks after birth. The foal may not eat much at first but will gradually increase intake as it grows and becomes accustomed to the creep. A creep ration also makes it possible to wean the foal earlier and easier if desired. It is extremely important that a creep ration be well balanced with respect to protein, calcium and phosphorus, since this is a critical stage of growth for the foal. The ration should also be highly digestible and palatable. It should contain 18 to 20 per cent of good quality protein, 0.8 per cent calcium, and 0.6 per cent phosphorus. A useful creep ration might consist of:

40 per cent cracked corn.
30 per cent rolled oats.
23 per cent soybean meal.
3.5 per cent molasses.
1 per cent dicalcium phosphate.
1 per cent limestone.
1 per cent trace-mineralized salt.
0.5 per cent brewer's yeast.

The rations given should meet the requirements of horses as listed in Table 6. The requirements are also listed in Table 7 as nutrient concentrations in the diet.

REFERENCES

1. Maynard, L. A. and Loosli, J. K.: Animal Nutrition. 6th Ed. New York, McGraw Hill, 1969.

TABLE 6. Nutrient Requirements of Horses on the Breeding Farm*

Classification	TDN (kg)	Crude Protein (kg)	Digestible Protein (kg)	Calcium (gm)	Phosphorus (gm)	Vitamin A Activity (1000 IU)	Daily Feed (kg)
Stallions, open mares, mares in early gestation	3.7	0.6	0.3	23	14	12	7.5
Mares, last 90 days gestation	4.2	0.8	0.4	34	23	22	8
Lactating mare, first 3 months	6.4	1.4	0.8	50	34	27	11
Lactating mare, 3 months to weaning	5.5	1.1	0.6	41	27	22	10
Nursing foal (3 months of age)	3.1	0.9	0.6	33	20	6	5
Requirements in addition to milk	1.6	0.4	0.3	18	13	0	2

*Adapted from the National Research Council, Subcommittee on Horse Nutrition, Nutrient Requirements of Horses, 1978. For horses of about 500 kg (1100 pounds) mature weight.

TABLE 7. Nutrient Concentrations in Diets for Horses on the Breeding Farm*

Classification	Diet Proportions				Crude Protein (%)	Calcium (%)	Phosphorus (%)	Vitamin A Activity (IU/kg)
	GOOD HAY		AVERAGE HAY					
	CONCENTRATE (%)	ROUGHAGE (%)	CONCENTRATE (%)	ROUGHAGE (%)				
Stallions, open mares, mares in early pregnancy	0	100	20	80	8.5	0.30	0.20	1600
Mares, last 90 days of gestation	25	75	40	60	10.0	0.45	0.30	3000
Lactating mare, first 3 months	50	50	60	40	12.5	0.45	0.30	2500
Lactating mare, 3 months to weaning	25	75	40	60	11.0	0.40	0.25	2200
Creep feed	100	0	100	0	16.0	0.85	0.60	—

*Adapted from the National Research Council, Subcommittee on Horse Nutrition, Nutrient Requirements of Horses, 1978.

2. National Academy of Sciences: Nutrient Requirements of Horses. 4th Ed. Washington, D.C., National Academy of Sciences, 1977.
3. Roberts, S. J.: Veterinary Obstetrics and Genital Diseases. 2nd Ed. Ann Arbor, Mich., Edwards Bros. Inc., 1971.
4. Robinson, D. W. and Slade, L. M.: The current status of knowledge on the nutrition of equines. J. Anim. Sci., *39*: 1045, 1974.

Equine Herpesvirus 1 (Rhinopneumonitis) Abortion

D. MITCHELL

Animal Diseases Research Institute (Western), Lethbridge, Alberta, Canada

CLINICAL SIGNS

Equine Herpesvirus 1 (EHV-1) infection can cause a wide range of clinical syndromes. Although differences in tissue affinity of EHV-1 strains have been demonstrated,[2] it should be considered a pantropic virus. Respiratory disease and abortion are the most common clinical signs, but neurological disease is not uncommon. Unlike bovine herpesvirus 1 (the causal agent of IBR-IPV in cattle), EHV-1 is not usually associated with vulvovaginitis. In horses, coital exanthema, the condition most closely resembling IPV in cattle, has been shown to be caused by an antigenically distinct strain of herpesvirus (EHV-3).

Respiratory disease and fetal infection are only infrequently seen in the same group of animals concurrently, and the majority of aborting mares have no previous history of respiratory illness. Neurological disturbances and abortion may occur in the same group of animals concurrently.[3] The severity of neurological signs varies from acute, with paralysis and death, to mild, with only transient ataxia. The incidence of abortion in groups of susceptible mares is not uncommonly as high as 60 per cent but may be as low as 1 to 2 per cent, presumably depending on the degree of exposure, the virulence of the infecting strain of virus and the immune status of the animals at risk. EHV-1 abortions rarely occur before the sixth month of pregnancy, and the majority occur between the ninth month and term. Many infected fetuses and foals are born alive but usually die soon after birth. Affected foals have been known to survive up to 2 weeks after parturition and mildly infected animals may survive for longer periods.

DIAGNOSIS

As EHV-1 is widely disseminated in all countries in which horse breeding is practiced, it should be considered as a possible cause whenever an outbreak of abortion occurs in mares during late gestation or whenever foals are born at term but fail to survive the first few days of life. Macroscopic findings observed at postmortem examination in aborted fetuses are often sufficient to confirm a clinical diagnosis. The most striking of these are generalized edema, excessive quantities of straw-colored fluid in body cavities, focal lesions of hepatic necrosis and hemorrhages varying from petechial to ecchymotic. A conclusive diagnosis must be based on demonstration of histological changes and isolation of the virus from fetal tissues. The fluorescent antibody technique has also been used for demonstration of viral antigen. Serological tests alone are of little diagnostic value because many normal animals show titers, peak titers often occur before the act of abortion and individual levels of serum antibody are extremely variable.

VACCINATION

Despite extensive efforts to develop a safe and reliable artificial immunization procedure, EHV-1 remains a serious cause of fetal and neonatal mortality in many countries. Early studies performed on a variety of inactivated tissue vaccines failed to indicate any protective effect, and it was not until the report of "planned infection" with live hamster-adapted virus that some apparent protective immunity was demonstrated.[4] This vaccine (Pneumabort) was administered intranasally but retained most, if not all, of the virulence of field strains and could be given safely only to mares that were either not pregnant or in the early stages (up to 3 to 4 months) of pregnancy. In Kentucky, a significant reduction in the overall incidence of EHV-1 abortion was claimed using a two-dose regime in Thoroughbred studs during July and October. Subsequently, an attenuated live virus vaccine was developed in Germany that was claimed to give equally good protection and could be administered to mares at any stage of pregnancy without harmful effect.[6] This vaccine (Rhinomune) was subsequently produced and licensed in North America. Shortly thereafter a second attenuated live virus vaccine (Rhinoquin), produced in monkey tissue culture cells, was also made available in North America, with the claim that it could be administered safely to mares at any stage of pregnancy.

Unfortunately, there have been an increasing number of reports from diagnostic laboratories of confirmed EHV-1 abortions in vaccinated mares. One laboratory in Ontario reported examining 69 fetuses between December, 1976, and May, 1977. Thirty-six, from 11 breeding farms, were diagnosed as having EHV-1 infection, and 34 of these were aborted by mares reported to have been vaccinated. In most cases, vaccination had been carried out several months before abortion occurred, and it was presumed that the abortions were caused by field strains of virus. Contact between horses from other farms and mares in the latter half of pregnancy often preceded these "vaccine" breaks. The physical stresses associated with such movements are likely to contribute to the recrudescence and excretion of latent virus in stressed individuals and to exposure and infection of susceptible contact animals.

CONTROL AND PREVENTION

Despite concerns expressed regarding our incomplete understanding of the mechanisms involved in protecting the fetus against EHV-1 infection,[7] the major prophylactic emphasis in North America and some other countries has been directed toward immunization of the mare before breeding or during early pregnancy. Although it may be argued that immunization with the live or modified live virus vaccines just mentioned has reduced foal losses, as indicated, they will not always provide adequate immunity to prevent abortion in mares exposed to virulent strains of field virus and may in some cases be a contributing factor in precipitating fetal losses.

In this context, it is interesting to note the experience of investigators in countries such as Britain[5] and Australia[1] where live virus vaccines have not been used. Despite widespread serological evidence of EHV-1 infection in the horse population of these countries, EHV-1 abortion has not been a significant problem. In Canada and the United States, on the other hand, despite extensive use of artificial immunization programs EHV-1 abortion is still a serious concern. This is no doubt due in some measure to differences in virulence and tropism of EHV-1 strains. Furthermore, the facts that the licensed vaccines previously listed were all derived from aborted fetuses and that herpesvirus infection once introduced into an animal is usually permanent, together with the observation that this virus can pass from the respiratory tract to the fetus even in the presence of serum neutralizing antibody, indicate that stimulation of humoral antibody levels may be of limited value in preventing fetal infection and that live virus vaccines may well have contributed to spread of this disease.

In the light of present knowledge and experience, it is, therefore, unwise to rely on artificial immunization alone to prevent EHV-1 abortion. Further research is required to improve our understanding of herpesvirus immunity and to develop safer and more reliable vaccines. The latter objective may not be easily achieved, and in the meantime, it is recommended that veterinarians advise clients to implement the following procedures in order to reduce the risk of EHV-1 abortion in their mares:

1. When practical, all pregnant mares on the farm should be segregated and not brought into contact with horses from other premises before foaling. The late stages of pregnancy (6 months or more) are the most critical.

2. Every effort should be made to protect mares in late pregnancy from exposure to stress or other factors (e.g., administration of corticosteroids) that might cause recrudes-

cence of latent virus. The risks incurred in transporting pregnant mares, particularly those of nervous disposition, and of bringing outside horses into contact with groups of pregnant mares must also be weighed against operational requirements. If artificial insemination were to be permitted on the farm, the reduction in such movements would greatly diminish the hazard of spreading this, as well as other, infections.

3. If a confirmed EHV-1 abortion occurs on a farm, every effort should be made to isolate the aborting mare and all in-contact horses. This physical isolation should be accompanied by implementation of strict hygienic precautions and quarantine procedures to limit spread of infection until foaling is completed. Because of the long period of time that may elapse between initial infection and abortion (3 to 16 weeks), additional cases of fetal death in in-contact mares can be expected. Vaccination in the face of an outbreak is unlikely to be of value and may, in fact, be contraindicated.

CONCLUSIONS

Although EHV-1 has been recognized as perhaps the most serious infectious cause of equine fetal mortality in North America for the past 30 years, extensive research has failed to provide a completely satisfactory method of prophylaxis. The live and modified live virus vaccines developed to date have proved to limited value, and further

study on immunizing products is required. It is suggested that, whether or not artificial immunization is practiced, every effort should be made to initiate management procedures designed to reduce the risk of exposing susceptible pregnant mares to infection.*

Note: At the time of preparation of this manuscript, claims on behalf of Rhinomune for the prevention of abortion have been retracted and Rhinoquin has been voluntarily withdrawn from the market because of adverse reactions.

REFERENCES

1. Bagust, T. J.: A review of viral infections of horses. Aust. Vet. J., *48*:520, 1972.
2. Burrows, R. and Goodridge, D.: *In vivo* and *in vitro* studies of equine rhinopneumonitis virus strains. Proceedings 3rd International Conference on Equine Infectious Diseases, Paris, S. Karger, Basel, 1973, pp. 306–321.
3. Charlton, K. M., Mitchell, D., Girard, A. and Corner, A. H.: Meningoencephalomyelitis in horses associated with equine herpesvirus 1 infection. Vet. Pathol., *13*:59, 1976.
4. Doll, E. R., and Bryans, J. T.: A planned infection program in immunizing mares against viral rhinopneumonitis. Cornell Vet., *53*:249, 1963.
5. Jeffcott, L. B. and Rossdale, P. D.: Practical aspects of equine virus abortion in the United Kingdom. Vet. Rec., *98*:153, 1976.
6. Mayr, A.: Vaccination of horses against equine herpesvirus 1 infection. Proceedings 2nd International Conference on Equine Infectious Diseases, Paris, S. Karger, Basel, 1969, pp. 43–45.
7. Studdert, M. J.: Comparative aspects of equine herpesviruses. Cornell Vet., *64*:94, 1974.

Contagious Equine Metritis

DAVID G. POWELL
Michigan State University,
East Lansing, Michigan

An outbreak of genital infections among Thoroughbred mares in the Newmarket area of England during 1977 posed a challenge to research scientists and to veterinarians specializing in equine stud practice. Investigations revealed that the disease is caused by a hitherto unidentified bacterial pathogen. The outbreak served to re-

emphasize the important role that bacteria play in the etiology of animal disease at a time when studies have tended to concentrate on the causative role of other agents.

HISTORY OF THE 1977 OUTBREAK

During April, 1977, a large public stud farm in the Newmarket area reported that an unusually large proportion of bred mares were returning to estrus after a shortened diestrous period. In some mares this was associated with obvious clinical signs of an acute endometritis and cervicitis accompanied by a profuse purulent vaginal discharge originating from the uterus. There were no signs of systemic involvement, and young nursing foals remained healthy. Stallions that had bred affected mares remained clinically normal although the disease was transmitted venereally.

Bacteriological examination of vaginal exudate on horse blood agar under aerobic conditions failed to demonstrate a possible pathogen. Attempts to isolate a specific virus, mycoplasmal organisms, trichomonads or chlamydial organisms also failed. By the first week of May nearly 50 mares on the stud farm were affected, and it was decided to stop breeding. Similar cases were also reported on other stud farms in the area. Swabs cultured anaerobically yielded several strains of *Bacteroides fragilis*, but these were considered to be opportunist rather than primary pathogens. Cervical swabs that were taken from acute cases, placed in Stuart's transport medium and cultured on chocolate (heated blood) agar under microaerophilic conditions resulted in the growth of gram-negative coccobacilli after 48 hours incubation. Swabs taken directly from the cervix were observed to contain gram-negative coccobacilli that were indistinguishable from similar organisms in the culture. A heavy and, in most instances, pure growth of the organism was isolated from 9 of 10 mares and was considered to be the putative pathogen, based on this initial evidence.

Attempts to culture the same organism from stallions proved more difficult because after 24 hours the culture plates became heavily overgrown with normal genital flora such as *Proteus* sp., coliform bacilli, *Staphylococcus aureus*, micrococci and fecal streptococci. A selective medium was developed incorporating streptomycin, which inhibited the growth of contaminating organisms but allowed the gram-negative coccobacilli to be identified. Using the selective medium the organism was identified from six stallions 42 days after they had stopped breeding mares. It was also shown that the disease could be reproduced by inoculating pure cultures of the coccobacilli through the cervix of clean pony mares in estrus.

Within the Newmarket area several infected stud farms discontinued breeding, but other stud farms in which the disease was present continued to breed mares following prophylactic treatment of mares and stallions. By the end of the breeding season it was estimated that approximately 200 mares and 23 stallions on 29 stud farms were involved in the Newmarket outbreak. The disease was not diagnosed among horses in any other part of England or in any other breed of horse apart from the Thoroughbred. During July of 1977 it was reported that in Ireland cases of genital infection had occurred among Thoroughbred mares, from which similar gram-negative coccobacilli had been isolated. During the same summer a number of countries including the United States, Canada, Australia and New Zealand banned the importation of horses from Britain, Ireland and France, although contagious equine metritis was subsequently diagnosed among horses in Australia during 1977 and in the United States in 1978. In September a Code of Practice to control the disease during 1978 was published in Britain by a scientific committee established by the Horserace Betting Levy Board.[2]

DISTRIBUTION OF CONTAGIOUS EQUINE METRITIS (CEM)

CEM was confirmed among Thoroughbred horses in England, Ireland and Australia during 1977 and in Kentucky in the United States during 1978. The disease has been confirmed among Thoroughbred and other breeds of horses in France during 1978. There is circumstantial evidence to suggest that CEM was present in Ireland in 1976 and France in 1977.

ETIOLOGY

The causal agent of CEM has been investigated in detail by Taylor et al.,[8] who examined the organism in a wide range of cultural and conventional biochemical tests. They found it has a DNA base composition of 36.1 per cent GC and is susceptible to a wide range of antimicrobial agents. The organism is a fastidious, gram-negative, non-acid-fast coccobacillus that is very unreactive in biochemical tests. In conventional tests only the oxidase, catalase and phosphatase tests were positive. Dependence on neither X nor V factors could be demonstrated, but some stimulation of growth by X factor was observed. The organism could not be identified with any known species but Taylor et al.[8] proposed the organism as a new species of the genus

Hemophilus: H. equigenitalis type strain NCTC 11184 (61717/77).

In addition to the streptomycin-resistant strain that has been isolated in Europe, recent reports from the United States suggest the presence of a streptomycin-sensitive strain that may have been introduced as the result of the importation of an infected stallion from France during the summer of 1977. A number of gram-negative coccobacilli that closely resemble the contagious equine metritis organism (CEMO) have recently been isolated from the genital tract of mares and stallions, but on detailed bacteriological and biochemical examination they do not appear to be the same organism.

TRANSMISSION

Field and experimental studies indicate that the disease is spread primarily by venereal transmission, although a number of mares have been infected that had not been bred. In this circumstance, the evidence suggests that the handling of the genital tract of infected mares by stud personnel and the use of contaminated instruments used to examine mares were responsible for the spread of contagious equine metritis (CEM).

PATHOLOGY

Studies in the pathology of CEM have recently been reported by Platt *et al.*[4] They observed that under experimental conditions the principal effects of the disease in the mare appear to be confined to the uterus, in which infection is associated with necrosis and shedding of endometrial epithelium and an intense inflammatory response. Cervicitis and sometimes vaginitis were also observed. Elsewhere in the reproductive tract there were minor changes in the fimbriae of the fallopian tubes, but salpingitis was not a feature. In experimentally infected pony stallions, as in Thoroughbred stallions infected during outbreaks of the disease, there was no reaction to local infection, with the organism persisting on the skin and mucosal surfaces of the external genitalia for an indefinite period.

DIAGNOSIS

Currently the diagnosis of CEM is confirmed by the isolation of the coccobacillus from the genital tract of a mare or stallion. Clinical signs are not always present, although the profuse nature of the discharge and the contagious nature of the disease may lead a clinician to suspect CEM. The recommended sites to swab in the genital tract of the mare are the cervical canal or endometrium and the clitoral fossa, which will include the clitoral sinus. The cervical/endometrial swabs should be taken during the early estrous phase of the cycle. Sites to swab in the male are the urethra, urethral fossa and penile sheath plus a sample of the pre-ejaculatory fluid. The swabs should be placed immediately in Stuart's or Amies' transport medium and sent to the laboratory as quickly as possible, preferably within 24 hours. The coccobacillus generally takes 48 hours to culture in the laboratory, but it is necessary to incubate the plates for 6 days before a negative result can be given.

Other tests in addition to the bacteriological examination of swabs may be utilized, although no one test is able to guarantee a 100 per cent accurate result. The examination of endometrial smears stained either by trichrome[10] or Gram's stain to demonstrate the presence of inflammatory cells and bacteria are examples of such tests. The use of endometrial biopsies to observe the extent of uterine damage[6] is another example.

The presence of antibody in equine sera following CEM infection in the mare has been reported by Benson *et al.*[1] They described reactions in agglutination and antiglobulin tests in sera from infected horses, suspected cases and negative controls. A complement fixation test was used extensively during the outbreak of CEM in Kentucky as an aid to diagnosis.

TREATMENT

Experience from the 1977 Newmarket outbreak suggests that infected mares may be classified into three categories: those cases that recover spontaneously without treatment, those that recover after treatment and those from which the organism continues to be isolated despite treatment. Clinical cases have been treated using a wide variety of antimicrobial agents given by topical or parenteral routes or by a combination of both. A commonly applied treatment for mares includes intrauterine infusion with benzyl penicillin or ampicillin daily for up to 5 days, although the efficacy of this treatment has been difficult to assess.

A satisfactory treatment of stallions involves a thorough cleansing of the external genital organs using a chlorhexidine surgical scrub followed by liberal application of 0.2 per cent nitrofurazone ointment on at least three occasions, either daily or at intervals of 2 or 3 days. Particular attention should be paid to the cleansing and dressing of the folds of the penile sheath and the cavities of the urethral fossa. The majority of stallions accept this procedure quite readily. At present there is a lack of substantiated scientific information about antimicrobial therapy in the mare (dosage, route and duration of use), which is required to prevent problems associated with drug resistance, toxicity and development of a carrier state.

EPIDEMIOLOGY

The breeding of Thoroughbred horses destined to be trained for flat racing is an international activity. Mares visit stallions in distant countries, and stallions are transported across the equator so that they are able to cover mares in the Northern and Southern hemispheres within a period of 12 months. As a result of the increased international movement of horses, which usually occurs by air, the risk of infectious disease being introduced into a susceptible population has greatly increased. On the public stud farm at which the disease was first reported, there were mares that had been on stud farms in six countries during the preceding year.

It is probable that the causal agent of CEM was present in the equine population before 1977. O'Driscoll et al.[2] described an outbreak of venereal infection among Thoroughbred horses in Ireland during 1976 that was clinically and epidemiologically similar to CEM. Before the 1977 outbreak, it was unusual for swabs taken from the genital tract of mares to be examined under anaerobic or microaerophilic conditions. Therefore, a mare with a uterine discharge may have harbored the organism of CEM, even though a negative bacteriological result was obtained with a swab examined under aerobic conditions.

Timoney et al.[9] reported the isolation of the contagious equine metritis organism (CEMO) from experimentally infected pony mares for a considerable period after challenge, and similar findings were reported by Powell and Whitwell[5] among in-foal and barren Thoroughbred horses following natural infection.

In the majority of these natural infections, CEMO was isolated from the clitoral area, including the clitoral sinus,[7] and it is therefore important to examine this area in detail in those mares with a history of the disease. CEMO has also been isolated from the placentae of several known CEM-positive foaling mares,[5] emphasizing the importance of maintaining strict standards of hygiene in the foaling box, especially with mares that have been covered by a positive stallion. A single case of the isolation of CEMO from the penile sheath of a colt foal born to a positive mare has been reported.[7]

The antiseptic precautions practiced on stud farms during the 1977 outbreak appear to have been ineffective in preventing the spread of infection. The introduction of aseptic principles involving greater use of disposable and sterile equipment should act as an effective barrier to the spread of infection.

CONTROL

The Codes of Practice published in Britain and Ireland to control CEM have emphasized the importance of early diagnosis of the disease and the standards of hygiene necessary on the stud farm. The Codes recommend an extensive bacteriological screening program of mares and stallions to identify infected animals. Only after infected animals have been treated and found not to harbor the organism may they then become involved in the breeding program. Recommended stud farm hygiene includes the use of disposable gloves by personnel handling the genitalia of mares and stallions and sterile instruments for the examination of each mare.

Before it can be confidently stated that CEM can be controlled or possibly eradicated, further information is required about the pathogenesis of the disease. Bacteriological screening is the method currently in use to identify animals with positive results, but it has the disadvantage that false negative results may be obtained. In order to reduce this possibility, it is important that swabs are taken in the correct manner and from the appropriate sites and that the procedure is repeated on more than one occasion.

The available evidence suggests that the prevalence of CEM is low, although as the techniques for the culture of the organism become more widely applied, it is possible that the organism will be isolated from equine populations that at present are considered free of the disease. Should the current methods of control prove ineffective in preventing the spread of CEM, the limited use of artificial insemination or the development of a vaccine may require active consideration.

REFERENCES

1. Benson, J. A., Dawson, F. L. M., Durrant, D. S., Edwards, P. T. and Powell, D. G.: Serological response in mares affected by contagious equine metritis 1977. Vet. Rec., *102*:277, 1978.
2. David, J. S. E., Frank, C. J. and Powell, D. G.: Contagious metritis 1977. Vet. Rec., *101*:189, 1977.
3. O'Driscoll, J., Troy, P. T. and Geoghegan, F. J.: An epidemic of venereal infection in thoroughbreds. Vet. Rec., *101*:359, 1977.
4. Platt, H., Atherton, J. G. and Simpson, D. J.: The experimental infection of ponies with contagious equine metritis. Equine Vet. J., *10*:153, 1978.
5. Powell, D. G. and Whitwell, K.: The epidemiology of contagious equine metritis (CEM) in England 1977–1978. Proceedings Second International Symposium on Equine Reproduction (in press).
6. Ricketts, S. W., Rossdale, P. D. and Samuel, C.: Endometrial biopsy of mares with contagious equine metritis 1977. Equine Vet. J., *10*:160, 1978.
7. Simpson, D. J. and Eaton-Evans, W.: Developments in contagious equine metritis. Vet. Rec., *102*:488, 1978.
8. Taylor, C. E. D., Rosenthal, R. O., Brown, D. F. G., Lapage, S. P., Hill, L. R. and Legros, R. M.: The causative organism of contagious equine metritis 1977; proposal for a new species to be known as *Haemophilus equigenitalis*. Equine Vet. J., *10*: 136, 1978.
9. Timoney, P. J., McArdle, J. F., O'Reilly, P. J. and Ward, J.: Infection patterns in pony mares challenged with the agent of contagious equine metritis 1977. Equine Vet. J., *10*:148, 1978.
10. Wingfield-Digby, N. J.: The technique and clinical application of endometrial cytology in mares. Equine Vet. J., *10*:167, 1978.

Surgery of the Equine Reproductive System

J. T. VAUGHAN
Auburn University, Auburn, Alabama

THE MALE HORSE

Surgery of the reproductive system of the male horse is classified according to anatomy and etiology. Anatomically, the penis, prepuce, scrotum and testes constitute the organs important to a discussion of surgery. Inasmuch as it is impossible to differentiate certain processes, such as diseases of the penis from disorders of the urinary system or cryptorchidism from disorders of the abdominal cavity, there are instances in which the discussion may border on other systems. Etiologically, the principal concerns involve injuries, infections (including parasitisms), neoplasms, hernias, congenital anomalies and surgical complications.

Penis and Prepuce

Injuries

Injuries occur during breeding, fighting with other stallions, falling on fences and stall partitions and in various other ways. One of the most serious injuries to the breeding stallion is a kick to the erect penis by a poorly restrained mare. Severe contusions cause hemorrhage and intense inflammatory edema of both penis and prepuce. In contrast to the internal hematoma of the penis in the bull, the parallel injury in the horse usually produces hemorrhage external to the tunica albuginea.

The immediate result of the rapid congestion and edema of the injured part is acute paraphimosis, characterized by an inability to retract the turgid (*vis à vis* tumescent) organ into the prepuce. In fact, the obstacle to retraction may be the inflammatory swelling in the preputial laminae (posthitis) even more than the inflammation of the penis proper (balanitis). Inflammatory swelling and hemorrhage are complicated further by edema of stasis and gravitation caused by the restricted venous and lymphatic drainage in the pendulous state. Also, it seems likely that stagnation of blood in the sinusoidal spaces of the corpus cavernosum penis and corpus spongiosum urethrae is as aggravating a factor in traumatic balanoposthitis as it is in the flaccid paralysis associated with adverse reactions to the phenothiazine-derivative tranquilizers.

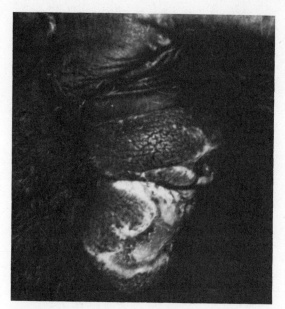

Figure 1. Chronic ulcerated paraphimosis.

Delay in re-establishment of circulation allows for clotting and organization of humoral elements of inflammation, leading quickly to chronic prolapse and either a protracted course of recovery or a refractory condition that may require preputial reefing, surgical retraction (the Bolz technique) or even amputation of the penis.

To mark the progression from acute to chronic paraphimosis, the doughy character of the pitting edema undergoes gradual induration. The thin, glossy skin of the swollen part becomes dry and inelastic, and patchy excoriations develop into indolent ulcers. In this irritated state, the ability to retract the penis may return before the desire to do so. Recovery is predicated in terms of weeks and usually proceeds apace with epithelialization and reduction of scarring (Fig. 1).

Recovery may be interrupted at any point by localized or generalized pathological findings that prevent the normal telescoping of the prepuce and penis. If the problem is focal, a simple elliptical excision of the scar and closure of the wound under suture may be all that is required. If the problem is circumferential and limited to the dermis, a preputial reefing operation is indicated, but this still falls within the classification of revisional skin surgery. If the problem is generalized and involves the penis as well as the prepuce, the two surgical options (after conservative care has been exhausted) are the penis retrac-

tion operation (Bolz technique) and the penis amputation. In both instances, the patient is a gelding or a candidate for gelding in that the subsequent use of the horse as a stallion has been, of necessity, relinquished.

Abrasions of the penis result from exposed breeding sutures used to protect the Caslick closure of the vulva in mares that have been operated on for pneumovagina. Strangulation of the collum glandis may occur with an ill-fitting stallion ring. Obstruction of the urethra may stem from a dissecting hematoma of the sinusoidal tissues of the penis. Rupture of the bladder and urine peritonitis may be a further complication. Disruption of the urethra may produce regional urine cellulitis. Chronic irritation, with or without infection, may result in varices, ulcers and granulomas of the urethra that are manifested as dysuria and hemorrhage on ejaculation (hemospermia). Lacerations and puncture wounds of the penis may also compromise the course of the urethra. Misdirected castration surgery and/or postoperative infections not infrequently cause paraphimosis and other injuries, however unintentional, to the penis and prepuce.

Nonoperative Management. Treatment of acute paraphimosis is directed at early reduction of the edema by promoting improved circulation by massage, hydrotherapy and suspension of the prolapse to relieve the pendulousness. The skin should be protected against maceration with emollients. Pre-existing infections, such as in castration wounds, should be treated vigorously. As soon as mechanically possible, the penis and internal laminae of the prepuce should be manually returned to their normal, retracted position and retained there by a stallion supporter or an improvised nylon mesh bag. This material permits uninhibited urination and is easily cleaned. Alternative, although less desirable, methods include the use of a cylindrical pessary and of retention sutures in the external orifice of the prepuce. Systemic antibiotics, anti-inflammatory drugs and diuretic agents (to reduce edema) are discretionary. Tranquilizers are specifically contraindicated. Stallions should be isolated from mares, preferably out of sight and sound.

Conservative treatment of chronic paraphimosis follows the general guidelines for the acute form, except that greater effort must be directed toward keratolysis of dry, thickened skin; gradual healing of ulcers and excoriations; and resolution of indurated subcutaneous tissues. Retention of the penis in traction should be encouraged and daily care conscientiously maintained until function is restored, bearing in mind that, if nonoperative methods fail, surgery is the alternative. Salvage of a useful stallion is the incentive for much nursing care.

It should be emphasized that free urine output should be confirmed if necessary by catheterization and that until the horse is observed in the natural act of urination, this function should never be taken for granted. The stallion should also be studied carefully upon his first return to the breeding shed. Hemospermia may be inapparent at all other times than on intromission and ejaculation. Prior history of this disorder requires urethroscopy and contrast radiography. Chronic, bleeding lesions of the urethra require special attention for diagnosis as well as treatment. Ascending tract infections must be cultured and urethral mucosal scrapings examined for cytological findings. Granulomas, varices and ulcers can be treated by debridement, curettage or cautery either transurethrally or by urethrotomy. Retrograde medication with infusions or suppositories may be used in conjunction with systemic treatments, such as urinary antiseptics and pH alterants (which are ordinarily acidifiers in herbivores). Sexual rest is mandatory. Exercise *ad libitum* or regulated at the halter is helpful to reduce edema and prevent its return.

Management of sharp wounds of the penis and prepuce should follow the principles that apply to injuries of the hollow organs in general, i.e., provide decompression to areas of occlusion, relieve obstructions (such as encroaching hematomas, abscesses, granulomas), prevent ascending tract infections (especially when the external sphincter has become incompetent) and prevent cicatricial strictures upon healing. Drainage catheters should be used with scrupulous regard for asepsis. If a catheter is left indwelling, it is imperative that a one-way (exit) valve be used to prevent aspiration of air and the attendant contaminants. Even so, it is good practice to change catheters every 24 to 48 hours to avoid accumulation of urine salts. If the catheter is used for bougienage, care should be taken to avoid provoking fresh hemorrhage from

the site of stricture (the wound site). However, if hemorrhage does occur, the catheter should be left in place and sterile irrigations administered until bleeding is controlled so that blood clots are not retained in the bladder and urethra. Even with relatively little special attention, the urethra shows a remarkable capacity for healing if physiological rest and daily hygienic wound care are provided.

Neoplasms and Parasitisms

Neoplasms and parasitisms are discussed in the same section because of gross similarities that require careful diagnostic considerations. Neoplasms may be organized as epithelial or mesenchymal lesions. Epithelial tumors of the hair-bearing skin surface of the external prepuce reflect the same distribution as tumors of the skin anywhere else on the body, such as sarcoids, melanoma, mastocytoma, hemangioma and squamous cell carcinoma. However, the most common tumor of the penis and internal laminae of the prepuce of the horse is the squamous cell carcinoma. Typical lesions are sessile, cauliflower-like growths, often multi-focal, with a gross appearance that may be confused with sarcoid or the benign squamous papilloma of the equine genitalia. Squamous cell carcinoma of the penis and prepuce is slow growing at the outset, and circumscribed lesions can usually be successfully removed surgically by local excision or cryotherapy. Later, deeper invasion of the penis with the possibility of metastasis to the superficial inguinal lymphatics and the lungs makes radical excision necessary. There is, in addition, the predictable tendency to recurrence.[12, 27, 42]

Representative of the mesenchymal tumors of the prepuce and penis is the rare fibrosarcoma. This is not an important group from the standpoint of incidence.[27]

The most significant of the tumor-like lesions is the chronic granuloma caused by the larval migrations of *Habronema* species. This form of granulomatous habronemiasis must be differentiated from squamous cell carcinoma, squamous papilloma and sarcoid in order to establish a rational basis for treatment. Although each type bears identifying features, and much could be said to support the gross morphological diagnosis, a final decision should always depend on the biopsy made in the histo-

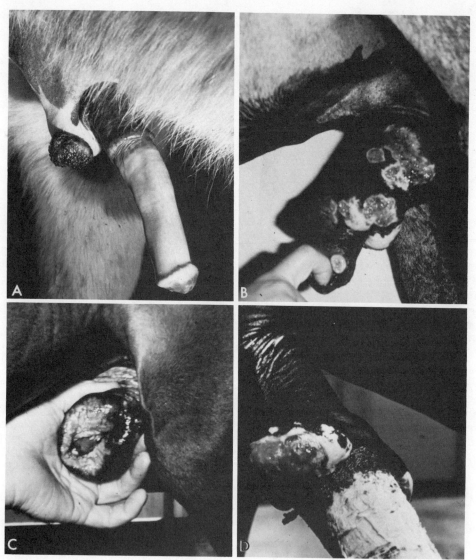

Figure 2.   Habronemiasis granuloma. *A*, Preputial orifice; *B*, preputial ring and inner laminae; *C*, glans penis and urethral process; and *D,* preputial ring.

pathology laboratory. This may be made on a sample or on the lesion *in toto,* in which case the completeness of the excision can frequently be assessed (Fig. 2).

Habronemiasis lesions show a propensity for the urethral process and the preputial ring. The surface of the granuloma may or may not be ulcerated, but oftentimes appears as a raw, red proliferation. Numerous caseous, mulberry-shaped masses are found on the cut surface, which are indistinguishable from the Bollinger's granules seen in botryomycosis. These are surrounded by eosinophilic, histiocytic and lymphocytic infiltrations. The parasite itself may occasionally be demonstrated in the cut paraffin section.

The diagnosis of space-occupying lesions of the penis and prepuce is also confused by the misleading appearances of carcinoma and the occasional occurrence of other diseases. Once it starts to spread, squamous cell carcinoma can cause fixation of the penis within the prepuce (phallocrypsis). It can result in deep-seated abscesses that fistulate to the outside and mimic the inguinal abscess of strangles or other varied causes. Of course, the familiar surface ulcerations and raw, red granulations of superficial carcinoma may closely resemble the *Habronema* granuloma.

Representative of less common diseases of this anatomical region is the microfilariasis attributed to *Onchocerca* and *Se-*

taria species that causes swollen genitals and "erysipelatoid" lesions of the prepuce with dry, crusted and fissured skin and firm, pendulous swellings of the prepuce.[58] Another example that has been described was a spirochete infection of the prepuce and penis, suspected of being caused by the genus *Treponema*. This infection was characterized by multiple circumscribed gummatous lesions and irregular shallow ulcers through the external and internal folds of the prepuce and extending onto the free body of the penis. Spirochetes were found in the semen, and the left testis was observed to be slightly indurated, both findings reminiscent of syphilis in man.[47]

Nonoperative Management. Common lesions frequently treated by means in addition to or other than surgery are sarcoids, *Habronema* granuloma and squamous cell carcinoma. Sarcoids possibly have the greatest diversity of treatments, including the induction of immune response by initial sensitizing injections followed at weekly intervals by repeated infiltrations around the tumor base of bacillus Calmette-Guérin (BCG), tuberculin or bovine transfer factor, with anticipated regression or remission of the lesion during the ensuing weeks. Escharotic therapy has been used with Tn. podophyllin 25 per cent in pine tar applied topically once daily until the lesion gradually sloughed or regressed under eschar. Topical 5-fluorouracil in propylene glycol has been applied daily to the open site of surgical excision as an antimetabolite to reduce the incidence of recurrence. Electrofulguration is an older modality of treatment that has met with varying success. Cryotherapy is a somewhat more recent method that has been widely used in the 1970's, with enthusiastic acceptance by many, for the dual reasons that the local immunity to the viral agent of sarcoid was thought to be enhanced while, at the same time, the frozen lesion was undergoing a slough.

Habronema granulomas, once treated by either thermocautery or surgical excision, are now recognized to be vulnerable to organophosphate medication. It is common practice to treat small lesions topically and large ones both topically and systemically with trichlorfon. The topical form can be prepared by mixing approximately 4.5 gm of trichlorfon in 4 oz. of nitrofurazone cream. This is applied once daily if the lesion is left open and every several days if

the granuloma is placed under bandage. In the context of the present discussion, the first method would have more frequent applications. Systemic medication can be given by mouth as a calculated anthelmintic dose of trichlorfon or by vein at the dosage rate of 22 mg/kg of body weight diluted in 1 to 2 liters of sterile physiological saline solution and administered by slow intravenous drip. Atropine and pralidoxime chloride should be on hand in the event that adverse reactions due to organophosphate toxicity require an antidote.

Nonoperative treatment of squamous cell carcinoma of the penis and prepuce may include radiation therapy by gamma sources such as radon implants placed in the tumor bed following surgical excision. However, this form of treatment is not ordinarily used. By the same token, it would not be inappropriate to use conventional radiotherapy on sites of deeper invasion or on lymphatic metastases, but such instances are thought to be infrequent. Cryotherapy has been reported as successful in treating localized lesions.

Operative Surgery of the Penis and Prepuce

Surgical procedures involving the incised approach include the total or partial circumcision of prepuce (known as the reefing operation), the surgical retraction and fixation of the penis and the amputation of the penis.

Reefing Operation (Posthioplasty). Although posthioplasty is commonly used to refer to total circumcision, it is correct to include partial posthetomy in this discussion. Indications are extirpation of the circumscribed neoplasms that are confined to the dermis, revision of chronic scarring of the prepuce that has resulted from repeated *Habronema* parasitisms, extensive removal of the prepuce necessitated by chronic intractable posthitis and, in rare instances, posthioplasty for congenital anomalies of the prepuce and penis.

Although for different reasons, the objective of both procedures is restoration of the telescoping function of the concentric elastic sleeves that facilitate extension and retraction of the penis. The prepuce is divided into internal and external reflections that are readily opposed by scars, granulomas, neoplasms and other such space-occupying lesions. The surgery consists of the removal of the obstruction and the ap-

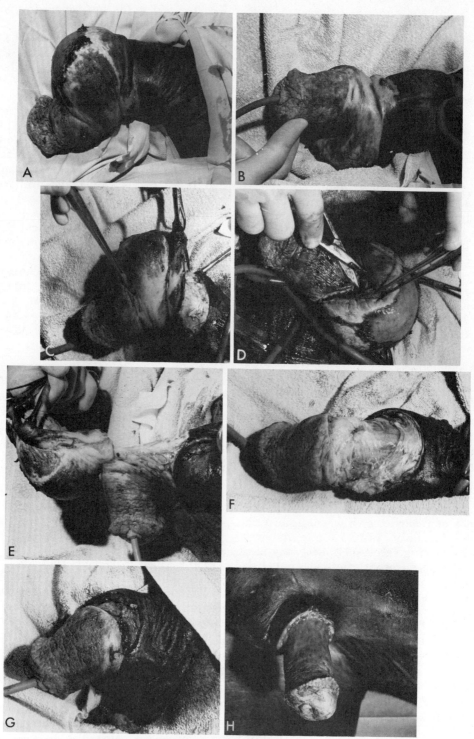

Figure 3. The reefing operation. *A*, Chronic scarring and ulceration of preputial ring; *B*, catheter and tourniquet in place; *C*, dissection of proximal annular incision; *D*, dissection of distal annular incision; *E*, removal of surgical specimen; *F*, ready for reconstruction; *G*, suture closure; and *H*, completed operation.

position under suture of the neighboring normal prepuce. Excision may be in the form of an ellipse for circumscribed lesions or a circle in the case of circumferential lesions, e.g., extensive granuloma scar of the preputial ring. Limited reefing will salvage the use of a breeding stallion. Extensive reefing places such future service in doubt. There are no established safe minimums to use as guides; therefore, discretion of the surgeon must be exercised in each case (Fig. 3).

Success depends on optimum healing with minimal scarring and early return to function. These are insured by control of sepsis and hemorrhage and by accurate reconstruction under suture. The patient is restrained under general anesthesia in dorsal recumbency and prepared for aseptic technique. The urethra is catheterized, and the penis is fixed in forward extension by a traction tape secured around the collum glandis. Surface ulcerations or other breaks in the skin should be disinfected. Use of a tourniquet is optional but advantageous in the face of chronic inflammatory engorgement. Gum rubber tubing secured proximal to the site is satisfactory. The lesion is bracketed by skin incision. The dissection plane is the loose subcutaneous fascia external to the tunica albuginea of the penis. Scissor dissection is helpful. Bleeders should be controlled as identified, loosening the tourniquet periodically for this purpose. The lesion should be isolated from the dissection to prevent contamination by micro-organisms, tumor cells or the like and removed from the field as soon as possible. Suture reconstruction is done in two layers. The subcutaneous fascia is approximated by multiple simple interrupted sutures of 0 medium chromic surgical gut. No attempt is made to quilt fixation points to the underlying tunica albuginea. The skin is closed with interrupted mattress sutures (vertical or oblique) taken with 00 polypropylene. If the suture line is long, it may be permissible, in the interests of time, to close the skin with a continuous vertical mattress suture pattern that is cut and tied at each quadrant. This minimizes the constricting effect of an uninterrupted circular suture line.

Postoperative care should include daily wound hygiene and topical medication as needed and systemic antibiotics for prophylaxis, since it is impossible to render the surgical site free of contaminants. Stallions should be isolated. Skin sutures are left in for 10 to 14 days.

Surgical Retraction of the Penis (Phallopexy). When conservative care has not resulted in recovery of spontaneous retraction and when posthioplasty is not the answer, phallopexy offers an alternative to amputation. The advantages are a simpler procedure with less chance of postoperative complications such as hemorrhage, dehiscence, delayed healing and urethral constriction. The candidate should be a gelding with complete resolution of the castration. Premature phallopexy in the incompletely healed castration site is inadvisable. All nonoperative efforts to reduce the morbid swelling of the penis should have been exhausted. Infection should be controlled, and physical placement of the penis into the prepuce should be possible. Surgical revision of scar tissue may be done in advance or at the same time, although the former is preferred. Epithelialization of ulcerated skin should be essentially complete.

The patient is restrained in dorsal recumbency under general anesthesia with the hindlegs in passive abduction. Strained positions caused by forced abduction predispose to obturator nerve injury. The penis is catheterized, but is neither fixed in traction nor tourniqueted. The field is prepared for aseptic technique. A skin incision 10 cm long is made on the median raphe just behind the castration scar. The loose, subcutaneous fascia is separated by blunt dissection to expose the penis, which is pulled up into the incision sufficiently to expose the annular thickening at the point of attachment of the internal lamina of the prepuce to the free body of the penis. This lies at the forwardmost extent of the plane of dissection. The procedure should be done without unduly disrupting the loose tissue bed of the penis so that vascular and lymphatic pathways remain as little disturbed as possible. The retraction required causes slight sigmoidation of the penis, but dysuria has not been a reported complication. A traction suture of noncapillary synthetic material is placed in the annular thickening on each side of the urethra (identified by catheter location), avoiding entry of the preputial cavity. The suture ends are brought through the skin alongside the incision with eyed needles and then are retained by passing them through a short length of polyvinyl laboratory tubing used

790 *SURGERY OF THE EQUINE REPRODUCTIVE SYSTEM*

as a suture splint. The suture ends on each side can then be pulled in sufficient tension to retract the glans penis into the external preputial orifice. The ends are tied in a bow knot or can be held together by a small clamp so as to permit adjustment of tension and, thus, extent of retraction after the horse regains his feet. It is important to be able to regulate the position of the glans so that it is concealed but not so deeply retracted as to cause urine scald inside the prepuce. This adjustment is difficult to estimate when the patient is lying on his back. After placement of the traction sutures, the loose adventitia is closed with interrupted sutures of fine surgical gut. A Penrose drain is optional. The skin incision is closed with interrupted vertical mattress sutures of polypropylene.

Postoperative care consists of providing daily local wound hygiene and discretionary antibiotic therapy. The site can be kept clean more easily if the patient is restrained standing and given regular exercise at the halter. The use of fly repellents will reduce any self-irritation that might be caused by much switching of the tail between the legs. The traction sutures can be removed after 14 days. Recently gelded horses and those that retain some stallion behavior should be separated from both mares and stallions during the first 2 to 4 weeks. Evaluation should be made after this time in order to allow for recession of swelling and soreness.

Amputation of the Penis (Phallectomy). The common indications for amputation are squamous cell carcinoma of the glans or free body of the penis and intractable paralytic paraphimosis. In the circumscribed carcinoma *in situ,* limited excision may be successful; however, once the lesion has invaded the tunical layer, amputation is necessary. If there is palpable or visible evidence of lymphatic spread or of phallocrypsis, *en bloc* resection offers an alternative to euthanasia. Radiation therapy may also be tried.

The preferred method of management of unresponsive paraphimosis is phallopexy; however, if morbid swelling of the penis (phalloncus) or other changes are so extensive as to prevent mechanical retraction, the last resort must be amputation.

The patient is restrained in dorsal recumbency under general anesthesia. The penis is catheterized, pulled into forward traction and tourniqueted. The field is prepared for aseptic technique. Using the method described by Williams,[17a] a site is chosen well above the pathological process, and a triangular section of skin, subcutaneous fascia, smooth muscle and corpus spongiosum overlying the urethra is carefully dissected away from the urethra. The base of the triangle (3 cm) corresponds to the cross-sectional plane of amputation. The two sides of the triangle (4 cm) represent the bilateral reflections of the urethra as it is spatulated over the cut surfaces of the corpus spongiosum. The apex of the triangle points backward. After the urethra has been exposed, the ventral wall is split and sutured to the skin sides of the triangle with multiple simple interrupted sutures of 00 polypropylene or possibly synthetic surgical gut (polyglycolic acid), which seems to hold up well in the presence of moisture. Closely spaced sutures are necessary to prevent worrisome hemorrhages from the corpus spongiosum, particularly during the immediate postoperative time. The V-shaped spatulation is a safeguard against cicatricial stricture of the urethra after healing.

Once the sides of the urethra are sutured, the remainder of the penis is amputated at the line established by the base of the triangle. The plane of transection is directed slightly craniad from ventral to dorsal, so that urine flow will be diverted downward during the natural act. Before the urethra is sutured in this plane, the individual bleeders must be identified and ligated. Due to chronic hyperemia of the pathological process, some of the vessels are greatly engorged and may require transfixation ligatures. Others may be safely cauterized by electrofulguration. The cut surface of the corpus cavernosum penis can be closed by placement of sutures in the tunica albuginea. It is customary to include the cut edge of the urethra in this layer. Interrupted sutures are preplaced to insure even spacing and to avoid puckering the closure. The first suture bisects the circular cross-section of the penis, passing through the urethra and the tunica albuginea at the center of the urethral groove, up over the corpus cavernosum, down through the dorsalmost centerpoint of the tunica albuginea and thence through the skin. The suture ends are held together with a small clamp while succeeding sutures are placed. The second and third sutures divide the halves into quarters. The next four sutures divide the quarters into eighths, and so on. When enough sutures are preplaced, they are tied in the same sequence. When done properly, the skin is evenly apposed to the urethra, and hemorrhage upon release of the tourniquet is negligible. Nevertheless, it is not unusual for some minor bleeding to occur for the first few postoperative days, particularly during the act of urination. Indwelling catheters are unnecessary. Prophylactic antibiotics are discretionary but usually advisable. If still exhibiting stallion behavior, the patient should be isolated from mares. Healing should be complete in 14 to 21 days.

Complications of phallectomy include hematoma of the suture line, which causes partial or complete dehiscence, and resultant healing by granulation, which may or may not be further complicated by exuberant granulation. This may necessitate debridement or reamputation. Wound infection and urethral stricture are the other important complications.

En Bloc Resection. If invasive or metastatic carcinoma is evident, radical inguinal dissection is sometimes considered as an alternative to euthanasia. Preparation is the same as for simple amputation, except for the tourniquet. The penis may or may not be fixated in retraction (phallocrypsis). Radical dissection differs from the simple form in that the entire prepuce and free body of the penis are removed together with the superficial inguinal lymph glands on both sides — all in one mass. In keeping with good technique of tumor dissection, skin incisions and dissection planes should be located well into normal neighboring tissue, and venous and lymphatic drainage pathways should be controlled and mobilized early in the dissection to prevent further spread at the time of surgery. The surgical specimen should be draped and isolated from accidental contact with normal host tissues, and changes of gloves, linens and instruments should be made as indicated to minimize chance of spread. Amputation of the penis in the perineal region necessitates a urethrostomy, done in much the same way as the operation in the male of the bovine and ovine species. The stump of the penis is sutured into the skin incision so as to permit spatulation of the urethra to the skin. Due to the extensive dissection and unavoidable areas of dead space, Penrose drains are required. For the same reasons, wound hygiene, a clean stable, prophylactic antibiotics and regulated exercise are necessary. All tissues, both preoperative specimens and the surgical specimens, should be submitted for biopsy. Consideration should be given to the feasibility of radiation therapy with the understanding that only in selected cases with access to appropriate clinical facilities would such management be proposed.

Scrotum and Testes

Castration of the normal and the cryptorchid horse and surgical management of complications of castration account for the majority of operative surgery in this region. Correction of hernias, revision of anomalies and production of teasers round out the list.

Castration (Orchiectomy)

Candidates for elective castration are selected on the basis of disposition, trainability and breed characteristics. The operation can be done at any age, although there are advantages for deferment to postpuberty so that the gelding displays masculinity. Selection of bloodstock should depend upon performance testing as well as conformation, and this cannot be well determined until maturity in most cases. For these reasons, a case is made for elective castration no earlier than 2 years of age, although it is conceded that there may be perfectly valid reasons for earlier castration in the individual horse.

In the temperate as well as the subtropical zones, castration by the open method is best done during the cooler months of the year because of the lesser aggravation by insects and the somewhat reduced incidence of wound infection during these seasons. In much of the southern border of the United States and in the nations to the south, screw worms continue to be a problem, necessitating special aftercare of all surgical wounds.

Castration of horses is well established as a field procedure, i.e., one that does not require the use of an operating room or a period of hospitalization. Even when performed at a clinic, the horse is usually treated as an outpatient. This is basically a matter of economics, and the current safety record for general anesthesia of horses has not changed this fact. For so long as this remains the case, the great majority of horses will be operated by the open wound method, with certain complications such as eventration, wound infection and hemorrhage accepted as calculated risks.

Anesthesia. The great change that the procedure has undergone in the past 20 years is the widespread acceptance of humane technique, using either local or general anesthesia. Even the advantages of succinylcholine chloride in speed and physical restraint have not obscured the central fact that its use does not abolish pain. Hence, neuromuscular blockade does not have universal approval, and those who follow this practice continue to find it necessary to justify its existence. There are, of course, other risks associated with suppression of respiration and plasma cholinesterase levels.

Whether the patient is restrained in standing or recumbent position is a matter of choice by the owner or veterinarian. The use of the double-sideline casting harness has been virtually abandoned in light of advanced anesthetic pharmacology. It is debatable if standing castration is much faster than that using the ultrashort general anesthetics, such as thiamylal sodium. The objectionable floundering during induction and recovery periods is less of a problem with the use of combinations of tranquilizers and muscle relaxants for preanesthetic and anesthetic medication. Certainly, cryptorchidectomy and management of hernias, hemorrhages and the like are sufficient reasons for having the capability to do castrations under general anesthesia. The defensible arguments for standing castration include the controllable patient with bilateral testicular descent and no evidence of history of scrotal hernia. Lack of needed assistance and use of facilities unsuitable for safe induction of general anesthesia may have added bearing on the choice. Perhaps the only justification for the use of succinylcholine chloride in castration is for management of the uncontrollable horse, in which case attempts to anesthetize the animal by slower intravenous infusion or by local infiltration would place the personnel at unnecessarily high risk of injury.

Examples of acceptable local anesthetics are mepivacaine hydrochloride and lido-caine hydrochloride 2 per cent solution (with epinephrine). As with most methods, there are at least three alternative methods of infiltration: direct infiltration of the spermatic cords at the superficial inguinal ring, infiltration by long needle (15 cm) of the spermatic cords and infiltration of the testicular parenchyma. In the last mentioned method, anesthesia of the cord occurs by diffusion. Profound skin anesthesia at the sites of scrotal incision usually requires direct subcutaneous infiltration except in the first-mentioned technique, in which scrotal anesthesia may result if enough anesthetic is distributed. Needle sizes vary from 18 to 23 gauge according to the preference of the operator and the sensitivity of the patient. The amount of anesthetic varies from 10 to 30 ml per side, depending on the size of the testis and cord.

General anesthetic, tranquilizer and muscle-relaxant combinations are subject to even wider variation. These include acetylpromazine, promazine, xylazine and diazepam (tranquilizers), pentazocine (analgesic), glyceryl guaiacolate (muscle relaxant), sodium thiopental and thiamylal sodium (barbiturate anesthetics), ketamine hydrochloride (nonbarbiturate anesthetic), halothane and methoxyflurane (inhalant anesthetics) and meperidine hydrochloride (narcotic analgesic).

An example of a combination anesthesia for a 454-kg horse would be 30 to 40 mg of acetylpromazine IV followed in 20 minutes by 2 gm of thiamylal sodium and 50 gm of glyceryl guaiacolate in 1 liter of 5 per cent dextrose solution given rapidly (12- to 14-gauge needle) by gravity flow IV injection. The animal's fall should be controlled by snubbing a strong halter rope to a wall ring or equivalent with a dally (as opposed to a knot) so that tension can be tightened or loosened according to need. The hindquarters can be directed by holding the tail during the casting. If the calculated dose is given and the injection is arrested at that point, surgical anesthesia is provided for 15 to 20 minutes, with a struggle-free recovery. If, on the other hand, the unexpected occurs, such as scrotal eventration, the IV infusion can be resumed by slow drip and the patient maintained under surgical anesthesia for up to an hour or so with little problem. If complications required general anesthesia much beyond an hour, considerable advantage is gained with halothane anesthesia and the capability to give mechanical assistance to ventilation.

Other combinations that have been reported are:[41]

1. Acetylpromazine (0.04 mg/kg) IV followed by glyceryl guaiacolate (100 mg/kg) and thiopental (4 mg/kg) IV.

2. Xylazine (1 mg/kg) IV followed by same as above.

3. Xylazine (1 mg/kg) IV followed by thiopental alone (same dosage).

4. Xylazine (1 mg/kg) IV followed by ketamine (2.2 mg/kg) IV.

5. Diazepam (0.2 mg/kg) IM and xylazine (1 mg/kg) IV followed by ketamine (2.2 mg/kg) IV.

Operative Technique. Despite many variations, all orchiectomies follow a common technique. First, it should take advantage of anesthesia. Second, it should be done with a scrupulous regard for asepsis. This may be only a halo of cleanliness in a generally germy environment, and field procedures cannot duplicate the controlled situation of the operating room. Nevertheless, it should be assumed that all castrations benefit from a surgical scrub of both the site and the surgeon and that aseptic technique is practiced in every way possible.

In the open wound method, orchiectomy is done through the ventral scrotum, and the most common approach is made through two parallel skin incisions lengthwise over the two testes. The incisions should be equidistant from the median raphe and extend the full length of each testis, through the dartos and to the scrotal fascia. Care should be exercised to avoid opening the parietal tunic (tunica vaginalis parietalis) until after the testis has been freed from the scrotum to midway up the extra-abdominal spermatic cord. The dissection plane is the scrotal fascia. Then, an incision is made through the parietal tunic over the cranial pole of the testis and extended upward along the exposed spermatic cord. The testis is prolapsed from the vaginal cavity through this incision, at the same time everting the caudal sac of the parietal tunic over the fingertips so as to provide a handle on the tunic to oppose the retractile action of the external cremaster muscle. The testis now hangs suspended by the mesorchium and visceral pedicle composed of the testicular artery, veins, lymphatics, nerves and ductus deferens. In preparation for amputation, the mesorchium is perforated by the fingertip, and the opening is enlarged sufficiently to admit the jaw of the emasculator. The visceral (or vascular) pedicle is divided separately and apart from the musculofibrous component of the spermatic cord, which prevents stretching the testicular artery at the time of emasculation and minimizes serious hemorrhage (all other things being equal). After the musculofibrous cord is divided with the emasculator, remaining loose tags of scrotal fascia are trimmed to prevent obstacles to drainage.

Minor hemorrhage stops spontaneously if the wound is undisturbed and the horse is kept quiet for a few minutes. If hemorrhage continues, the wound should be explored for the source, most often the testicular artery. If this is the case, the artery should be ligated immediately by slipping a snare ligature of No. 2 chromic gut over kidney forceps (Stille vessel clamps or equivalent) used to cross-clamp the arterial stump. If circumstances do not permit ligation, the alternative is sterile gauze packing retained with sutures or clips in the scrotal incision. The adjunctive use of systemic exogenous clotting factors such as conjugated mare estrogens may be of value.

Postoperative care includes tetanus immunization, wound hygiene and regulated exercise to facilitate drainage from the open wound. Insect irritation can be controlled by use of topical insect repellents around the wound. The use of topical and systemic antibiotics is optional, depending on the cleanliness of the environment and the reliability of the attendants. Given an either/or choice, liberal exercise in a clean surrounding would be of greater benefit than antibiotics and no exercise. Usually, however, we are faced with a compromise choice.

Observation during the healing period is emphasized. The greatest risk is during the initial 24-hour postoperative period. In one series of 371 cases, small intestinal eventration occurred in 11 horses. Seven eventrations happened within 2 hours, one in 4 hours, two in 24 hours and one 6 days later. Although this accounts for only a small number of the total cases, it must be remembered that 11 elective procedures turned into emergencies with an ominous mortality rate of 63.6 per cent.[30]

In addition, hemorrhage of consequence can also take place during the first postoperative day, as a rule, but there are unusual instances of late-occurring hemorrhages after the first day. One case of hemorrhage followed heavy exercise that was allowed prematurely in the first convalescent week.

Penile paralysis from adverse reaction to the use of a phenothiazine tranquilizer (promazine, acetylpromazine) becomes a major problem if unattended for even 12 hours. In fact, if recovery of retractility of the penis fails to occur within 4 to 8 hours, the use of a suspensory should be considered without further delay.

Unusual edema of the scrotum and prepuce, with or without paraphimosis, may herald wound infection and should receive early attention. A sudden fever rise may indicate wound infection, or it may mean no more than putrefaction of a retained blood clot in a poorly drained wound. Such infections can lead to chronic complications, namely, champignon (a streptococcosis of the spermatic cord stump), botryomycosis (a staphylococcosis of the cord) and aggravated paraphimosis, even penile paralysis. Septicemia and peritonitis are representative of acute complications. Survivors of either group must be subjected to further surgery upon localization of the wound infection for incision and drainage of the inguinal abscess and debridement of the purulent sinuses and chronic inflammatory granulomas of the cord stumps.

Primary closure castration technique is done with the patient restrained in dorsal recumbency under general anesthesia. Aseptic surgery is presumed. The skin incision is oriented with the spermatic cord, extending upward to the proximity of the superficial inguinal ring. The incision is deepened through the parietal tunic into the vaginal cavity, exposing the visceral components of the cord. The incision is extended sufficiently to permit exteriorization of the testis and adnexa (after cutting the gubernacular ligament). The visceral cord is then ligated and amputated, and the stump is returned to the vaginal cavity. The parietal tunic is closed with gut sutures, then the fascia is closed and, finally, the skin. Operative time for both sides is about 30 minutes. Aftercare includes moderate regular exercise, tetanus prophylaxis and discretionary use of antibiotics.[29, 34]

Cryptorchidism

The transabdominal migration of the fetal testis during the first 9 months of gestation may be attributed to both testicular migration and differential growth of the fetus. An example is the testicular hypertrophy due to increasing numbers of interstitial cells up to about 7 1/2 months of gestation, after which regression occurs (to a greater degree in the right testis than in the left). Distally, the testis is attached to the inguinal region by a column of mesenchyme known as gubernaculum, divided into intra-abdominal and extra-abdominal parts, as it descends into the peritoneal eversion forming the vaginal process. For the first 8 1/2 months, these structures grow at nearly the same rate, except that the caudal gonadal ligament (forerunner of the proper ligament of the testis) lengthens more rapidly than the gubernaculum (future ligament of the tail of the epididymis), which causes a wide separation between the caudal pole of the testis and the cauda epididymis. This accounts for the fact that the cauda epididymis may occupy the vaginal process inside the inguinal canal as early as the fifth month of gestation. Owing to the length of the caudal gonadal ligament, hypertrophy of the fetal testis, small diameter of the vaginal ring and lack of tension on the gubernaculum, descent of the testis through the inguinal canal does not occur until the eleventh month, by which time testicular regression and differential development of the vaginal process (producing increased tension on the gubernaculum) combine to usher the testis into the inguinal canal where it resides until after birth. This is in contrast to the human, in whom the testes reach the scrotum by the end of the eighth month of gestation.[24, 44, 50, 52]

The cause of maldescent remains unresolved and, indeed, may be due to several factors. Studies in the human have proposed (1) defective hypothalamic-pituitary axis and deficiency of luteinizing hormone, which fails to explain the more commonplace (3 to 5 times) unilateral cryptorchidism; (2) mechanical defect, i.e., gubernacular abnormality; (3) genetic factor, based on familial and inherited tendencies; (4) defect in the testis itself, resulting in a deficiency of the testicular production of androgens, which influence the ductus deferens, epididymis and gubernaculum during descent (or a defect in the end-organs themselves, resulting in a different response to testicular androgens), which may offer the best answer for unilateral cryptorchidism and (5) testicular dysgenesis based on abnormal testicular chromosomes.[50]

In the horse, abdominal cryptorchidism shows an interruption of development at the 5-month fetal stage, with or without descent of the cauda epididymis.[52] Despite the effectiveness of human chorionic gonadotropin (HCG) in the treatment of undescended testes in man,[50] use of HCG for treating abdominal cryptorchidism in the horse is considered unjustified by some.[52] Clinical impressions tend to support this claim and increase the dependence on surgery for rectifying the problem.

Prevention, on the other hand, appears to rest on the public conscience, which shows an amazing disregard or ignorance of the fact that equine cryptorchidism is considered to be an inherited abnormality. Although in other species it is classified as a recessive trait, the disorder in horses in reputedly a dominant inheritance.[31, 48] Interestingly, of 29 equine breed associations reporting to the AVMA Council on Veterinary Service (published in 1976) on unacceptable surgical procedures for eligibility and qualification for registration with the respective breed association, only one, the Appaloosa Horse Club, Inc., specified "surgical correction of cryptorchidism or monorchidism." Only two, the Spanish-Barb Breeders Association and the American Suffolk Horse Association, specified surgical correction of hereditary defects or procedures that mask hereditary defects. The National Trotting and Pacing Association, Inc., and the United States Trotting Association specified "surgical correction of inguinal or umbilical hernia, without castration."[5] In a retrospective study of 350 cases of cryptorchidism seen over a 14-year period at a large midwestern United States university clinic, 49 per cent of the cases were observed in Quarter Horses, as compared with 4 per cent for American Saddle Horse, 3.7 per cent Arabians, 3.1 per cent Standardbred and 1.4 per cent Thoroughbred.[54] Unacceptable surgical procedures reported by the American Quarter Horse Association were "removal of white spots, cosmetic ear surgery and tail surgery."[5]

Analysis of cases has revealed the probabilities of distribution. Of a series of 350 cases, 59.4 per cent of the cryptorchid testes were abdominal,[54] which compares favorably with another series of 417 cases in which 60.2 per cent were abdominal.[35] Unilateral cryptorchidism in the two series ranged from 86 per cent of 350 cases to 93 per cent of 417 cases, 7 to 14 times the incidence of bilateralism, an even higher statistic than for humans. Unilateralism favored the left side from 53 per cent of 350 cases to 65 per cent of 417 cases, except for the fact that in position, the inguinal retention occurred more commonly on the right side (58 per cent of 350 cases). Conversely, 75 per cent of the abdominal retentions occurred on the left side, reminding us of Smith's observation that the regression of the hypertrophied fetal testis appeared to be slower on the left side.[35, 52, 54]

Diagnosis. Diagnosis of cryptorchidism has long been a source of speculation and much discussion. Since known castrates may exhibit stallion behavior[8, 13] and since many candidates for cryptorchidectomy have histories of previous (unsuccessful) surgery, the patient is not infrequently presented as a diagnostic problem. Short of exploratory surgery, the common diagnostic approaches include: (1) external palpation of the scrotum and superficial inguinal rings, (2) pelvic palpation *per rectum* and (3) laboratory testing for plasma androgen concentrations.

External palpation is done to detect the retractile testis lying just outside the superficial inguinal ring, the inguinal testis that is occasionally palpable through the ring or the scarred stump of the spermatic cord. The horse must be controllable, and relaxation of both horse and examiner is necessary. The examination may be facilitated by prior tranquilization or sedation of the patient.

Palpation *per rectum* places the same premium on cooperation. Correct diagnosis on the basis of this method has been reported in as many as 88 per cent of 350 cases that were confirmed at the time of surgery.[54] Objectives are palpating the testis *per se* or the ductus deferens entering the vaginal ring or noting the absence of the same. It is not difficult to trap the cryptorchid testis against the wall of the caudal abdomen by carefully sweeping the region of the deep inguinal ring with the hand in the relaxed rectum. The soft, hypoplastic testis can be felt to slip under the fingertips or the edge of the hand as it passes from the linea alba upward toward the vaginal ring. A full bladder will interfere and may necessitate catheterization or voluntary urination before the examination can be completed. Palpation of the vaginal ring just cranial to the pelvic inlet is done most easily by feeling the caudal abdominal wall from the midlateral region downward to detect the slitlike opening in the parietal peritoneum. If the epididymis has descended into the vaginal process, the ductus can be felt entering the ring. Absence of pulsations differentiates it from the external pudendal artery. Of course, this does not obviate the possibility that the testis may still reside in the abdomen, but it does at least insure the chances of retrieval by a noninvasive procedure (in the sense of peritoneal cavity).[3, 4, 46, 54]

Laboratory assay of androgen levels in the plasma has become a useful way to detect the presence of testicular tissue in questionable animals, particularly those not yielding easily to physical examination and those with a history of previous surgery. The test is based on the Leydig cell elaboration of testosterone in increased amounts in response to the injection of human chorionic gonadotropin (HCG); hence, the frequent reference to the HCG test. The procedure calls for the comparison of testosterone levels in paired plasma samples harvested from heparinized blood drawn at 0 minutes and 30 to 120 minutes after the intravenous injection of 6000 to 12,000 IU of HCG.[13, 14, 16] Testosterone and other plasma androgens are measured by either competitive protein-binding assay (CPBA) or radioimmunoassay (RIA).[3] Basal concentrations of testosterone in the stallion range widely from <100 pg/ml to >1500 pg/ml. In one study of known geldings, the values averaged 15.3 pg/ml. In previously castrated animals that were presented as "false rigs" (ostensible cryptorchids), the mean basal concentration of testosterone was 17.7 pg/ml. In true cryptorchids the comparative mean was 423 pg/ml. Between 0 and 120 minutes following intravenous injection of 12,000 IU of HCG, testosterone levels in the plasma of the stallion experienced a 4- to 30-fold increase. In geldings, the highest concentrations were from about a 1.5- to 3-fold increase above the average. The comparative figures for "false rigs" did not differ significantly from that for geldings. This has also been shown to be true for castrates with intact epididymides ("proud cut").[16, 17] In contrast, HCG response in cryptorchids demonstrated greater than a 3-fold increase of the mean within 30 minutes postinjection.[16] The technique varies somewhat in human testing, in which the child is given HCG, 2000 IU daily for 4 days, and plasma assay is run on the fifth day. If normally responsive gonads are present, there may be as much as a 10-fold increase over baseline. The point is made, however, that any rise in the testosterone level after HCG treatment is evidence of functioning testicular tissue until proved otherwise.[50] It has also been observed that individual cryptorchid horses with low initial testosterone concentrations show a tendency to respond more to HCG than those with higher initial concentrations.[16]

Other work has sought to compare the total estrogen levels in plasma of male horses; levels were significantly higher in the bilaterally cryptorchid animal and higher in the animal with a cryptorchid testis than in one with a scrotal testis in unilaterally cryptorchid animals. The lowest levels were in the gelding. Thus, it was hypothesized that simultaneous measurement of total estrogen and androgen levels in horses may be a more useful method to determine the presence of viable testicular tissue than the HCG test.[23]

Operative Technique. The undescended testis can be approached through (1) the inguinal canal, (2) the ventral abdominal wall (paramedian) or (3) the lateral abdominal wall (flank). Experienced and ardent advocates can be found to support the advantages of each. It may be safe to say that if sufficient numbers of patients are presented under varied circumstances, one might justify the use of all three.

INGUINAL APPROACH. With the patient restrained under general anesthesia in dorsal recumbency and prepared for aseptic surgery, a skin incision approximately 10 cm long is made over and aligned with the superficial inguinal ring. Accidental injury to the large subcutaneous branches of the external pudendal vein should be avoided. The inguinal fascia is separated with the fingertips, and the inguinal canal is explored for the vaginal process and contents or for the scarified stump of spermatic cord of the castrate. Notation of skin scar and inguinal fibrosis raises expectation of the latter, but only the demonstration of all the components of the spermatic cord, including ductus deferens, vessels, tunica vaginalis and external cremaster muscle, should serve to cancel the further search for the retained testis. In not a few instances, the epididymis is amputated in the mistaken belief that it is a hypoplastic inguinal testis. In such cases, the testis is retained in the abdomen and usually requires invasion of the peritoneal cavity.

If the vaginal process is encountered, it should be grasped by forceps and retracted to permit incision, revealing the gubernaculum, epididymis and ductus deferens. The incision can be lengthened by either scissor or fingertip toward the vaginal ring, and gentle traction on the epididymis will produce the small, soft testis most often found.[3, 59] A characteristic feature is the increased length of the caudal gonadal ligament (proper ligament of the testis) separating the caudal aspects of the testis and epididymis.

If search fails to yield the vaginal process or if it is thought to be inverted, the forceps technique of Adams can be employed to grasp the gubernaculum through the rudimentary vaginal process (presumed to exist). Curved 10-inch Foerster sponge forceps are manually guided into the deep (internal) inguinal ring to the peritoneal covering of the vaginal ring. The partially opened jaws are pressed carefully into the vaginal process and closed, so as to grasp a small fold of the process. Care must be taken not to tear the peritoneum. The inverted process is retracted into the canal until it can be seen. Palpation through the process will reveal the cordlike gubernaculum. A small incision in the process can be made safely with Mayo dissecting scissors, and access is thus provided for grasping the gubernaculum, retraction of which produces the epididymis and finally the testis.[3]

Alternatively, the index and middle fingers can be introduced through the vaginal ring to grasp the gubernaculum, epididymis or ductus deferens.[39, 53] Retrieval of the testis follows retraction of these structures. The procedure is facilitated by dietary reduction of colon bulk and by elevation of the hindquarters (using differential padding or an inclined plane). A variation of this technique is to perforate the medial muscular wall of the inguinal canal just inside, or just outside, the superficial inguinal ring. In the latter case, the aponeurosis of the external oblique muscle must also be perforated. In all three instances, the search is conducted in much the same way. In the event the limited exploration is unsuccessful, the coned fingers are used to enlarge the opening so as to admit the hand. The pelvic inlet is explored for the respective ductus, leading from the ampulla in the genital fold above the urinary bladder, over the lateral ligament of the bladder to the epididymis of the retained testis. It is advantageous to use the right hand to explore the left canal and the left hand to explore the right canal so that the palm and flexor surfaces of the fingers face medially and backward.[53] If it is necessary to introduce the hand in small subjects, it is better to use the paramedian or flank approach to avoid unnecessary disruption of the inguinal canal. This is also advisable if the testis is tumorous and too large to deliver through the canal.[15, 35]

The exteriorized testis and epididymis can be amputated with angiotribe forceps and ligature or simply with an emasculator. If the funiculus is too short to permit exteriorization, a chain écraseur can be used. Lacking that, a snare ligature can be slipped over the retracting forceps and tightened around the funiculus inside the abdomen. Blunt pointed scissors can be manually guided into the abdomen to amputate a safe distance from the ligature. On other occasions, an emasculator has been manually introduced inside the abdomen, but great caution must be exercised to avoid accidental injury to the bowel or mesentery.

Following orchiectomy, the wound is closed under suture in three layers. The superficial inguinal ring, which is a slit in the aponeurosis of the external abdominal oblique muscle, is closed with either surgical gut or polyglycolic acid (PGA) synthetic No. 2 gut double-strand, in a simple continuous pattern. The secret in the strength of the repair is to initiate the row beyond the cranial end of the ring and terminate it beyond the caudal end to avoid unnecessary distraction and tension on the end knots. A flat hernia needle is used to facilitate manual placement without breaking asepsis, which occurs inevitably when sharp-pointed needles are so used. The distance from needle hole to ring margin is staggered to avoid common stress lines. The pattern is vertical, i.e., perpendicular to the principal direction of fibers. Approximately six bites are necessary to close the ring. Slight adduction of the corresponding thigh during the closure reduces the distraction of the ring margins.

The second suture layer consists of interrupted gut or PGA sutures in the inguinal fascia, and the third layer is a row of interrupted mattress sutures of noncapillary nylon or polypropylene in the skin incision. Primary closure of cryptorchidectomy incisions is axiomatic if aseptic procedure has been followed. The only excuse for packing such wounds today is the presence of gross contamination, which may occur in the field procedure but should never be accepted as a part of the surgical plan. If the primary closure is done as described, herniation, eventration or abscess are not anticipated sequelae.

Postoperative care is the same provided for any such procedure that involves the abdominal wall and peritoneal cavity, whether "invasive" or not. The horse should be allowed the use of a private box stall with clean bedding, fresh water and light hay. Hand-walking can be started the first 24 hours after surgery and gradually increased as soreness subsides. Paddock exercise *ad libitum* may be permitted by the second or third day, if the horse is confined to a private paddock. Skin healing should allow suture removal in 10 days. Tetanus immunization is mandatory, and use of prophylactic antibiotics is discretionary.

PARAMEDIAN APPROACH. Preparation and restraint parallel that described for the inguinal approach. A 10-cm longitudinal skin incision is made 6 to 8 cm off the midline and alongside the external preputial orifice. Because it is extensile, the incision can be readily extended caudad for easier access to the region of the deep inguinal ring. Parenthetically, this is much the same approach as used for access to surgery of the urinary bladder in the male. This plane of dissection is deepened progressively through the superficial and deep abdominal fascia, the conjoined aponeuroses of the external and internal abdominal oblique muscles (superficial sheath of the rectus) and the longitudinal fibers of the rectus abdominis muscle. The aponeurosis of the transversus abdominis muscle (deep sheath) can be incised in the same longitudinal plane, which transects its fibers, or it can be split transversely with its fibers, employing the principle of a grid incision. The fatty layer of fascia transversalis lies just underneath and covers the final layer, the peritoneum, which is perforated to admit the hand. Again, exploration is facilitated by reduced bulk in the colon and the elevation of the hindquarters. The wound margins can be retracted manually or mechanically, according to the surgeon's preference. The retrieval of the testis follows the same procedure as described previously. An advantage of this method is that bilateral abdominal testes can be removed through the one incision, with some slight preference expressed for the left paramedian incision in such cases. It may be necessary, however, to use écraseur for other remote access techniques for the contralateral testis. A disadvantage is that its use is confined to the abdominal cryptorchid, necessitating accurate preoperative diagnosis.[15, 35]

Closure of the incision is subject to some variation. Peritoneal suture is optional. The deep sheath of the rectus should be closed with gut or PGA sutures. However, this layer will support very little tension, and continuous sutures must be preplaced, tensing several bites at once to avoid tearing the thin aponeurosis. The main purpose of this layer is to keep the fat of the underlying tissue out of the ensuing closure. The next layer is taken in the superficial sheath and provides the major support. Although gut has been used successfully, it is my preference to use a nonabsorbable synthetic (nylon, Dacron or polypropylene) in a continuous, imbricating mattress pattern (modified Mayo), starting and finishing beyond the ends of the incision to eliminate the weakpoint of knot-break strength. Care should be taken to exclude fat and muscle from the overlapped interface of aponeurosis. The edge is sutured down with a continuous row of the same suture. The superficial abdominal fascia is closed with interrupted sutures of gut placed in reverse so as to invert the knots. The skin is closed with interrupted mattress sutures of a noncapillary synthetic. Aftercare is the same as previously described.

FLANK APPROACH. This method is performed as a field procedure on the standing horse under sedation and local anesthesia. As with the paramedian approach, its use is confined to the abdominal cryptorchid, and the location of the testis must be known beforehand. The flank site also offers an alternative approach for access to the unilateral testicular tumor (commonly teratoma). In this case, surgery is usually done on the patient restrained in lateral recumbency under general anesthesia because of the obvious benefits afforded by relaxed abdominal musculature. Inasmuch as only grid incisions are made in the lateral abdominal wall, delivery of large masses through such incisions is mechanically impractical, if not impossible, in the standing patient.

The practicality of the standing operation, however, is that both in the horse undergoing surgery for abdominal cryptorchidism and in the mare for ovariectomy the procedure can be performed satisfactorily in the field without the facilities or assistance required for responsible administration of general anesthesia. It has been adopted as a routine approach by many practitioners who prefer this method especially for the retention of a unilateral abdominal testis. Therefore, any balanced discussion of the subject requires its inclusion.

Sedation is provided by tranquilization (see discussion under Castration) with or without sedation by intravenous chloral hydrate, 7 per cent solution or stronger concentrations combined with magnesium sulfate. Local anesthesia is by line infiltration or inverted L field block of the incision site with 2 per cent lidocaine or mepivacaine. Preoperative medication with intravenous hydrocortisone sodium succinate suppresses the noxious effects on circulation when the peritoneal cavity is invaded in the conscious horse.

A 15- to 20-cm transverse skin incision is made in the midflank, equidistant from the last rib and the tensor fasciae latae. The superficial fascia is divided in the same plane. The external oblique muscle is divided in the direction of its fibers running caudoventrad from the rib. The internal oblique muscle is divided in the cranioventral direction. The transversus abdominis muscle is divided in the plane of the skin incision, and the peritoneum is perforated with the fingertips. At this point, additional local anesthetic can be used topically to give deeper anesthesia of the peritoneum. The left hand, with the palm upward and backward, is used to explore the left side; the right hand, the right side. Upon entering the peritoneal cavity the palm of the hand, turned upward to locate the kidney, is passed caudally to identify the mesorchium, which extends from the region behind the kidney caudoventrad toward the inguinal canal. This leads directly to the testis. If a visceral mass makes this difficult, the pelvic inlet can be explored for the ductus deferens (see earlier discussion). When located, the testis is exteriorized for emasculation. Again, in the case of the short funiculus, écrasement or blind emasculation may be required. In the case of misadventure in removing an inguinal testis, there is every likelihood that successful removal will require a second approach through the inguinal canal. In the bilateral abdominal cryptorchid, it is possible, but difficult, to remove both testes through the one side, and the procedure does require a remote amputation.[57]

The flank wound is closed easily with individual layers of simple interrupted gut sutures to appose the separated planes of muscle and to obliterate dead space. The peritoneum is not sutured. The superficial abdominal fascia should be closed carefully with No. 2 gut interrupted sutures. The skin incision is apposed with interrupted mattress sutures of noncapillary synthetic material. Aftercare parallels that of the other approaches.

Scrotal Hernia

Inguinal hernia occurs in both sexes and may be congenital or acquired, emergency or elective, reducible or strangulated, correctable or irreparable, inherited or not. Heritability[48] remains somewhat of a moot issue in some cases, such as whether the mature stallion that herniated while breeding a mare may have had a predisposing weakness since birth. Although some surgeons have performed scrotal herniorrhaphy without castration,[7] the practice borders on malpractice and of course is in express violation of the rules of several breed associations.[5] The lay public should be able to look to the profession for guidance in such matters, and if we vacillate on the issues, the layman can scarcely be expected to do better. Herniorrhaphy without castration is certainly no technical feat and nothing to brag about; rather it is something to explain and show cause for. In such instances as the breeding stallion, if there has been no evidence of scrotal hernia as a familial problem, correction with retention of the testes may be justified, but the records should clearly show the conditions that dictated such a decision.

Hernia may first appear in the newborn in which there is defective development of the inguinal canal. The hernial ring is large, and the contents can be easily reduced with very little concern for strangulation. In fact, if the foal strains at the bowel movement, e.g., meconial obstipation, the worry is that the hernia will enlarge. Surprisingly, if there is no such complication, some of these hernias will correct themselves spontaneously. This does not reduce the need for vigilance against strangulation but does argue the case for watchful waiting. Meanwhile, in the absence of other problems, the foal grows stronger, muscles gain tone, anesthetic risk diminishes and tissues will provide better support to sutures if surgery is necessary. Such individuals should be marked for castration whenever the proper time arrives. The only justification for delaying castration is to allow for development of masculine traits.

The visible and reducible hernia is known, and treatment is elective. There should be little problem in dealing with these. It is the obscure hernia, recurrent or not, that causes problems either as a complication of castration (eventration)[30] or as a strangulation. Although inguinal or scrotal swelling is not a consistent feature of scrotal hernia, if there is a history of such (characterized by occurrence and disappearance) in the candidate for castration, time should be taken to palpate *per rectum* for enlargement of the vaginal rings prior to surgery. If this is suspected, primary closure of the castration wound is warranted.

The strangulated hernia is presented as an acute colic, characteristically of small intestinal locus. It need not be in a breeding stallion, although if such signs occur directly after breeding, strangulated hernia should be assumed until proved otherwise. Some cases are difficult to diagnose because there may be no externally visible or palpable evidence of the hernia. The entrapped limb of small intestine (usually the case) may be confined to the inguinal canal. Even on palpation *per rectum*, it can be misdiagnosed as torsion of the spermatic cord. However, this does not alter the course of action, which is surgical invasion of the inguinal canal. One instance of this diagnosis is recalled with some embarrassment, as it was made at the time of an exploratory laparotomy through the linea alba. This serves to underscore the importance of a searching palpation *per rectum* on every case when possible.

Herniorrhaphy Procedure. It should be understood that the preoperative preparations will range across the full spectrum of possibilities already alluded to; therefore, the discussion of the procedure simply addresses the mechanics that are common to all.

The patient is restrained under general anesthesia in dorsal recumbency and prepared for aseptic surgery. The skin incision is made over the superficial inguinal ring and extended downward over the scrotum for the distance required by the size of the hernia. Complicating adhesions will necessitate more extensive dissections. The tunica vaginalis parietalis is freed from scrotal fascia by blunt dissection, and the hernial contents are "milked" back into the peritoneal cavity. A time-honored method of doing this and simultaneously retaining the reduction until ligated is to twist the tunica (with the testis in the fundus of the sac) on itself, winding up the cord as it were, to obliterate the vaginal cavity and force the intestines out. This presumes the hernia to be reducible. Then, the cord is ligated with transfixation at the level of the superficial ring. The cord is transsected, and the stump is allowed to retract into the inguinal canal. The closure of the ring and other layers parallels that described for inguinal cryptorchidectomy.

If the hernia is irreducible, the parietal tunic must be opened, incarcerated intestines freed of adhesions and decompressed of gas or fluids and the hernial ring enlarged if necessary to permit return of the hernial contents to the abdomen. If the hernia is strangulated, the preferred course is decompression of the intestine (if required) and return to the abdomen. If viability of the gut has been compromised, resection is necessary. It may be possible to extend the contents sufficiently to provide room for this. The alternative is to reduce and return the devitalized bowel to the abdomen and exteriorize it through a ventral laparotomy. The justification is that the architecture of the inguinal canal is preserved, undesirable traction on bowel and mesentery is avoided, and resection and anastomosis can be done without tension. In such cases, the inguinal canal and abdomen must be treated as contaminated, and appropriate safeguards such as drains and prophylactic antibiotics should be used.

Reconstruction of the canal has been described previously.

Space-Occupying Lesions of the Scrotum and Testes

A differential diagnosis should consider the major possibilities: (1) orchitis, which in turn may be sterile and possibly accompanied by seroma or hematoma or septic with abscess; (2) cyst of the testis, e.g., hematocyst; (3) effusion of the vaginal cavity, e.g., hydrocele and hematocele; and (4) neoplasm.

Orchitis may result from trauma, such

as a kick, or from infection, although the latter is somewhat less frequent a cause in the horse than in other domestic species.[48] Fluctuation is not a reliable diagnostic feature in such cases because of the tension under the tunica albuginea as well as the plaque of scrotal edema that so often overlies the testis. Therefore, differentiation of seroma, hematoma and abscess will likely depend upon needle aspirates and signs of leukocytosis, fever and pain, if not ultimately upon surgical incision for drainage.

The cystic testis may present a problem in the abdominal cryptorchid as well as the horse with a scrotal testis. In the former case, much of the parenchyma has been displaced by serous fluid, which may account for an increase in size by several times that of the normal gonad. Paracentesis may be effective in reducing it sufficiently so that it can be removed through an inguinal approach. In the animal with a scrotal testis, a hematocyst is usually the result of trauma, and the physical findings are that described under Orchitis.

Serous effusion of the vaginal cavity or hydrocele in the horse is more common following castration and is characterized by a painless, noninflammatory, fluctuant swelling that gives the appearance of a scrotal testis. Paracentesis yields clear peritoneal fluid. Hematocele is the presence of whole blood, usually clotted, in the same space and is thought to be caused by trauma.[25]

Neoplasms of the equine testis are uncommon, but do occur with sufficient frequency to be a diagnostic consideration. Teratoma is the most important testicular tumor in the horse, and the equine accounts for the greatest incidence of this tumor type among the domestic animals. Teratomas are composed of multiple tissues foreign to the part in which they arise, e.g., bone, cartilage, skin, hair, epithelial ducts, dentigerous cyst formation, mammary tissue and nerves. They may be bilateral, occur during the first 5 years of age, and affect the cryptorchid testis in as many as 25 per cent of the cases.[12, 42] The large size of some lesions necessitates laparotomy for successful removal.[18]

Other neoplasms of the equine testis include seminoma, Sertoli cell tumor and interstitial cell adenoma, all rare but reported, usually in the older stallion.[42] Unilateral lesions may be removed and the fertility of the horse salvaged if the opposite testis is normal.[25]

Surgical management of these masses is by incision and drainage or resection. Techniques employed are those used for castration and cryptorchidectomy as well as for complications of these operations.

Vasectomy and Epididymectomy

Production of teasers for the breeding industry has used various methods, including penile deviation (retroversion),[6] epididymectomy[19] and vasectomy.[49] The advantage of the retroversion is that accidental intromission is prevented; however, the method has not been adopted for general use since its description 24 years ago.[6] The epididymectomy has stimulated some interest, but there is concern about the likelihood of sperm granuloma. A technique of vasectomy that can be performed as field surgery has been proposed more recently.[49]

The patient is restrained in lateral or dorsal recumbency under intravenous general anesthesia and prepared for aseptic surgery. A skin incision is made over the caudomedial aspect of one testis near the median raphe of the scrotum and is aligned with the oblique course of the ductus deferens in its ascent from the cauda epididymis to the spermatic cord. The incision is deepened through the dartos, fascia and parietal tunica vaginalis to open the vaginal cavity. The ductus is exteriorized and a 2-cm section excised, double-ligating the cut ends with 00 silk to prevent sperm granuloma. The tunic is closed under fine gut suture, and through the same skin incision the scrotal septum is opened along the medial side of the opposite testis for access to the other ductus deferens. The vasectomy is repeated on the second side, and the tunic, septum, fascia and skin are closed in separate layers. Sequential semen evaluations have shown the disappearance of all viable spermatozoa by the sixth postoperative week.

THE FEMALE HORSE

Surgery of the reproductive system of the female horse is classified by anatomy and etiology. According to surgical access, the female reproductive system can be divided into the cranial tract, including uterus and ovaries, and caudal tract, comprised of the vulva, vagina and cervix. Other systems are involved secondarily. The rectum and colon may be sites of injury or prolapse. The urinary system is subject to obstruction, disruption and malposition. Iliac and uterine arteries may be the source of spontaneous hemorrhage associated with advanced pregnancy. Any component of the system may be affected by neoplasia, surgical infections and congenital anomalies.

Injuries

The caudal tract, including rectum, vagina and intervening perineum, is most vulnerable to injuries, especially those due to foaling. Other less frequent causes are accidental injury to the rectum during manual examinations of the pelvic and abdominal viscera or accidental injury to either the rectum or the vagina by the stallion (misdirected intromission or mismatched size), by overly forceful correction of dystocias and as the result of sadism. These injuries may be retroperitoneal and confined to the pelvic cavity, or they may extend by perforation into the peritoneal cavity. A second, but no less important consideration, is the transmural migration of sepsis from foci of infection in the pelvis into the peritoneal cavity. Therefore, a pelvic abscess that results from a retroperitoneal injury of the rectum or vagina may extend with little opposition into the peritoneal cavity and result in a localized pubic or inguinal abscess or a generalized peritonitis.

Injuries to the cervix and uterus are almost invariably dystocial, although not a few of them are iatrogenic. The cervix is either stretched or torn, and as with a sphincter injury, valvular function is compromised. The uterine injury takes the form of rupture or of hemorrhage. Somewhat different from hemorrhage following the other injuries, consequential hemorrhage from uterine vessels (intra- or extramural) is usually spontaneous and preparturient.

Displacements

Complications of pregnancy and parturition are uterine torsions, rectal and uterine prolapses, eversions of the urinary bladder and eventrations through ruptures in the rectal prolapse or through vaginal tears. All are associated with tenesmus except uterine torsion. Of course, rectal prolapse can occur in either sex and from causes other than parturition.

A more insidious displacement is that of splanchnoptosis in the older pluriparous mare, in which the normal caudoventrad slope of the vagina changes to horizontal or cranioventrad. This, in turn, opposes the natural outward gravitation of urine and results in vesicovaginal reflux with retention of voided urine in the vaginal fornix. Selected animals may respond to urethroplasty, which creates an extension of the urethra beyond the dividing line of outflow versus inflow.

Space-Occupying Lesions

Neoplasms, cysts, abscesses, hematomas and seromas account for the majority of these lesions. Diagnosis is established on the basis of paracentesis and biopsy as well as physical characteristics and location.

Neoplasms

Neoplasms are divided into those of the female tubular genital tract, the ovaries, the cutaneous perineum and the mammary gland. Tumors (neoplasms and cysts) described in the mare have included adenoma of the uterine tube (oviduct); paramesonephric (Müllerian) duct cysts of the fimbria; fibrosarcoma, leiomyosarcoma and lymphosarcoma of the uterus and cervix; cystic hyperplasia of the endometrium; lymphangiectasia in the ventral part of the body of the uterus in aged mares; mesonephric duct cysts of the mesometrium and myometrium; squamous metaplasia of the surface endometrium in pyometra; squamous cell carcinoma, malignant melanoma, fibrosarcoma, hemangioma and hemangiosarcoma of the vagina and vulva; and carcinoma of the mammary gland.[37, 42, 43]

Tumors of the ovary of the mare receive the most attention owing to their relatively greater incidence and to their effects on fertility and psychological behavior. The most common by far is the granulosa cell tumor of sex cord-stromal origin.[11, 38, 42, 45] This tumor is typically unilateral and may be diagnosed fortuitously or upon examination because of infertility or of abnormal behavior, as might be characterized by hypersecretion of estrogen and/or androgen.[33, 42] Teratoma is the second most common tumor and can be presumptively diagnosed on palpation *per rectum* by its hardness and irregular surface (having points and edges). Malignant tumors are represented by cystadenocarcinomas and secondary (metastatic) lymphosarcomas. The only common ovarian cysts in the mare are the subsurface epithelial (germinal) cysts and parovarian cysts of the mesovarium and mesosalpinx. Graafian follicle cysts are of clinical importance in the cow and sow, but not in the mare, as is so frequently misdiagnosed.[45]

Focal lesions of the uterus are occasionally confused with early pregnancy on palpation *per rectum*. Examples are muscular atrophy, focal myometrial atonia, myometrial lymphatic lacunae and endometrial cysts. These are mainly diagnostic problems and fall more in the province of theriogenology than surgery; however, reference to surgical removal of endometrial cysts has been made.[33]

Abscess

The abscess of greatest clinical importance is the pelvic abscess, which usually originates from injury to the vagina or rectum and less frequently is caused by wounds to the base of the tail or the perineum. Abscesses are usually suspected on the basis of a stormy course marked by fever, pain, straining, pelvic phlegmon (often apparent in the perineal region), constipation and dysuria. Additionally, there may be the history of a penetrating or lacerating injury. Pelvic examination may require epidural anesthesia and general sedation. Paracentesis is confirmatory. One case revealed adhesions of the colon to the vagina around a necrotic core and a fecal fistula perforating into the vaginal floor. The mare had recently been delivered of a dystocia.

Hematoma and Seroma

Hematoma and seroma occur in the walls of the uterus and vagina and are associated with advanced pregnancy and the trauma of difficult birth. Circumscribed hematoma of the vaginal wall may be confused with vascular tumors and varices. Hematocyst has been diagnosed in the ovary, but great care must be exercised to avoid mistaking this for the unilocular cystic granulosa cell tumor. Pelvic hematoma has been seen in the barren mare. This is due to spontaneous rupture of vessels and also to laceration or rupture of the pelvic vasculature, e.g., the obturator artery by sharp bone splinters and pelvic fracture. The significance of hematomas extends the full range of the spectrum from incidental findings to life-threatening events.

Physiological Surgery

Not fitting any pathological classification of diagnoses but constituting important categories of what has been called physiological surgery are the cesarean section (cesarotomy) and the bilateral ovariectomy for purposes of neutering. Indications for cesarotomy are the immutable dystocias that do not lend themselves to fetotomy. These include the transverse lie or presentation of the fetus during labor when the long axis of its body crosses the long axis of the maternal body, and cases in which the ends of the fetus may occupy both horns of the uterus. Certain fetal monsters may pose problems for nonoperative means of delivery, such as the hydrocephalus in which a greatly enlarged calvarium may resist the most strenuous efforts to reduce the size to one compatible with the pelvic diameter. Perosomus and multiple arthrogryposis are examples of other monsters.[48] An occasional indication for cesarotomy is for delivery of the live foal when normal birth is prevented by pelvic deformity, uterine torsion or other mechanical obstacles or in the emergency delivery from a mare that has just died.

Bilateral ovariectomy is performed for neutering the mare valued only for work to eliminate the undesirable periods of estrus and also to correct the ungovernable behavior of the chronic nymphomaniac. It is important to the prognosis to understand that although bilateral ovariectomy assures sterility, it does not promise altered behavior. The prospects are favorable in the normal mare and in the mild type of chronic nymphomania. In the severe type, viciousness and other unacceptable behaviors are apt to be so ingrained as to make the mare incorrigible even after surgery. The risk of injury to life and limb of personnel and the undesirable influence on other livestock may dictate euthanasia as the practical alternative. Recovery of desirable traits in nymphomaniac mares has been quoted as 60 per cent successful after spaying. Interestingly, the ovaries recovered from such mares may display no abnormalities or may be small and atretic, as opposed to the enlarged follicular cysts that often attend nymphomania in cows.[48]

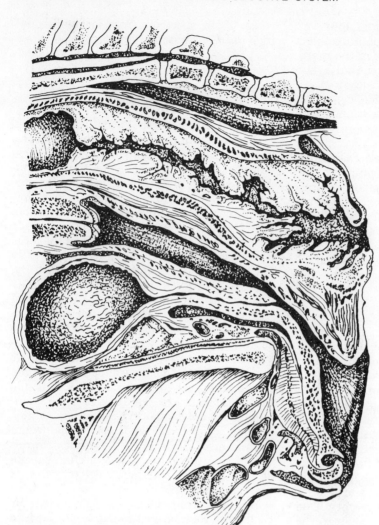

Figure 4. Sagittal section of the pelvic cavity and viscera of the mare, emphasizing the relative positions of the segments of the caudal tubular tract of the genital system to the rectum and anus above and the urinary bladder and urethra below. (Redrawn from Nickel, R., Schummer, A., Seiferle, E. and Sack, W. O.: The Viscera of the Domestic Mammals. New York, Springer-Verlag, 1973, p. 362.)

Surgery of the Caudal Tract

Procedures fall into two categories: (1) revision or reconstruction of structural defects (lacerations, sphincteric incompetence, fistulae, splanchnoptosis, adhesions, displacements and anomalies) and (2) extirpation and drainage of space-occupying lesions (neoplasms, cysts, abscesses and hematomas). The vulvovaginal procedures account for the majority of such operations. These include (1) episioplasty (Caslick operation) for faulty conformation and first and second degree injuries to the dorsal commissure of the vulva and the perineal body and (2) reconstruction of third-degree perineal lacerations and rectovaginal fistulae (Fig. 4).

Foaling injuries to the caudal tract are graded first, second or third degree in order of increasing severity. First-degree injuries involve the mucosa of the ceiling of the vestibule and the dorsal commissure of the vulva, including the skin. Disruption of underlying muscle bundles is minimal. Second-degree injuries involve stretching or disruption of the vulvovestibular musculature, especially in the perineal body but sparing the rectal floor and anal sphincter. Third-degree injuries occur usually in the primipara when hard labor contractions force the foal's foot upward at such an angle as to catch in the dorsal transverse membranous fold of the vaginovestibular junction. If the foot is retrieved and the malposition is corrected in time, only a fistula results. If not, the foot (feet) extends through the rectovaginal septum into the rectal lumen and in the ensuing course of labor traumatically divides perineal body, anus, vulva and cutaneous perineum.

Episioplasty

The Caslick operation was initially introduced as a means to reduce the size of the mucocutaneous cleft of the vulva to prevent aspiration of air associated with ascending tract infections. However, the concept of this operation has since been expanded to include repair of the compromised function of the constrictor muscles of the vulva and vestibule, which serve, together with the labia, as the first line of defense against the environment, especially around the perineum. One has only to compare the vulvovestibular characteristics of the normal tract with that of the chronic windsucker to appreciate the functional deficit in the latter case. When the labia of the normal tract are parted (overriding the constrictor vulvae muscle), the constrictor vestibulae still provides closure of the vestibule. This is especially apparent by the closure effected at the vaginovestibular junction just craniad to the urethral orifice and at the site of the hymen. The efficacy of this function in the young, healthy mare has been demonstrated time and time again by the ability of some animals to be bred successfully despite third-degree perineal lacerations or rectovaginal fistulae that were located caudad to the vaginovestibular junction. In the chronic windsucker, however, the vulva may stand open; or if closed, the simple act of parting the labia will usually provoke aspiration of air, as no effective valvular action remains in the vestibule.

One of the common causes of pneumovagina is the injury to the perineal body sustained at parturition, particularly the dystocia that produces a first- or second-degree laceration. The circular muscles forming the sphincters of the anus, vulva and vestibule cross each other in the rectovaginal septum, and the primary intersection of the decussating bundles of smooth muscle is the perineal body.[26] On sagittal section, the cut surface has roughly the shape of a right-angle triangle, with the base being the cutaneous perineum, the hypotenuse the ceiling of the vestibule and the perpendicular the floor of the rectum.[44] When these muscle fibers are disrupted ("lacerated"), they retract on themselves. Despite the rapid healing that results from granulation and epithelialization, spontaneous reunion of sphincters does not occur, and the function is either diminished or lost altogether. The first line of defense to the outside environment has been violated, and restoration usually requires reconstructive surgery.

Successive parturitions may be expected to add to problems that were minimal at the outset; therefore, pneumovagina is more of a problem of the aging mare than of the young animal. Not infrequently, the sagging viscera (splanchnoptosis) associated with gradual stretching of mesometrium and enlargment of the abdominal cavity is an attendant feature, which may necessitate urethroplasty concurrently with episioplasty. Other contributing factors include malnutrition, parasitism, dysmasesis and other chronic problems that cause a deterioration in the constitution, resulting in weight loss and generalized atony of smooth and skeletal musculature. The desired outcome from reconstructive surgery is partially dependent upon the successful management of the constitutional disease.

The complexity of surgical repair somewhat parallels the grade of injury or conformational defect. The conventional Caslick operation suffices for the majority of juvenile windsuckers (racing fillies) and mares with comparatively minor malconformation of the vulva, e.g., inversion of one labium, separation of labia or sloping perineum. Using local anesthesia, the edges of the labia are infiltrated with 2 per cent lidocaine hydrochloride. A narrow (6 to 8 mm) strip of mucous membrane is removed with scissors from the mucocutaneous junction at the edges of both labia from the dorsal commissure down to a level just below the bony floor of the pelvis. The raw margins are apposed with a single row of simple continuous suture using 00 polypropylene monofilament swaged on a general closure needle (or the equivalent).

The repair will approximate a fraction of the vulvar cleft and is subject to the degree of correction required by the individual animal. Closure should not be so extensive, however, as to cause dysuria. Also, if breed association regulations require a natural cover, the opening must be sufficient to allow for intromission. It is customary to culture or biopsy the uterus and to treat for existing infections prior to doing the Caslick operation, although treatment by intrauterine infusions through a vaginal cylinder can continue to be done after the surgery. In this case, as in breeding, the repair can be protected from accidental dehiscence with a single mattress tension suture (breeder's stitch) of 0.6-mm Vetafil sutures (or equivalent) taken at the lowest point of the closure. Skin sutures are removed upon healing in about 10 days. The breeder's stitch is removed when treatments are discontinued or upon termination of breeding. The closure line should be opened, usually with scissors or a blunt-pointed bistoury, just prior to foaling. If the mare foals through the unopened Caslick closure, irregular tears may result, and the repair is unnecessarily complicated.

Episioplasty for second-degree injuries and more extensive defects requires special dissection and reconstruction of the perineal body and ceiling of the vestibule as well as the dorsal commissure of the vulva. The operation is done on the standing patient, tranquilized and restrained in stocks. Local anesthesia is provided by epidural injection of approximately 6 to 7 ml of 2 per cent lidocaine or mepivacaine hydrochloride in mares weighing approximately 450 kg. If additional anesthesia is required, local infiltration of the ischiorectal region will usually suffice. No change in feeding routine is necessary since the rectum is not involved; therefore, this repair can be scheduled at the convenience of the surgeon, paying attention to the condition of the specific tissues and of the total patient.

The objective of the dissection is to expose a triangular area of the dorsal aspect of the defect to conform to the sagittal sectional area of the perineal body or to the amount that has been disrupted in the estimation of the surgeon. Exposure for the submucous resection requires dorsal retraction of the tail and dorsal commissure and bilateral retraction of the labia. The lines of incision through the mucous membrane can be drawn with the scalpel in the shape of the right-angle triangle previously described. The mucous membrane is elevated by tissue forceps and scissor or scalpel dissection for a distance of 10 to 15 cm craniad from the edge of the labium. This should approximate the length of the vestibule and reach the vicinity of the vaginovestibular junction. Suture closure of the triangulated field starts in the forwardmost depths of the wound with interrupted bites of 0 or 00 surgical gut or polyglycolic acid (PGA) placed in a quilting pattern out to the line of mucosal incision.

A variation is described by Gadd[22] in which the submucous resection is done in a continuous field, finally removing a V-shaped gore to create the desired area for apposition. The cut edges of mucosa are closed in the initial line of sutures, and the exposed face of the perineal body is approximated with successive rows of buried interrupted sutures using 0 or 00 PGA sutures or equivalent.

Skin closure for reconstruction of the commissure defect is made with 00 polypropylene in an interrupted vertical mattress pattern. Aftercare consists of tetanus immunization, systemic antibiotic therapy for 72 hours, maintenance of wound hygiene and removal of skin sutures in about 10 days. Natural breeding can resume when uterine cultures are negative.

Repair of Third-Degree Perineal Lacerations

Surgery involving the rectum requires adjustment of the diet so that the bowel movement becomes soft and reduced in volume. Painful or difficult defecation (dyschezia) is as responsible as errors of technique for surgical failure. Straining on defecation subjects the wound repair to excessive tension, and dehiscence results. Crash diets and laxatives are used to soften the feces but are less preferred than natural means, notably pelleted feeds, which have a tendency to produce a softer bowel movement, and bran mashes, long used for this effect. The advantage of pelleted feeds is that they furnish a balanced ration. On the other hand, if the mare is in constitutionally good health when placed on a diet, no adverse effects will result from feeding bran mashes for the 3 weeks usually required. It is also recommended that the change from the regular feed to pelleted feed or bran mash be done gradually over at least a period of 1 week to prevent any digestive disturbance that might otherwise occur. The day of surgery is scheduled at the discretion of the surgeon when the bowel movement is judged to be sufficiently soft and reduced in volume for the procedure. It must be kept this way for at least 2 weeks postoperatively, accounting for a total time of about 3 weeks on a restricted diet. Twenty-four hours prior to surgery, the mare is given a 1-gallon mineral oil gavage, and feed is withheld for the last 12 hours. It is misinformed to suggest that mineral oil is contraindicated because of possible interference with healing. This is no more the case than suggesting that intestinal resection and anastomosis is precluded in animals with intestinal obstruction that have been treated for colic with mineral oil. Nevertheless, the idea crops up from time to time, usually to support the argument for saline cathartics or dihydroxyanthraquinone. Suffice it to say, the argument strains the evidence.

The second requirement for successful surgery is the health of the tissues at the wound site. At the time of initial injury, the tissues are somewhat atonic and edematous in preparation for parturition. Although commonly referred to as a laceration, the tissues are not sharply divided but are literally torn apart, oftentimes in eccentric planes. If there is a delay of as long as 4 to 6 hours between the time of injury and the repair, the tissues become even more edematous and desiccated on the surface. Irregular tags of tissue become devitalized, and the superficial layers become infected. Repairs attempted at this time will not be very successful. Careful observations of both natural and experimental wounds show that 3 to 4 weeks are required for the host's natural defense and repair mechanisms to return the tissues to a degree of health to support primary healing of an elective surgical procedure. Therefore, if circumstances do not favor reconstruction at the time of injury, the next opportunity occurs about 1 month later. Then, if the foal survived the delivery, there is the choice as to whether or not to subject the youngster to the enforced confinement necessitated by the strict diet imposed on the mare, as well as to the hazards, noxious influences and nosocomial infections to which foals are so susceptible. Sound judgment opposes this option in favor of postponing the surgery until the foal is weaned, which may be done as early as 3 to 4 months of age with the help of milk formula and dietary supplements for the suckling. By waiting an additional 6 to 8 weeks beyond the earliest advisable date, the wound will have undergone further healing by contraction and differentiation. The defect at 12 weeks is significantly smaller than at 4 weeks, and the tissues are better able to respond to surgery. The same thing is true of rectovaginal fistulae, which may reduce in diameter to a surprising degree in even 1 month, improving the chances for successful repair. In fact, some fistulae may heal spontaneously during the waiting period.

The surgery is done with the animal standing, preferably using restraint provided by stocks. The rectum is emptied by hand and cleansed with a mild antiseptic wash that is safe for use on mucous surfaces. A low enema can be used but should precede the epidural block. Local anesthesia is by epidural injection as previously described under Episioplasty. One injection usually suffices for the 1 to 1 1/2 hours required by surgery. Some like to leave a spinal needle indwelling for addi-

tional anesthetic, if needed. The tail is wrapped and reflected dorsally. The defect is retracted laterally by tension sutures placed in the margins of the old wound and anchored in the hairline over the ischiatic area on either side. The kickboard, sides of the stocks and the hindquarters peripheral to the field should be draped (Fig. 5).

The defect extends caudally from the vaginovestibular junction in the ceiling of the vestibule in almost every case. The field should be well lighted to facilitate dissection and suturing. The dissection is made in a frontal plane starting in the shelf, which is the remains of the rectovaginal septum in the forwardmost part of the defect. The shelf should be split from side to side, leaving the rectal floor as thick as possible to support suture closure. Dissection by both scissors and scalpel is aided by placing the tissues in tension with forceps. The plane started in the shelf is continued around on either side at the line of junction of healing of the rectal and vaginal mucosa, recognizable by the slight difference in color of the two mucous membranes. This junctional incision is deepened into the sides of the defect sufficiently to free rectal and vaginal (vestibular) flaps on each side that can be brought together in the middle without tension. Inattention to this most important step is thought to be a common cause of failure. The bilateral dissection is extended to the cutaneous perineum with a modification in the posterior half, consisting of a triangulated submucous resection over the cut face of the perineal body, as described under the repair of second-degree perineal lacerations in the section on Episioplasty. This part of the dissection can be deferred until the anterior half of the wound has been reconstructed under suture. This insures a fresher and less contaminated tissue surface for suture closure.

The suture pattern in the cranial part of the dissection is the modified Goetze pattern, after Straub and Fowler.[56] All these sutures are interrupted, nonabsorbable, noncapillary synthetic sutures placed no more than 1 to 1.5 cm apart with a curved needle. The first two sutures are placed as vertical mattress bites ahead of the defect, so as to create a fold in the margins of the defect that will merge smoothly into the apposed surfaces. Closure of the defect is made with a six-bite vertical suture that starts in the left vaginal flap at least 3 cm from the margin; goes directly upward into the left rectal flap,

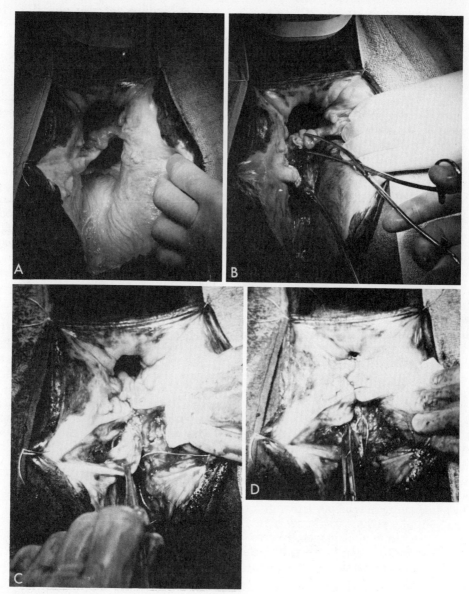

Figure 5. Reconstruction of the third-degree perineal laceration. *A*, The surgical field retracted and draped; *B*, dissecting the shelf; *C*, bilateral dissection undergoing reconstruction—placement of the first bite of the modified Goetze suture; *D*, placement of the second bite; *E*, placement of the third bite; *F*, placement of the fourth bite; *G*, placement of the fifth and sixth bites; *H*, manual tension on suture with hand ties; *I*, quadrantal apposition of the rectal and vaginal components of the reconstructed septum; *J*, progressing closure of the rectal fault; *K*, closure of the fault in the anal sphincter; and *L*, completed reconstruction of the perineum.

Illustration continued on opposite page

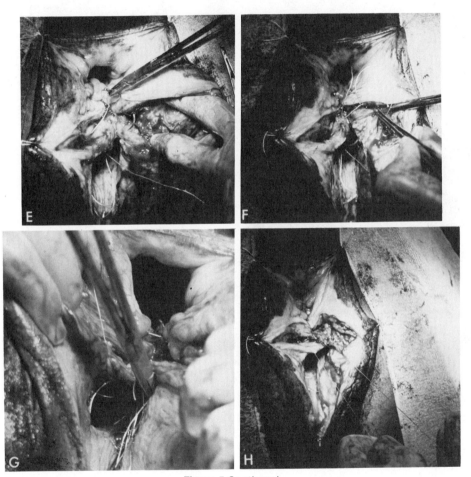

Figure 5 *Continued.*

Illustration continued on following page

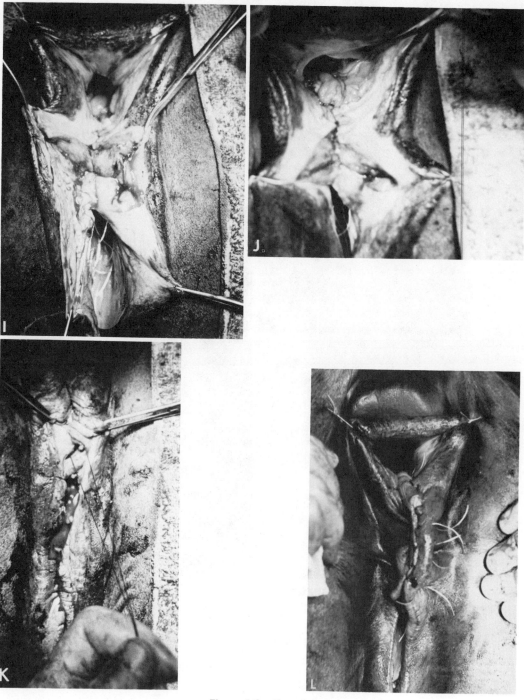

Figure 5 *Continued.*

emerging at the submucosal margin *without* perforating the mucosa; re-enters the right rectal flap at the same spot, emerging at least 3 cm from the margin; goes directly downward through the right vaginal flap, 3 cm from the margin; and then turns medially to pass through the near margins of the vaginal flaps to be tied by hand (not instrument) on the left side of the now apposed vaginal defect. The suture material should have tensile strength sufficient to permit ties snug enough to effect intimate apposition of the rectal margins with *no* exposed suture, either visible or palpable. Failure to do this may cause fistulization or total dehiscence of the repair. The principle of repair is much the same as that required by a milk fistula or laceration through the teat canal of a dairy cow.

Repair of the perineal body, exposed by the triangular submucous resection, is the same as described for the second-degree laceration except that the wound in the rectum and anus must be closed. The use of Ob-Gyn gut or PGA gut in this area gives a stronger, longer-lasting closure; however, others report the successful use of buried polypropylene sutures.[55] The cutaneous perineum is repaired as described under Episioplasty. The skin sutures and the nonabsorbable synthetic sutures tied inside the vagina (vestibule) are removed in 11 to 14 days. No anesthetic is required for the usual case. The reconstruction is completed in one operation. Despite variations in wound characteristics,[28] it has not been necessary to resort to the phased procedures[1, 2] to achieve primary healing.

Postoperative care consists of the use of prophylactic antibiotics for 5 to 7 days, mainly to guard against stitch abscesses that might predispose to fistulae. Pelvic phlegmon and fascial abscess have not been common problems. Dyschezia is an occasional problem in the mare that may have been operated on for the second or third time, but this complication can usually be averted by reducing the colon content and maintaining a laxative bowel movement during the 2 weeks after surgery. This is not an inconvenience to either the mare or the manager.

Splanchnoptosis and urine reflux are unusual in the primipara; therefore, it is anticipated that the majority of such cases that benefit from primary healing on the first try can be returned to breeding. It is a consideration, however, to provide attendance on successive parturitions.

Repair of Rectovaginal Fistula

Preparation parallels that for repair of the third-degree laceration. The dissection is made in the frontal plane in its entirety. The skin incision extends from side to side between the buttocks and midway between the anus and the vulva. Thereafter the perineal body and rectovaginal septum are split sideways in the same fashion, so as to separate the rectum from the vagina (vestibule) to a point 2 to 3 cm beyond the fistula. The thickness of the rectal floor is maintained at the expense of the vaginal roof. The rectal fistula is closed transversely, i.e., at right angles to the long axis of the rectum, which is in alignment with the principal lines of stress when the rectum contracts in peristalsis. This is done in essentially the same way as the Heineke-Mikulicz operation for pyloroplasty, by preplacing a series of interrupted Lembert sutures (0 or 1 surgical gut or PGA). The first suture bisects the fistula, the next two divide the halves into quarters and the next four divide the quarters into eighths until intimate closure has been effected. The sutures are tied in the same sequence. This is repeated on the vaginal fistula except that the closure is oriented on the longitudinal rather than the transverse plane. After both fistulae have been closed, the divided septum and perineum are reunited with a series of interrupted fine gut sutures placed out to the cutaneous perineum, which is closed with mattress skin sutures. There is little tension on this part of the reconstruction, and high tensile strength sutures are not required. Postoperative care is the same as for the third-degree laceration.

There are occasional references made to conversion of fistulae to third-degree lacerations for use of repair techniques adapted to the latter injury. This is justified if the fistula has healed (see earlier description) and still remains so large as to impose an unusual tax on the conventional fistula repair. In such cases, the perineum that remains intact may be a narrow isthmus of tissue, which makes the wound a fistula only in a technical sense. Oftentimes this is the result of previous unsuccessful attempts to reconstruct a third-degree laceration. Therefore, in these instances, conversion to a full-fledged third-degree laceration is merely a technicality. However, if the characteristics of the fistula do not conform to these exceptions, the defect should be operated as a fistula in accordance with the principles of Forssell described more than 50 years ago.

Urethroplasty

For relief of splanchnoptosis and urine reflux only two surgical procedures are currently known — the episioplasty and the urethroplasty. The first operation was introduced more than 40 years ago[10]; the second, less than 10 years ago.[40] Since then, both procedures have been adopted by the industry and have undergone some modifications.

The urethroplasty is a revisionary technique for caudal extension of the urethra[9] in the mare that has been rendered infertile at least partially as the result of vesicovaginal reflux with retention of voided urine in the vaginal fornix. Chronic cervicitis and endometritis are the expected consequences. Understandably, the competence of the vulvovestibular closure and the morphological condition of the endometrium must be carefully assessed[32] before predicting the benefits of urethroplasty. This done, the mare is prepared and anesthetized for pelvic surgery in the standing position, as described in the previous section. The labia are retracted by stay sutures or self-retaining retractors. Two procedures have been described.

The Monin technique[40] fixes the transverse membranous fold overlying the external urethral orifice in a posterior position by denuding the lateral edges of the retracted fold and suturing these edges to similarly denuded recipient sites along the sides of the floor of the vestibule. Caution is observed to provide a channel large enough to prevent dysuria. Intimate apposition of tissue avoids fistula formation. A continuous suture pattern with 00 polypropylene, Ob-Gyn gut or PGA material is satisfactory. Prophylactic antibiotics are recommended. A healing time of about 2 weeks is required. Success is based on the disappearance of urine pooling in the cranial vagina. Treatment of endometritis and correction of vulvovestibular incompetence must be managed separately, often concurrently for return of breeding soundness.

The Brown technique[9] may be likened to the surgical separation of the rectum from the vagina in the reconstruction of the third-degree perineal laceration. The shelf is the membranous fold overlying the urethra. This is split from side to side, extending the incision bilaterally along the sides of the vestibular floor backward to about 3 cm from the labial margins. The plane of dissection is deepened to free flaps, dorsal and ventral, of mucous membrane. These flaps are then brought together in the middle by two or three layers of suture to construct a membranous extension of the urethra back to the vulvar cleft. Number 00 polypropylene or PGA suture material in continuous mattress patterns is used to appose the cut mucous edges in eversion. The third (optional) layer can be used in the submucosa between the two mucosal layers for added support in case there is tension on the suture line. Postoperative procedures are the same as for the Monin technique. Breeding thereafter has been accomplished by both natural and artificial means.

Repair of Vaginal Adhesions and Anomalies

Partitioning defects of the vagina occur as congenital anomalies as well as traumatic adhesions. They may be two-dimensional or three-dimensional, longitudinal or transverse. They cause diagnostic problems and may or may not be surgically remediable.

Longitudinal bands in the sagittal plane are usually identified as persistent median walls of the embryonic Müllerian duct system. They may be discovered fortuitously upon a routine examination, and since they may present a mechanical obstacle to breeding or foaling, these bands should be excised. This is done most simply under local or no anesthesia with long-handled dissecting scissors to sever the band at its junctions with the vaginal floor and ceiling. Hemorrhage is negligible, and healing occurs by second intention.

Transverse, two-dimensional partitions may be congenital or acquired. The persistent hymen is the congenital form, usually broken by the first breeding or speculum examination, and rarely requiring surgery. The imperforate hymen is uncommon, may be attended by mucometra or at least some accumulation of mucous secretions and detritus and, in such cases, requires surgery. Traumatic adhesions may mimic imperforate hymen in every respect, with the possible exception of bacteria in the trapped secretions. This may justify the designation, in some cases, of pyometra, although the typical example of pyometra includes adhesions of the cervix rather than of the vagina.

Demonstration of the two-dimensional characteristics may be done by palpation *per rectum* and *per vaginam* as well as by needle test puncture and aspiration. Under local anesthesia and suitable preoperative preparation, the partition is incised from quadrant to quadrant, and the four flaps of redundant tissue created by the cruciate incision are excised by scissors, scalpel or electric scalpel. Retraction of the labia and illumination of the field are essential. If a large volume of mucus and/or exudate has been trapped in the uterus and vagina, tenesmus may be a prominent clinical sign and may require heavy sedation as well as epidural anesthesia to facilitate surgery. Also, it may be advisable to drain such accumulations by indwelling catheter or release incision as part of the preparations for surgery. This, in itself, may suffice to control the violent straining. If dysuria is an attendant problem, an indwelling balloon catheter may also be desirable. If the urinary catheter is to remain postoperatively, it should be fitted with a one-way valve (such as a split latex glove-finger) to prevent aspiration of air and contaminants into the bladder — the unavoidable cause of ascending infection if this feature is overlooked.

Three-dimensional adhesions must be distinguished by medical history from the segmental aplasia of the tubular tract that is seen occasionally. Since neither problem is common, diagnosis may be confusing, unless it is established that the patient is or is not a maiden mare. The only likely explanation for an acquired defect other than injury by dystocia would be by breeding or a malicious act (sadism).

Correction is accomplished either by restoration of the pre-existing lumen or, when this is not possible, by ovariohysterectomy. Mechanical breakdown of adhesions must be done under local anesthesia on the standing patient with the organs suspended *in situ* and free of the intra-abdominal pressures present in the recumbent position that displace and compress the pelvic viscera. Alternatively, recumbent positioning would require cranioventral tilt to displace the abdominal viscera forward. Fibrolysis is primarily by scissors dissection, spreading and cutting, as adhesions are distinguished from the vaginal wall. The urethra should be identified by catheter and the bladder exhausted to avoid accidental injury. The rectum should be emptied and cleansed somewhat to permit periodic palpation *per rectum*. The dissection must be followed closely by manual palpation to maintain proper orientation with the cervix, which is, of course, obscured from view in such cases. The tract should be re-entered manually at regular intervals during the

convalescence to prevent cicatricial constriction and recurrence of adhesions before epithelialization is complete. Hysterectomy for segmental aplasia with mucometra is discussed under the surgery of the cranial tract.

Repair of Prolapses

Prolapses of the caudal tract can be ranked in order of importance as rectal, uterine and vesical. Rectal prolapses may or may not occur as complications of urogenital disease, but usually result from some cause of straining, such as dystocia or pelvic irritability, e.g., an inflammatory or a space-occupying lesion. Rectal prolapse in the mare is initially of little more consequence than is a case of aggravated hemorrhoids in man and, if the cause is countered at this time, may amount to treatment for proctitis. If neglected, the problem increases to sizable prolapse of the rectum, which, in turn, can lead to prolapse of the small colon. The ominous fact is that when this occurs, all but the minor prolapse of short duration must be considered for amputation and anastomosis. The segmental blood supply to the terminal small colon and rectum resembles that of the esophagus in that collateral circulation is comparatively poor, and if the tissue bed and terminal mesocolon are sufficiently disrupted so as to compromise the blood supply, infarction results unless the involved bowel is resected. For this reason, replacement of sizable rectal prolapses and pure-string suture of the anus are not high on the list of successful treatment modalities in the horse. Certainly, if this "conservative" course of management is elected, the condition of the rectum and of the total patient should be carefully monitored for at least the postoperative week.

When amputation is the choice, the technique should follow closely the principles of intestinal anastomosis. The procedure is performed under epidural anesthesia if possible, and the site of anastomosis is near the cutaneous anus. It is common practice to place stay sutures crossing the diameter of the bowel at the four quadrants. These are tied as mattress sutures and serve to stabilize the tissues for further dissection and to orient even suture placement. It may be necessary to open the prolapse lengthwise for a distance to provide access to the interior wall for accurate suturing. An interrupted mattress pattern is used circumferentially, with enough sutures to prevent constriction of the lumen.

Although 00 or 0 gut or PGA suture can be used, a technique used in cattle may be followed, employing a 0.4- to 0.6-mm synthetic nonabsorbable suture tied tightly so as to create a slough of the diaphragm of tissue at the site of amputation 10 to 14 days postoperatively. Alternatively, a cylindrical plastic prolapse ring, drilled with a series of holes around its circumference, is introduced into the prolapse and sutured in place with the same type of sutures designed to slough by 14 days. The sutures pass through the holes in the cylinder in a mattress pattern and are tied on the outside. The prolapse is amputated just beyond the sutures. The plastic cylinder maintains patency of the rectum during the healing time and then is voided upon sloughing of the sutured diaphragm of tissue. Prophylactic antibiotics, laxatives by gavage (mineral oil and dioctyl sodium sulfosuccinate) and dietary changes are required during convalescence.

Uterine Prolapse. Advice on the management of this relatively infrequent problem parallels that given for rectal prolapse in that much advantage is gained by early attention. Once again, the controversy regarding epidural anesthesia in the mare should be laid aside, since its use is very beneficial to suppress straining, particularly in the hot-blooded breeds. The concurrent use of tranquilizers, sedatives and narcotics is certainly indicated to quell sensitivity, but nothing controls pelvic origin tenesmus so effectively as epidural anesthesia.

Scrupulous toilet of all exposed surfaces should also consider the time limitations and irritation factors. The race is against development of thrombosis of the engorged and stagnated uterine vasculature, after which replacement of the organ is a somewhat futile effort since infarction and death are the likely sequelae. Amputation of the gangrenous uterus in the mare should be done when the need is evident, but it ranks among the truly heroic procedures, with opportunity for success very slight. Treatment of shock is the major factor. In the replacement procedure in the horse, as in any species, care should be taken to insure that the retroverted tips of the horns are repositioned completely and that thought is given to mural as well as intraluminal hemorrhage. The conjugated estrogen products of equine origin were developed for control of just such hemorrhage in the human female and, barring a major arterial injury, are indicated for such need in the mare.

Recurrence of prolapse following replacement seems not to be the problem in the mare that it is in cattle; however, the continuation of tranquilization for a time thereafter is indicated with the proviso that it be in agreement with blood pressure and any premonitory signs of shock.

Vesical Prolapse. Displacement of the urinary bladder takes two forms — extrusion through a break in the floor of the vagina and prolapse (eversion) through the urethra. The latter is more frequent in the mare, although both are uncommon. As with other prolapses, the principal causes are increase in intra-abdominal pressure, primarily during terminal gestation and parturition, and straining, usually precipitated by the presence of a mass in the pelvis or by pelvic irritability. For these reasons and because of the short and distensible urethra of the female, vesical prolapse is a gynecological problem, most often associated with pregnancy.[21, 36] However, there may be other contributing causes such as acute distention of the bowel from intestinal obstruction, whether due to mechanical or paralytic ileus.[20]

Diagnosis is based upon recognition of the retroverted or everted bladder lying in the floor of the vestibule and protruding through the vulva. In the rare retroversion, the urethra is blocked and urine flow prevented. The distention must be evacuated by paracentesis before the bladder can be returned. If the peritoneal reflection in the pelvic cul de sac is unbroken, the principal risk is pelvic abscess. The defect in the vaginal floor should be freshened and repaired under suture if feasible in consideration of the duration and nature of the injury. An indwelling urinary catheter with a one-way valve would be a further consideration. Antibiotics that reach effective levels in the urine would also be indicated.

The true prolapse, commonly referred to as an eversion, is recognizable by its mucous surface and the two elevated openings of the ureters that appear on the dorsal surface of the organ near its neck. Inflammatory swelling in the bladder wall may cause some retardation of urine flow from the ureters and perhaps even some ureteral distention, but no obstruction exists beyond that. For this reason, a chronic form of vesical prolapse has been described in which the bladder could not be returned and amputation of the corpus vesicae beyond the ureteral orifices was successfully accomplished. The healed stump returned to the vestibule, and the ureters discharged directly thereinto.[21]

In the more typical case, the acute prolapse that occurs around the time of parturition should receive immediate care while it is still possible to reduce the edema in the bladder wall sufficiently to return the everted organ through the urethra. This requires patient manipulation and gentle massage under epidural anesthesia to suppress straining. If replacement is difficult and the bladder wall is friable, urethral sphincterotomy may be helpful. After replacement, prevention of recurrence is the problem, suggesting the need for an inflatable, indwelling balloon catheter of a capacity of 100 ml or more (such as a human rectal retention catheter). Also, chronic cystitis requires long-term urinary antibiotic therapy. Control of straining by use of tranquilizers, sedatives and narcotics is necessary.

Repair of Cervical Lesions

Lesions of the cervix include (1) injuries sustained during foaling (rupture of muscle fibers and tearing of the mucosa), (2) consequences of chronic inflammation (cervicitis with adhesions or chronic granuloma due to persistent bacterial infection) and (3) congenital anomalies (e.g., segmental aplasia or incomplete development). When dystocial injuries of the cervix impair its function as a valve to close the tube between the vagina and uterus, the disorder is referred to as an incompetent cervix and may constitute a cause of infertility. The condition may be remediable if healing is attended by recovery of muscle tone or if discrete tears ("lacerations") can be freshened and reconstructed under suture. The latter may be done through a metal speculum (bivalve or trivalve) in some mares, or without speculum in others. A Knowles cervical forceps can be used as effectively for retraction of the cervix in the mare as in the cow, bringing the cervix into the reach of conventional instruments for dissection and suturing. Without this, the structure is all but inaccessible. Even so, suturing is difficult and oftentimes done blindly. Old defects that encompass no more than one-quarter of the circumference can be freshened with a long-handled scalpel, exerting forceps traction on the cervix to facilitate more accurate dissection. Interrupted sutures of 0 or 1 Ob-Gyn gut or PGA material must be placed with circular, cutting edge or trocar point needles. If retraction of the cervix is inadequate for the length of conventional needle holders, the Knowles forceps can be used for this purpose as well as for a tissue forceps. If the defect is more extensive than 45°, the chances of successful surgical reconstruction are greatly reduced. Also, the interior lumen of the cervix does not lend itself to such external methods of repair. However, the external os for a distance of about 3 cm inward is accessible for such procedures.

Sometimes the cervix is badly stretched with no apparent surface disruption, and the mare may appear unresponsive to treatment. These animals should be examined and treated as required for endometritis, pneumovagina and urine pooling and then turned out to pasture or returned to physical work with the best general health maintenance possible. In some animals in which local treatment of the organ system is to no avail, the recovery of overall muscle tone will be attended by recovery of cervical function.

When chronic cervicitis results in adhesions, pyometra may be the ensuing complication. To treat or to prevent this may require the use of an indwelling cannula to maintain cervical patency and to provide continuous drainage of the uterus when needed. An acceptable item in standard supply is the inert plastic cannula and inflatable cuff used for barium enema in the human to perform contrast radiography of the rectum. The rectal retention cannula is self-retaining in the mare's cervix when the cuff is inflated inside the body of the uterus. The cannula can be fitted with flexible plastic laboratory tubing to provide the length necessary to drain outside the vulva. The exit end is covered with a glove-fingertip valve to prevent aspiration of air and reflux of exudate. If fitted with a sealable second-lumen infusion tube, the uterus and cervix can be irrigated or infused on an as needed basis without disturbing the drainage tube. However, it is advisable to change drainage tubes at least once every 48 to 72 hours. Latex or red rubber tubes should be changed more frequently, partly because of the tendency to build up crystals of urine salts and adherent deposits of exudate.

Chronic granuloma of the cervix is an infrequent lesion and, based on very limited experience, is regarded as resistant to treatment. It is a space-occupying lesion palpable *per rectum* and should be viewed with concern as far as future breeding soundness. Diagnosis is based upon biopsy. When due to *Staphylococcus*, it has been assigned the name botryomycosis of the cervix, after the comparable condition seen in postcastration infection of the stump of the spermatic cord.

Of the several types of congenital anomalies seen in the cervix of the domestic animals, two have been observed in the mare — complete aplasia with no lumen whatsoever and incomplete development of the muscular walls with a lumen but no effective sphincter. As mentioned earlier in this section, segmental interruption of the tubular tract predisposes to either mucometra or pyometra, necessitating hysterectomy if luminal patency cannot be established. Both degrees of aplasia are permanent conditions of unsoundness to be regarded more as diagnostic than therapeutic problems.

Surgical Management of Space-Occupying Lesions

Neoplasms of the caudal tract are most often the malignant melanoma in the gray horse and squamous cell carcinoma in horses with white skin areas. Both types metastasize by blood and lymph, although metastasis is slow at first, and cutaneous as well as mucosal sites may provide the origin for the primary tumor. Complete surgical excision with a generous margin of normal tissue remains the most reliable and most practiced modality for the circumscribed lesion with no known metastasis. Evidence of regional or remote spread is usually regarded as a contraindication for surgery. When radiation therapy is used for such surface lesions, it is in conjunction with surgical excision. No special surgical techniques have been developed as standardized approaches to such lesions in the mare.

Cysts are usually of the mucous retention type. They are due to displaced embryonal remnants in the walls of the tubular tract and are rarely of clinical importance. When drainage is required, liberal excision is done to evacuate the contents and to permit cauterization or dissection of the lining.

Hematoma of the vaginal wall must be differentiated from hemangioma, and if not enlarging or associated with varicosities, it may be managed simply by incision and evacuation or, if small, left undisturbed. If continued hemorrhage is anticipated, particularly of a major artery in an undisclosed location, the best course may be one of watchful waiting. Conjugated estrogens may be given. Opinion is divided as to the value of paren-

teral fluids in cases of truly consequential hemorrhage in the parturient or preparturient mare. Absolute quiet and judicious use of sedatives are advised. Unless the exact source of the hemorrhage is known (and is surgically accessible) much dependence is still placed on spontaneous arrest, as in the case of uterine arterial hemorrhage into the mesometrium or uterine wall.

Abscesses involving the caudal tract are, in the majority of cases, pelvic abscesses. Frequently originating through wounds in the vaginal wall, the lesion ranges from a small, focal abscess to a dangerous pelvic phlegmon, not only causing dyschezia and dysuria but also threatening peritonitis and septicemia. Tenesmus is a prominent clinical sign, and if the vaginal wall is broken, eventration may even result. It should be remembered that the pelvic fascia is confluent with the fascia transversalis of the abdominal wall, and there is no barrier to extension of infection other than the humorocellular host defenses. Transmural migration of infection to the peritoneal cavity occurs freely. Therefore, pelvic cellulitis of an infectious nature should be treated as a systemic problem as well as a local one.

Once the process has localized and an abscess has formed, an attempt is made to locate the most direct and the most benign drainage route. Pelvic examination *per rectum* and *per vaginam* requires epidural anesthesia to control straining. Confirmation of the abscess and identification of contents are made by paracentesis and examination of the aspirate. The three avenues most often employed for drainage are the vaginal, perineal and abdominal routes. The superficial abscesses located on the floor or sides of the pelvic canal can be drained through incisions made in the perineum or vaginal wall. Deepseated abscesses that extend to or beyond the pubic brim may require drainage through an incision in the caudal abdominal wall in the inguinal or pubic regions. In this case, an exploratory laparotomy can be done concurrently to determine the best location. The drainage path is made through the retroperitoneal fascia so as to avoid direct soilage of the peritoneal cavity. It may be possible to place a through-and-through drain (fenestrated tube or Penrose drain), exiting at a remote point such as the perineum, in order to allow irrigation of the abscess. Antibiotic therapy is based upon the infectious organism and whether the process is contained within the region or not. As with any acute and consequential pelvic disease, maintenance of normal urination and defecation is a primary consideration.

Operative Surgery of the Cranial Tract

Surgical procedures commonly performed on the cranial reproductive tract of the mare are the ovariectomy, detorsion of the uterus and cesarean section. Much less often done is the ovariohysterectomy for pyometra, neoplasia or anomaly. All these share the involvement of the peritoneal cavity, whether by colpotomy for the vaginal spay or by laparotomy in the flank or ventral body wall. Otherwise, the techniques vary widely, even those with the same objective.

Ovariectomy per Colpotomy

The patient is restrained in stocks and prepared for pelvic surgery as previously described. The classic vaginal spay, as it has been practiced for many years, involves a stab incision through the vaginal fornix performed under epidural anesthesia on the standing mare. In order to do this safely, it is imperative that the bladder and rectum be empty, the colon contents reduced and the vagina free of infection. Also, the mare must stand quietly without straining. The mare is stimulated to balloon the vagina by infusing 1 liter of warm saline solution. A knife (scalpel or bistoury) is carried into the ballooned vagina, and an incision is made through the vaginal wall in the upper right hand quarter of the fornix at the 1:30 position. The knife is removed, and Mayo dissecting scissors are carried in to make a stab through the vaginal incision so as to perforate the peritoneum in the cul de sac. The scissors are removed, and the gloved hand is introduced by deliberately stretching the incision one finger at a time until the coned hand is admitted to the peritoneal cavity. A gauze sponge saturated with lidocaine is carried in the palm to wrap around the ovarian pedicle for local anesthesia. The sponge is removed, and the chain loop of the écraseur is carried in. The ovaries are resected one at a time with the chain loop, removing each ovary into the vagina as amputated.

The greatest caution should be taken to insure that only the ovary passes through the loop — not mesentery or intestine (Fig. 6). At the moment of écrasement, the mare must not be allowed to make sudden movements lest the pedicle be torn, causing severe hemorrhage. Before leaving the site, the cut stump should be palpated gently to detect arterial hemorrhage. If all goes well, the mare is removed from the stocks after a few minutes and is placed standing in cross-ties in an individual stall. She should be monitored for signs of shock or straining, since the two major concerns during the first postoperative hours are hemorrhage and eventration. The preoperative fast can be broken and the mare allowed to eat light hay and bran mash or pelleted feed. Prophylactic antibiotics should be continued for 5 days as a safeguard against peritonitis. The mare should be hand-walked at the halter at regular intervals during the day but should be restrained standing in cross-ties otherwise for the first 5 days until all risk of eventration is past. The vaginal wound may be expected to heal by second intention in 2 weeks.

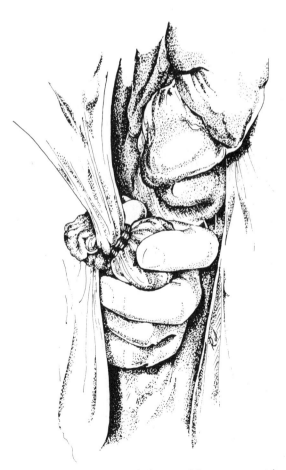

Figure 6. Placement and closure of écraseur around ovarian pedicle.

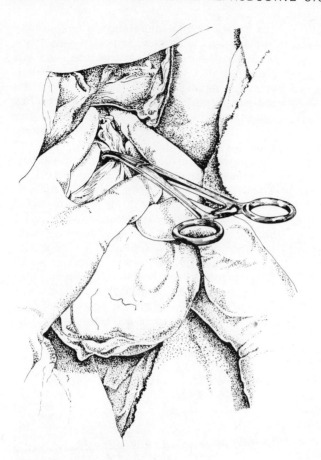

Figure 7. Exteriorization of ovarian tumor through grid flank laparotomy.

Ovariectomy per Laparotomy – Grid Flank Technique

This approach is most often used for removal of a single diseased ovary too big to be removed *per vaginam*. The procedure can be done under local anesthesia on the standing patient if the ovary is not too large or under general anesthesia with the patient in lateral recumbency if the patient is difficult to manage or if problems are anticipated with exteriorization and hemostasis.

The technique for grid flank laparotomy is essentially the same as that described in Cryptorchidectomy, with the exception that incision dimensions may be somewhat greater. The lower flank permits more flexibility of tissue planes and can be used for access and delivery of the larger tumors, while still having the advantages of a grid approach. This recommendation is emphasized by the fact that one of the sites of choice for the cesarean section is the Marcenac incision, which is a grid approach through the low flank.

Upon entry into the abdomen, the ovary is easily located in proximity to the respective flank, especially if tumefied. To aid exteriorization, cystic tumefactions of the ovary can be aspirated. Solid ones can be elevated to the abdominal incision to permit the placement of vulsellum forceps and/or heavy gauge guy sutures (e.g., umbilical tape) in the tough, fibrous cortex of the ovary. This allows the surgeon to use external traction on the enlarged ovary while manually retracting the separated muscle planes. Delivery of the ovary to the outside puts considerable tension on its attachments and caution must be taken to avoid accidental rupture of the blood vessels, which are often engorged owing to the chronicity of such lesions (Fig. 7). In the process of dissecting the mesovarium and associated structures, it is important to control the ovarian arteries and veins by double transfixing ligatures before dividing the proper ligament of the ovary. This acts as a safeguard against abrupt or inadvertent stretching of the vasculature. Once the vessels are safely ligated and the mesovarium, uterine tube (oviduct) and ligament are transected, the stump of the pedicle is examined carefully for hemorrhage before returning it to the abdomen. If the opposite ovary is to be removed from the same side, there should be provision for intra-abdominal écrasement if the ovary is small. If it is pathological, and the blood supply is therefore increased, remote écrasement without ligation is inadvisable. The closure and aftercare of the abdomen parallel that of the flank cryptorchidectomy incision.

Ovariectomy per Laparotomy–Ventral Abdomen Technique

Approach through the ventral paramedian or midline incision requires general anesthesia and dorsal recumbency. It is justified on the basis of preference or in the case of a very large tumor that would tax the limits of a grid incision. The ventral incision is extensile and can be started small for exploration and lengthened as needed.

The midline incision is made on the linea alba and gives maximum exposure and access to either side. The tissue planes incised are skin, superficial abdominal fascia, linea alba, the fatty fascia transversalis and peritoneum. Upon entry into the abdomen, the tumor is handled in the same way as described in the flank approach. Suture closure of the peritoneum is optional, and opinion is somewhat divided as to its desirability. If done, the peritoneum can be effectively closed with a continuous suture of No. 0 or 1 gut placed in bootlace fashion and tensed during the patient's inspiration. The incision in the conjoined aponeuroses at the midline is closed by preference with a continuous oblique modified Mayo imbricating mattress suture pattern taken with doubled strands of a high tensile strength nonabsorbable synthetic suture material. The overlapping margin is fixed securely to the superficial sheath of the rectus muscle with a second row of continuous suture taken with a single strand of the same material. The superficial abdominal fascia is closed with a third row of No. 2 chromic gut placed in an interrupted mattress pattern and tied with inverted knots. The skin is closed with a fourth row of interrupted horizontal or oblique mattress sutures of any acceptable noncapillary, nonabsorbable material. A stent bandage is oversewn and, if desired, a protective support bandage (corset) applied over that. Healing allows removal of the skin sutures in 14 days.

The paramedian incision is usually made 4 to 8 cm lateral and parallel to the midline over the respective ovary. The tissue planes incised are the skin, superficial abdominal fascia, superficial sheath of the rectus abdominis (comprised of the deep abdominal fascia and the conjoined aponeuroses of the external and internal abdominal oblique muscles), the musculature of the rectus abdominis (with intersecting tendinous inscriptions), the deep sheath of the rectus abdominis (aponeurosis of the transversus abdominis muscle), the fatty fascia transversalis and the peritoneum. The superficial sheath and muscle belly of the rectus are always opened longitudinally and coincident with the skin incision. The fibers of the deep sheath run transversely and are cut by a longitudinal incision. For this reason, some prefer separating the fibers of the deep sheath transversely, in the manner of a grid incision, continuing then with a longitudinal incision of the peritoneum. This is an acceptable alternative; however, the argument strains the evidence. The deep sheath is a very thin, weak layer that contributes little to the strength of the closure of the ventral laparotomy, while restricting exposure and limiting access. Also, the grid defeats the purpose of using an approach through the ventral abdomen to take advantage of the extensile feature of ventral longitudinal incisions. Therefore, it seems more practical to use the through-and-through paramedian incision made in the same sagittal plane. Ovariectomy is routine.

Closure of the paramedian incision approximates that of the linea alba except for the muscle mass. Closure of the peritoneum is as previously described. The deep sheath is closed with horizontal mattress bites if incised (longitudinally) and with vertical sutures if separated (transversely). No sutures are placed in the muscle fibers of the rectus abdominis muscle. The superficial sheath provides the major support and is closed by preference according to the technique described for the linea alba with a two-layer overlapping mattress suture. Because of the close attachment of the underlying muscle, however, it is necessary to free the undersurface of the superficial sheath on the overlapping side so that a fascia-to-fascia healing interface is created. Muscle or fat interposed between the fascial overlap will weaken the eventual union and predispose to dehiscence and herniation. Some care should be taken when reflecting the muscle from the rectus sheath to avoid unnecessary hemorrhage from the multiple vascular branches of the superficial abdominal arteries that perforate the rectus sheath. Once the incision in the sheath is repaired, the superficial abdominal fascia and skin are closed according to the previous description. Aftercare is also the same.

Detorsion of the Uterus per Laparotomy

Torsion of the uterus occurs less frequently in the mare than in the cow, but it is a more serious problem in the mare, owing to the relatively greater difficulty in correction and the lower survival rate. In one compilation of more than 50 cases in the mare and more than 400 cases in the cow, the mortality rate in the mare was greater than three times that in the cow.[48, 51, 64] This may be due partly to the high percentage of success with the nonoperative technique of reduction by rolling the cow with a torsion versus the much more frequent need in the mare for surgical reduction per laparotomy. Physical problems of restraint and patient safety can't be compared when one considers the basic difference in casting a cow with a rope squeeze, rolling her over in fully conscious recumbency and allowing her to jump up to her feet, as opposed to casting a mature mare, which, in this modern age, means either general anesthesia or the use of some profound muscle relaxant or neuroleptic that may last for at least 15 to 20 minutes before the mare is able to regain her feet, somewhat unsteadily. Add to this the vulnerability of the uterus of the mare to rupture as a result of such manipulations or to break and hemorrhage spontaneously to a consequential degree, and it is understandable why uterine torsion in the mare is regarded with more gravity than in the cow.

Diagnosis is based upon careful examination of every case of colic or malaise seen in the pregnant mare, especially during the last 4 months of gestation. Labor contractions are usually absent because the fetus cannot be presented into the pelvis so long as the torsion exists. On manual examination of the pelvic canal *per rectum,* the torsion can be palpated as either a clockwise (more prevalent) or a counterclockwise rotation by feeling the broad ligaments (mesometrium) of the uterus pulled into tense bands crossing the uterus dorsally from right to left or left to right. The actual twist of the uterine body may be less readily detected. The common dorsosacral position of the term fetus may have assumed a dorsopubic posture, unless of course the torsion has increased from 180° to 360° or greater. On examination *per vagin-*

am, contorted folds may be apparent or palpable in the fornix.

It is possible that the cervix may have dilated and that the torsion is not great enough to prevent introduction of the hand. Herein lies a hazard. In such cases, the torsion may go unrecognized, and the temptation is to provide an assisted delivery by external traction. If this is attempted in a torsion of 180°, for example, the odds are great that the uterus will be ruptured by the effort and that the mare will die early from hemorrhage or later from peritonitis. Therefore, be on guard against hasty conclusions at the time of such pelvic examinations, and if torsion is present, do whatever is necessary to correct it.

Although no great confidence has been placed in rolling the mare, there will be some cases in which the method is justified. The mare is cast on the side toward which the torsion is directed and then turned rather quickly in the direction of the twist, with the objective of turning the body around the uterine axis, counting on inertia in the gravid uterus to keep the fetal position constant while the maternal position changes. The surgeon may elect to follow the course of events with one hand in the vagina, holding onto a part of the fetal anatomy if the cervix is open. Rolling may need to be repeated several times. If it is unsuccessful or if this method is not used, the alternative is manipulation through a grid flank laparotomy in the standing mare, done under local anesthesia as described for the flank cryptorchidectomy.

Although both sides have been used successfully, there seems to be some reason for approaching the torsion from the side toward which the twist is directed. One paramount consideration is that correction is best accomplished by pushing rather than pulling. Therefore, if the uterus is twisted to the right, entry through the right flank would permit pushing the gravid horn back over the uterine (or somatic) axis. This is facilitated by elevation of the gravid horn from underneath by manually lifting with one arm while pushing with the other to cause the displaced horn to roll back over. Great care should be exercised to avoid perforating or tearing the uterine wall by overzealous efforts, remembering that the tissues may have been rendered somewhat friable.

Once the torsion has been corrected, there is still concern for the blood supply, which may have been strangulated long enough to cause thrombosis, which will result in infarction of the gravid horn and very probably death of the mare. In torsions that approximate parturition, it must be determined whether labor will be affected. If the mare has gone full term, has come to milk and is dilated, the decision may be to assist delivery, either by induction of labor with oxytocin or by more direct manually assisted delivery.

In the event the torsion cannot be corrected per flank laparotomy or if that alternative is not appropriate to the circumstances, the last resort is cesarean section, and incorrectable uterine torsion is a justifiable indication for this procedure.

Cesarean Section

Proper emphasis dictates that cesarean sections should be done only when the fetus cannot be delivered by either mutation of malposition or fetotomy or when the latter technique would be unduly injurious to the mare or would unnecessarily sacrifice a live fetus. These considerations stress the importance of prompt assessment and quick action while the fetus is still alive or before the dam develops further complications. Treatment for shock should be presumptive, and regardless of clinical signs, administration of parenteral fluids and prophylactic antibiotics should commence with preparations for surgery. The use of adrenocortical steroids and antihistamines is discretionary but should be considered in light of the frequency of shock and laminitis in such cases. If a mechanical respirator and oxygen are available, they should be readied for use.

Hypotensive tranquilizers and barbiturate anesthetics are generally contraindicated if the fetus is alive or if the mare has been greatly stressed. Vandeplassche has recommended the combination of epidural anesthesia to suppress tenesmus and relax the abdominal wall, intravenous glyceryl guaiacolate to induce relaxation of skeletal muscle necessary for recumbent positioning and local infiltration for incisional anesthesia.[60-63] Low level halothane by inhalation is also well tolerated and eliminates the need for continuous drip glyceryl guaiacolate, which tends to retard recovery owing to its calcium-binding action. The use of inhalation anesthesia also makes possible simultaneous mechanically assisted ventilation. The principal advantage of the glyceryl guaiacolate method is that it is readily available

for use in the field for emergency purposes such as this, and if inhalation equipment must be dismantled and transported for such use, the time lost in the process may be the margin between fetal life and death. Therefore, it is necessary that the alternative method be available and familiar to the surgeon. The calcium-binding effect of intravenous glyceryl guaiacolate can be countered by the cautious infusion of 10 to 20 per cent solution of calcium borogluconate during the postanesthetic recovery period, being careful to monitor heart action all the while.

The choice of incisions for cesarean section is somewhat a matter of preference between the low flank grid through an oblique incision and the ventral midline incision. Both have been used widely and should provide alternative methods. The chief criticisms of the ventral technique are vulnerability of the incision to disruption, greater compromise of the pleural space and interference with respiration due to the intra-abdominal pressure on the diaphragm and the occasional inadvertent production of obturator paralysis by failure to support or suspend the weight of the hindlegs hanging in abduction. The major criticism of the grid technique is comparatively smaller exposure, requiring greater retraction, and perhaps some risk of radial nerve paralysis in the dependent foreleg. To stretch a point, the anesthesiologist argues the case of the congested downside lung and the poorly perfused upside lung caused by protracted lateral recumbency. Needless to say, these disadvantages can be met and minimized by use of precautionary methods and competent technique.

The low flank oblique incision, often referred to as the Marcenac approach, is directed caudoventrad from a point midway the costal arch along a line extending backward and downward to a point inside the fold of the flank. The left side is usually preferred owing to the mobility of the bowel on that side, as opposed to the capacious cecum and fixed limbs of the colon on the right side. The superficial abdominal fascia is incised in the same plane. The deep abdominal fascia, recognizable by its yellow, elastic fibers, runs at a right angle to the incision and must be incised or separated. The fibers of the external abdominal oblique muscle and aponeurosis are separated in the direction of the incision, and the underlying aponeurosis of the internal oblique muscle is separated as it runs at a right angle to the incision. The transversus abdominis muscle runs in a transverse direction that splits the right angle between the oblique muscles and is also separated in the direction of its fibers. The upper edge of the rectus abdominis muscle is encountered in the lower extremity of the incision and must be retracted downward. The fatty fascia transversalis and peritoneum are incised in agreement with the skin incision, and all the muscles are retracted sufficiently to permit the elevation of the tip of the gravid horn of the uterus into the incision.

Manipulation of the uterus follows the methods advocated in detorsion of the uterus. Undue pulling and tugging on one part may cause a weakening or rupture of the uterine wall. Posterior presentations place the fetal head and forelegs in the uterine tip and require proportionately longer incisions for delivery than when the feet and hocks of the hindlegs are encountered in the anterior presentation.

Incision of the uterus should be on the greater curvature and should avoid the tip near the junction with the uterine tube (oviduct). The contents should be handled as contaminated and carefully drained to the outside. The use of plastic laparotomy drapes placed so as to protect the laparotomy wound margins from contamination will reduce the number of postoperative wound infections and insure stronger repairs. This becomes of special importance in ventral midline incisions.

The live foal should be laid alongside the mare with the umbilical cord left intact until the foal is breathing normally and pulsations in the umbilical vessels have stopped. Then, the cord should be broken or severed at the slight constriction a few centimeters away from the cutaneous navel. This should be done without tugging roughly on the site of attachment to the foal, which may predispose to umbilical hernia. If the foal is alive, the placenta may be difficult to remove and should be left inside the uterus. If the foal is dead, the membranes should be removed if possible. The cavity of the uterus should be medicated with an antibiotic compatible with that used systemically.

Closure of the uterus should take account of the problem in achieving adequate hemostasis along the cut margins of the uterine incision. Because of the diffuse placentation in the mare, ligation of discrete bleeders in a few locations is inadequate to control mural hemorrhage, which continues to cause bleeding into the lumen of the uterus after a conventional closure. This has been recognized as a significant cause of maternal mortality. The use of a continuous interlocking suture, through all layers of the uterine wall and around the entire margin of the incision, has been recommended for control of this problem and has been credited with much of the reduction of mortality rate in one series of 71 cases.[60-63] After placement of this row, the uterus is closed with inverting rows of Lembert or Cushing suture pattern of No. 1 chromic gut or PGA swaged on a curved atraumatic needle. Care is taken to exclude any remaining placenta from the suture lines. The uterus is cleansed and returned to the abdomen.

Closure of the grid incision is effected by placement of simple interrupted or continuous sutures in each plane of muscle or fascia independently. The superficial abdominal fascia and skin are closed as previously described. Upon completion, oxytocin, 20 IU, is given intravenously to aid in expulsion of the remaining placenta, fluids and detritus. If the membranes are retained beyond the fourth postpartum hour, 50 IU of oxytocin diluted in one liter of physiological saline solution is given intravenously by continuous drip over 30 to 60 minutes.[60-63]

Thereafter, the treatments already initiated for complications described should be maintained as needed until the mare's condition is rated safe. This may include manual disruption of early adhesions by palpation of the uterus *per rectum* on the fourth day, lavage and siphonage of the uterus if an unusual accumulation of lochia occurs, administration of small doses of oxytocin if involution is slow, maintenance of a laxative diet for constipation, continuation of antibiotics for infection, attention to the wound and constant alertness for signs of peritonitis, hemorrhagic shock, laminitis and metritis.[60-63]

Ovariohysterectomy

If chronic pyometra has made the mare permanently barren, if the uterus is the site of localized neoplasia or if there is segmental aplasia of the cervix with mucometra, and if the mare is otherwise sound for work, ovariohysterectomy is justified.

The procedure is done through the ventral midline with the patient under general anesthesia in dorsal recumbency. The hindlegs should be supported by side cushions or suspended in semiflexion from above. Preoperative antibiotics are advisable. The approach is the same as described for cesarean section. The ovarian and cranial uterine blood supply is controlled by double ligation as the mesovarium and mesometrium are dissected. This allows both ovaries and uterine horns to be resected *en bloc*. At this point, they are exteriorized and packed off to guard against accidental contamination of the peritoneal cavity during the subsequent amputation. The uterus is retracted sufficiently to expose the uterine body, which is tourniquetted (with gum rubber tubing or equivalent) as close as possible to the cervix. A second tourniquet is placed near the bifurcation, leaving at least an 8-cm space between the two tourniquets. The uterine body is transected within this space, closing the stump with double-layer inverting sutures according to Parker-Kerr technique and oversewing to insure seal against contamination. The surgical specimen (uterus and ovaries) is removed from the field along with any soiled drapes. As the remaining tourniquet is loosened, care is taken to ligate any bleeders originating from the bilateral urogenital arteries that supply the caudal uterus. Once hemostasis and asepsis are secured, the field is cleansed and undraped, and the abdominal incision is closed as described under cesarean section. Aftercare is routine. If the procedure has gone according to plan, recovery should be relatively uneventful but prudence dictates that the mare's condition be monitored carefully for the first 2 postoperative weeks.

REFERENCES

1. Aanes, W. A.: Surgical repair of third-degree perineal laceration and rectovaginal fistula in the mare. J.A.V.M.A., *144*:485, 1964.
2. Aanes, W. A.: Progress in recto-vaginal surgery. Proceedings of the Nineteenth Annual Convention of the American Association of Equine Practitioners, Atlanta, 1973, pp. 225–240.
3. Adams, O. R.: An improved method of diagnosis and castration of cryptorchid horses. J.A.V.M.A., *145*:439, 1964.
4. Ashdown, R. R.: The anatomy of the inguinal canal in domesticated mammals. Vet. Rec., *75*:1345, 1963.
5. A. V. M. A. Council on Veterinary Services: Council report — Unacceptable surgical procedures applicable to domestic animals. J.A.V.M.A., *168*:947, 1976.
6. Belonje, C. W. A.: The operation for retroversion of the penis in the stallion. J. South Afr. Vet. Med. Assoc., *27*:53, 1956.
7. Bignozzi, L.: Surgical treatment of scrotal hernia in foals and yearlings, without orchectomy. Tijdschr. Diergeneeskd., *98*:1025, 1973.
8. Bishop, M. W. H., David, J. S. E., and Messervy, A.: Some observations on cryptorchidism in the horse. Vet. Rec., *76*:1041, 1064.
9. Brown, M. P., Colahan, P. T., and Hawkins, D. L.: Urethral extension for treatment of urine pooling in mares. J.A.V.M.A., *173*:1005, 1978.
10. Caslick, E. A.: The vulva and vulvo-vaginal orifice and its relation to genital health of the Thoroughbred mare. Cornell Vet., *27*:178, 1937.
11. Clark, T. L.: Clinical management of equine ovarian neoplasms. J. Reprod. Fertil. (Suppl.) *23*:331, 1975.
12. Cotchin, E.: A general survey of tumours in the horse. Equine Vet. J., *9*:16, 1977.
13. Cox, J. E.: Surgery of the Male Reproductive Tract in Large Animals. Published by the author, University of Liverpool Veterinary Field Station, "Leahurst," Neston, WIRRAL, L64 7TE, Merseyside, England, 1977.
14. Cox, J. E., and Williams, J. H.: Some aspects of the reproductive endocrinology of the stallion and cryptorchid. J. Reprod. Fertil., (Suppl.) *23*:75, 1975.
15. Cox, J. E., Edwards, G. B., and Neal, P. A.: Suprapubic paramedian laparotomy for equine abdominal cryptorchidism. Vet. Rec. *97*:428, 1975.
16. Cox, J. E., Williams, J. H., Rowe, P. H., and Smith, J. H.: Testosterone in normal, cryptorchid and castrated male horses. Equine Vet. J., *5*:85, 1973.
17. Crowe, C. W., Gardner, R. E., Humburg, J. M., Nachreiner, R. F., and Purohit, R. C.: Plasma testosterone and behavioral characteristics in geldings with intact epididymides. J. Equine Med. Surg., *1*:387, 1977.
17a. Danks, A. G.: Williams' Surgical Operations. Published by the author. Ithaca, N.Y., 1945, pp. 84–87.
18. DeMoor, A., and Verschooten, F.: Paramedian incision for the removal of abdominal testicles in the horse. Vet. Med./Small Anim. Clin., Nov., pp. 1083–1086, 1967.
19. Dietz, O., Gangel, H., and Richter, W.: Die Sterilisation des Ebers und des Hengstes. Mhefte Vet. Med. Leipzig, *29*:906, 1974.
20. Donaldson, R. S.: Eversion of the bladder in a mare. Vet. Rec. *92*:409, 1973.
21. Frank, E. R.: Veterinary Surgery, 7th Ed. Minneapolis, Burgess Publishing Co., 1964, pp. 292–294.
22. Gadd, J. W.: The relationship of bacterial cultures, microscopic smear examination and medical treatment to surgical correction of barren mares. Proceedings of the Twenty-first Annual Convention of the American Association Equine Practitioners, Boston, 1975, pp. 362–368.
23. Ganjam, V. K., and Kenney, R. M.: Androgens and oestrogens in normal and cryptorchid stallions. J. Reprod. Fertil. (Suppl.) *23*:67, 1975.
24. Getty, R.: Sisson and Grossman's Anatomy of the Domestic Animals, Vol. 1, 5th Ed., Philadelphia, W. B. Saunders Co., 1975, pp. 531–541.
25. Gygax, A. P., Donawick, W. J., and Gledhill, B. L.: Hematocoele in a stallion and recovery of fertility following unilateral castration. Equine Vet. J., *5*:128, 1973.
26. Habel, R. E.: The perineum of the mare. Cornell Vet., *43*:249, 1953.

27. Hall, W. C., Nielson, S. W., and McEntee, K.: Tumours of the prostate and penis. Bull. World Health Org., *53*:247, 1976.
28. Heinze, C. D., and Allen, A. R.: Repair of third-degree perineal lacerations in the mare. Vet. Scope, *11*:12, 1966.
29. Hoffman, P. E.: Castration of normal and cryptorchid horses by a primary closure method. Proceedings of the Nineteenth American Association of Equine Practitioners, Atlanta, 1973, pp. 219–223.
30. Hutchings, D. R., and Rawlinson, R. J.: Eventration as a sequel to castration of the horse. Austral. Vet. J., *48*:288, 1972.
31. Jones, W. E., and Bogart, R.: Genetics of the horse, East Lansing, Mich., Caballus Publishers, 1971, pp. 241–278.
32. Kenney, R. M.: Cyclic and pathologic changes of the mare endometrium as detected by biopsy, with a note on early embryonic death. J.A.V.M.A., *172*:241, 1978
33. Kenney, R. M., and Ganjam, V. K.: Selected pathological changes of the mare uterus and ovary. J. Reprod. Fertil. (Suppl.) *23*:335, 1975.
34. Lowe, J. E., and Dougherty, R.: Castration of horses and ponies by a primary closure method. J.A.V.M.A., *160*:183, 1972.
35. Lowe, J. E., and Higginbotham, R.: Castration of abdominal cryptorchid horses by a paramedian laparotomy approach. Cornell Vet. *59*:121, 1969.
36. Lundall, R. L.: The urinary system, in Oehme, V. W., and Prier, J. E. (eds.): Textbook of Large Animal Surgery. Baltimore, The Williams and Wilkins Co., 1974, p. 459.
37. McEntee, K., and Nielsen, S. W.: Tumours of the female genital tract. Bull. World Health Org., *53*:217, 1976.
38. Meagher, D. M., Wheat, J. D., Hughes, J. P., Stabenfeldt, G. H., and Harris, B. A.: Granulosa cell tumors in mares — A review of 78 cases. Proceedings of the Twenty-third Annual Convention of the American Association of Equine Practitioners, Vancouver, 1977, pp. 133–145.
39. Merriam, J. G.: Inguinal approach to equine cryptorchidectomy. Vet. Med./Small Animal Clin., Feb., pp. 187–191, 1972.
40. Monin, T.: Vaginoplasty: A surgical treatment for urine pooling in the mare. Proceedings of the Eighteenth Annual Convention of the American Association of Equine Practitioners, San Francisco, pp. 99–102, 1972.
41. Moore, J. N., Johnson, J. H., Tritschler, L. G., and Garner, H. E.: Equine cryptorchidism: Presurgical considerations and surgical management. Vet. Surg., 7:43, 1978.
42. Moulton, J. E.: Tumors in Domestic Animals, 2nd Ed., Berkeley, University of California Press, Berkeley, 1978, Chapt. 10.
43. Moulton, J. E.: Tumors in Domestic Animals, 2nd Ed., Berkeley, University of California Press, 1978, Chapt. 11.
44. Nickel, R., Schummer, A., Seiferle, E., and Sack, W. O.: The Viscera of the Domestic Mammals. New York, Springer-Verlag, 1973, pp. 351–392.

45. Nielsen, S. W., Misdorp, W., and McEntee, K.: Tumours of the ovary. Ch. XV, Bull. World Health Org., *53*:203, 1976.
46. O'Connor, J. P.: Rectal examination of the cryptorchid horse. Irish Vet. J. *25*:129, 1971.
47. Osborne, V. E.: Genital infection of a horse with spirochaetes. Austral. Vet. J., May, pp. 190–191, 1961.
48. Roberts, S. J.: Veterinary Obstetrics and Genital Diseases (Theriogenology). Published by the author, Ithaca, N. Y., Distributed by Edwards Brothers, Inc., Ann Arbor, Mich., 1971.
49. Selway, S. J., Kenney, R. M., Bergman, R. V., Greenhoff, G. R., Cooper, W. L., and Ganjam, V. K.: Field technique for vasectomy. Proceedings of 23rd Annual Convention of the American Association of Equine Practitioners, Vancouver, 1977, pp. 355–361.
50. Shapiro, S. R., and Balazs, I. B.: Current concepts of the undescended testis. Surg. Gynecol. Obstet., *147*:617, 1978.
51. Skjerven, O.: Correction of uterine torsion by laparotomy. Nord. Vet. Med., *17*:377, 1965.
52. Smith, J. A.: The development and descent of the testis in the horse. Vet. Ann., *15*:156, 1975.
53. Stannic, M. N.: Castration of cryptorchids. Mod. Vet. Pract. Dec., pp. 30–33, 1960.
54. Stickle, R. L., and Fessler, J. F.: Retrospective study of 350 cases of equine cryptorchidism. J.A.V.M.A., *172*:343, 1978.
55. Stickle, R. L., Fessler, J. F., and Adams, S. B.: A single stage technique for repair of rectovestibular lacerations in the mare. Vet. Surg., *8*:25, 1979.
56. Straub, O. C., and Fowler, M. E.: Repair of perineal lacerations in the mare and cow. J.A.V.M.A., *138*:659, 1961.
57. Swift, P. N.: Castration of a stallion with bilateral abdominal cryptorchidism by flank laparotomy. Austral. Vet. J., *48*:472, 1972.
58. Thomas, A. D.: Microfilariasis in the horse. South Afr. Vet. Med. Assoc., *34*:17, 1963.
59. Valdez, H., Taylor, T. S., McLaughlin, A. and Martin, M. T.: Abdominal cryptorchidectomy in the horse, using inguinal extension of the gubernaculum testis. J.A.V.M.A., *174*:1110, 1979.
60. Vandeplassche, M.: Caesarean section in the horse. *In* Grunsell, C. S. G., and Hill, F. W. G. (eds.): The Veterinary Annual, Bristol, John Wright, 1973, pp. 73–78.
61. Vandeplassche, M.: Caesarean section in the mare. Vet. Rec. *96*:412, 1975.
62. Vandeplassche, M.: Embryotomy and cesarotomy. *In* Oehme, F. W., and Prier, J. E. (eds): Textbook of Large Animal Surgery, Baltimore, The Williams & Wilkins Co., 1974, pp. 521–537.
63. Vandeplassche, M., Bouters, R., Spincemaille, J., and Bonte, P.: Caesarean section in the mare. Proceedings of the Twenty-third Annual Convention of the American Association of Equine Practitioners, Vancouver, 1977, pp. 75–80.
64. Wheat, J. D., and Meagher, D. M.: Uterine torsion and rupture in mares. J.A.V.M.A., *160*:881, 1972.

section **IX**

FELINE

Consulting Editors

EMERSON D. COLBY
and
NICKOLAS J. SOJKA

The Cat in Evolution

EMERSON D. COLBY
Dartmouth Medical School, Hanover,
New Hampshire

The feline ancestor, in common with the Canids and other small carnivores, was derived from an animal called Miacis that over millions of years developed into two distinct groups called Holophoneus and Dinctis. The group Holophoneus contained the Smilodon or saber-toothed tiger that disappeared at the end of the great herbivore era. Animals from the group Dinctis developed specialized adaptations over tens of thousands of years and have resulted in the family Felidae as we know it today.

Man probably became associated with the cat during the Stone Age. As time evolved, the cat was used for fishing and for hunting wild birds. Its primary use down through the centuries has been that of rodent control, and the fortunes or misfortunes of the cat have revolved significantly around this activity.

The cat has been revered and worshipped (Egypt, about 1500 to 1000 B.C.) by common people as well as by royalty. Witness creation of the diety of the cat-goddess Bastet. Cats were embalmed and buried in special cemeteries that have been unearthed in modern times. It is thought that cats found throughout the world came originally from Egypt and that they were established in many countries by armed invasion and commerce because they were used to control rodent populations near food depots on land or at sea.

During the Middle Ages, cats were offered as sacrifices. As late as 1484, a decree by Pope Innocent VIII denounced the cat and all who gave it homage, and thus many cats were destroyed. The introduction of the plague-carrying black rat into the European community with the return of the Crusaders probably saved the cat from extinction in Europe.

Reverence for the cat by Japanese royalty nearly ruined the silk industry by making it fashionable to follow the example of royalty, who preferred to keep cats confined for breeding purposes and to walk them on a leash. Because of this, the silk industry was being consumed by an increasing mouse population and was eventually saved by a government decree in the year 1602 liberating the feline population.

When Louis Pasteur discovered the microbe in the mid-nineteenth century, dogs were discarded as household pets in favor of the more fastidious cat, and the breeding industry called for a wider variety of the feline species in order for cats owners to be fashionable. Breeds and varieties have resulted from this nineteenth century activity and have led to today's cat shows, the first of which was held in the state of Maine in 1860. The first official English show was held at the Crystal Palace in London in 1871.

Selective breeding has produced many breeds, both long- and short-haired, as well as some that are hairless and some with the curled or Rex mutation. Whatever the breed or phenotypical appearance, we should continue to remind ourselves that history, past and present, controls the destiny of the cat and that we as humans should respect the feline species, especially as we try to regulate its reproductive destiny.

REFERENCE

1. Pond, G.: The Cat Encyclopedia. New York, Crown Publishers, Inc., 1972, pp. 354–358.

Laparoscopic Determination of Ovarian and Uterine Morphology during the Reproductive Cycle

*DAVID E. WILDT and
STEPHEN W. J. SEAGER*

*Baylor College of Medicine/Texas A & M
University, Houston, Texas*

To completely comprehend reproductive function, it is advantageous to understand the sequence of morphological events occurring on the ovary. Ovarian morphological observations have conventionally been documented by laparotomy or necropsy. These methods, however, generally do not allow monitoring of ovarian activity repeatedly within the same animal. Consequently, it has been difficult to perform detailed studies on the consecutive events associated with ovarian follicular development, ovulation, luteinization and corpus luteum development and regression.

LAPAROSCOPIC TECHNIQUE

Laparoscopic techniques, used extensively in a variety of species, have been adapted in this laboratory for use in the domestic cat. The advantage of laparoscopy is that only minor surgical intervention is necessary, requiring simply a small midline skin incision for insertion of a laparoscopic telescope. Auxiliary instruments can be used through accessory abdominal cannulae to manipulate internal organs and measure ovarian anatomical structures. The details of the technique of laparoscopy in the cat have been published elsewhere. In brief, each animal is anesthetized for laparoscopic examination. Queens are given an intramuscular injection of ketamine hydrochloride (Ketaset), 20 mg/kg, and acepromazine, 0.18 mg/kg. Each animal is restrained in a supine, head-down position at a 30° angle. The posterior abdominal region is surgically prepared. A midline incision (1 to 2 cm) is made near the umbilicus, and a trocar cannula unit is inserted through the incision and into the abdominal cavity. The trocar is removed, and the laparoscope is inserted through the cannula (Fig. 1). The laparoscope is attached to an illumination source by means of a flexible fiberoptic cable. A Verres needle probe (graduated in millimeters) is inserted through the skin and into the abdominal cavity at a site 4 to 8 cm lateral to the midline. This instrument is used to manipulate internal organs or tissue and to obtain precise measurements of ovarian structures. Photographs of reproductive organs are taken using a camera attached to the laparoscopic telescope by means of a specialized adapter. At the end of the examination, the instruments are removed and the incision sutured. Laparoscopy is less traumatic than laparotomy and can be performed routinely in individual animals at 1 to 2 day intervals for as long as 3 weeks with no adverse physical effects.

OVARIAN AND UTERINE MORPHOLOGY

Laparoscopy is readily adapted for observation of the reproductive organs in the cat. Upon initial observation, the body of the uterus and the paired extended uterine horns are visible (Fig. 2). In the adult anestrous queen, uterine horn tissue appears smooth and pink in color and measures 3 to 4 mm in width. Uterine morphology changes dramatically as the queen demonstrates sexual receptivity to the male. The uterus becomes pale pink to gray in color and appears turgid. The uterine horns tend to coil slightly and increase in width to 5 to 7 mm. In the event that ovulation occurs, pseudopregnancy is characterized by the horns remaining swollen, convoluted and very pale gray to white in color. As ovarian activity declines, the appearance of the uterus gradually returns to that observed in the anestrous state.

On laparoscopic examination, each uterine horn can be observed cranially and laterally to the base of each uterine horn. The ovary of the cat is located in a pocket of

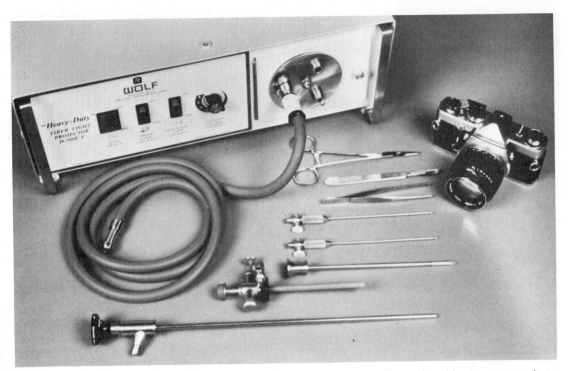

Figure 1. Laparoscopic equipment including laparoscope, light source, fiberoptic cable, trocar cannula assembly, Verres needles, and camera.

peritoneum, the ovarian bursa or fimbria (Fig. 3). The tortuous oviduct begins near the cranial pole of the ovarian bursa, courses caudally along the bursa's lateral plane and

is continuous with the cranial end of the uterine horn. During anestrus little observable oviductal activity is detected. However, as the queen demonstrates sexual receptivity

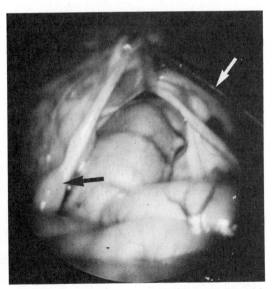

Figure 2. Reproductive tract of queen as viewed by laparoscopy. The Verres needle proble (white arrow) elevates the left uterine horn and ovary (black arrow).

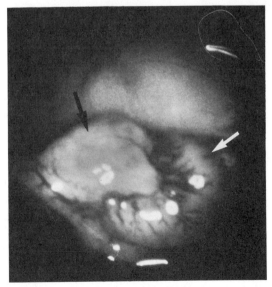

Figure 3. The right ovary (black arrow) covered by the vascular ovarian bursa (white arrow).

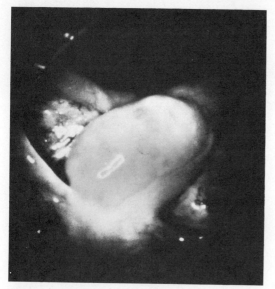

Figure 4. Quiescent or anestrous ovary. The ovarian bursa is held from the ovarian surface with the Verres needle probe.

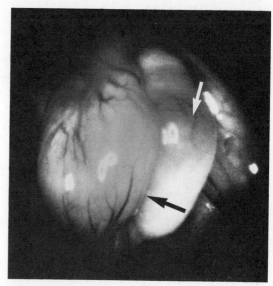

Figure 6. Ovary with a mature follicle with surface vessels (white arrow). Vascular ovarian bursa (black arrow) adjacent to ovary.

to the male, the oviduct can be noted to contract dramatically, exhibiting considerable peristaltic activity.

The ovarian bursa is attached laterally to the dorsal suspensory ligament of the ovary. This translucent tissue is highly vascular and normally completely encompasses the ovary. Since the fimbria is not attached to the medial portion of the suspensory ligament, it can be gently removed, using the Verres needle probe, to expose the ovarian surface (Fig. 4).

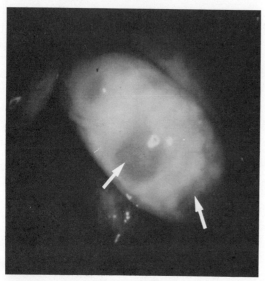

Figure 5. Ovary during estrus with mature, slightly raised vesicular follicles (arrows).

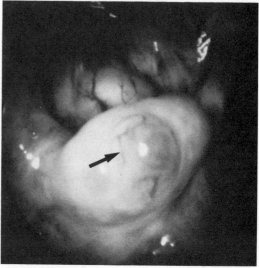

Figure 7. Ovary containing a vesicular follicle just prior to ovulation. Vascularity evident at follicular base (arrow).

The ovaries of the queen are oval-shaped organs, grayish-white in color. During anestrus each ovary is generally smooth, often having no visible structural activity (Fig. 4). Queens that begin to show a relaxed and receptive attitude toward the male but that disallow copulation are designated as being in proestrus. The ovary of the proestrous queen is characterized by clear grayish areas with indistinct boundaries visible at random locations on the ovary. These areas, 0.5 to 1.5 mm in diameter, are distinctly different in coloration in relation to the remainder of the ovarian surface. As estrus approaches and the queen allows mating, these areas develop into distinct fluid-filled preovulatory follicles (Fig. 5).

Follicular development in the cat is a rapid occurrence, with most follicles developing to the vesicular stage within a 24 to 48 hour interval. Most follicular development occurs during the 48-hour interval just prior to the first day of estrous behavior. The queen ovary always contains mature follicles on the first day of exhibited estrous behavior. Vesicular follicles are spherical in shape, contain convoluted vascular patterns within the follicular wall and generally are flattened or protrude slightly above the ovarian surface (Fig. 6). Mature follicles measure 2.5 to 3.5 mm in diameter.

Ovulation has not occurred spontaneously in any animal examined. Only queens that were mated or artificially induced by injecting gonadotropin drugs ovulated. Follicles that fail to ovulate regress gradually to a nondetectable state over a 3- to 7-day period. As ovulation approaches, the follicular dome becomes clearer in appearance while the base of the follicle becomes heavily vascularized (Fig. 7). Often prior to ovulation, a clear grayish stigma will form in the center of the follicular dome (Fig. 8). Ovulation is a gradual process culminating in the release of a yellowish-gray cumulous mass that can often be observed adhering to the ovarian surface. As in certain other species, ovulation in the cat is accompanied by considerable hemorrhaging at the follicle site and an inward cratering of the follicle dome.

Luteinization and maturation of the corpus luteum occur over a short interval, 24 to 36 hours. The developing corpus luteum is opaque in appearance and changes gradually in color from a dark red to an orange

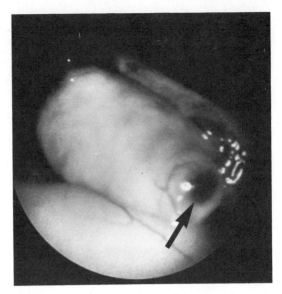

Figure 8. Ovary containing ovulatory follicle on its lateral pole. Note the dark stigma forming at the dome of the follicle (arrow).

yellow color. The mature feline corpus luteum is raised above the ovarian surface, contains a flattened dome and increases only slightly in diameter, to a maximum of 4.5

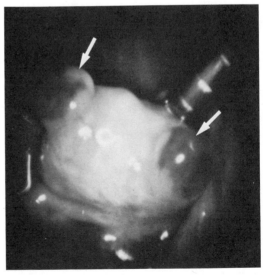

Figure 9. Ovary with two maturing corpora lutea (arrows).

mm (Fig. 9). Each corpus luteum gradually regresses in size to a small, yellowish, flat luteal scar that sometimes remains visible on the ovarian surface for as long as 6 weeks.*

---

*This research is supported in part by a grant from the Ralston Purina Company, St. Louis, Missouri.

REFERENCES

1. Dukelow, W. R., and Ariga, S.: Laparoscopic techniques for biomedical research. J. Med. Primatol., 5:82, 1976.
2. McClure, R. C., Dallman, M. J. and Garrett, P. D.: Cat Anatomy: An Atlas, Text and Dissection Guide. Philadelphia, Lea and Febiger, 1973.
3. Wildt, D. E., Kinney, G. M. and Seager, S. W. J.: Laparoscopy for direct observation of internal organs of the domestic cat and dog. Am. J. Vet. Res., 38:1429, 1977.

The Estrous Cycle and Pregnancy

EMERSON D. COLBY
Dartmouth Medical School,
Hanover, New Hampshire

THE ESTROUS CYCLE

The cat is a seasonally polyestrous animal with two to three cycles per year. There is generally more than one estrous period during any given cycle, and there is not a single cycle common to all females. Geographical location and breed may have considerable influence on the length and timing of the cycle of the female. The first estrous period, or periods, may be brief and may go unnoticed by the owner. Discharges and vulvar swellings are usually absent.

Puberty in the domestic female cat is generally given as 7 to 9 months, but it has been known to occur as early as 5 months and as late as 12 months. Many purebred cats tend to reach puberty later than the domestic cats, 9 to 12 months being the accepted average.[10] The male cat matures slightly later (1 to 2 months) than the female. Animals kept in a free-roaming environment may reach sexual maturity earlier than their housebound counterparts. Older cats may show irregular cycling habits as age progresses but may continue to produce offspring, with declining numbers of offspring per litter as well as only one litter per year.

Estrus may first be noted by a change in behavior. There is little or no characteristic swelling or bleeding in the vaginal area. Frequent squatting to urinate may be observed. Raising the tail head and flagging in response to handling may be evident.

The breeding season is usually recognized as being from late December to early January through the early part of September. Breeding data taken from a number of authors would indicate that the first cycle will occur from January to March, the second cycle from April to early July and the last cycle during late July through early September. Again, variations may occur between different latitudes as well as among various breeds. It is known that light will affect the estrous cycle, which probably accounts for the early onset of estrus in some females late in December or early in January. In the absence of the male for breeding purposes, the cycle will last approximately 7 to 10 days followed by a quiescent period of 2 to 3 weeks prior to the next cycle.

MATING

The queen is always taken to the cage of the male. If this process is reversed, the male may show no interest in the female and may spend time examining the new surroundings. Posturing and postmating activity have been described by Voith (see following article).

Receptivity to the male usually lasts from 1 to 4 days. Aged cats are more irregular in their cycling habits, have shorter periods of receptivity and are less likely to deliver viable term fetuses. The optimum breeding time of the naturally cycling female is thought to be between 1 and 8 years of age. Beyond that time the litter may be fewer in number, and there may be an increase in the number of stillborn fetuses.

Coital activity is brief, but the female may be bred again within 5 to 10 minutes by the same or a different male. The relative size of the male and female may have a bearing on the success of the mating and the time that it may take. Thus, when choosing mates, some consideration should be given to the relative size of the animals. Certain males that consistently have difficulty breeding because the female is either too large or too small for a successful rapid coital act may eventually become poor animals to keep at stud, owing to a lack of interest in the female. Similarly, a male that experiences difficulty in mating may give up and refuse to cover the female. The activity of the male while trying to cover the female could be enough to induce ovulation although the lack of intromission has failed to deposit the semen necessary for fertilization.

Females that are kept in colony situations may react differently when in estrus from those housed singly in separate cages. Females may be induced to cycle by having close contact, caged or free-roaming, with those females that are naturally cycling. The amount of light should receive consideration, as 14 to 16 hours of daylight will increase the percentage of cats that are naturally cycling when compared with a 12-hour light cycle. When inducing cats by the use of exogenous hormones, it is recommended that the animals be caged individually, with or without an increased light cycle. The vaginal smear of the cat demonstrates four phases of the estrous cycle: anestrus, proestrus, estrus and metestrus. The true anestrous period is generally thought to be from October to mid-December. Each phase has distinct vaginal cytological findings. If breeding occurs, the estrus period may last from 1 to 4 more days. Ovulation occurs about 24 hours postmating, and the sperm are capable of fertilization for approximately 50 hours after coitus. Approximately 5 days are needed for normal passage of the fertilized egg from the oviduct to the uterus. Implantation occurs between days 11 and 14. Corpora luteal regression takes place between 40 and 44 days; the cat is unique in this respect in that pseudopregnancy will also terminate at this time.

Catnip (*Nepeta cataria*), when presented to a cat, causes behavioral patterns similar to those exhibited by the estrous female.[13] There is currently no evidence to indicate that physiological changes associated with natural estrus can be elucidated by the presence of catnip.

Synchronization of estrus in the feline species is rarely required. If necessary, it may perhaps best be accomplished by housing estrous females with those that may not be cycling. It is strongly recommended that when estrous induction is required, the animals should be housed (caged) separately and not in a colony situation. Successful induction of estrus is poor when attempted on queens living in a free-roaming situation.

Postpartum estrus does occur in some cats, although it is brief and may go unnoticed. It may occur within 24 hours after kittening. The normal estrous pattern will appear 2 to 3 weeks after the removal of the kittens.

VAGINAL SMEAR

The vaginal smear[7] is perhaps the best way to accurately determine the estrous cycle of the cat.

The animal must necessarily be restrained when vaginal smears are taken. Although one person can effectively make the smear, it may take longer and require some struggling, which could make subsequent attempts more difficult. Assistance will minimize trauma to the vaginal mucosa, thus making the cellular detail observed in the smear more representative of the true reproductive state of the animal. The animal is usually grasped by the scruff of the neck and forced down on her elbows. The hindquarters can then be elevated and the vaginal orifice rapidly identified and entered. As the vagina is visualized, its condition should be noted. If the medicine dropper technique is used before the fluid from the vagina is placed on the slide, it should be checked for clarity, turbidity or evidence of blood. A variety of stains may be used, but most commonly a 1 per cent solution of new methylene blue is placed on the slide for 5 to 10 minutes or a Wright's stain may be used in a manner similar to that of staining a blood smear. If the smear is to be examined wet for cellular detail or evidence of sperm, a drop of 0.25 per cent solution of toluidine blue may be added to the smear and a coverslip used for microscopic examination. The cellular detail and numbers of cells may be roughly proportional to the degree of agitation used when making the smear. The anestrous smear usually contains fewer cells, which are of the parabasal type with no red blood cells and zero to a few leukocytes. The proestrous smear will contain parabasal cells that are becoming more cornified and the nuclei more pyknotic (Fig. 1). No red blood cells are present, but a few leukocytes may be noted. The estrous smear (Figs. 2 and 3) is typified by many cells, mostly of the cornified type with pyknotic or absent nuclei. There is no proven way to predict pregnancy by the use of the vaginal smear.

Toward the end of estrus and the beginning of metestrus, white blood cells appear and may remain for several days. The basic cell type of the vaginal wall returns to that of the parabasal cell. If the cat is not to recycle but is to enter its true anestrous period, the cell type will be that of the parabasal cell, with only a few being exhibited.

The most gentle and successful method of obtaining the smear is the flushing action made by a blunt medicine dropper, but even this, if handled improperly, can remove layers of cells from the vaginal wall. It must be remembered that either of the methods used can cause ovulation in the cat, which is a postcoital ovulator. One should not attempt to correlate the vaginal cytology of the estrous cycle of the dog with that of the cat. Although there are similarities in cellular detail, the differences are sufficient to confuse the uninitiated.

If postmating vaginal smears are used to determine a successful coitus, one must remember that semen will be destroyed by making the smear. It is recommended that if these smears are to be made, they can be prepared an hour or so after a mating and still prove that mating took place. One should observe the queen before making this smear, as some queens will mate only once if timid. A smear made immediately postcoitus could diminish the chances for a successful pregnancy.

OVULATION

The cat normally ovulates only in response to coitus. Ovulation is not triggered by excitement, exhibited during the height of the estrous period but by afferent impulses originating in the area of the vagina or cervix uteri.[15] Fertile and sterile matings, manipulation of a glass rod at the cervix uteri, roughness at the time of making the vaginal smear or rough handling of the perineal area during estrus are all means of inducing ovulation. Ovulation has been known to occur following a mating in which intromission did not occur.

A time lag of about 24 hours occurs between vaginal stimulation and the act of ovulation.[15] During this time, it can be shown that, as in other species, there is a release of luteotropic hormone that peaks at the time of rupture of the follicles and the release of mature ova.

Hemorrhage does not occur in the follic-

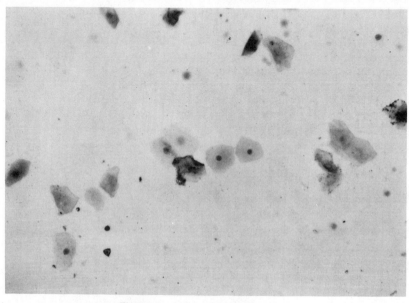

Figure 1. Late proestrous smear.

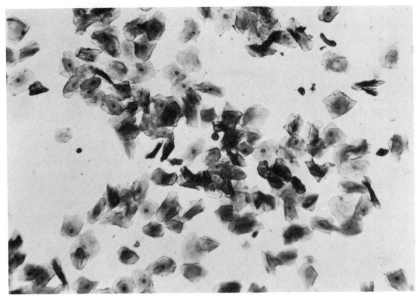

Figure 2. Estrous smear.

ular cavity, but a deep invagination of the follicular wall occurs. The corpora lutea from each follicle immediately become active and reach peak progestin activity by day 16 or 17. Progesterone activity begins to decline after 20 days and continues until 40 to 44 days, which is indicative of the end of pseudopregnancy.

Luteinizing hormone (LH) is occasionally used to initiate ovulation in the female cat when it can be determined that insufficient hormone is produced by the cat.[11] In this case, 50 international units (IU) given intramuscularly may be satisfactory. Human chorionic gonadotropin (HCG) may also be used to accomplish the same end in the cat, and doses of 100 IU are usually employed and given once, intramuscularly, immediately after the first mating. Care must be taken in storing these hormone prepara-

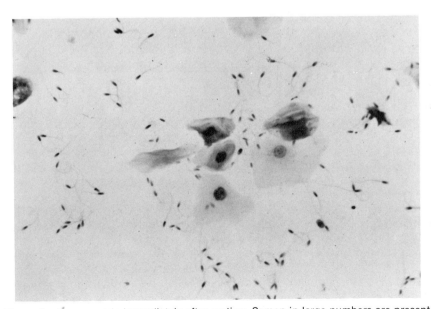

Figure 3. Smear made immediately after mating. Semen in large numbers are present.

tions, and freezing will prolong the life of the individual sample. Should discoloration of the material be observed, it should not be used. The hormone preparations may be reconstituted with sterile water or normal physiological saline solution. Excessive use of pregnant mare serum gonadotropin (PMSG), which has an LH contaminant, may release the ova.

IMPLANTATION

Subsequent to ovulation the egg requires 5 to 6 days to reach the uterus.[8] At that time it is in the 8-cell stage. This knowledge, gained recently, is the basis for a method of postmating inhibition of pregnancy developed by Herron and Sis[10] using estradiol cypionate (ECP) 40 hours after coitus. Implantation is thought to occur between 11 and 14 days, and slightly later if the estrous period is prolonged naturally or as a result of exogenous hormone induction.

DIAGNOSIS OF PREGNANCY

The diagnosis of pregnancy by manual palpation prior to the fourteenth day is not likely. Between the fourteenth and seventeenth day, the implantation sites within the uterus attain the size of a small marble and are firm. At about 21 to 25 days a more linear swelling may be noted and the uterus has enlarged and will be much softer to palpate. Between 25 and 50 days only the experienced person may correctly diagnose a pregnancy by palpation unless there are a considerable number of fetuses resulting in continued distention of the abdominal cavity. Beyond 50 days the fetus may be felt through the wall of the uterus.

There is considerable danger if manipulation of the uterus is rough. Absorption or abortion can occur, depending upon the state of the pregnancy. The optimum time for palpation would be between 17 and 21 days. After 50 days the fetal head is the most prominent feature palpated.

Radiographic diagnosis of pregnancy is safe and may be made at about 38 days,[1] depending upon the skill used in taking the radiograph. Utilizing a method of alizarin red staining (a red stain bound to calcium deposits), it may be noted that calcium is being laid down as early as 25 days but will

not appear radiographically.[3] By knowing the pattern of ossification of the fetus or by using a marker of known length, one could approximate the gestation age of the fetus; i.e., at 41 days the radius and ulna are visible, and at 43 days the tibia, fibula, ilium, ischium and occipital bones of the skull may be visualized. At about 55 days, the axioskeleton may be readily visualized.

Ultrasound techniques have been used to diagnose pregnancy in the queen, but are not as satisfactory as in the bitch.[2] There is currently no laboratory test available utilizing blood or urine of the cat for the purposes of pregnancy diagnosis. Human testing systems cannot be used. Ovarian and uterine morphology may also be determined by laparoscopy.[16]

During the last 5 to 7 days of gestation it is difficult to determine fetal tissues by palpation. This is primarily due to the secondary characteristics of approaching parturition in the queen, such as mammary enlargement, development of the nipples and rigid distention of the abdominal wall, especially when numerous fetuses are present.

Other signs indicative of pregnancy at the time of impending parturition may be vulvar enlargement, occasional mucus at the vaginal orifice and behavioral changes, which may be marked by seclusion or by attachment to a particular person. Whatever the means used to diagnose a pregnancy, care must be taken when handling the animal.

Pseudopregnancy (Pseudocyesis, False Pregnancy)

In the absence of a fertile mating, no luteal phase will ensue. If, however, ovulation is induced by sterile mating, the making of a vaginal smear or induction by manipulation with a glass rod, corpora lutea will form and uterine endometrial change may be observed. Corpora lutea under these conditions will begin to involute at approximately 20 days and become nonfunctional at 41 to 44 days, at which time the signs of false pregnancy rapidly begin to subside.[6] Because of the early cessation of false pregnancy, the secondary signs noted in other species rarely develop (i.e., mammary enlargement, behavioral changes and so forth). Should mammary gland development occur, the queen may allow young other than her own to suckle.

Hormonal therapy to induce early reduction of the false pregnancy is not recommended. Should it be so desired, repositol progesterone (1 mg/lb of body weight) or repositol diethylstilbestrol (1/4 mg/lb of body weight) may be given and repeated in a week, if deemed necessary.[15]

Further evidence of the length of the luteal phase during pseudopregnancy was provided by Pappe et al.,[12] who used assays to follow the variations in the levels of plasma progestins. Pseudopregnancy was declared when the plasma progestin level rose above 1 mg/ml, followed by a sustained increase, and was declared ended when the level fell below 1 mg/ml of plasma. Using these criteria the mean length of luteal activity was found to be 36.5 days. This correlates with observed luteal activity and the end of pseudopregnancy at about 40 days.

GESTATION

This will vary with the breed of the cat.[14] It is generally thought that the gestation period is from 63 to 65 days in length. Cats have been known to deliver and raise healthy kittens when giving birth as early as 59 days or as late as 71 days. Variations in gestation times may be related to breed differences and the number and physical size of the fetuses present. Certain cats within a particular breed may consistently require cesarean delivery. A complete history must be taken to determine variations from the norm within a specific breed that would indicate the proper time for such an artificial delivery.

The type of placentation in the cat is endotheliochorial, indicating that the maternal connective tissue and epithelial layers are missing. The gross shape of the placenta is zonary.[4]

Mammary development begins several days prior to parturition, with visible growth evident during the last 72 hours. Milk may often be expressed from the teat 24 hours prior to parturition. The mammary development in the cat is dependent upon estrogen influence for ductal growth and upon progesterone for lobular alveolar growth. It does not appear that an interaction of the two hormones in the form of a ratio is necessary for development of mammary tissue, as in other species such as the cow.[4]

PARTURITION

The mechanism of parturition has not been studied in the cat. Hormonal inter-relationships are essentially unknown. In spite of this, it is perhaps safe to say that the cat does not differ significantly from other species. If this is the case, the termination of pregnancy is based primarily on the ratio of circulating estrogen to progesterone, with estrogen levels rising close to the time of parturition and progesterone levels decreasing. The inter-relationships of these hormones, along with the action of oxytocin, need considerable study in the cat in order to pinpoint the mechanisms required for the termination of pregnancy. The part played by the placenta, the mechanism of action of the myometrium and the activity of the pituitary during the act of parturition in the cat also need considerable study.

In general, the domestic cat needs little help at the time of parturition. For those animals with a history of previous parturition problems, a prepartum examination is recommended. At this time the fetuses can be palpated, positions within the uterus identified and general body condition of the cat noted. Radiography is perhaps the only way that the exact number of fetuses may be determined, especially if they are several in number. The bladder should be evacuated prior to such an examination, as a full bladder will interfere with palpation and could be damaged in the process. If the examination is performed within an expected 2 to 3 days of the time of parturition (based on a known breeding date and previous history), one could expect to see mammary development, and the glandular element should be included in the examination. Within 24 hours prior to birth, milk can usually be expressed from the nipples.

Before recommending a prepartum examination, one should remember that the cat will usually seek seclusion immediately prior to giving birth. Therefore, transportation to a clinic or other strange surroundings could be detrimental to the normal course of birth of the kittens, either by delay or by premature birth. It is this author's observations, and those of others,[8, 14] that using a normal gestation period of 63 to 65 days, kittens born more than 3 days prior to the norm have had a less-than-even chance of survival. When making such a judgment, one must remember that the cat breeds more than once per day and for more than 1 day during the normal heat period and that there is a 24-hour delay in ovulation because the cat is a postcoital ovulator. These factors and others may influence a shift in the mean gestation period of 63 to 65 days. Consideration of these factors is also necessary if one is to determine the proper time to perform a cesarean section for the purpose of removing healthy, viable young. The tonal quality of the uterus may be determined by digital palpation, and assistance in delivery may also be aided in this manner.

The delivery of young in the cat may be spaced minutes or hours or even days apart, the latter again depending on the length of the estrous period and the time period in days over which the female was bred. Thus, several kittens may be born, with additional kittens appearing days later. The queen and kittens should be examined soon after parturition has ceased to determine the status of the animals. Use of oxytocin to aid parturition or to induce milk flow is rarely necessary in the cat. On occasion, kittens have been found closely tied together by one or more umbilical cords (Fig. 4), which has necessitated the sacrifice of some kittens because of ischemia of a foot or leg to the point where it

cannot be saved. Although these particular births have not been observed, it is reasonable to believe that the kittens were expelled in rapid succession. All had been cleaned by the queen and were viable but were tied into a ball by the umbilical cord.

The queen should be watched closely after parturition to determine if sufficient milk is available for the number of kittens born and to observe the vagina for signs of continued bleeding. If temperatures are to be taken, one should remember that the queen's temperature should be close to normal but that the kittens' normal temperature is low immediately after birth (see Growth Patterns, Fetal and Neonatal, page 850). If the queen continues to bleed postpartum and does not provide care for the kittens, retained placental membranes may be the primary cause and oxytocin may be given. However, a thorough examination of the queen is essential prior to the administration of oxytocin to insure that tears in the uterine or vaginal wall are not the cause of the bleeding.

Twinning may occur in the cat but is difficult to identify. This would be evidenced most characteristically by mirror image color patterns. There is evidence that twinning does occur, although the literature does not indicate that blood supplies have been traced. More often than not when suggested twinning is noticed, one of the fetuses is dead and often in the process of mummification.

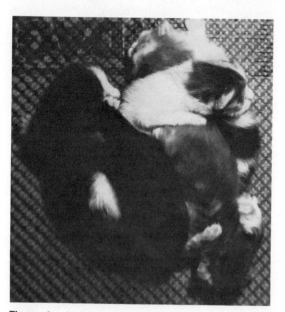

Figure 4. A single umbilical cord (not visible) tying together five kittens 20 minutes old.

REFERENCES

1. Boyd, J. S.: The radiographic identification of the various stages of pregnancy in the domestic cat. J. Small Anim. Pract., *12*:501, 1971.
2. Burke, T. J.: Fertility control in the cat. Vet. Clin. North Am., 7:715, 1977.
3. Colby, E. D. Personal observations.
4. Cole, H. H. and Cupps, P. T.: Reproduction in Domestic Animals. 2nd Ed. New York, Academic Press, 1959, p. 429.
5. Dawson, A. B. and Friedgood, H. B.: The time and sequence of preovulatory changes in the cat ovary after mating and mechanical stimulation of the cervix uteri. Anat. Rec., 76:411, 1940.
6. Foster, M. A. and Hisaw, F. L.: Experimental ovulation and resulting pseudopregnancy in anestrous cats. Anat. Rec., 62:75, 1935.
7. Herron, M. A.: Feline vaginal cytologic examination. Feline Pract., 7:36, 1977.
8. Herron, M. A.: Feline reproduction. Vet. Clin. North Am., 7:715, 1977.
9. Houdeshell, J. W. and Hennessey, P. W.: Megesterol acetate for control of estrus in the cat. Vet. Med./Small Anim. Clin., 72:1013, 1977.
10. Herron, M. A. and Sis, R. F.: Ovum transport in

the cat and the effect of estrogen administration. Am. J. Vet. Res., *35*:1277, 1974.

11. Langman, B. A.: Breeding and reproduction disorders. J. Small Anim. Pract., *5*:504, 1964.
12. Pappe, S. R., Schille, V. M., Seto, H. and Stabenfeldt, G. H.: Luteal activity in the pseudopregnant cat. Biol. Reprod., *13*:470, 1975.
13. Palen, G. F. and Goddard, G. V.: Catnip and estrous behavior in the cat. Anim. Behav., *14*:372, 1966.

14. Prescott, C. W.: Reproduction patterns in the domestic cat. Aust. Vet. J., *49*:126, 1973.
15. Stein, B. S.: The genital system. *In* Catcott, E. J. (ed.): Feline Medicine and Surgery. 2nd Ed. Santa Barbara, Cal., American Veterinary Publication, 1975, pp. 303–354.
16. Wildt, D. E., Kinney, G. M. and Seager, S. W. J.: Laparoscopy for direct observation of internal organs of the domestic cat and dog. Am. J. Vet. Res., *38*:1429, 1977.

Female Reproductive Behavior

VICTORIA LEA VOITH

University of Pennsylvania, Philadelphia, Pennsylvania

Problems related to reproductive behavior of female cats can be found at opposite ends of a spectrum. Lack of recognition of normal reproductive behavior is as common as the occurrence of maladaptive behaviors. Some owners either misinterpret behavior associated with estrus and breeding as pathological conditions or do not attach any significance to or notice changes in the behavior of their animals. On the other hand, abnormalities do occur in surprising numbers when cats are subjected to selective breeding in controlled situations.

NORMAL BEHAVIOR ASSOCIATED WITH ESTRUS

A female cat at the time of estrus will make her condition known to the male. The queen usually increases her vocalizations and may urinate more frequently. Owners may notice that their cats are more restless and have an increased desire to go outside. Some female cats in estrus become more affectionate toward their owners, but occasionally a queen becomes aggressive toward humans. Owners may also notice an increased number of male cats in the vicinity of their home.

A receptive female, in the presence of a male cat, usually crouches on her elbows, elevates her pelvis, deviates her tail and treads with her back legs (Fig. 1). However, a female cat does not necessarily limit her display to male cats. Sometimes the sight of a familiar person will also evoke these behaviors. Generally, however, she must be tactilely stimulated before exhibiting sexual responses. When stroked along her back and at the base of her tail, she raises her pelvis. She will deviate her tail if its base is tactilely stimulated and will tread with her hind legs in response to being stroked in the perineal region. Grasping the female's neck will generally facilitate these movements and sometimes initiate them. If a cat is unfamiliar with an individual or is afraid of people in general, she may not exhibit any receptive signs, even if grasped by the neck and physically stimulated. However, she still may respond to a male cat.

Many cats naturally display affection by approaching, rubbing against a person and elevating their pelvis. Only if such displays are out of character for an individual animal may these actions be an indication of estrus. A cat that normally engages in these behaviors may perform them with greater intensity and frequency when she is in estrus.

Demonstration of sexual behavior several weeks following breeding does not always mean that the cat did not conceive. It has been estimated that 10 per cent of cats that are pregnant can manifest sexual behavior. Superfecundation can occur at this time.

Queens will come back into estrus during the fourth to sixth week of lactation and can conceive at this time.

UNDESIRABLE BREEDING BEHAVIOR

It is necessary that some female cats be acclimated to the breeding area. A female may repel the male if she is intimidated by strange surroundings. This problem can usually be circumvented by placing her in

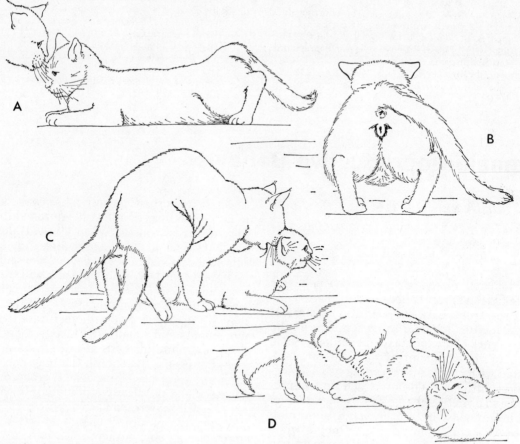

Figure 1. *A* and *B*, The typical posture adopted by the queen in full estrus. Note the flexion of the limbs, lordosis, and deflection of the tail. *C*, Tom holding the queen during intromission. *D*, Postcoital rolling by the queen. (From Scott, P. P.: *In* Hafez, E. S. S. (ed.): Reproduction and Breeding Techniques for Laboratory Animals. Philadelphia, Lea & Febiger, 1970, pp. 192–208.)

the breeding area for a few hours daily several times prior to actually being introduced to the male.

A sexually inexperienced female cat may retreat from the approach of a male. To minimize this possibility and to reduce the probability of her developing a habit of repelling the advances of a male, an experienced stud cat should be used the first several times that the queen is serviced.

Sometimes an estrous queen aggressively rejects a male cat. An effective remedy for such a situation, if an experienced stud cat is being used, is for a person to physically stimulate the queen and induce her to display sexual behaviors. The person then continues to hold her head, allowing the male to breed her.

Partner preferences, as well as discrimi-

nation against specific individuals, have been observed in many mammalian species, including cats. If an estrous female persistently avoids one male, it is still possible that she will readily accept another.

COPULATORY BEHAVIOR

The neck grip of the mounted male usually stimulates the female to elevate her pelvis, deviate her tail and tread with her back legs. If not, the alternating stepping movements of the male's hind feet or the strumming of the female's thorax with his front feet will cause the female to perform these behaviors. The treading of the female's back legs may be a signal for pelvic thrusting and intromission by the male. Frequently used males do not always require lordosis and treading by the female before beginning pelvic thrusting and attempting intromission.

When the male cat has intromitted, the female usually emits a cry and pulls away from the male. As she twists free, she turns, swatting at him and then vigorously engages in rubbing and rolling on the floor. The male watches her. For several minutes she will repel subsequent advances of the male and may scratch and bite a person attempting to pick her up. After copulation, she usually licks her genital area. As the rubbing and rolling subside, she frequently reaches out and touches the male with her paw, approaches him or visually solicits him by assuming a lordosis and treading posture. Soon she will permit the male to mount again. Copulation will occur several times during one breeding session. The female cat is in estrus 4 to 8 days and will copulate several times each day.

ABORTION

Environmental stress in any form can result in abortion. Not only can a long shipment, such as across country, result in abortion but sometimes moving a cat from her home area to a different location, particularly if it is inhabited by unfamiliar cats, will result in this as well. Cats transported during the last trimester of pregnancy are particularly likely to abort. The female generally removes all evidence of the abortion by consuming the fetuses, fetal membranes and fluids and by meticulously grooming herself. Because of her assiduous behavior, abortions are frequently undetected.

QUEENING

The process of parturition may take a few hours to 24 hours. If the queen has recently been moved to a new area or otherwise disturbed by her environment during parturition, she may neglect her kittens. A queen should be familiarized with her surroundings prior to parturition. Preferably, the area should be isolated from other cats and excessive environmental activity. Visual barriers, such as paper covering the cage or a large cardboard box for the queen to hide in, can be utilized to give the cat a feeling of seclusion.

Cats have been known to seek out the owner during queening. With such cats, it is advisable that the owner stay with the queen while she is delivering. After parturition is completed, the queen is generally sufficiently attached to her offspring that the owner can leave without the cat following and deserting her kittens.

POSTPARTURIENT BEHAVIOR

During the first 24 to 48 hours the cat may not leave her kittens to eat, drink, defecate or urinate. If food and water are not close by, she may prolong her fast or reduce the amount of time she spends eating. A litterbox or access to an appropriate place to eliminate should be close by. Initially, an effort should be made to make it easy for her to care for her essential needs. After 7 to 8 days the cat will stay away from her kittens for longer intervals than previously.

The first 20 days or so following parturition, the mother initiates contact with the kittens. During the first week she is particularly fastidious about retrieving stray kittens. Generally a queen responds only to distress cries of kittens. She can watch with moderate interest a nonvocalizing kitten that is desperately trying to reach her, and she will make no effort to retrieve it. By the time the kittens are 10 to 14 days old, the mother is less motivated to retrieve a stray kitten but may "thrill" (a low pitched vocalization) to it or reach out with a paw to give it direction as it struggles to find the nest. At about 21 days both the kittens and the mother are equally initiating contacts, and the mother begins spending progressively longer time away from the nest. At 1 month of age the kittens are able to eat, and the mother will begin to resist nursing attempts of her offspring.

Normally, kittens disperse from their mother as they approach adulthood. However in domestic situations, if a kitten has continual access to its mother, it may persist in nursing until it is several years old. If an owner suspects that a queen is not going to totally wean her kittens, it is advisable to separate the mother from her offspring for a few weeks to stop lactation.

Precautions should be taken to prevent a tomcat's access to kittens. Infanticide by males is not an uncommon practice among domestic cats.

Handling and petting kittens for a few minutes each day for the first days after birth can accelerate their physical development. Laboratory experiments indicate that neonatal kittens that are frequently handled are less emotional in novel or exciting situations as adolescents. One can hypothesize that the adult cat, handled as a kitten, is more likely to adjust to novel situations such as the show-ring, crowds and so forth.

Handled neonatal laboratory rodents are reported to be more resistant to physical stress as adults. However, this resistance depends upon the type of stress and the kind of disease to which the animal is exposed. The effect is variable among strains within a species, and handled animals are sometimes less resistant to some diseases and stresses as adults. The long-term effects of neonatal handling on cats is unknown.

It is known that laboratory-reared cats that have frequent contact with people throughout kittenhood are less excitable, easier to work with and adjust better to changes in their environment than are cats that were rarely handled as kittens.

ADOPTING ALIEN KITTENS

Lactating queens readily adopt alien kittens the same age as their offspring. The likelihood of a female accepting foreign kittens is inversely proportional to the differences in ages between her present litter and the foreign kittens. Usually a mother cat will accept kittens within 2 weeks of age of her own. Mixing litters of kittens that vary greatly in size and strength is not advisable. Large kittens can prevent small kittens from access to the mother. Utilizing a foster mother is the optimal way to raise an orphan kitten.

ORPHAN KITTENS

Orphan kittens can be raised successfully provided physical, nutritional and behavioral needs are met. If a foster mother is not available, orphaned kittens should be kept together rather than separated. Not only does the interaction with other kittens reduce the possibility of the development of abnormal behaviors but may also enhance survival for unknown reasons. One laboratory experiment reported a much higher mor-

tality rate in isolated kittens versus motherless kittens being raised in a group.

If kittens are deprived of nursing a lactating female for several days, there can be a delay of several hours before they initiate nursing when again given access to the queen. The delay is not due to a loss of sucking reflex, unless the kitten has been raised in isolation from birth to 3 weeks of age, but is related to difficulty in locating and responding to the mother's nipple. The longer the separation and the older the kitten, the greater the delay in initiating sucking.

There are several ways of feeding orphan kittens. They can be fed via a stomach tube, from a bottle with a small nipple or from a syringe equipped with an adapter. Kittens can also learn to feed themselves from an artificial mother.

Small infant feeding tubes can be passed into the stomach through the mouth of the kitten. The laryngeal reflex is usually sensitive enough to prevent the tube from entering the trachea. Particular care must be exercised when intubating 1- to 2-day-old kittens. Passing a piece of tubing long enough to reach the stomach usually assures that the tube is in the digestive tract and not in the respiratory system.

When using a bottle, it is essential to have a large enough patent hole to allow the kitten to suck easily. Simply punching a hole in the nipple with a needle rarely works because a rubber flap remains that hampers the effectiveness of the sucking of the kitten. Burning a small hole 1 mm in diameter in the nipple with a hot needle provides a smooth-edged opening of sufficient size to allow the kitten to regulate the flow of milk easily. If a plastic bottle is used, slight positive pressure can be applied manually. As the kitten gets older, the opening of the bottle can be enlarged to accommodate gruel.

Some kittens readily learn to suck on a conversion adapter that can be attached to a syringe. With this method, milk is slowly injected into the mouth manually. Whenever fluid is being manually forced into the kitten's mouth, it should be done very slowly, allowing the kitten to swallow frequently. Should the kitten gasp for a breath it is likely to aspirate the fluid into its lungs.

Artificial mothers have been used to raise orphan kittens from birth. The apparatus is in the form of a U-shaped vessel covered with cloth. A nipple allows the kitten to suck a formula available at a controlled temperature. Initially the kittens have to be manually placed in the U and guided to the nipple. If enough tactile cues are present, within 3 days kittens orphaned at birth are able to crawl up into the brooder and locate and attach independently to the nipple. If the apparatus does not provide enough tactile cues, the visual system of the kittens may have to develop before they are able to locate and utilize the apparatus.

The younger a kitten is, the more rapidly it learns to suck from an artificial nipple. Kittens over 40 days of age will chew on, rather than suck on, an artificial nipple. If the opening of a nipple is appropriately designed, kittens 1 to 2 days old will begin nursing within a few minutes. Older kittens may take up to 15 minutes to begin actively sucking on a nipple. Day-old kittens can tolerate about 1 ml of fluid at a feeding. Each day thereafter, they can accommodate an additional 0.5 ml until a maximum of 10 ml is reached. The ideal frequency of feeding the orphan is 12 times a day for the newborn and gradually diminishes to four to six times a day for the month-old kitten. Kittens are able to drink from a dish and eat soft food at 4 weeks of age.

Queens spend considerable time grooming the entire kitten. Grooming by the mother cat not only stimulates urination and defecation but may facilitate the development of the eyes and ears as well as supplying a general sensation of mobility or enhancement of peripheral circulation. Orphan kittens should be stimulated to urinate and defecate during the first 2 to 3 weeks of age. Stroking the anogenital area with moist cotton or soft paper towels readily stimulates the kitten to eliminate. The facial and body grooming may also have a functional significance, and therefore it is probably beneficial to provide these same sensations to orphan kittens.

Young kittens depend upon behavioral means to regulate their body temperature during the first several weeks of life. If a queen is not available to warm the kittens, the ambient temperature must be raised sufficiently to keep the kittens warm. This is particularly important if the kitten is by itself and cannot curl up with other kittens to keep warm.

Deprivation experiments in which kittens are isolated and raised with minimal handling in restricted environments from a very early age generally result in adults that are more fearful and emotional than cats that were raised with their mothers. However, raising an orphan kitten need not mimic a deprivation experiment. Orphan kittens should frequently be handled, petted and picked up — but only for short periods of time. When they are older, they should be played with frequently. If an orphan is without littermates, it should be exposed to members of its own species, particularly its peers, as often as the opportunity presents itself. This is done to minimize the chance of development of abnormal reproductive behaviors in adulthood.

Orphans raised with littermates or with other cats have a high likelihood of developing into normal adults.

REFERENCES

1. Daly, M.: Early stimulation of rodents: A critical review of present interpretations. Br. J. Psychol. *64*:453, 1973.
2. Kling, A., Kovach, J. K., and Tucker, T. J.: The behaviour of cats. *In* Hafez, E. S. E. (ed.): The Behaviour of Domestic Animals. 2nd Ed. Baltimore, The Williams and Wilkins Co., 1969, pp. 482–512.
3. Konrad, K. W. and Bagshaw, M.: Effect of novel stimuli in cats reared in restricted environment. J. Comp. Physiol. Psychol., *70*:157, 1970.
4. Meier, G. W.: Infantile handling and development in Siamese kittens. J. Comp. Physiol. Psychol., *54*:284, 1961.
5. Rosenblatt, J. S., Turkewitz, G. and Schneirla, T. C.: Early socialization in the domestic cat as based on feeding and other relationships between female and young. *In* Foss, B. M. (ed.): Determinants of Infant Behaviour. New York, John Wiley and Sons, Inc., 1961, pp. 51–74.
6. Schneirla, T. C., Rosenblatt, J. S., and Toback, E.: Maternal behavior in the cat. *In* Rheingold, H. L. (ed.): Maternal Behavior in Mammals. New York, John Wiley and Sons, 1963, pp. 122–168.
7. Scott, P. P.: Cats. *In* Hafez, E. S. E. (ed.): Reproduction and Breeding Techniques for Laboratory Animals. Philadelphia, Lea and Febiger, 1970, pp. 192–208.
8. Seitz, P. F. O.: Infantile experience and adult behavior in animal subjects. II. Age of separation from the mother and adult behavior in the cat. Psychosom. Med., *21*:353, 1959.
9. Wilson, M., Warren, J. M. and Abbot, L.: Infantile stimulation, activity and learning by cats. Child Devel., *36*:841, 1965.

The Male Reproductive System

NICKOLAS J. SOJKA

University of Virginia, Charlottesville, Virginia

ANATOMY

The reproductive tract of the male cat is a simplified system compared with that of most other mammalian species. It consists of testes, epididymides, ducts, prostate, bulbourethral glands and penis.

Of the common domestic animals, only boars and cats have the scrotum located caudal to the thighs, and caudal and ventral to the ischiatic arch. The testicles of the healthy adult male cat are slightly ovoid, firm and small (1.2 to 2.0 cm long and 0.7 to 1.7 cm wide). Prior to puberty, the testicles are free to move up and down the inguinal canal. Unlike most other species, the ampullar region of the ductus deferens of the male cat is not glandular and the seminal vesicles are absent. The prostate is characterized by lamellar corpuscles in the capsule. The penis of the cat has no bulbus glandis. It is short and has a terminal cap containing numerous spines (papillae) pointing toward the base. Unlike most other species, the feline penis points caudally and downward (retromingent).

Puberty in the male lags slightly behind that of the female. It is subject to great individual variation and is commonly accepted to occur when the male reaches about 2.5 kg of body weight or 8 to 10 months of age. After reaching puberty, males are fertile throughout the year.

PHYSICAL EXAMINATION

In examining prepuberal male animals, it will be noted that the distance between the urethral and anal openings is greater than in females and that the area is furred. In the adult male, any tenderness or softness observed during examination of the testes can be indicative of a pathological condition and should be examined further for a source of trauma, such as a bite wound. Very few cases of infections or tumors of the reproductive tract have been reported in male cats.

Sertoli cell tumor of the testes is rare in the cat, with few verified cases reported in veterinary literature. As previously mentioned, most cases of orchitis are the result of cat bite wounds. Poor nutrition and specific vitamin deficiencies can result in either reduced libido or functional infertility. Examination for penile hair rings should accompany any evaluation of males presenting persistent, abnormal mating behavior. Reluctance to copulate and inability to ejaculate may result from urinary calculi lodged in the urethra. Such calculi are common in male cats but are uncommon in frequently used breeders.

Laparoscopic techniques for intra-abdominal examination of the cat have been published[3] and may be of assistance in the further evaluation of suspect conditions.

If a male has been caged with a female during her estrus, he will often exhibit a weight loss over the course of several days due to failure to eat adequately. As with certain other species, it is recommended that the female be brought to the male. If the female is screened for estrus by behavioral manifestations and cytological examinations, the matings should be supervised because she may not fully accept the male and may demonstrate this by swatting him. Less mature and inexperienced males can become "shy breeders" that are even beyond the point of being retrained after this type of encounter.

Male cats are subject only rarely to any type of congenital reproductive tract defect, possibly because of their somewhat simplified system. Unilateral cryptorchidism is more common among males than is bilateral cryptorchidism. The latter usually results in a sterile animal, one that does not develop either the ability or the desire to breed. On the other hand, a male with only one testicle descended (unilateral) is more likely to mature normally in both behavior and ability to fertilize. Hormonal treatment to remedy such conditions is discouraged since treatment is only rarely successful and, if successful, may result in the production of additional defective animals. The male tortoiseshell cat (Klinefelter's syndrome) is uncommon and in theory cannot exist, as the yellow color is linked to the female X chro-

844

mosome. Several have been reported to be XY/XXY and rare fertile males are believed to be XX/XY. Sperm abnormalities may also be congenital, but this is a self-limiting condition since reduced fertility, unless altered by artificial insemination (AI) procedures, limits the number of carrier offspring.

Any systemic infection accompanied by fever, malnutrition or heavy parasitism will interrupt libido and spermatogenesis. Recent developments in immunization can greatly minimize viral and secondary bacterial problems in cats by the use of rhino-tracheitis, calicivirus and panleukopenia vaccines.

REFERENCES

1. Loughman, W. D., Frye, F. L. and Congdon, T. B.: XY/XXY bone marrow mosaicism in three male tricolor cats. Am. J. Vet. Res., *31*:307, 1977.
2. Whitehead, J. E.: Neoplasia in the cat. Vet. Med., *62*:44, 1967.
3. Wildt, D. E., Kinney, G. M., and Seager, S. W. J., Laparoscopy for direct observation of internal organs of the domestic cat and dog. Am. J. Vet. Res., *38*:1429, 1977.

Male Reproductive Behavior

VICTORIA LEA VOITH

University of Pennsylvania, Philadelphia Pennsylvania

In the feral or wild state the domestic cat, *Felis catus,* and its ancestral stock, *Felis libyca,* are relatively asocial animals except for mother-offspring relationships, territorial disputes and the coming together of animals for reproductive purposes. They are, however, almost constantly in communication with members of their species. The yowling of a male cat announces his presence to other males and to females. The cries of an estrous female signal her readiness to the males living in adjacent territories. Information may also be transmitted by pheromones in secretions from cheek, anal and tail glands and in urine sprayed by males and, occasionally, by females.

Flehmen behavior is frequently seen in both sexes. Flehmen is theorized to be a method of assessing odors via the vomeronasal-olfactory system. A cat engaged in flehmen remains motionless, holding its mouth open about 1 cm for 1 to 5 seconds (Fig. 1). This particular method of assaying olfactory information is associated with investigation of inanimate objects and the atmosphere, as well as of other cats. Flehmen could easily be a means by which the solitary cat is kept informed of the presence and reproductive status of other cats in the vicinity.

NORMAL COPULATORY BEHAVIOR

An uninhibited, experienced male cat will approach a female, touch her nose and then investigate her rear quarters. If she is sexually receptive, the male emits a cry, grasps her neck and mounts her. If the estrous female has not already elevated her pelvis upon being grasped by the neck, she does so in response to the strumming of her thorax by the male's front feet. She also treads with her back feet, which probably serves as a stimulus for pelvic thrusting and intromission by the male. After the male ejaculates, he releases or relaxes his hold on the female. She frees herself, turning, spatting and swatting at the male. He then watches her engage in postcopulatory displays and grooms his penis. When the female's afterreaction subsides, he usually mounts and breeds her again. Copulation generally occurs several times during one breeding session.

Neck Grip

The male must have a secure grip on the female's neck to prevent her moving out from under him as he begins to intromit. An inexperienced male or a male unfamiliar with his surroundings will frequently let go of the female's neck the moment she begins to cry. Some males simply have idiosyncrasies such as releasing the neck grip after mounting, letting go of the female's neck

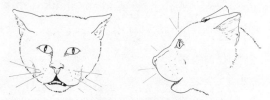

Figure 1. A cat engaged in flehmen remains motionless, holding its mouth open about 1 cm for 1 to 5 seconds.

and grooming her or even mounting a very receptive female without ever attempting a neck grip. Sometimes a female will remain in the position of lordosis and treading although the mounted male does not have a neck grip. However, once the tom begins to intromit, the female will move away from him. In such cases, the female may emit a cry and engage in a mild afterreaction, although ejaculation has not taken place. If breeding is not observed, hearing the copulatory cry of the female, particularly a short cry, is not assurance that a successful copulation has taken place. A sustained cry of several seconds is more likely to correspond with the longer period of complete intromission and ejaculation.

Appropriate positioning of the neck grip is necessary to permit intromission. A short-bodied male may not be able to serve a long-bodied queen. With experience, however, some males learn to adjust the placement of their neck grip caudally and are able to copulate successfully with a longer-bodied female.

An inexperienced male often inappropriately grasps the female's neck. He may grab her throat or the lateral aspects of her neck. After a proper grip he may remain perpendicular to her rather than mounting her. If he does mount, his grip may be too far forward or backward to achieve intromission. He is also likely to release her as soon as she begins to resist him. After several exposures to receptive females, these problems usually disappear.

Pelvic Thrusting

Inexperienced males may engage in sporadic pelvic thrusting for 30 minutes before achieving intromission or letting go of the female. As the male gains experience, the time spent mounting and in pelvic thrusting

decreases. Many experienced and frequently used male cats will service a receptive female in less than 5 minutes.

When a male that has been a successful and relatively expeditious breeder begins to engage in long bouts of pelvic thrusting without achieving ejaculation or intromission, he may have a hair ring around his penis. If a male does not groom his penis after copulation or if his grooming is inadequate, hairs from the back of the female, accumulated during pelvic thrusting, can form a ring around the male's penis. The hair ring can easily be removed manually, and the male will then be able to intromit and breed successfully.

Acclimation

A newly acquired male cat, even though a proven stud, is unlikely to engage in breeding behavior until he has adjusted to his new living situation. It may take 1 to 4 weeks before he feels secure in his surroundings. Constant intimidation by other males may suppress a cat's libido. Providing a tom with his own territory out of harassment's way may facilitate his breeding activity.

Diurnal Cycles

Under natural conditions cats generally engage in breeding activities during the night. To facilitate breeding in a colony situation, the cats can be maintained on a 12-hour cycle that is reversed, so that during normal working hours the cats are in the dark phase.

TRAINING THE STUD CAT

The first 10 to 15 times that a novice male cat is placed in a potential breeding situation the conditions should be optimal. Initial adverse experiences with a female can prolong the training of a male as a stud or permanently render him useless for selective breeding purposes. Aberrant neck grips; stepping on the female; prolonged mounting times, with or without pelvic thrusting, and releasing the female too quickly when intromission is achieved are common behaviors of inexperienced males. Therefore, the females used for training should not only be known to be receptive but should be extremely tolerant as well. Maintenance of a few ovariohysterectomized females with such generous temperaments is a worthwhile investment for a private individual as well as for an institution desiring to breed specific male cats. The spayed females can be brought into behavioral estrus for 14 to 28 days with two subcutaneous injections of 100 mg of estradiol cypionate (Depo-Estradiol) administered 48 hours apart. Because of the possibility of estrogen-induced bone marrow suppression, the spayed cats should not be kept on hormonal treatment for prolonged periods of time and should occasionally be monitored by hematological studies.

If a tomcat has experienced many successful breedings, he will tolerate subsequent rebuffs and even severe attacks by a female without losing sexual interest. If a male cat loses interest in females because of adverse experiences, it would be best to start his training over again with an estrogen-induced female known to be extremely receptive. It may take several introductions and pairings with such a female before he again initiates any sexual behavior.

Conditioning a male to anticipate a sexually receptive female so that he breeds her almost immediately saves many hours of observation time. It also prevents having to put the animals together overnight without direct observation of the breeding activities. A specific area, designated solely for copulatory activities, allows the male to associate encountering only receptive females in this area. A small, bare room with a window for observations is ideal. The male should first be acclimated to this area. Then daily or every other day a routine sequence of procedures should be followed until the cat becomes conditioned to anticipating the breeding activities: The male is first placed in the chamber, followed by the known receptive female. After the male has bred her several times, the female is first removed, then the male. Initially, it may be necessary to leave them together for several hours before breeding occurs. When this sequence has been repeated for a total of 10 to 15 times, the novice male usually knows why he is being placed in the test area and breeds the female within a few minutes. Males can become conditioned to a set routine of breeding to the extent that when taken from their home area into the breeding region, they will walk into the test area and wait expectantly.

PREFERENCES

Males may demonstrate partner preferences as well as discrimination against specific females. A male may be persistently uninterested in one receptive female but will readily respond to others.

MASTURBATION

Masturbation has been observed in intact and castrated male cats. Cats will masturbate by using the edge of a bowl or clothing. The cats engage in pelvic thrusting, penile erection, penile spasms and emission of fluids.

HORMONAL AND ENVIRONMENTAL INFLUENCES

Castration usually eliminates copulatory behavior of male cats, although males in laboratory settings have demonstrated the ability to retain copulatory behavior for years postcastration. However, even these males exhibit impairment of breeding activity, as reflected in decreased frequency of copulation and prolonged mounting times.

Castration is approximately 90 per cent effective, regardless of the age of the cat, in eliminating the reproductive-related behaviors of spraying, roaming and fighting. Since spraying is testosterone-dependent in most male cats, medications containing androgens may instigate spraying behavior in castrated male cats. Withdrawal of these drugs should eliminate this behavior.

Environmental factors can also influence spraying behavior. The presence of numerous cats in the household or neighborhood promotes spraying activity. The incidence of spraying may be higher during the reproductive season.

Most males that persist in spraying after castration will cease when treated with synthetic progestins. A single 5 mg/kg subcutaneous injection of medroxyprogesterone acetate (Depo-Provera) is usually effective within 24 hours. If the animal does not respond, a repeated dose a week later is recommended. The length of effectiveness of a single or repeated dose varies from several weeks to months. Although it is commonly used, one should note that medroxyprogesterone acetate is not marketed for use in cats in some countries.

Megestrol acetate tablets (Ovaban, Ovarid) can also be used to inhibit spraying in castrated male cats. An effective therapeutic regimen is 5 mg of megestrol acetate daily *per os* for 1 week or until the spraying ceases. The frequency of administration is then reduced to every other day for a week and then every third day for a week, followed by increasing subsequent time intervals of administration by 1 day until a minimum dosage schedule is obtained. Many cats stabilize at 5 mg every 7 to 14 days. If after 14 days a cat has not responded to the initial megestrol acetate loading dose of 5 mg *per os* per day, the medication should be discontinued because it is unlikely that the compound will be of therapeutic value. Sometimes a cat that has not responded to one synthetic progestin will respond favorably to another.

Mastoplasia as a sequela to progestin therapy has been observed in male cats, as well as females. A reversible aspermatogenesis occurs when an intact male cat is under the influence of progestins. These hormones should not be used in high doses in intact female cats because of possible uterine pathology.

A small percentage of male cats persist in spraying despite any of the methods of treatment just discussed. Bilateral ablation of the medial preoptic nuclei in the hypothalamus, utilizing stereotactic neurosurgical techniques, will reduce the spraying behavior of these individuals.

REFERENCES

1. Hart, B. L. and Barrett, R. E.: Effect of castration on fighting, roaming and urine spraying in adult male cats. J.A.V.M.A., *163*:290, 1973.
2. Hart, B. L. and Peterson, D. M.: Penile hair rings in male cats may prevent mating. Lab. Anim. Sci., *21*:422, 1970.
3. Hart, B. L. and Voith, V. L.: Changes in urine spraying, feeding and sleep behavior of cats following medical preotic-anterior hypothalamic lesions. Brain Res., *145*:406, 1978.
4. Rosenblatt, J. S. and Aronson, L. R.: The decline of sexual behavior in male cats after castration with special reference to the role of prior sexual experience. Behavior, *12*:285, 1958.
5. Scott, P. P.: Cats. *In* Hafez, E.S.E. (ed.): Reproduction and Breeding Techniques for Laboratory Animals. Philadelphia, Lea and Febiger, 1970, pp. 192–208.

Feline Semen Collection, Evaluation and Artificial Insemination

NICKOLAS J. SOJKA
University of Virginia, Charlottesville, Virginia

SEMEN COLLECTION

Collection of semen for analysis or artificial insemination, or both, can readily be accomplished using an artificial vagina (AV) (Fig. 1). A male with sufficient libido and a temperament malleable to frequent handling can be trained to mount a "teaser" queen or even the technician's hand in some cases (Fig. 2) and allow his penis to be guided into the AV for ejaculation. Colony-raised males that have been separated from females prior to puberty are often less likely to develop into good breeders. Four to 5 days are usually necessary for a male to develop an acceptable environment suited to optimum interest in mating or AV collection following washing of the caging in which males are housed individually.

Semen may also be collected via electroejaculation. The male is restrained and the perineal region is exposed. The apparatus used by Lang[1] for the squirrel monkey is commonly used for male cats. This method produces a "split" ejaculate, one portion sperm-free and the other sperm-rich.

The AV method is less traumatic in that it does not call for restraint of the animal or use of any equipment that is in any way uncomfortable for him. Also, the equipment used is far less expensive and may be used easily by one technician with a minimum of training. The preference for whole or "split" semen is at the discretion of the user, but there can be no doubt that the metabolism of the sperm will vary according to the method used. Procedures that should be commonly practiced with both collection methods are

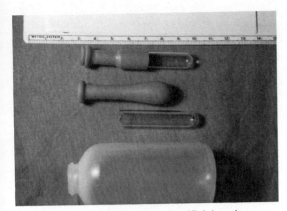

Figure 1. Components of artificial vagina.

avoidance of (1) contamination by urine, water or extraneous chemical substances; (2) temperature shock and (3) exposure to direct light. All of these hazards either immobilize the sperm or radically alter their metabolism.

Many of the procedures for handling cat semen have been adapted from these routinely used for the collection of semen from farm animals. For rapid evaluation and/or immediate use in artificial insemination, the method of Sojka *et al.*[4] that utilizes physiological saline has the advantages of being both simple and successful. After the ejaculate has been collected into an AV maintained at 44 to 46°C, the semen is diluted with 0.1 ml of saline (0.9 per cent sodium chloride) and a sperm count is made.[2] The semen is further diluted with saline to give a final sperm count of about 50×10^6 sperm per ml when it is to be used for artificial insemination.

Long-term storage of frozen cat semen has also been shown to be possible. Several extenders are being evaluated to determine which provides the best protection for the longest period of time. Preliminary results indicate that it will be possible to maintain frozen cat semen in a chemically defined medium, thus reducing the poor visibility and large sample-to-sample variability encountered with the use of egg yolk extenders.

SEMEN EVALUATION

Semen may be evaluated in a variety of ways. Sperm concentration and the degree and type of motility can be easily determined using a Fuchs-Rosenthal hemocy- tometer and a microscope. The number of spermatozoa counted in 16 small squares on this hemocytometer is an estimation of the number of spermatozoa in 0.2 cu mm of whole or diluted semen. Live-dead analysis and gross morphological abnormalities can be observed using eosinaniline blue and Giemsa staining.[3] Various physiological techniques allow evaluation of metabolic processes. The selection of which techniques to employ is at the discretion of the user, but there are several commonly accepted parameters for all species. Any evaluation should include these determinations: semen volume, per cent normal (rapid, progressive) motility, sperm concentration and per cent abnormal forms. All of these parameters have a direct bearing on the fertilizing ability of a semen sample (Table 1).

The average ejaculate volume for male cats has been observed to be 0.04 ml and contains 56.5×10^6 sperm. Males can be ejaculated two to three times per week without diminution of libido or sperm concentration.

ARTIFICIAL INSEMINATION

Sperm suspensions (whole semen, extended semen or frozen extended semen) to be used for artificial insemination may be deposited in either the anterior vagina or posterior cervix using a 0.25-ml syringe with a 20-gauge needle bulbed at the tip or tipped with 1-cm polyethylene tubing. Concentrations of from 5×10^6 to 3×10^8 sperm in 0.1 to 0.2 ml of diluted semen have been successfully inseminated into queens showing both behavioral estrus and vaginal cell cornification.

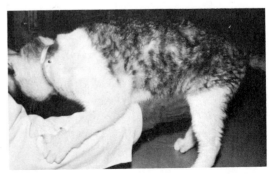

Figure 2. Collection of semen with artificial vagina without "teaser."

TABLE 1. *Characteristics of Cat Semen*

Cat Identification	Number of Ejaculates Collected	Volume of Ejaculate (ml)	Sperm per ml of Ejaculate ($\times 10^8$)	Total Sperm per Ejaculate ($\times 10^8$)	Percent Motile	Percent Abnormal Forms	Semen pH
A–713	4	0.01–0.05	12.66–28.60	0.13–1.43	40–80	1–6% cytoplasmic droplets, 2–10% club tails	7.0–7.4
E–815	4	0.01–0.02	20.35–37.40	0.20–0.49	50–65	1–3% cytoplasmic droplets, 1–2% club tails	7.3–7.6
B–892	4	0.02–0.05	18.37–51.01	0.30–1.11	95–100	1–7% cytoplasmic droplets, 1–5% club tails	7.1–7.9
D–804	4	0.03–0.07	5.13–19.18	0.27–1.34	35–95	0–1% cytoplasmic droplets, 1–3% club tails	7.1–7.4
A–849	4	0.03–0.12	0.96–13.20	0.03–0.53	80–95	0–4% cytoplasmic droplets, 0–4% club tails	7.3–8.2
F–819	4	0.03–0.11	6.71–26.45	0.74–1.16	60–100	0–4% cytoplasmic droplets, 0–1% club tails	7.0–7.9
AVERAGE	24	0.04	17.30	0.57	78	1.6% cytoplasmic droplets, 2.1% club tails	7.4

REFERENCES

1. Lang, C. M.: A technique for the collection of semen from squirrel monkeys (*Saimiri sciureus*) by electroejaculation. Lab. Anim. Care, *17*:218, 1967.
2. Rothschild, L.: Counting spermatozoa. J. Exp. Biol., *26*:388, 1950.
3. Saacke, R. G.: Proceedings of 3rd Technical Conference, Animal Reproduction and Artificial Insemination. Chicago, National Association of Animal Breeders, 1970.
4. Sojka, N. J., Jennings, L. L. and Hamner, C. E.: Artificial insemination in the cat (*Felis catus L.*). Lab. Anim. Care, *20*:198, 1970.

Growth Patterns, Fetal and Neonatal

EZRA BERMAN

Environmental Protection Agency, Research Triangle Park, North Carolina

The complicated and usually coordinated process of growth begins shortly after fertilization of the ovum and, in the strictest sense, does not end until death. Growth is expressible in terms of morphological units, i.e., body mass or linear measurements. There are a variety of physiological changes, as well as behavioral and functional alterations, that are not only contributory but part and parcel of this grand process.

Growth is looked upon as normal matura-tion. However, the clinician should be aware of pathological states in which growth is abnormal and detrimental.

FETAL GROWTH

The clinician is sometimes called upon to make value judgments as to the degree of maturity of fetuses. If the fetus has normal morphological findings and little postmortem change, the weekly age can be accurately determined by measurement of the crown-rump length and observation of external characteristics. Table 1 contains fetal data from observed breedings in scientific production colonies that occurred within 3 hours by single sires. The crown-rump lengths and weight values are from Nelson and Cooper.[4] The external characteristics are personal observations by the author on a different group of cat fetuses. Of the three criteria in Table 1, the external characteristics would prove most useful clinically as an estimation of fetal age.

Frequently, the clinician is presented with a suspected case of superfetation in which a single fetus of a litter appears relatively immature but normal in all other respects. This condition has been reported in case histories,[1, 3] but the sexual lives of the animals involved were not fully controlled. In the scientific production colony just noted, fetuses that might ordinarily be considered superfetations were found in pregnancies of single breedings. The characteristics of the pregnancies detailed in the case histories and the singly bred pregnancies were similar: a relatively immature but normal sole living fetus among littermates seemingly 3 weeks older. Both the physiological improbability of superfetation and the comparability of suspected cases with cases showing normal gestational variability lead us to believe that superfetation in the cat will remain theoretical.

POSTNATAL GROWTH

At birth the kitten's growth is totally dependent upon the amount and quality of available nutrition (milk supply), the presence of transmissible diseases in littermates and environmental conditions. Body weight, because of its convenience as a measurement, has been a conventional criterion of growth. Periodic weighing is the most common assay for continuing health and growth. A number of sources contain growth tables of the body weight of the cat. A body weight age curve is not included here because of the difficulties associated with any attempt to compare weight curves among a cat colony, cattery, pet environment or clinical situation. In the absence of any chart, three rules may be applied:

1. A kitten gains 7 to 10 or more gm per day.
2. Any loss of weight is a detrimental sign.
3. Birth weight (male or female) is approximately 100 gm $\pm$ 10 gm.

HEMOGRAM

The blood values in Table 2 were obtained from kittens born in the outdoor scientific colony mentioned previously. The kittens used were from observed pairings with known birthdates, with no more than two kittens from any litter included in the compilation. Values given are means and standard deviations. Erythrocyte and leukocyte concentrations were determined using an automatic particle counter, hemoglobin determination was by the cyanmethemoglobin method and cell volume determination by microhematocrit. No significant differences could be found between male and female values, and all data were pooled. It may be concluded from Table 2 that the kitten is

TABLE 1. *Weight, Length and General External Characteristics of Aged Feline Fetuses**

Fetal Age (days)	Weight (gm)†	Crown-Rump Length (cm)†	N†	Characteristics
21	0.16 ± 0.09	1.48 ± 0.32	18	–
28	0.89 ± 0.2	2.43 ± 0.46	17	Opened eyes and ears, digits without claws
35	4.98 ± 1.2	4.73 ± 0.90	19	Closed eyes and ears, claws
42	17.8 ± 5.6	7.24 ± 1.07	21	Vibrissae follicles
49	40.7 ± 6.5	9.54 ± 0.90	18	Fine body hair without pattern or color
56	75.6 ± 15.0	11.7 ± 0.8	21	Full body hair with color and pattern
63	102 ± 24.6	13.8 ± 1.03	18	–
65 (birth)	97.1 ± 23.1	13.7 ± 0.92	78	–

*Values are mean and standard deviation. N = number of fetuses.
†Data from Nelson, N. S. and Cooper, J.: Growth, *39*:435, 1975.

TABLE 2. *Hemograms of Young Felines**

Variable	Days of Age									
	0	7	14	28	42	56	70	84	105	120
Number of fetuses	32	5	18	17	9	13	13	9	13	13
Erthyrocytes ($\times 10^6$/cu mm)	5.87 0.71	4.35 0.93	3.97 0.51	4.33 0.42	5.74 0.41	5.85 0.72	6.23 0.46	7.03 1.16	6.74 0.79	7.14 0.56
Hemoglobin (gm/100 ml)	15.7 2.6	11.3 1.8	7.9 0.8	6.9 0.7	8.6 1.0	8.5 1.1	9.3 0.8	10.4 1.7	10.0 1.1	10.8 0.8
Packed cell volume	42 10	27 7	20 2	19 2	24 2	24 3	26 3	29 5	29 3	31 3
Mean corpuscular volume (cu microns)	71 12	62 5	52 5	44 3	43 1	40 3	41 3	42 1	43 3	43 3
Mean corpuscular hemoglobin (pg)	26 3	26 2	20 2	16 1	15 2	15 1	15 1	15 1	15 1	15 1
Mean corpuscular hemo-globin concentration (%)	38 4	43 5	39 2	37 1	36 3	36 2	36 3	36 1	35 3	35 1
Plasma total protein (gm/100 ml)	4.1 0.9	4.8 0.2	4.3 0.5	4.8 0.4	5.1 0.5	5.2 0.6	5.5 0.6	6.4 0.8	5.8 0.5	5.8 0.3
Platelets ($\times 10^3$/cu mm)	185 85	420 92	491 152	561 159	542 128	561 187	552 242	578 146	612 163	535 187
Leukocytes ($\times 10^3$/cu mm)	12.2 3.7	10.2 4.0	12.9 7.2	13.2 6.7	10.6 4.6	14.2 6.6	15.7 3.9	15.0 6.9	16.8 5.8	16.8 6.5

*Values are mean and standard deviation.

anemic, especially between 2 and 4 weeks of age. The anemia is described as a condition of below-normal concentration of erythrocytes or hemoglobin or both. The low erythrocyte number and low hemoglobin concentration seen in the young kitten is not a pathological condition but a normal state. The hemogram in Table 2 indicates conversion from values of fetal existence to adult values and is influenced by many factors such as body water, nutrition and activity. The clinician should consider the age of a kitten when its hemogram is made available for diagnosis.

BODY TEMPERATURE

The neonatal kitten has a limited ability to sustain its body temperature under adverse conditions during the first few days of life. Temperatures of kittens recorded immediately following birth and daily for 1 week (Table 3) show that care should be taken to prevent environmental exposure for up to 1 week of age.

BEHAVIOR

The behavior of young kittens is a function of their age. Suckling is initiated within minutes to hours of birth, depending on prior maternal experience and the difficulties of the labor. Nursing occupies up to 70 per cent of the queens' time, but this decreases to 20 per cent after 5 weeks; the queen is so occupied because of the individual and successive patterns of suckling by the kittens at an early age. For its first few days, the kitten tends to nurse from a single nipple. The kittens are confined to a maternity area during the first 3 weeks of life.

At 12 days of age the eyes open. Consumption of semisolid or solid food begins at approximately 3 weeks, as the maternal bond is broken. Walking and self-grooming now

TABLE 3. *Rectal Temperatures of Newborn Cats in an Outdoor Colony*

Day of Age	Rectal Temperature			Number of Fetuses
	MEAN (°C)	MEAN (°F)	S.E.	
Birth	36.0	96.8	0.3	3
1	36.6	98.0	0.5	11
2	37.4	99.3	0.3	11
3	37.4	99.3	0.3	11
4	37.4	99.3	0.3	11
5	37.9	100.3	0.2	11
6	37.8	100.1	0.2	11
7	37.7	99.9	0.2	8

begin, followed by climbing at about 4 weeks of age.[2]

If artificial fostering is expected to occur, the kitten should be introduced to the bottle as soon as possible. The earlier in life this occurs, the easier and quicker the kitten will succeed in its feeding. Even at 1 to 2 weeks of age, the kitten will try to avoid a bottle nipple. This can later become an exhausting struggle for both kitten and handler. When introducing feeding by bottle, caution should be exercised so that the mouth is not flooded; inspiration pneumonia may be caused by an eager or frustrated handler.

REFERENCES

1. Jepson, S. L.: A case of superfetation in the cat. Am. J. Obstet., *16*:1056, 1883.
2. Kling, A., Kovach, J. K., and Tucker, T. J.: The behaviour of cats. *In*: Hafez, E. S. E. (ed.): The Behaviour of Domestic Animals. Baltimore, The Williams and Wilkins Co., 1975.
3. Markee, J. E., and Hinsey, J. C.: A case of probable superfetation in the cat. Anat. Rec., *61*:241, 1935.
4. Nelson, N. S. and Cooper, J.: The growing conceptus of the domestic cat. Growth, *39*:435, 1975.

Feline Nutrition

RICHARD D. KEALY

Ralston Purina Company, Checkerboard Square, St. Louis, Missouri

INTRODUCTION

Cats have several inherent biochemical and social differences that set them apart from other species. It is imperative that we understand these characteristics if we are to maintain the norm in nutrition for the feline.

Some of the characteristics are as follows: Cats are occasional eaters and seldom, if ever, eat all of their daily food at one sitting. Cats have a very keen sense of taste and can perceive flavor components at thresholds far below that of humans. Cats eat slowly and discriminately, as opposed to dogs, which eat rapidly and voraciously. Cats are true carnivores and typically prefer to eat meat. Cats are uninhibited eaters and seldom are influenced by the presence of man.[10] Cats exhibit an unusually high protein requirement compared with other species. Cats are water conservers and are seldom observed drinking. Even though this is true, the *water:food ratio* approximates that of other species. Cats have a unique kidney characterized by unusually high vitamin A storage,[11] excretion of a sulfur amino acid called felinine[10] and excretion of a magnesium ammonium phosphate crystal called struvite.[18]

COMMERCIAL DIETS

The average cat owner is frequently confused by the barrage of commercial products available that range from dry to semimoist to canned meat-type diets. These diets can be formulated to provide the nutrient requirements of the cat during any phase of its life.

The American Association of Feed Control Officials (AAFCO) regulates the labeling of pet foods. Certain of these regulations enforce standards for nutritional quality of pet foods. Specific commercial-type claims for pet food products are as follows:

1. Complete and balanced nutrition.
2. Complete and balanced nutrition for gestation/lactation.
3. Complete and balanced nutrition for growth.
4. Complete and balanced nutrition for adult maintenance.

These label claims are ranked from strongest to weakest. "Complete and balanced nutrition" insures that the pet food manufacturer has provided evidence to the AAFCO indicating that the product will support normal reproduction (gestation/lactation) in adult cats and normal growth of kittens. Overall, it assures one that the product will support all phases of the cat's life. Other claims support only specific phases of the cat's life cycle. These are self-explanatory by the titles.[1]

Dry, semi-moist and canned diets can support normal growth and reproduction provided the nutrients are balanced. Table 1 provides applied nutrition information along with estimated food consumption for a 5-kg cat.

NUTRITIONAL REQUIREMENTS

Water

Most cats originated from arid or semi-arid regions. They are seldom observed drinking and have a tendency to concentrate their urine. The latter is perhaps related to water-conserving characteristics of the kidney. It has been suggested that cats derive a rather high percentage of their water from conversion of body fat to water and carbon dioxide. Work involving labora-

tory cats has suggested that the *water:dry food ratio* is approximately 2:1, which is similar to other species.[10]

Protein

Cats require dietary protein as a source of essential amino acids. Essential amino acids are those that cannot be synthesized at a sufficient rate to maintain normal growth, reproduction and/or maintenance. The amino acids essential for monogastric animals are as follows: arginine, histidine, isoleucine, leucine, lysine, methionine, phenylalanine, threonine, tryptophan and valine.

Cystine and tyrosine have a sparing effect on methionine and phenylalanine, respectively. At this point, we must assume that the aforementioned essential amino acids are also essential for the feline. Cats excrete rather large amounts of the amino acid felinine in the urine.[19] Felinine is apparently synthesized in the kidney. The biosynthetic function of this amino acid is unknown. Cats also have an apparent inefficient conversion of tryptophan to niacin, which is unique to the species.[4, 9]

The specific amino acid requirements for the feline are unknown. For that reason the general protein requirement of the feline will be discussed. Cats exhibit a very high protein requirement compared with other species.

The protein requirement for growth has been reported to be as high as 37 to 43 per cent[5] to as low as 30 per cent in dry foods.[12]

A level of 30 per cent of a high-quality protein will support normal growth and reproduction.[10]

TABLE 1. *Caloric Requirements and Estimated Food Consumption for a 5-Kg Cat*

	Food		
	DRY	SEMI-MOIST	CANNED
Protein (%)	30.0	25.0	14.0
Fat (%)	10.0	27.0	8.0
Carbohydrate (%)	38.0	28.0	1.0
Moisture (%)	10.0	30.0	75.0
Estimated digestible kcal/kg of food	3,620	2,750	1,320
Estimated food consumed/day (gm)*	76	100	208

*Based on caloric needs of a 5-kg cat using a requirement of 55 digestible kcal/kg of body weight.

TABLE 2. *Sources of High Quality Protein for Cats*

Ingredient	Protein (%)	Moisture (%)	Protein (Dry Matter Basis) (%)
Tuna fish	25	70	83
Liver	20	60	50
Milk	3.5	87	27
Poultry meat meal	65	8	71
Meat and bone meal	50	8	54
Fish meal (Peruvian)	65	8	71
Corn gluten meal	60	8	65
Soybean meal	48	8	52

Sources of high quality protein for cats include tuna, liver or milk. Combinations of proteins also provide resultant quality proteins. Commerical diets combine meat meals, fish meals, gluten meals, oil meals and other protein sources to provide a high-quality protein (Table 2).

Carbohydrate and Fat

The cat does not have a specific carbohydrate requirement, and it is questionable if there is a fat or fatty acid requirement. However, the cat does require energy. Energy values of 4, 9 and 4 kilocalories per gram for protein, fat and carbohydrate, respectively, will be utilized in this text as estimated digestible caloric values. Adult cats require 55 digestible calories per kg of body weight. Growing kittens require 2 to 3 times the adult requirement per kg of body weight. The greatest requirement is at birth and then declines until 1 year of age, when the adult requirement becomes 55 digestible calories per kg of body weight.

Carbohydrate is utilized well by the cat, provided it is processed correctly. Proper cooking of the carbohydrate renders the starches and dextrins available to the digestive system. Pencovic and Morris[14] observed that finely ground or cooked grains exhibited starch digestibility coefficients of 88 to 97 per cent.

Sucrose, glucose and cooked starch compounds are all well utilized by the cat. However, these are generally unpalatable to cats, owing to their sweetness and/or powdery texture. Boiled rice or potatoes provide a bland flavor plus texture and are good sources of supplemental carbohydrate. These sources contain about 85 per cent carbohydrate on a dry matter basis. High levels of lactose are not tolerated by the cat; however, no data are available on specific limits.

There is no evidence for a fat or essential fatty acid requirement for the feline. Therefore, it must be assumed that fat serves only as a source of essential calories. Cats utilize saturated and most unsaturated fats equally well with digestibility coefficients almost always exceeding 85 per cent for this nutrient. Bleachable fancy tallow, pork lard, corn oil or soybean oil are all satisfactory fat sources.

Highly unsaturated fats of fish oils have been associated with a syndrome called steatitis. Steatitis is characterized by yellow to brown discoloration of the adipose tissue, rough haircoat, emaciation, anemia, motor weakness, terminal spasms and coma.[3] The syndrome is especially prevalent in cats fed tuna fish for long periods of time. Inclusion of vitamin E in tuna at 68 IU/kg of diet has afforded complete protection.[9]

Vitamins

Many of the vitamin functions, deficiency symptoms and requirements of the feline are similar to those of other species. These will not be reviewed but will be cited in Table 3.

Certain vitamins, however, have different roles in the feline. The feline specifically has a requirement for preformed vitamin A, since it lacks the ability to convert β-carotene to vitamin A.[2, 8]

Cats also exhibit higher concentrations of vitamin A in the kidney than other species.[11] Liver concentrations appear to re-

TABLE 3. *Functions, Deficiencies, Requirements and Therapeutic Dosages of Various Vitamins for Cats*

Vitamin	Function	Deficiency	Requirement/ kg Dry Food	Commercial Source*	Concentration	Recommended Daily Therapeutic Dosage†
Vitamin A	Dim light vision	–	15,000 IU	Vitamin A acetate	500,000 IU/gm	5 mg
				Vitamin A palmitate	250,000 IU/gm	10 mg
Vitamin D	Metabolism of calcium and phosphorus	Muscular weakness	1,000 IU	Cholecalciferol (vitamin D_3)	400,000 IU/gm	1 mg
Vitamin E	Biological antioxidant	Steatitis in conjunction with fish oil	136 IU	dl-alpha tocopherol acetate	250 IU/gm	1 gm
Vitamin K	Blood clotting	–	–	Menadione sodium bisulfite	100%	0.5 gm
Thiamin	Energy metabolism	Convulsions	4 mg	Thiamine hydrochloride	100%	2 mg
				Thiamine mononitrate	100%	2 mg
Riboflavin	Energy metabolism	Anorexia	4 mg	Riboflavin	100%	2 mg
Pyridoxine	Transamination	Convulsions, kidney stones	2 mg	Pyridoxine hydrochloride	100%	1 mg
Niacin	Metabolic reactions	Tongue inflammation	40 mg	Nicotinic acid	100%	15 mg
				Niacinamide	100%	15 mg
Pantothenic acid	Energy metabolism	Fatty liver	5 mg	d-pantothenic acid calcium salt	100%	2.5 mg
Biotin	Fatty acid synthesis	–	NR	d-biotin	100%	2 µg
Folic acid	Metabolic reactions	Macrocytic anemia	NR	Folic acid crystalline	100%	4 µg
Choline	Phospholipid synthesis	Fatty liver	3,000 mg	Choline chloride	100%	1,500 mg
Vitamin B_{12}	Nerve transmission	–	NR	Vitamin B_{12}	100%	0.25 µg

*Source of vitamins—ICN Life Sciences Group, 26201 Miles Road, Cleveland, Ohio.

†This is the recommended amount per 5 kg of body weight in the feline. These levels should be fed no longer than 14 days since they represent averages. Cats should be placed on a complete and balanced diet after this period.

TABLE 4. *Sources of Calcium and Phosphorus for Cats*

	Calcium (%)	Phosphorus (%)	Ratio
Steamed bone meal	26	13	2:1
Dicalcium phosphate	23	18	1.3:1

flect dietary levels of vitamin A, whereas kidney concentrations do not. It is possible that the kidney is a point of vitamin A storage. There has never been any strong evidence for an excessively high vitamin A requirement at 25,000 IU/kg of diet, as cited by the National Research Council.[13]

Thiamin deficiency has occurred in cats fed certain species of raw fish (carp and salt water herring) containing a thiamin-destroying enzyme called "thiaminase." Thiaminase was destroyed by cooking the fish. Deficiency symptoms included anorexia, ataxia, circus movements, head ventroflexion, loss of righting reaction, convulsions, prostration and death.[17]

The niacin requirement of the cat is confounded by the fact that cats have the inability to convert the amino acid tryptophan to niacin.[9] This is in contrast to most species, which are considerably more efficient in the conversion. This characteristic, however, has not had a profound effect on elevating the niacin requirement.

Minerals

There has been a marked deficiency in published work on the mineral requirements of cats. Calcium deficiency was produced in cats by Scott *et al.*[16] Deficiency resulted in signs of osteogenesis imperfecta

but not in rickets. No phosphorus deficiency information is available. The minimum requirement for calcium and phosphorus on a dry basis is estimated at 1.0 and 0.8 per cent, respectively.

Processed bone meal or dicalcium phosphate provide excellent sources of calcium and phosphorus to cats. Both provide these minerals in satisfactory ratios (Table 4).

Cats exhibiting calcium and/or phosphorus deficiency may be supplemented with either processed bone meal or dicalcium phosphorus at a level of 0.5 gm/kg of body weight. A source of vitamin D_2 or D_3 is necessary for calcium and phosphorus metabolism.

Table 5 cites minerals, functions and signs of deficiency based on data from other species. No requirements will be cited, since there is insufficient data available.

Ash

Ash is a general term referring to the noncombustible portion of food. The crude term "ash" frequently makes it appear to be an adulterant. However, this is not the case since it contains essential minerals for the health and well-being of cats. Without these ash components, life could not be sustained.

TABLE 5. *Functions and Deficiencies of Various Minerals for Cats*

Mineral	Function	Deficiency
Calcium	Bone structure	Osteogenesis imperfecta
Phosphorus	Bone structure	–
Potassium	Fluid balance	Paralysis
Sodium	Fluid balance	–
Magnesium	Bone calcification	Ataxia
Iron	Synthesis of hemoglobin	Anemia
Copper	Synthesis of hemoglobin	Anemia
Manganese	Bone formation	–
Zinc	Skin and hair synthesis	Keratitis
Iodine	Part of thyroid hormone	–

Another misconception is that ash predisposes to feline urolithiasis (FUS). This has not been the case with the typical ash that is consumed in cat foods. Also studies by Dickenson and Scott[4a] and work at the Ralston Purina Company have indicated that ash at 30 or 24 per cent, respectively, did not cause urinary problems.

Rich *et al.*[15] reported that urinary calculi and urolithiasis occurred with increasing frequency as dietary magnesium was increased to 0.75 or 1.0 per cent (dry basis). This, however, is an unusually high magnesium concentration, representing five-fold or more of that found in a commericaltype diet. The most promising work on urolithiasis has indicated that feline herpesvirus (CAHv) is relevant to the onset of feline urolithiasis.[6]

SUPPLEMENTATION

Supplementation is necessary only when there is a nutrient deficiency. There is no need for supplementation when a complete and balanced diet is fed. Certain supplements are potentially harmful. Vitamin A should not exceed 6,000 IU/day/cat, and vitamin D should not exceed 1000 IU/day/cat. Calcium and phosphorus intake should not exceed 3 and 2.5 gm/day, respectively. As previously mentioned (see Carbohydrate and Fat), a fatty acid requirement has not been established for the feline for skin or haircoat condition.

Supplements such as wheat germ meal, wheat germ oil, brewers' yeast and cottage cheese can be fed with relative safety, provided they are necessary.

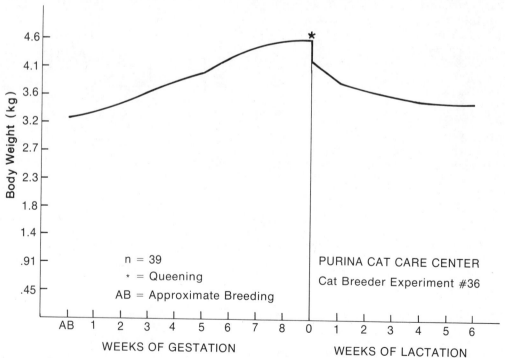

Figure 1. Chart showing weight changes of queens during gestation and lactation.

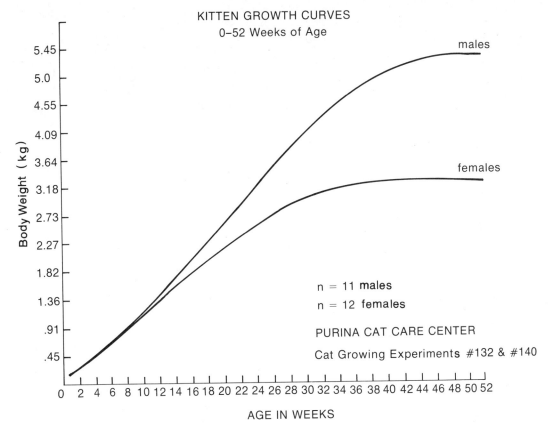

KITTEN GROWTH CURVES
0–52 Weeks of Age

males

females

n = 11 **males**

n = 12 **females**

PURINA CAT CARE CENTER

Cat Growing Experiments #132 & #140

AGE IN WEEKS

Figure 2. Chart indicating kitten growth curves.

FEEDING FOR BREEDING AND GESTATION

The specific nutritional needs for the breeding tom and queen have not been established. Essential amino acids and most B-vitamins are not stored and must be replenished daily for optimal performance. Use of the nutrient standards for growth are recommended until such time as more specific reproductive data are available.

The breeding queen requires a balanced ration prior to breeding. A 5-kg cat requires 275 kcal of digestible energy. After 6 weeks of gestation the caloric requirement is elevated approximately 25 per cent (to 345 digestible kcal per day). During lactation there is an additional requirement, increasing 100 per cent to 550 digestible kcal per day at 6 weeks of lactation. This, of course, inclines linearly. It is extremely important that queens do not reject their food during the first trimester of pregnancy.

Queens exhibit a linear type of weight gain during gestation amounting to 30 to 40 per cent. The weight loss at parturition is less dramatic, usually amounting to less than 10 per cent of preparturition weight. During the 6 weeks of lactation the normal queen returns to the original prebreeding weight. These data are cited in Figure 1 and are based on feline reproductive studies conducted at the Purina Cat Care Center.

A healthy kitten weighs approximately 100 gm at birth. The weight should increase by approximately 100 gm/week for the first 26 weeks of life. Kittens depend on queen's milk for the first 4 weeks of life. At 4 weeks of age they are able to eat part of the queen's food. Food at this time should be moist, highly digestible, highly nutritious and of rather soft texture for ease of eating.

Figure 2 illustrates normal kitten growth during a 12-month period. Body weight is maximized at approximately 40 weeks of age in the female and at 50 weeks in the male. The divergence between male and female body weight occurs at approximately 10 weeks. At this point the difference in the growth rate between male and female kittens continues to increase until 52 weeks.

It is necessary for kittens to receive supplemental food after 4 weeks since lactation is frequently insufficient to support a litter after 4 weeks of age. Dry foods should be fed with 50 per cent added water at this stage. Certain human baby formulas or livestock milk replacers have been used successfully at this stage.

FEEDING FOR GROWTH

Kittens should be taken from the queen when they reach 6 weeks of age. It is necessary to provide a soft food during this period. This may include canned food; a soft-moist product in small particles or a dry food in small particles fed moistened. Such food is essential until 10 weeks of age. Afterwards, as teeth develop, there is less concern about texture.

REFERENCES

1. Association of American Feed Control Officials: Official Publication, pp. 164–176, 1977.
2. Ahmad, B.: The fate of carotene after absorption in the animal organism. Biochem. J., *25*:1195, 1931.
3. Coffin, D. L. and Holzworth, J.: "Yellow fat" in two laboratory cats: Acid-fast pigmentation associated with a fish-base ration. Cornell Vet. *44*:63, 1954.
4. De Castro, F. T., Brown, R. R. and Price, J. M.: The intermediary metabolism of tryptophan by cat and rat tissue preparations. J. Biol. Chem., *228*:777, 1957.
4a. Dickenson, C. D. and Scott, P. P.: Failure to produce urinary calculi in kittens by the addition of mineral salts derived from bone meal to the diet. Vet. Rec., *68*:858, 1956.
5. Dickenson, C. D. and Scott, P. P.: Nutrition of the cat. Protein requirements for growth of weanling kittens and young cats maintained on a mixed diet. Br. J. Nutr., *10*:311, 1956.
6. Fabricant, C. G.: Viral induced feline urolithiasis. Am. J. Vet. Res., *38*:1837, 1977.
7. Gershoff, S. N., Andrus, S. B., Hegsted, D. M. and Lentini, E. A.: Vitamin A deficiency in cats. Lab Invest., *6*:227, 1957.
8. Gershoff, S. N. and Norkin, S. A.: Vitamin E deficiency in cats. J. Nutr., 77:303, 1962.
9. Jackson, R. W.: The excretion of kynurenic acid by members of various families of the order Carnivora. J. Biol. Chem., *131*:469, 1929.
10. Kealy, R. D.: Unpublished data, 1977.
11. Lowe, J. S., Morton, R. A. and Vernon, J.: Unsaponifiable constituents of kidney in various species. Biochem. J., *67*:228, 1957.
12. Miller, S. A. and Allison, J. B.: The dietary nitrogen requirements of the cat. J. Nutr., *64*:493, 1958.
13. National Research Council: Nutrient Requirements of Laboratory Animals. *Nutrient Requirements of the Cat.* Number 10. Washington, D. C., National Academy of Sciences, 1972.
14. Pencovic, T. A. and Morris, J. G.: Corn and wheat starch utilization by the cat. J. Anim. Sci., *41*:325, 1975.
15. Rich, L. J., Dysart, M. I., Chow, F. H. C. and Hamar, D.: Urethral obstruction in male cats: Experimental production by addition of magnesium and phosphate to diet. Feline Pract., *4*:44, 1974.
16. Scott, P. P., Greaves, J. P. and Scott, M. G.: Nutrition of the cat: Calcium and iodine deficiency on a meat diet. Br. J. Nutr., *15*:35, 1961.
17. Smith, D. C. and Proutt, L. M.: Development of thiamine deficiency in the cat on a diet of raw fish. Proc. Soc. Exp. Biol. Med., *56*:1, 1944.
18. Sutor, D. J., Wooly, S. E. and Jackson, O. F.: Crystalline material from the feline bladder. Res. Vet. Sci., *2*:298, 1970.
19. Westall, R. G.: The amino acids and other ampholytes of urine. The isolation of a new sulphur-containing amino acid from cat urine. Biochem. J., *55*:244, 1953.

Suppression/Induction of Estrus in Cats

EMERSON D. COLBY

Dartmouth Medical School,
Hanover, New Hampshire

SUPPRESSION OF ESTRUS

A variety of compounds, hormones and hormone analogs have been tried in the cat for the express purpose of suppressing estrus. The results have been variable, perhaps because two effects are desired using only one agent, i.e., estrous suppression and early abortion or resorption after an unsatisfactory mating. The suppression of estrus should be dealt with as a separate entity, and in doing so, one must realize that many, if not all, of the compounds currently used in the United States are not approved for use in the cat and therefore should be administered with caution and with the agreement of the animal's owner.

The results of these treatments are variable in that they may well suppress the overt clinical signs of estrus while delaying the return of the animal to the estrous state for variable lengths of time. There are recorded side effects that may be undesirable, such as cystic endometrial hyperplasia (CEH)-pyometra complex as well as long-delayed estrous cycling. The preparations are summarized in Table 1 but are briefly described as follows:

Provera (medoxyprogesterone acetate)[5] has been used at a dose level of 5 mg/day given orally. The cat will usually refuse mating within 24 hours. Continuing this dosage for another 2 to 4 days is recommended in order to create a depo effect. A single injection of 25 to 100 mg will also effect the same result. Estrus will usually return after a period of 2 to 4 months. The hormone acts by causing a reduction in the activity of the ovary and by effectively reducing the size of the reproductive tract. Subsequent pregnancies have not been impaired by the action of this progesterone ester.

Orgasterone (methyloestrenolene)[7] will prevent or suppress estrus in the female cat within 1 to 2 days by giving 15 to 30 mg/day (5 to 10 mg t.i.d.) orally for 5 to 7 days. Normal fertile estrus may return after 2 to 3 months.

Ovaban (megestrol acetate)[12] may also be used when given at the rate of 5 mg for 3 days to control the signs of estrus and then administered at a dose of 2.5 to 5 mg once per week for 10 weeks to keep the cat in anestrus. The usually reported undesirable side effects of the treatment are related to weight gain. Other side effects may include diarrhea, listlessness, urine odor, temperature change, mammary enlargement, hair color change and pyometra (listed here in order of decreasing incidence). It should be noted that the treated females should be isolated from males for the first 3 or more days of the treatment, as the drug may aid conception if mating occurs during this time.

DMA (delmadinone acetate)[13, 15] has been shown to control or suppress the estrous cycle in the cat. It has been used with both an oral and a subcutaneous treatment regimen and has been observed to be successful in preventing estrus for periods of up to 12 months. The treatment regimen for estrous control is given as 0.25 to 0.7 mg/kg of body weight orally once per week or 2.50 to 5.0 mg/kg of body weight subcutaneously twice a year. For estrous suppression the oral dose is 0.50 to 1.0 mg/kg body weight daily for 6 days or 2.6 to 6.75 mg/kg body weight in one or two subcutaneous injections in 24 hours. (One should examine the package insert for a more complete explanation.)

Mibolerone (dimethylnortestosterone) has been used for the suppression of estrus in the cat[1] but not without some problems associated with increased thyroid weights and clitoral enlargement and subsequent formation of cartilaginous or osseous baculums. At the present time Mibolerone is not recommended for estrous suppression in the cat.

Abortion may be induced in cats over 40 days of gestation by the use of THAM salt, an $F_{2\alpha}$ prostaglandin, at doses of 0.5 to 1.0 mg/kg of body weight. THAM-$F_{2\alpha}$ may also induce early parturition during late gesta-

TABLE 1. *Preparations for Suppression of Estrus in Cats*

Product	Manufacturer
Chorionic gonadotrophin (HCG)	Sigma Chemical Company, St. Louis, Missouri
Delmadinone	Syntex Pharmaceuticals Ltd., Maidenhead, Berks, England
Estradiol cypionate	Upjohn Company, Kalamazoo, Michigan
FSH-P	Burns-Biotech, Oakland, California
Gestyl (PMSG)	Organon Laboratories, West Orange, New Jersey
Luteinizing hormone	Burns-Biotech, Oakland, California
Orgasterone	Organon Laboratories, West Orange, New Jersey
Ovaban	Schering Corporation, Kenilworth, New Jersey
Provera	Upjohn (Glaxo), United Kingdom
Utonex	Upjohn Company, Kalamazoo, Michigan

tion.[15] Detrimental side effects have not been noted or reported.

The use of a hormone preparation to prevent pregnancy after mismating is not uncommon. A variety of preparations have been used. Side effects in each case should be a consideration before administering the hormones.

Repositol diethylstilbestrol has been used as an abortifacient in the female cat and may be recommended at the level of 2 mg given on day 2 and repeated on day 10 following coitus.[10] It should be remembered that continued use of diethylstilbestrol can lead to a poisoning situation.[6] High levels and daily dosing may produce lesions in the liver, heart and pancreas. Diethylstilbestrol is detoxified by the liver.

Pilocarpine[14] has also been reported as preventing estrus in the cat when given orally and thus should not be used for treating other disorders in animals that are naturally cycling with the intention to breed. The side effects of this compound should be thoroughly examined before its use can be contemplated.

Recent work done by Herron and Sis[11] indicates that prevention of estrus after mismating in the cat may be successfully

accomplished by the use of proper amounts of estradiol cypionate (ECP) when given at the proper time — timing is important. The action is either by a process called tube-locking or by the flushing action that estrogens exert on the uterus. The work is based on the fact that the normal transit time of the ovum from ovary to uterus is known to be 3 to 5 days and that the cat is an induced ovulator. Thus coitus and ovulation are known to be separated by approximately 24 hours.

In effect, in this study the ovum was retarded in its movement to the uterus so that it was in the degenerate stages at the time of entry. The action of estrogen also retards the development of the uterine endometrium when contrasted with the endometrium of nonestrogen-treated cats. The dose of ECP given was 250 μg intramuscularly 40 hours after coitus.

In subsequent work[4] it has been noted that pregnancy has been prevented by using 250 μg of ECP intramuscularly up to 5 days following an undesirable mating.

The thesis for this work has been based on knowledge available for animals of other species, especially the rabbit,[9] also a postcoital ovulator. In the rabbit, small doses of estrogen caused expulsion of ova from the reproductive tract and large doses caused tube-locking, thus effectually bringing about destruction of the egg.

The side effects of the use of ECP in the cat are usually related only to some continuance of the estrous behavior. However, larger doses of ECP than those just listed may cause what appears to be induction of the CEH-pyometra complex, so care should be taken when handling the compound.

It is not recommended that hormones be used to prevent the unwanted pregnancy. Both the interaction of hormones and their circulating levels at certain times during the estrous cycle are not known, although these factors are currently being investigated. Until it is firmly established how the female cat responds to the administration of exogenous hormones, one should utilize considerable caution when these preparations are used.

INDUCTION OF ESTRUS

The induction of estrus may be accomplished by several means. It has been observed that many cats will begin to cycle in response to those cats already exhibiting estrus. A large percentage of these animals will begin to cycle within a few days of each other. The lengthening of light cycles 14 to 18 hours per day[17] is also known to induce queens to cycle. The response to lengthening the light cycle is not immediate but may be noted over a period of several weeks.

Cats may be brought into estrus by the use of a variety of exogenous hormones.[3, 14, 20]

The administration of hormones under these conditions must be judicious, for it is easy to overstimulate the ovaries, producing large numbers of follicles that may not contain mature ova, or to produce cystic follicles.[3, 19] Excessively long periods of heat may be observed when overdoses of certain hormones are given. Methods of artificial induction in general produce an estrous period that may exceed the length of the natural cycle by 2 to 4 days.

As previously stated, it should also be recognized that many of these preparations are not recommended for use in the cat in the United States (see Table 1), and thus such advice must be given to the owner of the animal when these compounds are to be administered.

Hormonal treatment may also be used successfully to initiate estrus in cats that have not previously exhibited heat or in those that tend to cycle irregularly.

Pregnant mare serum gonadotropin (PMSG)[21] has been used successfully under these conditions following a specific dose regimen[2, 3] (Table 2). This hormone is given intramuscularly, using 100 IU on the first day and 50 IU each day thereafter for 5 to 6 days. If the female is induced during the natural breeding season, the dosage may be reduced to 25 IU as estrous behavior becomes apparent by observation of behavior with and without handling. The use of PMSG in cats less than 1 year of age may produce cystic ovarian follicles. PMSG is currently obtained as an experimental preparation (Table 1) when used in the cat. There are several preparations available, but variation in actual dosage units per vial or ampule may occur when assay methods are not similar. It is considered best to use a preparation of PMSG that has a high ratio of units per milliliter of sample so that the unit volume injected is small. Table 2 gives the dosage regimen followed when PMSG is used to initiate estrus. The results are usually 80 per cent efficient.

All injections are given intramuscularly in the thigh using a tuberculin syringe and a 22-gauge needle. Young cats, less than 1 year of age, have a tendency to produce small cystic follicles and exhibit estrus but will not breed if the dosages are excessive. Superovulation may also be an unfavorable result. PMSG is primarily of a follicle-stimulating hormone (FSH) character but does have a luteinizing hormone (LH) component, which, if given in excess, could result in ovulation. Older cats beyond the prime of their reproductive activity, 5 years or more, can be induced and mated successfully using PMSG, but they tend to produce fewer young and may be less predictable in their response to the hormone.

When induction of estrus is performed correctly, the litter size has approximated the natural birth rate of four kittens per litter. The system seems to work best in females that are between 1 and 5 years of age. Although there are no data to substantiate it, clinical observation would appear to indicate that continuous induction of estrus in the female cat will shorten the reproductive life that would be expected under natural conditions.[18]

Certain queens, either cycling naturally or when induced, will fail to exhibit estrus even when handled. They can usually be

TABLE 2. *Induction of Estrus in Cats by PMSG*

	Day							
	1	2	3	4	5	6	7	8
Calendar Months				PMSG (IU)				
December–January	100	50	50	50	50	50	50	50
February–August	100	50	50	50	50	25*	25*	25*
September–November	100	50	50	50	50	50	50	50

*In cats near estrus (behavior), dose decreased until bred.

bred when placed with a male that is familiar with breeding when given an estrous female.

It is necessary that a queen be handled more than once daily during an induction period for demonstrating evidence of estrus. An attempt should be made to have the queen assume the breeding posture by grasping behind the neck and stroking the tail head and perineal area.

PMSG has been used successfully to induce estrus and cycling in cats that have no previous breeding history or that have had estrus terminated for extended periods of time following use of other hormones to terminate estrus or pregnancy. The CEH-pyometra complex can be a result of excessive hormone therapy using PMSG or other estrogenic substances.

Estrogens (50 μg of estradiol benzoate or 0.25 mg of estradiol cypionate) will initiate estrus in most queens when given intramuscularly. Estrogens when given in excess may be toxic to the cat. No more than 8 mg of estrogens should be given within any continuous 4-month period.[20] Testosterone may also be used to initiate estrus in the cat when given intramuscularly at the level of 20 mg/day. Excessive use of estrogens or testosterone may initiate estrus that will last for 2 to 4 weeks unless natural or artificial coitus is performed.

Follicle-stimulating hormone-pituitary (FSH-P) has recently been used to induce estrus in the domestic cat.[23] The effective dosage of FSH-P was 2.0 mg injected daily intramuscularly until the queen exhibited signs of typical estrus. It is recommended that FSH-P not be administered for longer than 5 days because of the hyperstimulative effects of the gonadotropin. Cats treated with this regimen of FSH-P exhibited estrus between 4 and 5 days, with the estrous period lasting an average of 6.2 days. On days 1 and 2 of estrus, 250 IU of human chorionic gonadotropin is given intramuscularly. Follicle rupture was observed by laparoscopy in 11 (91.7 per cent) of the 12 cats involved. Mean litter size in queens treated with FSH-P has been 5.8 kittens. It is interesting to note that queens treated with FSH-P and inseminated with frozen semen have delivered viable offspring.[16]

When hormonally induced cats are presented for breeding, the best results are noted when the queens are bred at least twice on each day of estrus for a period of up to 4 days.

Current evidence points to the fact that female cats should be older than 1 year of age when hormones are used in order to expect a reliable response. A complete history should be obtained for all animals, including information about other hormonal defects. Parasitism and low-grade bacterial infections should not be evident, nor should cats be induced when in the presence of other cats exhibiting clinical signs of panleukopenia or upper respiratory tract disease. Before induction of estrus with hormones, the cat should be proved to be feline leukemia-negative.

REFERENCES

1. Burke, T. J., Reynolds, H. A. and Sokolowski, J. H.: A 180-day tolerance-efficacy study with Mibolerone for suppression of estrus in the cat. Am. J. Vet. Res., *38*:469, 1977.
2. Colby, E. D.: Feline reproduction. American Animal Hospital Assoc., Scientific Proceedings, 1977 pp. 141–144.
3. Colby, E. D.: Induced estrus and timed pregnancies in the cat. J. Lab. Anim. Care, *20*:1075, 1970.
4. Colby, E. D.: Personal observations.
5. Colton, M. W.: Progestational hormones in pet practice, indications, agents and doses, precautions. Mod. Vet. Pract., June, 1965, pp. 53–56.
6. Dow, C.: The pathology of stilbestrol poisoning in the domestic cat. J. Path. Bacti., *LXXV*:151, 1958.
7. Gerber, H. A. and Sulman, F. G.: Use of progestative hormones for prevention of heat, pregnancy and sexual disturbances in dogs and cats. Refu. Vet., *24*(3):154, 1969.
8. Gerber, H. A., Jochle, W. and Sulman, F. G.: Control of reproduction and of undesirable social and sexual behavior in dogs and cats. J. Small Anim. Pract., *14*:151, 1973.
9. Greenwald, G. S.: Species difference in egg transport in response to exogenous estrogen. Anat. Rec., *157*:163, 1967.
10. Herron, M. A.: Feline reproduction. Vet. Clin. North Am. 7:715, 1977.
11. Herron, M. A. and Sis, R. F.: Ovum transport in the cat and the effect of estrogen administration. Am. J. Vet. Rec, *35*:1277, 1974.
12. Houdeshell, J. W. and Hennessey, P. W.: Megestrol acetate for control of estrus in the cat. Vet. Med/Small Anim. Clin., *72*:1013, 1977.
13. Jochle, W.: Progress in small animal reproductive physiology, therapy of reproductive disorders, and pet population control. Folia Vet. Latina, *IV*:706, 1974.
14. Mintschev, Von P.: Suppression of estrus in cat. Zuchthygiene, fortflanzyngsstoerungen und Besamung der Haustiere, 7:120, 1963.
15. Nachreiner, R. F. and Marple, D. N.: Termination

of pregnancy in cats with prostaglandin F$_{2\alpha}$. Prostaglandins 7:303, 1974.

16. Platz, C. C., Wildt, D. E. and Seager, S. W. J.: Pregnancy in the domestic cat after artificial insemination with previously frozen spermatozoa. J. Reprod. Fertil., 62:279, 1978.

17. Scott, P. P. and Lloyd-Jacob, M. A.: Reduction in the anoestrus period of laboratory cats by increased illumination. Nature (London), 184:2022, 1959.

18. Sojka, W.: Personal communication.

19. Starkey, W. F., and Lathem, J. H.: Ovarian cysts in immature female cats following pregnant mare serum hormone administration. Anat. Rec., 86:401, 1943.

20. Stein, B. S.: The genital system. In Catcott, E. J. (ed.): Feline Medicine and Surgery. 2nd Ed., Santa Barbara, Cal., American Veterinary Publication, 1974. pp. 303–354.

21. VanTeinhoven, A.: Reproduction Physiology of Vertebrates. Philadelphia, W. B. Saunders Co., 1968, p. 167.

22. Wildt, D. E., Kinney, G. M. and Seager, S. W. J.: Laparoscopy for direct observation of internal organs of the domestic cat and dog. Am. J. Vet. Res., 38:1429, 1977.

23. Wildt, D. E., Kinney, G. M. and Seager, S. W. J.: Gonadotrophin induced reproduction cyclicity in the domestic cat. J. Lab. Anim. Sci., 20:301, 1978.

Obstetrics, Surgical Procedures and Anesthesia

BARBARA S. STEIN
Chicago Cat Clinic, Chicago, Illinois

DYSTOCIA

Primary uterine inertia and secondary uterine inertia are the most common causes of dystocia in the feline. Obese primigravid queens may never completely develop second stage labor contractions because of poor muscle tone. Fetal passage is further impeded by intrapelvic and perivulvar fat deposits. Secondary uterine inertia is frequently encountered in the older multiparous queen if parturition is very labored or prolonged, or both. Some of the kittens may have already been successfully delivered by the queen, but she is unable to continue and the uterus is atonic. Occasionally, passage of the last kitten or kittens may be hastened before complete uterine inertia occurs if the dorsal vaginal wall is "feathered" or digitally stroked.

In cases of either primary or secondary uterine inertia, ecbolic drugs should be used with caution to avoid uterine rupture. Subcutaneous or intramuscular administration of oxytocin (3 to 5 units USP) will usually stimulate uterine contractions. Theoretically the uterus may be further sensitized to this hormone by the concurrent intravenous administration of 5 ml of 10 per cent calcium gluconate. Additional amounts of oxytocin at the same dosage may be administered 30 to 45 minutes after the first injection. Cesarean section is indicated if no productive contractions occur within ½ hour after the second injection of oxytocin.

Fetal dystocia due to size, presentation or physical monstrosity may also occur. Particularly if there is a combination of early secondary uterine inertia, loss of amniotic fetal fluids and awkward presentation of the fetus, lubrication of the vagina with sterile viscous solutions such as light mineral oil or nitrofurazone (Furacin) solution may be very helpful. The lubricant is introduced via soft flexible plastic or rubber tubing into the vagina and advanced as far anterior as the cervix. However, if uterine rupture is suspected, this procedure is contraindicated.

If the fetus is partially expelled and primarily within the vagina, light lubrication plus a firm grasp of the fetus with a dry gauze sponge should aid delivery.

Delivery of the fetus by manipulation and instrumentation is done primarily with the queen's health at stake. Rather than risk endometrial trauma or uterine rupture by the use of forceps instrumenation, an ovariectomy hook may be more safely utilized. It is positioned with the hook portion directed dorsally and held parallel and adjacent to the middle finger of the operator. The open tip of the hook should rest against the middle fingernail as it is introduced into the queen's vagina and uterus. If the kitten is in a posterior presentation, the tail is grasped in the hook with the finger and gentle traction is applied in a dorsocaudal direction. Once the fetal pelvis clears the maternal pelvis, the direction of applied pressure should be ventrocaudal.

If the fetus is being presented in a dorsosacral position, the hook and finger are placed in the fetal mouth, the hook is redirected into the soft area between the mandible and the middle finger is pressed in the open portion of the hook, creating a pincer-like grip on the mandibular symphysis. Dorsocaudal pressure is applied until the fetal head is past the pelvis, and then the direction of pressure is changed to ventrocaudal until the fetal pelvis clears the queen's pelvis.

If the queen's bladder or colon is distended, evacuation will be required before employing either ecbolic therapy or manipulative techniques for dystocia.

CESAROTOMY

Cesarean section is not commonly required in the feline species primarily because great disproportion in body size rarely occurs between male and female. However, as certain breeds of cats with their accompanying physical and psychological idiosyncrasies have become more popular, e.g., Persian, Manx, Siamese, so has the need for cesarean section increased in frequency.

Indications. As in other species, there are no exact criteria for establishing when and if a cesarean section is required. Because cesarotomy has been necessary for one queening does not require that all future pregnancies be terminated in the same manner. The possibility of cesarean section should be considered in the following instances of dystocia: (1) strong nonproductive contractions exceeding 3 hours' duration (2) weak contractions that never develop into true second stage labor even after the use of pitocin (3) passage of bright to dark red vaginal discharge without the onset of labor and (4) continuation of intense contractions 2 to 4 hours after the delivery of the first kitten or kittens. Judicious use of ecbolic drugs and manipulative techniques should precede surgical intervention.

Anesthesia. The type and amount of anesthesia administered to the queen will be directly related to the degree of fetal depression at the time of surgical delivery. Inhalation anesthesia is preferred and may be induced by use of halothane and nitrous oxide delivered through an anesthetic chamber, followed by intubation and maintenance of these same agents. One of the main advantages of this type of anesthesia is that the queen is awake very soon after surgery so that nursing may begin.

Alternatively, ketamine hydrochloride administered intravenously at 5 to 10 mg/kg will provide sufficient relaxation for intubation and surgical preparation. If necessary, this may be supplemented with very low levels of halothane (0.5 to 1 per cent) and nitrous oxide, or if the queen is sufficiently sedated, only the administration of local anesthesia to the surgical site may be necessary.

Surgical Procedure. A midline incision is begun 1 inch anterior to the umbilicus and extended caudad approximately 3 to 4 inches. Care should be taken to avoid incising engorged mammary tissue so as to minimize milk leakage into the surgical site. A slightly shorter incision is made through the linea alba to expose the abdominal viscera. The distended uterus is usually immediately visible just beneath the peritoneum. The uterus is gently removed from the abdominal cavity, and both horns are laid out so as to determine the total number of fetuses present.

A longitudinal incision into the uterus is made over the ventral surface immediately posterior to the cornual bifurcation and may be extended craniad for a short distance on one uterine horn. If there is a kitten just caudad to the cervix toward the vagina, it should be delivered first. Then systematic removal of fetuses from each horn should occur, with caution exercised to be sure the cranial-most fetuses are delivered.

As the fetus is gently manipulated to the cervical incision area, the body of the kitten can best be grasped with a dry sterile gauze sponge. Steady upward and outward pressure is applied to the fetus so that fetal placental detachment occurs at the same time. Once removed from the maternal placenta, the kitten and its placenta are handed to an assistant who is then able to open the amniotic sac enclosing the kitten (if the sac is still present) and stimulate respiration. In most instances, the kitten only needs to be briskly rubbed with a dry towel and its mouth cleared of mucus to induce spontaneous respiration. A hemostat should be applied approximately 1 inch away from the umbilicus until such time as a proper suture may be placed. If the fetus becomes prematurely detached from its placenta at the time of delivery, the surgeon should also be certain to manipulate and deliver the fetal placenta as well.

In cases of newborn respiratory depression, the respiratory passages may be further cleared of mucus by grasping the kitten firmly in both hands, with the kitten facing away from the assistant, and then swinging sharply in a downward arc. Further stimulation may be provided by administering 1 drop of doxapram hydrochloride (Dopram) topically under the tongue. External artificial respiration should also be employed. Even if a kitten appears to be lifeless after all these measures, it should be maintained in a warm environment for an additional 15 minutes before final pronouncement of stillbirth.

Immediately after cesarean delivery of all kittens, a healthy uterus will undergo spontaneous involution. If this is not evident to the surgeon by the time suturing is to occur, 5 units of pitocin, intramuscularly (IM), should be administered to the queen. If the uterus still remains atonic, ovariohysterectomy is indicated.

The uterus should be closed with an inverting pattern using 3-0 chromic gut. The peritoneal, subcutaneous and skin closures are routine.

Supportive Care. Routine use of intravenous fluids (lactated Ringer's solution with 5 per cent dextrose) during surgery will definitely hasten the postoperative recovery of the queen so that she is willing and able to nurse. The use of antibiotics is governed by the condition of the queen preoperatively, her previous reproductive history and the status of the uterus at the time of surgery.

UTERINE RUPTURE

Although uncommon, rupture of the uterus may occur during (1) late pregnancy caused by extrinsic trauma; (2) parturition due to dystocia, forceful manipulative techniques or injudicious use of ecbolic drugs; (3) postparturition due to acute necrotizing metritis and (4) cases of pyometra.

Clinical Signs. Vomiting, depression, anorexia, fever and abdominal pain are usually the early signs of uterine rupture. Although the condition should be considered life-threatening, occasionally uterine rupture may occur following which the cat survives without medical attention. This fact is verified by several reports of partially resorbed ectopic fetuses along with old uterine scars and adhesions found at the time of routine ovariohysterectomy.

Treatment. If uterine rupture is suspected, prompt exploratory laparotomy is indicated. When the queen involved is a valuable breeding animal, it may be possible to perform unilateral ovariohysterectomy to save her reproductive capacity. However, in most instances complete ovariohysterectomy is performed.

Because the cat is usually in severe distress and possibly in shock, inhalation anesthesia is preferred. The abdominal cavity should be treated for peritonitis due to uterine rupture by rinsing with either warm saline or lactated Ringer's solution, and water-soluble antibiotics should be instilled. Nongut suture material such as fine-gauge stainless steel or Dexon should be used to close the abdominal incision. Some surgeons may also prefer the use of an abdominal Penrose drain for several days to minimize complications associated with peritonitis.

Intensive supportive care, including administration of intravenous fluids, electrolytes and antibiotics, should be utilized. Further antibiotic therapy is continued for 2 weeks.

UTERINE TORSION

Uterine torsion is a rare complication of late pregnancy, although it may also occur in cases of pyometra. The cause is unknown. Only one horn of the uterus is usually involved and is twisted on its long axis to a variable degree of rotation (90° to 360°).

The signs of uterine torsion are usually acute and reflect severe abdominal pain. Anorexia, depression, restlessness, fever and vomiting are common, along with signs of straining as if to defecate or urinate. The presence of a vaginal discharge is variable. There may be a history of normal delivery (24 to 48 hours prior) of healthy or stillborn kittens.

If the condition goes undiagnosed, the cat usually develops signs of shock, i.e., subnormal temperature, pale mucous membranes and polypnea.

Diagnosis. Abdominal palpation will elicit pain. The uterus is usually difficult to palpate, partially owing to ascitic distention from venous stasis and occlusion. Provided the cervix is sufficiently dilated, vaginal examination may be diagnostic if the caudal aspect of the rotated cornu can be palpated.

Radiographic examination will reveal a markedly enlarged uterus filled with air or fluid densities, or both.

Treatment. Exploratory laparotomy should be performed as soon as uterine torsion is suspected. Inhalation anesthesia and intensive supportive care (administration of intravenous fluids, electrolytes, antibiotics and corticosteroids) are imperative, as most deaths are a result of shock or massive placental hemorrhage. Complete ovariohysterectomy is recommended. However, if the queen is a valuable breeding animal, it may be possible to remove only the affected cornu and corresponding ovary.

UTERINE PROLAPSE

Complete or partial uterine prolapse usually occurs within 48 hours after parturition of either the multiparous or primiparous queen. In some instances, one uterine horn may be prolapsed while the other is still gravid. The cause is unknown, but most often the condition is seen in queens experiencing prolonged tenesmus accompanying dystocia.

The diagnosis is made by the obvious presence at the vulva of one or two turgid, erythematous, tubular structures that may be encrusted with feces, placental membranes or litter. As the queen continues to strain, she will intermittently turn to lick the prolapsed organ, resulting in further ulceration and hemorrhage. Painful abdominal palpation and progressive signs related to shock will ensue if prompt care is not available.

Treatment. The duration of the prolapse will determine therapy. If the uterus appears viable and the prolapse has occurred within an hour, manual reduction may be attempted. Inhalation anesthesia, including nitrous oxide, is preferable for maximal relaxation. After gentle cleansing with a mild antibacterial wash and rinsing with warm saline solution, a water-soluble lubricant is applied to the uterus. With the queen on her side or in dorsal recumbency, gentle manipulation with a sterile gloved finger may reduce the prolapse. If the uterus is too edematous for replacement, a cold 50 per cent dextrose solution should be applied topically for a short period to reduce swelling.

Once the uterus is replaced within the abdomen, its position may be confirmed by abdominal palpation. With the cat's hind legs elevated, each cornu should be infused with an antibiotic-estrogenic solution (Utonex) delivered via soft flexible plastic or rubber tubing. No vulvar sutures are required, as prolapse is not reported to recur in the cat. Routine follow-up systemic antibiotic therapy is indicated. Most queens may be bred again after 6 months without complication.

If the uterus has been prolapsed for several hours or no longer appears viable, surgical treatment is required. Once a laparotomy has been performed, a combination of internal and external manipulative efforts may be required to replace the uterus, followed by routine ovariohysterectomy.

In severe cases in which the uterus is too edematous to be drawn back into the abdomen at the time of laparotomy, the uterus should be incised on the ventral surface, distal to the cervix, and the freed portion returned to the abdomen for ligation and removal. The remainder of the prolapsed portion may be excised vaginally after ligating the uterine vessels and applying a purse-string suture to the uterine stump. Both ovaries should also be removed before closing the abdomen with 3-0 nongut suture (Dexon, stainless steel wire). Routine supportive care consisting of administration of intravenous fluids, electrolytes and antibiotics should be sufficient to return the queen to her litter and allow nursing within a few hours.

PYOMETRA

Pyometra is a debilitating metestrous uterine disease of the middle-aged or older cat. The exact pathogenesis of pyometra is unknown but apparently is directly related to repeated progestational dysfunction.

Clinical signs are variable in intensity, as pyometra may temporarily be self-limiting for several estrous cycles. To clarify this statement, the cat that is actively cycling will have a brief period of anestrus followed by proestrus during which estrogenic influence on the uterus will again occur. This may result in dilation and relaxation of the uterus and stimulation of myometrial contractions causing evacuation of uterine contents. A pattern of recurring pyometra may produce cyclic signs. That is, during the luteal phase of metestrus when the uterus is filled with purulent exudate, the cat will be typically ill. As the uterus evacuates, the queen's health will improve, although it will not completely return to normal.

Pyometra in the feline rarely produces the dramatic clinical signs that it does in the canine. Partial anorexia, mild polydipsia, depression and occasional vomiting may be the only abnormalities noted by the owner. As the abdomen becomes more distended, the owner may be unaware of gradual generalized weight loss. Even when a vaginal discharge is present, it is often overlooked by the owner because of the cat's fastidious grooming habits. In later stages the cat may appear cachectic, except for an enlarged abdomen, and be uremic, unable to walk and severely dehydrated.

Diagnosis. Abdominal palpation of the enlarged uterus is not painful but must be done with caution to avoid rupturing the organ. Radiography will confirm the presence of a homogeneous fluid density within the greatly distended cornua.

Laboratory data are variable, depending upon the stage of the disease and the degree of depression exhibited by the cat. An absolute neutrophilia is usually present unless the condition is prolonged or recurring, in which case the white blood cell count may be normal or decreased. A normocytic, normochromic anemia exists in 50 per cent of cats with pyometra. As is typical for any debilitating disease, laboratory evaluation of renal and hepatic function should also be made.

Differential Diagnosis. A differential diagnosis should include uterine rupture, uterine torsion, ascites due to hepatic or renal dysfunction or severe malnutrition, peritonitis from rupture of a viscus organ, normal pregnancy, feline infectious peritonitis and diabetes mellitus.

Treatment. Ovariohysterectomy is the treatment of choice in cases of pyometra. Inhalation anesthesia and strict supportive care (administration of intravenous fluids, electrolytes and antibiotics) are required to minimize surgical complications and hasten recovery.

REFERENCES

1. Collins, D. R.: A simple obstetrical technic for assisting with fetal delivery. Vet. Med./Small Anim. Clin., *61*:455, 1966.
2. Dow, C.: Experimental uterine infection in the domestic cat. J. Comp. Path. 72:303, 1962.
3. Stein, B.: The genital system. *In*: Catcott, E. J. (ed.): Feline Medicine and Surgery. 2nd Ed. Santa Barbara, Cal., American Veterinary Publications, 1975.

Infertility and Disease Problems

EMERSON D. COLBY
Dartmouth Medical School,
Hanover, New Hampshire

INFERTILITY

Infertility in the female cat may be related to a wide variety of factors that may range from environmental and behavioral problems to infectious diseases or genetic-related conditions. The diagnosis of a fertility problem should always begin with a complete history and physical examination.

History

Preferably, all of the following should be included:

1. Reproductive problems related to parentage (tom and queen).
2. Condition of the animal as a kitten.
3. Progress of littermates.
4. Vaccination history.
5. Disease - related problems — feline leukemia virus (FELV), feline viral rhinotracheitis (FVR), hemobartonellosis, panleukemia and so forth.
6. Method of housing.
7. Nutrition.

8. Amount of other feline contact, male and female.

9. Medical treatments for previous or current disease conditions.

10. Hormonal therapy or other similar treatment.

11. Surgical procedures.

12. Dates of estrus and length of previous cycles.

13. Abnormal estrous cycle.

14. Previous pregnancies, vaginal discharges.

15. Sexual behavior.

16. Male receptivity.

17. Stress factors — environmental or otherwise.

18. General status of sire (tom).

Physical Examination

The physical examination should include the following items, especially if a reproductive problem is presented:

1. General body condition.

2. Presence or absence of ecto- and endoparasites.

3. Routine hemograms.

4. Blood profiles.

5. Urinalysis.

6. Abdominal radiograph.

7. Vaginal cytological examination.

8. Urogenital examination.

9. Test for infectious diseases — FELV, feline infectious peritonitis (FIP), hemobartonellosis and so forth.

Entering the abdomen to determine the cause of a reproductive disorder is a rare diagnostic procedure in the cat. However, this may be done by laparoscopy[16] or by laparotomy under general anesthesia should the history and general physical condition warrant such examination. At that time biopsies may be taken, if necessary, and the urogenital tract may be thoroughly examined.

Queens show a variety of patterns associated with poor reproductive performance. These may be related to complete lack of estrus in the maturing animal, nonrepetitive estrous periods following an initial cycle, failure to cycle following a difficult parturition and so forth. It is helpful to establish this pattern if at all possible.

Early or late estrous patterns may be related to the age of the animal and the time of the year in which it was born. Some kittens are precocious and show estrus as early as 4 months of age, while the larger breeds may not come into season until they are well over 1 year old. Adequate light, nutrition and contact with actively cycling queens may also influence this reproductive pattern. Mammary gland development may also appear at an early age without signs of estrus. This usually occurs when sexually immature animals have had close association with cycling or nursing queens. Regression of the mammary tissue usually causes no problems, but the presence or development of mammary tissue at a time other than parturition should not be a cause for radical mastectomy without proper diagnosis to determine the presence or absence of neoplastic disease.

Queens have been known to have what might be called a silent heat period that may go unnoticed. This may occur in the young, maturing animal or in the older, proven females. Estrus under these conditions may be detected only by proper handling of the cat or by placing her with a breeding male. Nymphomania may occasionally be observed in female cats and may not be related to cystic follicles on the ovary. Cystic follicles have been noticed in cats that have had kittens delivered by cesarean section but that have had no obvious indication of the presence of the cysts.[4] Cystic follicular endometrial hyperplasia degeneration may also result in a nymphomania-like syndrome. Nymphomania may also be related to behavior or to an improper surgical procedure following which a portion of the ovary is left within the abdomen.

Levels of circulating hormones associated with reproduction in the cat are not yet available, although data are currently being processed by some investigators. Until techniques using small serum plasma volumes to determine the levels of circulating estrogens and progesterones are perfected, there will be many unanswered questions concerning the various reproductive problems of the female cat.

SPECIFIC PROBLEMS IN THE FEMALE CAT

Cystic Endometrial Hyperplasia-Pyometra Complex

The cystic endometrial hyperplasia complex is not uncommon in the cat and is often associated with pyometra or pyometritis. Either of the conditions may be the cause for lack of estrus and subsequent pregnancy. This may be difficult to confirm diagnostically unless abdominal entry is allowed. Cystic endometrial hyperplasia (CEH) may be the result of a natural but improper estrous cycle. It may also be caused by the use of exogenous hormones used to induce estrus and has been associated with the use of progestational hormones. Whatever the cause, the only successful treatment is ovariohysterectomy. The condition may be observed in queens of all ages, although it is perhaps more common in proven females having had one or more litters. The cysts are variable in size and usually fill both uterine horns. The fluid, if uncontaminated, is clear and gives the appearance of small fluid-filled sacs attached to the uterine mucosa (Fig. 1). Pyometra, subsequent to CEH, may be related to the state of the animal with relation to circulating levels of estrogen. This would allow for some dilation of the cervix, with the pyometra being of an ascending type.

Pyometra, either alone or as a sequela to CEH, is most commonly caused by *Escherichia coli*,[9] although staphylococci and streptococci are also found. Pyometra caused by other bacteria is not common but may occur. A low-grade pyometra (if one can be allowed to define the condition in those terms) may occasionally be noted at laparotomy or autopsy. Such a condition is difficult to diagnose and may take the combined efforts of laboratory analysis and radiography to be proved. There may be no visible evidence of the pyometra if the cervix is closed, thus preventing passage of the telltale fluid.

Therefore, the quantity of fluid may be extremely small. There are reports of flushing the uterus in these cases using an estrogen solution or an antibiotic-estrogenic solution (Utonex) with successful subsequent pregnancy. However, pyometra is not an uncommon sequela to the pregnancy. It has been shown that bacterial growth may be limited under conditions in which circulating estrogen levels are high.[5] Any progestogen therapy would certainly be contraindicated.

Fulminating pyometra, which may be defined in the traditional terms of acute, subacute and chronic, requires considerable attention and is probably best treated if possible, by ovariohysterectomy. The cervix is usually open, and although it may be successfully flushed, considerable danger is involved because of the condition of the uterine wall. In some cases the wall may be paper-thin, resulting in rupture when under the pressure of attempted flushing. Since return to successful reproductive activity is questionable, removal of the tract by surgical means is indicated.

The CEH-pyometra complex has also been initiated by the indiscriminate use of hormones to bring the cat into estrus or to keep it out of estrus. Because the sexual activity of the cat has not yet been correlated with known facts about the circulating hormone levels, as determined by radioimmunoassay or other means, it would be unwise to use hormone preparations to control the estrous cycle of the cat in this manner. Similarly, preparations used for other species and for other conditions and those not approved for

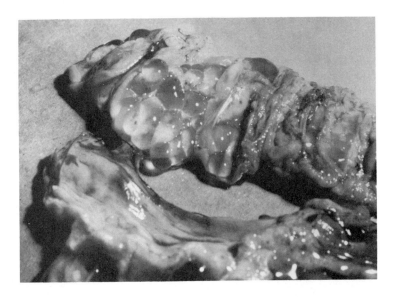

Figure 1. Cystic endometrial hyperplasia — CEH.

use in the cat in the United States may invite unwarranted reproductive problems.

Pseudopregnancy

Pseudopregnancy in its true form may be induced in the cat by sham mating with a sterile male, by inserting a glass rod into the vagina and stimulating the cervix, by the making of a vaginal smear or even by handling the cat roughly in the perineal area during the height of the estrous period. Although pseudopregnancy in the cat is rather well defined and lasts approximately 40 to 45 days, induction of the condition to eliminate estrus in the queen is not recommended. This is because of the possibility of inducing the CEH-pyometra complex and its complications, which would not necessarily become evident until near the end of the pseudopregnancy period.

Non-infectious and Infectious Problems

A number of causes of abortion, both infectious and noninfectious, may be related to complications of pregnancy.[11] Noninfectious causes may be poor nutrition, trauma, abnormalities of the genital tract of the queen, fetal abnormalities, endocrine disturbances and behavioral problems. Any of these may result in abortion or resorption. If it can be established that repeated abortions are occurring approximately at the same time in each case, the abortions may be due to either premature regression of the corpora lutea or their improper development. In such cases repositol progesterone may be given intramuscularly at doses of 0.5 to 1.0 mg/lb of body weight beginning 7 to 10 days prior to the expected time of abortion and discontinued 7 to 10 days prior to the expected time of parturition.[15] It is important to know the date of the last breeding in these cases. Excessive use of progesterone may result in masculinization of any female kittens.

The etiology of prolonged estrous periods is not currently known. One might suspect excessive follicular activity, cystic follicles or treatment with hormones having estrogenic potential. Mating in such cases does not always shorten the estrous activity. Exploratory surgery to determine the cause may not provide the answer but may eliminate the estrous activity, for reasons not yet determined. If surgery is performed on the estrous cat, barbiturate anesthesia is contraindicated, as it is known to block ovulation in the cat.[13]

Vaginitis

Vaginitis can be a cause of infertility as well as a cause for refusing to accept the male during a given estrous period. Vaginitis has been noted in conjunction with coital injury and excessive mating and has occurred secondary to uterine problems such as pyometra that is due to a definable bacterial entity. Excessive licking by the female may be the first sign of a problem if no secretions are noted. If secretions are present, they may be serous or mucoid, and bacterial cultures are indicated. Queens that have prolonged heat periods and breed frequently should be checked for signs of vaginitis. Flushing with antibiotic or warm sterile saline solutions to control infections, concomitant with parenteral therapy, is indicated. Breeding should be stopped.

Treatment

Treatment of pregnant cats with biological products should be handled with great care. Depending upon the stage of pregnancy of the queen, abortion, mummification, stillborns and other anomalies may be noted. It is not specifically known which products in particular are hazardous to the health of the fetus, other than those already reported. The most significant of these may be griseofulvin, which causes multiple teratogenic effects in the kitten. It is unwise to vaccinate pregnant queens, as viruses have predilections for the most rapidly growing tissues and thus may result in fetal anomalies that may not be apparent until the kitten is several days or several weeks old.

Disorders of the Mammary Glands

Mammary gland problems are occasionally reported. These may be related to lactation failure that has been successfully corrected by the administration of progesterone (1 mg/lb of body weight),[14] lactational tetany that has been treated with calcium (Calphosan), 5 ml given intravenously and/or subcutaneously,[1] and benign mammary hypertrophy[12] that may regress without treatment and that should be treated conservatively before a radical mastectomy is performed.

Feline Viral Rhinotracheitis

Feline viral rhinotracheitis (FVR) may cause fetal mummification in the very young fetus and stillborns or abortions if present during the late stages of gestation. It is commonplace to note abortions of some viable and some stillborn fetuses in cats that exhibit symptoms of the respiratory disease complex. Pregnant cats that are presented with this disease complex should be treated symptomatically with regard for the fetus. Human care, good housing and adequate nutrition are essential for the survival of the fetus. This author has had a modicum of success preserving pregnancy in cats exhibiting FVR by the use of methylprednisolone acetate (Depo-Medrol) and antibiotic therapy.

Panleukopenia

Panleukopenia is known to cause abortions, stillborns and early neonatal deaths and has the added problem of having a teratogenic effect, resulting in cerebellar hypoplasia.[10, 13] The virus attacks the central nervous system of the fetus during late gestation and also attacks the neonatal kitten. Death may not ensue, but the virus will result in ataxia and often in a woodpecker-type eating syndrome as the animal matures. There is no treatment. Vaccination during pregnancy is not recommended.

Feline Leukemia Virus

Feline leukemia virus (FELV) has been associated with fetal resorption, abortion and, in particular, infertility. Queens having a history of infertility with no estrous cycling should be checked for the presence of this virus. It is not recommended that antibody-positive animals be bred, as the reproductive problems may continue should the animals be induced to cycle. FELV has been associated with the fading kitten syndrome in which the kittens exhibit thymic atrophy and thus may be immunologically incompetent.[8]

Toxoplasmosis

Active toxoplasmosis infections[6] may cause abortions, but it is not known whether this is a primary or secondary complication. Toxoplasmosis has not yet been proved to pass the placenta in the cat, and indeed the kitten may receive the parasite immediately after parturition or through the milk.

Breeding Failures

There may be many causes of mating failure. Some of the more common are mating before the queen is in full estrus, use of an untrained or novice male, attempting to mate a queen with a male that she will not accept, short-bodied males used to cover long-bodied females and vice versa, timid queens and so forth. A common mistake made by many breeders is failure to observe the act of coitus by leaving the male and female together for a period of hours or days. Unless vaginal smears are made and observed for semen, mating cannot be proved under these circumstances.

Congenital Problems

There are a wide variety of congenital malformations that have appeared in the literature. Many of the kittens are born with normal littermates, and the history of the queen is either incomplete or insignificant. In cases in which it is known that the queen received no medication during pregnancy, the cause of the fetal anomaly is left entirely to conjecture. However, one should always attempt to obtain a complete history in order to prevent such births if these can be determined to be drug-related.

THE MALE CALICO CAT

In order to have both black and orange in the coat color, a cat must have two X chromosomes. Thus, the normal male with a sex chromosome constitution of XY in all cells cannot have both black and orange in the coat color. Conversely, if a male does have both black and orange in the coat, he must have two differerent X chromosomes occurring in the body. This can happen in one of several ways. Frequently the orange and black coat is associated with an XXY cell line and sterility of the individual. This is not always true, however, and male cats with black and orange coats may be fertile. Thus, black and orange coloration simply denotes the presence of an abnormality in the sex chromosome constitution or the occurrence, which is always abnormal, of combinations of two or more normal cell lines providing two or more different X chromosomes to that individual. There is no way to determine from the coat color what the chromosome constitution is or whether the individual is sterile or fertile. Extensive chromosome studies are required to delineate the mechanism by which the unusual orange and black coloration has occurred. This subject has been amply discussed by Centerwall and Benirschke[2, 3] and studied by Wurster-Hill.[17]

REFERENCES

1. Cartwright, C.: Lactational tetany in cats. Panel Report. Mod. Vet. Pract., September, 1973, p. 95.
2. Centerwall, W. R. and Benirschke, K.: An animal model for the XXY Klinefelter's syndrome in man: Tortoiseshell and calico male cats. Am. J. Vet. Res., *36*:1275, 1975.
3. Centerwall, W. R. and Benirschke, K.: Male tortoiseshell and calico (T-C) cats. Animal models of sex chromosome mosaics, aneuploids, polyploids, and chimerics. J. Hered., *64*:272, 1973.
4. Colby, E. D.: Personal observations.
5. Dow, C.: Experimental uterine infection in the domestic cat. J. Comp. Path., *72*:303, 1962.
6. Dubey, J. P.: Toxoplasmosis. Pract. Vet., Winter, 1978, pp. 10–14.
7. Foster, M. A. and Hisaw, F. L.: Experimental ovulation and resulting pseudopregnancy in anestrous cats. Anat. Rec., *62*:75, 1935.
8. Herron, M. A.: Feline reproduction. Vet. Clin. North Am., 7:715, 1977.
9. Joshua, J. O.: Some conditions seen in feline practice attributable to hormonal causes. Vet. Rec., *88*:511, 1971.
10. Kilham, L., Margolis, G. and Colby, E. D.: Cerebellar ataxia and its congenital transmission in cats by feline panleukopenia virus. J.A.V.M.A., *158*:888, 1971.
11. Leni, D.: Proceedings of the Feline Health Symposium. New York State College of Veterinary Medicine, June 5, 1976.
12. Mandel, M.: Benign mammary hypertrophy. Vet. Med./Small Anim. Clin., *70*:846, 1975.
13. Margolis, G., Kilham, L. and Davenport, J.: A model for virus induced reproductive failure: Theory, observations and speculation. *In* Benirschke, K. (ed.): Comparative Aspects of Reproductive Failure. New York, Springer-Verlag New York Inc., 1966, pp. 350–360.
14. Mosier, J. E.: Common medical and behavioral problems in cats. Mod. Vet. Pract., October, 1975, pp. 699–702.
15. Stein, B. S. The genital system. *In* Catcott, E. J. (ed.): Feline Medicine and Surgery. 2nd Ed. Santa Barbara, Cal., American Veterinary Publications, 1975, pp. 303–354.
16. Wildt, D. E., Kinney, G. M. and Seager, S. W. J.: Gonadotropin induced reproduction cyclicity in the domestic cat. J. Lab. Anim. Sci., *28*:301, 1978.
17. Wurster-Hill, D. H.: Personal communication.

OVINE

Consulting Editors

E. D. FIELDEN
and
A. N. BRUERE

876

Selection for Reproductive Performance and Hereditary Aspects of Sheep Reproduction

A. L. RAE

Massey University, Palmerston North, New Zealand

INTRODUCTION

Improvement in the reproductive performance of the ewe is a major requirement in a wide variety of sheep enterprises. Except under harsh environmental conditions in which multiple births may lead to high lamb mortality or place the life of the ewe at risk, increased litter size will contribute substantially to the efficiency and profitability of sheep production. Indeed, the continuing existence of sheep farming in many countries is now dependent on producing sheep with a substantially increased reproductive rate.

A higher reproductive rate also is important because it results in a larger number of young sheep being available for selection and thus leads to accelerated genetic gain in other productive traits.

MEASUREMENT OF REPRODUCTIVE PERFORMANCE IN THE EWE

Reproductive performance may be measured in many ways. Because emphasis is on selection for reproductive performance, the measures used have to be made on the individual ewe under near-normal conditions of flock management. For this purpose, the usual measure is reproduction rate, which is defined as the number of lambs weaned per ewe per year. It is a function of fertility (whether or not the ewe lambs, fecundity (the number of lambs per pregnancy) and survival (the ability of the lamb to survive to weaning). Reproductive rate is thus a complex trait, its variation resulting from effects contributed by the ewe, the ram and the lamb and the interactions among them.

GENETIC AND PHENOTYPIC PARAMETERS OF REPRODUCTION RATE IN THE EWE

In Table 1, the range of estimates for the repeatability and heritability of reproduction rate and its components, fertility, fecundity and survival, is summarized.

It is concluded that: (1) both heritability and repeatability are generally low for all traits, although there is some evidence that heritability of the number of lambs born at the second lambing in Merinos is distinctly higher than at the first lambing; (2) the number of lambs born per ewe has a slightly higher heritability than the number of lambs weaned per ewe and (3) fecundity has, in most cases, higher repeatability and heritability than fertility, i.e., selection for lambs born is likely to be more effective than selection *against* barrenness.

The limited information available on genetic correlations between reproduction rate and other traits indicates a positive relationship to yearling body weight and probably a near zero relationship to fleece weight.

The reproduction rate and all its components are markedly influenced by the age of the ewe and by differences in environmental conditions from year to year. It is desirable that these nongenetic factors should be eliminated when making comparisons for selection purposes between the performances of different sheep within the flock. This is achieved by expressing each ewe's annual record as a deviation from the average re-

TABLE 1. *Range of Estimates of Genetic Parameters for Reproduction Rate and Its Components*

Trait	Repeatability	Heritability
Lambs weaned per ewe	0.03–0.25	0.03–0.22
Lambs born per ewe	0.05–0.30	0.03–0.35
Fertility	0.08–0.18	0.03–0.12
Fecundity	0.04–0.30	0.04–0.26
Survival	0.03–0.15	0.02–0.10

production rate of her contemporaries (i.e., the ewes in the flock of the same age and in the same year). Thus, if a ewe in her 3-year-old lambing weans two lambs and all 3-year-old ewes in the flock in the same year averaged 1.3 lambs weaned, her record would be $(2-1.3) = +0.7$ lamb.

DIRECT SELECTION FOR REPRODUCTION RATE

In selecting for improved reproductive performance, it is necessary to assess the breeding value of the young ewes and rams for reproduction rate in order to choose those that will enter the flock. In this context, the breeding value of an individual is an estimate of the average reproduction rate of the daughters of that individual. Since reproduction rate can be measured only in the ewe, the records for predicting the breeding value of the young rams and ewes (if they have not yet had a lambing) must come from female relatives such as the dam, grandams, half-sisters and daughters.

Records of the Dam

The dams of the young rams and ewes born in a particular year will differ in age, in the years over which they have had lambing records and in the number of such records. The first two effects are eliminated, as shown earlier, by expressing each record as a deviation from the average performance of the contemporaries. These deviations are then averaged. The breeding value of the son or daughter is thus predicted:

$$BV = \frac{\frac{1}{2} kh^2}{1 + (k-1)t} \text{ (average deviation)}$$

In this equation, h^2 is the heritability, t is the repeatability of reproduction rate and k is the number of records included in the average deviation. The breeding value (BV) is expressed in terms of the number of lambs born or weaned (as the case may be). Its mean over the flock is expected to be zero.

Records of the Grandams

The records of the paternal grandam are easily included in the prediction of breeding value along with those of the dam, the coefficient in the prediction being one-half that just given for the dam. Use of the records of

the maternal grandam is more complicated because some of the information that these supply is already contributed by those of the dam.

Records of Half-Sisters

Some of the young rams will have half-sisters that have had lambing records in the flock. The prediction of breeding value from this source is:

$$BV = \frac{\frac{1}{4} nh^2}{1 + (n-1)\frac{1}{4}h^2} \text{ (half sister's average deviation)}$$

Here, n is the number of half-sisters in the average deviation. This information will usually be added to the estimate of breeding value obtained from the dam's records to give a useful increase in the accuracy of prediction.

Records of Daughters

With a sex-limited trait of low heritability, one would expect the average records of the daughters of a sire to be a valuable estimator of his breeding value. The progeny test is certainly the most accurate assessment of the breeding value of a ram. However, it substantially increases the generation interval on the sire side (in most cases from about 2½ to about 4½ to 5½ years) because of the time required to get the daughters' records. Thus, progeny testing is likely to be worthwhile only when progeny-tested rams can be used widely by artificial insemination.

Relative Accuracy of the Various Methods

The accuracy of the various methods of selection can be compared by using the correlation between the records used and the true breeding value. Using a heritability of 0.10 and a repeatability of 0.15, the following correlations are found:

One record of dam	0.16
Average of three records of dam	0.24
Average of four records of dam	0.26
Average of five records of dam	0.28
Average of three records of dam plus average of three records of paternal grandam	0.27
Average of three records of dam plus average of three records of maternal grandam	0.26

Average of three records of dam
plus average of 20 half-sisters   0.38

With the possible exception of the last method, the generation interval is unaffected.

INDIRECT SELECTION

Because improvement of reproduction rate by direct selection is often slow and because it is costly and sometimes difficult to measure, the study of more easily measured traits that are related to reproduction are of interest.

Although there is evidence of a phenotypic correlation between face cover and reproduction rate, the genetic correlation is small and of little value for indirect selection. The same is true of the degree of skin fold in Australian Merino sheep. The genetic correlation between yearling body weight and reproduction rate is being used in combination with the lambing records of the dam in New Zealand, but the genetic relationship appears to vary from breed to breed and needs more investigation.

Several promising possibilities are being investigated at present. They are: (1) determining the ovulation rate by endoscopy, (2) measuring the number of estrous cycles before the first mating, (3) measuring luteinizing hormone and follicle-stimulating hormone levels and (4) assessing testis growth.

CONCLUSION

When records of the lambing performance of the dam are available and all selection is devoted to reproduction rate, selection experiments have shown rates of gain in the number of lambs born per ewe to be of the order of 0.01 to 0.02 per year. Thus, heritability and the size of the selection differentials that can be achieved are sufficiently large to allow a useful selection response.

Under conditions of extensive husbandry in which no records of relatives are kept, choosing twin-born rams and ewes is a possible approach to selecting for reproductive rate. This is equal in accuracy to the use of one record of the dam.

Usually, the objectives in improvement of a breed will include other traits in addition to reproduction rate. In these circumstances, selection index procedures to give suitable weighting to the traits included in the objective will commonly be used.

REFERENCES

1. Bradford, G. E.: Genetic control of litter size in sheep. J. Reprod. Fertil. (Suppl.), *15*:23, 1972.
2. Land, R. B.: Physiological studies and genetic selection for sheep fertility. Anim. Breed. Abstr., *42*:155, 1974.
3. Rae, A. L.: National sheep breeding programmes — New Zealand. Proceedings 1976 International Congress on Sheep Breeding. Perth, Western Australian Inst. Technology, 1976, pp. 33–39.
4. Turner, H. N.: Genetic improvement of reproduction rate in sheep. Anim. Breed. Abstr., *27*:545, 1969.

Mating Management and Health Programs

A. NEIL BRUERE

Massey University, Palmerston North, New Zealand

Sheep are to be found in the most diverse climates. They are husbanded at latitudes relatively near to the North and South Poles, where the breeding season is short and only the hardy breeds survive, and in semi-desert areas where the breeding season is longer but survival is also difficult during prolonged drought periods. In some countries, housing and hand feeding are practiced; while in others, greatly improved pastures, which are available to sheep the year round, have produced animals of exceptionally high productivity.

It is difficult, therefore, to give a precise account of management for so diverse a geographical range to which a wide variety of breeds have been adapted. However, it is possible to give a general picture of sheep management, some of which will apply to one area more than to another. The annual pattern of sheep husbandry is shown in Table 1. The seasons are referred to in a general way, and the approximate months of

TABLE 1. *Calendar of Sheep Farm Events*

Season	Northern Hemisphere	Southern Hemisphere	Operation
Midsummer	June July August	November December January	Ewe and ram shearing Weaning Ewes on lower plane of feed Attend to foot conditions (foot rot)

Late summer	August
	
	September
		March
		
		April
			Dipping
			Flushing
			Ring crutch prior to mating
			Chlamydial vaccination
			  (enzootic abortion)
			Drenching—dose selenium;
			  sensitizing clostridial vaccinations
			Mating (tupping)

Autumn or fall	September October November	April April–May May	Reduce feed (mob stocking) Begin winter feeding Dose iodine (if endemic goiter area) or feed brassicas
Winter	November February	June July	Dose selenium, copper, iodine Vaccinate booster clostridial vaccines
Spring	March April May	August September October	Crutch, prelamb shearing Lambing, early lambing ewes segregated Docking (tailing, castration, ear marking) Vaccinate lambs if necessary for clostridial diseases, scabby mouth Where endemic—blue tongue Drench lambs (*Nematodirus*) Louping ill vaccination (ovine encephalomyelitis)

the year are given for the Southern and Northern hemispheres, respectively. Obviously the nearer one goes to the equator the less demarcated are the seasons, the longer the possible breeding season and the less it may be necessary to provide special feeding conditions.

Some countries have diseases that do not occur in others, so that any references to vaccinations and medication are to cover what may be considered the major international aspects of sheep health. This includes the prevention of trace element diseases, clostridial diseases, principal viral diseases, foot diseases, and endo- and ectoparasitism.

Ewes are usually shorn prior to or soon after weaning, and the plane of feeding is reduced to cause a rapid cessation of lactation and also to prevent the animals from becoming too heavy before the mating season. As the breeding season approaches, the feed supply is increased slightly to "flush" the ewes by increasing the body weight and the ovulation rate. Ewes are now selected for their mating flocks and are mated on a flock basis with from 2 to 3 per cent of rams, or less under some circumstances. However, in the case of pedigree animals, ewes are mated in smaller groups to individually selected rams.

It is now common practice in some countries to use vasectomized (teaser) rams to stimulate overt estrus. In addition, mating rams are frequently harnessed with tupping crayons that identify individual ewes as they are served by the ram.

The crayon color is usually changed every 14 to 15 days, just short of the average estrous period. Rams are usually mated to the ewes for four breeding cycles, and frequently in the case of wool breeds or dual-purpose breeds of sheep, a down ram is used for the final cycle so that late lambing ewes can be culled from the flock. In addition, the progeny of such ewes are slaughtered and are not kept for breeding.

Prior to mating, sensitizing vaccinations against enterotoxemia and tetanus should be given. This is indicated for ewes that have not previously been vaccinated and when a long passive immunity is intended for the lambs. Also at this stage, trace elements such as selenium should be given to the ewe, and pretupping drenching, as prac-

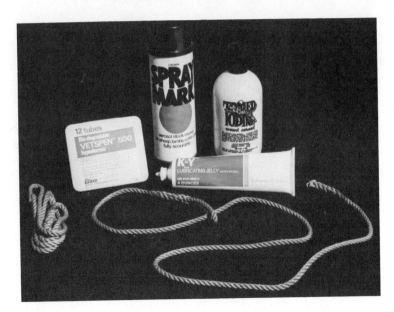

Figure 1. Lambing kit containing obstetrical jelly, antibiotics, nylon lambing cords, identification sprays and antiseptic.

ticed in some countries, should be carried out. Dipping and spraying for ectoparasites is usually undertaken before mating. In many countries this is compulsory.

Management during pregnancy is aimed at providing a lower plane of nutrition during the second and third months, followed by a steady increase for the final 2 months (see following article). In the last month of pregnancy, ewes may be given annual booster vaccinations against tetanus and enterotoxemia. Other clostridial diseases, namely black leg and malignant edema, should be covered at this period. Final doses of selenium and iodine should also be given to ewes within the last 2 months of pregnancy in areas where deficiency occurs (see following article and Perinatal Lamb Mortality, page 918).

Before lambing, ewes are either crutched or prelamb shorn and sorted into early and late lambing flocks from either crayon color marks from tupping or from udder development. In some countries, lambing ewes are carefully shepherded either in small flocks or in enclosures where they are hand fed. Under these conditions, considerable attention is given to individual ewes and all dystocia cases are treated. Alternatively, in many sheep areas where labor costs are high, "easy-care" sheep are being developed. Under the easy-care system, the labor input is reduced and lambing supervision is minimal. Easy-care sheep must have a reduced incidence of dystocia and are also selected for good mothering ability. They must be well exercised and their diet carefully regulated during late pregnancy to reduce the incidence of fetal dystocia.

When intensive and assisted lambing is carried out, lambing kits (Fig. 1) containing obstetrical jelly, antibiotics, nylon lambing cords, identification sprays and antiseptic are invaluable.

Tailing and castration of lambs (docking) usually takes place at 2 to 3 weeks of age, and in most areas lambs are weaned between 10 and 14 weeks of age. In some countries, creep feeding is practiced before weaning and early weaning is carried out.

Feeding Sheep for High Reproductive Performance

W. J. PRYOR

Massey University, Palmerston North, New Zealand

PLANNING FOR GOOD NUTRITION AND REPRODUCTION

Providing proper management and nutrition of sheep for maximum reproduction is important. Nutrition affects the speed with which either the lamb or the hogget can reach the so-called critical reproductive weight for its breed. This will determine whether it can be mated before 1 year of age (hogget), as a two-tooth (about 18 months), as occurs in New Zealand, Europe and some other countries, or whether it must wait before being mated at an older age, as is necessary in more arid environments.

Further, the nutrition of the ewe itself is a vital factor for immediate reproductive performance and, to some extent, reproductive performance of the progeny, as nutrition affects birth weight and survival.

Climatic conditions will determine whether there is sufficient good pasture or browse available during the normal period of pregnancy for the particular breeds of sheep of the area concerned. In arid countries, the odds of inadequate range or pasture growth due to poor rainfall can be sufficiently low to justify regular planning of supplementary sources of feed. Likewise, the expected feed deficiencies of winter can be similarly gauged. In these situations, supplementary feed may be provided by saved pasture or conserved roughage and/or concentrates. In extreme cases such as persistent drought, complete hand-feeding may be necessary.

In these situations the amount of feed to see the ewe through pregnancy and lactation can be calculated and should be held as a reserve. In Australia the cost of hand feeding may not justify its use; thus, sheep are not hand fed and numbers may die.

Pregnant ewes can consume a wide variety of supplementary feeds, although they need gradual introduction to high-grain diets. Wheat feeding alone has given disappointing results and cannot be recommended as a total diet, notwithstanding the fact that in some countries wheat is the cheapest form of energy for animal feeding during drought years.

Ewes that are unaccustomed to supplements will not automatically accept them, and it may take a period of many weeks before adequate intake occurs. A number of methods can be used to train ewes to take supplements, including: (1) confinement of the sheep and feeding in small areas; (2) use of coachers, usually sheep that have been fed supplements previously and (3) use of highly palatable feed, e.g., alfalfa (lucerne) on top of other feeds. Because of higher present-day labor costs, there is a trend toward "easy-care" sheep, which may modify any feeding program for ewes.

USE OF CONDITION SCORING

Obviously the condition of the ewe reflects its past and present nutrition. However, the appearance of unshorn sheep can be misleading. To overcome this, the use of condition scoring can be used in planning ewe management and nutrition. Condition scoring is done in sheep by palpating the vertical and lumbar spines and associated structures of the vertebral column. By this simple method the amount of fat covering this region can be estimated and scores ranging from 1 (poor) to 5 (very fat) allocated.

A system used in Australia and New Zealand is as follows:

Grade 1. The spinous and transverse processes are sharp, the fingers pass under the transverse processes and it is possible to feel between the processes.

Grade 2. The processes are smooth and rounded. The fingers can be passed under the transverse processes with pressure.

Grade 3. The spinous processes are smooth and rounded and have only a small elevation. Individual bones can be felt only by applying pressure. Firm pressure is needed to feel over the ends of the transverse processes.

Grade 4. Spinous processes can be detected only by firm pressure. The ends of transverse processes cannot be felt.

Grade 5. The spinous processes cannot be detected, nor can the transverse processes. The eye muscles (iliopsoas and psoas minor) are very full and fat.

In general it is desirable that ewes be fed to attain a score of 4 at mating. They must not be grossly overfat, as may be the case with a condition score of 5.

NUTRITION OF THE EWE

Effect of Nutrition on Lamb Productivity

The effects of nutrition on wool growth are many and varied. Restricted feed intake during pregnancy reduces the total number of both primary and secondary follicles in the lamb's skin. These numbers are determined before birth. Although the number of fibers cannot be altered after birth, postnatal nutrition can affect adult wool weight by making the wool fibers longer and thicker. Thus, adult wool production may be only very slightly depressed by nutritional effects during fetal life.

The birth weight of lambs is influenced by ewe nutrition. Generally speaking, the growth rate of lambs is favorably affected by the initial birth weight, i.e., lambs of greater birth weight gain their critical weight earlier. Thus, good prenatal and postnatal nutrition of the ewe will increase the likelihood of a successful two-tooth mating of its progeny.

Effect of Nutrition on Subsequent Reproduction

This is not too important when annual mating only is carried out, as any untoward effects of poor nutrition at this time can be overcome by improved feeding nearer to the next mating.

Nutrition and Ovulation Rate

Both the plane of nutrition and the body condition of the ewe have a major effect on the number of ova shed. The practice of providing improved nutrition at mating time, known as flushing, should be carried out, although it is probable that the attainment of good ewe body weight is more important than an actual rise in the plane of nutrition during mating. Experience in New Zealand indicates that the grazing of alfalfa (lucerne) in high-fertility flocks may reduce the lambing percentage, so that it is recommended that ewes be transferred to alternative pasture, if available, during the flushing and mating period. The present belief is that an estrogen-like compound is involved in this depression of fertility.

Nutrition in Early Pregnancy

It is probably wise to try and keep the body weight of ewes at the mating level for the first month of pregnancy, after which some body weight loss can occur without affecting the subsequent lambing percentage. A 5 per cent weight loss (which corresponds to a 15 per cent reduction in energy needs) for from 1 to 3 months of gestation is quite acceptable, attained by either providing poorer pastures or supplements or higher stocking rates. This additionally helps to reduce the likelihood of overfat ewes carrying multiple fetuses during late pregnancy and the development of pregnancy toxemia.

Nutrition in Late Pregnancy

Because 70 per cent of weight and 80 per cent of energy and protein deposition of the fetus and its membranes occur in the last 2 months of pregnancy, nutrition must be good. It is likely that when multiple births are imminent, depression of the ewe's abdominal space occurs, making it difficult to meet dietary needs by medium- or low-quality roughage sources alone. A higher energy feed is therefore required. Increased energy is needed both to insure proper growth and wool follicle development of the fetuses and to avoid the negative energy balance that, in the case of fat ewes with multiple births, can lead to pregnancy toxemia (see page 903). There is frequently no need to consider protein requirements when green pasture is available (see Table 1). However, in late pregnancy higher crude protein diet levels, up to 14 per cent, will increase nitrogen retention and therefore, particularly with complete hand feeding, extra protein should be supplied.

Mineral Considerations

If the diet contains legume, either as hay or in pasture, in practice there is rarely a need to provide any calcium supplements. Supplemental phosphorus will rarely need to be provided to pregnant ewes either, unless levels in the feed are much lower than usual.

An insufficient level of copper in the ewe's diet that is due to a simple deficiency or to a high molybdenum and/or sulfate level can lead to enzootic ataxia (swayback) in lambs. In such situations copper may be given to the ewe in an injectable form, e.g., 50 mg of copper-calcium edetate subcutaneously at about midpregnancy, but in some countries this is not widely recommended because of the risk of copper toxicity. On a long-term basis, copper sulfate can be added to fertilizer and the land topdressed at a rate of 5.7 to 11.25 kg of copper sulfate/hectare. Copper supplementation needs to be undertaken with care, as sheep are very susceptible to copper toxicity. In areas where white muscle disease in lambs may occur, the ewe should be provided with 5 mg of sodium selenate either

by injection or orally just prior to mating and again about 1 to 2 months before parturition. This prevents early embryonic loss and congenital white muscle disease in endemically selenium-deficient areas.

In some parts of the world where goiter is endemic, it is necessary to provide iodine to the pregnant ewe in the third or fourth month of gestation. This is best done by oral dosing of individual ewes with 250 mg of potassium iodide.

Nutrition and Lactation

Lactation places the highest energy requirements on ewes, particularly if there are multiple births. Nutrition should be at its best at this time to insure maximum milk production. Milk production is affected to some extent also by preparturient nutrition.

If feed supplies are a serious problem at this stage, consideration should be given to early weaning of the lambs, since it is possible to save 30 per cent of total ewe and lamb energy requirements by doing this, although labor needs are increased.

TABLE 1. *Daily Nutrient Requirements and Rations of Sheep in Moderate Condition*

Body Weight (kg)	Metabolizable Energy (Mcal)	Crude Protein (%)	Suitable Ration
EWES:			
Maintenance			
50	2.0	8.9	1.0 kg of ration A*
70	2.4	8.9	1.2 kg of ration A
Early gestation			
50	2.2	9.0	1.1 kg of ration A
70	2.8	9.0	1.4 kg of ration A
Late gestation			
50	3.6	9.3	1.7 kg of ration A
70	4.4	9.3	2.1 kg of ration A
Early lactation (singles)			
50	4.9	10.4	2.1 kg of ration B†
70	5.9	10.4	2.5 kg of ration B
Early lactation (twins)			
50	5.6	11.5	2.4 kg of ration B
70	6.6	11.5	2.8 kg of ration B
Replacement lambs and yearlings			
30	2.9	10.0	1.2 kg of ration B
50	3.0	8.9	1.5 kg of ration A
RAMS:			
100	5.6	8.9	2.8 kg of ration A

*Ration A—67 per cent good meadow hay, 33 per cent barley grain or 12 per cent higher intake of meadow hay only.

†Ration B—45 per cent good meadow hay, 55 per cent corn (maize).

SPECIFIC NUTRIENT NEEDS OF BREEDING SHEEP

Various international authorities publish nutritional needs for sheep. Table 1 provides recommended intakes expressed in metabolizable energy (ME) units, plus crude protein. The table is slightly modified from the National Research Council report.[2] ME units are also used by the Agricultural Research Council of the United Kingdom.[1] It should be clearly understood that such tables serve as a good guide only and can be modified by a number of factors, including previous nutrition, bodily condition, breed of sheep and climate.

These levels should be increased when sheep are in poor condition or are being maintained in very cold conditions. They should be reduced for overfat sheep.

Requirements for sheep other than the weights listed can be reasonably well estimated by taking values proportionate to the animals' weight, e.g., for each 60 kg of body weight take the mean value for 50 and 70 kg.

Protein needs are generally met quite easily by pasture or supplements, although in total hand feeding during late pregnancy or lactation, the listed protein requirements as shown in Table 1 should be supplied.

Examples of two suitable, practical rations are shown in Table 1, but other feedstuffs can replace the ones suggested, so long as this is done on an energy basis and adequate protein and minerals are also supplied. Note particularly that in late pregnancy and lactation, roughage sources alone are often inadequate as the sole diet.

Table 2 gives the ME and protein values of some feeds that can be used.

Table 3 attempts to show what percentage of nutrient needs ought to be given as a supplement, as pasture conditions vary. This can be a rough guide only.

NUTRITION OF THE RAM

The first sperm can be collected at about 5 to 6 months of age, and normal fertility is established at about 7½ to 9 months of age, depending on breed. However, the onset of puberty, which varies with breed, is delayed by undernutrition.

In the ram, testis size, which is highly correlated with spermatogenic activity, responds to nutrition. It is known that sperm production can be increased by a male flushing. This is especially important both under natural mating conditions and when semen is to be collected for artificial insemination programs. The flushing of rams is best done by providing a high-protein supplement for about 8 weeks before mating starts. This can be done either by grazing rams on good pasture during this period or by providing up to about 2.5 kg of good alfalfa (lucerne) hay per day or about two-thirds this quantity of good quality sheep nuts. It has been shown that fertility of rams has been seriously reduced when they have been without green feed for approximately 6 months. When a vitamin A supplement is required for rams, 1 million IU should be injected about 7 weeks before mating, at commencement of mating and 6 to 8 weeks later on if the mating period is still continued.

TABLE 2. *Nutrient Content of Some Sheep Feedstuffs*

Feedstuffs	Metabolizable Energy (Mcal/kg)	Crude Protein (%)
Pasture:		
Leafy pasture	0.4–0.5	2–4
Hays and straws:		
Alfalfa (lucerne)		
Hay	1.5–1.9	11–16
Meadow hay	1.4–1.8	6–12
Oat or barley straw	1.4	4
Wheat straw	1.1	1
Silage:		
Maize silage	0.7	2.4
Pasture silage	0.4	2.8
Roots and crops:		
Turnips	0.3	1.2
Chou moellier	0.4	1.8
Grains:		
Barley	2.7	10
Corn (maize)	2.8	9
Oats	2.4	10
Protein concentrates:		
Linseed meal	2.5	36
Soybean meal	2.6	42

TABLE 3. *Percentage of Ration Required as Supplement for Varying Pasture Conditions*

Period	Pasture Condition			
	GOOD	FAIR	POOR	NIL
Late pregnancy	Nil	25%	50%	100%
Lactation	Nil	35%	60%	100%

It is widely believed that overfat rams or those in very poor condition lack libido and are of low fertility, although studies of nutritional effects on ram growth and fertility are very limited. Probably obese males lack mating ability, especially in the hot months, but their semen quality should not be impaired. Limited data on the consequences of moderate undernutrition showed no significant effects in winter but a small decline in morphology, longevity and sperm count in summer. Libido appeared unaffected.

REFERENCES

1. Agricultural Research Council: The Nutrient Requirements of Farm Livestock, No.2 Ruminants. London, Agricultural Research Council, 1965.
2. National Research Council: Nutrient Requirements of Sheep. 5th Ed. Washington D.C., National Academy of Sciences, 1975.

Artificial Rearing of Lambs

D. M. WEST

Massey University, Palmerston North, New Zealand

The starvation/exposure complex has been reported as a major cause of perinatal lamb mortality, accounting for the death of approximately 10 per cent of the total lamb crop. Much of this loss could be prevented by the use of artificial rearing systems providing food, shelter and warmth. Traditional hand rearing methods involve bottle feeding lambs several times per day with warm cow's milk over a 10 to 12 week period. This requires considerable time and labor and often results in poorly grown lambs.

Alternative systems of rearing newborn lambs utilizing milk replacers, self-feeding devices and early weaning have been developed. Although some sheepmen are using these, their full potential for efficient artificial rearing has not yet been realized.

LIQUID MILK–FEEDING PERIOD

Colostrum Milk

Before the lamb can be introduced to the artificial rearing system, it is essential that the newborn animal has colostrum, whether natural or artificial. Colostrum milk serves three functions: it is laxative; it has special nutritive value with a high content of fat, protein and vitamins and it has a protective function because of the antibodies it contains. Cow's colostrum is a satisfactory substitute for ewe's colostrum and can be frozen and stored ahead of the time that it is needed. In the event that natural colostrum cannot be obtained by the newborn lamb, a synthetic colostrum consisting of 750 ml of cow's milk, one beaten egg, one teaspoon of cod liver oil and two teaspoons of sugar may be fed. Although this substitute is better than no colostrum, it does not provide the lamb with protective antibodies.

Milk Replacer

Any synthetic milk must be based on whole milk or its byproducts, as the young lamb possesses only those enzymes capable of digesting the nutrients found in whole milk. Milk replacers in powder form that can be reconstituted to a liquid by adding water prove the most satisfactory. For optimum growth, the composition of lamb milk replacers should be within the ranges listed in Table 1.

This formula contains relatively high fat and low lactose levels compared with cow's milk. Because of the high fat content, mixing is facilitated by adding the powder to a small quantity of warm water, premixing and then adding the balance of required water. Mixing 1 kg of milk replacer powder with 4 to 5 liters of water creates a solution

TABLE 1. *Composition of Lamb Milk Replacers*

Ingredient	Percentage Range (Dry Basis)
Crude fat	30–32
Crude milk protein	22–24
Crude fiber	0–1
Lactose	22–25
Ash	5–10

similar to ewe's milk in total fat and solids and results in the lambs' obtaining sufficient nutrients without excessive consumption of liquid. In an *ad libitum* feeding system, 1 to 2 liters of the liquid milk replacer will be consumed daily by each lamb.

SOLID FEEDS

Roughage should be offered to the lambs within 1 week of their being started on liquid milk replacer. Although only a limited amount of solid feed will be consumed, the lambs become familiar with such feeds, and this aids in the development of rumen function, which is essential when early weaning is to be accomplished. Good quality leafy hay has proved satisfactory for this. Water should be available *ad libitum* during the milk feeding period.

WEANING

For artifical rearing of lambs to be economical, early weaning from the relatively costly liquid milk replacer is essential. To assure optimum performance upon early weaning, it is important that the lambs have consumed solid feed during the liquid milk–feeding period. Under these circumstances, lambs can be weaned abruptly at 4 to 5 weeks of age to a palatable diet of concentrate. The postweaning growth check is reduced if the concentrate ration is available to the lambs before weaning and if, following weaning, they are kept in a similar environment for about 1 week.

POSTWEANING DIET

The lamb passes through two stages in becoming a functional ruminant. The first phase, from birth to 21 days of age, is the nonruminant phase. The second phase is from 21 to 56 days of age and is termed the transitional phase. During this phase, the lamb is developing the physiological, histological and metabolic characteristics of a functional ruminant. Thus, the diet formulation for the lamb during the transitional phase remains somewhat speculative. If the aim of the artificial rearing system is to rear lambs to pasture-feeding stage, grass should be incorporated into the diet soon after the lamb has been weaned from the liquid milk replacer. The balance of the lamb's requirements during the transitional phase would be met by a concentrate ration fed *ad libitum*. By about 56 days of age, the lambs should experience little difficulty in functioning as mature ruminants and can be changed to all grass feeding.

However, if the lambs are being reared indoors to slaughter weight, they would be maintained on the concentrate ration.

The concentrate ration should have a relatively high protein level. Lambs fed rations containing 17 to 19 per cent protein have significantly greater weight gains than when lower protein levels are fed. Urea is not an especially valuable replacement for preformed protein in the diets of early weaned lambs, and only levels providing not more than 10 per cent of the total dietary nitrogen can be tolerated without a marked depression in performance.

The other nutrient of major concern is energy, which in ruminant diets is usually adjusted by changing the ratio of roughage to concentrate. Young lambs have a higher maintenance requirement than older lambs, so to obtain maximum performance it is necessary to feed high-concentrate diets. Lamb weight gains are increased and the feed required per pound of grain is reduced by decreasing the amount of roughage in the diet to about 10 per cent. Below this level, little improvement in performance is noted. If the roughage is finely ground and the diet pelleted, levels of roughage above 10 per cent can be fed.

The composition of one such diet is shown in Table 2.

TABLE 2.   *Ingredient Composition of Postweaning Lamb Diet (Loose Mix)**

Ingredient	Per Cent
Ground, shelled corn	50.0
Soybean meal, 44 per cent crude protein	20.0
Alfalfa meal	25.0
Animal fat	3.0
Dicalcium phosphate	1.0
Ground limestone	0.5
Salt, trace mineralized	0.5
Vitamin A	5000 IU/lb

*Adapted from Glimp, H. A.: J. Anim. Sci., *34*:1085, 1972.

REFERENCES

1. Frederiksen, K. R.: Artificial rearing of lambs. Proceedings — Symposium on Sheep Industry Development Program, Sheep for Profit through Intensive Management. Paducah, Kentucky, June 20–22, 1972.

2. Glimp, H. A.: Effect of diet composition on performance of lambs reared from birth on milk replacer. J. Anim. Sci., *34*:1085, 1972.
3. Hinds, F. C.: Feeding for growth from early weaning to market. Proceedings — Symposium on Sheep Industry Development Program, Sheep for Profit through Intensive Management. Paducah, Kentucky, June 20–22, 1972.

Development of the Female Reproductive Tract, Oogenesis and Puberty

W. R. WARD

University of Liverpool, Leahurst, Neston, Wirral, England

The female reproductive tract develops in the sheep embryo in a fashion similar to that of other domestic species. There is little of special interest to the clinician; intersex conditions are far more common in goats and pigs, as are freemartins in cattle. Of interest in the sheep are the pigmented caruncles and fallopian tubes (oviducts) present in the embryo. The embryology of the Merino sheep has been documented by Cloete.[1]

OOGENESIS

Oogenesis, the formation and development of the egg, begins in the embryo and is completed when a spermatozoon penetrates the zona. As in most mammals, primitive germ cells become oogonia, which multiply by mitotic divisions to form oocytes (whose number cannot increase) in the embryonic ovary. The primary oocytes, with 54 chromosomes, begin meiosis in the embryo, and at the time of birth, most have reached diplotene — the fourth of the five stages of prophase, which is the first of the four stages of meiosis. When the sheep is in estrus, a small number of oocytes (one to three in most breeds) resume meiosis while the surrounding follicles (graafian follicles) enlarge. By the time the follicle has reached its maximum size of 10 mm, the oocyte has completed meiosis to produce a first polar body,

which is discarded, and one secondary oocyte, with 27 chromosomes. A second meiotic division passes through a rapid prophase but is arrested in metaphase until after ovulation. Observation by laparoscopy shows that, as in other species, ovulation is not explosive but involves a slow trickle of fluid with some blood from the follicle. Fertilization in the fallopian tube stimulates resumption of meiosis to form the egg nucleus and the second polar body.

PUBERTY

Puberty in the female sheep occurs in the first or second year of life. Suffolk lambs born early in the year reach puberty at the beginning of the breeding season; those born later reach puberty toward the middle of the season at 6 months of age; lambs born later still do not achieve puberty until their second year.[2] Merino ewes in Australia first demonstrate estrus in February or March, during declining day length, at ages ranging from 5 to 9 months.

Lambs reared on a high plane of nutrition reach puberty earlier than those on a low plane. This is partly a reflection of the tendency to reach puberty only above a certain body weight and partly a direct effect of nutrition on the reproductive system.

It is generally believed that at puberty the female sheep ovulates without overt estrus and displays estrus at the time of the next ovulation. In a small group of ewe lambs, however, measurement of progesterone concentration in peripheral blood showed that there was no ovulation until the time of the first estrus detected by a ram. Lambs only 8 weeks old are able to ovulate when treated with pregnant mare's serum gonadotropin (PMSG) and human chorionic gonadotropin (HCG). Spontaneous estrus and ovulation, however, appear to depend on the initiation of hypothalamic activity by estrogens.

REFERENCES

1. Cloete, J. H. L.: Prenatal growth in the Merino sheep. Onders. J. Vet. Sci. Anim. Ind., *13*:417, 1939.
2. Hammond, J., Jr.: On the breeding season in sheep. J. Agric. Sci., *34*:97, 1944.

The Breeding Season and the Estrous Cycle

W. R. Ward

University of Liverpool, Leahurst, Neston, Wirral, England

THE BREEDING SEASON

In common with many mammals, most breeds of sheep breed during a restricted period of the year. It is presumed that the young are thereby born at a time of year when they have the best chance of growing to maturity. Sheep begin to breed when the days are shortening and are sometimes classed as "short-day breeders" in contrast to "long-day breeders," such as the mare. The breeding season for sheep extends for about equal periods both before and after the shortest day of the year.

Movement of sheep between Northern and Southern hemispheres is followed by adaptation to the appropriate breeding season. That the length of daylight is an important factor in the time of the breeding season was demonstrated by regulation of artificial lighting in housed sheep.[4] Decreasing periods of light at a time of year when sheep were normally anestrous induced estrous cycles, and this remains a method of producing more than one crop of lambs a year in housed sheep. Yeates[4] found that the actual length of the daily light periods was not important, thus showing that breeding was not dependent upon a critical total amount of light. The annual breeding season is not controlled by an intrinsic rhythm.[3]

The level of nutrition exerts some effect on the time of onset of breeding in sheep. The effect can be measured when the differences in diet have ended almost 12 months earlier and when differences in body weight between experimental and control ewes have disappeared.

The time of onset of the breeding season varies from year to year. In field conditions it is difficult to correlate the variation with nutrition, temperature or other factors. In laboratory conditions, however, it was found that ewes maintained at 7°C began breeding 30 to 40 days earlier than ewes at normal ambient temperatures of 27 to 32°C.

The length of the breeding season clearly differs among breeds. In general, breeds of mountain origin have short seasons, while lowland breeds have longer seasons. The season remains roughly symmetrical about the shortest day, however. The Merino and Dorset Horn have very long breeding seasons, and in countries near the equator some breeds are capable of breeding all year.

During seasonal anestrus the pituitary contains large amounts of follicle-stimulating hormone (FSH) and luteinizing hormone (LH). The ovaries contain small numbers of large follicles, but corpora lutea (indicating ovulation) are found only at the end of the anestrous period. In the middle of the anestrous season, gonadotropin-releasing hormone produces ovulation, without overt estrus, and the resultant corpus luteum is short-lived.

THE ESTROUS CYCLE

The estrous cycle lasts for 16 to 17 days during the middle of the breeding season but varies widely at the beginning and end of the season, when longer cycles are common. Estrus lasts about 36 hours (Fig. 1).

On the day before estrus, one or more follicles grow rapidly, and the concentration of 17β-estradiol in the blood increases

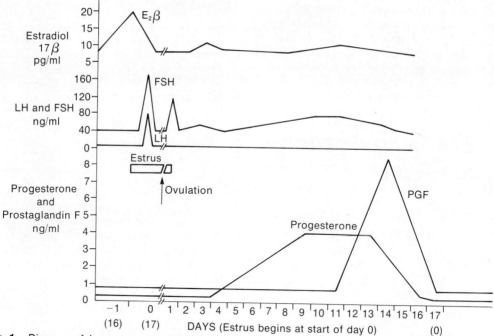

Figure 1. Diagram of hormone concentrations during estrous cycle of sheep. (Prostaglandin F in uterine vein blood; other hormones in jugular vein blood.)

from about 10 pg/ml to 20 pg/ml. The estrogen causes behavioral estrus. Other effects of the estrogen include stimulation of the production of a small amount of cervical mucus, erythema of the vulva and the growth of thick, stratified squamous epithelium in the vagina. These changes are of limited value to the clinician, and the usual indication of estrus is marking of the ewe by a harnessed ram.

Estradiol stimulates release from the pituitary of LH, partly stimulated by hypothalamic gonadotropin-releasing hormone (GnRH). The concentration of LH in the blood rises to a peak of about 80 ng/ml 10 hours after the beginning of estrus, and then both LH and estradiol concentrations fall rapidly. LH stimulates ovulation, which occurs about 14 hours after the LH peak, i.e., about 24 hours after the beginning of estrus. Throughout the rest of the estrous cycle, the LH concentration remains very low, 2 to 3 ng/ml.

At the same time as the LH peak, FSH reaches a maximum of about 170 ng/ml and then falls rapidly. Unlike LH, it rises to a second peak 24 hours after the first. After estrus, FSH concentration is elevated at day 3 and from days 8 to 12 to about 80 ng/ml and declines to about 40 ng/ml before the next estrus. The function of the

rises in FSH concentration during the sheep's estrous cycle is not clear. It is usually stated that FSH stimulates growth of follicles. There is growth of follicles (which undergo atresia) between 6 and 9 days after estrus and 13 and 15 days after estrus. The two obvious peaks of FSH are, however, ill-timed to be regarded as causing follicular growth.

Synthetic GnRH stimulates release of physiological amounts of LH and FSH. The mechanism of the separate release of FSH without LH at the end of estrus in the sheep is not yet understood. It is possible that more than one hypothalamic factor controls the release of the gonadotropins.

The corpus luteum secretes progesterone from 3 days after estrus and produces maximum concentrations of about 4 ng/ml from 9 to 13 days after estrus. During this period, endometrial glands are stimulated to grow in size and complexity.

If no embryo is present in the uterus on the twelfth day, the corpus luteum later regresses and estrus recurs. On the twelfth day in the nonpregnant (and pregnant) ewe, prostaglandin-$F_{2\alpha}$ ($PGF_{2\alpha}$) increases in concentration. In the nonpregnant sheep, $PGF_{2\alpha}$ reaches a peak on the fourteenth day, at a concentration in the uterine vein of about 10 ng/ml. $PGF_{2\alpha}$ is established as the luteolysin in the sheep and reaches the corpus luteum by means of the close apposition of the uterine vein and ovarian artery.

The corpus luteum shows histological evidence of regression on the fifteenth day. By day 16, the concentration of progesterone is basal (< 0.2 ng/ml). This fall in progesterone concentration stimulates estradiol secretion by the growing follicles, and the absence of progesterone permits stimulation of gonadotropin release by estradiol. Progesterone is also believed to be a necessary precursor for the production of estrous behavior by the estradiol.

Among other hormones, androstanedione is produced in large amounts by the follicle and is probably important in the control of gonadotropin release. Prolactin is released throughout the cycle, but particularly at estrus. Prolactin and LH together are able to maintain the corpus luteum in ewes hypophysectomized just after ovulation.

REFERENCES

1. Hammond, J., Jr.: On the breeding season in the sheep. J. Agric. Sci., *34*:97, 1944.
2. Pant, H. C., Hopkinson, C. R. N. and Fitzpatrick, R. J.: Concentration of oestradiol, progesterone, luteinizing hormone and follicle-stimulating hormone in the jugular venous plasma of ewes during the oestrous cycle. J. Endocrinol., *73*:247, 1977.
3. Perry, J. S.: The Ovarian Cycle of Mammals. Edinburgh, Oliver & Boyd, 1971.
4. Sadleir, R. M. F. S.: The Ecology of Reproduction in Wild and Domestic Mammals. London, Methuen, 1969.
5. Yeates, N. T. M.: The breeding season of sheep with particular reference to its modification by artificial means using light. J. Agric. Sci., *39*:1, 1949.

Pregnancy and Parturition

R. J. FITZPATRICK

University of Liverpool, Leahurst, Neston, Wirral, England

PREGNANCY

After fertilization, the ova remain in the fallopian tubes for about 4 days and then enter the uterus at the 8- to 16-cell stage. Attachment occurs between 14 and 18 days, which means that the blastocyst, before being attached, is able to prevent the regression of the corpus luteum, possibly by inhibition of the luteolysin released from the uterus at day 12 or 13 if the ewe is not pregnant. The corpus luteum of pregnancy initially secretes progesterone, but the developing placenta takes over this function. After about the fiftieth day, pregnancy is not terminated by ovariectomy or by administration of luteolytic doses of prostaglandins.

In the first half of pregnancy there is rapid growth of membranes and accumulation of fluids. Ossification of the fetus, sufficient for radiological diagnosis of pregnancy, is established by day 50. During the second half of pregnancy, growth of the fetus dominates, e.g., its weight doubles during the last month. It is toward the end of this phase of exponential fetal growth that the incidence of pregnancy toxemia is greatest. There is a proportionate increase in uterine blood flow from about 100 ml/min when the ewe is nonpregnant to 1500 ml/min near term, and almost the whole of this increase is cotyledonary (placental) flow. The placental circulation is sufficiently developed by 60 days to permit pregnancy diagnosis by ultrasound techniques. Body temperature drops about 0.5°C during the last 48 hours before lambing, and a fall to below 39.2°C has been proposed as a method for selecting which ewes are due to lamb within the next 2 days.[9] This method is 80 per cent effective.

UTERINE CONTRACTIONS AT TERM

In the last 2 weeks of pregnancy, the previously quiescent uterus shows infrequent, nonpropagated contractions of low amplitude (10 mm Hg) of about 5 minutes' duration once every hour. The frequency increases slightly, but only in the last 12 to 24 hours before delivery does this activity become coordinated and regular, although still of low amplitude. Eventually, approximately 2 to 8 hours before birth, contractions and relaxations follow without pause, the amplitude increases to 20 mm Hg and the ewe is in advanced first-stage labor. In twin pregnancies, one horn, often the larger, is dominant in initiating contractions, and the fetus of this side first engages the cervix, which is now compliant and semi-relaxed and yields to the pressure exerted by the distended membranes and fetus. Stretch receptors of the cervix and vagina are activated, and the expulsive pressure is increased by two reflexes: (1) the release of oxytocin, which augments myometrial contractility to pressures of 40 mm Hg and (2) the contractions of abdominal muscles, which are thus precisely superimposed on uterine contractions. The ewe is now in second-stage labor, and birth follows in a few minutes. Immediately after delivery, separation of the placenta by tearing of the tiny villi commences, and the placenta is finally delivered in a few hours. Powerful rhythmic contractions continue, probably under the influence of prostaglandins, during the third stage and for several days afterward in order to discharge the final necrotic placental shreds and the lochia.

MYOMETRIAL CONTRACTILITY

The contractility of the myometrial cells, as with all muscle cells, is finally precipitated by a rise in intracellular free calcium ions, which activate the contractile protein. Although this is relevant to the inertia of hypocalcemia in the ewe, hormones are the more interesting variables, affecting the contractile mechanism at a slightly earlier stage. Chief amongst these are progesterone, which inhibits this mechanism, and the prostaglandins, which stimulate it. Parturition effectively begins when the concentration of circulating progesterone falls and that of prostaglandins rises.

THE ENDOCRINE CONTROL OF LABOR

The changes of hormone secretion before birth have been thoroughly studied in sheep,[4] and in this species it is now well established that the fetus influences its own birth (for review see references 7 and

8). The sequence of events starts with activation of the hypothalamus and pituitary of the fetus by a mechanism as yet unknown. It is, however, certain that about 5 days before birth, adrenocorticotropic hormone (ACTH) is secreted and stimulates the fetal adrenal glands to liberate cortisol. Cortisol acts on the steroid-secreting cells of the fetal cotyledon, which for most of pregnancy have been actively secreting the progesterone essential for the maintenance of the pregnancy. Cortisol induces an enzyme, 17α-hydroxylase, which, in effect, switches steroid production from progesterone to estrogen.[1, 6] Fetal estrogen (sulfated esterone) crosses the placenta, where it becomes unconjugated estradiol. At the same time, the clearance rate of progesterone increases.[2]

The change to estrogen dominance over progesterone is important in several respects but particularly in the production of prostaglandin-$F_{2\alpha}$ ($PGF_{2\alpha}$) in the cells of the myometrium and maternal placenta. Unconjugated estrogens promote the synthesis of $PGF_{2\alpha}$ in sheep, whereas progesterone inhibits this; conversely, the enzymatic degradation of prostaglandins is enhanced by progesterone throughout pregnancy but is depressed by the dominance of estrogen during the last few days before birth. Thus, the endocrine changes promote the production of $PGF_{2\alpha}$ and also of PGE_2 both of which are powerful stimulants of uterine muscle. Uterine contractions themselves then facilitate the further release of the intracellular lysosomal enzymes that synthesize prostaglandins, and the whole process becomes self-perpetuating.

The ultimate effect of uterine contractions in combination with cervical relaxation and other changes is to advance the fetus into the cervix and anterior vagina, which will elicit the reflex release of oxytocin. This will augment the myometrial contractions, with the liberation of even more prostaglandins, so that the whole sequence takes on a cascading effect. The significance of this and the reflex-synchronized abdominal effort is to increase the efficiency and decrease the duration of second-stage labor, which is when the risks of anoxia and other hazards are maximal. That each uterine contraction outlasts the accompanying abdominal spasms is also important in maintaining uterine "tone," without which a flaccid uterus could be damaged by compression against the fetus and would also be everted with the fetus at the moment of birth.

SOFT TISSUE CHANGES AT BIRTH

Parturition is more than mere contraction of the uterus. The increase in expulsive force must be coincident with decrease in resistance, which, for practical purposes, means softening of the collagen of the cervix uteri and pelvic ligaments. Changes in these ligaments have been studied in sheep by Bassett,[3] and recent studies on the sheep cervix by Fitzpatrick[5] have revealed that the dense collagen that normally makes up most of the wall changes dramatically at the very end of pregnancy. Both the total amount of collagen and its concentration fall and there is a very marked increase in water. Histologically, the collagen bundles become disaggregated and the fibrils dispersed, almost certainly because of the loosening of the chemical bonds of the mucopolysaccharides (which form the cement of collagen) under the influence of estrogens, prostaglandins and possibly relaxin. Such changes increase the compliance (stretchability) of the cervix over a matter of hours but are reversed again after birth within a very few days. The control mechanism is certainly endocrine in origin, but in the sheep little of this is understood as yet, beyond knowing that PGE_2 and possibly $PGF_{2\alpha}$ are effective after progesterone concentrations have fallen and estrogen concentrations have risen.

REFERENCES

1. Anderson, A. B. M., Flint, A. P. F. and Turnbull, A. C.: Mechanism of action of glucocorticoids in induction of ovine parturition: Effect on placental steroid metabolism. J. Endocrinol., *66*:61, 1975.
2. Ash, R. W., Challis, J. R. G., Harrison, F. A., Heap, R. B., Illingsworth, D. V., Perry, J. S. and Poyser, N. L.: Hormonal control of pregnancy and parturition. *In* The Barcroft Symposium on Fetal and Neonatal Physiology. Cambridge University Press, 1973, p. 551.
3. Bassett, E. G.: Some effects of endogenous hormones on muscles and connective tissue with special reference to the ewe. Proc. N.Z. Soc. Anim. Prod., *23*:107, 1963.
4. Chamley, W. A., Buckmaster, J. M., Cerini, M. E., Cumming, I. A., Goding, J. R., Obst, J. M., Williams, A. and Winfield, C. G.: Changes in the levels of progesterone, corticosteroids, estrone, estradiol-17β, luteinizing hormone and prolactin in the peripheral plasma of the ewe during late pregnancy and at parturition. Biol. Reprod., *9*:30, 1973.
5. Fitzpatrick, R. J.: Dilation of the uterine cervix. *In* The Fetus and Birth. Ciba Symposium No. 47. Amsterdam, Elsevier, 1977, p. 31.
6. Flint, A. P. F., Goodson, J. D. and Turnbull, A. C.: Increased concentrations of 17α,20α-dihydroxypregn-4-en-3-one in maternal and fetal plasma near parturition in sheep. J. Endocrinol., *67*:89, 1975.
7. Liggins, G. C., Fairclough, R. J., Grieves, S. A., Kendall, J. Z. and Knox, B. S.: The mechanism of initiation of parturition in the ewe. Rec. Prog. Hormone Res. *29*:111, 1973.
8. Liggins, G. C.: Parturition in sheep. *In* The Fetus and Birth. Ciba Symposium No. 47. Amsterdam, Elsevier, 1977, p. 3.
9. Winfield, C. G. and Makin, A. W.: Prediction of the onset of parturition in sheep from observations of rectal temperature changes. Livestock Prod. Sci., *2*:393, 1975.

Fertilization Failure

H. M. CHAPMAN

Murdoch University, Murdoch, Western Australia

Although fertilization is a complex process, failures are relatively uncommon, and a fertilization rate of greater than 90 per cent can be expected in ewes mated to fertile rams under natural mating conditions.

Fertilization takes place in the oviduct of the ewe and begins about 3 hours after ovulation with the penetration of the egg by a capacitated spermatozoon. The egg is activated, male and female pronuclei are formed and these are replaced by two haploid groups of chromosomes that unite to give the diploid chromosome number in the new zygote. Ova can remain viable for 10 to 25 hours following ovulation, and sperm can live for about 24 hours in the genital tract of the ewe.

DIAGNOSIS OF FERTILIZATION FAILURE

Diagnosis of fertilization failure is difficult. Records of returns to service are useful, although a ewe that is served and returns to service at the normal interval (16 to 20 days) may in fact have conceived but suffered early embryonic loss before day 12 or 13 (discussion in following article) and the ewe that is mated and produces one lamb may have had two ovulations with fertilization of only one of the two eggs.

Ewes can be slaughtered at 2 to 3 days postcoitus, or alternatively a laparotomy can be done at this time and ova flushed from the tract and classified as either fertilized or nonfertilized. At the same time a check can be made for genital tract abnormalities. The fertilization rate is calculated as a percentage of the ova shed (from counts of corpora lutea).

FACTORS ASSOCIATED WITH FERTILIZATION FAILURE

Failure of fertilization can result when ovulation is delayed or fails to occur. These effects are likely to be important at the beginning of the breeding season. There is good clinical evidence to suggest that low cobalt or copper levels may be associated with infertility and irregular estrous cycles in sheep, and it is well known that the effects of inanition, including failure of estrus, are more pronounced in young, growing animals. Inability of ova or sperm to fertilize can occur if the gametes are defective. Ova may have structural abnormalities that are due to faulty maturation of the oocyte, genetic or environmental factors or failure of polar body extrusion. Fragmentation of eggs is common in immature and superovulated animals. Any damage to the spermatozoon may impair its capacity to migrate and survive in the ewe's reproductive tract. Aging of ova, either as a result of delayed ovulation or in association with delayed breeding, may result in fertilization failure. This can happen if ewes are bred too late following estrus and is likely to occur if artificial insemination is used. Similarly, fertilization failure can occur when spermatozoa are aged, whether this aging takes place in the ewe's reproductive tract (as a result of poor synchronization of ovulation

and mating or insemination) or in storage (as with frozen semen). Sperm motility is affected, and sperm lose their viability.

Lowered conception rates are often reported at first service following a course of progesterone or progestogens, as used in estrous synchronization in either cycling or anestrous ewes. These drugs interfere with sperm transport and survival, resulting in fertilization failure.

A specific type of infertility can occur when ewes graze pastures containing estrogenic compounds, such as are found in alfalfa (lucerne) and certain clovers. Temporary "clover disease" affects ewes mated on green estrogenic clover (*Trifolium subterraneum*), and permanent disease affects ewes after prolonged estrogen ingestion. Clover disease can be diagnosed by weighing cotton wool plugs that have been in the vagina of a ewe in estrus for an hour. Plugs from ewes grazing estrogenic pastures are heavier than those from ewes on other pasture. The spinnbarkheit test (length to which a thread of mucus can be drawn out between two glass slides) is also a useful diagnostic test. In clover disease the mucus becomes thinner and more watery, and sperm movement to the cervix is impeded, resulting in low fertilization rates in affected ewes. Cysts are seen on postmortem examination of the cervix and uterus in permanent clover disease cases.

High ambient temperatures (35° C plus), especially during and after estrus, have an adverse effect on fertilization, as sperm quality is lowered and abnormal ova may be produced.

Fertility at the first estrus following embryonic death is often severely depressed because ovulation occurs in some ewes before resorption and uterine involution are complete; sperm transport is affected, and thus conception does not occur.

Infertility resulting from fertilization failure may be brought about by semen of poor quality, as occurs in many diseases of rams (see Semen Collection and Evaluation, page 944). Exposure of ewes at mating to *Brucella ovis* infection may interfere with ovulation, conception, implantation, or embryonic survival. In addition, ewes mated with *B. ovis*-infected rams sometimes develop vaginitis and cervicitis, and such ewes may have reduced fertility at subsequent matings. In some individual ewes the application of stress has been shown to reduce the efficiency of sperm transport, and this is more apparent after matings with exhausted rams or following inseminations with diluted ejaculates.

Any condition leading to the obstruction of the genital tract of the ewe and preventing the union of sperm and egg will cause fertilization failure. However, abnormalities of the genital tract, either developmental (e.g., intersex conditions) or acquired (caused by trauma or infection) are not a common cause of infertility in the ewe.

Two viral conditions occasionally associated with failure of conception are contagious ecthyma (scabby mouth) and ulcerative dermatosis. Both diseases can cause painful lesions on the vulva, and affected ewes tend to avoid coitus. Low conception rates may also result in flocks in which ewes have blowfly strike, especially if it involves the crutch area. The affected animals may refuse to mate because of the irritation and pain caused by the maggots.

TREATMENT AND PREVENTION

It is important that the percentage of rams used is adequate to insure that every ewe is served. Many factors affect ram performance (see Examination of the Ram for Breeding Soundness, page 936), and these, as well as fertility differences among rams, farm topography, feed availability and even the breed of sheep concerned, must be taken into consideration when deciding on the number of rams per flock of ewes to be mated. In most situations, 2 rams per 100 ewes will be adequate, but 1 per cent of rams may be satisfactory if active, healthy, mature rams are used and provided returns to service are carefully monitored. This means that every ram must be fitted with a harness and marking crayon. In many areas where a low percentage of rams is used, spot semen tests are performed during mating. A sample of semen is aspirated from the vagina of a ewe immediately following coitus and is examined microscopically. Some stock owners consider this type of test to be very helpful in detecting rams of lowered fertility.

Under extensive conditions of husbandry or when the fertility of either rams or ewes is depressed, such as when ewes are grazing estrogenic pastures, a higher proportion of rams should be used (4 to 6 per 100 ewes).

In areas where clover disease is a problem, it may be necessary to stock wethers only, but these should be given alternate grazing until the pastures have dried out (dry clover is not estrogenic). The problem can be lessened if the proportion of grass in the pasture is increased or, alternatively, if the potent subclovers are replaced by low-estrogen strains.

Conception rates following synchronization treatments can be improved if the time interval between mating and ovulation is very carefully controlled and if greater numbers of spermatozoa are provided, either by inseminating with fresh semen or by using an excess of rams in natural service (up to 6 per 100 ewes).

Local antiseptic emollient dressings can be used to treat or prevent secondary bacterial infection and soften the scabs of sheep suffering from contagious ecthyma. If only a few ewes are infected, these should be isolated, and the remainder should be taken to a clean paddock and vaccinated.

No specific treatment is available for ulcerative dermatosis. It may be prevented, however, if rams with lesions on the prepuce causing posthitis are not run with ewes during the breeding season.

Short-term relief from blowfly strike can be obtained by clipping the wool around the anus and vulva and applying insecticide. In Merino and other heavily-fleeced breeds it may be necessary to perform Mules operation to increase the area of smooth skin around the vulva and anus.

The use of genitally sound rams for breeding cannot be overemphasized; this aspect of fertility is discussed in Examination of the Ram for Breeding Soundness, page 936.

REFERENCES

1. Adams, N. R.: Clover disease in Western Australia. *In* Tomes, G. J., Robertson, D. E., and Lightfoot, R. J. (eds.): Sheep Breeding. Proceedings International Congress Muresk. Perth, Western Australian Institute of Technology, 1976, p. 424.
2. Blood, D. C. and Henderson, J. A.: Veterinary Medicine, London, Bailliere Tindall, 1974.
3. Hancock, J. L.: Fertilization in farm animals. Anim. Breed. Abstr., *30*:285, 1962.

Prenatal Loss

H. M. CHAPMAN

Murdoch University, Murdoch,
Western Australia

Prenatal loss is the term used to refer to deaths occurring over the full period of pregnancy. This loss can be subdivided into embryonic deaths (losses of fertilized ova and embryos up to the end of attachment) and fetal deaths (losses from the time of attachment until parturition).

Although embryonic deaths are an important source of pregnancy wastage, they may have little effect on lambing percentage. This is because the majority of such deaths occur during the first 13 to 18 days of gestation so that most ewes return to service and are remated. That is, the effect of embryonic death in a flock is to spread lambing and reduce twinning rates, although some ewes may be barren if the joining period is not long enough to allow for returns to service.

Estimates of losses occurring in the absence of any identifiable cause (basal loss) vary, but on average about 20 to 30 per cent of fertilized ova are lost during pregnancy, the majority before 28 days gestation. Losses attributable to specific factors (induced loss) are added to this basal loss. From 1 to 5 per cent of fetal deaths (abortion) are usually accepted in a flock, but higher levels than this should be investigated.

DEVELOPMENT OF THE CONCEPTUS

Following fertilization the zygote begins to divide, and the blastocyst enters the uterus 3 to 4 days after ovulation at the 16- to 32-cell stage. Attachment of the blastocyst is a gradual process that begins about day 15 and is completed by day 40. The fetal cotyledons appear by day 22 and gradually fuse with the maternal caruncles to form the placentomes. The trophoblast elongates very rapidly from day 12, and by day 14 it is about 10 cm in length. By 34 days the major tissues, organs and systems are formed, and growth and maturation of the fetus continue until parturition.

Various methods are available for estimating the developmental age of an ovine fetus: determinations of crown-anus length (50 to 100 days), brain weight, long bone length and number of appendicular ossification centers (50 days to term) and correlations between embryo morphology and days of gestation.

FACTORS ASSOCIATED WITH PRENATAL LOSS

Although the cause of much prenatal loss is uncertain and possibly inevitable, various factors are known to increase losses above the basal level (Fig. 1).

Severe undernutrition lasting from 1 to 3 weeks during the first month of pregnancy may cause measurable losses of embryos. In some experiments increased duration of undernutrition and in others very low ewe body weights have been associated with higher embryonic loss. High planes of nutrition (200 per cent of maintenance ration) in the preimplantation period have been associated with increased embryonic loss in certain breeds, e.g., Merino. The physiological basis of these nutritional effects on embryo survival is not known. Undernutrition during the last 2 months of pregnancy can result in losses of ewes due to pregnancy toxemia and in the consequent prenatal death of lambs.

Selenium deficiency causes embryonic death at 3 to 4 weeks postconception.

Abnormally high embryonic losses have been reported in ewes bred both early and late in the breeding season.

Continuous high temperatures (sufficient to raise rectal temperatures to 40° C) in the first week after mating will usually kill all embryos, but if the environmental temperature decreases at night, these losses are reduced to about 35 per cent, that is, when diurnal variation in temperature occurs, heat stress is probably a minor cause of reproductive wastage.

Several plant and chemical poisons are known to cause prenatal loss in sheep. Nitrates may occasionally cause abortion in ewes if consumed at levels that cause a significant methemoglobinemia. *Zygadenus* poisoning causes abortion, and up to 80 per cent of pregnant ewes may abort if locoweeds (*Astragalus* and *Oxytropis* spp.) are grazed or fed as hay. Embryonic deaths may occur in ewes fed toxic amounts of *Veratrum californicum*. Embryos are most susceptible

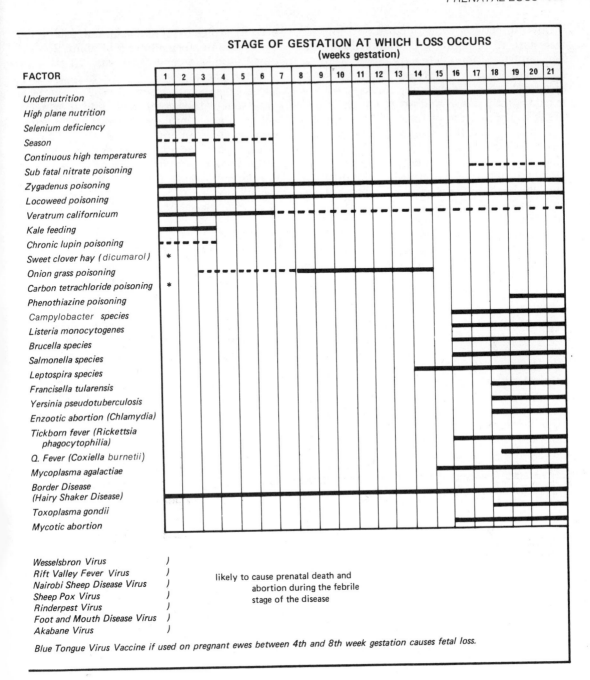

FACTOR	STAGE OF GESTATION AT WHICH LOSS OCCURS (weeks gestation)																				
	1	2	3	4	5	6	7	8	9	10	11	12	13	14	15	16	17	18	19	20	21
Undernutrition																					
High plane nutrition																					
Selenium deficiency																					
Season																					
Continuous high temperatures																					
Sub fatal nitrate poisoning																					
Zygadenus poisoning																					
Locoweed poisoning																					
Veratrum californicum																					
Kale feeding																					
Chronic lupin poisoning																					
Sweet clover hay (dicumarol)	*																				
Onion grass poisoning																					
Carbon tetrachloride poisoning	*																				
Phenothiazine poisoning																					
Campylobacter species																					
Listeria monocytogenes																					
Brucella species																					
Salmonella species																					
Leptospira species																					
Francisella tularensis																					
Yersinia pseudotuberculosis																					
Enzootic abortion (Chlamydia)																					
Tickborn fever (Rickettsia phagocytophilia)																					
Q. Fever (Coxiella burnetii)																					
Mycoplasma agalactiae																					
Border Disease (Hairy Shaker Disease)																					
Toxoplasma gondii																					
Mycotic abortion																					

Wesselsbron Virus	)	
Rift Valley Fever Virus	)	
Nairobi Sheep Disease Virus	)	likely to cause prenatal death and
Sheep Pox Virus	)	abortion during the febrile
Rinderpest Virus	)	stage of the disease
Foot and Mouth Disease Virus	)	
Akabane Virus	)	

Blue Tongue Virus Vaccine if used on pregnant ewes between 4th and 8th week gestation causes fetal loss.

* Stage at which loss occurs not known.

- - - - Loss likely to occur at this stage.

Figure 1. Prenatal loss in sheep.

at 14 or 15 days postcoitus and may die and be resorbed or survive malformed and die perinatally. There is some evidence for an increase in early embryonic death in ewes fed kale. Chronic lupin poisoning (lupinosis) has been associated with fetal death and abortion, as has sweet clover hay containing dicumarol, and onion grass (*Romulea bulbo-codium*) has been implicated both in early losses and in abortions midway through pregnancy. Abortion has been recorded in ewes dosed with carbon tetrachloride and in those given phenothiazine during the last 3 weeks of pregnancy.

Most infectious conditions have their effects late in pregnancy, and specific organisms appear to play a very small role in embryonic death in sheep. Hairy shaker disease (border disease) may cause embryonic death, fetal death and abortion, perinatal death and the birth of hairy shaker lambs. The diagnosis of this disease is made on the basis of clinical signs and specific histopathological studies of the central nervous system of hairy shaker lambs in an infected flock. Other infectious causes of abortion are discussed later in this section.

It is unclear as to whether ovulation rate affects embryo mortality. Results from superovulated or litter-bearing sheep may not be applicable to single or twin ovulators, as uterine capacity may be the limiting factor. It has been estimated that partial loss of pregnancy (one of two embryos) may occur in up to 50 per cent of ewes.

The condition of the gametes at the time of mating is known to affect embryonic mortality. Aging of gametes and consequent cytogenetic abnormalities that result in early embryonic loss can occur because of poor synchronization of mating and ovulation. High levels of embryonic loss have also been recorded consequent to the use of frozen semen and semen from heat-stressed rams.

FATE OF DEAD EMBRYOS AND FETUSES

The fate of dead embryos and fetuses depends upon their stage of development and cause of death. Dead embryos are usually resorbed while dead fetuses can be either aborted or mummified.

EFFECT OF PRENATAL DEATH ON EWE FERTILITY

The presence of an embryo in the uterus about day 12 or 13 of the estrous cycle prevents regression of the corpus luteum. In the absence of an embryo, the corpus luteum starts to degenerate about day 14. If an embryo dies before day 12 or 13, the corpus luteum regresses, the ewe comes into estrus about day 17 (i.e., within the normal cycle length) and most ewes have a normal conception rate when remated. Embryos that die after day 13 prolong the secreting life of the corpus luteum, resulting in extended estrous cycles (e.g., embryonic death on day 15 results in a cycle length of about 25 to 30 days), and the conception rate at the next mating is often low. Estrus may occur in these ewes before resorption of the embryo, autolysis of the membranes and uterine involution are complete, so that sperm transport or attachment, or both, are affected. The practical result is that many ewes fail to conceive to a second service, or if the joining period is too short, the ewes do not receive a second service.

DIAGNOSIS AND MEASUREMENT OF PRENATAL LOSS

The occurrence of prenatal loss is difficult to diagnose. A farmer may complain of having a low lambing percentage, but this problem may be compounded by anestrus, low ovulation rate, fertilization failure, embryonic death and abortion, as well as by perinatal deaths.

The simplest direct method for determining the extent of prenatal loss is to slaughter a sample of the flock at 2 or 3 days following service to determine the number of ova shed (count the corpora lutea) and the percentage fertilized (classify ova as fertilized or nonfertilized and calculate the fertilization rate as a percentage of ova shed). The rest of the flock is left to lamb. If it is assumed that the sample fertilization rate and the lambing result are representative of the flock, prenatal deaths can be expressed as a percentage of fertilized ova that do not result in full-term lambs. The point at which losses occur can be determined by slaughtering at intervals throughout pregnancy, e.g., days 2, 18, 30 and 140. In addition, a sample is allowed to lamb. Because of the large number of sheep that need to be slaughtered, this method is impracticable except in a research situation.

Various alternative approaches are possible: laparotomy or endoscopy at day 2 or 3 then radiography after day 80 (count fetuses) or laparotomy at 3 days (count corpora lutea) then record returns to service up to 20 days (ram with harness). This method gives an estimate of fertilization failure plus embryonic death occurring before day 13. Subsequent returns to service represent later embryonic death, and the lambing result is also recorded. Because the fertilization rate is not known, the results are expressed as the percentage of ova shed that are not represented by full-term lambs.

Laparoscopy can be used instead of laparotomy to enable counts to be made of corpora lutea and has an advantage in that the procedure has very little effect on reproductive performance. There is some evidence to show that laparotomy can have a deleterious effect on fertility, and manipulations of the reproductive tract soon after mating may affect survival of ova from multiple ovulations.

Indirect estimates of prenatal loss can be made from flock data but are of limited value. Good mating and lambing records are needed, and ewes need to be identified. Fertilization failure or embryonic loss before day 12 or 13 can be suspected if a ewe is served and returns to heat at the normal interval. Embryonic death has probably occurred if a ewe has been served and returns to heat with a long interestrous period (20 days or more). If a ewe has been served and does not return to service but does not produce a lamb, it is possible that (1) it conceived and the embryo(s) or fetus(s) were later resorbed or aborted, (2) it failed to conceive and exhibited silent heat at the next ovulation, (3) it failed to conceive and then entered anestrus or (4) it failed to conceive but because of the length of the joining period did not get the opportunity to be remated. Many ewes will be recorded as having lambed, but this result does not distinguish between ewes with one ovulation producing one lamb and ewes with double ovulations producing one lamb. From a practical point of view, it is the latter losses that are important.

The diagnosis of infectious abortion is discussed later in this section.

TREATMENT AND PREVENTION

Until more is known of the reasons why apparently normal fertilized ova develop for a period and then die, the prospects for reducing basal embryonic losses are not great. Some control can however be exerted over many of the factors known to be associated with induced prenatal loss.

Management procedures should be adjusted in order to achieve high body weights before mating (to increase ovulation rate) and to provide adequate nutrition for the first 3 weeks and last 2 months of pregnancy. If it is necessary to restrict feed intake, this should be done only from weeks 4 to 12 of gestation. In view of the higher embryonic mortality rates recorded in ewes of low body weight, overstocking should be avoided. Embryonic mortality due to selenium deficiency can be prevented by administration of 5 mg of selenium (11 mg of sodium selenite) orally to ewes and rams 1 month before the rams are put out with the ewes. Plant poisonings can be prevented if breeding ewes are grazed on pastures free of the plant in question, or alternatively, if this is not possible, ample supplementary feed (e.g., hay) should be provided to minimize the desire to eat these plants. Nitrate poisoning can be prevented if crops are fed in the mature state only and if grazing of pregnant animals on rapidly growing pastures is avoided.

Anthelmintics other than phenothiazine and carbon tetrachloride should be used in the pregnant ewe.

Although the relationship between stress and embryonic mortality is not clear, it is probably wise to avoid physical stress, fright, heat stress and so forth during mating and pregnancy. In this respect it is particularly important to insure that mating flocks are undisturbed. Sheep should not be excessively "dogged" during mating, and strangers should not be allowed into the paddocks being used for mating.

Some control of hairy shaker disease can be achieved by retaining those ewes that have produced affected lambs in the breeding flock and mixing replacement breeding stock with these in the hope that the replacements will become infected and immune before pregnancy.

The length of the joining period should be sufficient to allow ewes a second service.

Although little is known regarding genotypic effects and prenatal mortality, it is possible that genetic variation for this does exist. It may be possible to select for embryo survival and so improve reproductive performance in sheep.

REFERENCES

1. Edey, T. N.: Prenatal mortality in sheep: A review. Anim. Breed. Abstr., *37*:173, 1969.
2. Edey, T. N.: Embryo mortality. *In* Tomes, G. J., Robertson, D. E. and Lightfoot, R. J. (eds.): Sheep Breeding. Proceedings International Congress Muresk. Perth, Western Australian Institute of Technology, 1976, p. 400.

3. Quinlivan, T. D., Martin, C. A., Taylor, W. B. and Cairney, I. M.: Estimates of pre- and perinatal mortality in the New Zealand Romney Marsh ewe. J. Reprod. Fertil., *11*:379, 1966.
4. Richardson, C., Hebert, C. N. and Terlecki, S.: Es-timation of the developmental age of the ovine fetus and lamb. Vet. Rec., *99*:22, 1976.
5. Roberts, S. J.: Veterinary Obstetrics and Genital Diseases. 2nd Ed. Ann Arbor, Mich., Edwards Bros. Inc., 1971.

Pregnancy Diagnosis in the Ewe

D. M. WEST

Massey University, Palmerston North, New Zealand

The accurate prediction of pregnancy in ewes would greatly add to the efficiency of sheep farming. A reliable technique for the early detection of pregnancy and the diagnosis of multiple fetuses would enable the culling of barren ewes and the appropriate feeding of pregnant ewes for the remainder of gestation.

The useful techniques for pregnancy diagnosis can be grouped under two headings: (1) aids to diagnosis and (2) most reliable methods of diagnosis.

AIDS TO DIAGNOSIS

Use of a Harness and Crayon on the Ram

The use of a harness and colored crayon (Fig. 1) to detect mating patterns within a flock is almost a standard technique now. It is important to choose the crayon according to the weather conditions prevailing at the time of use, as sudden cold weather may prevent the crayon from leaving a mark. The harness must be carefully fitted to the ram, insuring that it is comfortable and is positioned correctly to mark the ewe. Problems of the harness chafing or slipping should be checked regularly, but these will be minimized if the rams have a fleece length of 1 to 2 cm. At intervals of 14 to 16 days the color of the crayon should be changed so that ewes returning to the ram are marked with a different color. Care must be taken in interpreting the results of crayon marking, as very light marks may go undetected and not all ewes that are marked necessarily produce a lamb.

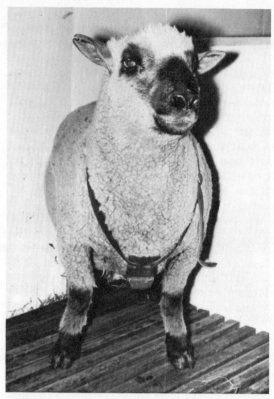

Figure 1. Ram with harness and crayon for marking ewes when serving.

Ballottement and Subjective External Examination

Pregnancy diagnosis by external examination and abdominal palpation is a useful technique in late gestation. It has been shown to be 80 to 95 per cent accurate in Merino ewes that are 90 to 130 days pregnant, the accuracy increasing with increasing gestational age. It is advantageous to withhold feed and water for 12 to 24 hours before diagnosis, especially when the ewes are in better condition. The ewe is held in a sitting position approximately 2 feet above ground level by an assistant. With one hand pressed against the left side of the ewe's abdomen, the operator ballottes the lower abdominal area with the fingertips of the other hand. Although the technique is simple and relatively fast (up to 200 ewes per hour), the number of fetuses cannot be determined accurately and this limits its usefulness.

MOST RELIABLE METHODS OF DIAGNOSIS

The most reliable methods of pregnancy diagnosis include: (1) vaginal biopsy, (2) radiology, (3) laparotomy and peritoneoscopy, (4) ultrasonic fetal pulse detector, (5) blood progesterone assay, (6) rectoabdominal palpation and (7) detection of pregnancy-specific antigens.

Vaginal Biopsy

The vaginal biopsy method was most favored by Richardson[5] in a review of pregnancy diagnosis in the ewe. Sections of vaginal mucosa taken from the wall of the vagina just anterior to the urethral orifice are examined histologically. The stratified squamous epithelium of the nonpregnant ewe is gradually replaced during early pregnancy by layers of cells that tend to be cuboidal in shape with accompanying changes in the nuclei and cytoplasm. The method has been found to be approximately 93 to 97 per cent accurate after 40 days gestation, rising to 100 per cent after 80 days. However nonpregnant ewes are more difficult to detect. Of 204 of these ewes, only 167, or 81 per cent, were correctly diagnosed as being nonpregnant. Multiple pregnancies are not indicated by vaginal biopsy, and this factor, plus the time delay and laboratory expense in arriving at a diagnosis, precludes its use in the field.

Radiology

Most investigators agree that for accuracy, radiography is the best method of pregnancy diagnosis. By 80 days gestation the fetal skeleton is well calcified, making the radiological diagnosis of pregnancy and fetal numbers relatively simple and accurate. However, radiological equipment with a capacity of 100 ma and 90 kv is required to minimize the blurring effect of the ewe's respirations by reducing the exposure time. Radiographing entire flocks is therefore im-

practical, as equipment of this capacity requires permanent installation.

Laparotomy and Peritoneoscopy

Lamond[4] demonstrated that pregnancy can be diagnosed in early gestation by the digital palpation of the uterus via a 5-cm paramedian laparotomy incision. At 4 weeks' gestation the pregnant uterus is tense, thin-walled and about 1 cm in diameter, extending beyond the pelvic brim. At 6 to 7 weeks the uterine horns are 5 to 10 cm in diameter and cotyledons can be detected. It is apparent that for diagnosis of pregnancy alone, digital palpation or direct observation of the internal genitalia would be highly accurate, but this would be of limited value in predicting multiple fetuses.

Ultrasonic Fetal Pulse Detector

The ultrasonic fetal pulse detector makes use of the Doppler phenomenon. Very high frequency sound waves are transmitted from a transducer, and the reflected signal is received back. If the rebound occurs from a moving object or moving particles, there will be slight differences between the transmitted and the received signal. These differences are amplified, and an experienced operator can distinguish between fetal and maternal components. In application, the transducer head is moved over the posterior abdomen of the ewe. It is helpful to remove the wool from the area and to use a lubricant to promote good skin contact. A modification of this method, in which the transducer is fixed on a probe and inserted into the rectum of the ewe, gives greater accuracy in detecting pregnancy during the second trimester.

The results to be expected from the ultrasonic devices are good for distinguishing pregnancy, with 100 per cent accuracy being quoted at 100 days gestation.[1] Detection of multiple fetuses was not possible with the rectal approach and was of relatively low order of accuracy when the instrument was used over the abdominal surface. Early hopes of the widespread use of ultrasonics in pregnancy detection in ewes have not been realized.

Blood Progesterone Assay

The development of rapid and sensitive assays of plasma progesterone in sheep has permitted the diagnosis of pregnancy with an accuracy of approximately 90 per cent by the twenty-eighth day of gestation. Furthermore, a success rate of 65 per cent has been claimed in predicting litter size at 90 to 105 days gestation, although this was achieved under optimal conditions of standardization. A similar method, measuring progesterone levels in milk, has been adapted for pregnancy diagnosis in cattle. It must be remembered that, with dairy cattle in particular, milk is readily available, and differentiation between single and multiple pregnancies is not required. Except for research purposes, progesterone assay for pregnancy diagnosis in sheep will be limited because of the cost, the time delay and the lack of sensitivity in differentiating singles from multiples.

Rectoabdominal Palpation

Pregnancy diagnosis by rectoabdominal palpation has been described by Hulet.[2, 3] It is recommended that the ewes be fasted overnight. The ewe is restrained on her back in a cradle, and a lubricated hollow plastic rod 1.5 cm outer diameter (OD) × 50 cm with a rounded tip is inserted into the rectum a distance of about 30 cm. With one hand on the posterior abdomen, the other hand guides the rod so that the distal end palpates the region that should accommodate the fetus. In early pregnancy (before 70 days) it is advantageous to have the ewe tilted forward so that the gut falls forward, away from the genitalia, but this is not necessary in later pregnancy. Virtually 100 per cent accuracy at 70 to 110 days after mating can be obtained in differentiating nonpregnant from pregnant animals. However, the overall accuracy rate in differentiating between single and multiple pregnancies is only about 70 per cent.

Rectoabdominal palpation has the advantages of immediate results, speed (approximately 120 ewes per hour) and economy. The disadvantages include the necessity of fasting the ewes overnight and the danger of inflicting internal injuries with the rectal probe. Losses from ewe deaths and abortions have been reported following the use of this technique.[6]

Detection of Pregnancy-Specific Antigens

Recently a technique has been described in which antigens specific to pregnancy in the ewe can be detected using a hemagglutination test. Hemagglutination occurred when rabbit anti-sheep embryo serum was added to a few drops of blood from ewes between days 6 and 50 of pregnancy, but not when added to blood from nonpregnant ewes, rams or wethers. The test offers very early detection of pregnancy, but its usefulness is limited at present because: (1) it cannot differentiate single from multiple fetuses and (2) the time delay of about 30 minutes for hemagglutination to occur requires identification and a further gathering of ewes.

CONCLUSION

The economic justification for the diagnosis of pregnancy in ewes in commercial flocks lies in the saving of supplementary feed to nonpregnant sheep and the efficient feeding of ewes carrying multiple lambs. However, for a technique to be acceptable, certain criteria must be attained. Equipment and materials should be inexpensive, and the diagnosis should be rapid, safe and accurate. After 100 days gestation an accuracy of almost 100 per cent in terms of pregnancy and 90 per cent in separating singles from multiples would appear to be reasonable goals. None of the techniques described can currently reach these criteria.

In contrast, there are very useful methods of pregnancy diagnosis for research purposes. These include vaginal biopsy, laparotomy, blood progesterone estimations and the detection of pregnancy-specific antigens, which achieve accuracies approaching 100 per cent early in gestation. By 80 days gestation the number of fetuses can be accurately determined by the use of radiology.

REFERENCES

1. Fraser, A. F., Nagaratnam, V. and Callicott, R. B.: The comprehensive use of Doppler ultra-sound in farm animal reproduction. Vet. Rec., *88*:202, 1971.
2. Hulet, C. V.: A rectal abdominal palpation technique for diagnosing pregnancy in the ewe. J. Anim. Sci., *35*:814, 1972.
3. Hulet, C. V.: Determining fetal numbers in pregnant ewes. J. Anim. Sci., *36*:325, 1973.
4. Lamond, D. R.: Diagnosis of early pregnancy in the ewe. Aust. Vet. J., *39*:192, 1963.
5. Richardson, C.: Pregnancy diagnosis in the ewe — a review. Vet. Rec., *90*:264, 1972.
6. Turner, C. B. and Hindson, J. C.: An assessment of a method of manual pregnancy diagnosis in the ewe. Vet. Rec., *96*:56, 1975.

Pregnancy Toxemia

A. NEIL BRUERE

Massey University, Palmerston North, New Zealand

Pregnancy toxemia (sleepy sickness, twin lamb disease) has been described in improved breeds of sheep for over 100 years. It is a disease mainly of twin-bearing ewes, who because of undernutrition during the latter stages of pregnancy are unable to maintain normal homeostatic mechanisms. Hypoglycemia and ketosis develop, producing a series of nervous signs that follow a distinct phyletic order depending on the degree of interference with normal brain function. Although many of the biochemical changes seen in pregnancy toxemia are not fully explained, for practical purposes it is now well known as a disease primarily attributable to poor husbandry. The statement by husbandmen that "pregnancy toxemia in sheep occurs when pregnant sheep are fed injudiciously and is prevented when they are fed judiciously" is perhaps an oversimplification but nonetheless is basically the clinical truth.

NUTRITION OF THE PREGNANT EWE

In order to understand the etiology, clinical signs, treatment and prevention of pregnancy toxemia, it is necessary to summarize the major aspects of digestion in the normal sheep and the sheep under the stress of advanced pregnancy. Probably about 70 per cent of the digestible energy of a sheep's ration is derived from the three important volatile fatty acids (VFA) — acetic, propionic and butyric. These are the end products of rumen microbial digestion of a variety of sugars, starch, cellulose, pentosans and pectins. Smaller amounts of energy may be derived from protein by deamination of amino acids.

The mean production of acetic, propionic and butyric acids for a 24-hour period is about 3.7, 1.0 and 0.7 moles, respectively. With the exception of β-hydroxybutyrate, all the VFA pass directly to the liver. However, acetate is mainly metabolized as energy for skeletal muscle, heart and kidney via the tricarboxylic acid cycle. Excess acetate is converted to fat. Propionate is converted to glucose in the liver and excess glucose-like acetate becomes available for lipogenesis in adipose tissue. The reverse process seen in fasting is lipolysis with the appearance of free fatty acids (FFA) in the circulation.

Glucose plays the key role in normal homeostasis of the ewe. Its significance increases dramatically with advancing pregnancy, as glucose forms the basis of energy metabolism of the developing fetus or fetuses (Fig. 1). The glucose requirement for a nonpregnant 50-kg sheep is approximately 110 gm in a 24-hour period.

STRESS IN LATE PREGNANCY

The survival of the ewe and her lambs during the terminal stages of pregnancy does not depend entirely on sudden stress such as inclement weather but basically on the degree of metabolic imbalance that the ewe can withstand before restoring homeostasis in the face of the ever-increasing demand for energy by the fetuses. Glucose and fructose form more than 70 per cent of the oxygen uptake of the fetus. Fructose is synthesized in the placenta, and the total fetal demand for glucose is about 8 to 9 gm/kg of fetus per day or about 30 to 40 gm per day for a single fetus. In twin-bearing ewes the requirement is much higher.

It is therefore easy to understand that the hypoglycemia of twin-bearing ewes on a low plane of nutrition is the result of this high fetal avarice for glucose. The fetuses produce an obligatory drain of the ewe's energy supply.

The ewe responds by restoring homeostasis in the following manner: Lipolysis replaces lipogenesis and FFA may appear in the circulation. However, in pregnancy toxemia FFA conversion to glycerol and glucose is incomplete, fatty infiltration of the liver becomes marked and ketone bodies of higher than normal levels appear in the blood. Protein is also metabolized, gluconeogenesis is increased and the ewe begins to lose body weight rapidly. A severe hyperketonemia now develops, together with the excretion of acetoacetic and β-hydroxybutyric

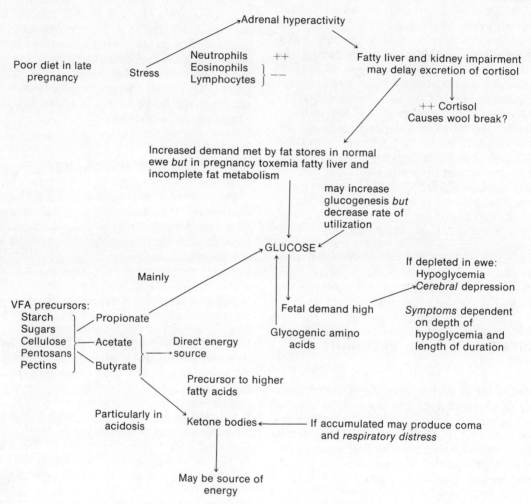

Figure 1. Possible cycle of events in glucose formation and relationship to symptoms of pregnancy toxemia in the ewe.

acids in the urine. The plasma bicarbonate level falls, and metabolic acidosis develops.

Other notable biochemical changes in the pregnant ewe under stress are adrenal hyperactivity and decreased insulin release but increased glucagon release. The hyperactivity of the adrenal, marked by a rise in cortisol levels of blood, may increase gluconeogenesis, but it also acts against the intended effect by inhibiting glucose utilization by the sheep. The hypoglycemia is therefore aggravated. The decrease in insulin release and the increase in glucagon release probably are an attempt to improve gluconeogenesis.

ETIOLOGY AND PREDISPOSING FACTORS

The exact etiology of pregnancy toxemia is unknown, but in general a rapidly declining plane of nutrition in the last 1 to 2 months of pregnancy in twin-bearing ewes is one of the major predisposing factors. Two syndromes, the starvation syndrome and the stress syndrome, are arbitrarily described. In the former, the symptoms are seen as a result of a prolonged period of low nutrition during which the ewe has lost considerable body weight. The latter refers more to the so-called overfat ewe who may not be able to metabolize sufficient food because abdominal space is usurped by fat and by two large fetuses. In either instance some severe trigger factor or stress finally hastens the onset of symptoms.

The following factors predispose to pregnancy toxemia:

1. Prolonged low plane of nutrition in ewes bearing twins. This eventually leads to the starvation syndrome, although under some circumstances a slow reduction in the plane of nutrition may not predispose to pregnancy toxemia unless there is a sudden change, such as bad weather. The explanation given for this is that "adrenal conditioning" is more likely to take place under such circumstances.

2. The overfat ewe bearing twins.

3. Sudden onset of inclement weather when ewes are denied shelter. In some countries prelamb shearing has caused severe outbreaks of pregnancy toxemia.

4. Sudden changes in nutrition. The pregnant ewe requires regular and consistent feeding, particularly in late pregnancy. It is also important not to alter any particular regimen suddenly.

5. Lack of exercise. It is believed that this may contribute to a poor appetite in the overfat ewe. Steady walking or daily movement on to supplementary feed often delays the onset of pregnancy toxemia.

6. Concurrent disease. Many diseases may predispose a sheep to pregnancy toxemia, e.g., foot rot, foot abscess, parasitic infestations and so forth.

7. Individual variation. Some ewes appear to be more resistant to pregnancy toxemia than others.

8. Age of ewes and tooth wear. In some situations ewes that have broken mouths or excessively worn teeth are retained in the mating flock. Such sheep are physically unable to meet the demand for hard grazing prior to lambing, particularly when carrying twins.

CLINICAL SIGNS AND DIAGNOSIS

The veterinarian, in addition to recognizing the signs of pregnancy toxemia in the individual ewe, must be able to assess the general state of health of the flock involved. From this assessment he can advise not only on the treatment of individual cases but also on the more important aspect of improving the nutrition of the other sheep, some of which may not be showing obvious symptoms but could be in the prodromal stage of the disease.

A history of the previous management and feeding will frequently lead rapidly to confirming a diagnosis of pregnancy toxemia. In addition, a close inspection of the flock may reveal sheep showing severe loss of condition (razor back) and wool pull, which is also common in the starvation syndrome. Driving the flock may also show up "stragglers" or sheep that are showing the first nervous signs of pregnancy toxemia. Such sheep will lag behind the flock or may even lie down.

Individual Sheep

The clinical signs in individual ewes are shown in a number of ways and usually follow a pattern that may be relatively brief or spread over a number of days.

Anorexia is a characteristic and early

sign. Intermittent eating may occur, and if the sheep's appetite can be stimulated, further development of the disease may be arrested at this stage. As anorexia advances, the sheep refuses to eat and even food placed in the mouth is briefly chewed and then dropped.

Nervous signs are quite variable but in general tend to follow a phyletic order as far as the brain centers are concerned. The more recently evolved brain centers, such as the cerebral cortex and the neocerebellum, are affected first. The nervous signs, as seen in order of development, are as follows (it must be borne in mind, however, that at any stage several of the signs may be seen):

1. Lagging behind the flock on driving.
2. Recumbency.
3. Teeth grinding.
4. Aimless wandering.
5. Apparent blindness (amaurosis) shown by walking into fences.
6. During recumbency, Kussmaul-Kien respiration is frequently seen (air hunger).
7. More terminally, as additional cerebral centers become involved, blindness, deafness and complete lack of response to stimuli develop.
8. Terminally violent nerve signs are frequently seen, including eye rolling, head tremor and jaw champing.
9. Occasionally some ewes abort their fetuses before advanced symptoms develop and have been known to recover.

The assessment of the stage to which clinical signs have developed bears considerably on the prognosis, and in general once the ewe refuses to eat, the prognosis for recovery is poor.

CLINICAL PATHOLOGY

There are four fairly constant biochemical changes in pregnancy toxemia, namely, hypoglycemia, hyperketonemia, delayed excretion of cortisol and terminal acidosis. The hyperketonemia produces ketonuria that can be detected early, but the main significance of these biochemical changes is their relationship to the various clinical signs. It is generally accepted that the nervous signs are related primarily to the developing and persistent hypoglycemia, and some believe the main lesion to be a hypoglycemic encephalopathy. It is also believed that the hyperketonemia and increased cortisol lev-

els may contribute to the more terminal nervous signs, as does the acidosis. It has been suggested that the wool break and pull so frequently seen in pregnancy toxemia are a result of prolonged cortisol retention. In the stressed starvation syndrome, the sheep usually displays a neutrophilia, a lymphocytopenia and varying degrees of hemoconcentration due to dehydration.

AUTOPSY

As a clinician, it is frequently necessary to explain the autopsy features of pregnancy toxemia to the owner of the affected flock in order to convince him of the serious nature of the disease. The gross autopsy features are as follows:

1. Multiple fetuses are almost invariably to be found in the uterus. In advanced cases they will have died before the ewe and may have undergone varying stages of autolysis.
2. One outstanding autopsy feature is the enlarged, fatty liver, which is usually quite friable. On histological examination, the liver cells are full of mobilized fat.
3. Kidneys are usually pale, and fat accumulation in the tubules is not uncommon. The histopathological features are those of uremia.
4. The blood vessels of the mesentery are usually distended and in early autopsies have a blue-hued appearance of cyanosis.
5. The adrenal gland is usually enlarged, particularly in the starvation syndrome. The cortex is usually dark, and the medulla is light in color.

PROGNOSIS

Any consideration of treatment, either for the individual ewe or for the entire flock, must be based on a careful prognosis. It should be emphasized to the sheep farmer that the current and future loss of production of the flock in which cases of pregnancy toxemia are occurring is a very real consideration. In general, the clinically affected animals are the danger sign that indicates that the husbandry of the flock needs careful assessment and improvement. In flocks in which a high incidence of pregnancy toxemia has occurred, it is likely that the rest of the flock will perform below its limit during that season. Lamb weights may be reduced at birth and the lambs may be less viable, lactation will be delayed in onset and may never attain its peak, mothering behavior of the ewe will be impaired and wool defects in the ewe will be more prevalent. Wool weights will invariably be reduced.

TREATMENT

The value of treating individual animals with pregnancy toxemia depends entirely on the degree to which the symptoms have progressed. In general, once anorexia becomes complete there is little chance of recovery. Treatments are many but are mainly applicable only in the relatively early stages following the onset of the clinical signs. Severely depressed and recumbent animals are better destroyed.

Glycerol, Glucose and Insulin

These materials are useful primarily in the early stages of the disease. Glycerol is given by mouth at the rate of 150 to 200 ml with water either daily or twice daily. Glucose may be given by intravenous injection; a dose of 250 to 500 ml of a 5 per cent solution is adequate. Some people recommend the use of insulin, 40 IU of a long-acting type given subcutaneously, to increase the usage of the glycerol and glucose. Such treatments, however, are expensive, particularly when large numbers of animals are involved.

The developing ketosis should also be treated with bicarbonate, which may be given with a balanced electrolyte solution to combat the concurrent dehydration and acidosis. The general recommendation is 1 to 3 liters of a balanced electrolyte solution containing 50 mEq/L of bicarbonate equivalents as acetate or gluconate.

The use of glucocorticoids to induce hyperglycemia seems to be of little value. In view of the already elevated cortisol levels in pregnancy toxemia, it is hard to rationalize their use.

Other forms of therapy practiced include cesarean section and the use of abortifacients. Once the fetuses have been removed, blood glucose frequently reaches normal levels and the ewe may recover very rapidly.

Some workers have reported on the force-feeding by stomach tube of ewes that have lost their appetite. Thin gruels and chopped grass can be fed in this way. However, the point remains that the main role of the modern veterinarian is to turn his attention to the yet clinically unaffected animals and to insure that in future years the husbandry of the flock is improved in order to prevent pregnancy toxemia.

PREVENTION

Rations for pregnant ewes have already been given (see page 882). The prevention of pregnancy toxemia requires that adequate fodder is stocked to insure that these recommendations can be achieved, particularly during late pregnancy. It is also important to see to such factors as exercise to insure adequate stimulation to appetite. Under all circumstances, any procedure, such as pre-lamb crutching, shearing and so forth, must be carried out in such a way as to reduce prolonged periods without fodder and to avoid hungry sheep facing inclement weather. Concurrent disease must be controlled, and those who are responsible for the management of the flock must be consistent with their husbandry and alert to any changes that are likely to reduce the ewe's intake of food.

REFERENCES

1. Kronfeld, D. S.: Ketosis in pregnant sheep and lactating cows. A review. Aust. Vet. J., *48*:680, 1972.
2. Reid, R. L. : The physiopathology of undernourishment in pregnant sheep with particular reference to pregnancy toxaemia. Adv. Vet. Sci., *12*:163, 1968.

Infectious Ovine Abortion

E. D. FIELDEN

Massey University, Palmerston North, New Zealand

Although sporadic cases of abortion and fetal mummification are regularly observed on sheep farms, the major causes for concern are those enzootics that occur from time to time and that lead to substantial loss of potential progeny, not only from abortion but also from perinatal death of lambs. Some of the agents concerned directly attack the fetus or placenta, or both, leading to what is often called a primary abortion. Others, because of the marked systemic disturbance caused to the ewe, result in secondary abortion. A list of agents that have been reported to cause prenatal loss, together with the reported stage of gestation at which the loss generally occurs, can be seen in Figure 1 of the article on Prenatal Loss, page 896. Further references are made to congenital infections and their relationship to perinatal lamb deaths in the article on Perinatal Lamb Mortality, page 918.

Two major problems confront the veterinarian faced with one of these outbreaks: first, the need to establish a diagnosis and second, control of the disease. Diagnosis is not difficult if one is aware of the type of problem that exists in the area with which you are concerned. Careful gross examination is made of several dead or dying lambs and their placentae (many characteristic lesions associated with diseases causing ovine abortion occur), and care is taken in selection and transport of specimens to a competent diagnostic laboratory. Control, both because of problems of cost and because of our limited knowledge of the epidemiology of many of these diseases, may be an entirely different matter. It would not be possible, within the limitations of this article, to deal comprehensively with all the infectious agents that may cause abortion and perinatal mortality in sheep. I have therefore selected and tabulated some of the more important conditions that have been described and have commented particularly on matters that are relevant to their diagnosis and control (Table 1 and Figs. 1 and 2). Further information concerning these diseases can be obtained from the references listed.

SELECTION AND TRANSPORT OF DIAGNOSTIC SPECIMENS

1. Reliable laboratory diagnosis depends on a correct selection of specimens that reach the laboratory in a satisfactory condition for processing. A comprehensive case history concerning the problem under investigation should be submitted with the specimens (see previous comment on the value of gross examination of dead and dying lambs and placentae).

2. Remember the cardinal law of diagnosis is that you have every chance of not finding what you don't look for! It is therefore generally better to submit too many samples rather than too few.

3. You should consult with your own diagnostic servicing laboratory personnel concerning their requirements regarding selection of diagnostic material and method of packaging and transport in your own particular area. Submission of the following material will generally permit diagnosis of known infectious diseases causing abortion in sheep to be made:

   a. Placenta including placental cotyledon — fixed and fresh.
   b. Fresh fetuses — chilled if they can be delivered rapidly to the laboratory — otherwise:
      (1) Fetal liver and lung — fresh and fixed.
      (2) Fetal abomasum and contents — fresh.
      (3) Fetal heart blood or exudate from body cavities, or both — fresh.
      (4) Fetal brain — fixed.
   c. Whole blood (only if specimen reaches the laboratory in 24 hours) or sera from affected ewes.
   d. Vaginal discharge from affected ewes — fresh.

4. Fresh material to be used for microbiological examination should be packaged individually in sterile containers to avoid cross contamination and should be chilled (use coolant packs and insulated containers). Deep frozen tissues are generally suitable for virological and most bacteriological examinations but not for histopathological studies.

5. Material for histopathological exami-

TABLE 1. *Infectious Diseases Causing Ovine Abortion and/or Perinatal Loss*

Disease	Transmission	Clinical Features	Gross Pathology of Fetus and Placenta	Diagnostic Aids
VIBRIOSIS:				
Campylobacter fetus var. *intestinalis* affects sheep. The same serotype occasionally affects cattle. Vibriosis is widespread and is regarded as an important cause of ovine abortion in Britain, the United States and New Zealand.	Ingestion, especially during last 2 months of gestation. Rapid spread occurs during close confinement of ewes during lambing.	Abortions in late pregnancy, stillbirths, birth of weak, infected progeny. The disease tends to occur in epidemic form every 4 to 5 years; seldom seen as cause of serious loss in same flock in successive years. Metritis may occur after abortion; other ewes die from peritonitis following retention of dead lambs.	Placentitis with edema and necrosis of cotyledons; cotyledons sometimes diffusely pale. The placental lesions are usually not as severe as with brucellosis. Fetus shows usual signs of intrauterine death with subcutaneous blood-stained edema and excess fluid in body cavities. In about 40 per cent of cases characteristic circumscribed necrotic foci 10 to 20 mm in diameter occur in the liver (see Fig. 1).	Culture and direct microscopy to identify organisms from placenta, fetal stomach contents and uterine discharge after abortion.

CONTROL OF VIBRIOSIS:
1. During an outbreak careful attention should be paid to hygiene if at all practicable. Thus, affected ewes (and their surviving lambs) should be isolated until genital discharges cease; dead fetuses, lambs and placentae should be burnt or destroyed with quicklime; the pen area or lambing site should be disinfected. Spreading out the ewes in advanced pregnancy over a wide grazing area reduces contact with infective material. Running both ewes in early pregnancy and those not yet bred with aborting ewes helps spread natural immunity in the flock.
2. The use of a formalinized vaccine of the same serotype as the organism causing the outbreak and/or the intramuscular injection of all in-contact ewes in advanced pregnancy with 300,000 IU of penicillin and 1 gm of dihydrostreptomycin may reduce losses *provided very early diagnosis is made.* The cost of such a procedure needs careful evaluation.
3. Although the prophylactic use of such a vaccine for all replacement ewes each year will confer a 2- to 3-year immunity, this may not be economically justifiable because of the cyclical nature of the disease on a property.

BRUCELLOSIS:				
Brucella melitensis affects sheep, goats and other species including man. It is recorded in continental Europe, the Mediterranean area, Africa, Central America and rarely in the United States. *Br. abortus,* particularly important in cattle and other species including man, only occasionally affects sheep.	Ingestion is main method, especially during the lambing period. Droplet inhalation and entry both through the conjunctival membrane and broken skin occasionally occur. Venereal transmission following natural mating is rare.	Abortions in late pregnancy, stillbirths, birth of weak, infected progeny. Congenital infections may persist throughout life (especially *Br. melitensis*). Systemic effects may be seen in the dam with fever, lameness (associated with joint swellings), sometimes central nervous system (CNS) signs.	Essential lesion is placentitis with edema and necrosis of cotyledons. The intercotyledonary membrane may be thickened, yellow-brown and leathery; cotyledons show yellow-brown necrotic areas, often with adjacent hemorrhage. Mucopurulent material may be adherent to the allantochorion. Fetus shows usual signs of intrauterine death.	Culture and direct microscopy to identify organisms that are plentiful in placenta, fetal stomach and vaginal discharge of ewe. Modified Ziehl-Neelsen technique is satisfactory for staining for direct microscopy. Complement fixation (CF) test on sera of aborting ewes.
Br. ovis affects sheep only and has been reported in Central Europe, South Africa, Western United States, Australia and New Zealand.	Method of natural transmission in ewes is not known. For spread of the disease in rams see page 941.	Pathogenicity for the ewe is low, and outbreaks of abortion have been reported only in New Zealand. *Br. ovis* is more important as a cause of ram wastage.	As above.	As above. (For diagnosis of the disease in rams see page 941.)

Table continued on the following page.

TABLE 1. *Infectious Diseases Causing Ovine Abortion and/or Perinatal Loss (Continued)*

Disease	Transmission	Clinical Features	Gross Pathology of Fetus and Placenta	Diagnostic Aids
CONTROL OF BRUCELLOSIS: 1. Test and slaughter policy can be used in areas where the disease is under control and appropriate testing of replacement stock can be undertaken. 2. Otherwise general hygiene at lambing and protection of ewes before first breeding using *Br. melitensis* (Elberg Rev. 1) or *Br. abortus* strain 19 vaccines. 3. For control of *Br. ovis* infections see page 941.				
SALMONELLOSIS (paratyphoid abortion): *Salmonella abortus ovis* is relatively uncommon but endemic in the south of England and parts of Europe. Other salmonella species, which are widespread throughout the world, may cause abortion in sheep, e.g., *S. dublin*, *S. typhimurium*, *S. oranienburg* and so forth. Salmonellosis can affect man.	Ingestion of contaminated food and water usually from a carrier animal(s). Ewes in late-pregnancy appear more susceptible. Over-crowding and other forms of stress favor an outbreak.	Abortions, stillbirths, birth of weak, infected progeny that usually die within 7 days of birth. Ewes show high fever before aborting; most recover but some die from metritis and/or septicemia. Some ewes and newborn lambs show diarrhea; in the lamb this is usually fatal. Where infection is endemic, abortions tend to be confined to the younger ewes.	No specific placental lesions have been reported. Aborted fetuses show usual signs of intrauterine death. Septicemia lesions may be seen in those lambs dying during or shortly after birth.	Culture of organisms from fetus, placenta and uterine discharge. Serum agglutination tests, where available, may be useful on a flock basis for identifying presence of the particular organism.
CONTROL OF SALMONELLOSIS: 1. Maintenance of a closed flock, avoidance of overcrowding and other stress situations and rodent control in areas where food contamination is a problem. During an outbreak normal hygienic precautions as described for vibriosis help reduce the rate of spread. 2. Mass treatment of exposed animals with drugs is generally disappointing and usually economically unjustified. Individual cases can be given 10 mg/kg of tetracycline per day until improvement occurs (fluid therapy in conjunction with, or even instead of, such treatment may be just as effective). 3. Vaccines given before unavoidable exposure of susceptible ewes to the disease have been suggested as being of value. Because of the natural immunity that develops following exposure to the disease, careful evaluation of the real merit of such vaccines is required.				
LISTERIOSIS: *Listeria monocytogenes* affects a wide range of animals, including man. It usually manifests as a meningoencephalitic form in adult ruminants, but abortions and perinatal lamb losses have been described in cattle, sheep and goats. The organism is probably worldwide but appears to be of most significance in North America, Iceland, Britain, Europe, Australia and New Zealand.	Portal of infection under natural conditions is not clear but ingestion, inhalation, conjunctival contamination and venereal transmission are all thought to occur. The organism is robust and survives well in soil and poor quality (high pH) silage; in such silage, active multiplication of organisms readily occurs.	Abortion may occur from the twelfth week of gestation on but is generally in late pregnancy. Affected lambs born alive generally die. Metritis commonly occurs, and a fatal septicemia may develop in both the ewe and lamb. The meningoencephalitic form of the disease is not often found with the abortion form in natural outbreaks of the disease. Ewes that survive generally do not abort again from this disease, and the total incidence of abortion in a flock rarely	Placental lesions may be similar to those for brucellosis but are generally less severe. In the fetus numerous gray-yellow abscesses 1 to 2 mm in diameter are often seen scattered throughout the liver and lung. Meningeal edema and congestion are commonly observed in the fetus.	Culture of organisms from fetal stomach, liver, placenta and uterine discharge. A fluorescent antibody (FAB) test to detect the organisms has been developed.

Apart from general hygiene in respect to disposal of aborted and dying lambs and isolation of affected ewes when cases occur, there is little that can be done to control the disease. Heavy feeding of spoiled silage should be avoided, but this is more likely to be associated with the septicemic form of the disease in feedlot lambs. Both killed and attenuated vaccines have been produced; their efficacy under field conditions remains to be evaluated, and no recommendation can be made at the present time.

BORDER DISEASE (hairy shaker disease):

Appears to be caused by a viral agent serologically related to the BVD virus. More than one strain may be involved. The disease has been described in Britain, America, New Zealand and Australia.

Probably by ingestion and inhalation of aerosols, but method of ewe to ewe transmission is not known. Vertical transmission from ewe to lamb during gestation is well established. Venereal spread cannot be excluded.

Losses of potential progeny at any stage during pregnancy and in the postnatal period occur. Infertility with a marked increase in barren ewes, fetal mummification and/or maceration, abortions, stillbirths and losses of lambs born alive are all features of the disease. When the fleece has developed, it tends to be hairy and may be pigmented. If born alive, lambs may show muscular tremors causing incoordination and difficulty in nursing.

Cotyledons tend to be small for fetal age; they occasionally show areas of focal necrosis (1 to 3 mm). Fetal mummification; hairy, pigmented coats if the wool has developed; fetus small for gestational age; muscular tremors and incoordination if lambs are born alive are all signs of the disease.

CNS shows hypomyelinogenesis. BVD neutralizing antibodies in serum of dam or lamb may help to differentiate the disease from enzootic ataxia.

CONTROL OF BORDER DISEASE:

No satisfactory recommendations concerning control can be made at present. Separation of sheep from cattle known to have BVD would appear to be a wise precaution.

The efficacy of vaccines in controlling the disease has yet to be evaluated.

TOXOPLASMOSIS:

Toxoplasma gondii affects a wide range of animals and man. It is widespread and has been reported in Australia, New Zealand, Britain, Turkey, USSR and North America. The same organism infects and behaves like a coccidian in cats, which are thought to be natural hosts. Other species such as sheep and man are regarded as secondary hosts. In these species the organism is found in two forms: (1) trophozoites, which are actively multiplying, invasive and found in the acute state of the disease and (2) cysts found in the chronic phase of the disease.

Congenital transmission from ewe to lamb is established, but the method of spread during an epidemic is not understood. Ingestion of food contaminated by cat feces may be responsible for spread of the infection.

Ewes infected in the earlier stages of pregnancy either resorb the embryo or fetal death and mummification (often only one of a twin pair) may occur. Infection in late pregnancy leads to abortion and perinatal losses of lambs. Many congenitally affected lambs survive. Disease in the adult is generally asymptomatic, occasionally CNS signs develop. In areas where endemic, only younger ewes usually lose lambs.

Gross lesions of the cotyledons (numerous gray-white foci 1 to 3 mm in diameter) are indicative of the disease (see Fig. 2). Not all cotyledons are equally affected, and such lesions should be differentiated from nonspecific calcification. Mummified fetuses may be seen; otherwise focal leukomalacia in the brain of stillborn lambs or lambs dying shortly after birth is a common finding — microscopy of brain sections is nearly always necessary to confirm this.

Histological examination of cotyledon to demonstrate focal areas of necrosis and organisms; histological examination of fetal brain to demonstrate focal leukomalacia. All serological tests relate poorly to clinical stage of the disease. Other immunological tests are being evaluated.

CONTROL OF TOXOPLASMOSIS:

Since the immunity that is induced following a natural infection leads to a reduction in subsequent losses of lambs, it has been suggested that unbred flock replacements should be exposed to aborting ewes to aid the development of natural immunity. Until more is known of the epidemiology of the disease in sheep flocks, no other forms of control seem to be practicable at present.

Table continued on the following page.

TABLE 1. *Infectious Diseases Causing Ovine Abortion and/or Perinatal Loss (Continued)*

Disease	Transmission	Clinical Features	Gross Pathology of Fetus and Placenta	Diagnostic Aids
ENZOOTIC ABORTION (EAE, chlamydial abortion): Caused by a chlamydial agent that affects sheep, occasionally goats and cattle, rarely man. Abortion-producing strains differ antigenically from strains producing polyarthritis (sheep and cattle) and ovine conjunctivitis. The disease appears to be of greatest importance in Britain, Europe and the Western United States.	Ingestion during the lambing period following contamination of food and surroundings by aborted fetuses, placentae and vaginal discharge. Spread is more rapid when ewes are confined; droplet inhalation may also occur under these conditions.	Late abortions, stillbirths and birth of weak, infected progeny. Since fetal death often occurs some time before abortion takes place, fetal mummification is commonly seen. Lambs with congenital infections usually abort during their first pregnancy; ewes infected in the last month of pregnancy may not abort until the next gestation period, i.e., latent infections occur. Ewes seldom abort more than once.	A chorionitis with the chorionic epithelial cells packed with elementary bodies appears to be the essential lesion. Since both gross and microscopic lesions are similar to those of ovine brucellosis, isolation of the actual organism causing the disease is imperative.	Placental smears and smears of vaginal discharge (but not fetal stomach) stained by the modified Ziehl-Neelsen technique. (FAB techniques provide more specific identification where available). Organisms can be cultured in yolk sac of embryonating chicken eggs. CF test of aborting ewes (of limited value).

CONTROL OF ENZOOTIC ABORTION:

1. During an outbreak all aborting ewes and weak lambs and their dams should be isolated until uterine discharges cease and surviving lambs are normal. Infected placentae, dead lambs and lambing areas should be handled as for vibriosis.
2. Although treatment of in-contact ewes with intramuscular oxytetracycline (12 mg/kg for 2 to 4 days) has been reported to have value in field outbreaks, it is doubtful whether the return justifies the cost. At the time of impending abortion, irreversible damage has already taken place.
3. Immunization with commercial killed vaccine of susceptible ewes before breeding appears to protect for at least 2 to 3 years. This may be justifiable in some areas where the disease is endemic and losses are severe.

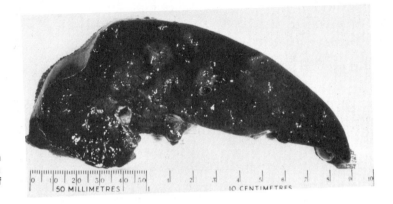

Figure 1. Necrotic foci in liver seen in about 40 per cent of lambs born dead or dying during an outbreak of ovine vibriosis.

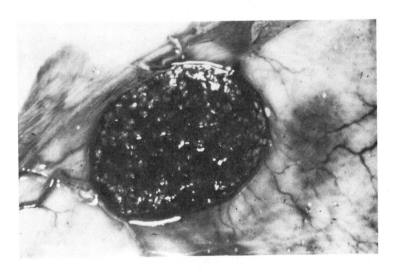

Figure 2. Characteristic necrotic foci seen in cotyledon during an outbreak of toxoplasmosis.

nations should be fixed in neutral solutions of 10 per cent formalin (1 volume of commercial formalin with 9 volumes of water) as soon as possible after collection. Brains, cotyledon and placental tissue should be fixed whole. Several slices of lung and liver (about 5 mm thick, using boundary zones including normal and abnormal tissue when this can be seen) permit better fixation for these specimens.

REFERENCES

1. Arthur, G. H.: Veterinary Reproduction and Obstetrics. 4th Ed. London, Bailliere Tindall, 1975.
2. Jensen, R.: Diseases of Sheep. Philadelphia, Lea and Febiger, 1974.
3. Manktelow, B. W.: Gross pathological features and laboratory diagnosis of infectious diseases of the sheep placenta and foetus. Proceedings of New Zealand Veterinary Association Sheep Society. 3rd Seminar. Massey University, 1973, p. 58.

Vaginal Prolapse

E. D. FIELDEN

Massey University, Palmerston North, New Zealand

Prolapse of the vagina (bearing trouble) consists of displacement of some organs or tissue, bringing about an eversion of part or all of the vaginal wall in such a manner that the mucosa is visible between the lips of the vulva. When the lateral and dorsal walls evert, the bowel is often involved; when the ventral wall everts, the bladder is often contained within the prolapsed mass. In the latter case, urine flow is generally obstructed. The majority of cases in sheep result in the whole, rather than just part, of the vaginal wall everting. The condition is not related to prolapse of the uterus but is sometimes associated with "ringwomb."

INCIDENCE AND SIGNIFICANCE

Vaginal prolapse in ewes occurs in most countries of the world but varies in frequency because of differences in husbandry and perhaps breed type. Thus, the incidence is low in Merino sheep run under extensive conditions, as in Australian and North American range country. However, in sheep farming areas of the North Island of New Zealand, where sheep of predominantly New Zealand Romney blood run on grass/clover pastures, the annual incidence may rise to 12 per cent in individual flocks. Most English breeds and their crosses seem susceptible; the greatest frequency is seen in mature ewes in advanced pregnancy. Occasionally, cases occur at or after lambing; many of these are relapses of cases occurring before lambing. Rarely is the condition seen in the maiden ewe unless she is grazing "estrogenic" pasture.

On an individual farm basis, prolapse of the vagina may result in significant losses since approximately 40 per cent of affected ewes either die following complications associated with the condition or are destroyed for humane reasons. Many of those ewes that survive experience difficulty in lambing and as a consequence have a high rate of stillborn lambs. As prolapse of the vagina has an established hereditary basis in the ewe and because risk of recurrence of the condition in the affected animal is high, surviving ewes are generally marked for culling and are lost to the breeding flock.

PREDISPOSING AND PRECIPITATING FACTORS

Although an hereditary predisposition to prolapse of the vagina has been proved by selection and breeding studies, it is still not entirely clear why some ewes suffer from the problem and others do not.

Predisposition to prolapse is greatest when tissues associated with the reproductive tract are slack, as occurs close to lambing. Therefore, there is an increased potential for displacement at this time.

If a predisposition exists, any factor leading to an increase in intra-abdominal pressure is likely to precipitate the disease. Advanced pregnancy, ewes with multiple fetuses, abundant lush feed, overfatness, topography of the grazing area (which affects the position that the ewe adopts when lying down to rest) and lack of exercise (when the ewe spends long periods in sternal recumbency) all contribute to such a situation.

DIAGNOSIS AND TREATMENT

Diagnosis is readily made by visual appraisal. Treatment involves restraining the animal, preferably with the hindquarters elevated; emptying the bladder (usually easily achieved by simple elevation of the prolapsed mass, thus overcoming the urethral occlusion); cleansing of the everted tissue with a nonirritant solution (physiological saline is preferable); lubrication with an obstetrical cream and replacement of the vaginal mass by gentle manipulation using the fingers and hands. Epidural anesthesia is rarely found necessary.

Once the vaginal mass is returned, it can be retained by means of a subcutaneous suture encircling the vulva (Fig. 1). This suture must be released before the ewe lambs. When the process of parturition is complete, the suture may be retied if the prolapse shows any tendency to recur. Otherwise, sutures are removed after lambing. Should straining be severe and if there is difficulty in retaining the prolapse, either immediate induction of parturition if the ewe is within 14 days of lambing (see page 967) or cesarean section should be considered.

Whenever a prolapse is replaced, the ewe should be identified (for future culling), and one injection of a long-acting penicillin such as Prolopen Hypodermic* should be given to help prevent complications, particularly those associated with clostridial infection.

If severe necrosis of the prolapsed tissue has occurred, amputation may be required to salvage the life of the ewe. Surgical procedures similar to those used for amputating a prolapsed rectum in any species are followed, with care being taken not to excise either the urethral orifice or any viscera that may be contained in the prolapsed mass.

PREVENTION AND CONTROL

Culling of affected ewes, together with disposal of their lambs for purposes other than breeding, should be the cornerstones of any control policy for this disease. Rams for use in the breeding flock should be selected from parents with no history of "bearing trouble."

---

*Prolopen Hypodermic (biodegradable): Glaxo Laboratories (New Zealand) Ltd., Palmerston North, N.Z. Each tube delivers sodium penicillin, 100,000 IU; procaine penicillin, 250,000 IU; and benethamine penicillin, 500,000 IU.

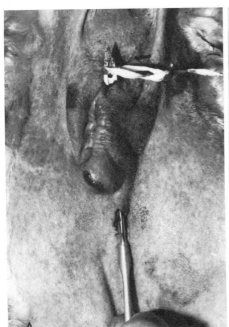 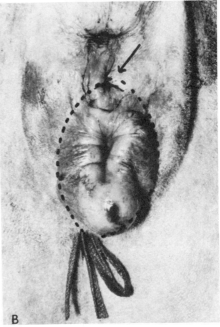

Figure 1. *A,* An umbilical tape-retaining suture being inserted with a 15 cm Gerlach's suture needle (Buhner method). A large half-curved cutting needle and a synthetic material such as Synthofil are equally suitable. *B,* Suture in position (dotted lines indicate its subcutaneous course). The arrow points to the area where the stab wound between the dorsal commissure of the vulva and the anus has been closed.

In addition, a management program should be devised in which the level of nutrition, degree of exercise and use of grazing land of different topographical types are all directed toward maintaining high productivity and avoiding producing any situation that might precipitate an outbreak of the disease. Methods of achieving this must depend on conditions that prevail on the individual farm.

REFERENCES

1. Arthur, G. H.: Veterinary Reproduction and Obstetrics. 4th Ed. London, Bailliere Tindall, 1975, pp. 124–130.
2. Davies, F. G.: The occurrence of vaginal eversion and allied disorders in fat ewes. Res. Vet. Sci., *11*:86, 1970.
3. McLean, J. W. and Claxton, J. H.: Vaginal prolapse in ewes. VII, The measurement and effect of intra-abdominal pressure. N.Z. Vet. J., *8*:51, 1960.

Dystocia

K. D. McSPORRAN

Wallaceville Animal Research Centre, Private Bag, Upper Hutt, New Zealand

Dystocia is commonly understood to mean difficult birth. Unfortunately, "difficult" in this context may be interpreted many ways. Therefore, it is important to insure that the problem does not stem either from excessive interference, which may result in the temporary cessation of labor, or simply from overzealous shepherding. In this article, dystocia refers to parturition that directly or indirectly results in injury to the lamb or the ewe.

Dystocia is often a major cause of lamb loss in the flock. Perinatal mortality may result from the direct effects of dystocia, e.g., hypoxia (see following article), or from the indirect effects, e.g., altered behavior of the ewe or lamb. The occurrence of dystocia varies both within and among breeds, often being high in lowland breeds selected for meat production, e.g., the Texel, Dorset Horn and Romney, but low in breeds such as the Merino and Scottish Blackface that are raised principally for wool production and are run under extensive systems of management. Such a situation has probably arisen from the reduced selection against dystocia as a consequence of intensive shepherding in lowland breeds, together with changes in the conformation brought about by selective breeding to improve carcass quality for meat production.

TYPES OF DYSTOCIA

The most common form of dystocia results from either a simple disproportion between the normally disposed* lamb and the maternal pelvis or a maldisposition of the lamb. The relative importance of each may vary greatly among flocks and breeds. Maldisposition of the lamb is common in sheep and is often associated with dystocia. Postural abnormalities involving the forelegs are most commonly encountered. Flexion of the shoulder with extension (more common), but also flexion, of the elbow accounts for the majority of these abnormalities. Posterior presentation with flexion or extension of the hip joint and, to a lesser extent, flexion of the neck with retention of the head is also important. Numerous other abnormalities have been recorded but occur only sporadically. Maldispositions do not all invariably result in dystocia. Unilateral shoulder flexion with extension of the elbow, a very common form of maldisposition, often simply prolongs parturition without resulting in dystocia. On the other hand, bilateral shoulder flexion with extension of the elbow and posterior presentation with hip flexion are less likely to be compatible with a normal birth.

A form of dystocia colloquially known as "ringwomb" and characterized by failure of the cervix to dilate occurs sporadically in sheep. The etiology of the condition is not clear but is probably related to a hormonal dysfunction affecting the cervix. A condition simulating "ringwomb" has been observed in ewes that have been treated with diethylstilbestrol or dexamethasone during late pregnancy. In the iatrogenic form of the disease, the lesion is apparently confined to

---

* Disposition relates to the orientation of the fetal axis and extremities and encompasses presentation, position and posture. Maldisposition is used to describe any abnormality in disposition.

the cervix, since uterine activity is indistinguishable from that of normal labor.

Dystocia associated with vulvar stenosis has been reported in Australia as one manifestation of a serious breeding problem of ewes grazing estrogenic subterranean clover pastures. Uterine inertia often results if the condition is undetected, and the mortality of ewes and lambs is high.

FACTORS INFLUENCING THE INCIDENCE OF DYSTOCIA

The ewe has an important influence on the incidence of dystocia, and the repeatability of the condition is reported to be high. A recent survey of 2500 births showed that in consecutive years 34 per cent of ewes that had been assisted to lamb during the previous year required assistance again, compared with only 16 per cent for those ewes that had not been assisted. It is probable that this effect is mediated to a large extent by the size of the pelvic inlet of the ewe. Differences in the area of the pelvic inlet have been demonstrated between ewes with and without histories of dystocia, and the area of the pelvic inlet has been correlated with the history of occurrence of dystocia in individual ewes. Parity of the ewe has little influence on the incidence of dystocia, despite the fact that parturition is often prolonged in the primiparous dam.

Lamb weight also has an important influence on the outcome of parturition. This was clearly demonstrated in a recent 9-year flock survey conducted by the author in which a high correlation was shown to exist between the annual incidence of assisted lambings and the mean birth weight of single lambs.

Maldisposition of the lamb is an important presenting cause of dystocia. Because maldisposition appears to be positively related to birth weight, it may be a manifestation of a disproportion in size between the ewe and the lamb, thus exacerbating an already difficult situation. In feral breeds the relationship between the size of the maternal pelvis and the size of the lamb is such that dystocia is uncommon and the absolute prevalence of maldisposition of the lamb is low (about 8 per cent). However, in breeds such as the Texel, disproportion between the lamb and the maternal pelvis occurs more frequently, dystocia is common and the incidence of maldisposition of the lamb is high (up to 43 per cent of all lambs born). Maldisposition of the lamb may result from the lamb's being unable, because of lack of space, to complete its conversion from a state of flexion, which has existed throughout gestation, to a state of extension, in preparation for parturition. Radiographs taken in the days before birth can demonstrate some of the maldispositions encountered at birth. Alternatively, maldispositions may be produced during the birth process by the repeated attempts of the ewe to force the lamb into the pelvic inlet. The explanation for the occurrence of posterior presentations is more uncertain, since the birth weight of the lamb appears to play little part in its development.

A high level of nutrition may increase the level of dystocia because of its effect on the birth weight of the lamb. However, it is difficult to determine to what extent nutrition is responsible for disproportion in size between the lamb and the maternal pelvis because it is only one of a number of factors involved. There is no evidence to support the view that nutrition plays an important part in determining the incidence of dystocia.

A sire effect on dystocia has been demonstrated in a recent study in which the disorder was found to be related to the birth weight of lambs within the sire groups.

REDUCING THE INCIDENCE OF DYSTOCIA

The incidence of dystocia in the flock can be reduced to a low level simply by the implementation of a selection policy that excludes all ewes assisted to lamb, together with their lambs, from the breeding flock. Such a policy has been adopted by a number of stud breeders in New Zealand with the result that the incidence of dystocia in their flocks is falling. On one large Romney stud farm the incidence is now consistently less than 2 per cent, and often less than 1 per cent, of all ewes lambing. Attempts to achieve this end by selecting for increased pelvic size have been thwarted by the poor correlation shown to exist between external pelvic measurements and internal pelvic dimensions. This is of little consequence, however, since selection, using the natural expression of a disparity in size between the lamb and the maternal pelvis (i.e., dystocia) as a criterion rather than pelvic measurements, is both practicable and effective as both lamb size and pelvic size are involved.

Attention should be paid to the nutrition of replacement breeding stock to insure that pelvic growth is not retarded by undernutrition. Such a situation can lead to increased dystocia in breeding ewes.

Selection of rams must also be considered, as the sire can have an effect on the incidence of dystocia irrespective of whether the same or a different breed of ram is used. Sires should be selected from flocks with a low incidence of dystocia and preferably from those with good individual performance records.

REFERENCES

1. Fogarty, N. M. and Thompson, J. M.: Relationship between pelvic dimensions, other body measurements and dystocia in Dorset Horn ewes. Aust. Vet. J., *50*:502, 1974.
2. McSporran, K. D.: Some aspects of dystocia in sheep, with particular reference to Romney stud ewes. Ph.D. thesis, Massey University, New Zealand, 1975.
3. Maaktgeboren, C., Bakker-Slotboom, M. F., Von Maren, M. J. and Stegeman, J. H. J.: Parturition in Texel sheep and Heath sheep, a contribution on the influence of domestication on birth. (Translated from the Dutch). Z. Tierzucht. Zucht. Biol., *88*:169, 1971.

Perinatal Lamb Mortality

K. G. HAUGHEY

The University of Sydney, Camden, New South Wales, Australia

Perinatal lamb mortality, defined as deaths occurring before, during or within 7 days of birth, is the major known source of wastage to the sheep industry. In Australia and New Zealand for example, the respective losses average 25 per cent and 15 per cent of lambs born, rising to as high as 45 per cent in individual grazing breeding flocks. Nearly all deaths occur during or within 3 days of birth. Losses vary greatly within and between flocks, districts and seasons.

ESTIMATION OF PERINATAL LOSS

Perinatal loss may be estimated directly or indirectly. Direct estimation involves counting the number of lambs born and expressing those dying as a percentage of the total born. This method is practicable only in closely shepherded lambing flocks in areas free from predators and scavengers. Indirect estimation involves "wet-drying" the breeding flock after lambing, i.e., the identification and removal of all ewes not rearing a lamb or lambs. "Wet-drying" can be carried out any time up to weaning but is more reliable when carried out within a few weeks of lambing, usually at lamb-marking. It is the most practical technique for estimating losses in large flocks

that are not intensively shepherded during lambing. The flock is classified into dry ewes (ewes that have failed to lamb) and lambed ewes. This latter group can be subdivided into those rearing a lamb, or lambs, and those losing all lambs.

The classification is based on the body condition and fleece quality of the ewe; the presence of "lambing stain," i.e., contamination of the posterior surface of the udder and hocks with the discharges resulting from lambing; udder development and the nature of udder secretions. Dry ewes have neither udder development nor "lambing stain" and usually show better body condition and fleeces than lambed ewes. Lambed ewes have enlarged udders, usually show "lambing stain" and have poorer fleeces and body condition than dry ewes. Ewes rearing lambs have full, resilient udders containing milk. The teats and adjacent areas are clean, soft and pliable as a result of the lamb's sucking activity. Ewes that have lost all lambs have variably developed udders with a tendency to cleavage between the two glands. The teats are stiff and dirty, with udder secretions ranging from normal to thin, watery or honey-colored viscous material. The perinatal mortality is represented by the number of ewes that have lost all lambs in relation to the total number of ewes that have lambed, expressed as a percentage. The estimate represents minimal loss because it does not take into account the extent of cross-mothering or situations in which one or both twins die. However, as 90 per cent of mortality occurs during or within 3 days of parturition, the estimate is a reliable reflection of minimal perinatal lamb mortality.

INVESTIGATION OF PERINATAL MORTALITY

Necropsy, supported by appropriate microbiological and histopathological examinations, is the simplest and most reliable method of determining causes of loss. An adequate sample (arbitrarily 50 carcasses that are representative of mortality throughout lambing) must be examined to arrive at a realistic assessment of the relative contributions that various entities make to total mortality. Table 1 lists the minimum number of carcasses required to detect a specific entity in at least one carcass with 95 per cent confidence, given a designated theoretical incidence in the flock.

Fetal membranes should be collected with dead lambs when possible because they are invaluable to the diagnosis of congenital infections. A knowledge of weather conditions during the previous 24 hours, i.e., hot, warm or cold; wet or dry; calm or windy; and a determination of the dead weight of lambs allow more reliable interpretation of necropsy findings. Dead weight often represents birth weight or is a reflection of birth weight of lambs dying within a few days of birth. High proportions of small lambs (<3 kg) succumb during cold or hot weather because of their relatively greater surface area, whereas large lambs (>4.5 kg) are more prone to dystocia. Birth weight is influenced by single or multiple births, nutrition during late pregnancy and genetic factors.

A full necropsy including examination of the central nervous system (CNS) is carried out using a systematic technique.[7, 11] Using this method, which classifies the time that lambs die relative to birth, the following groups can be recognized:

1. Anteparturient deaths — dying before the commencement of birth.
2. Parturient deaths — dying during birth or within a few hours of birth.
3. Postparturient deaths — dying more than a few hours after birth.

The classification is a valuable diagnostic aid as specific entities are more likely to occur in specific time-of-death categories (Table 2).

Examination of the CNS is mandatory because evidence of injury to the CNS resulting from trauma or hypoxia, or both, during birth is found in virtually all lambs dying during birth and in a high proportion of those dying after birth, notably those comprising the "starvation-mismothering-exposure" complex.

GENERAL NATURE OF PERINATAL MORTALITY

While the factors are certain to alter in different environments, Table 2 summarizes the findings from extensive investigations carried out in Australia and New Zealand.

Anteparturient deaths usually constitute an insignificant proportion (<2 per cent) of losses, leaving parturient and postparturient deaths to account variably for 25 to 75 per cent of losses, depending on the flock, district and season.

Lethal congenital malformations, specific nutritional deficiencies, predation and infections (both congenital and acquired after birth) usually account for less than 20 per cent of mortality occurring in the anteparturient, parturient and/or postparturient time-of-death classifications. At least 80 per cent of lambs die during or shortly after (and presumably because of) birth, or

TABLE 1. *Sample Size Required to Detect a Specific Pathological Entity in at Least One Carcass Given a Specified Flock Incidence**

	Flock Incidence (%)																		
	5	10	15	20	25	30	35	40	45	50	55	60	65	70	75	80	85	90	95
Number of carcasses to be examined	58	28	18	13	10	8	7	6	5	4	4	3	3	2	2	2	2	1	1

*p = 0.95.

TABLE 2. *Cause of Death in Relation to Time of Death Relative to Birth*

Cause of Death	Time of Death		
	BEFORE	DURING	AFTER
Incidence %	<2	75–25	25–75
Congenital malformations	+	+	+
Congenital nutritional deficiencies	+	+	+
Congenital infections	+	+	+
Birth injury	−	+	+
Infections acquired after birth	−	−	+
Predation	−	−	+
Starvation			
Mismothering	−	−	+
Exposure			
Miscellaneous	−	−	+

they die within the next few days. The latter are a particularly important group as they may constitute up to 65 per cent of losses. Superficially their necropsy is characterized by nothing more remarkable than extensive depletion of fat depots and an empty alimentary tract. Routine examination of the fetal CNS and definition of the lesions of cold injury have done much to resolve the pathogenesis of this large residual component.

COMMON CAUSES, DIAGNOSIS AND CONTROL OF PERINATAL MORTALITY

It is important to remember that there are many causes of perinatal lamb mortality, and carcasses often show lesions having more than one origin.

Birth Injury

Hemorrhage and congestion at single or multiple sites in and around the cranial and/or spinal meninges (the dura mater, arachnoidea and the pia mater) are the most common lesions found both in lambs dying during or immediately after birth and in those comprising the starvation-mismothering-exposure complex. In the parturient group, prevalence of one or more of these lesions approaches 100 per cent, whereas in the postparturient group it is a function of the proportion classified as the starvation-mismothering-exposure complex, as the lesions are almost invariably associated with evidence of cold injury

or starvation, or both. Male and female single and twin-born lambs are affected, and occurrence is not dependent on assistance during delivery.

Vascular lesions in the parturient group are often accompanied by other manifestations of trauma or hypoxia, or both, during birth. These include subcutaneous edema of the presenting portion of the fetus, abdominal hemorrhage derived from rupture of the liver or tearing of the liver capsule and subepicardial, subendocardial, subpleural and subcapsular thymic petechiae and ecchymoses.

The vascular lesions described have been interpreted as indications of injury to the more basic components of the fetal CNS. Such lesions have been induced artificially and their pathological significance demonstrated. Severe injury causes death during or immediately after birth, whereas less severe injury, by markedly impairing sucking activity, leads to rapid exhaustion of fetal energy reserves and death within 1 or 2 days, particularly under cold conditions. Variables implicated in the pathogenesis include the duration of second-stage labor, vigor of tenesmus, fetal-pelvic proportions and fetal blood gas status.

Prevention. In the author's experience, birth injury to the fetal CNS is the main cause of perinatal lamb loss. Perinatal loss by individual ewes tends to be repeatable mainly because of relative fetal oversize or small maternal pelvic size, or both. Individual sires exert marked effects on lamb survival. Deliberate culling of all ewes and their progeny having histories of lamb loss or lambing difficulty and the selection of sires born of ewes having lifetime histories of 100 per cent rearing success will probably lead to greatly improved lamb survival rates.

Cold Exposure

Small lambs are most susceptible to cold because they have relatively large surface areas from which to lose heat. Although heavy loss of newborn lambs occurs during severe, cold, wet, windy weather, a significant continuous loss occurs during "mild" weather. At about 28°C in "still" air (thermoneutral temperature) and at lower environmental temperatures during wet, windy weather, the newborn lamb maintains body temperature by shivering, catabolism of brown fat and reduction of heat loss by vasoconstriction.

The extent and time of onset of thermogenic activity are modified by the environmental temperature, wind velocity, birth weight and the thickness and dampness of the birth coat. When heat loss exceeds heat production for more than a short period, the lamb dies of hypothermia. Under blizzard conditions, death may ensue because heat loss greatly exceeds heat production despite adequate energy reserves. During less severe weather, lambs die because they are unable to replenish exhausted fetal energy reserves with milk owing to depressed sucking activity resulting from birth injury, aberrant maternal behavior or agalactia.

Experimentally induced lesions of cold exposure include catabolism of brown fat, subcutaneous edema of the distal limbs and adrenocortical changes.[9] Brown fat at the perirenal, pericardial and other sites is creamy-white or pink at birth or in newborn lambs exposed to environmental temperature above thermoneutrality. Below thermoneutral temperatures, brown fat depots are important sites of nonshivering thermogenesis as well as sources of triglycerides for use elsewhere in the body. Fat depletion occurs during exposure to cold and independently of starvation. In the process, the fat depots change to a red-brown color, the extent and duration of the rise in metabolism modifying the degree of color change. Varying degrees of yellow subcutaneous edema (up to 5 mm thick) invariably occur in the distal hind limbs and often at the base of the tail and the distal forelimbs. Changes in the adrenal cortex, including hypertrophy and focal hemorrhage, result from severe systemic stress. All these lesions occur to greater or lesser degrees in newborn lambs exposed to cold. They are more marked in lambs that died as a result of cold exposure.

Prevention. Although providing shelter mitigates losses from cold exposure, rational control measures also demand a reduction in birth injury, a common predisposing factor in the pathogenesis of exposure. The high cost of providing housing for lambing ewes often precludes its use. Prelamb shearing of ewes, thereby inducing them to seek and lamb in natural or specially prepared, cheap, low level shelters, shows considerable promise as a technique for significantly reducing lamb loss from exposure.[4]

Hyperthermia

Lambs born in hot, semiarid environments, particularly if they are small, often die from hyperthermia and dehydration. Their necropsy is characterized by severe dehydration, an empty alimentary tract, no color change of fat depots and intense leptomeningeal congestion. Dehydration is often caused or exacerbated by depressed sucking activity due to a prior birth injury to the fetal CNS.

Predation

Although primary predation is a constant source of low level loss under the extensive grazing conditions experienced in Australia, in isolated instances losses may be heavy. However, predation by wild animals and occasionally by birds may be overrated as a cause of lamb loss because lambs of low viability killed before death (secondary predation) and carcasses mutilated postmortem are included in the estimate. Death can be attributed to primary predation only when the carcass shows extensive and severe antemortem trauma and no other gross lesions. Fat depots will not be catabolized, and there will be evidence of milk absorption when the lamb has sucked. A substantial portion of the carcass should be skinned, as not only are external appearances misleading regarding the degree of mutilation but the nature of the mutilation may also indicate the predator species involved.

Deficiency of Essential Trace Elements

Congenital swayback, congenital goiter and congenital white muscle disease associated with deficiency of copper, iodine and selenium, respectively, are usually endemic to certain districts in which outbreaks may cause heavy mortality.

Prevention. Prevention of these main trace element deficiencies is possible by dietary supplementation, either by the use of top dressing or parenteral administration (see Feeding Sheep for High Reproductive Performance, page 882).

Infections

Although these may be important in isolated instances, the evidence at present (certainly in Australia and New Zealand) suggests that perinatal loss from this cause is relatively small on a national basis.

Congenital Infections

See Prenatal Loss, page 896, and Infectious Ovine Abortion, page 908.

Infections Acquired after Birth

A wide variety of bacterial infections have been associated with perinatal lamb loss. The prevalence rises with high grazing pressures and intensive husbandry systems such as shed-lambing. Most bacterial infections are acquired at or soon after birth, although their pathological manifestations may extend beyond the defined perinatal period.

Common pathogens include:

1. *Clostridium septicum, C. chauvoei* and *C. novyi,* manifested by gangrene around the umbilical stump and localized or generalized serofibrinous peritonitis.

2. *Pasteurella haemolytica* causes localized or generalized serofibrinous peritonitis often accompanied by pneumonia.

3. Infection by *Staphylococcus aureus, Streptococcus* spp., *Corynebacterium* spp., *Sphaerophorus necrophorus* and an unclassified gram-negative pleomorphic rod is manifested by pyemia with multiple puru-

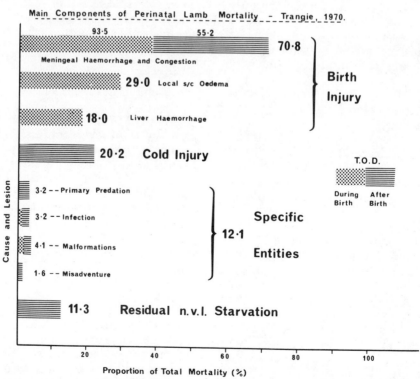

Figure 1. A representative example of the relative importance of various causes of perinatal lamb mortality in spring-lambing flocks in Southeastern Australia.

lent foci in the liver, kidneys, heart, lungs, muscles, joints and so forth.

4. *Escherichia coli* causes a variety of syndromes characterized by enteritis, polysynovitis, septicemia or leptomeningitis.

5. *Erysipelothrix insidiosa* and *Chlamydia* spp. infection are manifested by polysynovitis.

Diagnosis is confirmed by microbiological and histopathological examinations of appropriate specimens of whole carcasses. Annual vaccination of ewes within 3 to 4 weeks of lambing effectively controls losses due to *Clostridium* spp. by providing the lamb with a colostric immunity. Lethal congenital malformations usually constitute about 1 per cent of losses and are discussed in the following article.

CONCLUSION

Perinatal lamb mortality results from a summation of causes having environmental, genetic, nutritional, infective and managerial origins. The relative importance of various causes for a typical mortality occurring in New South Wales, Australia, is shown in Figure 1.

One hundred and twenty-four lambs that died during or within 7 days of birth were examined from a Merino flock in which 17 per cent of ewes lost all lambs born. The cause or causes of death were established in 89 per cent of carcasses examined. Many of these showed lesions of multiple etiology. Necropsy of the residual group, classified as no visible lesion (n.v.l.) starvation, was characterized by moderate to marked fat catabolism and an empty gut. Death in this group was attributed to starvation caused by aberrant maternal behavior or mismothering and mild cold exposure. Birth injury to the fetal CNS was the major component of mortality, affecting lambs dying during and after birth.

Methods of preventing these losses clearly depend on our ability to recognize the basic cause or causes of the lesions observed. In some instances, economic considerations will not permit appropriate action to be taken.

REFERENCES

1. Alexander, G.: Temperature regulation in the newborn lamb. III. The effect of environmental temperature on metabolic rate, body temperature and respiratory quotient. Aust. J. Agric. Res., *12*:1152, 1961.
2. Alexander, G.: Temperature regulation in the newborn lamb. IV. The effect of wind and evaporation of water from the coat on metabolic rate and body temperature. Aust. J. Agric. Res. *13*:82, 1962.
3. Alexander, G.: Energy metabolism in the starved newborn lamb. Aust. J. Agric. Res., *13*:144, 1962.
4. Alexander, G. and Lynch J. J. : *Phalaris* windbreaks for shorn and fleeced lambing ewes. Proc. Aust. Soc. Anim. Prod., *11*:161, 1976.
5. Alexander, G. and Williams D.: Temperature regulation in the newborn lamb. VI. Heat exchanges in lambs in a hot environment. Aust. J. Agric. Res., *13*:122, 1962.
6. Gemmell, R. T., Bell, A. W. and Alexander, G.: Morphology of adipose cells in lambs at birth and during subsequent transition of brown to white adipose tissue in cold and warm conditions. Am. J. Anat., *133*:143, 1972.
7. Haughey, K. G.: Vascular abnormalities in the central nervous system associated with perinatal lamb mortality: 1. Pathology. Aust. Vet. J., *49*:1, 1973.
8. Haughey, K. G.: Vascular abnormalities in the central nervous system associated with perinatal lamb mortality: 2. Association of the abnormalities with recognised lesions. Aust. Vet. J., *49*:9, 1973.
9. Haughey, K. G.: Cold injury in newborn lambs. Aust. Vet. J., *49*:555, 1973.
10. Hughes, K. L., Haughey, K. G. and Hartley, W. J.: Perinatal lamb mortality: Infections occurring among lambs dying after parturition. Aust. Vet. J., *47*:472, 1971.
11. McFarlane, D.: Perinatal lamb losses. 1. An autopsy method for the investigation of perinatal losses. N. Z. Vet. J., *13*:116, 1965.
12. Underwood, E. J.: Trace Elements in Human and Animal Nutrition. 3rd Ed. New York, Academic Press, Inc., 1971.

Congenital and Inherited Defects in Sheep

STANLEY M. DENNIS
Kansas State University,
Manhattan, Kansas

INTRODUCTION

Congenital defects, i.e., abnormalities of structure or function usually recognizable at birth, are primarily classified by the body system that is principally involved. More than 88 congenital defects, including 12 inherited lethals, have been described in sheep. Sheep have the highest incidence of craniofacial defects among domestic animals. Collectively, congenital defects cause economic losses by increasing perinatal lamb mortality, decreasing maternal productivity and reducing the value of viable defective lambs. Although the incidence of any defect in a flock may be low, the cumulative effect may be economically significant.

NATURE OF CONGENITAL DEFECTS

Congenital defects may affect a single structure or function, involve several body systems or combine structural and functional alterations. Defects may be lethal, semilethal or nonlethal and may affect all body structures and functions.

A defective lamb is an adapted survivor from a disruptive event at one or more stages in the complexly integrated process of embryonic or fetal development. Before the primary germ layers are formed, the embryo usually is not susceptible to teratogenesis, but during the critical period of early differentiation it becomes highly susceptible. After embryogenesis, the fetus becomes increasingly resistant to teratogenic effects. The estimated ovine embryonic mortality of 20 per cent suggests that unidentified lethal genes or chromosomal aberrations may be active during this critical period.

FREQUENCY

The frequency of congenital defects in sheep is difficult to assess. Because they are caused by genetic and environmental factors, the frequency of individual defects will vary with breed, breeding practices, location, year, level of nutrition, sex, parental age and other environmental factors. Based on studies in Australia, New Zealand and the United States, the incidence ranges from 0.2 to 2.0 per cent of all lambs born.

Body systems that were principally involved in a large number of defective lambs studied at necropsy included: musculoskeletal, 55.4 per cent; digestive, 12.7 per cent; cardiovascular, 9.7 per cent; urogenital, 8.0 per cent; central nervous, 6.0 per cent; special senses, 3.5 per cent; integument, 3.2 per cent and endocrine, 1.5 per cent. As determined by necropsy and survey findings in a large sheep population, the common congenital defects were (in alphabetical order): agnathia (missing lower jaw), arthrogryposis (rigidity of one or more limb joints), atresia ani, bowed forelegs, brachygnathia (undershot lower jaw), cleft palate, conjoined twinning, cryptorchidism, entropion, hernia, hypospadias (ventral urethral opening with bifurcated scrotum), interventricular septal defect, limb defects, microtia, partially bifurcated scrotum, perosomus elumbis (lack of lumbosacral vertebrae), polythelia (multiple teats), prognathia (overshot lower jaw), tail defects and torticollis.

EPIZOOTIOLOGY

Congenital defects in sheep are probably more common than reports indicate. Many defective lambs are not observed because of common ovine husbandry practices, and of those observed, many are not reported unless the number is high. This means that many sporadic cases, which would include most genetic defects, are not reported. Unless the rancher routinely examines the newborn dead lambs, most defects (i.e., semi- or nonlethals) will be observed during castration or other procedures, and lethal defects usually will be unrecognized.

CAUSE

Congenital defects are caused by genetic or environmental factors or by their interac-

TABLE 1. *Ovine Defects Reported to Be Inherited*

Defect	Mode of Transmission
Agnathia	Recessive
Alopecia	Recessive
Ancon dwarf sheep	Recessive
Anotia	Incomplete dominant
Arthrogryposis	Recessive
Blindness (microphthalmia to anophthalmia)	Recessive
Cerebellar ataxia	Recessive
Collagen dysplasia	Recessive
Cryptorchidism	Recessive
Dwarfism	Recessive
Earless and cleft palate	Recessive
Goiter	Recessive
Hyperbilirubinemia	Recessive
Lethal gray	Incomplete dominant
Luster mutant	Dominant
Muscular dystrophy	Recessive
Neuroaxonal dystrophy	Recessive
Paralysis	Recessive
Polythelia	Dominant
Rigid fetlocks	Recessive
Short ears	Recessive
"Wattles"	Dominant
Yellow fat	Recessive

TABLE 2. *Ovine Congenital Defects Suspected to Be Hereditary*

Adactyly
Anury
Atresia ani
Brachygnathia
Cerebellar atrophy
Cyclopia
Epitheliogenesis imperfecta
Entropion
Hernia
Holoacardius acephalus
Hypospadias
Hypotrichosis
Limb defects
Micrognathia
Micrencephaly
Osteogenesis imperfecta
Palatoschisis
Partially bifurcated scrotum
Perosomus elumbis
Persistent umbilical hemorrhage
Prolonged gestation
Pseudohermaphroditism
Syndactyly
Testicular hypoplasia
Ventricular septal defect

tion. Some defects are inherited, others are suspected to be, but the heritability of the majority of defects is unknown (Tables 1 and 2).

Genetic defects are caused by mutant genes or chromosomal aberrations. Most known genetic defects in sheep are autosomal recessives that occur in any environment (Table 1). Except for chromosomal aberrations, genetic defects occur in intragenerational patterns. Several chromosomal aberrations, i.e., variations in the normal number of chromosomes or structural abnormalities of individual chromosomes, have now been reported in sheep.

All genetic defects have their counterpart in environmentally induced phenocopies. The problem is to recognize which defects are genetic and which are environmental; this may be difficult in sheep.

Only a few environmental factors have been incriminated as teratogenic for sheep (Table 3).

DIAGNOSIS

When a defective lamb is born, the problem is whether the cause is genetic or environmental. Determining the cause is difficult because the etiological agent exerted its effects approximately 4 months before the defect is recognized. Even with several defective lambs, it is not easy to eliminate the possibility of disease, teratogenic plants or drugs or nutritional deficiencies. When affected ewes are restricted to a single flock or area, environmental factors are usually investigated first. Spontaneous epizootics of

TABLE 3. *Agents Reported to Be Teratogenic for Sheep*

Teratogenic Agent	Major Body System Affected
Viruses:	
Blue tongue	CNS
Bovine virus diarrhea	CNS
Akabane	CNS
Plants:	
Veratrum californicum	CNS and skeletal
Astragalus spp.	Skeletal
Oxytropis spp.	Skeletal
Trachymene spp.	Skeletal
Goitrogenic plants	Endocrine
Drugs:	
Parbendazole	Skeletal
Aminopterin	Skeletal
Nutritional:	
Iodine deficiency	Goiter
Copper deficiency	CNS and skeletal
Selenium deficiency	Muscular
Physical:	
Hyperthermia	CNS and skeletal
Irradiation	Skeletal

congenital defects are unlikely to be genetically induced.

Factors hindering diagnosis of congenital defects in sheep include defects not being reported, inadequate history, inadequate records and lack of interest in teratology by some veterinarians and diagnosticians.

History. A detailed history is necessary for diagnosing congenital defects and should include breed; geographical region; season; type of pasture and soil; exposure or suspected exposure to teratogenic plants, viruses or drugs; feeding and management practices; breeding records; health history of the flock; drugs used (routine or new) and congenital defects previously observed.

Diagnosing Genetic Defects. The basis for diagnosing genetic defects is that they tend to run in families. Mutant genes become evident over two or more generations by one of four major breeding patterns: dominant, incompletely dominant, recessive and overdominant. The patterns involve certain characteristic ratios of normal to defective progeny that form the basis for genetic diagnosis. Several factors prevent accurate diagnosis of hereditary patterns and ratios in sheep: rarity of particular defects, phenocopies, wide genetic diversity, inadequate breeding records and nonreporting or reporting only extreme cases. It is nearly impossible to have enough cases of many ovine defects to identify the hereditary pattern; the pattern must be repeated several times before it can be clearly identified. Genetic defects are differentiated from nongenetic defects by identifying supporting or contradictory evidence of a characteristic hereditary pattern or by establishing one or more nonhereditary patterns. Diagnosing a defect in a single lamb as being genetically induced is impossible.

Most known genetic defects in sheep are caused by recessive genes. They are usually characterized by a small number of defective lambs from normal-appearing parents. Recessive genes are insidiously perpetuated from generation to generation by normal carriers or by heterozygotes.

Test-mating of sheep to confirm genetic defects is impractical in commercial flocks. It is simpler to detect recessive defects by having all defective lambs reported.

Recommended Diagnostic Procedures. The following procedures are recommended for diagnosing congenital defects in sheep: encourage reporting of defects; re-

cord all defective lambs; obtain an adequate history; perform a detailed necropsy; collect serums from affected and in-contact ewes for viral serological examination; evaluate carefully for possible exposure to teratogens, especially during mating and early pregnancy; examine chromosomes of live defective lambs and analyze records for genetic cause.

PREVENTION

Determining whether the defect is genetically or environmentally induced is important, as proper identification indicates which control measures are applicable. It is essential to recognize inherited defects early to control their insidious spread. The difficulty of identifying normal carriers makes control of recessive defects virtually impossible.

To minimize the effects of congenital defects in sheep, the following are recommended:

1. If possible, establish an accurate diagnosis.

2. If this is not possible, regard all congenital defects as genetic until proved otherwise.

3. Do not breed defective sheep.

4. Eliminate defective lambs to keep recessive defects low.

5. Seek help from the regional diagnostic laboratory.

6. Encourage ranchers to report all defective lambs.

7. If the defect is environmentally induced, adjust the management program.

8. Report all defective lambs, as they serve as biomedical indicators of environmental hazards that may have public health significance.

9. Finally, take an interest in teratology.

REFERENCES

1. Binns, W., James, L. F. and Shupe, J. L.: Toxicosis of *Veratrum californicum* in ewes and its relationship to a congenital deformity in lambs. Ann. N.Y. Acad. Sci., *III*:571, 1964.
2. Binns, W., Keeler, R. F. and Balls, L. D.: Congenital deformities in lambs, calves and goats resulting from maternal ingestion of *Veratrum californicum*: Harelip, cleft palate, ataxia, and hypoplasia of metacarpal and metatarsal bones. Clin. Toxicol., 5:245, 1972.

3. Bruere, A. N.: The discovery and biological consequences of some important chromosome anomalies in the population of domestic animals. 1st World Congress Genetics Applied Livestock Production, Madrid. *I*:151, 1974.

4. Dennis, S. M.: A survey of congenital defects of sheep. Vet. Rec., *95*:488, 1974.

5. Dennis, S. M.: Perinatal lamb mortality in Western Australia. 7. Congenital defects. Aust. Vet. J., *51*:80, 1975.

6. Dennis, S. M. and Leipold, H. W.: Agnathia in sheep. External observations. Am. J. Vet. Res., *33*:339, 1972.

7. Dennis, S. M. and Leipold, H. W.: Diagnosing congenital defects in sheep. Zuchthygiene, March, 1976.

8. Ercanbrack, S. K. and Price, D. A.: Frequencies of various birth defects of Rambouillet sheep. J. Hered., *62*:223, 1971.

9. Leipold, H. W., Dennis, S. M. and Huston, K.: Congenital defects of cattle: Nature, cause and effect. Adv. Vet. Sci. Comp. Med., *16*:103, 1972.

10. Saperstein, G., Leipold, H. W. and Dennis, S. M.: Congenital defects of sheep. J.A.V.M.A., *167*:314, 1975.

Development of the Male Reproductive Tract, Spermatogenesis and Puberty

K. R. LAPWOOD

Massey University, Palmerston North, New Zealand

EMBRYOLOGICAL DEVELOPMENT OF THE REPRODUCTIVE ORGANS

Gonadal Development

As in other species, the testes of rams are derived from undifferentiated gonads on the ventromedial surfaces of the embryonic urogenital ridges. The undifferentiated gonad is covered by two or three layers of epithelial cells from which groups or strands of epithelial cells extend into the underlying mesenchyme. Primordial germ cells, presumably derived from yolk sac endoderm, are present in sheep gonads as early as the twenty-ninth day after conception. Histological evidence of the differentiation of gonads to testes first becomes apparent at 34 to 35 days with the appearance of the tunica albuginea. By the forty-second day of development, testis cords containing gonocytes and indifferent or supporting cells are formed, while interstitial cells are prominent between the cords. At this stage the gonocytes are centrally located within the testis cords and are surrounded by indifferent cells. Subsequent development of the sex cords involves a gradual increase in their diameter as a result of mitosis of both indifferent cells and gonocytes and an increase in the

amount of indifferent cell cytoplasm. The indifferent cells have poorly defined cell membranes and tongue-like processes that extend into the center of the sex cords. While the sex cords enlarge, the interstitial cells increase in number and develop eosinophilic cytoplasmic granules; such granules are present in most interstitial cells by the seventieth day of fetal life.

Testicular descent into the scrotal pouches occurs as a result of traction exerted by the gubernaculum. The gubernaculum shortens and also does not elongate at the same rate as the surrounding structures. In rams testicular descent is completed by the eightieth day of fetal life.

Reproductive Tract Development

Detailed analyses of the course of embryological development of the reproductive tract and accessory sex glands of rams do not appear to have been published. However, it is assumed that this course of development is unremarkable compared with development in other domestic species. One of the few points worthy of note is that the degree of ventral and anterior migration of the scrotum is extreme.

Regulation of Sexual Differentiation

Differentiation of the indifferent gonads and differential development of male, rather than female, reproductive tract primordia occur as a result of secretion of testosterone and androstenedione by the fetal gonads. In rams these two androgens can be detected in the testes from the thirtieth day of fetal life, and probably it is their secretion before the fortieth day of fetal life that determines sexual differentiation. In the absence of fetal androgen, potentially female structures such as the müllerian ducts develop, rather than male precursors such as the wolffian ducts. Fetal gonadal androgen secretion up to the fortieth to sixtieth day postconception also determines the sexual differentiation of adult sexual behavioral patterns and the sexual dimorphism of hypothalamic secretion. Androgen exposure at this critical stage abolishes the female-type cyclic control potential of the preoptic hypothalamic area so that male-type tonic control influences from the mediobasal hypothalamus become dominant. Fetal testicular androgen secretion reaches peak levels at about the seventieth day and then falls with the approach of parturition.

SPERMATOGENESIS

The Immature Testis

At birth, the testicular sex cords contain peripherally situated supporting cells and centrally placed gonocytes. Fibrous connective tissue located between the sex cords contains blood vessels and interstitial cells arranged in clumps or cords or singly. Prior to puberty only minor changes occur. Both gonocytes and supporting cells continue to multiply, and the gonocytes are transformed into prospermatogonia. During this transformation the number of nucleoli is reduced from two to four original nucleoli to one nucleolus, and nuclear dimensions increase. At the same time there is a reduction in the proportion of interstitial cells containing eosinophilic granules.

Pubertal Changes

Pubertal development of ram testicular germinal elements follows a uniform pattern despite slight breed differences in the ages and body weights at which particular changes are observed. Data from Ile-de-France rams indicate that when the testis

weighs 6 gm, prospermatogonia move to the basement membrane, transform into type A spermatogonia and then start multiplying rapidly. Primary spermatocytes are first seen in 12-gm testes (about 105 days of age), spermatids in 30-gm testes (120 to 125 days) and spermatozoa in 65-gm testes (140 to 150 days); full adult testicular weight is about 200 gm. At the same time as the gametogenic elements develop, the supporting cells transform into Sertoli cells. This transformation occurs just before the first appearance of spermatids and involves an increase in nuclear size as well as the extension of cytoplasmic processes between the germinal cells so as to provide points of attachment for spermatids. Seminiferous tubule lumen formation also occurs at about this time. During pubertal development, the size of groups of interstitial cells is reduced.

Testicular growth curves are sigmoid in shape, growth being slow in the first 2 to 3 months after birth; then becoming rapid between 2 to 3 and 5 months, when spermatogenesis is being established; then subsequently slowing. In fact, the time at which rapid testicular growth commences is better correlated with body weight than with age. Typically, prospermatogonia appear at a body weight of 15 kg, type A spermatogonia at 21 kg, and all spermatogenic cell types are present at 27 kg. However, there are breed differences in the exact body weight at which each stage commences.

Maximal efficiency of spermatogenesis does not occur until several months after the first appearance of spermatozoa. This is partly due to the variability in the onset of spermatogenesis within the seminiferous tubules, and partly due to an initial high rate of degeneration of spermatogenic cells. In rams this degeneration mostly affects intermediate spermatogonia and decreases with age. Adult spermatogenic production is not reached until testis weight is about 100 gm.

Spermatogenesis in Adult Rams

A detailed description of the histological course of spermatogenesis in the ram is beyond the scope of this article.

Using nuclear staining methods such as the Feulgen-hematoxylin technique, it has been shown that the spermatogenic cycle of the ram seminiferous tubules is divided into eight stages, each consisting of distinct associations or groupings of four to five generations of gametogenic cells. Generally in rams a stage in the cycle occupies an entire cross section of the seminiferous tubule. The period between successive appearances of the same stage in the cycle at a particular point in a tubule is 10.4 days, while the total duration of spermatogenesis in rams is 49 days.

Estimates of the daily sperm output of rams have been highly variable, ranging from 5.5 to 13.9 × 10^9 sperm/day. This deviation has been attributed to technical variations in methods of estimating daily sperm output, as well as to breed, age, individual and seasonal effects. Daily sperm output varies with testis size, which in turn varies seasonally. Seasonal effects are compounded because sperm production per gram of testis weight varies seasonally and is about 20 per cent lower in the nonbreeding than in the breeding season. Seasonal effects on spermatogenesis primarily result from seasonal variations in the daily photoperiod. However, extreme elevation of environmental temperature can disrupt spermatogenesis (the susceptible stage in rams is the pachytene stage of meiosis), so that the number of primary spermatocytes is reduced.

After release from the seminiferous tubules and passage through the rete testis, ram sperm spend 10 to 14 days in the epididymis undergoing the final stages of maturation.

PUBERTY

Puberty in the male may be defined as the time at which reproduction is possible, i.e., when spermatozoa are released. The course of gonadal development through the period of puberty has already been discussed.

Reproductive Tract and Accessory Organ Development at Puberty

The development of the reproductive tract and accessory organs is more highly correlated with physiological growth and testicular growth than with age. These as-

sociations in rates of growth occur mainly as the result of increased androgen secretion before and during puberty. Thus in ram lambs high correlations exist between the rates of growth of the testes and those of the epididymides, seminal vesicles, bulbourethral glands and ampullae and the concentration and total content of fructose and citric acid in ejaculates. Penile-urethral adhesions are broken down; adhesions first disappear from the urethral process, then from the glans penis and finally from the penile shaft. Failure of breakdown of penile adhesions may predispose to the development of ovine posthitis in wethers. Penile growth, particularly growth in circumference, occurs at or shortly after puberty. In horned breeds, horn growth precedes penile growth. Testicular androgens can also influence the rate of body growth so that ram lambs grow 3 to 8 per cent more rapidly than wethers if nutrition is adequate.

Neuroendocrine Induction of Puberty

Postnatal reproductive hormone secretion patterns of rams are becoming established. Plasma luteinizing hormone (LH) levels increase from birth to a peak at about 70 days of age and then decline. On the other hand, plasma follicle-stimulating hormone (FSH) levels peak at about 5 weeks. During the prepubertal period both gonadotropins are secreted in an episodic manner, and peak plasma LH levels are higher in rams of high fecundity breeds. However, because of the relatively low heritability of adult fecundity and because of low within-breed correlations between LH levels and fecundity potential of individual animals, measurement of prepubertal plasma gonadotropin levels is unlikely to assist in genetic selection for fecundity. Pituitary LH and FSH responses to exogenous gonadotropin-releasing hormone (GnRH) peak at approximately the same time as peak plasma levels are recorded.

Plasma testosterone levels are low after birth and then increase to peak levels at 5 to 9 months of age. Androstenedione always is secreted in low concentrations, and these levels decline during the first 2 months of age. Plasma prolactin concentrations are low in lambs born in autumn until a short sharp elevation occurs at 10 to 12 weeks of age; this peak coincides with the onset of spermatogenesis. In lambs born in spring, the normal seasonal elevation of prolactin secretion obscures any such peak.

The precise nature of the neuroendocrine interactions that trigger puberty are unknown. It is presumed that maturation of hypothalamic androgen-sensitive tissues is involved. This maturation probably takes the form of a decrease in sensitivity to androgen-negative feedback, which allows increased gonadotropin secretion to occur. The time course of pubertal development and endocrine changes can be modified by factors such as nutrition and photoperiod. Undernutrition inhibits body growth and reproductive development because pituitary secretion of gonadotropins is inhibited; consequently, androgen secretion is retarded. A declining daily photoperiod stimulates reproductive hormone secretion and may advance the pubertal endocrine surge slightly.

Endocrinology of the Adult Ram

In adult rams, LH, FSH and prolactin are secreted in pulsatile patterns, while peaks of testosterone secretion follow 30 to 60 minutes after each plasma LH peak. Under some conditions plasma prolactin levels are elevated nocturnally, but the other reproductive hormones are not secreted in a circadian pattern.

Marked seasonal fluctuations in mean plasma hormone concentrations are superimposed on these acute secretory patterns. Prolactin secretion shows the greatest seasonal variations, with peak levels occurring in midsummer and lowest levels occurring in winter. Subsequent to the peak of prolactin secretion, LH output is elevated in mid-to-late summer, while the seasonal peak of testosterone production follows in early autumn, coincident with the increase in libido at the commencement of the breeding season. Seasonal changes in the length of daylight contrib-

ute most to regulating seasonality of reproductive hormone secretion, probably as a result of influencing a retino-pineal-hypothalamo-hypophyseal-gonadal axis. Despite considerable between-breed differences in the extent of reproductive seasonality in ewes, breed appears to have little influence on the seasonality of hormone secretion in rams. Effects of factors such as temperature, nutrition and pheromones on hormone secretion patterns await more adequate investigation.

The functions of individual reproductive hormones have, in many cases, been difficult to elucidate. Testosterone regulates functions such as reproductive behavior, as well as maintaining anatomical and physiological integrity of the reproductive tract and accessory structures. LH controls testosterone secretion of the Leydig cells, and prolactin may function as a "permissive" or "conditioning" hormone that synergizes with the endocrine effects of LH and testosterone. The endocrine regulation of spermatogenesis in the ram is complicated and requires further study. Multiplication of gonocytes and supporting cells in the impuberal testes requires LH and FSH. Testosterone may also be involved in this control, as well as in regulating primitive type A spermatogonium production. This steroid also controls the meiotic divisions resulting in spermatid production, although the final stages of spermatid maturation probably require FSH secretion. LH affects spermatogenesis in postpubertal rams indirectly by its stimulation of androgen production.

REFERENCES

1. Courot, M.: Endocrine control of the supporting and germ cells of the impuberal testis. J. Reprod. Fertil. (Suppl.), *2*:89, 1967.
2. Drymundsson, O. R.: Puberty and early reproductive performance in sheep. II. Ram lambs. Anim. Breed. Abstr., *41*:419, 1973.
3. Ortavant, R., Courot, M. and Hochereau, M. T.: Spermatogenesis and morphology of the spermatozoon. *In* Cole, H. H. and Cupps, P. T. (eds.): Reproduction in Domestic Animals. 2nd Ed. New York, Academic Press, 1969, p. 251.

Normal Mating Behavior and Its Variations

R. J. HOLMES

*Massey University, Palmerston North,
New Zealand*

Sex behavior of the ram is dependent on both mating ability and libido (sex drive). It is not associated with either the production or the quality of semen.

There is wide individual variation in type and frequency of occurrence of the single components of mating. There are also many factors that can alter the degree of expression of the sex drive. It is therefore not appropriate, based on present knowledge, to arbitrarily divide activities into abnormal or normal. Mating behavior is not consistently sex-specific, and temporary reversal of roles commonly occurs. Male mating behavior is in general more elaborate than female, presumably because ritualization achieves an optimum time for ejaculation.

MATING BEHAVIOR IN THE RAM

The characteristic sequence of behavior associated with intravaginal ejaculation is as follows:

During the female sexual season, and to a lesser degree out of season, a free-roaming active ram moves about the ewes, identifying those in estrus, i.e., cooperating in standing to be mounted. If good conception rates are to be achieved, this activity is particularly important with low body weight females (which are less likely to seek out the male), with young ewes and when large numbers of ewes are spread over a wide area.

The direct approach to an individual ewe may be made from some distance and is a common sequel to the ram seeing the ewe urinate. The approach, with head and neck outstretched, is followed by nosing and possibly by licking of the vulvar area. If the female was not urinating when the approach was made, she will usually do so in response to a sexual challenge. This may be made on either a lying or a standing ewe. A recumbent ewe will be struck with a pawing action of the ram's forefoot (Fig. 1). In the case of a standing ewe, the ram will probably position himself behind her before striking (Fig. 2). The challenge can be associated with a low vocalization, tilting and lowering of the head, nibbling of wool, tongue-flicking, pushing with the shoulder and short forward darts with the head along the ewe's flank. This activity acts as a stimulus to the ewe, her response varying with her sexual state. The ewe's behavior affects the ram's subsequent response. After urinating, an anestrous female moves away, while the ewe in estrus stands still and turns her head toward the male, who commonly rests his chin briefly on her rump.

After nosing or licking urine, a characteristic posture called "flehmen" is adopted

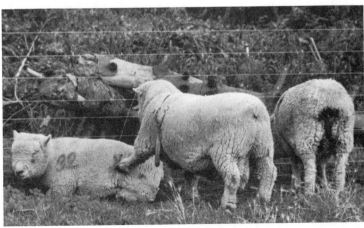

Figure 1. Ram foot-strikes recumbent ewe, which subsequently responds by standing and urinating. (Courtesy of K. R. Ross.)

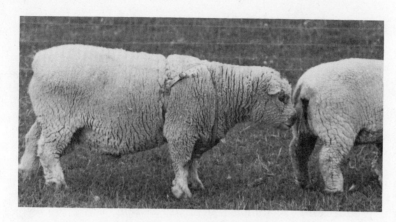

Figure 2. Southdown ram nosing urine stream from ewe. Ram is harnessed with crayon marker. Note characteristic posture of urination with flexion of spine. (Courtesy of K. R. Ross.)

(Fig. 3). The head and neck are usually raised, the mouth is opened slightly, the upper lip is curled upward and the nostrils are dilated. Rapid movement of air through the nostrils occurs, probably exposing the

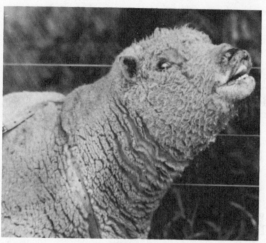

Figure 3. Flehmen posture of ram after nosing urine. (Courtesy of K. R. Ross.)

vomeronasal organ to olfactory constituents of the urine, which have sexual significance.

The reciprocal interaction between the sexes next results in the ram mounting the stationary ewe (Figs. 4 and 5). The mount involves the ram resting on the rump and consequently disturbing or marking the wool with any raddle or crayon attached to his sternum. This is the best indicator that mounting has occurred, but it does not indicate that either intromission or ejaculation has taken place. Rump markings are often seen on pregnant ewes; this does not necessarily mean that they have shown estrus. Rams often make opportunistic mounts on unreceptive females and leave a light mark during their brief encounter. Other rams apparently can serve without leaving any discernible mark at all — such a ram would not make a satisfactory "teaser" for use in identifying ewes in estrus.

Mounting is usually accompanied by pelvic thrusting and partial extrusion of the penis. Often a number of mounts occur be-

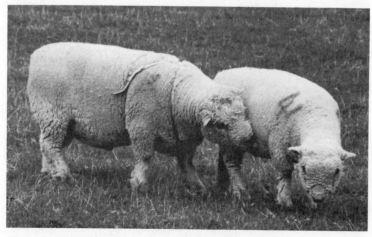

Figure 4. Southdown ram making a sexual challenge on Southdown ewe. Note orientation of bodies, rotation of ram's head and extension of his head, tongue and left foreleg. (Courtesy of K. R. Ross.)

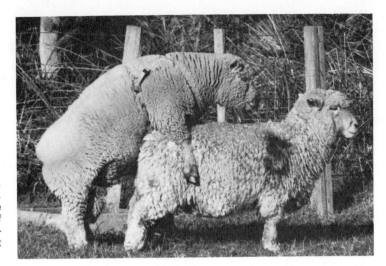

Figure 5. Southdown ram mounts a New Zealand Romney ewe in estrus. Note the distance between the animals' hindlegs and the lack of curvature of ram's lumbar spine, indicating that intromission has not occurred. (Courtesy of K. R. Ross.)

fore intromission, and these may be made without oscillating the pelvis or clasping the forelegs on the ewe's flanks. Contact of the glans penis with the vulva results in a distinctly greater thrust or a lunge, whereupon the hindlegs of the ram are brought right up behind the ewe. The back is curved to a greater degree. Ejaculation follows intromission in response to contact with the vagina, and the ram then dismounts. After service, the male usually stands quietly with the head low for a few seconds, then will either adopt a normal standing posture or begin grazing. Ewes interacting with the ram during this refractory period of the male are likely to be head-threatened and chased away (Fig. 6). At the end of the refractory period the ram may graze, lie down or begin to court the same or another ewe.

The sense of smell is not essential for males to determine the sexual state of the ewe, since he ultimately determines this by her characteristic posture and responses when she is in estrus.

Females that have been served usually receive little more than a nosing. Although some experienced rams are said to serve ewes only once when working among a large flock, females have been estimated to be served on average two to four times per estrus. Individual rams have been recorded as serving as many as 25 times in 9 hours. Masturbation is relatively uncommon in this species.

ONTOGENY

The basic level of sex drive characteristic of a ram appears to be determined *in utero* by the action of hormones on neural tissue. Mounting is shown by male lambs within

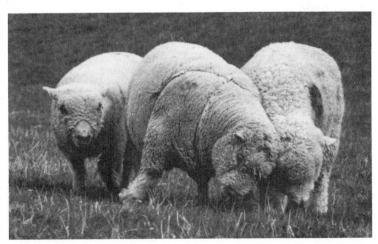

Figure 6. Ram head-bunts a ewe in response to her persistent courting immediately after intromission and ejaculation have taken place. (Courtesy of K. R. Ross.)

the first few weeks of life and thrusting within the first few months. Effective mating, which occurs at puberty, is a result of the greater activation of neural tissue mediating the full mating responses and can occur from 5 months of age. Males have a greater need for learning of sex behavior than do females, and there is therefore greater potential for modification by experience. Learning does not appear to be gained by association with a ram that is working.

Rearing of immature rams adjacent to cycling females does not increase testicular size, testosterone levels or sexual and aggressive activity, as it does for sexually mature yearling rams.

It is not uncommon for inexperienced males to be inactive initially for up to a month after introduction to the flock. On first becoming active, they show low mounting frequency, failure to intromit and a high mount:service ratio.

Libido is believed to increase during the first few years and gradually decline with age.

DOMINANCE

Dominance among a group of rams is determined by age, fighting ability, size and presence of horns. It is not necessarily associated with libido but is more an index of aggressiveness. The directions of the dominance relationship between pairs of rams may vary from year to year. Under usual husbandry situations dominance has not been found to have a major influence on male performance or flock fertility. The dominant male usually attempts to prevent subordinates from mating. The relationship can result in the subordinate not even attempting to mate when the dominant is in sight. Competition may increase the sexual activity of the dominant, although this is considered to have little effect under normal circumstances. Dominance can, however, be a significant factor when the dominant ram is infertile. Behavioral competency should therefore always be assessed when mating is limited to a small number of rams working in a small area.

ASSESSMENT OF MATING BEHAVIOR AND LIBIDO

Various indications of sex drive have been established. One index used is the number of mounts or services achieved in a limited time (e.g., 20 to 60 minutes) when the ram is penned with a group of four or five estrous ewes. However, one test does not allow for within-animal and between-day variation. A better measure is determination of the mean of three such tests conducted on different days with different females. It has been suggested that young rams so selected at 1 1/2 years of age, by serving more frequently and providing better coverage, may allow reduction in mating ratios without reducing flock fertility. It would be valuable also to simultaneously determine the mount:service ratio as an indication of mating dexterity or sex behavior efficiency. Young rams with lower sex drive show more mounts per service, and this characteristic does not improve with age.

The reaction times from introduction of the male and female to the first mount or service have also been used as a measure of sex drive; these are influenced by female behavior and the time since previous activity. The number of ejaculations before cessation of activity, i.e., sexual exhaustion, within a standard period is affected by habituation.

VARIATION IN SEXUAL ACTIVITY

Variation in sexual activity has been associated with many factors, one of the most important being the differences between individuals due to both inherited factors and experience. A positive relationship has been suggested between male libido and prolificacy of the ewes of the breed. Libido (number of services per unit time) changes little over several years, but mating dexterity (mounts:service ratio) is more variable. The number of mounts per given period increases with the number of estrous ewes present. Libido usually parallels female sexual activity within the year, but some breeds show little seasonal variation and no decline when run continually with ewes. Breeds differ in their response to a change in latitude; some show greater fluctuations in activity in the tropics and others show none.

Although the ram may be active throughout the 24-hour period, there are pronounced peaks of activity, mainly about sunrise and, to a lesser degree, sunset. Relatively high temperatures (mean daytime reading 27°C) reduce libido, but they have no apparent endocrinological effect. The loss of libido is probably an indication of discomfort because of overheating. Unless very severe, other types of inclement weather cause only minor disruption of sex activity.

Over a 17-day period a significant decline occurs in both the number of ewes served by a ram and the number of services per estrous ewe. During the mating season there is probably a decline in ram searching activity.

A high-protein diet does not improve performance, whereas undernutrition, sufficient to cause weight loss in 5 weeks, results in a significant reduction in services. Obesity is reported to increase reaction time. The factors involved in loss of male condition during the breeding period are not understood. There is no correlation between time spent eating and the number of estrous ewes present or the number mated. The energy expended in service is comparatively small.

ABSENCE OF MATING BEHAVIOR

In some instances, flocks of rams reared in sexual isolation from 3 months of age fail to respond sexually to adult cycling females. This is probably a dominance effect, and it would be reasonable to suppose the rams would serve those females over which they were dominant.

It is commonly suggested that rams may become inactive or sexually inhibited after adverse experiences; these have not been adequately identified. Painful conditions, e.g., foot rot and foot abscess, can be expected to reduce or eliminate mounting.

The reasons why many rams are inactive are not clear. Active rams immediately start searching for estrous ewes on introduction to a flock. Inactive rams show no obvious interest in females and attempt to remain in the company of other males, even avoiding ewes when separated from other males. The formation of all-male groups out of season, however, is characteristic of the species.

The role of thyroxine in the ram is not fully understood. Although it is apparently capable of increasing libido during the Australian summer, thyroidectomy made no difference to the libido of a small group of rams. Normal reproductive function is considered to require adequate circulating levels of thyroxine, and the possibility remains that a deficiency may be implicated in a loss of libido.

Treatment of intact but inactive rams with testosterone, human chorionic gonadotropin, p-chlorophenylalanine or pargyline has not been shown to have any beneficial effects on either mating behavior or libido in the ram. Although there may be an inherited basis for inactivity, this requires elucidation. One ram was reported to show adverse effects of inbreeding, reputedly an inability to recognize the olfactory signs of estrus.

The effect of inactive rams in the flock varies with conditions. It has been estimated that under intensive situations and when ewes require relatively few services for conception, up to 50 per cent of the males may be inactive before their presence is apparent. Conversely, 20 per cent of rams being inactive may result in markedly lowered conception rates under different circumstances. Young rams that do eventually become active mark fewer ewes, serve individual ewes on fewer occasions and serve fewer ewes per unit time.

MATING RATIOS

Effective mating ratios are influenced by the nature of the mating area and the age of both ewes and rams. Although one adult ram per 100 adult ewes is adequate on small, flat paddocks, a 3:100 ratio is required for adequate mating of 1 1/2-year-old ewes in the first cycle after introduction. As young rams (1 1/2 years old) mount and serve less frequently than older rams (2 1/2 years old), double the number of young males are required to achieve results equivalent to mature rams.

The size of the paddock also has a notable effect on the fertility of young females. It would be reasonable to suggest that more rams are required when there are many natural barriers that reduce visual contact.

A ratio of one adult ram to 50 ewes is usually considered a reasonable working figure under most conditions, but individual rams can serve 250 ewes within 6 weeks.

CONCLUSION

Present information does not allow a clear definition of normal mating behavior. Mating behavior needs to be considered in functional terms, and a ram's performance must remain the ultimate criterion of his mating fitness. However, it should be remembered that in controlling breeding, man may introduce and perpetuate inherited traits of behavior that reduce subsequent performance. At the present state of knowledge, therefore, a conservative approach seems to be justified, and if a ram's mating behavior is in doubt, it is better that he should be culled.

REFERENCES

1. Fraser, A. F.: Reproductive Behaviour in Ungulates. London, Academic Press, 1968.
2. Hulet, C. V., Alexander, G. and Havez, E. S. E.: The behaviour of sheep. *In* Hafez, E. S. E. (ed.): The Behaviour of Domestic Animals. 3rd Ed., London, Bailliere Tindall, 1975.

Examination of the Ram for Breeding Soundness

A. NEIL BRUERE

Massey University, Palmerston North, New Zealand

The veterinary inspection of rams for breeding soundness prior to either sale or mating is now practiced in many sheep-raising countries. As a result, considerable information has been recorded, and the incidence of disease affecting the genitalia of rams has been reported to be as high as 10.7 per cent in rams of all ages in Australia, rising to 35 per cent in aged rams. In New Zealand up to 20 per cent of ram lambs in some flocks have been rejected for unsoundness of the genitalia. Also as a result of these investigations, an extensive range of diseases and defects of the penis, prepuce, scrotum, testes and epididymides of rams has been documented. Many of these conditions affect the subsequent breeding performance and fertility of the ram either permanently or temporarily. The veterinarian involved in ram soundness examinations must have a wide knowledge of and experience with these diseases and must realize that in some instances their diagnosis, control, eradication and prevention are now possible, while in others we have a very poor understanding of either their etiology or transmission, let alone their control. The veterinarian should also recognize that he has an obligation to two different types of sheep farmer, the stud or pedigree breeder producing rams for sale to the commercial sheep farmer who, in turn, is aiming at maximum reproductive performance from his flock.

THE EXAMINATION

Whole-flock examination should be conducted with the rams in the standing position and should involve an examination of the scrotum and its contents and the prepuce. Rams that require more detailed examination should be tipped over.

Single-ram examination of pedigree and valuable animals should also include a general clinical examination. In either case a diagnosis of soundness or unsoundness may be supported by a semen test and other ancillary diagnostic aids.

Identification by either a wool or an ear tag of rams that have passed a veterinary examination may be useful for sheep that are destined for sale within a short time of examination. Technically a ram can *only* be guaranteed sound on the day of examination.

If a certificate is issued following either a whole-flock or a single-ram examination, it should state clearly what was done, e.g., an examination of the scrotum and its contents and prepuce or a full clinical examination. The results of other tests, if conducted, should also be included.

The timing of the ram examination is very important. Rams should be inspected regularly and well before the start of the mating season. In general two situations must be considered. First, the owners of stud or pedigree ram flocks and commercial ram-producing flocks have a particular responsibility to the sheep industry because they must supply rams that are not only of sound genetic background but also of good fertility and free from the major defects to be outlined shortly. In order that information can be gathered on the overall incidence of genital disease in a given stud flock, the first veterinary inspection of rams should take place soon after weaning. At least two to three inspections of rams between weaning and the two-tooth stage (1 year and 1 year, 6 months) not only acquaints the flock owner with any problems but also enables control measures to be initiated if disease is detected. Regular examination and record-keeping also provide important local and national data from which priorities for research can be established.

Second, in the case of flock rams at least one annual examination a month prior to mating will insure that animals are in rising health and free of known disease. Likewise, treatment and replacement of defective rams can take place in plenty of time to insure enough sound rams for mating.

CATEGORIES OF SOUNDNESS

For clinical differentiation the following categories of soundness or unsoundness are suggested for general use. A *genitally sound ram* is one that has no congenital, physical or genital abnormalities or any condition that in its progression will cause a ram to become incapable of service. A *fertile ram* is one that is able to serve and is capable, in the opinion of the examining veterinarian, of impregnating the ewes mated to him. A *certifiable ram* must be one that is both genitally sound and fertile, but for practical purposes of inspection three separate degrees of breeding soundness are recognized:

1. The *full sound ram*, which is free from all defects of the genitalia and, as far as can be gauged by clinical examination, is sound for sale and mating.

2. The *temporarily unsound ram*, which has some defect that can be treated and the ram restored to full soundness.

3. The *permanently unsound ram*, in which the defect or disease will permanently nullify or impair the performance of that ram.

SPECIFIC CONDITIONS CAUSING UNSOUNDNESS IN THE RAM

There are a number of conditions that contribute to genital unsoundness in the ram that, for descriptive purposes, are best dealt with in the order of the regions inspected.

The inspection usually begins with the prepuce and penis, followed by the scrotum, and finally the testes and epididymides are palpated through the scrotum. A full examination of the penis is not carried out in large numbers of commercial rams but is essential in valuable animals or those that are to be mated alone to selected ewes.

The Prepuce

Phimosis

Phimosis is recorded in some breeds of rams and may be detected either when the penis cannot be extruded or when ewes return to service or fail to produce lambs. It is generally accepted as a congenital condition causing permanent unsoundness.

Balanoposthitis or Pizzle Rot

The most common condition affecting the penis and prepuce of rams is balanoposthitis or pizzle rot. This disease is caused by a bacterium that grows profusely in alkaline urine, which is produced readily by sheep fed a protein-rich diet. It is seen very commonly in those countries in which such diets are produced by rapidly growing improved pasture. The causal bacterium produces ammonia from the urea excreted in the urine as a result of such a diet. The ammonia is the cytotoxic agent and has a direct scalding effect on the penis and prepuce, producing the characteristic signs of pizzle rot. The disease is venereal in nature and can be transmitted freely between ewes, rams, wethers and lambs. Cattle can also become affected and act as carriers.

This condition is easy to detect. The veterinarian should instruct the farmer about the nature of this disease and emphasize that it can be prevented. This can be done by insuring that infected animals are isolated from other mating animals. Such animals should be treated and cured well before mating. It is also highly desirable to eliminate the conditions under which the causative bacterium breeds. This can be done by keeping the male animals carefully shorn around the prepuce. Any stained wool from this area should be destroyed and not left to contaminate the environment. At certain times of the year it may be necessary to carefully restrict the diet of male animals in order to produce an acid urine, which will automatically clear minor external lesions of pizzle rot.

In the case of mild external lesions (posthitis), a few days of restricted diet with *ad libitum* water will usually effect a cure without topical medication. With severe internal lesions as well (balanoposthitis), it may be necessary to dose the ram with ammonium chloride (1 to 3 gm, two to three times daily) and in addition to irrigate the prepuce with suitable antiseptic solutions. In severe cases it may be necessary to incise the prepuce to allow drainage of urine and pus. In such severe cases, the urethral process and penis are frequently damaged, and the ram becomes permanently unsound.

The Penis

The examination of the penis of the ram requires the animal to be held in a sitting position with its forelegs held by an assistant. The examiner must then secure the penis near the sigmoid flexure with one hand and move it out of the prepuce, where it is held firmly by the other hand. The main defect of the penis is damage to the urethral process that occurs frequently during shearing. Its subsequent effect on fertility is largely unknown. Nevertheless, it does represent a defect and should certainly be noted in pedigree and valuable rams. Blockage of the urethral process by calculi is very common in some countries. As a result, the process frequently becomes necrotic and sloughs off. The necrosis can, and often does, extend to involve the glans penis as well.

The Scrotum

Three important features should be noted in the examination of the scrotum: wool length, the presence or absence of scrotal abscesses and chorioptic mange.

Wool Length

It is important to see that rams with woolly scrota (e.g., Romney, Merino, Corriedale) do not carry excess wool during the mating season. (Note that this is not an unsoundness as such.) Wool length can affect testis size, and an optimum length is about 0.5 to 1.0 cm at mating.

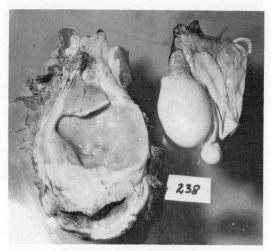

Figure 1. Penetrating scrotal abscess of the left testis. Note severe atrophy of right testis.

Scrotal Abscesses

These occur frequently in rams and are a common cause of both temporary and permanent unsoundness. They should be treated carefully, as they tend to extend to deeper structures and often permanently damage the genitalia (Fig. 1).

Chorioptic Mange

Chorioptic or scrotal mange is one of the primary diseases affecting the external genitalia of rams. The causative mites (*Chorioptes bovis*) live and feed on the skin of sheep, goats, cattle and horses. Their life cycle is about 3 weeks from the egg to the larval stage to the egg-laying female. The disease is not confined solely to the ram but is probably widespread in both sexes in most sheep flocks. The mites are usually found on the lower half of the body, particularly on the scrota of rams, around the dew claws, brisket and often on the poll. Many sheep have mites without mange, but when mange does occur, it is generally on those areas of the body on which the mites concentrate. Paradoxically, however, in individual sheep the extent of the mange is not necessarily related to mite numbers. Mildly infested sheep may have the most severe mange. Rams without lesions of chorioptic mange are just as likely to be infected with mites as those with lesions. Furthermore, rams with old inactive lesions may be free of mites.

Severe mange in the scrotum will reduce fertility and may even cause temporary or permanent sterility. Outbreaks of scrotal mange can be quite explosive and unpredictable and under suitable conditions will persist over long periods. Its control is therefore of considerable importance to the ram breeder.

From this summary of scrotal mange, the following implications can be drawn when considering ram soundness: First, lesions of chorioptic mange must be diagnosed as either active or inactive. Active lesions when rubbed usually produce a marked nibbling or biting response by the ram. Active lesions when scraped or interfered with leave a bleeding area or at least a noticeable hyperemia. Such areas may be pinhead size or larger. If such lesions are found, the ram is temporarily unsound and must be removed from the flock for treatment. Severe active or inactive lesions covering approximately more than half of the scrotum render animals totally unsuitable for mating during that season and may even render them permanently unsound. It is important to remember that all animals without lesions may carry mites, and this must be considered when advising the farmer on treatment and control.

Control and Treatment. Treatment can be applied either locally, i.e., to the affected scrotum, or generally, i.e., application by shower dip of a suitable parasiticide of which the organophosphorous compound diazinon is most widely used. Topical treatment is satisfactory for individual cases, but for flock treatment the use of shower dipping at the higher recommended concentrations of diazinon is highly efficient for both treatment and prevention.

The Testes

Testis Size

As many examinations will be carried out on ram hoggets (4 months to 1 year of age) actually completing puberty, it is pertinent to remember the following points: There appears to be a closer relationship between testicular growth and body weight than between testicular weight and ram age. When body weight increases beyond 20 kg, testicular weight increases at a greater rate, maximum growth taking place between 23 and 27 kg. Puberty is reached at approximately 140 days of age and at 35 kg of body weight.

However, there are wide between-breed differences (e.g., Suffolk, 112 days; Merino, 225 days). Increased testicular size implies increased spermatogenesis, and this is more so in younger than in older animals.

It must also be remembered that not uncommonly one testis in the ram descends before the other. Also there is frequently a size differential between testes during puberty that becomes inapparent at maturity. This must be considered carefully when rejecting young rams because of either hypoplasia or atrophy of one testis.

In the examination of the testis of the mature ram, we must insure that both size and tone are adequate. Testis size is related proportionately to the sperm output of the individual ram. The ram with large symmetrical testes that are free from defects is likely to produce semen of good quality. In fact, the manual examination of ram genitalia is now considered much more important and is generally more relevant to fertility prediction than a single semen examination. Semen examination, unless expertly executed, can lead to quite erroneous conclusions concerning the suitability of a particular ram for mating. Small testes are likely to produce semen of poor quality.

Hypo-Orchidism

It is clinically difficult to differentiate testicular atrophy from testicular hypoplasia unless the former is associated with an obvious defect such as concurrent epididymitis. Also, the inexperienced veterinarian must acquaint himself or herself with the seasonal variation in testes size, particularly noticeable in such breeds as the Romney. A sound ram at the height of the breeding season should have large oval testes that are firm to the touch and of equal size. The thin nonresilient testis is usually seen out of the breeding season or may be associated with poor health. Note also that remarkable changes in size and form can take place in the testis of the ram once mated.

The term hypo-orchidism has been coined to include both testicular atrophy and testicular hypoplasia. Distinct forms of testicular hypoplasia (Figs. 2 to 5) include:

1. Unilateral testicular hypoplasia.
2. Testicular hypoplasia due to cryptorchidism and monorchidism.
3. Primary micro-orchidism (XXY chromosomal complement).

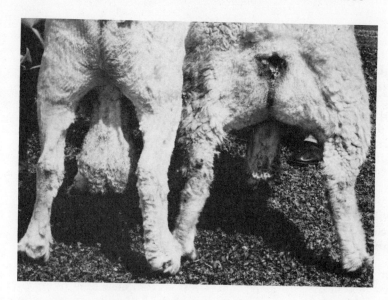

Figure 2. Scrotum and testes of a normal Romney ram (left) compared with those of a ram with severe testicular hypoplasia.

4. Micro-orchidism of unknown etiology.
5. Hypo-orchidism in association with segmental aplasia of the epididymis.
6. Bilateral epididymal spermiostasis and hypo-orchidism.
7. Hourglass testes and hypo-orchidism.
8. Hypo-orchidism and inguinal hernia.

9. Hypo-orchidism in association with varicocele.

Testicular atrophy can be seen in association with systemic disease and other physical and chemical factors. It can also be seen as a result of epididymitis, chorioptic mange and so forth. Therefore, extreme caution

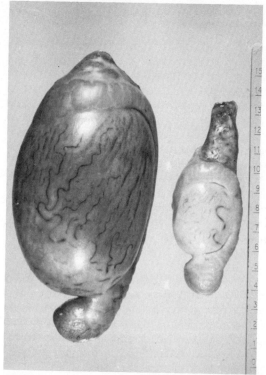

Figure 3. Testis of normal ram (left) and testis from ram of same age with primary micro-orchidism (right).

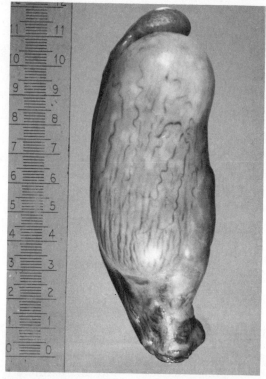

Figure 4. Hourglass testis caused by stricture of the tunica vaginalis testis.

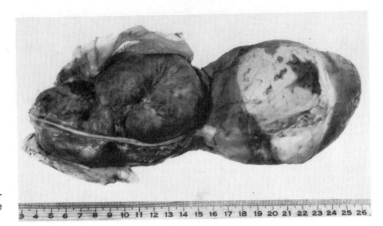

Figure 5. Testis of a ram and associated varicocele. The varicocele was intra-abdominal.

should be exercised when giving a decision on the soundness of a ram with hypo-orchidism. Many cases may have to be regarded as temporarily unsound and should be re-examined at a later date.

The many types of hypo-orchidism may need particular investigation to determine their etiology. For example, in valuable rams chromosome analysis may reveal individual cases of primary micro-orchidism in which rams have two X chromosome as well as a Y chromosome.

The Epididymides

Disorders of the epididymides are the most common cause of ram wastage, accounting for over half the rams rejected for genital unsoundness. There are several known bacterial etiological agents, of which the most common are *Brucella ovis*, *Actinobacillus* sp., *Corynebacterium* spp. and *Pasteurella pseudotuberculosis*.

The detection of palpable lesions of epididymitis presents few problems to the experienced veterinarian. The important factor is the diagnosis of the cause.

Brucella Ovis

Brucellosis of rams has been recorded in many sheep-raising countries of the world and is a major cause of epididymitis. Under some circumstances the organism can cause a placentitis with subsequent abortion in ewes, but as a cause of abortion in sheep its role is probably overemphasized. In many flocks the incidence of brucellosis is low, and the effect of the few rams with reduced fer-tility caused by epididymitis is offset by overmating, i.e., using 2 to 3 per cent of rams. However, in flocks in which the incidence among mating rams is high, there is good clinical evidence to support the belief that low fertility may result and that the lambing will be spread over a longer period than normal. The detection of affected rams and the control of this disease are therefore of considerable importance to sheep production.

Transmission. *Brucella ovis* may be transmitted from sheep to sheep by a number of ways. However, it would appear that rectal transmission from ram to ram, particularly young rams following sodomy, is the main means of spread in affected flocks. Rams may also acquire infection following passive venereal transmission from ewes, and some ewes may carry infection from one lambing season to the next. There is also evidence that suggests that some ram lambs may be born infected with *Br. ovis* and survive to infect other rams at puberty. *Br. ovis* may also be recovered for up to 10 days from the vagina of some ewes that abort or expel infected placentae, so that the postabortion estrus that normally follows 6 months later may be an important avenue of spread of brucellosis. However it is generally believed that the majority of ewes do not remain infected into the following mating season.

Diagnosis. Following active infection, palpable lesions of epididymitis can be detected within 5 weeks. At this stage the epididymis, usually the tail, will be hard and swollen, but as the lesions progress, the testis atrophies and the lesions attain relatively enormous size and frequently appear

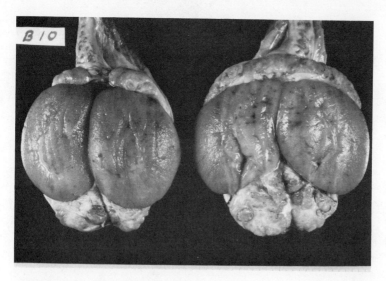

Figure 6. Acute epididymitis of the right testis caused by *Brucella ovis*.

larger than the atrophied testis itself. Lesions may be palpated in the body and the head of the epididymis as well as in the tail, and both testes are often affected. (Fig. 6).

A confirmed diagnosis of *Br. ovis* may be made in several ways. First it is possible to culture the organism from semen ejaculates obtained even from rams with nonpalpable lesions since *Br. ovis* resides in the secondary sex glands as well as in the epididymides. Semen culture is not absolutely reliable, and several ejaculates may need to be examined before either a positive or negative diagnosis may be made. The organism is acid-fast and stains readily by the Ziehl-Neelsen technique.

Second, autopsy of the affected ram and pathological and histopathological examination of the lesions will also be helpful but not completely diagnostic. Early lesions consist mainly of epithelial cysts with epithelial hyperplasia and fibrosis with lumen obstruction of the epididymides. The common lesion is a spermatic granuloma with rupture of the epididymal tubule and extravasation of spermatozoa. Testicular degeneration fibrosis and calcification are the usual sequelae.

The third and main aid to diagnosis is the complement fixation (CF) test for *Br. ovis*. This test is highly accurate in the hands of reliable operators. For the accurate diagnosis of infected rams, fresh serum samples need to be prepared and forwarded to a diagnostic laboratory as soon as possible, avoiding high temperatures. The CF test is, however, of no value in detecting affected animals if a vaccination policy of control has been introduced (see following paragraphs),

since CF antibodies persist in vaccinated rams for several years.

Control. There is no known therapy for *Br. ovis* in sheep; therefore, control either by detection and slaughter of affected animals or by vaccination is essential.

In pedigree and ram breeding flocks the regular inspection of all rams and sires for sale is essential. Once a diagnosis of brucellosis is confirmed, the regular use of the CF test for the detection of carrier animals is required for eradication. The use of this test will depend on the state of infection in the flock. Initially it may be necessary to repeat the screening of all rams twice a year, but once the incidence has been reduced, the annual testing of ram hoggets at about 10 to 12 months of age and of breeding rams at least 1 month prior to mating is probably adequate.

All rams to be introduced into the flock should be isolated and CF tested before contact with the main flock. A *Br. ovis* eradication scheme based on the CF test has been successful in markedly reducing the incidence of this disease in Tasmania.

In commercial flocks a full test and slaughter policy may not be acceptable. Good control of brucellosis can be achieved by vaccinating all rams without epididymitis. An oil-based vaccine is available that gives adequate protection for the breeding life of the ram. Rams should be in good health when vaccinated and must be injected at least 6 weeks prior to mating. Ram lambs are better vaccinated well after puberty but not during inclement weather. Vaccination is usually done by simultaneous use of the oil-based *Br. ovis* vaccine together with *Br. abortus* strain 19. It must be emphasized that vaccination precludes the detection of naturally infected animals by use of the CF test.

Control by the segregation of the different age groups of rams has been practiced prior to the development of the CF test and a vaccine. This produced some degree of success but necessitated the mating of each age group of rams with their corresponding age group of ewes. The management problems are obvious.

Actinobacillosis

There are reports from several major sheep-raising countries, Australia, New Zealand, South Africa and the United States, of a specific epididymitis of young rams caused by the organism *Actinobacillus seminis,* of which there are apparently many antigenically different strains. The organism has also been associated with a suppurative polyarthritis and posthitis in sheep.

Infection with *A. seminis* is seen as either an acute or chronic orchitis, epididymo-orchitis or epididymitis. The disease is usually very acute and mainly seen in ram lambs at or soon after puberty. It is occasionally seen in older rams but usually in the chronic form. The lesions are characterized by intense swelling and pain of the scrotal contents accompanied by a severe systemic reaction. Frequently lesions rupture to the exterior and discharge copious gray-to-yellow pus. Animals lose condition and death has followed in some instances (Fig. 7).

The chronic and more insidious epididymitis as seen in *Br. ovis* disorders also frequently follows *A. seminis* infection. The lesions are permanent and are detected easily on palpation of the genitalia.

Transmission. The method of transmission is uncertain. It is believed that between rams transmission may be by sodomy, but such venereal transmission is in doubt. It would appear that the organism may be transmitted by a variety of routes so that merely overcrowding young rams may be a major method of spreading the disease.

Control. Control of actinobacillosis is difficult. Clinically affected animals should be removed from the flock and slaughtered. The detection of carrier animals is also difficult, but a CF test has been shown to be valuable in South Africa. It is emphasized, however, that a number of antigenic strains need to be included in the test.

At present there is no vaccine available for the prevention of this disease. It is probable that vaccine production will be difficult because of the pleomorphic state of the organism.

Other Causes of Epididymitis

Other organisms (as just named) have been isolated from instances of epididymitis in rams; they are, however, relatively unimportant and sporadic in occurrence. In summary, it should be emphasized that in addition to the specific conditions described here, the general health and conformation of rams should be considered during a soundness examination. In some countries a full soundness examination includes evaluation of teeth, feet and other factors.

CONCLUSIONS

Genital disease of rams accounts for a high wastage in the sheep industry of most countries so that the examination of rams for breeding soundness has become an accepted and highly economical veterinary procedure.

Three broad categories of breeding soundness are now recognized for the ram: sound, temporarily unsound and permanently unsound. The examination requires a highly skilled and informed approach with the use

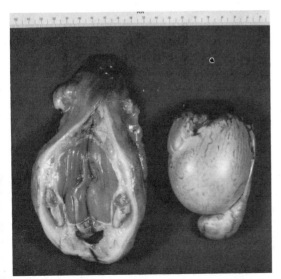

Figure 7. Chronic epididymitis and orchitis of left testis caused by *A. seminis.*

of a wide range of ancillary aids to diagnosis including semen examination and serological, microbiological, pathological and other special tests. There is an ever increasing demand from the sheep industries for sound, disease-free rams. The veterinary profession should be aware of the many new advances in knowledge of genital disease of sheep in order to be able to deal with this demand.

REFERENCES

1. Bruere, A. N.: Some clinical aspects of hypoorchidism (small testes) in the ram. N.Z. Vet. J., *18*:189, 1970.
2. Gunn, R. M. C., Sanders, R. N. and Granger, W.: Studies in fertility in sheep. Bull. Coun. Scient. Ind. Res. Melb., No. 148, 1942.
3. Hughes, K. L.: The epidemiology of *Br. ovis* infection. Proceedings of the New Zealand Veterinary Association Sheep Society. 2nd Seminar. Massey University, 1972, p. 55.
4. Miller, S. J. and Moule, G. R.: Clinical observations on the reproductive organs of Merino rams in pastoral Queensland. Aust. Vet. J., *30*:353, 1954.
5. Quinlivan, T. D.: Breeding soundness in the ram: A review of the proceedings and resolutions from two seminars held in 1964 and 1969. N.Z. Vet. J., *18*:233, 1970.
6. van Tonder, E. M.: Infection of rams with *Actinobacillus seminis*. J. S. Afr. Vet. Ass., *44*(3):245, 1973.
7. Watt, D. A.: Testicular abnormalities and spermatogenesis of the ovine and other species. Vet. Bull., *42*(4):181, 1972.

Semen Collection and Evaluation

ADRIAN P. RHODES
New Zealand Dairy Board, Hamilton, New Zealand

Semen is easily collected from the ram and provides a simple diagnostic method that may help evaluate the animal's reproductive status. It should be noted that this procedure is only one part of the total examination of the ram for breeding soundness. Semen collection and evaluation are also essential parts of the process of artificial insemination.

SEMEN COLLECTION

Semen can be collected from the dry vagina of a nonestrous ewe, by an artificial vagina or by electrical stimulation.

Artificial Vagina

An artificial vagina (AV) is illustrated in Figure 1. The temperature of the AV should be be between 41 and 44°C at the time of collection. The AV is lubricated with a sterile nontoxic lubricant, e.g., white petrolatum or K-Y jelly, and the pressure is adjusted via the tap. Rams are most easily trained to serve an AV during the breeding season. They should be handled frequently and quietly in the collection area and preferably hand-fed for a few weeks prior to training. They also vary considerably in their response to training, each animal requiring a slightly different technique.

Initially, estrous ewes are run with the rams in the collection area, and the rams are allowed to serve the ewes. Dominant rams may have to be removed. After the introductory phase, an estrous ewe is restrained in a crush, and one ram at a time is allowed into the collection area. This is then repeated with the semen collector present, the collector finally touching the ram's sheath. The AV is then introduced, the penis is deflected to the side by manipulation of the sheath, and the ram is allowed to serve the AV while in a rising motion. The ram should be given time to recover postservice before being taken quietly back to a different pen. Once rams are trained to serve an AV, subsequent collections are quick and several samples can be obtained in a short space of time.

This method is preferable to other methods of semen collection when maximum output is required over a period of weeks, e.g., in artificial breeding.

Electrical Stimulation

Rams respond well to electrical stimulation procedures for semen collection, and large numbers of untrained rams can be collected in a short period. Semen can be obtained at any time of the year from nearly

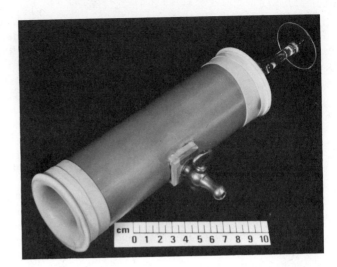

Figure 1. Artificial vagina suitable for collecting ram semen.

all rams. Electrical stimulation is therefore a good method for semen collection when evaluating rams for breeding soundness. A Nicholson transistorized electroejaculator suitable for this purpose is illustrated in Figure 2. Many other types are also satisfactory.

Rams to be electrically stimulated are best restrained on their sides with their hind legs tied back. A foot trimming cradle held in the horizontal position is ideal. The penis is extruded manually and is held in an exteriorized position with a gauze bandage so that the urethral process can be directed into a dry, clean, prewarmed, graduated glass tube. An assistant inserts the lubricated probe into the rectum, and the electrical stimulation is given for 3 seconds with a similar rest period between stimulations. If the ram has not ejaculated after 10 stimulations, the animal should be rested for 5 minutes and the process repeated. Some electrostimulators such as the Nicholson transistorized electroejaculator use a potentiometer rather than a simple make-and-break stimulus.

Semen volume and density are more variable with semen collected by electrical stimulation when compared with semen collected by the AV. However, the quality of the spermatozoa obtained by electrical stimulation is indistinguishable from that obtained with the AV at the time of collection.

Since spermatozoa production per gram of testis tissue is relatively constant in the ram, an estimate of testicular size should be made when assessing a ram's spermatozoa production potential.

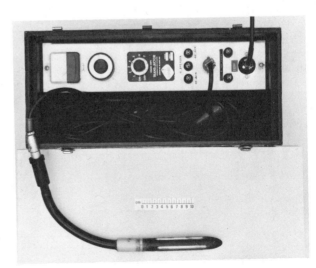

Figure 2. Nicholson transistorized electroejaculator assembled with ram probe (Nicholson Mfg., Inc., Denver, Colorado).

SEMEN EVALUATION

Routine Examination

A good microscope with a built-in light source and warm stage is a prerequisite for semen evaluation work. A simple warm box is also necessary. Ram semen is very sensitive to cold shock and many chemicals, and glassware should be thoroughly cleaned and prewarmed prior to contact with semen. Assessment of ram semen is usually limited to the physical parameters: volume, concentration, motility, percentage of live spermatozoa and spermatozoal morphological findings. In most circumstances more sophisticated semen quality tests do not help the veterinarian significantly in assessing the semen quality of individual rams. Immediately after collection the volume of semen can be read and an estimate of the concentration made by assessing the opacity of the sample (Table 1).

Actual spermatozoa counts can be made using a hemocytometer, the semen being killed and diluted with formal saline (9 gm of NaCl plus 10 ml of 10 per cent commercial formalin in 1 liter of distilled water).

A standard depth slide suitable for motility estimates can be made by gluing two coverslips about 1 cm apart to a glass slide. A drop of semen is transferred with a glass rod to the standard depth slide, covered with a coverslip and the motility assessed. The percentage of live motile spermatozoa can be readily estimated by diluting a small drop of semen with prewarmed normal saline on a plain glass slide and covering this with a coverslip. Care must be taken that semen and saline are at the same temperature.

Examination of the diluted sample will give an indication also of the morphological status of the sample and an indication of any cellular debris that may be present. For more detailed morphological assessment, a thin smear, prepared in the same manner as a blood smear, should be made. The smear should be allowed to dry overnight or should be fixed with low heat. Rose bengal is a commonly used morphological stain (combine 3 gm of rose bengal in 99 ml of distilled water plus 1 ml of 40 per cent formalin and sterilize). The slide is stained for 5 minutes and then washed gently in distilled water and dried. Spermatozoa can be classified as (1) normal; (2) immature — proximal and distal protoplasmic droplets; (3) having abnormalities that occur during spermatogenesis — piriform, small, large and twin heads; (4) having abnormalities that occur postspermatogenesis — tailless heads, broken necks, coiled, broken and severely returned tails and (5) having artifacts — returned tails.

Special Stains

Dead spermatozoa are eosinophilic while live spermatozoa do not normally take up supravital stains. The most commonly used live-dead stain is nigrosin-eosin. To obtain reliable results, great care is necessary in the use of supravital stains. Furthermore, the information adds relatively little to the estimate of the proportion of motile spermatozoa observed in a diluted sample. The procedure is not recommended for general use in the field but may be of use under controlled conditions, e.g., at artificial breeding centers.

A rapid repeatable estimate of acrosomal damage has recently been described using the Giemsa stain. The technique is not recommended for general use because of the exacting requirements of stain preparation and procedure. Furthermore, the significance of varying degrees of acrosomal damage in ram semen has not been clearly evaluated.

SEMEN QUALITY AND FERTILITY RELATIONSHIP

The usual reason for assessing a ram's semen quality is to assess the fertilizing capacity of that semen. With an unselected group of rams, approximately 50 per cent of the difference in fertility can be accounted for by difference in semen quality. However, when there is preselection, e.g., when rams are being used for artificial breeding, 20 per cent or less of the differences in fertility can be accounted for by differences in semen

TABLE 1. *Estimating Concentration of Semen by Assessing Opacity*

Degree of Opacity	Concentration (million spermatozoa/ml)	
Creamy	>2000	–
Thick milky	>1000	<2000
Milky	> 250	<1000
Watery milky	> 100	<250
Cloudy	< 100	–

quality. If the semen quality of a ram is high, one sample is enough to suggest that the fertilizing ability of this semen is likely to be satisfactory. If the semen quality is marginal, several samples may need to be taken to be sure that the sample is representative. Minimal requirements for satisfactory semen are milky semen, 60 per cent motile spermatozoa, moderate motility and less than 25 per cent abnormal spermatozoa. The different morphological abnormalities and the degree of degeneration give a good indication as to the severity of the reproductive dysfunction. Degenerate spermatozoa, spermatozoa with piriform heads and cellular debris all suggest severe dysfunction of spermatogenesis, while a high proportion of protoplasmic droplets in an otherwise normal sample may suggest that the reproductive process is in the recovery phase.

REFERENCES

1. Hackett, A. J. and Macpherson, J. W.: Some staining procedures for spermatozoa. A review. Can. Vet. J., *6*:55, 1965.
2. Watson, P. F.: Use of a Giemsa stain to detect changes in acrosomes of frozen ram spermatozoa. Vet. Rec., *97*:12, 1975.

Artificial Breeding Techniques in Sheep

S. J. MILLER
Warwick, Queensland, Australia

Artificial breeding has been utilized in sheep to extend the use of superior sires or to spread a specific character, such as "polledness," rapidly through a population. It has also been used to help in the speedy elimination of undesirable characteristics.

The economic importance of artificial breeding depends largely on the anticipated monetary return from using known superior sires that provide more rapid genetic gains or from overcoming infertility arising from certain causes in difficult environments, especially in the tropics. The likely results will depend on the skill of the operation and the way it is incorporated into any system of sheep breeding.

SELECTION AND MANAGEMENT OF RAMS

Artificial breeding programs should be conducted when ewes are cycling, i.e., late summer, autumn or early winter. However, in some environments rams may be infertile when needed unless precautions are taken. Thus, the events that occur 2 months prior to a program largely influence the results. Eight to 10 weeks prior to use, rams should be shorn, treated for internal and external parasites and wounds and have their feet trimmed. They should also be kept cool and should preferably be shedded and adequately fed. (Rations containing 10 to 12 per cent crude protein and 55 per cent total digestible nutrients in a mixture containing 55 per cent roughage and 45 per cent concentrate are satisfactory.) Two-tooth (1 1/2-year) rams should be segregated from older rams to avoid fighting and sodomy. Shedded rams become quiet and are easier to train to an artificial vagina.

During use rams should be penned individually while waiting their turn as semen donors. This prevents their mounting one another or fighting, and they quickly become accustomed to walking from pen to serving bail and back, saving considerable time.

SEMEN COLLECTION, DILUTION AND STORAGE

An artificial vagina is used to collect the semen, as this gives a maximum output over a period of time. Semen can be collected from most rams at least three times per day over a 17-day insemination period without a drop in semen quality. During an artificial breeding program, semen is assessed rapidly after each collection for volume, color, density and motility, and a visual estimate is made of live-dead ratios.

Semen is mostly used undiluted but can be diluted up to four-fold, depending on the initial concentration. The most common diluents used are whole, skimmed or reconstituted cow's milk that has been heated to 98°C for 10 minutes. Egg yolk, glucose citrate (15 per cent egg yolk; 0.8 per cent glucose anhydrous; 2.8 per cent sodium citrate dihydrate in glass-distilled water) has also been used successfully as a diluent. In practice, dilution rates greater than 1:2 are seldom used. Dilutions are made with the diluting solution at 30 to 35°C.

If not used immediately, diluted semen is cooled to 2 to 5°C over a 2-hour period and held at this temperature. Although some motility is retained for 14 days at this temperature, the fertilizing capacity decreases rapidly after 24 hours of storage, and semen should be used within this period.

Deep Frozen Semen

Preservation of semen by freezing has proved to be more difficult with rams than with bulls, and fertility rates comparable with those achieved by either natural mating or liquid semen techniques have still to be achieved.

Salamon and Visser[3] have conducted experiments on the effect of diluents, glycerol concentration, dilution rate and egg yolk concentration on sperm survival after freezing spermatozoa by the pellet method and storing the pellets at −196°C in liquid nitrogen. Thawed pellets frozen with raffinose-citrate-yolk-glycerol and used after 3 years resulted in a 50 per cent lambing. Lambings of 55 per cent have been achieved using pellet frozen semen in TRIS-glucose-yolk-glycerol diluent. Using dilutions of 1:2, a satisfactory diluent is: 360 mM of TRIS, 33.3 mM of glucose and 113.7 mM of citric acid (to adjust the pH to 6.98 to 7.0) mixed with egg yolk and glycerol so that the final volume of semen contains 12 per cent volume for volume (v/v) egg yolk and 4 per cent (v/v) glycerol. Semen is thawed in a tube at 37°C prior to use.

MANAGEMENT OF THE EWE FLOCK

Accurate and early detection of estrus is essential. Estrus in ewes is detected by va-sectomized rams (teasers) wearing harnesses with crayons (see Figure 1 in Pregnancy Diagnosis of the Ewe, page 900). Teasers should be young, healthy and free from disease. One per cent of vasectomized rams are joined with the ewes the day before insemination commences, and marked ewes are removed (drafted) that afternoon. These ewes are either discarded (as onset of estrus is not known) or else inseminated early the next morning to familiarize assistants with the task being undertaken and to test equipment. Only ewes with increased amounts of clear mucus are inseminated. Ewes are then drafted at 9 AM and 4 PM each day, the 9 AM draft selecting those ewes that came in estrus after the afternoon draft and the 4 PM draft selecting those ewes that came into estrus during the day. Using this teasing pattern, by far the greatest majority of ewes are presented within 12 to 24 hours after the onset of estrus, provided the teasers are efficient. Two teams of teasers are alternated every 3 days to insure this. Teasers may be inefficient when an increasing number of ewes with creamy mucus are presented. This indicates that estrus has terminated and that the teasers may not have been marking ewes early in estrus.

Ewes are normally held in a large yard with access to water between the morning and afternoon drafting to save remustering. This has no effect on fertility or body weights provided ewes are released to good feed following the afternoon draft. When large numbers (4000 to 5000 ewes) are handled in a 17-day program, well-designed facilities are required.

INSEMINATION TECHNIQUE

The ewe is generally restrained with her hindquarters elevated. Special cradles have been devised for this purpose, although simpler facilities can usually be utilized in the normal shearing shed (Fig. 1). When large numbers have to be handled, other operators will have the ewe backed up to a rail or strap and the inseminator standing in a pit. Either way, using two catchers, ewes can be inseminated at the rate of 100 per hour.

The instruments required are simple: a speculum, a head lamp, a Pyrex inseminating tube about 6 inches long and a 1-ml syringe that is attached with a 2-inch rubber

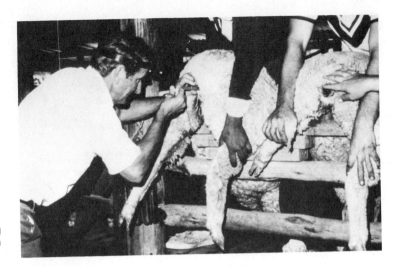

Figure 1. Method of positioning ewes for large-scale insemination program.

connector to the tube. Several types of speculums have been used, including the small duck bill type, a metal tube, a plastic speculum with a built-in light source and a Pyrex test tube with the end cut off at an angle (Fig. 2).

The latter instrument is preferred as it can easily be cleaned, reflects light from the head lamp well, gives a good view of the cervix and allows the operator to position the entrance of the cervix with the lip of the speculum. Plastic instruments are rather more difficult to clean, whereas glassware can be boiled and oven dried. Detergents and disinfectants should be avoided unless thorough rinsing with glass-distilled water is undertaken following the initial cleaning.

The ewe is restrained to limit movement. The speculum, lubricated with liquid paraffin, is inserted into the vagina by an assistant. The inseminator, using the 1-ml syringe, draws up 0.05 to 0.1 ml of semen into the inseminating tube, with a similar volume of air behind it. The tip of the inseminating tube is inserted into the cervical canal; this can usually be penetrated 1 to 3 cm if small-caliber nozzles are used. The long, tortuous canal and the firm cervical wall normally preclude deeper penetration. In old ewes either the annular folds of the canal may be prolapsed through the cervical

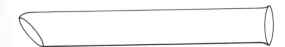

Figure 2. Diagram of Pyrex glass speculum made from a test tube (180 × 25 mm). Note lip at beveled end that is helpful in positioning entrance to cervix.

opening or there may be tissue tags at the opening, making the actual entrance difficult to find. Once the nozzle is in the canal, the plunger of the syringe is depressed and the speculum withdrawn before the tip of the inseminating tube is removed from the cervical os. This procedure allows the walls of the vagina to collapse, and the semen is retained in the cervical canal. It is important to insure that semen is deposited in the entrance of the cervical canal; if deposited only in the anterior vagina, larger volumes of semen and greater sperm numbers are needed to achieve comparable conception rates.

Timing of Inseminations

It has been clearly demonstrated that ovulation occurs about 30 hours after the onset of estrus, which lasts approximately 20 to 24 hours in the ewe. Ova survive in the fallopian tube from 4 to 10 hours. Spermatozoa need several hours to capacitate in the genital tract of the ewe; they may be recovered from the fallopian tube 5 minutes after insemination. Midestrus is therefore the optimum time for insemination, and in practical terms satisfactory results have been achieved when inseminations are performed 12 to 24 hours after the onset of estrus. If this procedure is followed, fertility levels will not be improved by reinseminating 12 hours later; a second insemination will improve conception rates 5 to 10 per cent when the first insemination was performed early in the estrous cycle.

The type of vaginal mucus present pro-

TABLE 1. *Relationship between Types of Mucus at Time of Insemination and Percentage of Ewes Lambing*

Stage of Cycle	Type of Mucus	Number of Ewes Inseminated	Ewes Lambing (%)
Early estrus	Clear and sparse	100	50
Midestrus	Clear and copious	200	68
	Cloudy and copious	103	65
Late estrus	Cloudy	108	55
	Creamy	90	32
Postestrus	"Cheese-like"	80	12

vides a good practical guide to the stage of the cycle at which insemination should be carried out (Table 1).

Ewes should be inseminated with a minimum of 50 million sperm in volumes of 0.05 to 0.1 ml of semen if satisfactory results are to be achieved (good quality ram semen should contain 150×10^6 sperm per 0.05 ml). Provided these standards are observed, good results can be achieved using diluted or undiluted semen.

Failures in sheep artificial insemination (AI) programs are mainly due to poor organization and technique. Thus, poor pretreatment of rams, failure to have adequate feed for ewes, inefficient teasing and unnecessary handling of ewes after insemination all lead to unsatisfactory results. Faults in technique commonly observed include lack of speed, failure to deposit semen in the cervical canal (particularly if too much air is used to expel the semen since this tends to blow the semen back into the vagina) and not withdrawing the speculum before the semen is deposited.

REFERENCES

1. Dun, R. B.: Artificial insemination of sheep. Aust Vet. J., *35*:256, 1959.
2. Morrant, A. J. and Dun, R. B.: Artificial insemination of sheep. Aust. Vet. J., *36*:1, 1960.
3. Salamon, S. and Visser, D.: Fertility of ram spermatozoa frozen and stored for five years. J. Reprod Fertil., *37*:433, 1974.

Estrous Synchronization and Control of the Estrous Cycle

T. D. QUINLIVAN

Animal Production Services, Waipukurau, New Zealand

Two considerations are necessary in programs designed to control the estrous cycle. The first depends upon the initial priming with progesterone/progestogen during the anestrous period, whereas the second, which is used during the breeding season, involves blocking ovulation in a simple manner and then producing an effective release at will. If natural service is to be used, estrus must accompany this release. Although this may not be essential when artificial insemination is employed (provided the time of ovulation can be accurately controlled), there is now evidence that conception rates are likely to be higher in ewes that exhibit overt estrus.

SYNCHRONIZATION TECHNIQUES AND THEIR APPLICATION

There is no universal technique that will cover all controlled breeding situations. Potential users must remember that estrous control programs are management tools only; the majority of failures occur because either the method is not adapted to the situation or the technique is used in circumstances in which it should not have been applied at all. For success it is necessary to recognize that several physiological states exist that are controlled by external and internal factors. For example, seasonal influences will determine whether the ewe is in her natural breeding season or in early, mid or late anestrus; her age will determine whether she is a pubertal lamb, maiden ewe or mature ewe, and her lactational state will determine whether she is dry because she has not been pregnant, dry because she lost a lamb postpartum or dry because she is either suckled or milked in the postpartum period. Each of the possible combinations must be considered separately in relation to such factors as dose and method of administration of progestogen, dose of pregnant mare serum gonadotropin (PMSG), number of spermatozoa used for insemination and whether fresh or frozen semen is used.

All the techniques described require the use of progestogens, whether in association with PMSG or not. The former may be given in the form of progesterone injections, Silastic implants or synthetic progestogens administered as intravaginal pessaries or in oral feed preparations.

Initiating Ovulatory Activity in the Anestrous Period

Systems designed to produce two lamb crops a year have been described. All require pretreatment with progesterone/progestogen for 12 to 16 days followed by the administration of PMSG within 24 hours after cessation of progestogen therapy. Table 1 details the treatment procedures for the three physiological states likely to be encountered.

The induction of estrus and ovulation does not constitute a problem if the dose of PMSG is modified according to breed and season, although the ratio of the conception rate to the induced estrus is variable in the spring and always lower than in the autumn. Poor results have been obtained when the technique is used with breeds that experience very deep anestrus. These seasonal influences may best be overcome by manipulation of the photoperiod.

Conception rates generally increase as the interval from parturition to service widens; some breeds perform better than others in this respect.[1]

The restoration of cyclic activity after parturition is strongly dependent upon lactation, and this influence persists even when estrus is induced by progestogen-PMSG treatment. To obtain a high proportion of ewes ovulating after hormonal induction, it is necessary to use a higher dose of PMSG for lactating ewes than that used for dry ewes. Furthermore, the conception rate is lower in ewes suckling more than one lamb. Early weaning, between 30 and 40 days postpartum, improves the conception rate to a level comparable with that obtained with nonlactating ewes.

Because of problems with size, alternative methods other than the intravaginal sponge have been tried for pubertal lambs. These include oral progestogens and Silastic Norgestomet (SC21009) implants, which exhibit an earlier onset of estrus after withdrawal — all treated lambs are served within 36 hours of removal.

One of the problems that occurs when ovulation activity is initiated in the anestrous period is associated with the high doses of PMSG that must be used. This causes considerable variation in both the number and spread of ovulations that result, and fertilization is subsequently affected because of variation in the age of ova. This leads to delayed embryonic development at 7 days and increased embryonic loss up to day 12. (Higher embryonic mortality between days 18 and 50 occurs in lactating ewes in the nonbreeding season also, but the reasons for this are at present not known.)

The anticipated results obtained from the treatment regimens shown in Table 1 should

TABLE 1. *Treatment Procedures for Initiating Ovulatory Activity in the Anestrous Period*

Physiological Status	Dose FGA* (mg)	Dose PMSG† (IU)
Dry ewe	40	400–800
Suckling ewe	40	500–800
Pubertal lamb	40	400–600

*Flurogestone acetate (Cronolone, Searle Laboratories).
†Pregnant mare serum gonadotropin.

result in an 80 per cent estrous rate and a pregnancy rate of 40 per cent to service at the induced estrus and 60 per cent to service one cycle later (i.e., returns to first service). Best results have been obtained when PMSG is administered at the time of cessation of progestogen treatment or 24 hours later.

Methods of Advancing the Time of Onset of the Normal Breeding Season

Hormonal Technique

Robinson[7] indicated that the progestogen-PMSG technique was effective in advancing the onset of the breeding season in British breeds of sheep. His results showed that progestogen treatment was required for 17 days, with PMSG (750 IU) administered at the time of sponge withdrawal. A 93 per cent estrous rate can be expected with PMSG treatment and 73 per cent without PMSG, and a lambing rate of 60 to 70 per cent can be achieved after two cycles with natural service. PMSG treatment may not always be necessary; this presumably depends on the physiological state of the particular ewe in respect to the onset of her own natural breeding season at the time the treatment is given.

Ram Effect

It has been well demonstrated that the presence of the ram prior to the commencement of the breeding season is of considerable value in achieving partial estrous synchronization. This joining can stimulate a considerable proportion of the flock to ovulate within a few days, the ovulation occurring without overt estrus. Normal estrous behavior is expressed at the following ovulation approximately 20 to 25 days after the introduction of the rams. However, if the ewes have already commenced ovulatory activity or are in deep anestrus, the ram effect will not operate. The use of the ram in this way has the following advantages:

1. The method is potentially cheap and requires a minimum of labor.
2. Partial synchrony may be useful if follow-up luteolysin treatments are to be used. At 10 to 14 days after ram introduction, a large proportion of the flock will be in the luteal phase of the estrous cycle. At this stage the corpora lutea that are present can

be destroyed by treatment with prostaglandin-$F_{2\alpha}$ ($PGF_{2\alpha}$) or one of its analogs.

3. An advancement in lambing dates can be expected.

4. If artificial insemination (AI) is to be used, the program can be timed to coincide with the first peak of estrous activity, and a large proportion of the flock may be inseminated within a week. Insemination may be restricted to this week if the flock owner wishes to inseminate only a certain number of ewes.

Control of the Time of Estrus, Ovulation and Lambing during the Breeding Season

There has been a general tendency to apply the principles used for the induction of breeding activity in the anestrous ewe to the cyclic animal. Various techniques are possible, and these have been reviewed by Robinson.[7] A universal problem has been the low conception rates obtained at first estrus after synchronization. This is primarily due to faulty sperm transport and can in part be overcome by using a dose of 200×10^6 sperm in a dense inseminate. A more practical solution, however, is to mate at the second estrus, when synchronization is still good and conception rates are indistinguishable from normal.

Use of Progesterone/Progestogens

Injections. Present recommendations show that if this technique is to be used, 12 mg of progesterone administered every 2 days for a total period of 12 days is adequate to provide good synchronization. Administration of PMSG (400 IU) on the day following the cessation of progesterone usage significantly advances and improves the precision of time of onset of estrus and ovulation. Fertility has been variable, ranging from a 13 to 80 per cent lambing rate after natural service or AI.

Oral Administration. The most commonly used oral progestogens are medroxyprogesterone acetate, MAP (Provera) chlormadinone acetate, CAP (Chlormadinone and flurogestone acetate, FGA (Cronolone). The minimum daily dose of CAP and MAP to completely inhibit estrus and ovulation is 1 mg/day. Overt estrus appears to be adequately suppressed during treatment but ovulation is not, and the percentage of con-

TABLE 2. *Dose Rates for Hormonal Treatment during the Breeding Season*

Physiological Status	Dose FGA* (mg)	Dose PSMG† (IU)
Dry cyclic ewe	30–40	0–400
Suckling ewe	30–40	400–600
Pubertal lamb	30–40	250–400

*Flurogestone acetate (Cronolone, Searle Laboratories).
†Pregnant mare serum gonadotropin.

eption rates to service at the first overt strus after progestogen withdrawal has een low, ranging from 23 to 38 per cent. Mauleon[5] reported the successful use of oral FGA at the rate of 8 mg/day followed by the administration of PMSG on the last day of treatment. He reported that 83 per cent of ewes cycled between 48 and 60 hours after treatment, with a mean conception rate of 50 per cent to AI at first estrus.

Intravaginal Pessary. This technique, following a 15-day insertion, leads to effective suppression of estrus and ovulation. Suggested dose rates are shown in Table 2. MAP has also been incorporated in intravaginal pessaries, and best results have been obtained with sponges containing 20 to 80 mg.

The intravaginal pessary technique has particular application in AI programs programs provided the following guidelines are met:

1. Intravaginal pessaries must be prepared using standardized controlled techniques that insure equal distribution of progestogen throughout the sponge.

2. Attention must be given to the nutritional requirements of both ewes and rams in the program, both prior to and during treatment.

3. If PMSG is used, it should be a standardized batch with known assay results. This is essential for accurate dose rate recommendations.

4. To spread the rate at which ewes come into estrus, it may be necessary to stagger the sponge insertion, using two periods separated by several days and for two durations (12 and 16 days).

5. If utilizing AI, only high quality semen must be used with a minimum dose per inseminate of 200×10^6 live sperm and with a maximum dilution rate of no more than 1:2.

6. When utilizing natural service, use 10 to 16 per cent rams to ewes.

7. The degree of synchronization at second estrus after withdrawal is good and fertility is normal. This is the most favored application of the technique in AI programs.

Subcutaneous Implants. Silastic Norgestomet implants have the advantage of continuous progestogen administration with a minimum of animal handling. The technique is characterized by a more rapid onset of estrus after progestogen withdrawal (Table 3), and ovulation after the commencement of estrus occurs earlier.

TABLE 3. *Estrous Synchronization after Various Routes of Progestogen Administration**

Route†	Interval between End of Treatment and Estrus (hours)					
	24	*36*	*48*	*60*	*72*	*84*
Oral FGA	–	–	29	54	4	4
Vaginal sponge	9	40	41	8	2	–
Norgestomet implant	51	49	–	–	–	–

*In all cases PMSG administered on the last day of treatment. Figures in body of table indicate percentage of treated animals responding at that time interval.

†Oral FGA, 8 mg/day; vaginal sponge, 40 mg FGA; Norgestomet implant, 3 mg of SC21009 implanted subcutaneously.

Use of Prostaglandins

As with progestogens, the reduced fertility at the estrus immediately following treatment with prostaglandins has also been a problem.

Single injection techniques have been described with the following results:

PGF$_{2\alpha}$, 15 mg on day 9 of cycle, 86 per cent in estrus 2 to 3 days after treatment.

PGF$_{2\alpha}$, 16 mg between days 7 and 11 of cycle, 66 per cent in estrus 2 to 3 days after treatment.

Luteal regression cannot be reliably induced in sheep by prostaglandins before day 5 of the estrous cycle, and this helps explain the incomplete response. Best results, in terms of estrus and conception rate, have been obtained using a double injection technique with 40 to 150 μg being administered intramuscularly on 27 and 17 days respectively prior to the introduction of 10 per cent of rams.[4] The estrous rate ranged between 85 and 93 per cent, and a conception rate of 45 to 65 per cent was obtained. The second synchronized estrus after treatment showed normal fertility. Additional work using 125 μg of chlorprostenol intramuscularly on day 10 after estrus, followed by a second injection of 125 μg 14 to 15 days later and insemination 64 to 70 hours after the last injection, resulted in a 41 per cent lambing rate.[2]

Increasing Ovulation Rate: The Chance of Multiple Births

Of the pituitary hormones, PMSG and horse anterior pituitary extract (HAP) administered near the end of the estrous cycle will regularly induce multiple ovulations in the ewe. Optimal results have been obtained when PMSG is administered on days 12 to 13 of the natural cycle. Pretreatment with progestogens requires the administration of PMSG at the time of cessation of progestogen treatment. The onset of estrus is earlier than that obtained when progestogens

alone are used. Effective dose rates range between 500 and 2000 IU depending on the body weight of the ewe. The highest doses may cause excessive luteinization of follicles and inhibition of ovulation.

Treatment with HAP for 3 days commencing on the twelfth day of the cycle gives optimal results with 60, 90 and 135 mg producing means of 4.3, 6.6 and 11.3 ovulations respectively. There is no excessive luteinization of follicles reported following the use of HAP in this way.

The superovulatory response of mature animals varies with breed, live weight, stage of estrous cycle, age, postpartum interval, season of year and plane of nutrition. Inconsistent results using pituitary hormones arise because of individual responses and between-batch variations. The number of ova obtained from successive superovulations in the same animal decreases because of refractoriness of the ovaries. The fertilization rate in superovulated ewes is low but can be corrected by the insemination of either larger numbers of spermatozoa or surgical insemination, i.e., intrauterine insemination by surgical means.

REFERENCES

1. Cognie, Y., Cornu, C. and Mauleon, P.: Proceedings from International Symposium on Physiopathology of Reproduction and Artificial Insemination in Small Ruminants. Thessaloniki, 1974, p. 33.
2. Fairnie, I. J., Cumming, I. A. and Martin, E. R.: Proc. Aust. Soc. Anim. Prod., *II*:133, 1976.
3. Gordon, I.: Third World Conference on Animal Production. *3*:34, 1973.
4. Lightfoot, R. J., Croker, K. P. and Marshall, T.: Sheep breeding. Proceedings International Congress, Muresk., Western Australian Inst. Tech., 1976, p. 449.
5. Mauleon, P.: Sheep breeding. Proceedings International Congress, Muresk., Western Australian Inst. Tech., 1976, p. 310.
6. Orskov, E. R. and Robinson, J. J.: Rowett Research Institute Annual Rep., *28*:116, 1972.
7. Robinson, T. J.: The Control of the Ovarian Cycle in the Sheep. Sydney, Sydney University Press, 1967.

Breeding Records

C. A. MARTIN
New Zealand Romney Sheep Breeders
Association, Feilding, New Zealand

An accurate recording system is most important for intensive pedigree breeding and for group breeding schemes. Exact knowledge of the overall performance and production of every ewe and ram must be available so that selection for improvement can be made.

MATING

Each year before the rams are joined with the ewes, a decision concerning mating is made for every ewe. Her pedigree and complete record of production are noted, and the appearance of the ewe is studied in conjunction with the rams, which are evaluated by similar criteria. When joining takes place, the system of using either ram crayons or paste in different colors is adopted so that at the end of mating the period in which every ewe will lamb is known and the sire of every lamb is defined. At this stage the final mating record can be completed.

LAMBING

Large ear tags with clear numbers inscribed or numbered neck tags make ewes readily identifiable during lambing without the need to handle each ewe. As soon as possible after each lamb is born, a permanent ear tag is inserted, thus providing a lifetime identification. Specially prepared field books are used for recording lambing data. The following are the main factors recorded: dam number, date of lambing, sire number taken from the identifying sire mark on the ewe and checked with the mating record, sex and status of the lambs and the serial numbers of the tags inserted. In some cases birth weights are taken, and more recently details relating to the type of birth are recorded, that is, whether the ewe was assisted or not.

WEANING

When lambs are weaned at about 10 weeks of age, the numbers and the weights of all lambs are related to their respective dams. By the use of a computerized system (which should be available to breeders), the maximum use can be made of these weights in assessing the productive values of the dams and the sires, and in these cases corrections can be made for date of birth, age of dam, sex and the rearing rank (single or multiple) of the lamb.

WOOL WEIGHTS

At hogget shearing (10 months to 1 year), when the young sheep are approximately 1 year old, fleece weights are recorded and become another valuable part of the hogget's basic record, as well as being noted on the dam's master record sheet. These wool weights are valuable in selection of the higher producing sheep to be retained in breeding flocks.

MASTER RECORDS

Every sheep in every breeding flock has a "master" record sheet, and these are assembled in numerical order in age groups. This record shows up to a five generation pedigree, and the lifetime performances of all females that appear in the pedigree are shown. The record for every ewe can show the date of each shearing and the weight of wool shorn. For every year that a ewe has been mated, the record will give the stud tag number of the sire, the estrous cycle in which she conceived, the date of lambing, the number and sex of the lambs born, the tag number allocated to each lamb, their weaning weights, the weight of wool at hogget shearing and, finally, comments on exactly what happened to each of the progeny each year. A ram sheet gives the same pedigree and wool information, and increasing numbers of breeders are assessing ram values based on the production of the ewes to which he is mated and on the performance of his dam, granddams and half sisters.

COMPUTERIZED RECORDING

Good recording is of maximum value only if analyzed properly and used efficiently. Because of the organization of the information on special lists for submission to a central record office, a computerized system is becoming an essential aid to sheep breeding. The computer input lists cover lambing, weaning and other live weights, wool weights, and details of the fate of every ewe that is deleted from the scheme. Outputs supply a whole-flock summary covering all aspects of production, an individual ewe summary, a sire summary and a two-tooth (1 1/2 year) selection list for rams and ewes based on the corrected weight of the lambs weaned by the dam together with the weight of wool produced by the two-tooth sheep itself. Formulas for establishing indices of production are established, taking into account the production and the commercial value of both meat and wool, so that the index figure shown against each two-tooth ewe and ram ranks them on productive capacity and becomes one of the most important aids in selection of superior sheep.

CONCLUSION

By using the system just described in New Zealand it has been possible to compare the improvement in lambing percentage achieved between a group of flocks (12,398 ewes) that were involved in a national flock recording scheme and a similar group of the same breed (15,131 ewes) that did not participate in any organized improvement scheme. In 7 years the improvement in the percentage of lambs weaned by those ewes that were included in the recording scheme was 17.7 per cent, whereas the performance of the other group had remained static. It would be possible to apply a similar system to improve sheep production in most countries.

Parameters of Reproductive and Productive Performance

C. A. MARTIN

New Zealand Romney Sheep Breeders Association, Feilding, New Zealand

In the investigation of the productive performance of any flock of sheep, it is essential to determine the levels of all factors that combine to give that performance. Soundly organized and executed survey procedures covering many flocks and large numbers of sheep under varying environments can provide a measure of the factors that are involved.

ONSET OF ESTRUS AND CONCEPTION RATES

In the mating of ewes to rams it is important to know the time and the rate at which the ewes come into estrus and the way in which they conceive. There will be varia- tions from district to district and between breeds. When the period of regular cycling is established, and sound rams are joined with their ewes at varying ratios depending on the type of country, in two estrous cycles (34 days) 99.4 per cent of all ewes will have mated with the rams, and of these, 15 per cent may return from the first mating. Given a normal situation in which 70 per cent of all ewes mate in the first round and 30 per cent in the second, 95 per cent of all ewes are apparently in lamb during the 34-day period. The density of lambing can be altered by the adjustment of the day that the rams are first joined with the ewes, e.g., early mating will give a slower coverage and a slightly higher return rate and, conversely, later mating will give a more rapid coverage and a lower return rate.

BARREN EWES

In a commercial flock situation, a 3.8 per cent level of barren ewes (dry/dry ewes or ewes that do not conceive) may be consid-

ered normal, but if this figure exceeds 5 per
cent, the causes should be investigated. In
defining the barren ewe problem when the
level is 3.8 per cent, 0.6 per cent of the ewes
involved would be those not covered by the
rams, 1.8 per cent would be ewes that took
the ram in each estrous cycle during which
the ram was available but did not conceive
and the other 1.4 per cent would be ewes
that were mated by the ram during one heat
period and did not return to service but subsequently did not produce a lamb.

ABORTIONS

The overall scale of ewes aborting does not
constitute a serious annual loss. In New Zealand, survey work over 15 years involving
50,000 ewes annually indicated an annual
loss of 1.12 per cent. On individual farms,
abortion losses, mainly in ewes in the
younger age groups, can be serious, and the
causes should be investigated (see Infectious
Ovine Abortion, page 908).

EWE DEATHS

By the examination of flock numbers normally kept by any sheep farmer for particular farming operations, it is possible to
assess ewe deaths during periods of the year.
Adoption of this procedure over a 5-year
period involving 1,461,223 commercial ewes
in 760 flocks in New Zealand showed an
annual ewe loss for all reasons of 4.6 per
cent, with the bulk of deaths occurring just
before and during the lambing period. In
stud flocks in which management factors are
optimal, ewe loss figures from 277,673 ewes
were 2.14 per cent during the same period.

EWES LAMBING AND TOTAL LAMBS BORN

When normal ewe loss factors are added
together, it is apparent that the combined
figure creates a very serious loss in potential
lamb production. The New Zealand Romney

TABLE 1. *Lambing Performance*

Factors of Performance	Per Cent
Ewes lambing singles	55.1
Ewes lambing twins	43.4
Ewes lambing triplets	1.4
Ewes lambing quadruplets	0.1
Single lamb deaths	9.8
Twin lamb deaths	9.4
Triplet lamb deaths	19.8
Quadruplet lamb deaths	25.0
Total perinatal lamb deaths	10.6

Survey Unit working with stud flocks over a
period of 12 years obtained the potential
lambing for this one breed by assessing the
total lambs born as a percentage of the ewes
that actually lambed (93 per cent). This figure of the potential varied annually from
142 to 149 per cent, with individual flocks
ranging from 105 to 182 per cent.

LAMBING PERFORMANCE

When the lambing performance of 44,018
ewes on 169 stud sheep properties was examined after the 1975 lambing in New Zealand, the factors of performance shown in
Table 1 were defined. The potential lambing
percentage from these ewes was 145.76 per
cent — the actual lambing percentage
(lambs that survived) in relation to all ewes
that were originally mated to the rams was
119.96 per cent. The reduction of 25.8 per
cent embraces all loss factors: barren, aborting and dead ewes and all lamb deaths.

CONCLUSION

Continuing survey projects must be designed to determine trends in the reproductive performance of both stud and commercial flocks. This work is important because it
establishes a baseline of knowledge that
aids the investigation of any facet of sheep
production.

Investigating Poor Reproductive Performance on a Flock Basis

T. D. QUINLIVAN

Animal Production Services, Waipukurau, New Zealand

Because of the diverse nature of sheep production throughout the world and the emphasis given to particular productive parameters (meat, wool, milk), values for acceptable reproductive rates for flocks vary. A multitude of management systems exist, and sheep populations have been extensively manipulated to meet certain market requirements (New Zealand, France) and to meet the demand for large-scale upgrading programs (Eastern Europe, USSR). Various breeds and their crosses have been developed to exist under extensive pastoral grazing conditions (Australia, South America, South Africa), semi-intensive systems (New Zealand) and highly intensive systems (United Kingdom, Europe).

Investigations designed to examine poor reproductive performance and the development of programs aimed at improvement of sheep reproduction rates must take into account economic and social considerations, the orderly application of proven farming techniques, the productive potential of a breed and the nature and limitations of the environment.

Reproductive performance in domestic species is a measure of the complex interaction between the animal unit and its genotype, the management systems imposed upon it and the environment under which it is run. The basis of any investigation into poor reproductive rate depends on reliable data collection, analysis and evaluation. It also requires a clear understanding of reproductive physiology of both the ewe and ram and a knowledge of the available techniques designed to examine specific aspects of the reproductive cycle. The investigator must then be capable of initiating programs aimed at correcting the problem and elevating the performance of the flock as a whole.

PROCEDURE

In order to proceed with the investigation of the reproductive performance of a flock, it is necessary to collect information concerning the following parameters: (1) ewe deaths, (2) barren (dry/dry) ewes, (3) aborted ewes, (4) ewes that lose all or some of their lambs, (5) lambs that survive, (6) ewes that lamb single births and (7) ewes that lamb multiple births.

These enable the investigator to determine the problem areas that are limiting flock production. The following points should be noted regarding data collection:

1. It is not always possible to collect accurately all the data required. Not only should the flock owner be directed to keep adequate records but also it may be necessary to establish an "observation flock" consisting of 10 per cent of the ewe population in equal age groups for detailed investigation by the veterinarian.

TABLE 1. *Mean Proportions of New Zealand Romney Ewes Based on Various Reproductive Parameters for Given Ranges in Lamb Marking Percentages**

Parameter (%)	Range in Lamb Marking Percentages						
	81–90	*91–100*	*101–110*	*111–120*	*121–130*	*131–140*	*141–150*
Ewe deaths	2.8	3.3	2.5	2.3	1.9	2.1	1.7
Barren ewes	12.4	8.7	6.7	5.8	4.7	3.4	2.8
Aborted ewes	1.0	1.0	0.7	1.1	0.7	0.7	0.5
Ewes lambing singles	68.5	60.6	56.7	50.8	46.3	40.5	37.1
Ewes lambing multiples	15.3	26.4	33.4	40.0	46.4	53.3	57.9
Lamb deaths	9.9	14.3	12.6	10.8	10.0	8.3	8.7
Ewes—lost all lambs	8.0	12.4	9.9	8.4	7.5	5.6	5.1

*Data from New Zealand Romney Survey, 1962–1972.

2. As it is desirable to examine between-year differences and thus flock trends over a period of years, particularly as they relate to breed changes and changes in management policies, every endeavor should be made to collect gross reproductive information for the previous 10 years. Basic counts of ewes, lambs and hoggets are possible at mating, crutching or prelamb shearing, lamb tailing and weaning, main shearing and dipping, and these can be manipulated to provide information about death rates and other aspects of performance.

3. Basic reproductive parameters for various sheep breeds are not readily available. Those presented in Table 1 show the mean values for reproductive traits of the New Zealand Romney breed over a 10 year survey period and are presented within lambing percentage ranges (percentage of lambs tailed/ewes to ram). Such data are subject to wide variation, but they do provide a standard of reference for at least one breed of sheep. Further data of this nature have been presented by Quinlivan and Martin.[4-7]

4. To establish basic property and flock information, the farming enterprise as a whole must be subjected to an examination of the factors likely to contribute to reproductive rate. The following information is recorded in such a way that it may be computerized:

Property Data. Routine data are collected concerning the property's size, annual rainfall, rainfall distribution, nature of the farming operation, terrain and height above sea level. The total stock-carrying capacity of the property is determined, as are such factors as periods of maximum grass growth, degree of land utilization, pasture improvement and winter supplementary feeding programs. Information is also recorded on the results of soil tests and herbage analyses as well as fertilizer application policies and the number of labor units. Environmental hazards that are likely to affect production are also noted.

Flock Data. Apart from breed definition, reproductive performance is defined on the basis of age group comparisons, with data required on the incidence and source of those females that for various reasons fail to rear lambs. Thus, the incidence of barren ewes, lost lambers and ewe and lamb deaths is recorded. Data are also recorded on the various factors known to influence reproductive performance: (1) ram soundness and freedom from disease; (2) basis of ram selection; (3) basis of female selection and factors considered in ewe culling; (4) number of rams used, date and length of mating; (5) incidence of confirmed disease outbreaks and (6) vaccination and drenching programs. Additional data required include wool production (kg per hectare and kg per animal shorn) and times and proportions of lambs drafted for slaughter.

Facilities exist within these data programs to collect 10 years of information concerning the parameters under investigation. Once these data have been collected and evaluated, limitations to flock productivity can be determined.

TECHNIQUES FOR EXAMINING REPRODUCTIVE PERFORMANCE

Flock Sample

If the basic data available from the flock owner are inadequate or if it is necessary to examine the entire reproductive cycle in more detail on the property, it may be necessary to establish an "observation flock" consisting of 10 per cent of the ewe population in equal age groups. The management of the flock initially must relate to that of the main flock as a whole and once established may be used to demonstrate the application of various techniques aimed at improving reproductive rate. If established, the following data can be recorded from this flock:

1. Analysis of premating management.
2. Premating body weight and condition scoring of ewes.
3. Ram soundness.
4. Analysis of coverage and conception by age group.
5. Analysis of postmating management and body weight and condition scoring changes during pregnancy.
6. Laboratory investigation of all abortions.
7. Autopsy of all ewe deaths.
8. Age group comparison for:
   a. Barren (dry/dry) ewes.
   b. Wet/dry ewes.
   c. Assisted ewes.
   d. Ewes lambing:
      (1) Live singles.
      (2) Dead singles.
      (3) Live multiples.
      (4) Dead multiples.

9. Autopsy of all dead lambs during the prenatal period and between birth and tailing and tailing and weaning.

10. Ewe age group comparisons for the percentage of lambs tailed and weaned.

11. Examination of the factors affecting lamb thrift from lambing to weaning.

12. Weight distribution of lambs at weaning.

13. Analysis of lamb drafting percentages of lambs for slaughter.

14. Wool production by ewe age groups.

Analysis of these data should provide a clear definition of the main production-limiting problems. It may then be decided to investigate more fully certain aspects of production. A detailed description of such procedures has been given by Moule.[3]

The Ram

The rams must be free from disease and other mechanical faults likely to affect conception rate (see page 927).

The Ewe

See previous articles, pages 891, 918, 924, 955, and 956. In addition, premating body weight and condition score should be determined and the following data obtained:

1. Analysis of breeding data.
2. Ovulation rates.
3. Fertilization rates.
4. Sperm transport.
5. Estimates of embryonic mortality.
6. Pregnancy diagnosis.
7. Lamb mortality.

TECHNIQUES FOR CORRECTING LOW REPRODUCTION RATES

The following are the main points of a program aimed at improving flock health and production that could be applied universally. The methods described relate specifically to within-breed improvement. The use of cross-breeding is not considered. The techniques employed are based on the premise that within any ewe population the full range of productive merit exists. By the systematic removal of the poorer producing sheep and by the use of sires with a high production potential, subsequent generations should show increased production.

Once a diagnosis of the main factors limiting flock production has been reached, the flock is then placed on a basic improvement program. Emphasis is given to those techniques that are known to improve the already defined problems.

Ram Selection. All rams must be genitally sound and derived from recorded stud flocks, which themselves are exhibiting high levels of performance (see page 877).

Mating Policy. The following points must be followed in the mating policy:

1. The date of joining is determined to coincide with the known period of maximum reproductive efficiency for the breed and the geographical location. The final decision depends upon likely feed availability during pregnancy, anticipated weather patterns at lambing and the time of lamb drop relative to patterns of spring pasture growth.

2. The ratio of ewes to disease-free, selected rams must be optimal and will depend on paddock sizes, terrain and time of breeding season.

3. Restricted mating for 34 to 40 days is practiced. Follow-up harnessed rams identify late lambers.

Under this mating system it is anticipated that at least 95 per cent of ewes should be pregnant at the end of a 34 to 40-day period when the rams are joined with the ewes at or near the height of the breeding season (see page 962).

Feeding Policies. Nutritional aspects of flock performance must be monitored carefully (see page 882).

Ewe Culling Policies. The following classes of stock are removed from the main breeding flock annually. They are either slaughtered or removed to a second flock with another breed of ram. The initial anticipated proportion of ewes falling into each of these classes is as follows:

Ewes mated after 34 to 40 days	5%
Barren (dry/dry) ewes	4%
Assisted ewes and their female progeny	6%
Wet/dry ewes	9%
Ewes that fail to rear lambs to weaning (lambs lost birth to weaning)	2%

Assuming a 5 per cent death rate from mating to lambing on the average, approximately 30 per cent of ewes at the commencement of a program either could be unproductive or could demonstrate undesirable performance characteristics.

Ewe Selection. The ewes in the main breeding flock consist of two groups. The first group includes those ewes that successfully reared lambs to weaning the previous year, less those culled for age, poor wool and other defects. The second group consists of maiden ewes entering the flock for the first time. These will eventually be the progeny of ewes and rams selected by performance. The parameters used, in combination, in maiden ewe selection are:

1. Hogget estrus — detected by vasectomized rams.
2. Evenness of wool and freedom from faults.
3. Yearling or premating body weight, or both. Levels set for premating weights are:
   a. below 43 kg — culled.
   b. 44 to 46 kg — may qualify if numbers insufficient.
   c. Above 46 kg — qualify for entry into the main flock.

Disease Control. Disease control programs are based upon the disease problems detected by property district patterns, and the economics of vaccination, drenching and other veterinary procedures.

Results. With the application of this type of program to a low production problem, the following general effects should be noted:

1. Significant reduction in ewe and lamb mortality.
2. Improved thrift, particularly of young sheep.
3. Improved conception rates to restricted mating programs.
4. Reduced incidence of barren ewes because of the selection criteria (hogget estrus, body weight) used for maiden ewes.
5. Reduction in the proportion of lost lambs and assisted ewes.
6. Thus, increased lamb marking percentages, particularly in maiden ewes, due to an improved total lamb drop and a lower incidence of nonproductive females.
7. Higher average lamb weights at slaughter.
8. Improved wool weights.

REFERENCES

1. Anonymous: Feeding the ewe. British Meat and Livestock Comm. Sheep Improvement Service Tech. Report No. 2, 1975.
2. Coop, I. E.: Proceedings N.Z.V.A. Sheep Society. 2nd Seminar. 1972, p. 8.
3. Moule, G. R.: Field Investigations with Sheep—A Manual of Techniques. Melbourne, C.S.I.R.O., 1965.
4. Quinlivan, T. D. and Martin, C. A.: Survey observations of the reproductive performance of both Romney stud and commercial flocks throughout New Zealand. I. National Romney stud performance. N.Z. J. Agric. Res., *14*:417, 1971.
5. Quinlivan, T. D. and Martin, C. A.: Survey observations on the reproductive performance of both Romney stud and commercial flocks throughout New Zealand. II. Lambing data from an intensive survey in stud flocks. N.Z. J. Agric. Res., *14*:858, 1971.
6. Quinlivan, T. D. and Martin, C. A.: Survey observations on the reproductive performance of both Romney stud and commercial flocks throughout New Zealand. III. National commercial flock performance. N.Z. J. Agric. Res., *14*:880, 1971.
7. Quinlivan, T. D. and Martin C. A.: Oestrous activity and lamb production in the New Zealand Romney ewe. Aust. J. Agric. Res., *22*:497, 1971.

Castration

M. D. COPLAND

Department of Agriculture and Fisheries, Naracoorte, South Australia

Most ram lambs not required for breeding are castrated to facilitate controlled breeding and to produce a more valuable carcass. The operation is usually performed at the time the tail is docked by using rubber rings, the Burdizzo instrument or a knife. In general, one specific technique is no more advantageous than any other. Partial methods of castration have been described but appear to offer little practical advantage.

The necessity for castrating ram lambs destined for the fat lamb market is questionable since these lambs are slaughtered before puberty and, particularly if feed is not limiting, the entire lamb produces the heaviest and leanest carcass.

CASTRATION OF THE RAM LAMB

Rubber Ring Method

Using an Elastrator, rubber rings are placed around the neck of the scrotum, dorsal to the testis. Avascular necrosis ensues, and the scrota and testes slough after 3 to 4 weeks. The method requires minimal preparation but incurs a greater risk of tetanus and the possibility of fly strike. Faulty technique may result in only partial castration. The older a lamb is when castrated with rubber rings, the greater is the risk of failure and the possibility of reduced growth rates.

Burdizzo Method

The Burdizzo instrument effectively deprives the testes of their blood supply by crushing the spermatic cords. Each cord is held in a lateral position and placed between the jaws of the instrument, which are then closed. Care should be taken not to include the median septum, as this may result in sloughing of the scrotum. Preferably each cord is crushed twice.

The method has the advantage that the skin remains unbroken and the procedure is bloodless. Failures may be common if the instrument is improperly adjusted or is in a state of disrepair.

Open Method

A sharp knife or scalpel is used to incise the scrotal sac and vaginal tunic along their posterior and ventral margins. Each testis is then extruded and removed, either by scraping and then severing the cord with the knife or by pulling.

Untoward sequelae that may follow this method include local infection, hemorrhage and the possibility of fly strike. Such sequelae may be minimized by adopting sound hygiene procedures and by castrating only young lambs in clean temporary yards.

CASTRATION OF THE ADULT RAM

Adult rams may be castrated with the Burdizzo instrument in a manner similar to that described for the lamb or by the open method. When using the open method, local analgesia or general anesthesia may be used. General anesthesia may be obtained with pentobarbital, 20 mg/kg, or with the shorter-acting but more expensive steroid CT1341 (Saffan), 0.3 ml /kg. Hemostasis is essential because of the greater blood supply to the adult testis. This may be achieved either by using crushing emasculators or preferably by using a transfixing ligature aroung the spermatic vessels. The effect of either method on subsequent performance has not been evaluated.

Vasectomy

M. D. COPLAND

Department of Agriculture and Fisheries, Naracoorte, South Australia

Rams are usually vasectomized to detect ewes in estrus and/or to provide ewes with a ram stimulus prior to the onset of the *physiological* breeding season.

To implement an artificial insemination program it is necessary to detect ewes in estrus. The number of vasectomized rams required is approximately 2 per cent of the ewes to be inseminated. After vasectomy, the rams are divided into two groups that are then used alternately every 3 days.

Many studies have shown that the practice of joining vasectomized rams with breeding ewes for 14 days prior to the joining with fertile rams leads to an early onset of the breeding season and to a degree of synchronization during the resultant lambing. The degree of synchronization may not always be predictable because of differences between years in the onset of physiological breeding activity. Claims have been advanced that vasectomized rams are not as effective as entire rams in producing this ram stimulus.

Even though sperm may be seen in the ejaculate of vasectomized rams for some months after the operation, the rams are rendered sterile within 2 weeks of surgery. Farmers should be advised not to use the rams during these 2 weeks and to permanently identify them to avoid any confusion between them and entire rams. The veterinarian should consider the possibility of subsequent litigation and, if necessary, should take the precaution of obtaining histological confirmation of the tissue removed during the operation.

OPERATIVE PROCEDURE

An assistant secures the ram in right lateral recumbency with the left hind leg extended and restrained anteriorly. After the usual skin preparation, local anesthesia is infiltrated into the spermatic cords and the skin over their caudal margins. The left side of the scrotal neck is then firmly grasped between the thumb and the fingers of the operator's left hand (Fig. 1). A 5-cm incision is made through the anesthetized skin, dartos muscle and fascia. Any loose fatty tissue present is blunt dissected away from the cord, which is then exteriorized using the index finger of the operator's left hand. By rolling the cord between the thumb and index finger, the vas deferens will be felt as a thick-walled tube that can be isolated and immobilized beneath the vaginal tunic (Fig. 2). A small incision (1 cm) is made through

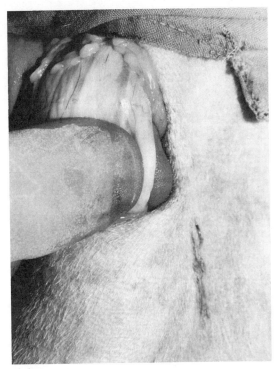

Figure 2. The vas deferens immobilized between the index finger and thumb prior to incising the vaginal tunic.

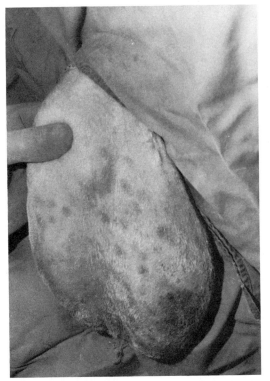

Figure 1. The posterior aspect of the testes, showing the left spermatic cord restrained by the operator's left hand prior to incising the skin.

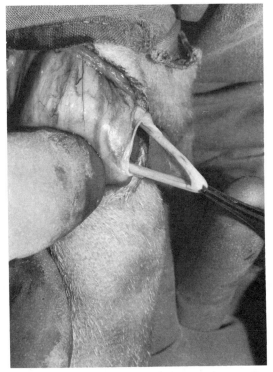

Figure 3. The exteriorized loop of vas deferens prior to ligation and removal.

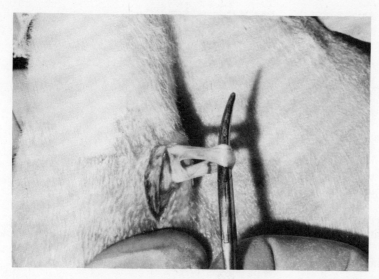

Figure 4. The posterior aspect of the testes, showing the small incision required to exteriorize a loop of the vas deferens by the alternative method.

the tunic over the vas deferens, and a loop of the duct is withdrawn (Fig. 3). Two ligatures approximately 3 cm apart are placed around the duct, and the segment in between is removed. After replacing the cord, the skin is sutured. Similarly, a section of the right deferent duct is removed by using the right hand to hold and immobilize the duct and the left hand to incise the tunic.

With experience, this procedure may be expedited by locating and immobilizing the ducts externally by palpation through the scrotal skin. All tissues external to the duct

are then excised over a distance of 1 to 2 cm, and a loop of the duct is removed without having to exteriorize the spermatic cord from the incision (Fig. 4).

REFERENCES

1. Louw, B. P., Marx, F. E. and Yates, G. D.: The influence of vasectomized rams on the lambing pattern of spring-mated Corriedale ewes. S. Afr. J. Anim. Sci., 4:167, 1974.
2. Trengrove, R. B.: Vasectomy of rams under field conditions. J. S. Afr. Vet. Med. Ass., 36:119, 1965.

Obstetrical Procedures

K. D. McSPORRAN

Wallaceville Animal Research Centre, Private Bag, Upper Hutt, New Zealand

CORRECTION OF DYSTOCIA

Correction of many of the common forms of dystocia in sheep may be achieved by adhering to a few general principles:

1. *Asepsis.* A mild antiseptic solution is used for disinfecting the vulva of the ewe, the hands of the operator and any cord used for traction.

2. *Lubrication.* A water-based obstetrical lubricant should be used liberally in any intervention.

3. *Repulsion of the lamb.* Repulsion is often necessary before correction of a maldisposition can be attempted (see Dystocia in the Flock, page 916). Bilateral elbow flexion (elbow lock position) is one of the few maldispositions that can be corrected without first repelling the lamb; simple traction is usually sufficient. Repulsion is most easily achieved if the hindquarters of the ewe are raised. It may be necessary to tie the hind legs of the ewe to a support to do this if you are in the field without assistance. Proprietary lambing cradles achieve the same result.

4. *Correction of maldispositions.* Once adequate repulsion has been achieved, the maldisposition of the lamb is corrected by retrieving the retained head or limb so that the lamb comes to lie in anterior or

posterior presentation with extended posture. Tearing of the uterine wall by the fetal hooves can be avoided by cupping these in the hands during manipulations.

5. *Traction.* Sufficient traction may often be applied simply by grasping the presenting parts. However there are occasions when it is necessary to use rope snares. This occurs especially when traction must be applied to more than one of the fetal extremities lying in the uterus or anterior vagina. I have found nylon rope of approximately 5-mm diameter to be suitable. Loops may be spliced in the ends to allow variable loops to be formed for grasping the fetal limb or head.

6. *Drugs.* I have found uterine spasmodics and spasmolytics to be of no value in treating ovine dystocia. Synthetic oxytocin, 5 to 10 IU intramuscularly, may be of value to contract the postpartum uterus and assist in involution. Triplopen* is routinely administered following obstetrical manipulations.

---

*Combination of benzyl, procaine and benethamine penicillin. Total of 1 megaunit subcutaneously given in the neck region.

SPECIAL PROCEDURES

Functional stenosis of the vulva associated with estrogenic pastures may require the use of an *episiotomy* to deliver the lamb.

Nondilation of the uterine cervix (ringwomb) is usually an indication for *cesarean section*. However, recently some success has been reported with the use of an ultrasonic vibrator.[1] This instrument has not been used by the author but may find application in areas where the number of such cases is high.

Total *fetotomy* is not practicable in sheep, but removal of a fetal extremity such as the head (simple decapitation at the allanto-occipital joint) may be used to permit repulsion and repositioning in difficult cases.

REFERENCE

1. Turner, C. B.: Cervical vibration as a method of treating partial dilation of the ovine cervix. Vet. Rec., *93*:598, 1973.

Cesarean Section

M. D. COPLAND

Department of Agriculture and Fisheries, Naracoorte, South Australia

The literature contains a number of references to the cesarean operation in the ewe. These show that in this species the operation was developed primarily for the relief of ewes suffering from partial dilation of the cervix (ringwomb) and less commonly for other obstetrical complications that preclude successful delivery *per vaginam*. The latter include relative and absolute fetal oversize, emphysema, fetal monsters and hydrallantois.

In many cases, because of the high cost of the operation, the economic benefit to the farmer is only marginal. Indirectly, this may have the advantage that the veterinarian is more likely to be presented with the ewe at the clinic, where better facilities may exist, rather than having to carry out the procedure on the farm.

Vaginal prolapse and pregnancy toxemia have been listed as other possible indications for cesarean section; however, greater success and economic benefit may accompany the induction of parturition with glucocorticoids in these cases.

ANESTHESIA

In selecting an anesthetic technique, the indications for the operation, the available facilities and the viability of the lambs need to be considered. All general anesthetic techniques incur some risk of regurgitation, and many depress the fetus. General anesthesia may, however, be the method of choice when obtaining gnotobiotic lambs by hysterectomy. In the author's experience, the use of the steroidal anesthetic CT1341 (Saffan), 0.2 to 0.3 ml/kg, for the induction of anesthesia, together with minimal concentrations of halothane and oxygen for maintenance, is accompanied by little depression. In general, however, local analgesia is preferred, and the administration of a local anesthetic by any one of several techniques such as local infiltration, inverted L block, paravertebral injections and epidural injections have all proved satisfactory for this purpose. Should it be necessary, tranquilization may be achieved with diazepam (Valium) 0.2 mg/kg.

OPERATIVE PROCEDURE

The available facilities and the viability, position and number of lambs present at the time of surgery should be considered when selecting the site for the abdominal incision. Most surgeons would probably utilize an approach through the left flank, although the midline, paramedian, right and left dorsoventral and oblique abdominal incisions have all been successfully used.

Adopting normal surgical procedures, an incision of approximately 15 cm is made through the abdominal wall and into the peritoneal cavity. The most accessible extremity (often the hind limb) or the head of the lamb is then palpated within the uterus and gently manipulated through the incision. The uterine wall is incised in a relatively avascular region, avoiding any cotyledons. The incision should be made over a sufficient length to enable easy manipulation and rapid delivery of the lamb. Prolonged manipulation of the lamb *in utero* should be avoided, as this may stimulate the lamb to breathe amniotic fluid, which is often contaminated with meconium. When more than one lamb is present, an attempt is made to deliver the remaining lambs through the same incision. If this proves difficult, the other uterine horn is incised. Unless readily removable, the fetal membranes are left *in situ*.

The uterine and abdominal incisions are then closed in accord with general surgical principles.

LAMB RESUSCITATION

After the lamb is delivered, amniotic fluid is "milked" from the muzzle, pressure is applied over the thorax and any fluid present in the pharyngeal region is aspirated. If the lamb does not breathe after 2 minutes, an endotracheal tube (4-mm diameter) is inserted, and intermittent positive ventilation is initiated. A severely depressed lamb is characterized by failure to breathe, a heart rate of less than 100/min and poor withdrawal reflexes. These lambs are usually acidotic, and the intravenous administration of sodium bicarbonate (5 mEq) and glucose (5 ml of a 10 per cent solution) should be considered. Once breathing, the lamb is dried, placed in a warm environment (37°C) and allowed to suckle its mother or, if this is not possible, is fed colostrum.

POSTOPERATIVE SEQUELAE

Included in the literature are reports of 191 ewes subjected to cesarean section because of obstetrical complications. Seventy-six per cent of these ewes survived the operation, and 69 per cent of 85 lambs alive at delivery were successfully reared. It is likely that better results could be anticipated in ewes subjected to elective cesareans.

Postmortem findings for 13 ewes that died after the operation showed severe endometritis in every case and delayed uterine involution in most cases. Other findings recorded were delayed uterine healing, retained placenta and septic peritonitis.

No records are available regarding the subsequent breeding performance of ewes after cesarean section although, as with cattle, some depression in fertility is to be anticipated.

REFERENCES

1. Copland, M. D.: The effects of CT1341, thiopentone and induction-delivery time on the blood-gas and acid-base status of lambs delivered by caesarean operation and on the onset of respiration. Aust. Vet. J., *53*:436, 1977.
2. Hopwood, J. B.: Bacterial flora of the genital tract of ewes undergoing caesarean section. J. Comp. Path., *66*:187, 1956.

Parturition Induction

W. C. WAGNER

Iowa State University, Ames, Iowa

Although glucocorticoids will induce parturition in the pregnant ewe, this procedure is not widely used in the sheep industry at the present time. The period during which ewes are responsive to this form of therapy is quite short, and irregular results occur when induction is attempted before day 140 of gestation.

The dosage of glucocorticoids is slightly less than for cattle, usually 10 to 20 mg/ewe of dexamethasone (or an equivalent dose if another corticosteroid such as flumethasone is used). Bosc[1] has reported that administration of 8 or 16 mg gives equal results, with lambing occurring about 42 hours postinjection when the sheep were treated on day 144. The latent period is prolonged if the dose is lower or if pregnancy is at an earlier stage. Retention of fetal membranes has not been reported as a serious sequela, and neonate survival seems to be satisfactory provided induction is during the last week of gestation.

Very little information has been reported on the use of prostaglandins for parturition induction in sheep. Abortion can be induced with luteolytic prostaglandins, but only before day 50 of gestation. In late pregnancy, it is not practicable to induce parturition with either oxytocin or prostaglandins by intravenous infusion (as in man), and these are minimally effective, or even dangerous, if given as a single injection.

REFERENCES

1. Bosc, M. J.: The induction and synchronization of lambing with the aid of dexamethasone. J. Reprod. Fertil., *28*:347, 1972.
2. Emady, M., Noakes, D. E., Hadly, J. C. and Arthur, G. H.: Corticosteroid-induced lambing in the ewe. Vet. Rec., *95*:281, 1974.

section XI

CAPRINE

Editor

MARY C. SMITH

Caprine Reproduction

MARY C. SMITH

New York State College of Veterinary Medicine, Ithaca, New York

The domestic goat, *Capra hircus*, has much in common with the sheep and cow. For many years it has either been neglected completely or mentioned in passing, as if it were identical in all respects to the sheep. This section represents an attempt to identify what is known and experimentally verified about reproduction in the goat, as reported in the Western literature. When information about a particular subject is not included, the reader is referred to the sections on cattle or sheep elsewhere in this book.

THE FEMALE REPRODUCTIVE SYSTEM

Anatomy

The ovaries of the goat are variable in shape. They may be round, oval, elongated or heart-shaped. The longest dimension is approximately 2.2 cm in European goats, and the weight of each ovary varies from 1.8 to 3.5 gm, depending on the presence and number of corpora lutea. (It should be noted that there are many breed differences in the reported dimensions of the reproductive tract.) The ovaries are smooth and shiny. Large follicles near the surface (up to 1.2 cm diameter) often have a bluish tinge, while the corpus luteum gives the ovary a pink appearance. When several large follicles are present, the ovary may resemble a cluster of grapes. The right ovary is generally more active than the left. Polynuclear and polyovular follicles are common in the goat's ovary, but only in primordial stages. Very rarely is more than one viable ovum present in the follicle at the time of ovulation. Parovarian cysts in the bursa and mesosalpinx have been observed.

The uterine tubes (oviducts) are long and sinuous, and the uterine horns are also long and coiled. Approximately 115 to 120 caruncles with a concave surface, arranged in four rows in each horn, are very distinct, even in virgin does (Fig. 1). Older, parous animals commonly have melanin pigment in the caruncles and intercaruncular endometrium. The short body of the uterus joins with the firm and fibrous cervix. The cervix has a number of transverse folds or rings, often about five, and is commonly 5 to 6 cm long. Microscopic coiled cervical glands within the cervix produce mucus.

The average length of the vagina is 7.3 cm, and the vestibule is an additional 3.6 cm long. A suburethral diverticulum is present on the floor of the vagina, and occasionally Gartner's ducts located ventrally on each side of the vagina are distended with thick, yellowish mucus. The vestibular glands have received little or no attention. Black pigmentation may be present in the vestibule. The clitoris normally should not be visible between the lips of the vulva. A large clitoris suggests that the doe is actually an intersex.

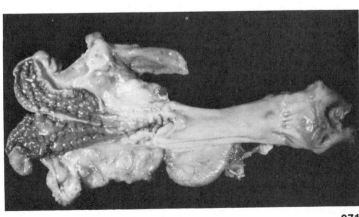

Figure 1. Normal female reproductive tract, opened longitudinally to expose vagina, cervical rings and caruncles. (Courtesy of Dr. K. McEntee.)

Clinical Examination

Clinical examination of the female goat's reproductive tract is limited by the impossibility of rectal examination in most animals. Laparoscopy has been used experimentally to allow observation of the ovaries and uterus in the living goat. After tranquilization with 2.2 mg/kg of promazine hydrochloride, the animal is restrained on her back in a V trough. Under local anesthesia, a pediatric laparoscope is inserted through a trocar cannula. The abdomen is inflated with 5 per cent carbon dioxide in air or nitrogen, and a 5 mm tactile probe is used to manipulate the internal organs and expose them for observation. Examination with the animal in the standing position is usually very unrewarding, especially without abdominal insufflation and without the use of a tactile probe. For further details, the reader is referred to the article by Dukelow et al.[7]

For the average practitioner who would not have a laparoscope, an exploratory midline or flank laparotomy under halothane anesthesia would be faster and easier. Visualization, palpation, acquisition of biopsy samples and specimens for culture of the uterus and examination of the ovaries are readily accomplished. The intrapelvic position of the nongravid organs will hamper an ovariohysterectomy unless the incision is made as close as possible to the udder.

The vagina and cervical os can be examined either digitally or with a speculum, after careful cleaning of the vulva. See Artificial Insemination (page 994) for details about the use of the speculum. If a short piece of rubber tubing is attached to a pipette, vaginal or cervical mucus can be aspirated for closer observation or culture.

Examination of the vulva is easy and should not be neglected. Neoplasms, ectopic mammary tissue, pox virus lesions and staphylococcal dermatitis may be evident. In addition, a slight reddening and swelling of the vulva often accompany estrus.

Puberty

The well-fed female of one of the Swiss breeds commonly reaches sexual maturity and begins to show estrus at 6 to 8 months of age. In Pygmy goats, this may occur as early as 3 months and occasionally even doelings of the larger breeds cycle this young. Generally, breeding should be delayed until the animal has attained 60 per cent or more of its adult weight. Angora goats should weigh a minimum of 27 kg; larger dairy goat breeds should weigh 32 to 41 kg before breeding. If these guidelines are followed, higher conception rates and safer parturitions will be achieved.

The percentage of multiple births seems to vary with the population under study. Twins or triplets are usually more common than single kids, except in primiparous animals. Quadruplets are not rare. In Angora goats, at least, the ovulation rate is 20 per cent higher on the second heat than on the first heat of the breeding season. Fertilized ova commonly migrate to the opposite horn in multiple births, allowing better spacing of conceptuses.

Gestation

Although slight breed differences do exist, the average duration of gestation is generally reported as 5 months, or 150 days (varying from 147 to 155 days). The level of progesterone, which is produced almost entirely by the corpora lutea of the pregnant goat and not by the placenta, remains high until about 4 days before parturition. There is little or no tendency for multiple conceptuses to be born earlier than single kids.

THE ESTROUS CYCLE

Estrous Detection

During the normal breeding season (August to March, and especially October to December in temperate latitudes), goats are polyestrous. Near the equator, they cycle year round. The normal estrous cycle of the dairy goat is approximately 20 to 21 days, while Pygmy goats are variously reported as having from 18- to 24-day average cycles. The estrous cycles are usually more erratic at the beginning and end of the breeding season. Short cycles of less than 12 days, and often only 5 to 7 days, are quite common, especially in young does. One study reports that the second estrus of the close pair is not always ovulatory, and another report suggests that the first estrus in the pair is anovulatory. Estrus is occasionally observed during pregnancy.

Proestrus often lasts about 1 day. It is a period when the buck or teaser closely follows the doe, but she will not stand to be mounted. Estrus, or standing heat, lasts a variable time, often 12 to 24 hours. Metestrus is the time from refusal to mate until formation of one or more corpora lutea. Ovulation is variously reported to occur 12 to 36 hours after the onset of standing heat. Diestrus, the period of corpus luteum function, is the longest portion of the cycle.

A teaser or breeding buck is best able to elicit and detect signs of estrus in the doe. If a buck is introduced into the herd at the beginning of the breeding season, the does will show heat in an average of 8 days. Standing and riding behavior among does is not as common as with cows. Many does will not cycle visibly unless a buck or another source of the buck odor, such as a burlap bag that has been rubbed all over a buck, is present in the environs. A common method of heat detection for small herds is to rub a rag on a rank buck's scent glands, caudomedial to his horns, and store this rag in a tightly covered container. The buck jar is opened and presented warm to the doe each day; when in estrus, she will be very interested in the jar. If the buck himself is present, the two animals will stay close together. If separated, they will restlessly search the perimeter of their enclosures for a means of escaping.

The external genitalia may be more swollen, reddened and more moist during estrus, but these signs are not dependable with all does. Rapid side-to-side or up-and-down tail flagging is a good sign of heat that can often be detected in the absence of a buck. The behavior probably serves to spread odors from the doe's vulva to any nearby males. Restlessness and a tendency to be more vocal than usual are also commonly observed. Urination may increase in frequency. Milk production and appetite may decrease.

Vaginal smears have been used to identify the stage of the estrous cycle with only partial success. A rod or swab is twirled inside the vagina and then rolled across a glass slide. The resulting smear is fixed and stained by a Giemsa or Papanicolaou technique. The period of standing heat corresponds fairly well with the appearance of greater than 50 per cent desquamated eosinophilic polyhedral epithelial cells in the vaginal smear. These cells decline rapidly and are replaced by more basophilic and spherical epithelial cells, which continue to be present until just before the next estrous period. Metestrous leukocytes with compact nuclei appear in the smear at the time of ovulation. Vaginal cycles have been detected at the beginning of the season when the doe is still experiencing silent heats.

A speculum examination of the cervix may be more helpful in detecting estrus. At the beginning of heat, the vaginal mucosa is reddened and moist but little mucus is present. As heat progresses, a variable amount of transparent mucus is visible in the cervix and on the floor of the vagina. This mucus later turns cloudy and finally is cheesy white at the end of heat. Conception is best when the doe is bred at the stage at which her cervical mucus is cloudy and the cervical os is relaxed. Metestrous hemorrhage, as seen in the cow, is not reported to occur.

Estrous Synchronization

There are several indications for manipulating the estrous cycle of the doe. Breeding outside the normal season may be desirable for animals that have failed to conceive or have aborted or for a percentage of a commercial herd when maintenance of a steady production level is necessary. Many owners would find it convenient if estrus were to dependably occur when the buck could be available or when the doe could best be transported to him. Synchronization is also a helpful tool for ova transfer research.

Synchronization Outside the Breeding Season

Outside the normal breeding season, the average doe is not cycling, blood progesterone levels are very low (less than 1 ng/ml) and there is little ovarian activity. Hormones may be used in various dosages and combinations to induce follicle formation and ovulation. It has been reported that 400 IU of pregnant mare serum gonadotropin (PMSG) injected intramuscularly will bring dry does into estrus; 40 per cent of the animals studied became pregnant. Higher doses of 600 IU or more may be necessary when treating lactating does. Use of 500 IU of PMSG and simultaneous injection intramuscularly of 250 IU of human chorionic gonadotropin (HCG) has been superior to use of 750 IU of PMSG alone, as measured by the number of fertilized ova recovered by laparotomy. Heat commences 2 to 3 days after administration of the hormones.

Progesterone vaginal pessaries have been used with mixed results. There have been reports of adhesions of the pessary to the vagina in virgin does and of very poor fertility from the induced heat. Other studies conclude that flurogestone sponges implanted for 16 to 20 days can be used successfully outside the breeding season (40 per cent conception with artificial insemination) and that administration of 400 to 600 IU of PMSG 48 hours before sponge removal improves fertility. Increasing the number of live sperm per insemination also improves conception during the anestrous season.

A very small study achieved ovulation outside the breeding season by daily injection of 100 μg of gonadotropin-releasing hormone (GnRH) for 4 or 5 days. Heat began 2 days after the first treatment.

When hormones are administered for the purpose of ova transfer, higher doses of PMSG or of horse anterior pituitary extract (HAP) will stimulate the production of more follicles. The fertilized ova are collected approximately 3 days after insemination by flushing the reproductive tract from the fimbriae to an incision in the uterine horn or through the cervix. The ova are then transferred to a synchronized recipient. Normally, fertilized eggs enter the uterus 4 days after mating.

The transition from the anestrous state to the breeding season may be hastened by the introduction of the buck or his odor. Use of artificial lighting that decreases the hours of daylight during the spring will bring most of the herd into estrus at that time. If the goats are kept under artificial light for 14 to 18 hours per day for 3 months in midwinter and are then abruptly or gradually cut back to 6 hours of light per day, more than 50 per cent will conceive in the spring.

Synchronization during the Breeding Season

During the breeding season, synchronization may be achieved by resorption of the corpus luteum and shortening of a cycle or by overriding the goat's system with exogenous progesterone to prolong a cycle. Prostaglandins would appear to be the drug of choice for shortening the cycle. Prostaglandin-$F_{2\alpha}$ at a dose of 5 to 10 mg has brought a limited number of does into heat within 72 hours, but the optimum dosage and the ef-

fects on subsequent fertility need to be studied.

Progesterone to prolong the cycle can be supplied in several forms. When progestogen-impregnated vaginal pessaries are implanted for 16 to 20 days (sometimes with administration of 400 to 500 IU of PMSG at the time of sponge removal, with or without administration of up to 500 IU of HCG at the first signs of heat), ovulation has been successfully induced with 55 to 90 per cent fertility. Heat occurs 20 to 40 hours after sponge removal, and the mucopurulent vaginal discharge that is evident when the sponge is pulled does not interfere with fertility.

Oral 6-methyl-17-acetoxy-progesterone (MAP) at 50 mg/day for 16 days will bring does into heat on the third or fourth day after treatment ends, with acceptable fertility. Injectable progesterone, at 10 mg/day or 20 mg every second day, may also be used for 16 to 20 days.

Although fertility may be decreased somewhat on the induced heat no matter which technique is used, it will usually return to normal on the subsequent cycle.

Anestrus

The sexually mature doe should show cyclic estrus during the normal breeding season. Failure to do so may be a sign of diverse problems. The intersex condition must be strongly considered if the doe is naturally polled. The stimulatory effect of the buck odor for the doe has already been discussed; if the presence of a buck or a buck jar for 1 month does not result in observable estrus, pregnancy, pseudopregnancy, hydrometra, nutritional deficiencies or other factors causing anestrus may be present. The first three conditions are discussed elsewhere in this section.

Nutritional Influences

Starvation and parasitism usually appear together in goats and are important causes of reproductive failure, including anestrus. Good quality forage and adequate concentrates should be fed. Grass hays should be accompanied by 16 to 18 per cent protein grain, while 12 to 14 per cent protein will be sufficient when legumes are fed. Approximately 1.4 kg of good hay is needed per day. A rough rule for determining grain feeding is 0.5 kg of grain per kg of milk production. More will be needed if the hay is poor. Many novice goat owners do not understand the progressive decrease in forage quality that occurs throughout the summer. September-cut weedy hay does not supply enough energy and protein for survival, let alone for reproduction. Those does that do cycle at the beginning of the winter will often abort if severe undernutrition continues.

Parasitism

Animals that are malnourished are usually also parasitized. The physical appearance is often diagnostic; the goat is emaciated, pot-bellied, anemic and diarrheic and has a rough hair coat that fails to shed in the spring. Fecal examinations may confirm the diagnosis, but clinical signs may occur during the prepatent period. Thus, parasitism cannot be eliminated on the basis of a single negative fecal examination. Every possible effort should be made to separate feed from feces. Hay and grain should be offered in feeders that cannot be contaminated by fecal pellets. Manure should be removed regularly. Barnyard drainage and pasture rotation are important. When many animals are present on a small, wet pasture, worming every 4 to 6 weeks may be necessary. Thiabendazole at a dose of 50 mg/kg is safe at any time. Paste is preferable to drenches when administered by unskilled owners who might otherwise induce inhalation pneumonia. Boluses are available, but improper administration may cause injuries to the pharynx. The goat's milk is not suitable for human consumption for 4 days after thiabendazole administration. Tramisole at a dose of 8 mg/kg is commonly used to allow alternation of worm medicines. This drug, however, is not approved for goats, and safety and milk withdrawals have not been established. It is thus best to avoid tramisole in pregnant and lactating does.

Coccidiosis in goats becomes a serious problem under the same management conditions that encourage intestinal strongylids. Diarrhea is typically prominent, but tenesmus and bloody feces are rarely observed. Treatment is with oral sulfonamides for 3 to 5 days, at the recommended dosage level for sheep.

When goats are housed in groups, the social dominance hierarchy will also affect estrus. Subordinate does eat less, lose weight, are more susceptible to parasites because they are forced to eat contaminated leftovers and show fewer heats. Separate housing and feeding are desirable any time an individual becomes unthrifty. Such an animal should also be closely examined for dental problems.

Mineral Deficiencies

Parasite-free goats with adequate dietary energy and protein may still fail to cycle if mineral deficiencies are present. Phosphorus deficiency may be associated with anestrus. Copper, iodine and manganese are among the trace minerals known to influence estrus. If the exact deficiency cannot be identified, a trace-mineralized salt block should be supplied. Unfortunately, mineral requirements for goats are not yet established. Cattle salt blocks are used by default but may supply too little or too much of individual elements. In localities in which selenium deficiencies are known to occur, injectable vitamin E-selenium preparations may improve reproductive efficiency. The mechanisms by which selenium affects caprine reproduction are not yet understood.

Hormonal therapy may be indicated for anestrous nonpregnant goats with no recognizable pathological condition or husbandry deficiencies. See previous discussion of estrous synchronization for drug regimens.

PREGNANCY

Pregnancy Diagnosis

There are several important indications for pregnancy diagnosis in the goat besides satisfying the general curiosity of the owner. Goats frequently show signs of estrus during pregnancy, and the ensuing unnecessary trips to the buck cause both irritation and expense to the owner. Pregnant does should be given a 6 to 8 week dry period and fed increased grain to prevent pregnancy toxemia, while open does should be milked through until the next breeding season and do not need the additional grain. Finally, in problem animals or those with apparent prolonged gestations, pregnancy needs to be distinguished from hydrometra, pyometra or pseudopregnancy.

Cessation of heat cycles after breeding is the most common indication of pregnancy, but this is clearly not 100 per cent accurate. Pregnant goats may show false heats, and nonpregnant or pseudopregnant does may go out of heat for the remainder of the season. A buck or teaser fitted with a marking harness will often do a better job of detecting return to estrus than will the owner. Serum progesterone values less than 1 ng/ml on day 21 after breeding indicate that the doe is not pregnant.

Palpation of the cervix is a simple field technique originally developed for sheep by L. M. Koger of Washington State University. This technique may also be applied to does. The standing animal is examined by inserting one or two sterile, lubricated, gloved fingers into the vagina after cleansing the vulva. The nonpregnant anestrous cervix is very firm and conical with distinct folds; it projects into the vagina. After 30 days' gestation, the cervix begins to soften and becomes more blunt. After about 50 days, the weight of the gravid uterus pulls the soft cervix forward and over the brim of the pelvis, where it will remain out of reach until greatly advanced pregnancy. Thus, a firm, almost cartilaginous cervix palpated in a doe bred more than 50 days suggests a failure of conception, while a very soft cervix or inability to reach a cervix would support a tentative diagnosis of pregnancy.

Abdominal palpation is performed by standing behind the doe and attempting to touch both hands together through her body. Another method is to encircle the abdomen with both arms and lift upward. Ballottement is also attempted, especially in the lower right flank. Fasting the doe for 12 to 24 hours before these procedures is helpful. If water is first withheld and then cold water is offered to the doe, the kicking of the chilled fetus can sometimes be felt just anterior to the udder. Usually the fetus cannot be detected with any of these techniques before 100 days. During the last month of gestation, fetal movements can frequently be observed in the right flank. First fresheners may have visible udder enlargement by 2 1/2 months, but this is not dependable, as precocious udders are common in nonpregnant doelings. Relaxation of the sacrosciatic ligament is pronounced in advanced pregnancy.

Laparotomy has been used for pregnancy diagnosis with close to 100 per cent accuracy after 42 days gestation. The does are fasted for 12 to 18 hours, tranquilized and placed in dorsal recumbency. Local anesthetics are infiltrated into the linea alba anterior to the udder, or else general anesthesia together with placement of a cuffed endotracheal tube is used. Two or three fingers are inserted through a 5- to 6-cm incision to allow palpation of the uterus, placenta and fetus. If the ovaries are also examined, follicles up to 1 cm in diameter may be found to accompany the corpora lutea of pregnancy. The abdomen is closed with several mattress sutures. Antibiotics, both intraperitoneal and intramuscular, have been recommended.

For a single doe or research animals, radiology is a useful technique. Enlargement of the uterus has been detected radiographically by about 38 days, but this would not permit differentiation from other causes of fluid in the uterus. By the sixty-fifth day, the fetal skeleton is usually radiopaque. A 12-hour fast is helpful. Premedication with acepromazine (0.9 mg/kg) or xylazine (0.05 to 0.1 mg/kg) will provide restraint so that human exposure can be avoided, but effects on the fetus are not known and xylazine does cause uterine contractions in advanced pregnancy. The doe is usually positioned in lateral recumbency with her hip joints at the posterior edge of a 14 by 17-inch cassette. Careful measurement of abdominal thickness should be done in order to determine proper exposure factors. After the seventieth day, 100 per cent accuracy can be expected, and the number of kids can usually be determined as well.

Fetal electrocardiography has been used experimentally for pregnancy diagnosis in goats, but special preamplification equipment is needed. Two electrodes are placed, one on each side of the lower abdomen, after shaving the area and applying electrode paste. The right front leg or chest is used for attachment of the ground lead. Because of the necessary high amplitude, muscle tremors of a nervous goat or panting will preclude a satisfactory tracing. Accurate diagnosis has been possible after approximately 50 days gestation.

Hulet's rod technique of rectoabdominal palpation has been applied to the doe. Preferably after a 12 to 24 hour fast, the doe is placed on her back and a well-lubricated 1.5 by 50-cm plastic rod is inserted approximately 35 cm into the rectum. The anterior end of the rod is moved from the spine in an arc toward the abdominal wall. The rod is then returned to the dorsal aspect of the doe before commencing another arc. If the doe is 70 to 100 days pregnant, the gravid uterus

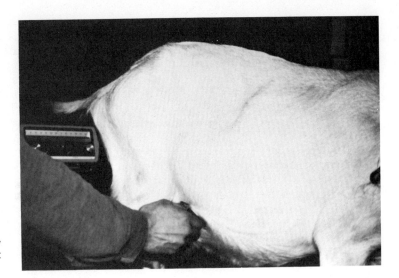

Figure 2. Ultrasound pregnancy detector, with sensor held against lower right abdominal wall.

can be palpated with the operator's other hand cranial to the pubis. If the doe is not pregnant, the end of the plastic rod is palpated instead. Many does are too nervous and wriggly to be safely examined by this technique.

With the advent of ultrasound techniques and portable machines, two new and safe methods of pregnancy diagnosis have become available to those who can afford the equipment. Doppler ultrasound pregnancy detection has been done with both intrapelvic and transabdominal techniques. A 5 MHz frequency seems to be superior to 2.25 MHz, at least in early gestation. A site immediately in front of the right udder or lateral to the left udder is clipped and lubricated with K-Y sterile lubricant or mineral oil. Data for goats are scarce, but apparently the fetal pulse, which is much faster than the maternal pulse, can be detected after 2 months' gestation. Another variety of ultrasound pregnancy detector uses echo detection (amplitude-depth). Lights on the scale indicate where waves are reflected from a fluid-filled structure. The sensor is coated with mineral oil and held against the lower right abdominal wall near the udder (Fig. 2). Hydrometra or pyometra cannot be differentiated from pregnancy with this technique. Once again, the exact time period for accurate use in goats has not been established, but based on a few personal experiences the period is approximately 60 to 90 days. Later in pregnancy, fetal volume increases and the fluid is harder to detect.

Induction of Parturition

Several drugs are available for the termination of pregnancy in does that are bred too young, mismated or severely affected by pregnancy toxemia. Normal parturition in the goat is associated with rising levels of prostaglandin-F (PGF) and 17α-estradiol, followed by a marked decline in progesterone concentration and the onset of uterine contractions. It has been proposed that the fetal pituitary-adrenal axis produces a high level of fetal corticosteroids, which in turn stimulates $PGF_{2\alpha}$ production by the endometrium or placenta. Prostaglandin-induced luteolysis is presumed by many to be the mechanism of inducing parturition, because the corpus luteum (CL) of the goat is essential for the maintenance of pregnancy. Ovariectomy is a dependable but obviously impractical way to induce abortion. After ovariectomy in the last trimester, 10 to 15 mg of progesterone injected intramuscularly daily will maintain the pregnancy.

Much of the research done by endocrinologists has been directed toward explaining the triggering mechanism for birth and has involved surgical intervention to permit fetal injections. These techniques are not applicable to routine clinical practice. Intramuscular injection of an experimental prostaglandin analog induces abortion within 2 to 2 1/2 days at any time during gestation. Limited clinical trials with the prostaglandin marketed for use in mares suggest that this will be a valuable drug for goats also. The literature lacks dosage data for goats, but 2.5 mg intramuscularly may be appropriate if the doe's response is similar, on a weight basis, to that of the cow.

Corticosteroids have been used to induce parturition in Angora goats. Prolonged high levels of corticosteroids during the second and third months of pregnancy have no effect. During the last trimester, a single dose of 250 mg of methylprednisolone acetate or daily doses of 100 mg of cortisol acetate for a week will sometimes, but not always, cause abortion or stillbirths. Dexamethasone at the rate of 20 mg IM on day 145 of gestation has been used to synchronize parturition in dairy goats. This treatment is ineffective if given more than 10 days before normal termination.

Estrogen at high dosages can induce either normal parturition or abortion in goats, depending upon the stage of gestation. Estradiol benzoate administered at the rate of 15 mg/day IM on days 147 and 148 of gestation has been used to synchronize parturition on day 149. Single or smaller doses will induce parturitions that are spread over a longer time period. Kids born more than 10 days prematurely are usually not viable.

Oxytocin levels do rise after parturition has begun, but no research has been reported concerning the possible use of exogenous oxytocin to stimulate parturition.

Periparturient Care of the Doe

Goats, like cows, need a 6- to 8-week dry period for best milk production during the following lactation. Does with a history of mastitis should be dry treated with half of a dry cow mastitis tube in each side of the udder. Culture and sensitivity testing will assist in choosing the appropriate antibiotics. Four weeks before the due date, the doe should receive tetanus and enterotoxemia vaccinations to boost her own and colostral immunity. This is also a suitable time for prophylactic vitamin E-selenium injections in localities in which white muscle disease occurs.

Pregnancy Toxemia

The pregnant doe should not be allowed to become fat. However, high-quality forage and increasing concentrates must be supplied during the last month of gestation to prevent pregnancy toxemia (ketosis). This is especially important for the doe carrying multiple kids; her energy demands are very high, and there is little room in the abdomen for feed. Early signs of pregnancy toxemia are twitching of the ears, muscular spasms and loss of appetite. Rapid respiration, ataxia, frequent urination, coma and death follow. Prevention requires feeding at least 0.25 kg of grain per day during the last month, and more if the hay is of poor quality. Even obese does will need the grain.

Ketone bodies in the urine are diagnostic of pregnancy toxemia. Most does will urinate shortly after getting up or after being released by the examiner. Blood glucose levels can be high, normal or low. Treatment must be given early if the doe is to be saved. Mild cases may be controlled by oral dosing with 3 mg/kg of glycerol or 60 ml of propylene glycol twice a day. More severely affected animals are given 200 ml of 5 per cent dextrose intravenously (avoid 50 per cent dextrose in goats), possibly with 40 IU of insulin administered subcutaneously. Recumbent animals should be treated with antibiotics and 25 mg of dexamethasone to combat endotoxic shock and stimulate parturition. Three liters of fluids given intravenously, together with 150 mEq of bicarbonate, will help to correct the severe dehydration and acidosis that accompany advanced cases. A cesarean section is indicated if the doe does not respond promptly to medical treatment.

Parturition

As normal parturition approaches, the udder fills. It is occasionally necessary to milk out the doe to relieve pressure in the udder. The vulva also enlarges. This is most noticeable in does with ectopic mammary tissue in the lips of the vulva. When parturition is imminent, the doe should be placed in a clean, well-bedded and roomy box stall. The water pail is removed to prevent accidental drowning of the kids.

The expectant doe is restless and may hollow out a nest. After parturition, she licks the membranes off the kid and may eat part of the placenta. There is no evidence for relative benefit or harm resulting from ingestion of the placenta. The kid is usually on its feet in 10 to 30 minutes. If the kid is left with its dam, it locates the udder after diffuse sucking activity. Once nursing begins, the kid wags its tail, and the doe sniffs underneath the tail. There is a critical period of about 2 hours after birth during which time the doe must be exposed to her kid if she is to accept it. Licking for 5 to 10 minutes is usually adequate for acceptance.

Care of the Kids

Most dairy goat owners separate the kids from the dams at birth. Brisk rubbing with a towel serves to dry the newborn and stimulate respiration. The colostrum is hand-fed with a pan or bottle, and a kid is never allowed to nurse a doe. Colostrum is very important for disease resistance in the neonatal kid. If deprived of colostrum, the kid's immunoglobulins do not reach normal levels for 8 weeks. Colostrum from an older doe on the premises should be frozen in ice cube trays and stored in plastic bags as an emergency source of colostrum for orphaned kids. One cube is thawed out and warmed for each feeding. If goat colostrum is not available, bovine colostrum may be substituted.

The navel of the newborn kid should be dipped in iodine solution. The kid is then placed in a warm, partially covered box. The doe will be less agitated if she can see the kid, even if nursing is not allowed.

Dystocia

Parturition begins with a 1- to 10-hour period of uterine contractions. Then, with the onset of abdominal press, the water bag suddenly protrudes through the vulvar lips. Within approximately 1 hour, the first fetus appears, and in 1 to 3 hours, all of the kids have been born. The umbilical cord usually breaks unassisted. Parturition concludes with the passage of the placenta within 2 hours after the birth of the last kid.

Anterior presentation occurs in 70 to 90 per cent of normal kiddings. A dorsosacral position and extension of the extremities should occur with either anterior or posterior presentations. Wild goats are reported to stand with the front end downhill to allow natural correction of an abnormal presentation. Dystocia occurs in the domestic goat in approximately 3 to 5 per cent of births, and most cases are handled, at least initially, by the breeder. The doe should be examined

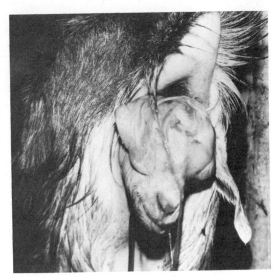

Figure 3. Dystocia due to retention of forelimbs.

internally if a kid has not been born after 1 to 1 1/2 hours of active labor or if labor stops once the water bag or an extremity is visible at the vulva (Fig. 3). If the doe is recumbent, she should be placed on her left side (rumen down) for examination. A standing animal is restrained by holding the head and the tail. The external genitalia are thoroughly washed with a mild soap, and a clean, preferably sterile gloved and lubricated hand is inserted into the vagina to determine the cause of the dystocia. Great care must be taken to avoid rupture of the fragile uterine wall. If straining interferes with the examination or with the correction of the dystocia, an epidural injection is given. An 18- or 20-gauge needle is used to introduce 2 to 5 ml of 2 per cent lidocaine between the last sacral and first coccygeal vertebrae.

Forced Extraction

If the cervix is dilated and the pelvic canal is of normal dimensions, the operator's fingers and, if necessary, a head snare are adequate to correct most malpresentations. It is often possible to deliver a kid with one leg still retained, and this is preferable to prolonged efforts at further mutation. If the head is swollen and protruding while the forelimbs are retained, amputation with a scalpel blade at the atlanto-occipital joint will be helpful, assuming the kid is dead. In the case of multiple kids, the operator must be careful to select both legs of the most accessible fetus before applying traction.

The constant use of lubricants such as 10 per cent boric acid ointment is imperative during manipulation and forced extraction. Soap is not a satisfactory lubricant.

The cervical canal often fails to dilate in the goat. Also, if the fetus has not been delivered in 2 to 3 hours, the cervix begins to close again. In either case, manual dilatation should not be attempted. It is usually ineffective and often results in rupture of the cervix or uterus. An immediate cesarean section, discussed in detail later in this section, is recommended for such animals. Some does with weak labor or incomplete dilation of the cervix will respond to a subcutaneous injection of calcium and magnesium solutions. An appropriate dose is 50 ml of a 20 per cent calcium borogluconate solution.

A cesarean section is also desirable if a valuable fetus is too large for the birth canal or if fracture and ankylosis of the tail obstruct the pelvic canal.

Fetotomy

A malformed, dead or emphysematous fetus that cannot be delivered by normal mutation and traction, even though the cervix is still open, is best handled by a subcutaneous fetotomy. A finger knife is convenient for this operation. An initial skin incision is made completely encircling the carpus and extending as far up the medial side of the leg as possible. After slight digital separation of the skin from the upper leg, the front limb is easily torn loose from the thorax. The procedure is repeated on the opposite extremity. The thorax can be compressed by working the hand beneath the skin and manually fracturing the ribs. Rotation of the neck and thorax will now cause the spinal column to fall apart in the lumbar region, leaving only the hind legs to be extracted. During the entire operation, the skin of the fetus protects the birth canal. Fetotome wire is much more dangerous to use and, if used at all, must be passed through a speculum for the protection of the doe. A douche of a warm disinfectant solution (tamed iodine or chlorhexidine) is helpful in cleansing the uterus after the fetotomy.

Hydrops of the pregnant uterus is a very rare condition in the goat. Hydrometra occurs more frequently, but animals with this condition are not pregnant.

Torsion

Torsion of the uterus is less frequent in goats than in cattle. The affected doe presents in unproductive labor. The condition may be diagnosed by careful palpation of the birth canal for spiral folds, unless only one horn is involved in the torsion. If the animal is not already moribund from an emphysematous fetus and sepsis, rolling is attempted to correct the torsion. If the uterus is torsed toward the doe's left side (counterclockwise), she is placed in left lateral recumbency and quickly rolled over her back onto her right side. Pressure on the abdomen with two hands or with a plank may help to fix the uterus while the goat is rotated. If the fetus can be reached *per vaginam*, one leg can be held while the doe is rolled. Another method of correcting uterine torsions involves suspending the doe by her hind legs and massaging the abdomen. If all these techniques fail, a cesarean section is indicated.

Vaginal Prolapse

Preparturient vaginal prolapse is another cause of dystocia. It often occurs 4 to 5 weeks

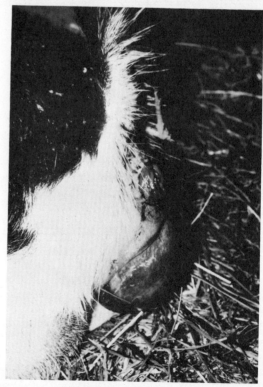

Figure 4. A preparturient vaginal prolapse, accompanied by a mild rectal prolapse.

before parturition. Initially, a red, smooth-surfaced protrusion of the vaginal wall is visible only when the doe is recumbent (Fig. 4). This may be mistaken for the water bag. Slight prolapses may be corrected by placing the animal in a stall with the floor slanting up toward the rear. A complete vaginal prolapse usually no longer returns to its normal position when the animal arises. With exposure, the vaginal wall dries out and becomes contaminated with feces and bedding material.

Replacement is attempted after cleansing and disinfecting the prolapsus. Elevation of the hindquarters is often helpful. If the presence of a full bladder within the prolapsus hinders replacement, elevation of the prolapsus toward the base of the tail will often open the urethra and allow urination. The vagina is then returned to its normal location. After epidural anesthesia, approximately four pairs of small umbilical tape loops are placed in the skin on each side of the vulva, but not in the vulva itself. The vulva is then laced closed with a length of gauze. The owner can loosen the lacing if parturition seems imminent and replace it if he is mistaken. Various trusses and vaginal retainers designed for sheep may also be tried in place of vulvar sutures.

After any dystocia, the uterus should be carefully examined for another kid or a laceration. Prophylactic antibiotics are placed in the uterus, and 5 to 20 IU of oxytocin is given parenterally to promote contraction. The placenta should not be disturbed unless it is no longer attached. A tetanus toxoid booster or 500 to 1500 IU of tetanus antitoxin is also advisable.

Cesarean Section

Cesarean section in the goat is easily performed, and the prognosis is good if the surgery is done early and there is no rupture of the vagina or uterus. Many different surgical approaches are acceptable. General anesthesia with halothane is perhaps optimum under hospital conditions. In the field, the goat may be tied on her right side on a ladder with her head downhill and her hind feet extended backward. An L-block of 1 per cent lidocaine permits a vertical incision in the left flank. The uterine horn is exteriorized, and tilting the ladder or table will help to prevent contamination of the abdomen when the uterus is incised along its greater curvature. If twins are present, an incision may be made in each horn. After removal of the fetus, antibiotic boluses are placed in the horn, and the uterus is closed with an inverting (Lembert) pattern of catgut. Abdominal closure is routine. Intramuscular antibiotics are given prophylactically for 3 to 5 days.

Uterine Prolapse

Prolapse of the uterus may follow parturition, especially in goats that are confined without exercise in separate stalls or that become hypocalcemic. The prognosis is good if the uterus has not been severely damaged. The uterus is thoroughly washed with warm water and a mild disinfectant solution. Then the hindquarters of the goat are elevated, and the hind legs are held apart by assistants. A towel is placed over the uterus to prevent perforation by the fingers during manipulation, and the uterus is then completely replaced to the tip of each horn. Antibiotics are placed in the uterus, and the vulva is sutured with a purse-string or several mattress sutures of umbilical tape. Epidural anesthesia will prevent both the pain associated with suturing and the tenesmus that sometimes follows replacement of the uterus. The sutures should be removed in 3 to 7 days. Administration of tetanus prophylaxis and 50 ml of subcutaneous calcium borogluconate solution complete the treatment.

Normal Involution

The postpartum uterus never returns to its original pregestational size. Involution is rapid. The placenta is normally passed within 1 to 2 hours after parturition. The length of the horns decreases by half during the course of the first day. By 1 week after parturition, the uterus weighs one-third of its immediate postpartum weight. The caruncles degenerate during the first week and are re-epithelialized by 3 weeks. The lochia, normally red and odorless, persists for a maximum of 3 weeks. The cervix is closed and uterine involution is complete by 6 weeks postpartum.

DISORDERS OF THE FEMALE REPRODUCTIVE TRACT

Metritis

Endometritis is a pathological condition in which the uterine mucosa is thickened and discolored and pus collects on the mucosal surface. The doe is typically febrile and anorectic. There may be a malodorous vaginal discharge. Metritis may follow dystocia, maceration of a fetus or retention of the fetal membranes. Pyometra occurs if the cervix is tightly closed and pus accumulates in the uterus.

Manual removal of the placenta should not be attempted unless the membranes are obviously no longer attached to the caruncles. Otherwise, perforation of the uterus or endometritis may result. The vulva should be cleansed and a sterile glove worn when a vaginal examination is indicated to ascertain the presence or absence of a retained fetus. The placenta is left undisturbed, and intrauterine boluses are used to limit bacterial growth. Intramuscular or subcutaneous penicillin-streptomycin or oxytetracycline should be administered until the placenta has dropped and the appetite of the doe has returned to normal. Oral antibiotics should be avoided; chloramphenicol in particular has been reported to cause a drastic drop in milk production. Diethyl stilbestrol should be used with caution as it has been associated (at an unspecified dosage level) with unresponsive nymphomania and lowered milk production.

Maceration of the fetus may occur early or late in gestation. Sometimes only a few bones and a small quantity of pus remain. It is possible for one fetus to mummify without the introduction of bacteria and for one or more normal fetuses in the uterus to continue to term. In these cases, a few bones may be passed with the placenta of the normal kid. If a large dead fetus is not expelled from the uterus during a dystocia, the cervix may be expected to close very quickly. Bacterial infection of the fetus is then life-threatening to the dam. When vaginal delivery or embryotomy is not possible, a cesarean section is indicated.

Endometritis may lead to permanent infertility if an ascending infection reaches the oviducts, causing salpingitis and occlusion.

Pseudopregnancy

Pseudopregnancy occurs rather frequently in the goat and is referred to as a "cloudburst." After what is approximately a normal gestation, the doe voids a large volume of cloudy fluid. The pre-existing abdominal distention disappears and lactation begins, but production is low. Subsequent fertility is usually normal.

The etiology of this condition remains obscure, and its sporadic occurrence makes scientific investigation difficult. Hormonal imbalances and early resorption of the fetus and membranes with continued fluid production have been proposed as possible causes. Some reported cloudbursts may represent spontaneous correction of a hydrometra.

Hydrometra

Hydrometra is a significant cause of infertility and abdominal distention in the goat (Fig. 5). The uterus is thin-walled and contains thin, clear fluid. Several liters of liquid may be present. An enlarged uterus without

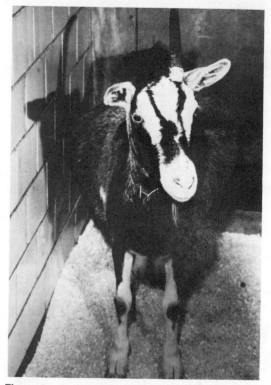

Figure 5. Abdominal distention due to hydrometra.

fetal skeletons is evident radiographically, and amplitude-depth examination for pregnancy will be falsely positive. Hydrometra is confirmed by transabdominal aspiration of uterine fluid and by laparotomy. After the majority of the fluid has been drained from the uterus through a surgical incision, further involution may be stimulated by the use of 0.5 to 1.0 mg of prostaglandin-$F_{2\alpha}$ every 12 hours for several days. If a laparotomy is not performed, prostaglandin alone may induce emptying of the uterus. The prognosis for later breeding is unknown.

Slaughterhouse studies frequently report cases of hydrometra but have failed to explain the condition. There is no confirmed association with cystic follicles, fetal remnants or membranes or cervical obstruction.

Cystic Follicles

A mature graafian follicle in the goat averages 1.0 cm in diameter. "Follicles" larger than 1.2 cm in diameter, and ranging up to 3.7 cm in diameter, have been reported from slaughterhouse material and classified as cysts of the ovary. The size distinction between follicle and cyst is clearly arbitrary. The cysts are shiny and bluish if thin-walled or are milky white if thick-walled. Histological examinations of these cysts have not been reported.

A clinical history of nymphomania may suggest the diagnosis of cystic follicular degeneration of the ovaries to the practitioner. If irregular estrous periods have occurred only with the end of the normal breeding season, they may be assumed to be physiological. If persistent or irregular estrus is observed during the period from October to December, the clinician may attempt treatment with 250 to 1000 IU of human chorionic gonadotropin given intravenously or intramuscularly. The efficacy of luteinizing hormone for the treatment of cystic ovaries in the goat is unknown. Progesterone therapy (10 mg/day for 18 days) or gonadotropin-releasing hormone (GnRH) might also be tried. Unless a laparotomy is performed, the diagnosis will remain tentative.

Several etiologies for cystic follicles have been proposed, but experimental data are not available. Heredity and a high calcium type of relative phosphorus deficiency have both been implicated in herds with frequent infertility problems. Heredity or excessive diethylstilbestrol treatment might explain some of the sporadic cases that present clinically as cystic follicles.

Intersexes

The intersex condition, or hermaphroditism, is a common cause of infertility in polled does. The affected animals are genetically female. The polled trait is dominant and completely penetrant, while the associated hermaphroditic trait is recessive, sex-linked and incompletely penetrant. If one parent is horned, the offspring will almost never be intersexes; a few exceptions have been recorded.

Some of the intersexes are phenotypically normal females; only dissection and histological study will disclose the presence of ovotestes rather than ovaries (Fig. 6). Others have a projecting, bulbous vulva or a clitoris

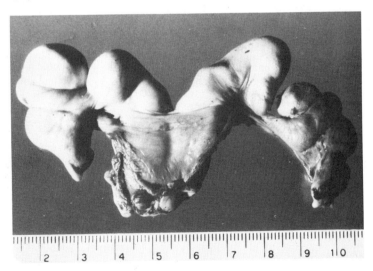

Figure 6. Uterus and ovotestes of an intersex goat.

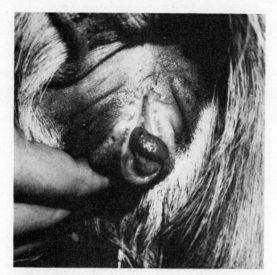

Figure 7. Enlarged clitoris of an intersex goat.

that is large enough to be visible externally (Fig. 7). The more masculine animals have a penile clitoris, shortened penis, hypospadias or hypoplastic testes. Variable development or degeneration of the mesonephric and paramesonephric ducts is also encountered. The masculine phenotypes in the spectrum are discussed under male infertility.

The use of a horned buck is the standard method of avoiding the condition. Horned and polled animals can be differentiated at birth. A whorl of hair precedes the hornbuds in the newborn kids; hornbuds are generally detectable within a few days on male kids but may not appear for several weeks on doe kids.

Caprine freemartins are rare but have been proved to exist by demonstration of XX,XY chimerism in cells of hematopoietic tissue. Anatomically, the freemartin cannot be distinguished from an intersex goat. Fertilization of a binucleate ovum by both an X-bearing and a Y-bearing spermatozoon gives a similar result, but all tissues may be expected to have both XX and XY cells.

ABORTIONS AND EARLY EMBRYONIC DEATH

The female goat that is not an intersex is normally a very fertile animal. There are, however, numerous reasons for failure of gestation. The incidence of embryonic mortality after multiple ovulations has been estimated from slaughterhouse material. Approximately 20 per cent of the ova either are not fertilized or undergo early resorption. There appears to be no simple way of estimating losses in does experiencing single ovulations. Clinically, early embryonic death is suggested when an animal fails to return to heat after breeding but later passes a cloudy white discharge.

Causes of Abortion

Plants. Several plants have been documented to cause abortion in goats. Angora goats abort when experimentally fed broomweed, *Gutierrezia microcephala*. The toxin is apparently a saponin. Feeding of false hellebore, *Veratrum californicum*, on the thirteenth and fourteenth days of gestation has caused embryonic death, abortion and cyclopian malformations. Presumably, many species of locoweed, *Astragalus*, also cause abortion in goats.

Medications. A number of worm medicines, including phenothiazine, tetramisole and carbon tetrachloride, have been reported by practitioners to cause abortion when administered in late gestation. Thiabendazole can be safely used at this time.

Nutrition. A chronic (6 months duration) and severe vitamin A deficiency has caused epizootic abortions in adult goats; kids in the same herd showed diarrhea, lacrimation and corneal opacities. Such a deficiency is caused by a diet limited to dry feed, by severe infestations with liver flukes or by coccidiosis. When parasitism is involved, general unthriftiness is evident. It should be noted that impending starvation due to malnutrition, parasitism, exposure, or a combination of these problems, will often induce abortion a few days before the doe herself dies.

Manganese deficiency causes abortion at 80 to 105 days of gestation, as well as low birth weights and paralyzed or deformed kids. Iodine deficiency is associated with stillbirths or weak and hairless kids. Sometimes the female kids are born dead and the males born alive, suggesting that there is a sex difference in iodine requirements. Once identified, abortions due to nutritional deficiencies can be easily prevented by appropriate supplementation of the diet.

Infectious Diseases. Many infectious diseases may cause failure of gestation. Some of these, brucellosis, leptospirosis, Q fever, enzootic abortion and mycoplasmosis, are discussed separately later in this section. Vibriosis and infectious bovine rhinotracheitis (IBR) are also considered separately, although these diseases probably have minimal significance in caprine reproduction.

Listeriosis is a common disease of goats. Signs vary from peracute deaths to brainstem central nervous system (CNS) disorders lasting several days to inapparent carriers. Silage feeding is not often involved in caprine listeriosis. A carrier or recovering animal may shed the organism in urine, milk or semen, as well as in nasal, ocular or vaginal discharges. Oral dosing of pregnant goats with *Listeria monocytogenes* causes abortion or stillbirth. There are no diagnostic fetal lesions, and maceration is often well advanced by the time expulsion of the fetus occurs. In natural herd outbreaks, abortion frequently occurs in the last month of gestation. The doe usually shows no illness prior to aborting but may develop a necrotic metritis and die soon afterward. Sometimes the organism localizes in microabscesses in the endometrium; the aborting doe aborts again if rebred soon after the initial infection.

Antibiotic therapy using high doses of penicillin or tetracycline is often to no avail if advanced encephalitic signs are evident. The intracellular location of the organism protects it. Prophylactic treatment of the remainder of the herd has been recommended to prevent new cases of either encephalitis or abortion. One such regimen involves administration of intramuscular tetracycline (3 mg/kg) for 3 days, followed by a week of oral tetracycline therapy. See Enzootic Abortion (page 1002) for dosages for prolonged tetracycline feeding.

Salmonella infections have caused outbreaks of abortion in some goat herds. Details of the clinical findings are not available.

Johne's disease, or paratuberculosis, in goats is a chronic condition characterized by unthriftiness, weight loss, diarrhea and parasitism. Antemortem diagnosis is very difficult; johnin tests are not very accurate and fecal cultures for *Mycobacterium paratuberculosis* require several months. Fecal smears are rarely positive. The complement fixation test is negative until late in the course of the disease. At necropsy, the intestinal mucosa is thickened but generally is less rugose than the mucosa in cattle affected by Johne's disease. Mesenteric lymph nodes may be edematous, caseated or calcified. Microscopic examination of the ileal mucosa and ileocecal lymph nodes for acid-

fast bacteria will confirm the diagnosis. Reproduction is generally poor when animals are noticeably affected. Failure of conception, abortions and weak kids have all been reported. There is no effective treatment; animals with positive fecal cultures should be culled.

Toxoplasmosis has caused herd outbreaks of abortions, mummified fetuses and neonatal deaths in goats. The fetuses are frequently decomposed; placental retention is common. The diagnosis is made by serum fluorescent antibody tests; high titers persist for several months after abortion has occurred. Control of the cat population on the farm may help to prevent toxoplasmosis in goats.

A syndrome of arthrogryposis and hydranencephaly has recently been reported in goats as well as in other domestic ruminants. The etiological agent is the Akabane virus, which is thought to be an arbovirus. So far, the syndrome has been recognized in Japan, Israel and Australia. Some deformed kids are aborted, while others go to term. The muscles of the affected limbs are reduced in volume because of hypoplasia and fatty dystrophy. Varying degrees of hydrocephalus are present in the cerebrum. Consideration should be given to controlling possible arthropod vectors. The initial infection appears to confer at least some immunity, such that the following gestation is uneventful.

Experimental inoculation of does in the second month of pregnancy with the agent of border disease sometimes causes abortion or ataxic and shaker kids. Placentitis occurs in the doe. Hypomyelinogenesis and hypergliosis of the CNS are present in the kids, but hair coat defects have not been observed.

It is clear that the diagnosis of abortion in goats is not an easy task; many different etiologies, each requiring special tests, need to be considered. Initial efforts should be directed toward obtaining a good clinical and nutritional history and submitting several fetuses and placentae to a diagnostic laboratory for culture and histological examination. Many of the possible agents will require special culture techniques. Serological tests should be used when available.

Goat × Sheep Hybrids

Goats have 60 chromosomes, while sheep have only 54. The two species readily inter-

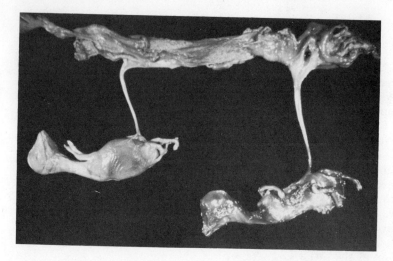

Figure 8. Mummified hybrid embryos resulting from mating of a ram with a doe. (Courtesy of Dr. K. McEntee.)

mate, and the resulting embryos have 57 chromosomes. Does bred to rams have greater fertility than is shown by ewes bred by bucks. Initial embryological development is apparently normal, but after about 1 month, hemorrhages appear in the hybrid embryo and its placenta. The maternal caruncle does not develop normally and fails to become concave. Round cells infiltrate the maternal tissue, indicating a possible immunological response. Platelets accumulate around subepithelial vessels in the placenta, and there is swelling of the endothelium; these changes suggest injury caused by antigen-antibody complexes. Hemolysins also have been reported in the maternal serum but have been discounted as the cause of embryonic death. The hybrid embryos generally die before 60 days gestation, especially during the sixth week (Fig. 8). Death usually occurs earlier, at about 3 weeks, in subsequent hybrid gestations. Substantiated reports of hybrids surviving are very rare, and usually the dams were experimentally desensitized in advance of breeding.

Reproductive Efficiency in Angora Goats

Reproductive efficiency has received more scientific attention in Angoras than in other breeds. Typically, efficiency under range conditions has been very low, with one large study indicating a kid crop of only 78.6 per cent dropped and 56.4 per cent raised. This is far below the potential for the breed.

The Angoras are seasonally polyestrous and often do not cycle until stimulated by the introduction of a male; a lag period before heat of approximately 8 days has been observed. Nutritional status is very important. Heavier, better conditioned does are more likely to have twins, while very small animals often fail to ovulate at all. Does selected for high mohair production and kept under typical range conditions are always under nutritional stress. The males also may be so undernourished or unthrifty that they lack libido. Predators and cold stress have a further serious effect on reproductive efficiency by decimating the kid crop; yet kidding in confinement is often not feasible.

The Angora breed, especially in South Africa, is also afflicted with a syndrome of habitual abortion. When extensive inbreeding has occurred, a flock incidence of abortion as high as 70 per cent has been recorded. By selecting for an extremely high level of hair production and by keeping the large does that produce mohair but not keeping kids for further breeding, breeding stock possessing altered metabolic priorities and low adrenal function have been selected. Low cortisol levels have been unintentionally achieved by selecting animals in which the inhibitory effect of cortisol on hair growth has been removed. These does produce more mohair and have significantly better breeding efficiency their first season; thus, their daughters are kept. Usually abortions do not occur until the fourth or fifth year of life. When these older does are stressed by rapid fetal development (especially at 90 to 110 days gestation), energy deficiency or inclement weather, abortions occur. The aborting doe shows adrenal atrophy, degeneration of the maternal placentome, regression of the corpus luteum of pregnancy and often follicular stimulation. The fetus, which is retarded in growth for its gestational age, is often anemic and shows adrenal hyperplasia and thymic involution. Surviving kids that will transmit the defect have a heavier, finer hair coat at birth. Older, habitually aborting does show adaptive changes, including enlarged pituitaries and adrenal hyperplasia. They will have higher than normal blood cortisol levels and cystic corpora lutea and may show clinical signs consistent with hyperadrenocorticism, such as abdominal distention and poor hair growth.

The means of controlling habitual abortion in Angoras is strict genetic selection. All aborters should be culled, or else subsequent surviving progeny may perpetuate the trait. Cull all does with stillborn or weak kids, as these are often an expression of the abortion tendency. Remove previous progeny of aborting does from the breeding flock. Carefully select bucks from strains free of the defect and give preference to bucks with well-developed testes.

In the United States, habitual abortion has not been as serious a problem as it has been in South Africa. Recommendations for improving caprine reproductive efficiency in the United States are aimed more at the nutritional status of the does. The shorn weight of yearlings should be at least 25 kg and of mature does a minimum of 34 kg at the beginning of the breeding season. Because hair-blind does usually fail to kid before they are 3 or 4 years old, open-faced does should be selected. Parasite control and supplemental feeding must be supplied when necessary to keep the flock thrifty. Shelter against inclement weather and predators should be provided for pregnant does and young kids.

Neoplasms of the Female Reproductive Tract

Information concerning the incidence of neoplasms of the doe's reproductive organs is scarce. One large granulosa cell tumor has been reported, and the author has personally seen a 1450-gm dysgerminoma in an aged doe (Fig. 9). Uterine adenocarcinomas, leiomyomas and fibromas, as well as adenomas and fibromas of the vagina and vulva, are infrequently seen. Numerous cases of lymphosarcoma have been reported in the goat, but there is no apparent predilection for the uterus.

Squamous cell carcinoma of the perineum is relatively common in animals with white or gray haircoats. These tumors are rounded, lobulated or ulcerated and may yield a foul exudate or become fly-blown. The squamous cell carcinoma must not be confused with the benign condition of ectopic mammary tissue in the vulva (Fig. 10). The animals with the latter anomaly show marked swelling and firmness of the vulvar lips just prior to each parturition; the swelling tends to regress completely in 60 to 70 days. Milky fluid containing fat globules can be aspirated from nodules that are within the vulvar lip but are unattached to either skin or mucosa. If desired, a biopsy is easily accomplished through the vaginal mucosa (Fig.

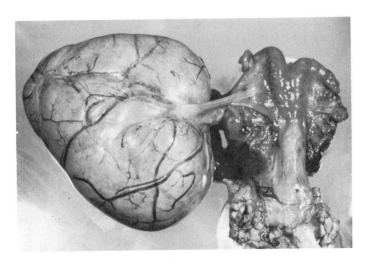

Figure 9. Dysgerminoma in a 16-year mixed breed doe. This ovarian tumor was detected by abdominal palpation prior to euthanasia.

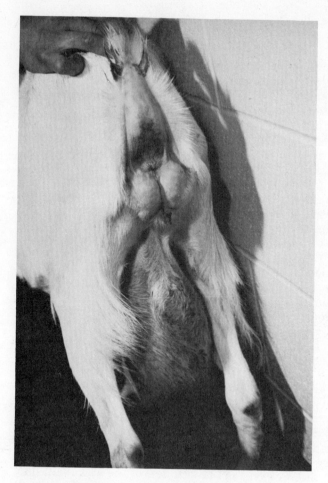

Figure 10. Postparturient vulvar enlargement due to ectopic mammary tissue.

11). Occasionally, the vulvar swelling is large enough to interfere with defecation and urination.

Warts and melanomas of the perineum may also occur in the goat.

THE MALE REPRODUCTIVE SYSTEM

Anatomy

The testes are normally present in the scrotum at birth and are positioned with the longitudinal axis vertical. The mature testes are quite large in proportion to the body weight, when compared with the testes of bulls. Approximately 15 to 20 efferent tubules collect spermatozoa from the rete tubules of the testis and join the head of the epididymis, which is located on the dorsolateral aspect of the testis. The body of the epididymis is located on the caudal aspect of the testis and slightly medial to it. Semen is stored prior to ejaculation in the tail of the epididymis, which is ventrally positioned.

The ductus deferens continues upward medial to the epididymis and passes to the abdominal inguinal ring adjacent to the spermatic cord. Blood vessels, nerves and tunics are also included in the cord. The testicular artery is greatly convoluted; its close proximity to the pampiniform venous plexus serves to precool the blood going to the testis. The ductus deferens continues from the internal inguinal ring via the genital fold to the caudal part of the bladder. The terminal part of the ductus widens into the ampulla, passes under the body of the prostate and ends as a slit-like opening on the side of the seminal colliculus.

The vesicular glands (seminal vesicles) (Fig. 12) are compact glandular organs with a lobulated surface whose paired excretory ducts open at the seminal colliculus just lateral to each ductus deferens.

The prostate is entirely disseminated and completely surrounds the urethra. It has

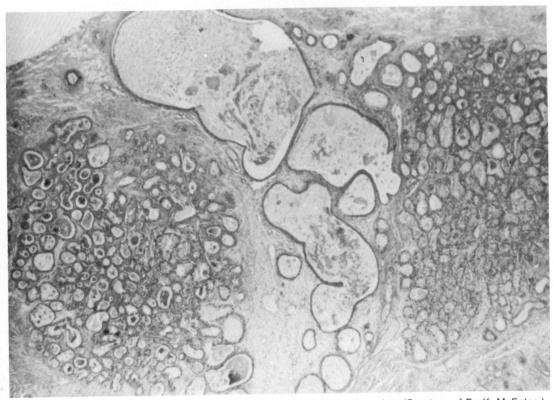

Figure 11. Histological appearance of ectopic mammary tissue in the vulva. (Courtesy of Dr. K. McEntee.)

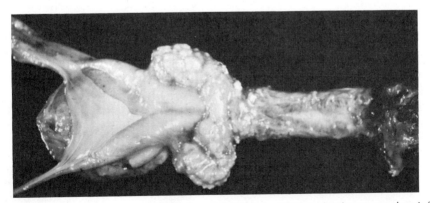

Figure 12. Internal genital organs of a normal buck; ampullae and vesicular glands are prominent. (Courtesy of Dr. K. McEntee.)

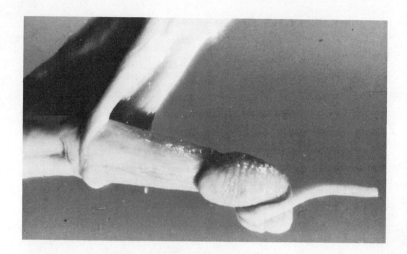

Figure 13. Normal buck's penis, showing urethral process.

multiple ducts that open into the urethra in rows proceeding caudally from the seminal colliculus. The bulbourethral glands (Cowper's glands) are relatively large but are covered by dense fibrous tissue and, in part, by the bulbospongiosus muscle. They open under a fold of mucous membrane that forms a blind pouch in the urethra.

The penis has a pronounced S-shaped sigmoid flexure, except when it is fully extended at the time of ejaculation. A very thick tunica albuginea encloses highly developed erectile tissue. The terminal portion of the urethra lies in a groove on the ventral surface of the corpus cavernosum penis. Here, a slightly twisted urethral process extends 3 to 4 cm beyond the glans penis (Fig. 13).

Clinical Examination

Only the scrotal contents and the penis can be conveniently examined on the live buck. Evaluation of the semen is discussed later. The examiner should position himself behind the buck with a hand on each side of the scrotum. Any dermatitis or skin wounds should be noted. The testes and epididymides are carefully palpated and compared. Each testis should be large, slightly egg-shaped and mobile within the scrotum. Its consistency should be firm, similar to contracted muscle. The normal epididymis is softer than the testis. The knot-like tail is the firmest part of the epididymis. Cryptorchid and hypoplastic testes are easily recognized, and every buck over 3 months of age should be examined for these conditions. Measurement of the circumference of each

testis or of the entire scrotum and comparison with a normal goat of the same age and weight will permit identification of hypoplastic testes, even if the examiner lacks previous experience in this diagnostic procedure. Sperm granulomas are most commonly palpated in the head of the epididymis but should not be confused with normal lobulations. They are hard lumps of variable size and may be bilateral or unilateral. If the granulomas are large enough to completely obstruct the epididymis, sperm stasis and a tense, fluid feeling will be initially present in the testis. The testis will then degenerate and become softer and smaller. In some cases of testicular degeneration, the testicular tissue becomes mineralized and thus feels gritty. The value or safety of testicular biopsy as a diagnostic procedure for evaluating bucks with fertility problems has not yet been reported. Infarction of the testis can be expected if large blood vessels in the tunica albuginea are injured during the surgical procedure.

The buck's rudimentary teats should be examined for evidence of gynecomastia. The prepuce and penis are examined for wounds, strictures and congenital abnormalities such as hypospadias, which are suggestive of the intersex condition. With the buck set up on his rump, massage of the preputial area may elicit protrusion of the penis to permit examination. The buck may be sedated with 0.05 mg/kg of xylazine, but great care should be taken when using this unapproved drug on valuable bucks. Special attention should be given to the urethral process in which urethral calculi commonly lodge. In some cases, stimulation with the electroejaculator may be necessary before the penis can be visualized.

If the buck is large and the examiner's hand is very small, rectal examination of the internal genital organs may be possible, but this procedure has not been reported in the literature.

Puberty

The rate of male sexual development seems to vary with breed, birth weight and nutrition. The initial growth of the sex organs is gradual for the first 3 months of life. Then, with the onset of spermatogenesis, the weight of the testes, epididymides and seminal vesicles increases rapidly. The spermatogenic cycle has been estimated to be 22 days in the buck kid, and mature spermatozoa are present in the epididymis by 3 1/2 months. Libido, it should be remembered, appears much earlier. The spermatogenic cycle of the adult buck has apparently not been studied.

The urethral process is initially located in a groove on the head of the glans penis. Separation from the glans and from the ventral wall of the prepuce begins at the distal tip of the process and proceeds toward the base, being complete by 4 months (Fig. 14). Separation of the penis from the remainder of the prepuce is usually not complete until after 5 months. These approximate times refer to milk goats under conditions of good nutrition; in these animals, fertile matings are easily possible by 5 1/2 months. Buck and doe kids should be routinely separated before 5 months of age to prevent early matings. Very large and fast-growing buck kids may mature earlier and should be separated by 3 months of age for maximum safety.

Male Sexual Behavior

Bucks show very obvious courtship behavior when in contact with estrous does. They nose the female's perineum and udder as well as the ground where she has recently urinated. The urine odors elicit the olfactory reflex of flehmen, in which the male extends his head and neck while retracting his upper lip. The buck also flicks out his tongue, strikes with a forelimb and makes low-pitched bleating sounds. He may butt the female's hindquarters or push them with his shoulders as a means of testing for heat. The female in standing estrus will remain still when urged to go forward. The buck then briskly assumes a position in direct line with and behind the female. False mounting may occur during courtship. Frequently the male spills urine on his own head and forelegs or licks at the stream of his urine.

The reaction time, from first contact with the teaser or estrous doe to coitus, is normally very short — less than 5 minutes — if the animals have not been together continuously. During the nonbreeding season, bucks may refuse service. Often this is associated with misalignment, in which the buck puts his head on the doe's hindquarters but his body is not in direct line with the doe's longitudinal axis. The partially impotent buck maintains this improper position for a long time. As libido improves with resolution of a temporary problem or passing of the seasons, the axis will gradually be corrected

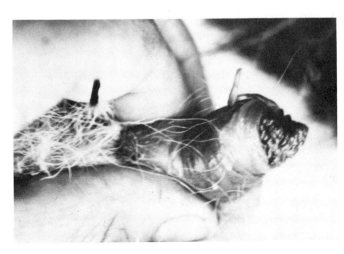

Figure 14. Partial separation of the urethral process and glans from the prepuce in a 3-month-old kid. Note the irregular surface of the glans.

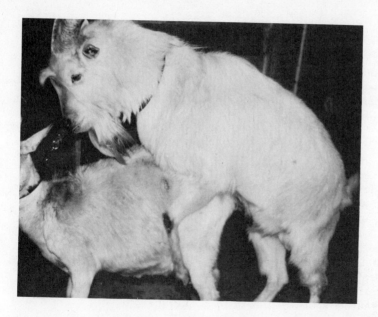

Figure 15. Buck mounting doe.

until the potent buck is once more properly aligned.

Mounting is rapid. The buck clasps the doe's body with his forelegs (Fig. 15) and rapidly searches out and enters the vagina with his penis. Coitus lasts a few seconds only, and the dismount follows immediately. Copulation can be repeated 20 times in a day.

The normal patterns of male sexual behavior are well established in kids housed in groups by the time they are 1 month old. Flehmen, perineal nuzzling and mounting occur, although the kid cannot extend his penis for several more months. If a male kid is raised in isolation, the animal may become imprinted on humans and mount the caretaker in preference to an estrous doe.

The male's typical and powerful odor, which emanates mainly from sebaceous glands caudomedial to the horns or bosses, stimulates a doe to show stronger heat than she would in the absence of a buck. Also, older and ranker males have a more positive effect than do young or descented bucks, and they will be sought out in preference by the average female. The buck whose scent, outside the breeding season, is more than his owner can tolerate can be made more presentable by trimming the beard and long facial hair, clipping the hair over the scent glands and wiping the crown of the head daily with a towel dampened with a mild disinfectant.

SEMEN COLLECTION, ARTIFICIAL INSEMINATION AND CASTRATION

Semen Collection and Evaluation

Examination of the buck for fertility requires collection and evaluation of semen. The preferred technique for collection is by use of an artificial vagina. A doe in natural heat or brought into estrus by subcutaneous injections of diethylstilbestrol (1 to 20 mg), estradiol (1 to 2 mg) or prostaglandin is used for a mount. Bucks can be trained to ejaculate with a doe that is not in heat or even with an inanimate object for a mount.

An artificial vagina used for a dog or ram is suitable for bucks. One can be made by using a 16-cm long, medium-hard canvas-back rubber cylinder 3.5 cm in diameter with a small tube or stopcock off one side. Automobile radiator hosing works well. A soft rubber liner, such as a bicycle inner tube about 23 cm long, is placed within the cylinder; each end is folded over the edges of the hard cylinder and held in place by rubber bands (Fig. 16). A rubber collection funnel with a glass test tube affixed is placed on one end of the cylinder. The artificial vagina is partially filled with water (50°C) by pouring the water into the space between the cylinder and the liner. The liner is then inflated with air to the appropriate pressure (a thumb can be easily inserted with slight pressure) (Fig. 17). The inner surface of the

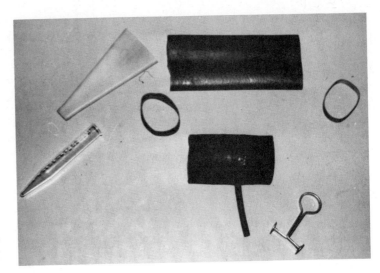

Figure 16. Components of a home-made artificial vagina, prior to assembly.

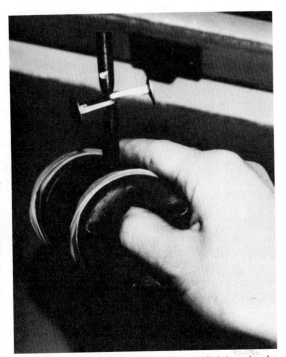

Figure 17. Testing pressure of the artificial vagina by thumb insertion.

liner is lubricated with a nontoxic substance such as sterile lubricating jelly. According to Herman,[16] the temperature of the artificial vagina during collection should be between 41 and 44°C, although lower temperatures have also been reported.

The doe's head is placed in a stanchion or is held by an assistant. The person collecting the buck, if right-handed, should kneel close to the doe's right flank. The artificial vagina is held in his right hand, at the side of the doe or between her hind legs, with its open mouth directed downward at a 45° angle. The extended penis is directed into the vagina by applying pressure on the preputial sheath (not the penis) with the left hand. Since the buck ejaculates rapidly, the semen sample is easily missed. Sometimes, the buck's urethral process rotates rapidly, causing semen to be sprayed in all directions. After ejaculation, the artificial vagina (AV) is turned open end up to allow the semen to drain into the tube.

Bucks may be collected by electroejaculation if they will not serve an AV or if a mount is not available. A commercial unit such as a Nicholson Trans-jector and a ram (boar) rectal probe are used. The buck may be restrained either standing or in lateral recumbency. After a warm 5 per cent salt (NaCl) solution enema, the lubricated probe is inserted into the rectum. Rhythmic stimulation lasting 2 to 5 seconds is begun with a peak voltage of 2 volts and a rest period between stimuli lasting up to 5 seconds. The voltage is gradually increased until ejaculation occurs, which will often be at about 8 volts. One report suggests the use of two initial 8-volt stimuli to cause extension of the penis before commencing regular stimulation at the lower voltage.

Another reported technique for semen collection is to place the buck in a quiet environment and lightly massage the end of the glans penis through the sheath. The massaging hand works toward the preputial opening as extrusion begins. The ejaculate may be collected with a funnel or an AV.

The volume of the ejaculate may be measured by using a graduated tube for collection. The fresh semen is immediately evaluated for motility by placing a drop of semen on a warm (37°C) glass slide on a warm microscope stage. A coverslip is applied, and mass motility is judged by an arbitrary system that assigns a rating of 0 to samples with no motility and a rating of 4 or 5 to samples with the most rapid forward motion, which appears as cloud formation. The percentage of sperm with forward motility is estimated to be from 0 to 100 per cent after dilution in warm physiological saline solution to provide a single layer of cells. The rating should be based on the microscopic field showing highest spermatozoal motility. A live-dead stain, such as eosin-nigrosin, is done, and 100 cells in the smear are counted. Another 100 cells are evaluated for morphological abnormalities such as coiled tails, tailless heads, large or small heads, midpiece defects or protoplasmic droplets. The sperm concentration is determined with a hemocytometer after dilution with a red blood cell diluting pipette, but concentrations can also be judged by optical density or by electronic counting methods.

The volume of an ejaculate collected by artificial vagina is variable but often averages between 0.5 and 1.0 ml in different studies. Concentrations of 2.5 to 3.0 billion/ml are normal. A motility of 85 per cent or higher is desirable and less than 60 per cent is unsatisfactory. Abnormal sperm totaling 3 to 15 per cent are commonly reported. Approximately twice the volume and half the concentration may be expected with electroejaculation.

There is some seasonal variation in semen quality collected by artificial vagina, with generally better semen characteristics during the normal breeding season. At this time, there is a concomitant higher urinary excretion of 17-ketosteroids. The buck's fertility is usually adequate for conception year round.

Artificial Insemination

Artificial insemination of goats has been performed with both fresh and frozen semen. For preparation of liquid semen, a volume of freshly collected semen is initially mixed with 2 or 3 parts of diluent in an Erlenmeyer flask in a 37°C water bath or at room temperature (if a water bath is not available). The flask of diluted semen is placed in a beaker of water of the same temperature and is then set in a refrigerator at 5°C. Final dilutions are done at refrigerator temperatures. A variety of diluents are satisfactory. Homogenized or skimmed cow's milk is usually readily available and can be used for dilution after holding at 95°C for 10 minutes and cooling to the temperature of the sperm solution. Although the importance of venereal vibriosis in goats has not been ascertained, 750 μg of dihydrostreptomycin per ml of diluent is often added. The dilution rate is determined by the volume of the ejaculate (V), the sperm concentration (C) and the percentage of motility (M).

$V \times C \times M$ = number of live, motile sperm. It is desirable to have 125 million live sperm per insemination, and it is difficult to introduce more than 0.2 ml of semen into the cervix, so a final concentration of 600 million to 1.25 billion/ml seems appropriate. The diluted semen is stored in 2-ml vials filled to the top and capped to exclude air. Semen stored at 4 to 5°C should be used within 48 hours.

If the semen is to be frozen, the initial dilution in skim milk is followed by dilution with an equal volume of 12 to 14 per cent glycerine to achieve a final glycerine concentration of 6 to 7 per cent. A period of 4 to 5 hours at 4°C is allowed for equilibration, and then the semen sample is frozen to −196°C (liquid nitrogen) using the same techniques employed for bull semen. After thawing, 100 to 125 × 10⁶ motile sperm are desired. Not all bucks' semen freezes well, and many samples will have to be discarded if good quality frozen semen is to be achieved.

Newer techniques involve washing the sperm twice in physiological saline to remove the seminal plasma immediately after collection. If washing is done, there is little or no subsequent decrease in motility following time in frozen storage.

Frozen semen may be transported from the large nitrogen storage tank to the doe in a good 1-quart thermos bottle, pretested and partially filled with liquid nitrogen. Two inches of nitrogen in the bottle will last 12 hours, after an initial 10-minute cooling period, if the top of the thermos is plugged with a paper towel. Just before use, the semen is thawed by placing it in a 37°C water bath for 10 to 15 seconds. Once thawed, it should be protected from cold shock and used within 15 to 30 minutes.

Deep cervical insemination is imperative if a good conception rate (greater than 70 per cent) is to be achieved. Double breedings, about 12 and 24 hours after standing heat is first detected, give the best results. Many means of restraining the doe have been devised. One of the simplest begins with stanchioning the doe on her milking stand. The inseminator rests one foot on the stand and drapes the doe's hindquarters across the horizontal part of his thigh. This elevates her rear parts slightly. A vaginal speculum with a light source is needed to locate the cervix. An inexpensive speculum can be made by taking a 22×175-mm Pyrex laboratory test tube for virgin does or a 25×200-mm tube for older does and heating it in a Bunsen burner flame to allow placement of a hole slightly off center at the end of the tube. The vulva is cleaned and the sterilized, lubricated speculum is inserted into the vagina. After the cervix has been visualized and aligned with the hole in the speculum, a bovine insemination pipette is inserted into the external os with the aid of a pen light. The pipette is then gently twisted and maneuvered past each of several cervical rings. The semen is deposited approximately 3 to 4 cm into the cervix, as determined by laying a spare pipette next to the first pipette and measuring the amount by which their outer ends are offset. The cervix acts as a reservoir for sperm.

It is considered advisable to pass a trial pipette before thawing the semen, as it is often impossible to penetrate into the cervix if the doe is not in exactly the right stage of estrus. Splashing the semen into the vagina is unsatisfactory and gives less than 30 per cent conception rates.

Artificial insemination (AI) is becoming more popular as semen from more good bucks is frozen and as AI clinics are available to teach the techniques to goat owners. Regulations need to be developed to control the quality of the frozen semen and to insure that it will not be a vehicle for the spread of diseases.

Castration

Goats are castrated for a variety of reasons. A male kid that is being raised for meat or mohair production or as a pet can be kept with the rest of the herd without fear of undesired matings. Also, the characteristic buck aroma is greatly subdued after castration. Goats that are castrated as adults retain their ability to ejaculate, often for a year or more, but the frequency of ejaculation decreases. Flehmen in response to female urine also decreases somewhat, and the wether becomes less attractive to females.

Several methods are commonly used. Laymen sometimes castrate young kids with elastic castration bands, but the method is inhumane. Tetanus prophylaxis is impera-

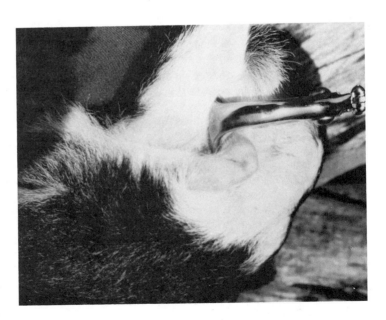

Figure 18. Castration of a young kid with the Burdizzo emasculatome.

tive; the doe is vaccinated during the dry period, or 200 units of antitoxin is administered to the kid. Tetanus prophylaxis is also advisable with the other methods, and the dose of antitoxin employed should be increased for larger animals. The use of a small Burdizzo emasculatome should be limited to young kids (Fig. 18); after just a few months, the testes become too large to be completely resorbed. Each spermatic cord should be crushed twice, while minimizing injury to the width of the scrotum. The end of the scrotum may be cut off with a scissors or a scalpel and the testes stripped out. An emasculator is necessary for hemostasis in all but the smallest kids. For adult bucks, separate U-shaped incisions may be made over the ventral aspect of each side of the scrotum.

A small kid may be restrained for castration by holding it upside down with all four legs held together. A standing position may also be used, with the tail pulled upward. Larger animals may be easier to handle if given xylazine at a dose of 0.1 mg/kg intramuscularly. A local block may be performed by injecting 0.5 per cent lidocaine into the cord or testis and into the skin where the initial incision is to be made. Care should be taken not to exceed 0.45 to 0.9 mg/kg of lidocaine, as toxicity, including opisthotonos and death, may result from higher doses. A fly repellent wound spray may be indicated but should be avoided in young nursing kids, as any abnormal smell may cause the rejection of the kids by the mother.

Teasers

When artificial insemination or planned mating is practiced, it is often convenient to have a teaser male in the herd that is able to stimulate and detect heat but that cannot successfully impregnate the doe. Ideally, to prevent the spread of genital disease, the teaser should also be unable to copulate.

A normal buck may be used temporarily as a teaser by simply fitting him with a harness and apron, available commercially for rams. If a marking harness is used, the owner can identify those does in heat with less frequent observations of the herd.

Several surgical procedures can be used to create permanent teasers, while maintaining libido in the buck. Bilateral vasectomy

can be performed, as is done with bulls or rams. A possibly simpler procedure involves the removal of the tail of the epididymis. The weaning or mature buck is secured in dorsal recumbency with its legs extended. The scrotum is washed with a mild disinfectant solution and rinsed. If desired, a small subcutaneous bleb of 2 per cent lidocaine may be placed before a 2.5-cm longitudinal incision is made through the skin and tunics over the tail of each epididymis. The epididymal tail is forced out through the incision, and a large portion of it is excised. The remaining severed portions of the epididymis are seared with a cautery unit or a piece of hot metal to reduce the likelihood of recanalization. The testis and epididymis are returned to the scrotum, the operation is repeated on the other side and the incisions are closed with sutures or wound clips to prevent periorchitis. Routine tetanus prophylaxis and antibiotics are desirable. Thirty days should elapse before the new teaser is used; this will allow for degeneration of sperm already in the tract beyond the epididymis, although most of the sperm will die sooner.

Because seminal fluids are resorbed in the head of the epididymis, obstruction or removal of the tail will not cause backpressure and testicular degeneration to the extent that libido is impaired. A spermatocele will form where the tail of the epididymis has been removed if ligation or cautery is not practiced. If this swelling later subsides, recanalization should be suspected. This may occur a year or more later.

A penile deviation procedure or a penectomy, using techniques developed for the bull, is possible. These methods have the advantage of preventing copulation, while, on the other hand, possibly resulting in decreased libido. If a buck's penis is surgically deviated to the right side, his semen can be conveniently collected with an artificial vagina.

Male goats may be sterilized by injecting 200 μg/kg of cadmium chloride into each testis. This is reported to cause total destruction of the germinal cells, although the interstitium eventually regenerates. Leydig cell tumors have been reported in other species. The cadmium or some other sclerosing agent, such as 10 per cent calcium chloride, may be injected into the tail of the epididymis. A dose of 1 ml per epididymis is suggested.

Probably the simplest and most reliable teaser is the intersex goat. Many of these, although genetically female, develop marked masculine odors and behavior. If an intersex goat with female or intermediate external genitalia is acquired, copulation and any concomitant spread of disease will be impossible.

INFERTILITY IN THE BUCK

In Germany, where much of the literature on goat reproduction originates, sterility is more common in the male than in the female goat. However, infectious causes of male infertility are almost unknown. Instead, significant problems occur that are due to genetically determined intersexuality, testicular hypoplasia, cryptorchidism, sperm granulomas and testicular degeneration.

Intersexes

Intersexes, or pseudohermaphrodites, occur quite commonly in the goat. The vast majority of these are genetic females; phenotypically they vary from being almost normal females to being almost normal males. The problem already has been discussed under female infertility. Some of these intersexes are so masculine in both external appearance and behavior that they can only be distinguished from normal males by karyotyping and examination of the semen. The XX testes usually do not produce germ cells in the seminiferous tubules after birth. Testosterone, however, is produced. There is normal male libido, and the seminal vesicles produce large amounts of fructose and citric acid. Other intersexes have an intermediate phenotype with hypoplastic testes, cryptorchid or inguinal testes or hypospadias as possible expressions of the condition.

Almost all hermaphrodites are polled. This is because the dominant gene for polledness is the same as or very closely linked to the recessive gene for hermaphroditism. This recessive gene has incomplete penetrance. A horned goat is expected to be homozygous for both the horned gene and the gene for normal fertility.

Sperm Granulomas

Sperm granulomas are a common cause of sterility in the buck. If one or more of the efferent tubules in the head of the epididymis end blindly, spermatozoa will migrate into the blind segments, undergo degeneration and release mycolic acid. While the initial lesion is merely that of sperm stasis and spermatocele formation, more advanced lesions have masses of spermatozoa in the interstitial tissue that are surrounded by histiocytes, lymphocytes, plasma cells and Langhans' type giant cells suggestive of tuberculosis. If the lesion is bilateral and large enough to obstruct the lumen of the epididymis, total sterility results. Sperm stasis with testicular edema is followed by degeneration and calcification of the testis (Fig. 19).

Careful examination by palpation or diagnostic castration of the epididymides of the affected goats will reveal firm granulomas in the head, body or tail of the epididymis. These vary in size from a pinhead to several centimeters in diameter and are usually, but not always, bilateral. Some of the granulomas escape detection by being located deep in the parenchyma of the epididymis. Typically the history reveals that the buck was once fertile but later became completely

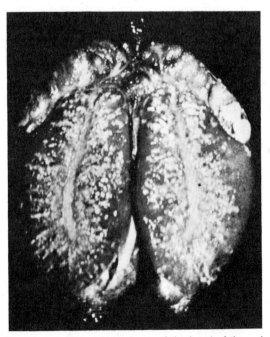

Figure 19. Sperm granuloma of the head of the epididymis, with degeneration and calcification of the testis. (Courtesy of Dr. K. McEntee.)

sterile, often quite suddenly. In these cases, spermatozoa will be absent from the ejaculate.

The etiology of sperm granulomas in the buck has received much consideration over the years. Experimental infection with *Escherichia coli* produced abscessation of the epididymis and sperm stasis, but naturally occurring cases do not show evidence of acute inflammation. Blind efferent tubules are more commonly believed to induce the lesion, just as described. Some bucks may be born with aplasia of a portion of the lumen of the epididymis, such that sterility is complete from the beginning. Current theories favor a genetic explanation for the failure of the mesonephric duct system to form properly. As with intersexuality, sperm granulomas are frequently associated with the polled condition.

It is very hard to interpret data from any study that is not accompanied by karyotypes when discussing male infertility. It has been proposed that the sterile males are actually completely transformed genetic females or, in other words, intersexes. Sometimes this is true, as in cases of testicular hypoplasia. On the other hand, there are numerous documented cases of XY polled males with sperm granulomas. Indeed, one study reports that approximately 50 per cent of homogeneous (PP) polled males will be completely sterile because of sperm granulomas. At least in the Alpine breed, the homozygous buck has a smooth head without scurs. The heterozygous buck has bean-shaped bony protuberances that often are surmounted by small, unsightly scurs. In the past, breeders have unintentionally selected for the homozygous condition while attempting to achieve a smooth head on a polled buck.

Control of spermatic granulomas as a cause of infertility in the buck should include selection of horned, or at least heterozygous, bucks, and careful palpation of all bucks before they are used for breeding. Affected animals should be eliminated from the herd or castrated.

Cryptorchidism

Not all cryptorchid goats are XX intersexes and, therefore, infertile. A form of cryptorchidism with possibly recessive inheritance has been well documented in Angora goats, in which intersexes are very rare. These animals are known as ridgelings.

In studies conducted in Texas, the right testis always failed to descend, while studies in South Africa invariably indicated that the left testis was retained. Occasionally, the opposite testis was also retained. Frequently, thin but strong membranous attachments, in addition to the gubernaculum, connect the small, degenerate internal testis to the internal body wall near the ilium and to loops of intestine. It has been postulated that it is these adhesions that interfere with descent that are inherited, rather than cryptorchidism *per se*.

A unilateral cryptorchid buck should never be used for breeding, even if the condition may not always be hereditary. (Bilaterally affected animals are sterile.) Siblings and dams should also be discarded from the breeding herd. In one experimental herd, strong selection pressure over the course of 20 years has reduced the incidence of cryptorchidism from 50 per cent to 0.8 per cent. The possible inheritance of the cryptorchid condition in breeds other than the Angora needs further study.

Testicular Degeneration

Testicular degeneration, or atrophy, is an important reason for loss of fertility in the buck. Not all cases are related to sperm granulomas.

Typically the testes are reduced in size by as much as one half. Shape also changes, so that the affected testes become small and spheroidal or else are reduced in horizontal circumference and assume an elongated appearance. The consistency either may become soft, with extensive tubular degeneration, or may become excessively firm, with testicular calcinosis. In some advanced cases, the head of the epididymis loses its normal lobulations. If the semen is examined, the density and motility of the spermatozoa will be found to be decreased. An increased incidence of sperm abnormalities such as separated heads and twisted midpieces will be found. Occasionally, testicular degeneration is preceded by a period of gynecomastia with milk production in 3 to 4 year old bucks.

There is no evidence that testicular atrophy is reversible and no known treatment. The buck should be replaced when his fertility is no longer acceptable. One study reports testicular degeneration induced by experimental *Trypanosoma vivax* infection;

therefore, tsetse fly control may prevent some cases in tropical countries. Selection of horned bucks is also indicated to decrease the probability of sperm granulomas as a cause of testicular degeneration.

Nutritional Influences on Fertility of the Buck

A diet adequate for normal growth and maintenance of general health is usually also satisfactory for reproduction. Very little experimental data are available. Overfeeding of energy may result in an obese, lethargic goat with poor libido. If the animal is kept on a poor diet, the volume of the testes will decrease but libido will usually remain until starvation is imminent. A severe protein deficiency will delay maturation of the testes and penis in young kids. In adults, sperm production will be adversely affected because spermatozoa are high in protein content.

The effect of trace mineral and vitamin deficiencies on male fertility in goats is largely conjectural. Presumably, iodine deficiency leading to goiter formation and poor body growth may be accompanied by decreased fertility. Likewise, a severe vitamin A deficiency may be expected to cause reversible atrophy of the testes and loss of libido. Testicular degeneration has been reported with vitamin E deficiency in goats, but details are not available. Finally, experimental zinc deficiency in goats, which requires a purified diet to be achieved, causes listless, weak, unthrifty animals with dry hair coat, alopecia and very small testes. In addition, many seminiferous tubules are lined only by spermatogonia. Thus, sterility can occur with zinc deficiency, but naturally occurring zinc deficiency is highly unlikely.

DISORDERS OF THE MALE REPRODUCTIVE TRACT

Posthitis

Posthitis (sheath rot or pizzle rot) due to a *Corynebacterium* infection is a problem when castrated goats are kept on a leguminous or high nitrogen diet. The Angoras are most commonly affected, probably because the castrates are kept for years for mohair production. Wethers tend to urinate within the sheath. The urea-hydrolyzing coryne-bacteria produce degradation products that are more irritating to the mucous membranes than normal urine is. Affected goats have an ulcerated or scabby prepuce. When the orifice becomes distorted or covered by scab, urination is accompanied by excessive straining.

Treatment with germicides is usually not effective. Prevention would include decreasing the protein in the feed and keeping males intact whenever practical. Testosterone implants have been used to prevent the problem in sheep in Australia, but these are not available in the United States.

Urolithiasis

Obstruction of the urethra by calculi is a common problem in castrated goats but also occurs occasionally in intact males. Any male goat of any age that is off feed or straining should be examined immediately to verify its ability to pass urine freely. Cases that are neglected for only a few days will progress to rupture of the bladder or urethra, uremia and death. If the buck is not observed to pass urine and the prepuce is not wet, a blood sample should be obtained to determine the creatinine level. The blood urea nitrogen (BUN) determination is not a dependable test in the goat, as animals may be completely obstructed and still have normal BUN values. Often the unobstructed goat will urinate promptly after being released from the restraint necessary to procure a blood sample.

Some cases of urinary obstruction may be easily diagnosed and treated because the calculus has lodged in the urethral process, where it can be visualized. The urethral process is snipped off with scissors and subsequent breeding is usually unimpaired. Unfortunately, many bucks have additional calculi in the bladder or are already obstructed proximally in the penis, often in the region of the sigmoid flexure. The dilated urethra on the midline of the perineum may be turgid, painful and pulsating. It may be impossible to exteriorize the penis of a wether that was castrated before the breakdown of preputial adhesions.

A wether with an obstruction proximal to the urethral process may simply be treated with a penectomy performed under general or epidural anesthesia. If it is hoped to save an obstructed buck for later breeding, a more complicated urethrostomy procedure will be necessary, and the prognosis is, at best, guarded.

If the animal has a distended abdomen, rupture of the bladder should be suspected. Palpation for a fluid wave and paracentesis 2 to 5 cm lateral to the prepuce will aid in the diagnosis. Abdominal surgery for repair of the bladder wall is indicated for these animals in addition to elimination of the inciting obstruction.

The cause of urolithiasis in goats has not been studied. Presumably, information gained from sheep should be applicable. The author suspects that many cases are related to feeding male goats a ration that is designed for milking animals and, therefore, is excessive in both calcium (Ca) and phosphorus (P). Ca:P ratios between 1:1 and 2:1 should be fed, but the total calcium requirement of the mature buck is only about 0.15 per cent of the diet on a dry weight basis. Thus alfalfa hay and dicalcium phosphate supplements should be avoided in the feeding of the adult male goat.

Neoplasms of the Male Reproductive Tract

Information concerning the incidence of neoplasms of the male reproductive tract is unavailable, with one exception. Adenomas of the adrenal cortex seem to be common in castrated male goats, especially in older Angoras. The neoplasms have been described as proliferative lesions of the cortex, containing abnormal cells (often polygonal or spindle-shaped) and growing in an unusual pattern. This tumor type is distinguished from the so-called nodules of hyperplasia, which are very common near the adrenal capsule of older goats. The adenomas vary in size from microscopic to 1 cm or more in diameter. They are frequently multiple or bilateral, and involvement of 13 to 22 per cent of the adrenals in castrates has been reported. Adrenal cortical adenomas are rare in female or intact male goats. Metastases and clinical signs are not reported. However, adrenal cortical inclusions have frequently been seen in the head of the epididymis, between the pampiniform plexus and vasa efferentia of both male and intersex goats. It is postulated that the castrated male goat lacks sufficient endogenous testosterone to inhibit pituitary gonadotropins, which mediate adrenal proliferation.

INFECTIOUS DISEASES OF GOATS

Brucellosis

Brucellosis is currently not a very important disease in goats in the United States, although it is highly significant in the Mediterranean area and in Central and South America. Sporadic outbreaks have been observed in the Southwest United States, with documented reports from Texas and Colorado.

Brucella melitensis is the principal cause of brucellosis in goats. *Br. abortus* has occasionally been isolated from goats. The two species cannot always be easily distinguished, as biochemical and serological tests may give differing results. Renoux[20] has proposed the name *Br. intermedia* for those isolates that share characteristics of both *Br. melitensis* and *Br. abortus*. There do not appear to be any published reports of *Br. ovis* infection in goats.

The organism enters through mucous membranes and may be found in any organ but tends to localize in the lymph nodes, udder and testes. Sexually mature goats are especially susceptible. Clinical signs include abortion, lameness, mastitis and orchitis. The first introduction of the disease on a farm will usually be accompanied by an abortion storm, with abortions being most frequent in the fourth month. The placenta is grossly normal. Few abortions will occur in later years, but some of the goats may remain sterile and have chronic uterine lesions. Many infected goats will be symptomless, and abortion does not occur under endemic conditions if the environment and management are good.

Usually infection of adults is lifelong, but some goats can recover from brucellosis. Apparently healthy kids from infected mothers are often infected, and normal newborn kids rapidly become infected if they drink infected milk. Often these very young infected kids will have negative serological tests. Opinions vary as to whether these kids will generally eliminate the infection before they are 4 months of age. Goats excrete the *Brucella* organisms in their milk even if they have not recently kidded. The milk from the same doe may give a positive culture result one day and a negative result the next. Brucellae may be excreted from the vagina of goats that have never kidded or aborted, and excretion continues for more than 3 weeks after parturition. Dust and soil are readily contaminated. Good data are not available on the probability of excretion in urine or feces.

Several diagnostic tests are available. Tube agglutination titers of 1:25 or higher are usually considered positive, while recently infected does may give negative reactions. The brucella card test has been used as a herd screening test. Whey agglutination tests are not sufficiently sensitive to detect infected goats. In one study, only 24 of 174 infected goats gave positive whey test results. A stained antigen test similar to the milk ring test has been successfully used; after overnight incubation, a radiated deposit of agglutinated antigen is visible on the bottom of the tube. True rings are rarely seen.

Cultures of milk, vaginal swabs, necropsy specimens and fetal tissues such as abomasal contents, spleen and placenta are routinely processed aerobically at 37°C. Higher CO_2 tension is needed for *Br. abortus.*

Vaccination is not practiced in the United States, where the incidence of caprine brucellosis in goats is so low that eradication by the test and slaughter method is a practical approach. If one animal in the herd is proved to be infected, the entire goat herd should be destroyed. If the owner refuses to permit elimination of the herd, testing and slaughter of all reactors should continue for several years before the herd is presumed clean. All new animals imported to an area or farm should have blood tests, and bucks should be tested before they are used for service. In parts of the country in which caprine brucellosis is essentially unknown, testing every 3 years is probably adequate. States adjacent to Mexico may find 6- to 12-month testing intervals to be more appropriate. Often the first indication of brucellosis in goats is the occurrence of undulant fever in humans consuming unpasteurized milk or cheese.

Leptospirosis

Epizootics of leptospirosis occasionally occur in goat herds. *Leptospira grippotyphosa* is the most frequently reported strain. A diagnosis based on clinical signs alone is often difficult. Icterus is not always present,

and most animals are afebrile. In the hyperacute form, the goats die of septicemia within 12 to 24 hours after the illness is first noticed. They go off feed and may hold their head down. Necropsy findings include anemia, an enlarged liver and enlarged, swollen kidneys. Goats with acute illnesses are sick from 1 to 3 days and show listlessness and inappetence before they die, manifesting vague nervous signs. The urine is often dark-red or brown, and abortions may occur. Goats with chronic illnesses are sick for about 1 week before they recover clinically without any treatment. The mucous membranes in these animals tend to be pale and icteric. The majority of infected goats become carriers without ever showing any signs and leptospiruria may last for at least 1 month.

Positive diagnosis can be made based on seroagglutination tests, dark field examination of the urine and culture procedures. Cultures of the liver and kidney are most apt to give positive results; blood, urine and milk may be injected intraperitoneally into white mice or guinea pigs and the liver and kidney of the laboratory animals cultured.

Treatment with 11 mg/kg of streptomycin intramuscularly twice a day for 3 days is usually effective in controlling the septicemia and preventing the carrier state, at least this is so in other species. Vaccination every 6 to 12 months with the appropriate strain (based on serological testing) should soon control the outbreak and prevent recurrences.

Q Fever

Q fever, or Queensland fever, is an infectious disease with a wide host range. Infected cattle, sheep and goats have been identified in Australia, Europe and North America, but these usually represent inapparent infections. Clinical disease is common only in man, in whom high fever, anorexia, malaise and interstitial pneumonia occur. The agent *Coxiella (Rickettsia) burnetii* localizes in the udder and placenta of domestic ruminants. The disease is spread by ingestion of the placenta or milk of the infected animal and by inhalation of contaminated dust. Several species of ticks can also transmit the disease, and dried tick feces on the skin of an animal is another potential source of infection to man. The rickettsial agent is resistant to drying, freezing and many disinfectants. Heating for 15 minutes at 65°C will destroy it, as will disinfection with 0.2 per cent formalin or 0.4 per cent phenol.

Goats generally show no signs of infection but excrete large numbers of organisms with the placenta and continue to excrete the agent in their milk for the entire period of lactation. Suckling transmits the infection to newborn kids, while ingestion of the placenta may infect others in the herd. Goats that inhale contaminated dust may develop nasal catarrh, a dry cough and bronchopneumonia. The organism can be demonstrated in conjunctival smears from these animals.

Occasionally, a goat herd may experience a large number of abortions that seem to be due to *Coxiella burnetii*. Examination of the placentae may reveal necrotic cotyledons with some thickening of intercotyledonary areas. Giemsa staining of the placentae will demonstrate large intracytoplasmic masses, 20 to 30 mμ in diameter, consisting of tightly packed organisms. Cotyledonary tissue, fetal abomasal fluid and maternal milk or blood is then inoculated intraperitoneally into guinea pigs or chick embryo yolk sacs to confirm the diagnosis. Complement fixation titers done on the sera of goats that have aborted are usually positive. It must be remembered that the same findings will be present in animals from herds in which Q fever is endemic, no matter what agent actually caused the abortions under investigation.

Burning placentae and aborted kids, general sanitation and pasteurization of the milk will help prevent infection of both goats and man. Tetracycline is commonly used to treat humans with Q fever, and streptomycin also inhibits growth of the organism. There do not appear to be any reports concerning the possible efficacy of tetracycline added to the feed of goats once an abortion storm due to Q fever has begun.

Enzootic Abortion

Enzootic abortion, also known as viral abortion, is caused by *Chlamydia*. The agent causes abortion in goats and sheep after 3 months and, most typically, during the last 2 weeks of gestation. The aborted fetus may be normal or slightly autolyzed, and the doe is generally clinically unaffected and has a normal hemogram. The placenta is passed promptly and subsequent fertility is normal; the doe usually does not abort again. During the parturition period, many goats and kids in the herd may show pneumonia; they cough and are listless, febrile and anorectic. Those that die show consolidated lungs and fibrinous peritonitis. Up to 10 per cent of the goats may show arthritis or conjunctivitis.

The chlamydial agent is excreted in the urine and feces as well as in uterine discharges. Dust in the pens becomes contaminated and remains infective for a long time. Infection is postulated to occur by ingestion or inhalation. Infected sheep may be a major source of infection for goats.

Diagnosis depends on examination of the placenta and fetus. The surface of the necrotic cotyledons should be scraped with a scalpel and the resulting smear stained with Stamp's, Macchiavello's, Giemsa or Ziehl-Neelsen stains to demonstrate numerous globular red elementary bodies (inclusions) in the epithelial cells. The use of stains is simpler than fluorescent antibody (FA) tests and is equally reliable. The fetal liver is sometimes enlarged and bright red; microscopic necrotic foci have been reported. The chorionic villi and endometrium show necrosis and leukocytosis as well as the presence of inclusions. Isolation of the chlamydial agent requires the use of embryonated eggs. Complement fixation (CF) tests are positive against the ovine viral abortion agent and ornithosis, with samples taken approximately 1 month after abortion. Goats having negative titers may excrete the agent in the feces, and goats with only intestinal chlamydial organisms may have positive titers.

Injectable oxytetracycline is recommended for treatment. Prevention of further abortions is attempted by feeding 100 to 250 mg of chlortetracycline per head per day continuously for the second half of gestation. If more convenient, the drug may be administered in the water instead of the feed. There is one report of good results with chloramphenicol and tetracycline used together, but dosages were not specified.

Vaccines are not yet available in the United States but have been used in Europe with good results, as indicated by a lowering of the abortion rate.

Mycoplasmal Infections

Mycoplasma causes several acute-to-chronic syndromes in goats. A variety of pleuropneumonia-like organisms have been isolated, but classification of the strains has been very difficult. Isolates that have different biochemical and growth characteristics and serological findings often produce similar clinical signs. Closely related strains may be very different clinically.

Contagious agalactia *(Mycoplasma agalactiae)* is one well-recognized syndrome in which a painful mastitis is frequently accompanied by fibrinopurulent arthritis and keratoconjunctivitis. Abortions are occasionally reported, but details are lacking. Sometimes cessation of lactation occurs in conjunction with the arthritis and conjunctivitis but without any swelling or tenderness in the udder. The mammary, ocular and articular forms appear to be spread by milk and exudates.

Contagious caprine pleuropneumonia *(Mycoplasma mycoides* var. *capri)* is a mycoplasmal infection that enters through the respiratory tract. Severe serofibrinous pleuritis and pneumonia occur but are usually unilateral. Systemic tetracyline or tylosin therapy may be useful in both agalactia and pleuropneumonia outbreaks.

Cases of granular vulvovaginitis have been reported in goats in India and have been reproduced experimentally by vaginal inoculation with *M. agalactiae*. After an incubation period of 11 to 34 days, mucopurulent exudate appears in the vagina. Multiple yellowish-white granular elevations develop near the clitoris, followed by epithelial necrosis and ulceration. Histological examination shows the lesions to be one of lymphocytic perivascular cuffs with diffuse lymphocytic and plasma cell infiltration in the lamina propria. Diagnosis of this syndrome is complicated by the fact that mycoplasmas have been isolated from the vagina of normal goats and that animals clinically affected with granular vulvovaginitis (both spontaneous and experimental cases) remain with negative serological titers for the mycoplasmal organisms. No treatments are reported.

Vibriosis

There is only one report available on vibrionic abortion in goats. Thus, it is misleading to give a general description of the disease. In the single verified case, a doe aborted at 115 days' gestation. Her appetite and milk production were good, and she showed no signs of metritis or systemic illness. Multiple necrotic foci 2 mm in diameter were visible in the liver of the fetus and *Campylobacter (Vibrio) fetus* was isolated in pure culture from the liver and stomach. However, the report does not specify whether *Campylobacter fetus* var. *venerealis* or var. *intestinalis* was involved. In the herd of 203 females, 19 abortions or premature births, mostly in young does, had occurred previously; the etiology of these abortions was not proved.

Vibriosis in goats, when it does occur, is probably similar to the *C. intestinalis* form of sheep rather than the *C. venerealis* form of cattle. Thus transmission would be expected to occur by ingestion rather than by sexual contact.

Infectious Bovine Rhinotracheitis

Although goats have been experimentally infected with the infectious bovine rhinotracheitis (IBR) virus, they are not considered a natural host. Their response is generally limited to pyrexia and mild clinical illness. The goats harbor the virus and develop antibodies.

A natural case involving severe respiratory disease and keratitis has been reported, but, to date, there is no evidence that the IBR virus has any effect on reproduction in goats.

REFERENCES

1. Barker, C. A. V.: Synchronization of estrus in dairy goats by progestin impregnated vaginal sponges. Can. Vet. J., 7:215, 1966.
2. Barker, C. A. V.: Penile deviation teaser bucks — A new development for dairy goat A/I. Dairy Goat J., 55:67, 1977.
3. Boyajean, D.: Intersexualité associée a l'absence de cornes chez la chèvre d'origine Alpine. Bibliographie signal étique. Ann. Génét. Sél. Anim., 1:447, 1969.
4. Corteel, J. M.: L'Insémination artificielle caprine: Bases physiologiques, état actuel et perspectives d'avenir. World Rev. Anim. Prod., 9:73, 1973.
5. Corteel, J. M.: The use of progestagens to control the oestrus cycle of the dairy goat. Ann. Biol. Anim. Bioch. Biophys., 15:353, 1975.
6. Corteel, J. M.: Production, storage and insemination of goat semen. Symposium Management Reproduction Sheep and Goats. Madison, Wisc., 1977, p. 41.

7. Dukelow, W. R., Jarosz, S. J., Jewett, D. A. and Harrison, R. M.: Laparoscopic examination of the ovaries in goats and primates. Lab. Anim. Sci., *21*:594, 1971.

8. Eaton, O. N.: An anatomical study of hermaphroditism in goats. Am. J. Vet. Res., *4*:333, 1943.

9. Eaton, O. N.: A semen study of goats. Am. J. Vet. Res., *13*:537, 1952.

10. Engum, J. and Lyngset, O.: Gynecology and obstetrics in the goat. Iowa State Univ. Vet., *32*:120, 1970.

11. Fraser, A. F.: A technique for freezing goat semen and results of a small breeding trial. Can. Vet., J., *3*:133, 1962.

12. Fraser, A. F.: Observations of the pre-coital behavior of the male goat. Anim. Behav., *12*:31, 1964.

13. Fraser, A. F.: Infertility in goats related to testicular atrophy. Trop. Anim. Hlth. Prod., *3*:173, 1971.

14. Hancock, J. L., McGovern, P. T. and Stamp, J. T.: Failure of gestation of goat × sheep hybrids in goats and sheep. J. Reprod. Fertil. (Suppl.), *3*:29, 1968.

15. Henning, M. W.: Q fever. J. S. Afr. Vet. Med. Ass., *24*:219, 1953.

16. Herman, H. A.: The Artificial Insemination of Dairy Goats. Columbia, Mo., American Supply House, 1972.

17. Lyngset, O.: Studies on reproduction in the goat. 1. The normal genital organs of the nonpregnant goat. Acta Vet. Scand., *9*:208, 1968.

18. Moore, N. W.: Multiple ovulation and ovum transfer in the goat. Proc. Aust. Soc. Anim. Prod., *10*:246, 1974.

19. Purcella, A. W.: A.I. (artificial insemination) of dairy goats. Dairy Goat J., *52*:3, Aug. 1974.

20. Renoux, G.: Brucellosis in goats and sheep. *In* Brandly, C. A. and Jungherr, E. L. (eds.): Advances in Veterinary Science, Vol. 3. New York and London, Academic Press, 1957.

21. Richter, J. and Gotze, R.: Tiergeburtshilfe. Berlin und Hamburg, Paul Parey, 1960.

22. Ricordeau, G., Bouillon, J. and Hulot, F.: Pénétrance de l'effet de stérilité totale lié au gène sans cornes P, ches les boucs. Ann. Génét. Sél Anim., *4*:537, 1972.

23. Shelton, M. and Groff, J. L.: Reproductive efficiency in Angora goats. Texas A & M Univ., B–1136, March, 1974.

24. Shelton, M. and Klindt, J. M.: A simple method of male sterilization for use with sheep and goats. Texas Agric. Expt. Sta. Res. Report, PR–3286, 1974.

25. Shelton, M. and Livingston, C. W., Jr.: Posthitis in Angora wethers. J.A.V.M.A., *167*:154, 1975.

26. Skinner, J. D., VanHeerden, J. A. H. and Geres, E. J.: A note on cryptorchidism in Angora goats. S. Afr. J. Anim. Sci., *2*:93, 1972.

27. VanRensburg, S. J.: Reproductive physiology and endocrinology of normal and habitually aborting Angora goats. Onderstepoort J. Vet. Res., *38*:1, 1971.

28. Whiting, R. D., White, B. M. and Stiles, F. C., Jr.: An epizootic of *Brucella melitensis* infection in Texas. J.A.V.M.A., *157*:1860, 1970.

29. Williams, C.: Selected causes of goat abortions. Proceedings, Sheep and Goat Practice Symposium. Fort Collins, Colorado, 1976.

PORCINE

Consulting Editor

A. D. LEMAN

Veterinary Services to Swine Breeding Herds

*A. D. LEMAN, H. D. HILLEY
and J. HURTGEN*

University of Minnesota, St. Paul, Minnesota

TABLE 1. *Actual and Feasible Goals for Breeding Herds*

	Gilts		Sows	
	ACTUAL	FEASIBLE	ACTUAL	FEASIBLE
Farrowings per year	1.4	1.7	1.7	2.3
Pigs weaned per year	9.2	12.7	12.9	19.6
Total pigs born per litter	8.8	9.4	10.1	10.5
Live pigs born per litter	8.1	8.9	9.2	10.0
Weaned pigs per litter	6.6	7.6	7.6	8.5

Veterinary services to pork producers have traditionally been centered in the farrowing house. Services to the breeding herd have usually been limited to specific vaccinations. Recent trends toward confinement of the breeding herd and toward swine farrowing complexes have placed new emphasis on efficient management of the breeding herd. Concurrently there are increased needs and opportunities for veterinary services. This paper attempts to briefly discuss many different opportunities for veterinary service to large breeding herds. It does not attempt to explain or document each opportunity completely. Rather it is intended to challenge practitioners to expand their capability for providing profitable service to pork producers.

Goals. Veterinarians can help their clients to establish reasonable short-term and long-term goals. General goals for the swine breeding herd are:

1. To produce the desired number of weaned pigs that have a high postweaning survival and an excellent growing efficiency.

2. To produce the desired number of pigs with minimal females, labor and cost.

3. To produce pigs that are free from diseases carried by the breeding herd, i.e., atrophic rhinitis, chronic pneumonia, internal and external parasitism and neonatal enteric colibacillosis.

Specific goals are useful only if they consider the feasibility of changing any reproductive parameter on the client's farm. An example of what can be done is shown in Table 1.

Other useful records and goals may include mean birth weight, mean weaning weight, first service conception rate and conception rate within 30 days after weaning.

Records. Without records, goals are useless. Veterinarians can help producers decide which records are useful and necessary to make critical management and veterinary decisions. Once the records are established, veterinarians should closely monitor the entries. They may also find it necessary to provide help in maintaining and analyzing the records.

Selection of Gilts. In addition to the usual concerns for conformation and growth rate, major consideration must be given to the underline of gilts. By selecting gilts with 12 to 14 evenly spaced and prominent nipples, both neonatal deaths and the number of very small pigs at the time of weaning can be reduced. Veterinarians can assist their clients in developing a system for selecting gilts. Gilt selection should begin in the farrowing house by permanent identification of gilts with superior underlines from large, healthy litters.

Selection of Boars. Some veterinarians are helping their producers to select boars, to reduce the probability of introducing new microbial agents via the boars and to identify boars with sound feet, legs and underlines. Incoming boars should be tested for antibodies to leptospirosis, brucellosis, eperythrozoonosis and pseudorabies. Their noses should be swabbed for *Bordetella bronchiseptica*. New boars should be tested for their susceptibility to porcine stress syndrome by using the creatine phosphokinase (CPK) card test. Veterinarians should insist that incoming boars be quarantined for at least 2 weeks, during which time they should be dewormed and sprayed at least twice for external parasites. By removing boar tusks every 4 months, veterinarians contribute to the safety of their clients.

Veterinarians should provide boar fertility examination services that assess sexual aggressiveness, sexual behavior and semen quality. In certain situations, vasectomized teaser boars may help to induce puberty in gilts.

Pregnancy Diagnosis. Pregnancy diagnosis is an integral part of monitoring breeding herd efficiency and providing early detection of problems. We personally choose to diagnose pregnancy in all the females whenever possible in order to get at least one opportunity to observe every female in the breeding herd. Observations are made concerning lameness, mastitis, mammary gland injury, soundness of underline, external parasitism and the nutritional state of the animals. Pregnancy diagnosis should be completed before 38 days following breeding so that nonpregnant animals can be returned to the breeding area prior to the second expected return to estrus.

Feed Additives. In many cases veterinary practitioners can save pork producers enough money to pay the veterinary service fee simply by proper utilization of antibacterials in the ration. There is no evidence that use of antibacterials throughout gestation will increase reproductive efficiency. The effect of antibacterials at breeding and at farrowing time is inconsistent. In most farm situations the choice of antibacterials depends almost entirely upon the disease problems that the veterinary practitioner diagnoses within the farrowing house, the nursery or the grow-finishing stage of pork production. For example, when atrophic rhinitis is judged to be a problem, adding sulfa to the lactation ration may reduce the vertical transmission of rhinitis-causing organisms from carrier sows to the pigs.

Vaccination Schedules. A breeding herd vaccination program should be the result of careful consideration of local and regional problems, the amount of exposure to the breeding herd and the disease history within the herd. In many large breeding herds, for example, the low incidence of leptospirosis and erysipelas makes these vaccinations questionable. When vaccines are judged to be necessary, veterinarians should recommend effective products and advise the client about least expensive sources. Vaccines and bacterins currently being used in breeding herds include transmissible gastroenteritis (TGE), *Escherichia coli*, lepto-

spirosis, erysipelas, rhinitis and mixed bacterins for control of mastitis-metritis-agalactia (MMA), pneumonia and enteritis.

Seasonal Infertility. Many large breeding herds experience a variety of reproductive problems in the months of July, August, September and October. By careful planning and by previous knowledge of the breeding herd, veterinarians can help reduce the seasonal infertility problem by encouraging producers to have a larger pool of gilts that can be bred during these months. By the appropriate use of hormones for inducing estrus, boar fertility examinations and early pregnancy detection, veterinarians can help minimize the cost of seasonal infertility.

Nutrition. Certain absolute nutritional requirements must be met in sows that are fed limited amounts of feed. For example, throughout pregnancy each sow should receive approximately 250 gm of protein, at least 15 gm of calcium, 10 gm of phosphorus and adequate vitamins and microminerals per day. In many parts of the United States, sows should receive vitamin E and selenium supplementation. Energy levels should be adjusted according to the weight gain of sows. Adjusting the level of feed intake in later stages of gestation will aid mammary development, and subsequent milking ability may increase the birth weight of pigs. Prefarrowing rations should be bulky or should contain a laxation substance such as magnesium sulfate (Epsom salts) to eliminate constipation that may occur in the sows. If the veterinary practitioner does not feel competent as a nutritionist, we strongly recommend the utilization of a nutritional consultant.

Disease Surveillance and Diagnosis. Veterinary practitioners must continuously monitor the breeding herd for internal parasites, external parasites, eperythrozoonosis and anemia. Every breeding herd should be tested at least twice per year for antibodies to eperythrozoonosis. Periodic fecal examinations for parasite ova and continuous monitoring for external parasites should be utilized. According to the Minnesota Disease Reporting System, mange is the most common disease in Minnesota swine. In order to control mange, thorough sprayings using lindane, toxaphene or malathion must be spaced 1 week apart, and not 2 weeks apart as is commonly believed. To eradicate external parasites from a breeding herd, we have found it necessary to spray the entire breeding herd every week for 6 consecutive weeks. Hemoglobin levels should be periodically monitored because sows with low hemoglobin values will have more stillborn and weak pigs.

By determining the severity of atrophic rhinitis, pneumonia and internal parasitism by slaughterhouse examination and post-mortem examination, the veterinarian can establish more precise feed additive and deworming programs for the breeding herd.

Artificial Insemination. Veterinarians should be prepared to provide information and counseling concerning artificial insemination. This is becoming increasingly necessary as breeding herd size increases and as people become more reluctant to transport boars because of such diseases as pseudorabies. Artificial insemination (AI) programs should reduce the number of boars required for breeding and the time spent on breeding herd management.

Client Education. Many successful veterinarians are basing their practice on providing new information to their clients. They teach the management of emergency obstetrical problems, the treatment of common diseases and the utilization of the most efficient sanitation methods. To base a practice on client education, the practitioner must be committed to a lifelong learning.

Most successful pork producers appreciate the opportunity to discuss problems and solutions with unbiased and educated observers. When payment to the practitioner is not dependent upon drugs and vaccines, veterinary consultation becomes even more credible.

Emergency Service. Properly managed breeding herds have minimal emergencies.

Conscience. Many pork producers know what is necessary for profitable production. Because of other time demands, however, the necessary details of successful production are sometimes not completed. Periodic visits by the veterinarian can be the necessary catalyst or reminder to get the tasks completed.

Preventive Medicine. Preventive medicine is not an accumulation of good ideas. It is not a "tried and true" formula for success and profitable production. It is not a recipe of routine ingredients that will solve all problems. Preventive medicine is the application of the least costly solutions to specific farm problems. It implies the need for continuous diagnostic effort and adjustment of prophylactic and therapeutic measures. Because much of the direct cost of preventive medicine involves feed additives, biologicals, injectable antibiotics and therapeutics and chemicals for parasite control, on each farm visit we utilize and update the forms that list all products and procedures used in the breeding herd and farrowing house. They provide a quick reference to our previous decisions and represent an obvious question and challenge for the current farm visit: "Which, if any, of these preventive medicine procedures is unnecessary or unprofitable?"

Normal and Aberrant Sexual Behaviors

JOHN B. MULDER
The University of Kansas, Lawrence, Kansas

Scientific studies concerning domestic animal behavior have been conducted primarily in the past 20 years. As a result, current detailed information is fairly limited. Furthermore, the normal behaviors of animals have been more thoroughly documented than their abnormal or aberrant behaviors. Therefore, the normal sexual behaviors of swine will be described in detail, with limited information provided about aberrant sexual behaviors.

NORMAL SEXUAL BEHAVIORS

Confinement Sexual Behavior

When a boar and sow in estrus are placed together in a small pen, courtship rituals and sexual behaviors are abbreviated. Sexual behavior under these conditions usually involves a short time period. The male mounts and ejaculates quickly without an elaborate demonstration of courtship behavior.

Free-Range Sexual Behavior

In pastured or free-living swine, elaborate courtship and sexual behavioral patterns are demonstrated. These will be presented as the swine progress from puberty and estrus to successful copulation. However, it must be remembered that all aspects of the described behaviors may not occur in all situations.

Boars frequently reach puberty before they are 7 months of age. The production of spermatozoa is usually not evident until they reach 10 to 12 months of age. Behaviorial puberty or sexual activity generally coincides with the age of spermatozoa production.

Most gilts initially come into estrus at 6 to 8 months of age. The normal estrous cycle requires 21 days, and there is little evidence to substantiate the belief that domestic swine have a definite breeding season.

The female becomes nervous several days prior to estrus and is frequently disturbed by minor incidents. She may leave the herd and follow any large moving object such as a feeding wagon or tractor. The vulva begins to enlarge 2 to 8 days before the onset of estrus. It becomes reddened and a mucous discharge appears.

Specific behaviors are displayed by the female during estrus. She goes to the boar and sniffs his anal and preputial areas. If the estrous female runs from the boar, he pursues her, attempting to herd her to a standstill position. During pursuit, he noses her sides, flanks and vulva. Additionally, he emits a series of soft gutteral grunts. These vocalizations have been termed the "mating song."

When the estrous female remains stationary, the boar presses his nose lightly against her head, shoulder or flank. Next, he proceeds toward her genital and anal region with increasingly more vigorous nuzzling. Often he places his head between her rear legs and with a quick upward jerk raises her hindquarters. At this point the boar grinds his teeth, moves his jaws from side to side, foams at the mouth and grunts continually. The boar emits urine in a rhythmic manner during this stage of sexual arousal.

As the courtship ritual continues, the female nuzzles the flanks and genitals of the boar. She may gently bite his ears. Generally, both partners remain in a head-to-head position for a time. The female may attempt to mount the boar. Frequent urination by the female occurs during this phase of courtship. The male is attracted by this behavior and sniffs the urine from the female.

When the female desires to mate, she stands rigid. This posture is called the "mating stance" or "immobility response." Durign this time of rigid posture, it is difficult to force the female to move. Both olfactory and auditory stimuli have been described as being responsible for the immobility response. The submaxillary gland of the boar produces the olfactory cues stimulating this response.

Behaviors of different boars vary during the immobility response. Some mount repeatedly before breeding. Others may mount only once and copulate. The frequency and duration of mounting are dependent upon the receptivity of the female, her ability to support the male and the dominance relationships among boars in the herd.

Once copulation begins, the boar seldom withdraws or dismounts. Copulation continues for a period of 4 to 5 minutes. The female generally stands immobile during this time. A boar may repeat mating with an estrous sow four to eight times over an interval ranging from 12 minutes to 15 hours.

If the courtship ritual of a male and female is interrupted by another boar, one of the courting pair may emit a threatening grunt and lunge toward the intruding boar. This generally provides sufficient warning and causes the intruder to flee. Thus, a fight seldom occurs.

During periods of high environmental temperatures, the sex drive is diminished and boars often refuse to mate. Mating activity usually ceases about midmorning and resumes toward dusk.

Detailed, careful observations during courtship or sexual behavior will detect males or females that do not breed. Thereby, loss of valuable reproductive time may be avoided and economic losses curtailed.

ABERRANT SEXUAL BEHAVIORS

Young, inexperienced boars frequently exhibit abnormal sexual behaviors. They may attempt to mount the female from her anterior or lateral side. Males that are reared apart from females may also show aberrant sexual patterns. Homosexual behaviors are common in all-male-reared boars.

Bizarre sexual objects are occasionally mounted by boars with high sex drives. These objects include feeding or watering devices, a bale of hay or straw or other objects available in their environment.

Presently, little is known about aberrant sexual behaviors in swine. Even less is known about their specific causes or methods for correction. Hopefully, additional controlled research studies will provide more

information and a better understanding of these behaviors.

REFERENCES

1. Baldwin, B. A.: The study of behaviour in pigs. Br. Vet. J., *125*:281, 1969.
2. Day, B. N.: Reproduction of swine. *In* Hafez, E. S. E. (ed.): Reproduction in Farm Animals. 2nd Ed. Philadelphia, Lea and Febiger, 1968.
3. Fraser, A. F.: Behavior patterns in pigs. *In* Fraser, A. F.: Farm Animal Behavior. Baltimore, The Williams and Wilkins Co., 1974.
4. Signoret, J. P., Baldwin, B. A., Fraser, D. and Hafez, E. S. E.: The behavior of swine. *In* Hafez, E. S. E. (ed.): The Behaviour of Domestic Animals. 3rd Ed. Baltimore, The Williams and Wilkins Co., 1975.

Hormonal Profiles in the Pig

ALLEN R. ELLICOTT
Clemson University, Clemson, South Carolina

Hormonal profiles in the pig vary primarily with the age, sex and reproductive status of the animal. Therefore, changes in the hormonal profiles will be discussed using these criteria. During the last decade, the use of a new type of hormone assay, radioimmunoassay, has allowed a fairly complete documentation of the hormonal profile in the pig. The average levels of hormones presented here may not agree closely with a specific laboratory's finding. They are designed rather to indicate a "physiological profile" and not absolute levels.

FETAL AND NEONATAL PERIOD TO PUBERTY

During the fetal and neonatal period of the female, plasma luteinizing hormone (LH) levels decline from about 3 ng/ml shortly before birth to about 0.3 ng/ml at 10 weeks of age.[2] However, plasma LH values in the male show no tendency to decline during the same time period, averaging greater than 2 ng/ml at 10 weeks of age.[2] A decline in plasma follicle-stimulating hormone (FSH), but not in plasma LH, also occurs in the female between 1 and 2 months of age and 4 and 7 months of age.[3, 4]

The levels of progesterone and LH in the fetus of both sexes are higher than in the sow just before parturition. This indicates that the fetal-placental unit can synthesize progesterone and LH. Progesterone concentrations of greater than 20 ng/ml are present in fetus before parturition. In the female neonate, these levels decline rapidly to about 5.5 ng/ml within 2 hours after birth. In the male neonate, progesterone levels decline to about 3.5 ng/ml during the first week of life, with a further decline to about 0.5 ng/ml by 10 weeks of age. During the first weeks of life the progesterone is primarily of testicular origin, as castration reduces these levels.[1] The levels of testosterone and its metabolite 5α-dihydroxytestosterone (5α-DHT) do not change significantly during the first 5 weeks after birth in the male. A significant increase in testosterone levels, from 1.5 ng/ml to 5.3 ng/ml, occurs from the first 5 weeks to the twelfth week of life, whereas the level of 5α-DHT increases from 0.3 ng/ml to 0.7 ng/ml during the same time period.

ADULT FEMALE

Estrous Cycle

As the gilt reaches puberty, cyclic changes in the hormonal profiles begin to occur. The average concentration of LH throughout the estrous cycle is 1.8 ng/ml.[4] A slight increase in LH levels near the time of estrus is probably responsible for the initiation of the process of ovulation. The average level of FSH throughout the estrous cycle is 7 ng/ml, with a slight increase occurring 2 or 3 days after the beginning of estrus.[3] The increases in LH and FSH levels observed near the time of estrus are physiologically, but not statistically, different from the average levels found throughout the remainder of the cycle.

Progesterone levels just prior to puberty average about 2.4 ng/ml, with erratic fluctuations of from 0.5 to almost 8.5 ng/ml.[5] After puberty, progesterone levels are low at estrus, about 0.5 ng/ml. Beginning on about day 3 after estrus, progesterone levels in plasma rise rapidly until day 7 or 8 and continue to rise at a slower rate until day 14 or 15 of a 20-day cycle.[4] A precipitous decline in progesterone concentration occurs on about day 15, with levels falling from 30 to 35 ng/ml to 1 ng/ml or less within about a 48-hour period. Plasma 17β-estradiol levels show a peak of from 55 to 80 pg/ml on the day preceding estrus or the day of estrus, then decline to levels of 5 to 20 pg/ml during the remainder of the estrous cycle.[5] The hormonal profiles during the estrous cycle of the pig are shown in Figure 1.

The level of progesterone in the plasma during the luteal phase of the estrous cycle is positively correlated with the number of corpora lutea. The administration of exogenous gonadotropic hormones will increase the ovulation rate. Therefore, the estrogen

levels in the plasma before ovulation and the progesterone levels after ovulation will be increased. No effect of gonadotropin administration on plasma LH levels before or during estrus has been observed.

Pregnancy

The cyclic changes in the patterns of hormone release are mainly absent during pregnancy. There is no marked decrease in the levels of plasma progesterone about day 15 after estrus, as is characteristic of the cyclic female. A slight decrease in plasma progesterone is found between days 15 and 25, with an increase near midpregnancy. Although progesterone levels are correlated with the number of corpora lutea, no useful correlations between progesterone levels and the number of live fetuses at day 25 have been reported. The administration of additional exogenous progestin has not been shown to increase the survival of embryos. Pregnancy can be maintained on as little as 4 ng/ml of progesterone, approximately 25 per cent of the normal level at midgestation.

Plasma LH levels remain low throughout pregnancy. Plasma estrogen levels during the first 25 days of pregnancy are similar to those found during the luteal phase of the estrous cycle. Unconjugated estrone and estradiol levels rise from baseline values at

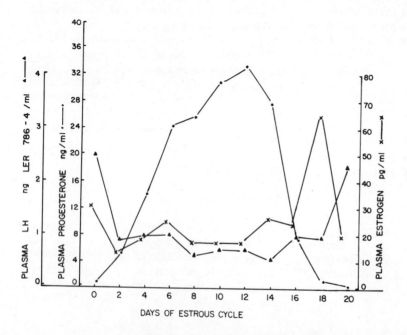

Figure 1. The average levels of progesterone, LH and estrogen throughout the estrous cycle in the gilt. (Redrawn from Hendricks, D. M., Handlin, D. L., Guthrie, H. D. and Skelley, G. C.: Animal Science Research Series 21, 1971, p. 9.)

day 80 to 2.5 ng/ml and 0.4 ng/ml, respectively, just before parturition.[5] Estrone sulfate, a conjugated estrogen, is detectable as early as day 16 of pregnancy. Two peaks of estrone sulfate, reaching levels of about 3 ng/ml, are found between days 23 and 30 and at parturition, respectively. Estrone sulfate is apparently secreted into the maternal plasma from the embryo.

Parturition

During the last 2 weeks of pregnancy, progesterone levels fall from about 15 ng/ml to about 10 ng/ml within 2 days of parturition.[1] These concentrations apparently decrease rather rapidly to levels of 3 to 4 ng/ml at the time of delivery. A further decline to levels of slightly more than 1 ng/ml occurs during the 24 hours following delivery. Total estrogen concentrations rise from levels of 2 ng/ml 10 days before term to a peak of approximately 7 ng/ml on the day before parturition. A rapid decline in estrogen concentrations to levels of less than 1 ng/ml occurs during parturition and continues for the next 24 hours.

Corticoid levels in the plasma of sows vary widely from sample to sample. Just prior to parturition, levels of 90 ng/ml have been reported.[1] After parturition is completed, levels are about 40 ng/ml, similar to those observed 3 to 10 days before parturition. Corticoids have been implicated as the possible mechanism by which the fetus controls the time of parturition in some monotocous ruminants. Recently a possible role of the fetal adrenal in controlling the time of parturition in the pig was shown. Decapitation of most of the fetuses in the litter led to a lengthening of pregnancy.

Lactation

During lactation, progesterone levels in the plasma average slightly above 1 ng/ml, estrogens average less than 0.2 ng/ml and corticoid levels fluctuate between 25 and 70 ng/ml. After the litter is weaned, the cyclic pattern of hormonal secretion characteristic of the estrous cycle is resumed.

ADULT MALE

In the adult male, no cyclic patterns of hormonal change occur, as is seen in the sow. No diurnal pattern in LH secretion was observed during a 24-hour period, averaging about 0.8 ng/ml of LH. Testosterone levels, however, were significantly lower during the night than during the day. Copulation significantly raised the average LH levels between 30 and 120 minutes following intromission. Testosterone levels showed no significant change in a 4-hour period after copulation.

CASTRATED ADULT

Castration of adult animals of both sexes leads to an increase in the average levels of both FSH and LH. The level of FSH is approximately twice as high following ovariectomy as during the estrous cycle, averaging about 15 ng/ml.[4] The LH levels increase from an average of 1.8 ng/ml during the estrous cycle to 2.6 ng/ml at 2 months following ovariectomy, with rather wide daily fluctuations.

Progesterone levels fall to about 0.8 ng/ml after castration of adult animals of either sex. The origin of this progesterone is thought to be the adrenal gland. Estrogen concentrations remain at low levels in the plasma after ovariectomy. No change in the average levels of corticoids has been observed following castration of either sex.

REFERENCES

1. Baldwin, D. M. and Stabenfeldt, G. H.: Endocrine changes in the pig during late pregnancy, parturition and lactation. Biol. Reprod., *12*:508, 1975.
2. Elsaesser, F., Ellendorff, F., Pomerantz, D. K., Parvizi, N. and Smidt, D.: Plasma levels of luteinizing hormone, progesterone, testosterone and 5α-dihydroxytestosterone in male and female pigs during sexual maturation. J. Endocrinol., *68*:347, 1976.
3. Rayford, P. L., Brinkley, H. J., Young, E. P. and Reichert, L. E., Jr.: Radioimmunoassay of porcine FSH. J. Anim. Sci., *39*:348, 1974.
4. Rayford, P. L., Brinkley, H. J. and Young, E. P.: Radioimmunoassay determination of LH concentration in the serum of female pigs. Endocrinology, *88*:707, 1971.
5. Shearer, I. H., Purvis, K., Jenken, G. and Haynes, N. B.: Peripheral plasma progesterone and estradiol 17-β levels before and after puberty in gilts. J. Reprod. Fertil., *30*:347, 1972.

Crossbreeding Programs

CHARLES J. CHRISTIANS
University of Minnesota, St. Paul, Minnesota

The heritability of a trait is that portion of the average superiority of the selected parents that is passed on to their offspring. Traits such as carcass merit and structural soundness are highly heritable and respond to individual selection. Production traits associated with growth and feed utilization are moderately heritable and can be improved by individual selection. Since progress is slower for these traits, individual performance records are essential. Reproductive traits such as litter size and birth and weaning weights have relatively low heritabilities and respond very little to individual selection.

In most herds, one sire is used for 20 to 25 females; more selection pressure is possible in the sire than in female selection. Traits that are highly heritable should be stressed in the sire as individual selection, whereas low heritable traits related to reproduction, should be stressed in the gilt by family selection. Fertility, sex drive and mating ability must be evaluated in the boar, and these respond well to individual selection. These selection tools are the primary means available to the seedstock producer.

Commercial producers can also use crossbreeding. One can combine desirable characteristics of different breeds and capitalize on heterosis. Heterosis is greatest for traits with low heritabilities.

When a boar of a different breed is mated to purebred dams, litter size is not significantly increased. Since the maternal breed in the original cross will influence litter size, breeds that are noted for large litters should be used as foundation females.

Even if litter size at farrowing is not increased, purebred sows will wean about 10 per cent more crossbred than purebred pigs. A greater survival rate results from heterosis responses in the crossbred pigs. A 24 per cent increase in litter weaning size can be expected when a crossbred sow is used. This improvement is due to an increased number of pigs born alive and greater baby pig survival to 21 days.

Pig survival and growth are the real benefits of a systematic crossbreeding program. When crossbred females are used, about 28 per cent greater 21-day litter weights can be realized per female exposed, as compared with purebreds.

Crossbred pigs reach market weight at an earlier age and have a slight improvement in feed efficiency as compared with purebred pigs. Even though traits of intermediate and high heritabilities are not greatly influenced by crossbreeding, overall efficiency can be improved by selecting superior parents. Real breed differences in male and female reproductive efficiency exist; therefore, choice of breeds appears to be critical in a crossbreeding program.

Comparing swine breeds accurately for all economically important traits is difficult. Although some crossbreeding experiments are being conducted to evaluate specific breed crosses, all breed combinations have not been adequately compared. Genetic breed composition and frequency of desirable gene combinations do change; therefore, evaluating breeds must be a continuous and endless process.

A comparison of published crossbreeding experiments indicates that Yorkshire females excel in birth and weaning litter size and 21-day litter weight. The Landrace female ranks high in her pigs' birth and weaning weight and 21-day litter weight. The Chester White female excels in 21-day litter weight per female exposed, which is a measure of overall reproductive efficiency (Table 1).

Crossbred sows of Yorkshire and Landrace breeding rank highest in all reproductive traits evaluated, and the combination of these two breeds is superior to any other breed combination. These results reflect the importance of the selection of one of the white breeds in the initial cross and their influence in total reproductive performance (Table 2).

Because of the increased possibility of disease contamination, most producers should retain their own crossbred females. The influence of sire breed on reproduction, therefore, must be evaluated. Of the breeds evaluated, the Yorkshire sire ranks high, as does the Yorkshire dam, for birth and weaning litter size and 21-day litter weight. In con-

TABLE 1. *Relative Reproductive Performance of Female Breeds**

	Breed					
Trait	BERKSHIRE	CHESTER WHITE	DUROC	HAMPSHIRE	LANDRACE	YORKSHIRE
Number of litters	19	145	348	393	44	379
Litter size born alive	87	99	89	84	94	100
Litter size weaned	83	95	86	84	89	100
Pig birth weight	82	81	94	94	100	82
Pig weaning weight	87	87	95	96	100	94
21-day litter weight	74	89	84	86	96	100
21-day litter weight /female exposed	84	100	78	94	89	94

*Composite results from Iowa, Oklahoma, North Carolina and Canada crossbreeding projects. Best breed performance is given score of 100 and compared with each breed. (From Christians, J. C. and Johnson, R. K.: Pork Industry Handbook, Extension Folder 361, St. Paul, University of Minnesota, 1978.)

TABLE 2. *Relative Reproductive Performance of Crossbred Females**

Female Breed Cross	No. of Litters	Litter Size Born Alive	Litter Size Weaned	Litter Size 21-day Weight	Litter Size 21-day Weight/ Female Exposed
Chester–Duroc	41	83	79	86	–
Chester–Hamp.	36	92	81	77	–
Chester–York.	37	97	87	86	–
York.–Land.	35	100	100	100	100
Hamp.–Land.	38	100	95	95	88
Hamp.–York.	192	91	87	87	81
Berk.–York.	33	90	85	83	93
Berk.–Land.	37	92	90	87	91
Berk.–Hamp.	36	81	77	76	74
Duroc–York.	193	93	85	82	85
Duroc–Land.	38	92	93	86	79
Duroc–Hamp.	205	86	82	79	76
Duroc–Berk.	39	93	82	79	77

*Composite results from Iowa, Oklahoma, North Carolina, and Canada crossbreeding projects. Best breed performance is given score of 100 and compared with each breed. (From Christians, J. C. and Johnson, R. K.: Pork Industry Handbook, Extension Folder 361, St. Paul, University of Minnesota, 1978.)

TABLE 3. *Sire Breed Influence on Reproductive Performance**

	Breed			
Trait	CHESTER WHITE	DUROC	HAMPSHIRE	YORKSHIRE
Numbers of litters	136	388	338	399
Litter size born alive	97	96	98	100
Litter size weaned	92	96	92	100
Birth weight	97	100	97	94
21-day litter weight	84	90	90	100
21-day litter weight /female exposed	89	91	81	100

*Composite results from Iowa, Oklahoma and North Carolina crossbreeding NC–103 project. Best breed performance is given score of 100 and compared with each breed. (From Christians, J. C. and Johnson, R. K.: Pork Industry Handbook, Extension Folder 361, St. Paul, University of Minnesota, 1978.)

TABLE 4. *Influence of Sire Breed on Various Production and Carcass Traits**

Trait	Breed			
	CHESTER WHITE	DUROC	HAMPSHIRE	YORKSHIRE
Number of litters	136	388	388	399
Production				
Days at 220 lb	96	100	98	98
Feed/gain	96	99	100	98
Carcass composition				
Length	99	99	100	100
Backfat	92	94	100	88
Loin eye area	94	97	100	93
Marbling score	100	100	76	76

*Composite results from Iowa, Oklahoma and North Carolina crossbreeding NC–103 project. Best breed performance is given score of 100 and compared with each breed. (From Christians, J. C. and Johnson, R. K.: Pork Industry Handbook, Extension Folder 361, St. Paul, University of Minnesota, 1978.)

TABLE 5. *Average Daily Gain and Feed Efficiency for Boars Tested to 220 lb at Central Test Stations**

Breed	No. of Boars Tested	Average Daily Gain	Feed Efficiency
Berkshire	310	96	94
Chester White	1017	92	96
Duroc	6334	100	100
Hampshire	4127	98	98
Landrace	172	93	90
Poland China	528	95	95
Spotted	1521	98	96
Yorkshire	3760	98	99

*Summary of 20 Central United States Test Stations. Best breed performance is given score of 100 and compared with each breed. (From Christians, J. C. and Johnson, R. K.: Pork Industry Handbook, Extension Folder 361, St. Paul, University of Minnesota, 1978.)

TABLE 6. *Carcass Traits (Adjusted to 220 lb) by Breed for Pigs Tested at Central Test Stations**

Breed	No. of Pigs Tested	Carcass Length	Backfat Thickness	Loin-Eye Area
Berkshire	184	96	87	91
Chester White	290	95	88	91
Duroc	1095	97	88	88
Hampshire	726	98	100	98
Landrace	153	99	78	89
Poland China	203	94	95	100
Spotted	574	97	86	95
Yorkshire	684	100	87	90

*Composite results from National Barrow Show and Minnesota Central Evaluation Stations. Best breed performance is given score of 100 and compared with each breed. (From Christians, J. C. and Johnson, R. K.: Pork Industry Handbook, Extension Folder 361, St. Paul, University of Minnesota, 1978.)

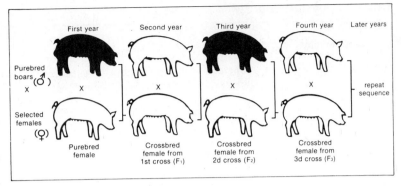

Figure 1. Two breed rotational cross system. (From Christians, C. J. and Johnson, R. K.: Pork Industry Handbook, Extension Folder 361, St. Paul, University of Minnesota, 1979.)

trast to the female breed evaluation, Yorkshire sires excel Chester White sires for 21-day litter weight per female exposed (Table 3).

The Berkshire, as a sire breed, ranks high in 21-day litter weight per female exposed when mated to Yorkshire or Landrace females. The Hampshire sire mated to the Landrace females excels in 21-day litter weight. Duroc sires influence pig birth weight and litter size weaned (Table 4). This advantage in weight is continued throughout the growth phase (Table 5). Crossbreeding provides an opportunity to reap the benefits of many genetic sources. An unplanned crossing program will not be successful. A crossbreeding system must be selected that will capitalize on heterosis, take advantage of breed strengths and fit the total management program (Table 6).

Two basic systems may be considered, namely, the rotational cross and the terminal cross. The rotational cross system combines two or more breeds in which a different breed boar is mated to the replacement crossbred females that are produced the next generation. The two-breed rotational cross (Fig. 1) is a simple program

in which two breeds are selected to complement each other. To capitalize on heterosis and other breed strengths, additional breeds can be added. The three-breed cross is probably the most used (Fig. 2). Using four or more breeds, the percentage of heterosis could be increased; however, management becomes very complicated.

The terminal cross system is well adapted to feeder pig production. A two-breed single or rotational cross female mated to a boar of a third breed producing the terminal market pig fits many of the feeder pig production requirements of reproductive efficiency in the crossbred female and fast growing, efficient pigs that produce superior carcass composition and quality.

The sire breed could be either a purebred or crossbred boar but should be of different breed composition than the crossbred female. Since no replacement gilts are retained from the terminal cross, the sire breed becomes less important, but the individual boar's performance becomes a key criterion of selection. Since only one breed of boar is used, females of different ages and groups can be mixed in the breeding groups.

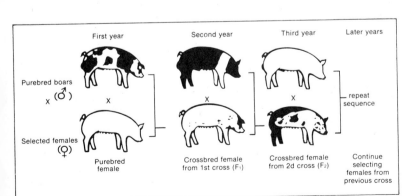

Figure 2. Three breed rotational cross system. (From Christians, C. J. and Johnson, R. K.: Pork Industry Handbook, Extension Folder 361, St. Paul, University of Minnesota, 1979.)

TABLE 7. *Inheritance of Swine Abnormalities*

Abnormality	Description	Mode of Inheritance
Bent legs	Front legs bent, fixed at front knee; causes farrowing difficulty; stillborn	Recessive
Clubfoot	Three symptoms: lower front legs thickened, hooves deformed; eczema on belly, spreads over body; giant alveoli cells in lungs result in difficult breathing	Recessive
Cryptorchidism	One or both testes retained in body cavity	Recessive and sex-linked
Goosestep	Pigs lift leg with jerk that often goes as high as the back	One or more recessive
Hairless	Inherited thyroid abnormality; hair follicles not normal	Two recessive
Hemophilia	Pigs normal at birth but bleed to death from induced wounds; full expression of trait occurs at 3 or 4 months of age	Recessive
Hernia	Scrotal (intestines come down inguinal canal into scrotum)	Two recessive
	Umbilical ("belly busts" wall weakness allows intestines to protrude)	Dominant
Hydrocephalus	Brain enlarged and much fluid accumulates in skull cavity; lethal	Simple recessive
Intersex	Both sex organs present; enlarged clitoris	Recessive
Inverted nipples	Nipples turn into belly wall instead of protruding; nonfunctional	Undetermined
Legless	Pigs born alive without legs and soon die	Simple recessive
Melanotic tumors	Moles or skin tumors highly pigmented and contain hair	Recessive
Muscle contracture	Lethal condition; front legs born stiff	Simple recessive
Paralysis	Hind legs have muscular tremors or are paralyzed; lethal	Recessive
Porcine stress syndrome	Stress; tail and muscle tremors; death	Recessive
Shaker	25 per cent incidence	Two-pair recessive
	A second type found in Landrace, in which only males are blind and shake	Sex-linked recessive
Syndactyly (mule foot)	One toe instead of two	Dominant
Thickened front legs	Front legs greatly swollen where connective tissue replaced muscle; lethal	Simple recessive

Although limited research information is available on the use of crossbred boars, indications are that crossbred boars are more aggressive breeders, have less leg soundness problems and improve overall breeding efficiency. A crossbred boar could combine those traits that may not be available in one straightbred breed.

Precaution must be taken in either a terminal or rotational crossing program so that the breed composition of the crossbred boar is different from the crossbred female. If a breed is repeated, an immediate reduction in heterosis will occur and will defeat the purpose of crossbreeding.

The forms of inheritance of swine abnormalities are summarized in Table 7.

Mating Systems and Boar Management

J. P. HURTGEN

University of Pennsylvania, Kennett Square, Pennsylvania

Many swine infertility problems are associated with poor boar management. Oftentimes, the particular system of mating used on a farm will predispose the herd or a group of females to a specific etiological cause of infertility or will frequently mask the etiology. Therefore, it is important that veterinarians and producers understand the mating system and methods of boar management being used.

SEXUAL DEVELOPMENT AND MATING BEHAVIOR

Coordinated sexual behavior and first ejaculation usually occur at 5 to 8 months of age. Age is more important than body weight in determining the onset of puberty. Normal precopulatory behavior between the male and female usually begins as nasonasal or nasogenital manifestations. This behavior may include grunting, grinding of the teeth, excessive salivation, rhythmic urinations, nuzzling of the female's flank area and sniffing of the perineum or head. Mock fighting and biting attempts may also occur.

The estrous female will usually seek out the boar and assume a characteristic immobile stance with arched back and erect ears. Even when the boar cannot be seen, courting grunts and sexual odor are sufficient to attract the estrous female. Therefore, estrous sows and gilts are frequently observed standing along the fence-line or gate nearest the boar pen. Boars, however, seem to detect the estrous female more readily by her behavioral activity (immobile stance) than by auditory, olfactory or visual stimuli.

Erection and protrusion of the penis occur after mounting. However, some boars will mount and dismount several times before copulating. After mounting, the boar thrusts until the tip of the penis penetrates the vulva. Following several intravaginal thrusts, the spiral end of the penis becomes fixed in the cervix and ejaculation begins. Muscular, wave-like movements over the perineum and rhythmic contractions of the anal sphincter occur during copulation. The average duration of ejaculation is 5 to 6 minutes.

Fertility gradually increases until boars reach about 12 months of age. Total sperm output and seminal fluid volume increase until the boar reaches 18 months of age, at which time the ejaculate consists of 20 to 100×10^9 spermatozoa in 200 to 400 ml of semen. The duration of the spermatogenic cycle in the boar is approximately 34 days plus an additional 10 days required for passage of spermatozoa through the epididymis.

BOAR SELECTION

The medical history from the herd of origin is important in selecting new boars. Breeding stock should be purchased from herds free of swine dysentery and transmissible gastroenteritis (TGE) within the past 6 months. The herd should also be free of brucellosis and pseudorabies, and individual animals should have negative results on serological testing for leptospirosis. Swine dysentery and TGE may be transmitted by recovered carrier animals. The breeder's herd should be observed for signs of lice and mange, lameness, atrophic rhinitis and chronic pneumonia. Herds with these disease problems should be avoided when purchasing breeding stock. Each group of boars should be purchased from one source in order to reduce disease and fighting among boars. Boars from litters affected by unfavorable genetic traits or traits that increase the degree of inbreeding should not be incorporated into a breeding program. Inbreeding decreases average litter size. Unfavorable genetic traits carried by boars include atresia ani, inguinal and umbilical hernia, myoclonia congenita and reduced libido.

Conception rate and litter size are influenced by the breed of the dam. Therefore, prolific breeds must be represented in the sow line of a crossbreeding program. Furthermore, individual boars within breeds directly influence conception rate and litter

1019

size. For every 10 per cent increase in conception rate, there is a concurrent increase in litter size of 1.2 pigs.

The number of boars required to achieve optimal fertility depends upon the age of the boars, breeding-pen size, weaning practices and mating system. Ideally, young boars (<12 months of age) should not be used more than once daily (maximum of five services per week). Because mating each female two or more times per estrus will improve conception rate and litter size, double mating is recommended. Sows come into a rather synchronous estrus 3 to 6 days after pigs are weaned. Therefore, if sows are weaned from their litter in large groups, the number of boars must be increased.

PRECONDITIONING BOARS

Boars should be purchased at least 6 weeks prior to service to allow a 2-week quarantine and a 4-week preconditioning period. Clinical observations indicate that boars should be at least 8 months old before routine usage. Upon arrival, new boars should be sprayed for external parasites. They should be observed for signs of swine dysentery and TGE during quarantine. Other pathogens carried by the boar are unlikely to be manifested during this time. Vaccinate boars with any vaccines and bacterins judged to be necessary for the herd. Treatment for internal parasites and a second treatment for external parasites should also be conducted during quarantine.

Approximately 1 month prior to breeding, an immunization program of controlled exposure to viral agents capable of causing reproductive failure should be initiated to establish common immunity among the breeding animals. Porcine enteroviruses and porcine parvovirus are of special concern. Because the epizootiology of these agents is not completely understood, methods by which this common immunity is established are empirical. Clinical evidence suggests that "fence-line" contact is insufficient for exposing all breeding animals; therefore, direct contamination may be accomplished by mixing boar fecal material with the feed of nonpregnant females and vice versa or by rotation of animals among pens. Pregnant sows and gilts should not be exposed to new boars. It is during this preconditioning period that each boar should be evaluated for breeding soundness or should be test-mated to a limited number of females in order to assess potential boar fertility. These females should be closely observed for return to estrus or possible pregnancy should be checked, using an ultrasonic device.

MATING SYSTEMS

Double mating is the servicing of an individual female twice, 12 to 24 hours apart, during the same estrus. This practice significantly increases conception rate and litter size. These benefits are probably due to breeding nearer the time of ovulation and to the frequent use of a different boar for the second service. Maximum conception rates are obtained when females are bred approximately 12 hours prior to ovulation. Heterospermic matings may result in improved fertility. Double mating, using different boars, may mask the effect of a low-fertility or sterile boar.

Pasture breeding, pen mating, hand mating and artificial insemination are breeding systems in use today. As the result of confinement and intensified production, pasture breeding is being replaced by other practices. The commonly used pen-mating system is a modification of pasture breeding. With these systems, a single boar or group of boars is placed in a pasture or pen with females for 23 to 45 (or more) days. It is hoped that estrous animals will be double mated, possibly with two or more boars. Various modifications of these practices include the rotation of boars between breeding pens at 8- to 24-hour intervals or removal of boars from breeding pens to assure sexual rest. Disadvantages to these systems are the inability of the manager to adequately identify serviced females, control the number of services per boar, observe mating behavior and libido or identify sire of offspring and fighting among strange boars. Some estrous females may fail to be serviced by the boars if pens or groups are large. The effect of social dominance by a boar on fertility and libido of subordinate males has not been investigated. However, observations in beef bulls indicate that one or two bulls may account for all pregnancies in a group of females.

In hand mating, estrous females are selected by the herdsman, frequently with the aid of a teaser boar, and taken to a breeding pen to be serviced. This practice allows close observation of mating behavior, accurate recording of breeding dates and controlled double mating; insures mating of all identified estrous females and allows control of services per boar per day. This system requires accurate heat detection and more labor by managers.

Artificial insemination utilizing both frozen and fresh semen is becoming more widely accepted for many reasons: increasing the use of superior, high fertility sires; preventing the introduction of disease from outside sources and spread within a herd; decreasing the number of boars; allowing the pooling of semen from two to four boars to maximize heterospermic mating at each insemination and facilitating the breeding soundness evaluation (including semen evaluation) of each boar at frequent intervals. Boar longevity is greatly enhanced because traumatic foot, leg and penile injuries are less frequent. Additionally, older boars may be used to service gilts or small females without risk. Demands on time and labor for heat detection, semen collection and insemination are increased, although synchronization of estrus, utilizing group weaning of sows and hormone therapy, greatly enhances an artificial insemination program. However, artificial insemination is accompanied by a series of factors critical to maintaining high fertility. Quality control must be practiced in the handling, storage and extension of semen. Osmotic pressure, pH and bacterial contamination of the seminal extender should be monitored periodically. Insemination technique must be closely ob-

served. Extended semen should be placed in the uterine body and a 50-ml minimal volume used. It is recommended that sows and gilts be inseminated two to three times during standing estrus, using 2 to 5×10^9 spermatozoa per insemination. It is expected that only boars of high fertility be used in an artificial insemination program.

REFERENCES

1. Dziuk, P. J.: Estimation of optimum time for insemination of gilts and ewes by double-mating at certain times relative to ovulation. J. Reprod. Fertil., *22*:277, 1970.
2. Koh, T. J., Crabo, B. G., Tsou, H. L. and Graham, E. F.: Fertility of liquid boar semen as influenced by breed and season. J. Anim. Sci., *42*:138, 1976.
3. Rasbech, N. O.: A review of the causes of reproductive failure in swine. Br. Vet. J., *125*:599, 1969.
4. Rodeffer, H. E., Leman, A. D., Dunne, H. W., Cropper, M. and Sprecher, D. J.: Reproductive failure in swine associated with maternal seroconversion for porcine parvovirus. J.A.V.M.A., *166*:991, 1975.
5. Signoret, J. P.: Swine behavior in reproduction. *In* Lucas, L. and Wagner, W. (eds.): Effect of Disease and Stress on Reproductive Efficiency in Swine. University of Nebraska Coop. Ext. Service, 1970, p. 28.
6. Strainslow, C. M. and Whitley, R.: Sexual inactivity effect on boar fertility. J. Anim. Sci., *40*:193, 1975.
7. Swierstra, E. E.: Duration of spermatogenesis in the boar. J. Anim. Sci., *26*:952, 1967.
8. Swierstra, E. E.: Effect of environmental temperature on semen composition and conception rates. *In* Lucas, L. and Wagner, W. (eds.): Effect of Disease and Stress on Reproductive Efficiency in Swine. University of Nebraska Coop. Ext. Service, 1970, p. 8.

Artificial Insemination

STIG EINARSSON
College of Veterinary Medicine,
Uppsala, Sweden

HISTORY

The very first inseminations of swine were performed in the Soviet Union. The development of procedures for practical field use of artificial insemination (AI) started about 20 years later. Technical equipment and suitable diluents were developed in several countries (e.g., Japan, England, France and Norway) during the 1950's. At present artificial insemination in pigs is used in many countries (e.g., Denmark, Finland, France, Germany, Holland, Japan, Norway, the Soviet Union, Sweden and the United States).

Much progress was made in 1971, as following the use of deep frozen boar spermatozoa, inseminated via the cervix, achievement of fertility was reported from Sweden and from the United States. This was accomplished by the development of procedures suitable for practical field work (see Long-term Preservation, page 1023).

GENERAL ASPECTS OF AI IN PIGS

Several advantages for utilizing artificial insemination in pigs can be listed, including:

1. Combining the best boars with the best sows within a breed.
2. Performing crossbreeding programs.
3. Improving health control by minimized spread of infectious diseases.
4. Permitting the performance of progeny tests for traits of low heritability.

METHOD OF ARTIFICIAL INSEMINATION

Selection of Boars

The recruitment of boars for AI should be done among the progeny from the very best boars and sows within breeds. In countries in which performance testing of young boars is adopted, the test period covers the interval when the boars weigh from 20 to 100 kg. Growth rates, feed conversion ratio, ultrasonic measurement of back fat thickness, leg quality and viability of the boars are the selection criteria employed. The best boars are thereafter trained to mount a dummy sow. Sexual drive and sperm quality and quantity, as well as fertility, are additional selection criteria recommended. Current questions concern how to judge and record the leg quality and the viability of the boars.

Ejaculation and Collection of Semen

Collection of semen is made when the boar is mounting a dummy sow, which should be satisfactory both to the operator and to the boar. As the dummy sow may be soiled with secretion from the prepuce of the boar and as bacteria may be transmitted from one boar to another, cleaning or disinfection, or both, of the dummy sow is therefore necessary when it is used for more than one boar.

Various types of artificial vaginas have been described, all of which make use of internal pressure to initiate ejaculation. Some are fitted with rubber bulbs to control pressure levels and provide pulsating pressure. Others make use of hand pressure or a spiral wire into which the boar's penis locks. The simplest procedure seems to be the gloved hand method. Ejaculation is evoked by maintaining a firm grasp on the spiral end of the boar's penis.

No collection of semen should be made until the fluid contents of the preputial sac are expelled, since contamination of semen with preputial fluid has an adverse effect on the spermatozoa. The duration of the ejaculation is long, and the semen is delivered in three fractions, namely, the presperm fraction, the sperm-rich fraction and the post-sperm fraction. The post-sperm fraction consists of gelatinous material and clear fluid from the accessory glands. Some boars produce intermittent sperm-rich fractions throughout the ejaculation. The volume of semen and the concentration of spermatozoa per ejaculate vary greatly, and the total number of spermatozoa per ejaculate varies between 10 and 100 billion sperm.

Semen should be collected in plastic bags enclosed in prewarmed (37°C) thermos flasks and covered with gauze for straining off the gelatinous material.

Semen Examination

Before dilution, the semen should be checked for its potential fertilizing ability. There is no *in vitro* method that gives a precise estimation of the fertility of the spermatozoa; however, the following laboratory tests are recommended: Estimation of *sperm motility* is probably the best method of determining the quality of fresh semen. The motility is estimated under a microscope at 300 to 400× magnification at 37°C. The motility of boar spermatozoa decreases quickly under anaerobic conditions, and estimation must therefore be made quickly. Semen with less than 70 per cent progressive motile spermatozoa should be discarded. *Sperm concentration* is most accurately estimated by hemocytometric counting. However, this is a time-consuming procedure, and many AI centers therefore use an absorptiometer that is calibrated for measurement of the sperm density. *Sperm morphology* should be checked for all boars selected for use in artificial insemination.

Semen Extenders

Semen extenders must afford protection against temperature and pH changes as well as provide a source of nutrients for the spermatozoa. Boar semen is amenable to extensive dilution. Therefore most commercial AI centers make an initial dilution of the semen, followed by final dilution at the time of insemination.

Most diluents currently used in swine AI are essentially based on glucose with added buffering material (citrate, bicarbonate or milk). If sodium bicarbonate or sodium citrate is used, potassium is added. Proteins in the form of egg yolk or milk proteins are sometimes added but do not appear to be essential.

Two widely used diluents in commercial swine AI are Illinois Variable Temperature (IVT) and edetate (EDTA) glucose. IVT, modified for boar semen by the French researchers Du Mesnil du Buisson and Dauzier, is saturated with carbon dioxide (CO_2). Liquid semen of good quality can be kept for 3 days in gassed IVT if stored at 18 to 22°C.

Recently, diluents that are thought to increase the life span of fresh spermatozoa up to 5 to 7 days have been introduced. Such diluents will improve the usefulness of fresh semen but will not eliminate the need for a suitable freezing method.

Long-term Preservation

Since 1970 a number of deep freezing methods for boar spermatozoa have been developed and described. Most of them are not practicable for large-scale use. However, three freezing methods developed in the United States, Germany and Sweden during 1975 and 1976 fulfill many of the requirements for a practicable deep freezing method. The semen is concentrated before dilution, and the diluted semen is frozen in plastic straws or as pellets. The pellets are packed in plastic tubes in liquid nitrogen according to dose. Each insemination dose contains 4.5 to 6.0×10^9 spermatozoa. Fertility results that are available are encouraging. A further minimizing of the number of spermatozoa per dose is desirable, however, to insure an optimum utilization of AI boars. A problem seems to be the difference in freezability of spermatozoa from different boars. Selection of boars for deep freezing of spermatozoa might therefore be necessary in the future.

Storage and Insemination

When using the modified IVT diluent, it is essential that the diluted semen remain saturated with CO_2 until used. Furthermore, the bottles of diluted semen must be stored between 18 and 22°C (absolutely not below 15°C). Immediately before the insemination the IVT-diluted semen is mixed with ungassed diluent up to the volume wanted.

The recommended number of spermatozoa per insemination dose varies between 2 and 10×10^9 spermatozoa. At present the most common dose is 2 to 3×10^9 spermatozoa.

Various types of insemination catheters are used in different countries. Disposable insemination equipment is attractive. However, the rubber spiral tipped catheter[3] is widely used. A thin-walled polyethylene bottle containing the semen is attached to the catheter, and the semen is allowed to flow in by gravity.

Time of Insemination

The average period of estrus in sows is about 48 hours. During the pre-estrous period the sows and gilts show signs of reddening and swelling of the vulva. During estrus the sows and gilts will stand rigid when pressure is applied to the back. Some females (up to 30 per cent of the gilts) will pass through estrus without giving a positive reaction to the back pressure at any stage. The presence of a boar facilitates the detection of estrus, however. Females should be inseminated only if they respond to the "back pressure test." Satisfactory fertility results are obtained if the sow is inseminated 10 to 30 hours from the beginning of standing estrus. Some sows will show signs of estrus for a longer period of time if a boar is close by. Heat control should be performed at least once a day.

Although the presence of a boar facilitates the detection of estrus, it can also make the detection of the optimum time for insemination more difficult. For determining the optimum time of insemination in the absence of a boar, an aerosol dispenser containing minute quantities of androgen steroids has been used to detect the signs of estrus.

It is recommended that gilts be inseminated when they have shown two estrus periods, whereas sows should be inseminated at their first estrus after weaning.

ESTROUS SYNCHRONIZATION

Estrous synchronization in sows and gilts is of great interest as it makes possible the insemination of several animals in the same herd on planned days. However, a satisfactory method is not available for practical use to date. Nevertheless, a disciplined weaning program utilizing considerable numbers of sows weaned on one particular day of the week (e.g., Thursday) will give a similar effect as estrous synchronization.

FERTILITY RESULTS

The fertility results with artificial insemination in swine under field conditions have varied. There are great differences in fertility between inseminators and between boars. The major problem, however, seems to be accurate detection of estrus in the herds. In herds with careful heat control and in which only females responding to the back pressure test have been inseminated, the conception rate, as well as the litter size, has been only slightly below that for natural service.

REFERENCES

1. Aamdahl, J.: Artificial insemination in the pig. Proceedings 5th International Congress on Animal Reproduction (Trento), *IV*:147, 1964.
2. Einarsson, S.: Deep freezing of boar spermatozoa. World Rev. Anim. Prod., *9*:45, 1973.
3. Melrose, D. R.: Artificial insemination of pigs — A review of progress and of possible developments. World Rev. Anim. Prod., *2*:15, 1966.
4. Polge, C.: Artificial insemination in pigs. Vet. Rec., *68*:62, 1956.

Seasonal Infertility in Swine

J. P. HURTGEN

University of Pennsylvania, Kennett Square, Pennsylvania

INTRODUCTION

A seasonal pattern of infertility has been identified in many countries, including the United States. Identification of this phenomenon is probably due to the increase in year-round swine breeding operations, increased use of individual animal identification and improved recording systems for swine. Although only limited research has been done on the effect of seasonal factors on reproduction, present reports agree on many features of this problem.

DESCRIPTION

Effect on the Female. Sows weaned during the months of July, August, September and October have a less synchronous, delayed interval from weaning to estrus. The incidence of postweaning anestrus may approach 50 per cent in some herds during these same months, whereas less than 10 per cent anestrus is observed for sows weaned from November to June. The duration of anestrus in individual sows has been observed to last for as long as 4 months. Postmortem examination of weaned, anestrous sows reveals that the ovaries are small and smooth and lack corpora lutea. Many follicles, ranging in diameter from 1 to 8 mm, may be present in the ovaries. No uterine pathological findings are present. Conception rates are also reduced for July through October matings. Conception rates of 70 to 90 per cent are expected for sows mated between November and June, but conception rates of 25 to 70 per cent are common for July through October matings. Therefore, an increase in repeat breeding occurs during late summer and early fall. Some workers have also reported an increase in the number of sows and gilts exhibiting estrous cycles of 24 days duration or longer. Therefore, this feature of seasonal infertility can easily be confused with the multiple etiologies associated with prolonged estrous cycles. Because of postweaning anestrus, lowered conception rates and estrous cycle aberrations during late July, August, September and October, a decreased farrowing rate is observed from November to early February.

It is currently thought that sows weaned from their first litter during late summer and early fall are more frequently affected by anestrus than are mature sows. Although not adequately researched, no particular breed susceptibility or resistance to seasonal anestrus and infertility has been reported. It is also suspected that litter size may be reduced for July to October matings.

The extent to which gilt reproductive efficiency is affected by seasonal factors appears less well defined, owing to a wide variety of management schemes for breeding gilts, lack of individual animal identification and inadequate record systems. However, it has been shown that gilts expected to reach sexual maturity during summer or fall months frequently have a delayed onset of puberty. I would also suspect decreased conception rates and estrous cycle aberrations to affect gilts 6 to 10 months of age during late summer and early fall.

Controlled environment studies have revealed an increase in the incidence of anestrus and silent estrus and a decrease in conception rates in gilts when environmental temperatures were elevated. Embryonic survival may also be jeopardized by ambient temperatures above 36°C during the first 14 days after service. Although light and relative humidity may be involved in a seasonal infertility pattern, these factors appear less well defined.

In my experience, the most salient feature of seasonal infertility affecting the female is that of extended periods of postweaning anestrus characterized by a lack of ovarian luteal tissue in sows weaned during August, September and October.

Effect on the Male. The role of the male in the July to October infertility pattern as it relates to decreased conception rates and prolonged estrous cycles is ill-defined, even though the effect of elevated ambient and testicular temperatures has been studied.

In boars subjected to ambient temperatures of 35°C for 8 weeks, total sperm/ejaculate, motility and fertility decreased. Boars housed outside during the summer (maximum temperature of 30 to 40°C) had decreased fertility and litter size compared with boars held in a temperature controlled facility (maximum temperature of 18 to 24°C). Local elevation of testicular temperature adversely affects spermatogenesis. The contribution of the boar to late summer and early fall infertility needs further investigation. The effect of ambient temperature fluctuations from May to November on semen quality and fertility in boars of all ages also needs further research.

DIFFERENTIAL DIAGNOSIS

Many conditions may mimic seasonal infertility because of the wide range of reproductive problems encountered. Postweaning anestrus can be associated with inadequate nutrition, lack of boar libido and deficient heat detection and management practices. Cystic ovarian degeneration also results in anestrus. Clinically, prolonged estrous cycles in serviced females are indistinguishable from early embryonic death, potentially caused by many factors. Delayed puberty in gilts also has multiple etiologies. Reduced farrowing rates may make one suspicious of bacterial or viral reproductive failure, boar infertility, poor breeding management and so forth.

DIAGNOSIS

A thorough history of the herd in question should include: time of year; onset of reproductive problems; monthly incidence of postweaning anestrus and farrowing in previous years; investigation of management practices surrounding weaning, estrous detection and mating; degree of boar libido; prior level of boar fertility; evaluation of the nutritional status of the herd; parity of anestrous and repeat breeder sows and incidence of delayed return to estrus in nonpregnant females. Anestrus due to deficient heat detection practices and pregnancy should be ruled out. Postmortem examination of the reproductive tracts from a representative sample of affected sows and gilts has proved extremely beneficial. Serum progesterone concentrations determined on paired serum samples taken 5 to 15 days apart from a representative group of anestrous sows or gilts will aid in differentiating sows and gilts with static ovaries from those with functional corpora lutea. Serum progesterone concentrations are less than 1 ng/ml only when corpora lutea are absent in the ovaries. Therefore, progesterone levels will be less than 1 ng/ml in sows during estrus or in sows with static ovaries. A thorough, systematic breeding soundness evaluation of boars in the breeding herd should also be conducted. Evaluation of the boar is discussed elsewhere in this section. It is recommended that boars with poor semen quality be excluded from the breeding herd until semen quality returns to normal.

PREVENTION AND TREATMENT

At the present time, it is thought that the majority of problems associated with decreased fertility from late July to October are due to elevated ambient temperatures that affect both the male and female. Therefore, it seems logical that managers of affected herds should attempt to reduce heat stress in both male and female, although adequate research has not been conducted in this area. Other stresses at weaning and breeding time should be avoided. Transportation of anestrous sows, rotation of anestrous and cycling sows and increased contact of these females with boars seem to be of little value. Pregnant mare serum gonadotropin, (PMSG), 500 IU, alone or in combination with a luteotropic hormone (250 IU of human chorionic gonadotropin, HCG), has been shown to induce a fertile, synchronous postweaning estrus in approximately 90 per cent of sows weaned from August through October. PMSG or PMSG and HCG are given on the day of or the day after weaning. Fertility of treated sows appears comparable to that of sows exhibiting spontaneous postweaning estrus during these months.

It may be advantageous for some small pork producing units to avoid August to October matings. In continuous breeding programs, this is not feasible. Therefore, it is recommended that additional gilts be selected for the breeding herd during July, August, September and October. The number of females needed to be serviced to attain a given number of farrowings 4 months later can be determined for each farm by dividing the number of desired farrowings by the farrowing rate experienced for that particular time period in previous years. For example, if 25 farrowings are desired for a particular week in January (or for the entire month) and if the particular farm has a conception (farrow) rate of 60 per cent for September matings, 42 females must be serviced in September. Weaned, anestrous (and, therefore, not serviced) sows are not included in the 42 females.

Only boars with normal semen quality should be utilized.

It is expected that further research will be forthcoming concerning the etiology, diagnosis, prevention and treatment of seasonal infertility in the gilt, sow and boar.

REFERENCES

1. Hurtgen, J. P.: Seasonal anestrus in a Minnesota swine breeding herd. Proceedings of the 4th International Pig Veterinary Congress, Ames, Iowa, 1976.
2. Liittjohann, R. M.: What we consider satisfactory reproductive performance. Proceedings of the American Pork Congress, Ames, Iowa, 1971, pp. 147–152.
3. Mavrogenis, A. P. and Robison, O. W.: Factors affecting puberty in swine. J. Anim. Sci., 42:1251, 1976.
4. Rasbech, N. O.: A review of the causes of reproductive failure in swine. Br. Vet. J., 125:599, 1969.
5. Sviben, S., Herak, M. and Vakovic, I.: Changes in the farrowing rate of sows mated during the individual months of the year and the calculation of the needed number of matings for a constant number of farrows. Proceedings 3rd International Pig Veterinary Congress, Lyon, France, 1974.
6. Swierstra, E. E.: Effect of environmental temperatures on semen composition and conception rates. In Lucas and Wagner (eds.): Effect of Disease and Stress on Reproductive Efficiency in Swine. University of Nebraska Coop. Ext. Serv., 1970, pp. 8–13.
7. Teague, H. S.: Effect of temperature and humidity on reproduction. In Lucas, L. and Wagner, W. (eds.): Effect of Disease and Stress on Reproductive Efficiency in Swine. University of Nebraska Coop. Ext. Serv., 1970, pp. 21–26.

Physical Examination of the Female and the Female Reproductive Tract

WAYNE L. SINGLETON
Purdue University, West Lafayette, Indiana

Careful physical examination of female swine is a useful tool in selecting potentially fertile breeding animals. Gilts with structural or genital abnormalities can be culled prior to breeding, thus eliminating the costs associated with the development of these animals to breeding age. Both a physical examination and a herd history derived from records of previous management, reproductive ability and health conditions are helpful in the diagnosis of reproductive failure in individual animals or in breeding groups within a herd. When indicated, internal reproductive organs should be recovered from slaughtered animals for a thorough examination. The clinician can often gain useful information from such an examination when other procedures fail.

EXTERNAL EXAMINATION

Structural Soundness

With the trend toward confinement rearing and breeding, structural soundness of females is becoming increasingly important. Soundness in replacement gilts is especially significant, since most structural faults and weaknesses are aggravated by age and confinement rearing. Special attention should be given to selecting gilts free from foot, leg and joint problems, which may impair their future reproductivity. A moderate slope to the pasterns provides the animal with a cushion to the foot and leg joints, enabling her to cope with solid surfaces in confinement. Gilts and sows with split hooves, sore pads or other foot problems should be culled because attempted treatments are often unsuccessful. Such problems may arise from abrasive or damp, slick flooring. These and other unsoundness traits may have genetic implications, and certain genetic lines may be more predisposed to them than others.

Too much slope in the rump area tends to make the animal more prone to unsoundness as she matures. A steep rump also displaces the vulva to a low position and angle so that boars often experience difficulties in entering the sow during mating.

Extreme muscling has been implicated as a characteristic of some females with reproductive problems — namely delayed puberty, low conception rate, farrowing difficulty and poor mothering ability. Again, the acceptable degree of muscling in females is difficult to define, but in general, females should be selected primarily for soundness and reproductivity rather than for carcass traits.

External Genitalia

Observing the vulva of replacement gilts at 5 1/2 to 6 months of age can help detect potentially sterile or slow breeding females. The most commonly observed abnormality is the "rosebud" or infantile vulva (Fig. 1). Field observations have revealed that an infantile vulva is usually accompanied by infantile uterine horns and nonfunctional ovaries. This condition is more frequently observed in confinement-reared gilts, but it occasionally occurs in field-raised females as

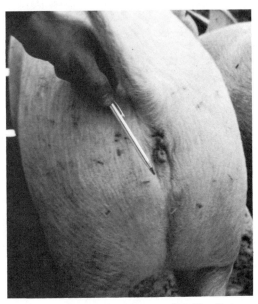

Figure 1. Eight-month-old noncyclic gilt with immature or "rosebud" vulva.

well. A higher than normal incidence of infantile reproductive tracts is usually observed in herds with above average muscling. Such gilts reared in confinement can sometimes be stimulated to develop sexually by moving them to new pens or outside lots (transport phenomenon) and by exposure to males. Treatment of gilts with 500 to 1000 IU of pregnant mare serum gonadotropin per gilt has also been successful in some herds. Treatment with exogenous hormones is not encouraged because of the possible implications involved in propagating females predisposed to this problem.

The "tipped vulva" is another abnormality that is less frequently observed (Fig. 2). Its relationship to future reproductive potential is unknown. However, the presence of an abnormally formed vulva may indicate an abnormal reproductive tract. It has also been observed that boars experience difficulty servicing gilts having this trait. Such gilts should be eliminated as potential breeding herd replacements.

Injuries to the vulva may occur from fighting or at parturition. Unless they are severe,

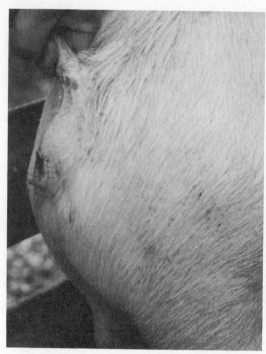

Figure 3. Atresia ani or imperforate anus.

they generally do not contribute to future reproductive problems.

Atresia ani or imperforate anus (Fig. 3) is a congenital defect observed in all breeds. In gilts, the rectum and vagina are joined, forming a rectovaginal fistula just anterior to the vulva. Males die because they are unable to defecate. Gilts defecate via the vulva. This condition is easily detected in newborn pigs if the animals are carefully observed. However, it is not uncommon for affected gilts to go unnoticed until breeding age or later. Inheritance of atresia ani is thought to be controlled by two pairs of dominant genes. It may also be caused by viral infections during early pregnancy.

Occasionally, an unusually large percentage of females within a group are observed to have red, swollen vulvas typical of females in estrus. This observation, when coupled with mammary development in nonpregnant females and barrows, indicates the presence of exogenous estrogenic substances in the feed. Diagnosis is often difficult because laboratory facilities are lacking or the feed source has been completely used before the effects are observed.

Mammary System

A sound underline is a fundamental characteristic to consider when evaluating a

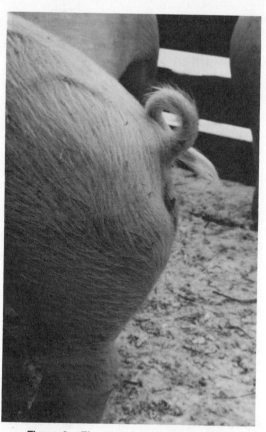

Figure 2. Tipped or "sky-hooked" vulva.

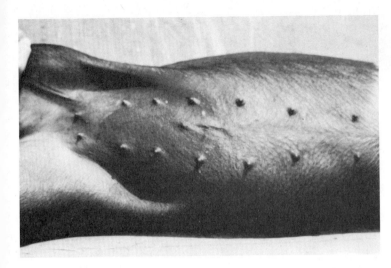

Figure 4. Four-month-old gilt with excellent teat placement. Note presence of three teats on each side in front of the navel.

female for reproductive potential. The underline should show at least six functional, well-developed and evenly spaced teats on each side, with three teats in front of the navel (Fig. 4). Gilts and boars having a blind teat (one that does not develop fully), a pin teat or an inverted nipple should not be considered as replacement animals (Figs. 5 to 7). Constant selection is required to maintain acceptable underlines in a breeding herd. Selection can be initiated soon after birth by observing the underlines of gilt pigs. Gilts with sound underlines and adequate teat numbers that were farrowed from productive dams can be ear marked for consideration as potential replacements when final selections are made. Although not proved experimentally, abrasive concrete flooring in farrowing crates or pens has been implicated as a causative factor in herds experiencing a greater than normal incidence of underline problems in young gilts.

INTERNAL EXAMINATION OF THE REPRODUCTIVE TRACT

Excellent descriptions of the normal reproductive tract and related changes during the estrous cycle and early pregnancy have been presented elsewhere in this book. Surveys conducted in the United States and Europe indicated that 5 to 10 per cent of all virgin gilts have abnormal reproductive tracts. Heritabilities of many abnormalities have not been estimated. Reproductive tracts from infertile animals or problem breeders are seldom recovered at slaughter. However,

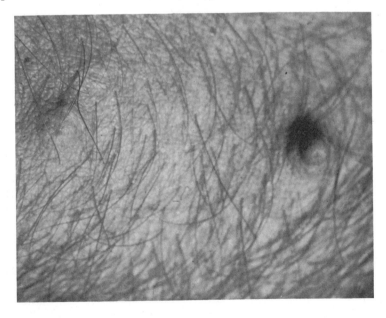

Figure 5. Note blind teat on left.

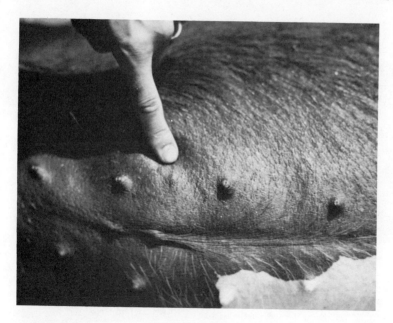

Figure 6. Pin nipple.

in herds having a high incidence of reproductive failures that are not diagnosed by other methods, examination at slaughter is recommended. Females should be tattooed for identification prior to slaughter so that the individual animal's reproductive history can be related to the observed reproductive tract disorder. Normal slaughter procedure is to sever the tract by a cut through the vagina. The abattoir personnel will usually remove the tract intact, if requested. If pathological study is indicated, a heavy string should be tied around the posterior end of the vagina to prevent contamination. The intact tract is then placed into a plastic bag with a numbered card corresponding to the tattoo identification. Specimens should then be packed in ice and transported to the laboratory for study.

For examination, arrange the tract on a tray with the dorsal side up (Fig. 8). Locate and observe each ovary. Some may be surrounded by the infundibulum; others will not. Count and record the number of follicles or corpora lutea. Externally trace each oviduct and uterine horn to the vagina, looking for occlusions, missing parts or adhesions. If pathological study is not indicated, an insemination apparatus may be used to inject fluid into the tract to facilitate detection of occlusions. After gross examination has been completed, open the tract beginning at

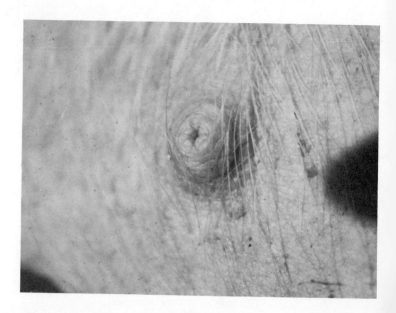

Figure 7. Inverted nipple.

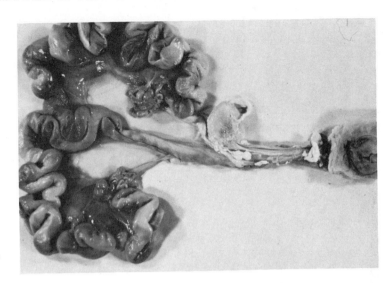

Figure 8. Intact reproductive organs from normal cycling gilt.

the vulva and continue through the cervix and each horn. Examine the uterine endometrium and note the presence and characteristics of any fluid or embryonic tissue.

ANATOMICAL AND HORMONAL ABNORMALITIES

Hydrosalpinx or Pyosalpinx. Hydrosalpinx and pyosalpinx refer to distention of oviducts with clear fluid and purulent material, respectively. These conditions occur more frequently in gilts than in sows and are caused by an occlusion or distention of the oviducts, usually bilaterally, which blocks the passage of spermatozoa and ova. It is thought that these disorders, as well as most other defects, result from abnormal embryonic development and may be hereditary. Females may show irregular or complete absence of estrus.

Blind Uterine Horn. The blind or unattached horn defect occurs unilaterally at a point between the anterior cervix and the posterior horn attachment (Fig. 9). Afflicted females will usually cycle normally. It is possible for pregnancy to occur in the patent side, but litter size is often reduced.

Unilateral Missing Horn. Complete absence or failure of one uterine horn to develop is observed infrequently. Females may cycle normally. Again, pregnancy is possible, but litter size is usually reduced.

Blind, Double or Missing Cervix. These abnormalities occur infrequent-

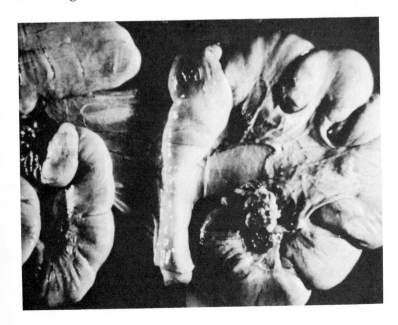

Figure 9. Blind or unattached left uterine horn.

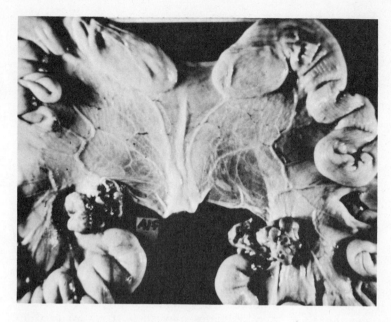

Figure 10. Tract with missing cervix. Normal ovaries indicate gilt cycled regularly.

ly. Females with these conditions cycle normally. If the blind or missing cervix condition exists, pregnancy will not occur because the passageway is missing (Fig. 10). Pregnancy can occasionally be achieved in females with the double cervix condition.

Infantilism. This is a common abnormality and is generally, but not always, associated with confinement-reared gilts (Fig. 11). It can be diagnosed externally by the

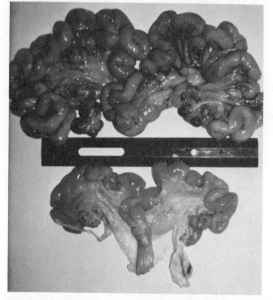

Figure 11. Reproductive tracts from two 8-month-old gilts of same age and from identical management conditions. *Top.* Normally developed tract from gilt that experienced two previous estrous cycles. *Bottom.* Immature tract from noncyclic gilt shown in Figure 1.

presence of a "rosebud" or immature vulva and the absence of estrus. The infantile tract is usually approximately 30 per cent of the size of a tract from a normally cycling gilt. The ovaries are often hypoplastic (butterbean size) and nonfunctional with numerous small follicles and no corpora lutea.

Adhesions. Adhesions have been observed in all areas of the reproductive tract but are more frequent in the oviduct and bursa. They are generally associated with intraperitoneal injections given too soon after birth or with improper injections later in life. Cyclic activity appears to depend upon the severity of the adhesions.

Intersexuality. Intersex pigs occur infrequently but are more predominant in the Yorkshire breed (Fig. 12). They are usually genetic females in which a portion of the reproductive tract has differentiated into its male homologue. A majority are inherited, with the mode of inheritance thought to be autosomal recessive accompanied by modifier genes. Exact classification must be done by combined chromosomal and anatomical study. Some individuals can be distinguished by the presence of an ovotestis, which may be internal or external, whereas others may be distinguished by the presence of a "sky hook" vulva, which contains erectile tissue. Some intersexes show male characteristics such as tusk development and mounting behavior. When possible, a pedigree study of such animals should be made and possible carriers removed from the breeding herd.

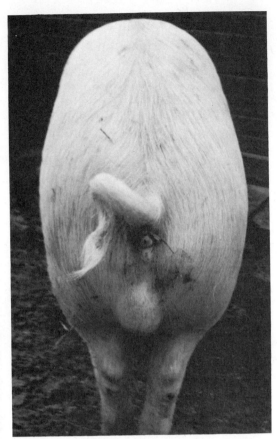

Figure 12. Intersex pig with descended ovotestis and "sky-hooked" vulva.

Cystic Ovaries. Much remains to be learned about cystic ovaries. They are distinguished by the presence of large cystic follicles or corpora lutea (Fig. 13). Sows or gilts with cystic follicles tend to show irregu-lar cycling with heat periods of slightly longer than normal duration. Enlargement of the clitoris has been observed in some cases. The cysts mainly secrete progesterone. They may be caused by partial or complete failure of ovulation or possibly by ingestion of mycotoxins or exogenous steroids. Under practical conditions, diagnosis in the living animal is difficult or impossible. Most attempts at treatment are ineffective.

SUMMARY

Systematic physical examination of the female and female reproductive tract and careful consideration of herd history records are useful when selecting potential breeding animals and when attempting to diagnose reproductive failures. Even though the state of the art is based as much upon practical experience and observations as upon scientifically proved facts, females that are selected on the basis of skeletal soundness, normal external genitalia and sound underlines are likely to be more productive than a randomly selected group.

Clinical examination of the internal reproductive organs recovered from nonbreeders at slaughter is helpful in identifying certain abnormalities and provides information needed for eliminating the genetic lines from which they originate. Methods of examining reproductive tracts in live animals, such as endoscopy, x-ray studies

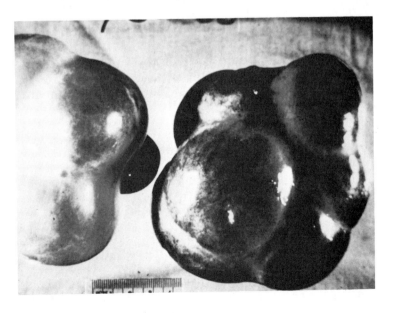

Figure 13. Cystic ovaries.

and laparotomy, are excluded from this discussion since they are still research techniques that have not been adapted to general use in the field.

Treatment of most nonpathogenic reproductive disorders has met with limited success. This is probably fortunate considering the apparent genetic basis for many of the structural and anatomical abnormalities that impair reproductivity. The importance of this discussion is not only in the treatment of such problems but also in creating an awareness of them so that the veterinar-

ian and swine producer can improve upon their ability to select potentially sound, productive females and to detect and cull sterile or problem breeders.

REFERENCES

1. Perry, J. S. and Pomeroy, R. W.: Abnormalities of the reproductive tract of the sow. J. Agri. Sci., *47*:238, 1956.
2. Rasbeck, N. O.: A review of the causes of reproductive failure in swine. Br. Vet. J., *125*:599, 1969.
3. Wrathall, A. E.: An approach to breeding problems in sows. Vet. Rec., *89*:61, 1971.

Evaluation of the Boar for Breeding Soundness

C. D. GIBSON
Michigan State University, East Lansing, Michigan

R. G. JOHNSON
Lake Region Veterinary Center, Elbow Lake, Minnesota

INTRODUCTION

The role of the boar in both swine breeding problems and good breeding programs is extremely important. It has been established that conception rate, pregnancy rate and litter size are all influenced by the boar. In order to perform successfully, a fertile boar must have normal libido and be able to mount the female, protrude the penis and penetrate the vagina and cervix in order to deposit semen. Semen quality has also been shown to be an important factor in high fertility rate and breeding capacity.[4, 5] The examination of the boar for breeding soundness should, therefore, include the assessment of libido and ability to mate and a semen evaluation.

HISTORY

A complete history should include the age and origin of the boar, as well as immunizations and previous disease problems. Information concerning origin also should include data pertaining to exposure to other

animals and premises, time spent in isolation and exposure to the present premises and its breeding animals. The history on boars currently in use should include the number of females serviced, conception rate and litter size.

PHYSICAL AND GENITAL EXAMINATION

The boar should be given a thorough physical examination, including evaluation of conformation and locomotor functions. Any defects should be noted, as they have been shown to greatly influence breeding capacity. The genital examination involves physical examination of genital organs, determination of libido and ability to mate and semen evaluation. All of these parameters must be considered during the course of the examination of the boar.

The testicles should be resilient, symmetrical and large. The libido should be determined by the precopulatory activity of the boar with an estrous female in his pen when the boar is separated from the other boars and females. Problems with libido may be associated with overwork, inexperience or high ambient temperature.[2, 3] The ability to mount the female, penetrate the vagina and lock the penis into the cervix is the next consideration. A physical evaluation of the penis and observation of any penile problems should be noted during the boar's attempts to mount and penetrate the vagina.

Penile problems include hypospadias, injuries and hemorrhage due to lacerations or abrasions, incomplete erection, persistent frenulum and balling of the penis in the diverticulum.[1] The persistent frenulum and balling of the penis, as well as injuries to the penis, can be corrected surgically in most cases. Complete evaluation and surgical correction of problems of the penis can be done under general anesthesia and electroejaculation.

Semen Collection

The next phase of the genital examination is semen collection. The three methods of semen collection are the gloved hand technique, the artificial vagina and electroejaculation. The artificial vagina is an accepted method, but equipment sanitization and cost make this method less practical than the gloved hand technique. Electroejaculation is unsatisfactory because libido and mating behavior cannot be evaluated and only a concentrated part of the sperm-rich fraction is collected. The electroejaculation method can be used in specialized cases in which artificial insemination is desired but semen cannot be obtained by natural mount because of arthritis, age or disease.

The gloved hand method is relatively easy to learn by the inexperienced clinician if a few guidelines are followed. The boar is allowed to mount the estrous female and to attempt several thrusting motions. The mounted boar should be approached quietly from the rear, without touching him and frightening him. The gloved hand should be closed to form a cone with the little finger tightly closed against the palm of the hand. The coned, gloved hand is placed anterior to the penis with the back of the hand against the body wall, and the boar is allowed to thrust into and through the coned hand. The penis is locked into the hand by tightly clasping the last two fingers around the tip and distal penis with the tip of the penis protruded through the closed hand (Fig. 1). One must be careful not to be too aggressive and tightly close the entire hand over the penis, since this will cause pain to the boar and he will dismount.

The inexperienced clinician must take care not to be overanxious and alarm the inexperienced boar by being too aggressive. If the boar is very shy and dismounts when

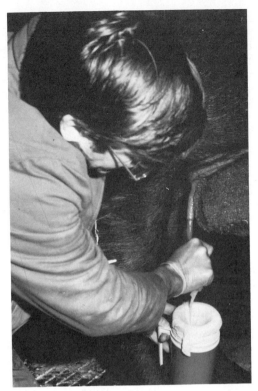

Figure 1. Collection of the boar by the gloved-hand method with a gauze-covered 37° C thermos bottle.

the attempt to grasp the penis is made, allow him to make several false mounts until he is aggressively attempting to lock up again. The occasional shy boar may not allow the penis to be locked into the hand even after several attempts. These shy animals can be collected by hand if the clinician will allow the boar to first enter and lock into the cervix and begin ejaculation. The penis then can be retrieved and locked into the hand at this time, if the retrieval of the penis is done quickly and smoothly in one motion. The shy boar will continue to ejaculate in most cases, and the rest of the ejaculate can be collected. Once the tip of the penis is firmly in the hand and is locked by the pressure of the last two fingers, ejaculation will proceed for 5 to 7 minutes.

A prewarmed thermos (37°C) covered by a double layer of coarse gauze is a convenient, economical collection vessel. The pre-sperm fraction, consisting of 5 to 15 ml of clear fluid, is usually ejaculated first. The gel fraction is expelled at intervals during the course of the entire ejaculation. The gel fraction is filtered out by the gauze because it coagulates the semen into a semisolid mass of gel and spermatozoa and interferes with the evaluation of semen quality. The sperm-rich fraction is a thick creamy color and may be ejaculated all at once or may be interrupted by a second ejaculatory wave of pre-sperm, seminal and prostatic fluid. One should be careful to collect all of the ejaculate possible and to let the boar complete the ejaculation and voluntarily withdraw the penis from the hand, dismounting of his own volition.

Semen Evaluation

In order to obtain a true evaluation of semen quality, several precautions need to be observed on the farm and in the laboratory. Temperature control at 37°C and protection of the semen from osmotic shock by water pH change, disinfectants and sunlight are required. All of the equipment (thermos, gloves, slides, stain, and glassware) should be clean, dry and warm (37°C).

Motility of spermatozoa should be observed microscopically as soon as possible after collection. Dilution of the ejaculate with isotonic saline or buffered 2.9 per cent sodium citrate will eliminate the wave motion phenomenon. Wave motion is due to concentration of sperm cells and will interfere with accurate evaluation of per cent motility and per cent progressive motility. Stained slides of the diluted and undiluted semen should be prepared immediately after semen collection. A 5 per cent nigrosin-eosin stain is available and allows some evaluation of per cent live sperm cells by selectively staining the dead and dying cells and leaving the viable cells unstained against a dark background. Live-dead evaluation is meaningless except under rigid laboratory control; however, this stain is excellent for morphological studies and can be used for this function. Other stains, such as new methylene blue, may be used as effectively as nigrosin-eosin for the morphological evaluation. The semen can then be transported to the laboratory for further evaluation.

Total volume and concentration of the ejaculate should be recorded. Gross determination of concentration can be obtained by observation of color, but the use of red blood cell (RBC) unipettes (1:200 dilution) and a hemocytometer is relatively easy and accurate. Coulter counter and spectrophotometric counting methods are good, if available. Total cells/ejaculate can be calculated by

TABLE 1. *Normal Semen Values*

	Young Boar (8–12 months)	Old Boar (over 12 months)
Volume	100–300 ml	100–500 ml
Concentration	10×10^9 minimum	$10–40 \times 10^9$
Motility	>85%	>85%
Progressive motility	>70%	>70%
Primary abnormalities	<10%	<15%
Secondary abnormalities	<10%	<15%
Free of blood, pus and foreign material	+	+

multiplying the concentration (sperm/ml) by the total gel-free volume.

A minimum of 100 cells should be evaluated, counted and categorized as normal cells or as cells with primary or secondary abnormalities as part of the morphological evaluation.

The primary abnormalities include all head and midpiece defects such as small, enlarged, double or misshapen heads; acrosomal defects; enlarged midpieces; double midpieces; proximal droplets; double tails and tightly coiled tails. Secondary abnormalities are defects that occur after the spermatozoa leave the testicle. These include distal protoplasmic droplets, bent tails and detached heads.[6] Abaxial midpiece attachments are not considered to be abnormal in the boar.

Normal semen values are shown in Table 1.

SUMMARY

The evaluation of a boar for breeding capacity must involve consideration of libido, mating ability and semen quality in order to be accurate. Semen quality is related to collection and handling techniques. Partial collection of the ejaculate caused by premature dismount will affect the total sperm count. The change in holding temperature, time and the presence of foreign material will result in the inaccurate diagnosis of poor spermatozoal motility. The libido and mating ability can be adversely affected by overwork or psychological trauma. Since the duration of the spermatogenic cycle is about 45 days, boars with unsatisfactory semen quality, poor libido or poor mating ability should be immediately separated and culled or reevaluated in 8 weeks.

REFERENCES

1. Adams, W. M.: Hormonal and anatomical causes of infertility in swine. *In* Lucas, L. and Wagner, W. (eds.): Effect of Disease and Stress on Reproduction Efficiency in Swine. University of Nebraska Coop. Ext. Serv., 1970, p. 16.
2. Christenson, R. K.: Effect of temperature on reproduction in the boar. Proceedings of the George A. Young Conference on Advances in Swine Repopulation, Lincoln, Nebraska, 1973, p. 3.
3. Dziuk, P. J.: Effects of isolation and confinement on reproduction in swine. Proceedings American Pork Congress. Des Moines, Iowa, 1971, p. 159.
4. Lehman, A. D. and Rodeffer, H. E.: Boar management. Vet. Rec., *98*:457, 1976.
5. Vente, J. P.: Investigations on boars. Proceedings 7th International Congress Animal Reproduction and AI, 1972, p. 370.
6. Zemjanis, R.: Diagnostic and Therapeutic Techniques in Animal Reproduction. 2nd Ed. Baltimore, The Williams and Wilkins Co., 1970.

Electroejaculation of the Boar

L. E. EVANS
Iowa State University, Ames, Iowa

DEVELOPMENT AND USE

Electroejaculation techniques have been described for use in the conscious[2, 3] and anesthetized boar.[1, 3] The latter method proved to be considerably safer and to provide a better sample for evaluation or insemination. Conscious boars are prone to rectal lacerations and other injuries caused by violent struggling during stimulation.

Electroejaculation may be used for collection of shy, mean, lame or injured boars that cannot be collected manually. Boars that are inexperienced in mating or lack libido and boars for which a suitable mount is unavailable can more readily be collected by electroejaculation.

Prior to anesthesia the boar should be given a physical examination. Skeletal or locomotor defects that might affect fertility should be noted. The general body weight and condition may reflect upon the management and fertility of the boar. Body weight and degree of conditioning will also influence the anesthetic dosage required for handling. Thin boars require relatively more anesthetic for induction, but they recover more quickly. Heavy boars require relatively less anesthetic per pound of body weight for induction, but they often require additional anesthetic, as the drug is redistributed to the fatty tissues.

Chronic pneumonia and porcine stress syndrome are the most common causes of death associated with electroejaculation. Death occurs most frequently during the recovery period. Boars suspected of having these diseases or those that have acute or chronic diseases should not be tested.

ANESTHESIA

With this procedure it is desirable to have an anesthetic agent that provides a rapid induction, good immobilization for 10 to 15 minutes and a short, smooth recovery period. Complete analgesia and muscle relaxation are not required. The ultrashort-acting barbiturates meet these requirements at relatively light dosage levels. They are simple and economical to use.

Thiamylal (Surital) has been used most frequently. The recommended dosage is 4.4 mg/kg up to 180 kg and 2.4 mg/kg thereafter. Maximum dosage should not exceed 8.0 mg/kg. Normally, 1 gm of Surital will give excellent results in a 350-lb (140-kg) boar. Additional doses can be given to prolong anesthesia for repeated collections or short surgical procedures, but the recovery period is usually longer and less smooth.

The marginal ear vein is the preferred route of administration, although careful injection into the anterior vena cava is equally effective. The danger of intra-arterial (carotid artery) or extravascular injections makes the latter route less desirable.

Approximately 75 per cent of the calculated dose is injected rapidly, and after 2 to 3 minutes the remainder is given to effect. A 1-inch, 20-gauge needle or butterfly catheter with an attached needle is affixed to the ear with a large hemostat. Backflow of blood from the needle assures proper insertion. Additional anesthetic can be administered through the subcutaneous abdominal vein. This large vein is located just lateral to the mammary papillae and can be distended by compression against the sternum.

A light plane of anesthesia is desirable. The pupils normally respond to light and may be in mid-dilation. Nystagmus normally does not occur unless deeper levels of anesthesia are reached. The boar should retain a mild-to-moderate response to pain. A relative overdose may cause temporary respiratory arrest, although it is normally of short duration. Artificial respiration by thoracic compression usually shortens this period.

Halothane anesthesia alone or following barbiturate induction works well for electroejaculation. Usually only a face mask is necessary for short periods of anesthesia.

Tranquilizer-sedatives such as xylazine (Rompun) alone or in combination with the dissociative agent ketamine (Vetalar) have been used experimentally for electroejaculation. Another dissociative agent, phencyclidine (Sernylan) has been used with limited success. The primary advantage of these products is the minimum restraint required for intramuscular administration. However, these agents generally have a prolonged recovery period, and electrical stimulation causes arousal and excitement. They are not currently approved for use in swine in the United States.

ELECTROEJACULATORS AND PROBES

Electroejaculators used in the bull are equally effective in the boar. Common models include the Nicholson Transjector, the Standard Precision Electronic and the Pulsator II. They vary in power from 30 to 45 maximum volts and 2 to 8 amp.

The success of electroejaculation is dependent upon the effectiveness of the probe to adequately stimulate the pelvic nerves and organs. The most effective probes are modeled after the old bull and boar probes.[3] These probes are constructed of flexible rubber hose approximately 35 cm long, 3.75 cm in diameter and affixed with 6 annular electrodes[2] (Fig. 1). The normal curvature of the hose approximates the pelvic arch in the boar. Although probes with straight longitudinal electrodes are considered to be better for use in the bull, none have been adequately devised for use in the boar. Use of the smaller straight ram probe has resulted in inconsistent and often unsatisfactory semen samples from the boar.

PREPARATION OF THE BOAR

Immediately after induction of anesthesia, the boar should be prepared for electroejaculation. Excessive fecal material should be removed from the rectum with a gloved finger, the anal ring should be lubricated and the probe inserted past the last ring, or approximately 25 cm.

The fluid contents of the diverticulum should be expelled by external digital pressure, and evidence of masturbation or infection should be noted. The long hairs around the opening of the sheath may be clipped to facilitate handling of the penis.

It is desirable to achieve protrusion of

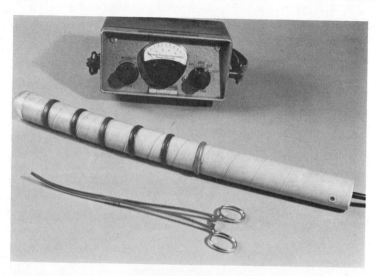

Figure 1. Boar probe and Bozeman uterine dressing forceps.

the penis prior to ejaculation. The penis may be exposed by manual manipulation of the prepuce while the boar is under light electrical stimulation. Pushing the opening of the sheath posteriorly will often exteriorize the penis. The glans penis may be guided toward the opening with the gloved index finger.

An alternative method of exposing the penis is by extraction with an atraumatic forceps. A Bozeman uterine dressing forceps (see Figure 1) is passed through the large portion of the prepuce with the curved end directed ventrally to miss the preputial diverticulum. The tip of the instrument is passed through the small opening leading to the narrow portion of the prepuce where the nonerect penis is located. The forceps is rotated 180° and opened. Once opened, the only unoccupied space within the narrow prepuce is between the jaws of the forceps. If the forceps has been inserted to the level of the glans penis, closure of the instrument engages the penis.

Boars under light anesthesia may resist extraction, but mild electrical stimulation will aid in protrusion of the penis. After protrusion, the penis is grasped with a sterile 4 × 4 gauze dressing and extended gently for examination and collection.

STIMULATION AND COLLECTION

Significant electrical stimulations can commence after a consistent respiratory rate has been established. Patterns of response will vary among individual animals, but older boars often require greater stimulation. Because muscle contractions often interrupt respiration, the stimulations should be spaced to avoid anoxia. Normally a boar is stimulated for 5 to 7 seconds and rested for 5 to 10 seconds or longer if necessary.

Initial stimulations are light, but they cause extension and rigidity of the rear legs. Later, with heavier stimulations, there is extension of the forelegs and some respiratory embarrassment. Each new stimulation should be introduced slowly to avoid muscle or skeletal damage. Boars that are suddenly released from stimulation may roll up on their sternum and become excited. It is generally best to avoid restraint of semiconscious boars. These boars should be further anesthetized or in-troduced and released from each new stimulation in a mild manner.

Ejaculation of clear fluids with or without mucus usually begins after three or four good stimulations. As the amplitude is increased, the sperm-rich fraction is normally seen after five or ten stimulations. This fraction is usually free of mucus and may reach 30 to 80 ml in volume if stimulation is continued. The boar will frequently ejaculate during the resting period or during the introduction to another stimulation.

Ejaculation of clear fractions or poorly concentrated sperm fractions should be followed by increased stimulations until the operator is satisfied that a representative ejaculate has been achieved. Occasionally, questionable boars are re-examined after a 10- to 15-minute rest period.

Failure to achieve proper stimulation may be due to insulation of the probe by fecal material, improper positioning of the probe, use of an inadequate probe or insufficient stimulation. It has been noted that boars may become refractory to electrical stimulation, particularly if the introductory period is prolonged. It has also been noted that excessively strong stimuli applied without an introductory work-up often yield small samples with considerable mucus intermixed.

ADVANTAGES AND DISADVANTAGES

Electroejaculation allows for collection of semen from boars that are unable or unwilling to mate. Sometimes a suitable female is not available, or the boar may lack breeding experience. These boars can be collected at the convenience of the evaluator if electroejaculation is used. The evaluator can more easily examine the penis and prepuce and palpate the testes of anesthetized boars. Samples collected by electroejaculation are often more consistent because they are primarily sperm-rich and are not dependent upon the boar's behavioral or sexual responsiveness.

A major disadvantage of electroejaculation is that the boar's libido and mating ability are not evaluated. The evaluator must rely upon the history obtained from the boar's handler. The possibility of death during anesthesia due to an accident or to individual idiosyncracies is small, but it demands serious consideration when valuable boars are involved. The death of boars with porcine stress syndrome may be to the benefit of the swine industry, but such deaths are often untimely and embarrassing to the evaluator. Owners should always be advised of the possible dangers when a general anesthetic is used.

REFERENCES

1. Adams, W. M., Clark, T. L. and Evans, L. E.: Electroejaculation of the anesthetized boar. Annual Meeting, A.V.M.A., mimeographed notes, 1969.
2. Clark, T. L.: Electroejaculation in the anesthetized and non-anesthetized boar. Proceedings International Pig Veterinary Society Congress, D.14, 1976.
3. Dzuik, P. J., Grahm, E. J., Donker, J. D., Marion, G. B. and Peterson, W. E.: Some observations on collection of semen from bulls, goats, boars and rams by electrical stimulation. Vet. Med., *49*:455, 1954.

Physiology and Pathology of Pregnancy

PHILIP J. DZIUK
University of Illinois, Urbana, Illinois

Following a fertile mating the sow maintains the pregnancy only if several conditions are met. Once the pregnancy has been established, it, in turn, will be interrupted only by a certain combination of circumstances. The apparent failure to conceive or the failure to produce a litter after an apparent conception is often the result of the normal physiology of pregnancy in the sow, perhaps combined with the effects of toxins or pathogens.

MAINTENANCE OF PREGNANCY

Effect of Numbers of Embryos. When only one to four embryos enter the pig uterus, the pregnancy is unlikely to be maintained. The next heat may be delayed a few days, so that the interval between a mating and the next heat will often be 25 to 27 days rather than the normal 21 days. This may occur in gilts that ovulate only a few eggs or that have less than five eggs fertilized as the result of a relatively infertile male.

Stage of Gestation and Intrauterine Migration. The uterus of the pig is bicornuate, with each horn being 1 to 2 m in length. Embryos can migrate freely from one horn to the other through the uterine body and do so in nearly every pregnancy. Embryos remain in the tip of each horn until day 5 or 6 of gestation. By day 7 they are about halfway to the body and reach it by day 8. At day 9 some have migrated to the horn opposite the horn of the origin. By day 12 migration stops. At this time embryos from each side are mixed with those from the other side. When embryos are restricted to the upper tip of the horns at day 4 and are then allowed to migrate again at day 11, migration and pregnancy are normal. When the restriction is not removed until day 12 or 13, migration does not resume and the pregnancy is not maintained. Restriction of intrauterine migration does not interfere with maintenance of pregnancy provided both uterine horns are nearly completely occupied.

Spacing and Distribution. Embryos are usually spaced approximately equidistant from each other in the uterus. When distribution is so uneven that one-third of one uterine horn is not occupied by embryos and placenta, the pregnancy is less likely to continue. When the unoccupied portion is two-thirds the length of one uterine horn, the pregnancy will rarely be maintained, even though there are a sufficient number of embryos in the remainder of the uterus. Gilts with congenital blind uterine segments and other conditions precluding nearly complete occupancy of the uterus will have normal estrous cycles and fertilized eggs but will return to heat regularly and never complete a pregnancy. Absence or surgical removal of a segment does not interfere with pregnancy.

Levels of Progesterone and Intrauterine Crowding. About 30 per cent of fertilized eggs are not represented by living fetuses at day 30. This loss is apparently not due to either an excessive level of progesterone or a deficiency of progesterone. Levels of progesterone associated with normal pregnancy are quite variable and are usually about twice the minimum required to maintain pregnancy. Administration of supplemental progesterone has not consistently influenced the proportion of embryos surviving. Ovariectomy at any stage of gestation will cause abortion in 36 to 48 hours, unless supplemental progesterone is given.

Intrauterine crowding of fetuses due to a very large number of fetuses or a reduction of uterine space is not associated with a reduction in the proportion of embryos surviving before day 30. However, from 30 to 45 days, the amount of space available to each fetus is critical. When the available space is just below optimum, the size of the fetus is reduced, causing a runt. When the space is further reduced, the fetus dies and becomes a mummy or may be completely resorbed. The incidence of runts is greatest for fetuses in the middle segment of each uterine horn, and mummies occur predominantly in the segment near the uterine body.

INTERRUPTION OF PREGNANCY

Removal of Embryos. Flushing the embryos from one uterine horn at day 4 or 10 stops the pregnancy even though live embryos still remain in the other horn. Flushing one horn at day 14 or 16 reduces the proportion of sows maintaining pregnancy. After day 16 there is no effect from flushing or killing the embryos in one horn on the continuation of pregnancy. Fetuses can be crushed in selected segments of the uterus, leaving only one or two fetuses. They will develop normally. At day 30 or later if all fetuses in both horns are killed by crushing them through the uterine wall, the remnants are resorbed but the sow does not return to heat. The corpora lutea are maintained, and the level of progesterone remains the same as in a normal pregnancy for 60 to 80 days. This helps explain often reported clinical signs of sows that were detected as being pregnant but that failed to produce a litter and did not return to heat. Agents that can kill fetuses are viruses, bacterial infections, toxins and materials with hormone-like action.

Estrogens. Estrogenic substances from feed contamination or molds are particularly insidious. The pig is very sensitive to even minute amounts of estrogen taken in over a short period. One injection of estrogen or one or two oral doses given during the early stages of development of the corpora lutea at days 2 to 12 will disrupt the pregnancy and may maintain the corpora lutea for 60 to 90 days. Contrary to what might be expected from an estrogen, the sow will not show heat, the vulva will not swell and a state of pseudopregnancy exists. Exposure to estrogenic materials later in pregnancy may not kill all the embryos but may cause a reduced litter size and an increased incidence of mummies and stillbirths. Following continuous treatment with estrogen, the contractibility of the uterus increases to the extent that fetuses are compressed, deforming the fetus. The front legs are embedded in the chest, the tongue protrudes and the fetus becomes spindleshaped, tapering sharply at each end.

PARTURITION

Initiation. The fetus apparently exerts a great deal of influence on the length of gestation. Decapitation or hypophysectomy of fetuses is associated with a very extended gestation; thus, the fetal head or pituitary effects initiation of parturition. Luteolytic materials such as prostaglandins will induce parturition when given near term. There is a slight negative relationship between litter size and length of gestation; thus, large litters are born somewhat earlier. There seems to be no local fetal-uterine-ovarian relationship on initiation of parturition. When ovaries are transplanted to the body wall or are otherwise functional but disconnected from the pregnant uterine horn, the length of gestation and the process of parturition are normal.

Anteroposterior Orientation and Order of Birth. Fetuses are presented from each uterine horn more or less at random. After birth of the first piglet, which may come from either the left or right horn, the chances are about 50:50 that the next pig will come from the same horn or the opposite one. The first portion of the litter is presented about equally in the anterior and posterior orientations. The last portion of the litter is presented primarily anteriorly. The incidence of stillbirth is greatest in the last three piglets born. A piglet is also more likely to be stillborn when there is a long time period between its birth and the birth of the preceding piglet.

REFERENCES

1. Dhindsa, D. S. and Dziuk, P. J.: Influence of varying the proportion of uterus occupied by embryos on maintenance of pregnancy in the pig. J. Anim. Sci., 27:668, 1968.
2. Polge, C. and Dziuk, P. J.: Time of cessation of intra-uterine migration of pig embryos. J. Anim. Sci., 31:565, 1970.
3. Reimers, T. J., Dziuk, P. J., Bahr, J., Sprecher, D. J., Webel, S. K. and Harmon, B. G.: Transuterine embryonal migration in sheep, anteroposterior orientation of pig and sheep fetuses and presentation of piglets at birth. J. Anim. Sci., 37:1212, 1973.
4. Webel, S. K., Reimers, T. J. and Dziuk, P. J.: The lack of relationship between plasma progesterone levels and number of embryos and their survival in the pig. Biol. Reprod., 13:177, 1975.

Locomotor Dysfunction Causing Reproductive Failure

RICHARD H. C. PENNY
University of London, London, England

INTRODUCTION

Lameness as a cause of reproductive failure in swine is not well documented in the literature. Yet few practicing veterinarians would disagree that under intensive systems of husbandry and management, lameness, of known or unknown etiology, is a common occurrence and is increasing in frequency.

Unfortunately, many lameness problems have not been well identified or quantified, and more research is obviously needed in this area. Also, in the polytocous species, reproduction is frequently not an "all or nothing" phenomenon, so lameness may contribute to problems associated with reduced litter size.

In breeding herds, a high culling rate for lameness, in either the breeding stock or stock reared for sale, can lower the projected output and thus jeopardize the economic viability of the herd. Lameness may also contribute to the problem of high preweaning mortality.

REASONS FOR CULLING SOWS AND GILTS

The literature regarding culling is not extensive. Table 1 shows some figures pertaining to culling breeding females, but increasing trends toward greater and greater intensification can markedly alter the disease picture.[1, 4, 9] It must also be remembered that mean figures do not indicate the severity of the problem on individual farms, and culling rates of breeding females for lameness as high as 18 per cent have been reported.

REASONS FOR CULLING BOARS

In the United Kingdom there is little information on the effective working life of the boar, although a mean (varying with the breed) of 12 to 18 months is suggested. A figure for Denmark of 447 days for natural mating and 319 days for artificial insemination (AI) is quoted.[11] In AI centers in the United Kingdom, locomotor upsets were the most common single reason for disposal of boars (Table 2); of 69 boars culled, 15 (21.7 per cent) were culled for lameness. Lameness could have contributed to other problems as well, e.g., poor service behavior.[7]

In the United States, lameness was listed as one of the four common causes of reproductive inefficiency in boars,[5] and "sick or lame soon after purchase" was the reason for 21.2 per cent of replacement boars according to the records of one large boar-breeding company.[8] Lameness of one form or another could have, and in some cases actually did, contribute to some of the other reasons for replacement (Table 3).

SPECIFIC DISORDERS OF LOCOMOTER DYSFUNCTION

"Leg Weakness"

Although this is a fairly well-documented clinical entity in rapidly growing pigs up to 100 kg of body weight, the exact etiology has

TABLE 1. *Reasons for Culling Breeding Females*

Cause	Anonymous (1964) (%)	United Kingdom Jones (1967) (%)	Australia Penny (1972) (%)
Poor milk supply and udder troubles	10.9	5.6	10.5
Lameness and paralysis	10.7	33.7	20.4
Failure to breed	21.8	32.3	25.0
Small litter size at birth	15.1	–	11.1
Poor weight gain to 8 weeks	5.4	–	–
Poor mothering ability	1.8	–	11.6
Prolapse of vagina/cervix/rectum	–	8.9*	7.1
Thin sows	–	–	3.1
Old age	6.0	8.1	–
Injuries and accidents	6.4	–	–
Miscellaneous causes	21.9	10.4	11.2
No. of sows culled	3306	124	352
Culling rate-breeding female %/year	33	27	20
Culling rate for lameness %/year	3.2	9.2	2.1

*Rectum only.

not been determined. However, it seems likely that a complex combination of factors is involved and that the various bone and joint lesions that have been reported[12] could well be an effect rather than a cause of "leg weakness."[3, 15]

In general the condition is most troublesome on farms and testing stations selecting for rapid rate of gain and good feed efficiency and on establishments where management, environment and hygiene are of a high order. Other precipitating factors are feeding *ad libitum,* restricting exercise and housing on concrete. Although some signs may be seen at an earlier age, the main features of abnormal angulation of the limb joints and a faulty leg action most commonly develop in animals between 35 and 80 kg of body weight. The forelimbs may be excessively straight, and adduction of the fore-

limbs at the carpus ("knock-knee" or "X legs"), hyperflexion at the carpus ("over at the knee") hyperextension of the phalanges or lateral angulation of the foot with marked separation of the toes may occur. In the hind limbs "sickle-hock" and hyperextension of the phalanges may be seen, and pigs are termed "down on their hocks."

Locomotor dysfunction is usually more severe in the hind limbs, and pigs may walk with a swaying action of the hindquarters or with a "paddling" gait. If pushed or when turning, they may collapse on their hind legs. Pigs may stand with an arched back with all four legs bunched together under the body, and they may show a stiff, stilted action of the front legs.

Treatment is of little value, although the following short-term measures have been recommended: restrict feed, provide exer-

TABLE 2. *Reasons for Culling Boars from AI Centers in the United Kingdom**

Cause	Breed			
	LARGE WHITE	LANDRACE	OTHER	TOTAL
Low fertility	1	3	1	5
Poor service behavior	3	8	–	11
Poor semen quality	7	2	–	9
Disease or injury	7	–	1	8
Locomotor upset	9	5	1	15
Old age	5	–	–	5
Small litter size	–	1	–	1
Unsatisfactory progeny test result	3	–	–	3
Hereditary defects in progeny	1	1	–	2
Miscellaneous	7	3	–	10
Total	43	23	3	69
Boars at risk	79	38	5	122

*Adapted from Melrose, D. R.: Vet. Rec., *78*:159, 1966.

TABLE 3. *Reasons for Replacement of Boars by a Breeding Company in the United States (Jan. 1970 to Dec. 1975)**

Cause	% Replacements
Mechanical difficulties or physical deformity preventing breeding	14.3
Breed but sows do not settle	9.1
Bleed from prepuce	6.0
Sick or lame soon after purchase	21.2
Boar will not try to breed	18.0
Physical defects: crooked legs, deformed feet, poor conformation	2.8
Boar too small or too large	2.5
Defective offspring, small litters	3.6
Slow or poor breeders	6.4
Other	16.2†

*Adapted from Nelson, D. A.: Proc. IPVS Congress, Ames, Iowa, D13, 1976.

†8.2 per cent of replacement boars died.

cise, take care when transporting and first using young breeding stock, avoid slippery floors or abrasive concrete, give adequate hoof care and provide a well-balanced diet containing sufficient vitamins and minerals.[3]

Although there is controversy about the heritability of some conformational characteristics of the feet and legs, careful selection for desirable traits is considered worthwhile.[3] Excessive development of the hams, stifle joints very wide apart and a narrow-waisted lumbar region seem undesirable characteristics. Long-term measures include an adequate genetic pool from which to select, selection for pigs that can withstand a high level of feeding and little or no exercise and selection for "good moving" pigs. Attempts should be made to define the most desirable conformational characteristics, and the breeding lives of pigs with the strongest constitutions should be extended whenever possible.[3]

Foot Rot

With the continuing trend toward more intensive systems of pig husbandry in confinement, foot lameness is being recognized as an increasing problem in many countries. Although infection may play an important part, it has been demonstrated that the primary erosive white-line and false sand-crack lesions, as well as bruising, can all be produced by housing pigs on floors of solid concrete or on concrete or aluminum slats. New so-called "green" concrete may be especially dangerous.[10, 16]

Breeding stock can be badly affected by both primary and secondary lesions, and foot problems can be a major reason for culling.[10] Infection may gain entrance to the hoof and the soft structures within, or the pedal bone or corono-pedal joint may become involved ("bush-foot"). Pus will then break out at the coronary band. Infection may also gain entrance to the tendon sheaths and so spread up the leg.

Antibiotic injections may help to resolve cases of bush-foot, but these are not specific and their main value may be to prevent pyemia. Topical applications of caustic agents in solution, such as 10 per cent formaldehyde or 5 per cent copper sulfate, are more satisfactory. Surgical removal of an infected claw can be tried, but the result is rarely an improvement on topical treatment and often is uneconomic.

A shallow foot-bath (containing 2 inches of formalin or 5 per cent copper sulfate solution and placed in some form of raceway or passageway), regularly used by the sows, is the best form of prevention. It should be used as frequently as possible, weekly preferably, but pigs with hyperkeratinization of the heel should not be treated unless the "corn" has been removed first.

Extra bedding, well-finished concrete and good pencil-edged slats may all help to control the condition, and turning affected pigs onto a "dirt" lot may resolve the problem temporarily. Although hereditary factors have not been conclusively proved, some sows seem better able to withstand confinement housing than others, so selection for good feet should be practiced. A variation in the calcium content of the hoof-horn among breeds has been demonstrated; colored horn contains more calcium than colorless horn, so breed susceptibility must be considered. Uneven claw size, particularly a smaller inside hind claw, is considered a hereditary characteristic and is thought to precipitate lameness. It should therefore be selected against.

Damage to Feet and Legs from Slatted Floors

Incorrectly designed and badly manufactured concrete slats and metal (punched, expanded or weldmesh) floors can cause injury to breeding stock housed in stalls or on tethers. Severe foot and leg injuries can be produced, and posterior paralysis and a high culling rate can result — up to 45 per cent in the extreme situation.[6, 14]

Major factors are sharp edges to the slats, particularly panel slats, due to poor casting and subsequent chipping in transport and installation or as a result of wear. Too wide a gap (more than 1 inch) and too narrow a slat (3 inches or less) are other possible undesirable characteristics. Narrow slats with too wide a gap or slot seem to give the pig a feeling of insecurity or instability, and an excessive proportion of edge to slat increases the trauma. Wider slats seem to "clean" fairly readily, provided the slope of the slat side is adequate, and pencil-edged triangular slats are under investigation as one way of insuring this.[2] Panel slats are, in general, unsatisfactory, and a pencil-edged slat is preferable.

A very high culling rate for lameness and paralysis may sometimes be seen in gilts that are tethered or stalled during pregnancy. A diagnosis cannot always be made, but loose housing the gilts, particularly if done early, may resolve the problem. Some authorities believe that gilts should not be stalled or tethered.

Fully slatted floors for piglets, at least during the first week of life, can cause damage unless covered with some material such as indoor/outdoor carpet, and expanded metal floors have also been incriminated if the mesh is too large or the metal badly finished. Severe foot injury, loss of supernumerary digits and tenosynovitis can lead to poor growth rate and a high mortality.[13]

Osteomalacia

Although rickets is an uncommon condition of pigs in the United Kingdom, osteomalacia producing a "downer" sow syndrome may be on the increase. Osteomalacia occurs in sows in mid to late lactation or when they are put to the boar. The main symptom is lameness and/or posterior paralysis, and the apparent paralysis may be the result of spontaneous fracture of the femur or vertebrae of the lumbosacral region.

The condition is not well understood, but a deficiency of calcium in the diet might be the most likely cause.

REFERENCES

1. Anonymous: PIDA sow wastage survey. London, PIDA, 1964.
2. Baxter, S. H. and Anderson, A. W. F.: A new reinforced concrete slat system for pig housing. Fm. Bldg. Prog., *46*:19, 1976.
3. Grondalen, T.: Osteochondrosis, arthrosis and leg weakness in pigs. Nord. Vet. Med., 26:534, 1974.
4. Jones, J. E. T.: The investigation of the causes of mortality and morbidity in sows in a commercial herd. Br. Vet. J., *123*:327, 1967.
5. Leman, A. D. and Dodeffer, H. E.: Boar management. Vet. Rec., 98:457, 1976.
6. Lunney, D. C. and Baxter, S. H.: Concrete slats in tethered sow stalls. Fm. Bldg. Prog., *36*:19, 1974.
7. Melrose, D. R.: A review of progress and of possible developments in artificial insemination of pigs. Vet. Rec., 78:159, 1966.
8. Nelson, D. A.: Boar management for the veterinarian. Proc. IPVS Congress, Ames, Iowa, D13, 1976.
9. Penny, R. H. C.: Some current thoughts on lameness in the pig. *In* Grunsell, C. S. G. and Hill, F. W. G. (eds.): Veterinary Annual. Bristol, Wright, 1972, p. 31.
10. Penny, R. H. C., Osborne, A. D., Wright, A. I. and Stephens, T. K.: Foot-rot in pigs: observations on the clinical disease. Vet. Rec., 77:1101, 1965.
11. Rasbech, N. O.: A review of the causes of reproductive failure in swine. Br. Vet. J., *125*:599, 1969.
12. Reiland, S.: Osteochondrosis in the pig. Thesis, Stockholm, Sweden, 1975.
13. Smith, W. J. and Mitchell, C. D.: Floor surface treatment to prevent lameness in suckling piglets. Fm. Bldg. Prog., *43*:17, 1976.
14. Smith, W. J. and Robertson, A. M.: Observation on injuries to sows confined in part-slatted stalls. Vet. Rec., 89:531, 1971.
15. Vaughn, L. C.: Leg weakness in pigs. Vet. Rec., 89:81, 1971.
16. Wright, A. I., Osborne, A. D., Penny, R. H. C. and Gray, E.: Foot-rot in pigs: experimental production of the disease. Vet. Rec., *90*:93, 1972.

Swine Leptospirosis

LYLE E. HANSON

University of Illinois, Champaign, Illinois

Leptospirosis is recognized primarily as a reproductive disease in swine, as the mild acute signs usually go unrecognized. The disease was first associated with swine because of its relationship to a disease in man called swine herders' disease.[6]

Leptospirosis in swine, as in other animals, is a disease caused by a number of serotypes. In the United States, four pathogenic serotypes, *Leptospira canicola, L. grippotyphosa, L. icterohaemorrhagiae* and *L. pomona,* have been isolated from swine.[7] Two other serotypes, *L. tarassovi* and *L. sejroe,* which have caused disease problems in swine in other countries, have been isolated from wildlife, but not from swine, in the United States.[1] Leptospires are motile, spiral, filamentous organisms with hooks at each end that require special techniques for visualization and cultivation. Live motile organisms can be observed with darkfield microscopy and dead organisms by special staining techniques. Leptospires can be cultivated at 30°C in special media that contain either serum or albumin.

EPIDEMIOLOGY

Leptospires are released primarily in the urine of infected domestic animals and wildlife. Swine, dogs and many forms of wildlife may be carriers for a year or more. Some serotypes, such as *L. pomona*, are usually transmitted directly between domestic animals but are also carried by wildlife. In contrast, *L. grippotyphosa* is primarily an infection of wildlife, with occasional transmission to swine, cattle, dogs and man. Swine usually become infected by leptospires entering through breaks in the skin when the pigs are in contact with contaminated surface water. The leptospires can survive for weeks in neutral surface water.

Venereal transmission also occurs, although it is not a common mode. Leptospires may be present in the semen during the acute stage, or the semen may be contaminated with infected urine during the chronic stage.

Food chain transmission is another mode of spread in swine, as ingestion of infected rats is a likely source of leptospires of the *L. icterohaemorrhagiae* serotype.

PATHOGENESIS

Leptospires enter either through abrasions in the skin of legs or body during contact with contaminated surface waters or through the mucous membranes of the eye or the gastrointestinal tract. The primary site of multiplication is in the visceral tissues, especially of the liver, spleen and kidneys. Bacteremias are usually detectable late in the incubation period and during the period of acute signs, most commonly 5 to 10 days following the initial infection. Both leptospiruria and agglutinating antibodies are usually detectable following the appearance of acute signs and persist from a few weeks to as long as 12 months. Shedding of leptospires in the urine may be constant or intermittent, without evidence of disease.

The acute signs, which vary from moderate elevation of body temperature to more evident signs that include hemoglobinuria, icterus and malaise, appear to be caused by toxin associated with the presence of leptospires.[2] Also, the acute lesions in the liver, spleen, lungs and kidneys are compatible with toxic reactions.

Chronic lesions become more extensive as the disease persists.[9] The lesions caused by cellular infiltration and proliferation of fibroblasts are compatible with an immunological reaction to the disease.

SIGNS

As previously mentioned, leptospirosis in swine is primarily recognized as a reproductive disease. Although acute signs occur, they are usually limited to a moderate elevation of temperature and inappetence lasting about 24 hours. In pregnant swine, leptospires migrate through placental tissue and infect the fetus during the acute phase of the disease. However, the abortion or stillbirths occur 1 to 3 weeks later.[3] Infections initiated late in the gestation period may cause delivery of weak pigs without stillbirths, although usually both stillbirths and weak pigs result from late-term infections.

Stillborn or weak pigs often appear anemic or icteric. Some live infected pigs, often weak at birth, may die during the first week, while others grow slowly and some develop normally, although infected with leptospires.

The most consistent lesions in porcine leptospirosis involve the liver and kidneys and vary from mild to severe, depending upon the duration of the infection. In the acute stage, hemorrhage in the renal cortex is the primary gross lesion, although more extensive changes of tubular necrosis and casts are often visible only on microscopic examinations.[2] Hemorrhages and white infarcts are both evident during the subacute stages of the disease. Interstitial nephritis, characterized by cellular infiltration of lymphocytes, plasma cells and fibroblasts and development of tubular casts, varies from mild in subacute cases to extensive in chronic disease. Tubular degeneration may be extensive in certain severe, acute and chronic infections. Glomerular changes vary from hemorrhage and edema early in the disease to a thickening of the Bowman's capsules and atrophy in the chronic stages. In swine that have persistent infections lasting from 6 to 12 months, the kidney lesions may become extensive, reducing the function of major portions of the kidney.[9]

The placental and uterine tissues from an aborted sow, although edematous, seldom contain major tissue changes. Leptospires often can be demonstrated in these tissues, although only minor changes are associated with their presence.

The tissues of aborted pigs are often edematous and icteric, and the body fluids are usually hemorrhagic. Kidney lesions may be present in the piglets but are not consistently evident.

The first recognition of leptospirosis in a swine herd is usually based upon the occurrence of abortions and stillbirths. A definitive diagnosis is dependent upon either serological or cultural confirmation. Serological tests consist of either a microscopic or plate agglutination test utilizing prevalent serotypes. Aborting sows usually have positive test results at the time of the abortion or within a few days of it. Serological testing of 10 per cent of the sows is recommended for a reliable herd evaluation. As the fetus is immunologically competent as early as 101 days, the fetal blood should be tested when available, as the demonstration of antibodies can be related to an infection.[4]

Leptospiral isolations can often be made either from the urine of adult swine or from stillborn or aborted swine fetuses. Isolations can be accomplished by inoculation of weanling hamsters or by direct culturing of the infected tissues or fluids, when free of contaminants, in special leptospiral liquid or semisolid media. The most widely used media are Stuart's, Fletcher's or bovine albumin polysorbate 80 solutions.[10] Although direct darkfield examination of urine or fetal fluids may give presumptive evidence of leptospirosis, a positive diagnosis should not be reported unless characteristic motility is observed.

CONTROL AND TREATMENT

The management on each farm should be evaluated so that all effective preventive measures can be instituted. As surface waters provide the most common means of transmission, susceptible swine should be fenced away from ponds, marshes and streams with which other livestock have contact. All new additions to herds should be demonstrated to have negative test results for the leptospiral sertoypes prior to their introduction into a herd. Rodent control should be a constant part of the swine management program.

Periodic testing of the sera of 10 per cent of the swine herds provides an ongoing evaluation of the leptospiral status of the herds. Initial infections ocurring during early gestation periods often go undetected unless serological tests are conducted.

Antibiotic therapy has been the most effective treatment for swine with acute leptospirosis. Dihydrostreptomycin at 25 mg/kg of body weight has been the most effective antibiotic in the treatment of both acute and chronic leptospirosis.[11] Dihydrostreptomycin accumulates in effective concentrations in the kidney and uterine tissues for longer periods than the other antibiotics. Although chlortetracycline and oxytetracycline have reduced the severity of acute signs and losses, they have been less effective than dihydrostreptomycin. However, precaution should be used in treating newborn pigs during an outbreak, as dihydrostreptomycin may cause respiratory depression, thereby reducing the pigs' ability to nurse. Antibiotics can be administered simultaneously with leptospiral bacterins, as they do not interfere with the antigenic stimulation of inactivated bacterins.

Oral administration of 200 gm/ton of feed of oxytetracycline or chlortetracycline has been an effective prophylactic procedure.[5] However, it must be recognized that the antibiotics are only effective during the period of administration.

Vaccination of breeding swine at 6-month intervals or of feeders at weaning time with appropriate leptospiral bacterins provides the most economical approach for most management situations.[7] As all pathogenic serotypes involving swine can also occur in wildlife, the maintenance of closed herds will not prevent the introduction of leptospirosis. Leptospiral bacterins are available for all the pathogenic serotypes (*L. canicola, L. grippotyphosa, L. icterohaemorrhagiae* and *L. pomona*) isolated from swine in the United States. As leptospirosis causes the greatest losses in pregnant swine during the third trimester, bacterins should be administered prior to or shortly after breeding or during the first trimester. For outbreaks occurring in continuous farrowing operations, vaccine can be administered along with streptomycin at 25 mg/kg to all sows. The antibiotic will control the new infections and protect the pigs until the bacterins have time to stimulate protective antibodies.

PUBLIC HEALTH ASPECTS

All leptospiral serotypes that are pathogenic to domestic animals are capable of producing disease in man. Precautions should be taken to protect the conjunctiva and skin from contact with urine or urine contaminated water. Leptospires may be shed in the urine of swine up to 1 year following the initial infection. Aborted fetuses and their membranes often contain leptospires; therefore, proper precautions should be followed in handling the tissues. The swine owners should be alerted to the public health dangers when the disease has been diagnosed in the herd.

REFERENCES

1. Alexander, A. D., Yager, R. H. and Keefe, T. J.: Leptospirosis in Swine. Bull. Off. Int. Epizoot., *61*:273, 1964.
2. Burnstein, T. and Baker, J. A.: Leptospirosis in swine caused by *Leptospira pomona*. J. Infect. Dis., *94*:53, 1954.
3. Fennestad, K. L. and Borg-Peterson, C.: Experimental leptospirosis in pregnant sows. J. Infect. Dis., *116*:57, 1966.
4. Fennestad, K. L., Borg-Peterson, C. and Bummerstadt, E.: Leptospira antibody formation by porcine foetuses. Res. Vet. Sci., *9*:378, 1969.
5. Ferguson, L. E., Lococo, S., Smith, H. R. and Hamdy, A. H.: The control and treatment of swine leptospirosis during a naturally occurring outbreak. J.A.V.M.A., *129*:263, 1956.
6. Gsell, O. R.: Etiologie der Schweinhuterkrankheit. Bull. Schweiz. Akad. Med. Wiss. *1*:67, 1944.
7. Hanson, L. E. and Ferguson, L. C.: Leptospirosis. *In* Dunne, H. W. and Leman, A. D. (eds.): Diseases of Swine. Ames, Iowa, The Iowa State University Press, 1975.
8. Langham, R. F., Morse, E. V. and Morter, R. L.: Experimental leptospirosis. V. Pathology of *Leptospira pomona* infection in swine. Am. J. Vet. Res., *19*:395, 1958.
9. Morter, R. L., Morse, E. V. and Langham, R. F.: Experimental leptospirosis. VII. Re-exposure of pregnant sows with *Leptospira pomona*. Am. J. Vet. Res., *21*:95, 1960.
10. Shotts, E. B.: Laboratory diagnosis of leptospirosis: *In* Johnson, R. C. (ed.) The Biology of Parasitic Spirochetes. New York, Academic Press, 1976.
11. Stalheim, O. H. V.: Chemotherapy of renal leptospirosis in swine. Am. J. Vet. Res., *28*:161, 1967.

Viral Reproductive Failure

WILLIAM L. MENGELING
National Animal Disease Center, Ames, Iowa

Virus-induced reproductive failure of swine can be broadly categorized into two clinical syndromes that are based on the presence or absence of maternal illness.

In syndrome I, reproductive failure is the result of a fatal infection of the embryo or fetus, and the dam remains clinically normal. Infection may occur by way of the genital tract, as with virus-containing semen, or transplacentally. The latter route is probably more common. Abortion is uncommon, and the usual sequela of prenatal death is resorption (embryo) or mummification (fetus). Fetuses are more likely to succumb if infection occurs early in gestation. Porcine parvovirus (PPV), porcine enteroviruses (PEV), Japanese B encephalitis virus (JEV) and, under certain circumstances, hog cholera virus (HCV) and pseudorabies virus (PRV) are associated with this syndrome. Since infection of the dam is subclinical, reproductive failure may go unsuspected until long after the death of the prenatal pig. Viruses other than PPV are rapidly inactivated during fetal mummification, thus often precluding an etiological diagnosis.

In syndrome II, reproductive failure is the result of maternal illness, with or without transplacental infection of the prenatal pig. Abortion is common, especially if disease occurs late in gestation. PRV, HCV and swine influenza virus (SIV) are associated with this syndrome. If transplacental infection has occurred, the virus may be isolated from aborted fetuses and neonatal pigs, as well as from affected dams.

TYPES OF VIRUS

Porcine Parvovirus

Porcine parvovirus is distributed worldwide, and the incidence of infection approaches 100 per cent among older breeding stock in areas of intensive swine production. Swine are the only known host, and the virus is maintained by subclinically infected swine carriers. The virus is also extremely resistant to inactivation. A single viral serotype has been recognized. The finding of PPV in boar semen suggests that in some cases apparent maternal infertility is due to infection with PPV at the time of copulation. On the other hand, there is no evidence that infection affects the fertility of the boar. Most cases of PPV-induced reproductive failure are caused by transplacental infection of the fetuses during approximately the first half of gestation. Within a few days after maternal exposure, virus and viral antigen are found in many maternal tissues and a viremia can usually be demonstrated. Despite extensive viral replication, the dam usually is clinically unaffected, although a mild fever and leukopenia may develop. Early in gestation the immunologically incompetent embryos or fetuses succumb to infection, whereas later, fetuses survive, at least in part resulting from the production of antibody and the consequent suppression of viral replication. Nevertheless, the virus may persist, replicate at a low level and be further disseminated at the time of parturition. No developmental anomalies of the fetus have been reported.

Virus can frequently be isolated from affected fetuses even if the fetus has mummified. However, direct examination of fetal tissues by immunofluorescent microscopy is the diagnostic method of choice, since viral antigen persists after virus inactivation. The virus produces cytopathic changes in cell culture, but several serial passages in mitotically active cells are often necessary before such changes are easily detected.

Although a vaccine is not presently available, the recognition of a single serotype indicates that vaccine development is feasible.

Porcine Enteroviruses

Porcine enteroviruses are distributed worldwide. The incidence of infection is known to be high; however, comprehensive serological surveys are difficult to perform because at least nine serotypes exist. Swine are the only known host, and the virus is maintained by subclinically affected swine carriers. Porcine enteroviruses have been isolated from boar semen and may be the cause of apparent maternal infertility when introduced into the female genital tract at the time of copulation. Moreover, infection of the boar has been shown to adversely affect semen quality. The pathogenetic mechanism for enterovirus-induced reproductive failure is similar to that of PPV. Although developmental anomalies have been reported, they are not a cardinal feature of the disease. Occasionally PEV can be isolated at term from tissues of affected pigs. The virus produces cytopathic changes in cell culture, and such changes are often obvious on initial inoculation of suspect material. Since four of the nine serotypes of PEV have already been incriminated in reproductive failure, an effective vaccine would have to be multivalent. A vaccine is not currently available.

Japanese B Encephalitis Virus

Japanese B encephalitis virus has been identified in numerous Asian countries. In the United States a few cases of encephalitis due to JEV have been recognized in persons who have returned from Asia. However, the virus has not become established in the United States. Subclinical epizootics occur among swine and other animal species, sometimes coincidentally with clinical epidemics of encephalitis in man and horses. A single serotype has been described. The virus is maintained by subclinical infections and is transmitted by mosquitoes. In temperate climates the virus overwinters in the mosquito. Infection has not been reported to affect the boar or to be directly transmitted by the boar.

The pathogenetic mechanism of JEV-induced reproductive failure is similar to that of PPV and PEV except that fetal developmental anomalies, e.g., hydrocephalus, are a common feature of the disease. Moreover, JEV clinically affects fetuses later in gestation than either PPV or PEV. The sequelae of late infection are stillborn pigs and weak pigs that die shortly after birth with lesions of nonsuppurative encephalitis. A tentative clinical diagnosis can be confirmed by virus isolation in mice (which develop encephalitis) or in cell culture.

Prevention can be accomplished by vaccination of breeding stock with modified live virus before gestation, by keeping stock away from the mosquito vector or by breeding so that gestation occurs during vector-free seasons.

Pseudorabies Virus

Pseudorabies virus is distributed worldwide, and the associated disease has been a serious clinical problem in swine in Europe, particularly Central Europe. Until the recent marked increase in the incidence of clinical disease in swine in the Midwest, however, few cases were reported in the United States outside of Indiana. In swine, infection is usually subclinical, with an overall incidence of infection estimated at less than 0.5 per cent. By contrast, fatal disease is the usual sequela of infection in other animals such as cattle, sheep, dogs and cats. The virus is maintained by subclinically infected swine carriers. Other reservoirs of infection have not been reported; however, feral animals, as well as dogs and cats, have been suspected of being disseminators of the virus from herd to herd. There is a single virus serotype.

The pathogenetic mechanism of PRV-induced reproductive failure has not been fully elucidated, but severe maternal disease and failure to isolate virus from affected fetuses suggest that transplacental infection is not a prerequisite for fetal death and abortion. On the other hand, transplacental infection has been reported. Histories of some naturally occurring cases indicate that reproductive failure also can occur as a result of transplacental infection in the absence of obvious maternal illness. Developmental fetal anomalies are not a feature of the disease.

A tentative clinical diagnosis can be confirmed by virus isolation from clinically affected dams. Isolation of PRV from affected fetuses or stillborn pigs is often unsuccessful, however, either because of the absence of transplacental infection or, in other cases, because of inactivation of virus after fetal death. Pseudorabies virus produces marked cytopathic changes in many kinds of cell cultures.

Prevention requires either isolation of susceptible stock during gestation or vaccination. Vaccines are available and are used extensively in some areas, but do not appear to contribute much to elimination of PRV. The present consensus in the United States is that all additions to a breeding herd should be free of antibody for PRV. The reason is that the presence of antibody indicates past exposure to PRV and the possibility that the animal is an immune carrier of the virus.

Swine Influenza Virus

Swine influenza virus has been reported in many countries of the world but seems to be more prevalent in the United States than elsewhere. In an extensive serological survey recently completed in the United States, approximately 20 per cent of swine serums, most from 6- to 8-month-old swine, contained antibody for the virus. Only one viral serotype is recognized, but minor antigenic differences exist. In addition to swine, SIV may sometimes infect man, and there has been much speculation as to the source of the virus causing the human influenza pandemic of 1918 and the more recent infection of man with a "swine-like" virus in New Jersey.

The role of SIV in swine reproductive failure is controversial and is based primarily on unconfirmed field observations and a few laboratory experiments. Consequently, the pathogenetic mechanism of putative SIV-induced reproductive failure is unclear but may be related to disturbed fetal nutrition during maternal respiratory illness. Transplacental infection has been reported. A tentative clinical diagnosis can be confirmed by isolation of virus from affected dams and perhaps from fetuses, if transplacental infection has occurred. The virus can be isolated

TABLE 1. *Selected Features of Porcine Reproductive Failures Associated with Viral Infection*

Feature	Porcine Parvovirus	Porcine Enterovirus	Japanese Encephalitis B Virus	Pseudorabies Virus	Hog Cholera Virus	Swine Influenza Virus
Transmission by copulation	Yes, but may not be most important means	Yes, but may not be most important means	No	Possible, but unlikely	Possible, but unlikely	No
Illness of dam	Subclinical to mild	Subclinical to mild	Subclinical to mild	Mild to severe	Subclinical to severe	Mild to severe
Maternal viremia and transplacental infection necessary for reproductive failure	Yes	Yes	Yes	No, but transplacental infection can occur	No, but viremia and transplacental infection are characteristic	No, but transplacental infection can occur
Most susceptible stage of gestation	Primarily first half	Primarily first half	Throughout, but most susceptible first half	Throughout	Throughout, but most susceptible first half	Unknown, but probably early
Incidence of abortion	Low or nil	Low or nil	Low or nil	High	Variable, depends on severity of maternal illness	Unknown
Embryonic and fetal death and stillbirth	Yes	Yes	Yes	Yes	Yes	Yes
Developmental anomalies	Not reported	Yes	Yes	Not reported	Yes	Yes
Demonstrable antibody in serum of neonate before nursing	Yes, common	Yes	Not reported	No	No	Yes
Likelihood of demonstrating virus and/or viral antigen at farrowing in: Dead fetus	Excellent	Poor	Poor	Fair	Poor	Poor
Live pig	Good, but difficult if pig also has homologous serum antibody	Fair	Fair	Fair	Excellent	Poor

in embryonated chicken eggs and in cell cultures.

A vaccine for swine has not been developed; however, if in the future swine are unequivocally identified as a source of influenza virus for man, a vaccine may be developed and used for public health reasons.

Hog Cholera Virus

Hog cholera virus is distributed worldwide but is notably absent from some countries such as the United States, England and Canada following eradication programs. There is a single serotype; however, antigenic variants have been reported. The virus is maintained by chronically affected swine and also has been disseminated by the use of modified live virus vaccines. Viremia is a feature of both clinical and subclinical hog cholera, thus providing ample opportunity for transplacental infection.

Abortion is a common sequela of severe maternal illness, whereas embryonic resorption, fetal mummification, developmental anomalies, stillbirth and weak pigs result from transplacental infection during mild or subclinical maternal illness. Virus and viral antigen can be detected in tissues of stillborn and weak pigs and sometimes in tissues of fetuses that die near term. Since HCV is not cytopathogenic, its identification in cell culture is usually made by immunofluorescent microscopy. Both inactivated and modified live virus vaccines are effective for immunization.

SUMMARY

Selected features of reproductive disease associated with each of the viruses previously discussed are summarized in Table 1.

Parainfluenza 1 virus, reovirus, foot and mouth disease virus, and vesicular stomatitis virus also have been incriminated as causes of swine reproductive failure. However, there is little information to suggest that these viruses play a major role.

REFERENCES

Porcine Parvovirus

1. Mengeling, W. L. and Cutlip, R. C.: Reproductive disease experimentally induced by exposing pregnant gilts to porcine parvovirus. Am. J. Vet. Res., *37*:1393, 1976.

Porcine Enteroviruses

1. Dunne, H. W., Wang, J. T., Clark, C. D., Hokanson, J. F., Morimoto, T. and Bubash, G. R.: The effects of *in utero* viral infection on embryonic, fetal, and neonatal survival: A comparison of SMEDI (porcine picorna) viruses with hog cholera vaccinal virus. Can. J. Comp. Med., *33*:244, 1969.

Japanese B Encephalitis Virus

1. Shimizu, T., Kawakami, Y., Fukuhara, S. and Matumoto, M.: Experimental stillbirth in pregnant swine infected with Japanese encephalitis virus. Jap. J. Exp. Med., *24*:363, 1954.

Pseudorabies Virus

1. Kluge, J. P. and Mare, C. J.: Swine pseudorabies: Abortion, clinical disease, and lesions in pregnant gilts infected with pseudorabies virus (Aujeszky's disease). Am. J. Vet. Res., *35*:911, 1974.

Influenza Virus

1. Mensik, J.: The immunologic behaviour of newborn piglets. I. Demonstration of antibodies to *Myxovirus influenza suis* in the precolostral serum of newborn piglets. Docum. Vet. Brno., 7:129, 1968.

Hog Cholera Virus

1. Johnson, K. P., Ferguson, L. C., Byington, D. P. and Redman, D. R.: Multiple fetal malformations due to persistent viral infection. I. Abortion, intrauterine death, and gross abnormalities in fetal swine infected with hog cholera virus. Lab. Invest., *30*:608, 1974.

Reovirus

1. McAdaragh, J. P. and Robl, M. G.: Experimental reovirus infection of pregnant sows. Proceedings International Pig Veterinary Society IV, DD.1., 1976.

Repeat Breeding in Swine

STIG EINARSSON

College of Veterinary Medicine, Uppsala, Sweden

GENERAL INTRODUCTION

The length of the average estrous cycle in female pigs is 21 days (±18 to 24 days). Sows that have conceived may occasionally show estrous symptoms 3 or 6 weeks, or both, after natural mating or insemination.

Return to service within 18 to 24 days after mating may be due to several factors. One is that the spermatozoa do not reach the site of fertilization in the oviducts. The most common cause for this is occlusion of the oviducts. Other reasons for return to service are failure of the spermatozoa to fertilize the ova or death of the ova after fertilization. Death of blastocysts within 12 days of fertilization is usually followed by the sow's returning to service within the normal 21-day cycle. The embryos, which at this stage of gestation are migrating freely within the uterus, may be too weak to survive, or adverse conditions may prevent them from implanting and developing further.

A prolonged heat interval (>24 days) occurs following embryonic loss 12 days or later postfertilization. There are several factors that may cause embryonic death at this stage of gestation. In addition, endocrine disturbances accompanied by ovarian cysts will sometimes cause prolonged heat intervals.

FREQUENCY OF REPEAT BREEDING IN NORMAL HERDS

Fertility can be expressed in different ways, of which 28 days nonreturn (NR) per cent and farrowing rate are the most common. The former is mainly utilized for boars used for artificial insemination but could also be valuable for boars used for natural service.

The average farrowing rate for sows mated at the first estrus after weaning is 80 to 85 per cent. The 28 days NR per cent exceeds the farrowing rate by 5 to 10 per cent. Thus under normal conditions about 10 per cent of the sows mated during their first postweaning estrus will return to service.

In herds using "traveling" boars, the farrowing rate is, according to available information, lower than in herds using their own breeding boars. The lower conception rate from "traveling" boars might be due to poor timing of services or to more frequent exposure to genital infections.

DIFFERENT CAUSES OF REPEAT BREEDING

Boar Infertility

In herds with severe infertility problems the boar, or boars, should always be suspected of having lowered fertility or sterility. Breeding and farrowing records are essential for the diagnosis. The review of the records should include the 28 days NR per cent after first service, farrowing rate and litter size as well as the incidence of irregular heat intervals and vaginal discharge after service. If possible, these records should be reviewed per month for the past 6 months.

Semen examination is recommended in all cases of suspected boar infertility. This is essential for a correct diagnosis of disturbances of testicular or epididymal function, or both. Different causes of boar infertility are presented elsewhere in this section, but one, namely testicular degeneration, will be mentioned here briefly. In addition to lowered sperm production and poor sperm motility, the semen of a boar with testicular degeneration is characterized by an increased frequency of immature and morphologically abnormal spermatozoa.

Occasionally, boars with apparently normal semen may be incapable of causing conception. Therefore, the results of the examination of semen samples and the clinical examination of the boar as a means of evaluating fertility should be judged with care. This is also the case when young boars suspected of infertility because of a low 28 days NR per cent are tested for semen quality. Usually 1 to 3 months have elapsed from the first mating by the boar in the herd to the andrological examination of the boar. In the meantime many of these boars suspected of immaturity have become sexually mature and have normal semen characteristics.

Female Infertility

Infection. Bacteriological as well as histopathological examination of the reproductive tract of repeat breeder sows has been carried out in several countries. Despite signs of endometritis at histological examination, the bacteriological findings have mainly been negative. In addition to return to heat, the clinical symptoms in cases of endometritis sometimes include a vaginal discharge. In these cases the microbiological culture sometimes results in isolation of *Escherichia coli* or different staphylococci and streptococci.

In living animals the samples should be taken from the anterior vagina by the aid of a vaginal speculum. To obtain a correct diagnosis in a problem herd, however, it is recommended that two or three sows be slaughtered. The specimens for culture should be taken directly from the uterus as soon as possible after slaughter.

Vaginal discharge may also be related to pathological conditions not localized to the uterus. Vaginitis and pyelonephritis may thus cause a purulent vaginal discharge.

No infectious disease that is strictly venereal in origin is known to occur in pigs. A venereal spread of *Staphylococcus aureus* in a herd with infertility problems was, however, reported in Denmark in 1955. At histopathological examination of the uterus, a chronic metritis was demonstrated in many sows served by an infected boar.

Ovarian Dysfunction. Endocrine disturbances are responsible for 20 to 50 per cent of the infertility problems among sows in herds with "normal" fertility. The frequency of ovarian cysts is higher during spring than during fall.

Vandeplassche and co-workers[5] demonstrated that cystic follicles are present in 10 per cent of sows. Half of these affected sows show no ovarian cyclic activity. The remainder have normally developing follicles or corpora lutea in combination with cysts.

A diagnosis of cystic ovaries is difficult to establish in the living animal. Rectal examination of the ovaries has been attempted in large sows but is difficult to

perform. According to Nalbandov,[1] sows with large luteinized cysts sometimes have an enlarged clitoris. This phenomenon has not been confirmed in later studies. Irregular heat intervals in sows belonging to herds with "normal" fertility may, however, be indicative of cystic ovaries.

Developmental Abnormalities. Developmental abnormalities of the genital tract occur frequently in female pigs. Approximately 5 per cent of gilts belonging to nonselected populations have been shown to have abnormalities that might potentially influence their fertility.

The ability to conduct a clinical examination of the internal genital organs is limited. Therefore abnormalities of the sexual organs are seldom diagnosed in the living animal. Gilts with repeated returns to estrus at regular intervals after mating should, however, be suspected of having abnormalities of their genital organs.

THERAPY RECOMMENDATIONS

Boar Infertility

Careful supervision of the boars and their services is important. Boars should not be used for breeding before having attained sexual maturity. After that time the boars can be used for services, but not too frequently. As soon as a boar is suspected of being sterile or having low fertility, he should not be allowed to serve any more sows.

Restitution of testicular degeneration takes a long time and is sometimes not possible. It is therefore usually preferable to slaughter a boar with diagnosed testicular degeneration.

Female Infertility

Infection. Diagnosis by microbiological testing is necessary before a recommendation for treatment can be given. If the diagnosis is a venereal infection spread by a boar, the boar should immediately be isolated from the rest of the breeding stock. Treatment of an infected boar is not recommended.

If possible, females with vaginal discharge should be isolated from breeding animals, at least until the cause is established. Sows with infection localized to the genital tract should be culled. Treatment of valuable animals could be tried, using antibiotics for several days. The results of such treatments are, however, not always encouraging.

Ovarian Dysfunction. Endocrine dysfunction accompanied by cystic ovaries is difficult to treat successfully in sows. Various types of hormonal treatments have been tried, e.g., progesterone, human chorionic gonadotropin and gonadotropin-releasing hormone, but the results of such treatments are not encouraging.

As stress is suspected as being a cause of the development of ovarian cysts in sows, management and environmental factors should be carefully checked.

REFERENCES

1. Nalbandov, A. V.: Anatomic and endocrine causes of sterility in female swine. Fertil. Steril., 3:100, 1964.
2. Paredis, F.: Onderzoekingen over vruchtbaarheid en kunstmatige inseminatie bij het varken. Medelingen Veeartsenijschool, Rijksuniversiteit Gent., 5:135, 1961.
3. Pomeroy, R. W.: Infertility and neonatal mortality in the sow. I. Lifetime performance and reasons for disposal of sows. J. Agric. Sci. Camb., 54:1, 1960.
4. Rasbech, N. O.: A review of the causes of reproductive failure in swine. Br. Vet. J., 125:599, 1969.
5. Vandeplassche, M., Spincemaille, J., Bonte, P. and Bouters, R.: Herd infertility in pigs. Proc. XIX World Veterinary Congress, Mexico, 1971, p. 441.
6. Wrathall, A. E.: Reproductive disorders in pigs. Commonwealth Agricultural Bureaux, Farnham Royal, Slough SL2 3BN, England, 1975.

Vaccination Program to Maximize Swine Reproductive Performance

M. R. WILSON

Ontario Veterinary College, Guelph, Ontario, Canada

For this article the reproductive period is taken as the time from conception through pregnancy to the end of the neonatal period. I have taken the latter to be the period up to the time that under normal conditions a suckling piglet starts to produce its own antibodies, that is, at about 10 days of age.

Vaccinations during the reproductive period are given for three reasons:

1. To protect the sow.
2. To prevent abortion or increased still-birth rate.
3. To protect the piglets passively from neonatal infections.

It is important to remember that more than 90 per cent of immunoglobulins in colostrum are obtained from the circulatory system of the sow, whereas more than 70 per cent of the immunoglobulins in milk are produced in the mammary glands. It follows therefore that if the objective is to induce protection against a systemic disease of the neonate or the sow, circulating antibodies must be induced in the sow. These are passed into the colostrum and transported to the circulation of the newborn piglets. Conversely, for optimal results, if protection against an enteric disease in the piglet is desired, theoretically, stimulation of the immune system in the sow's mammary glands should be attempted. Reliable and safe methods of effectively achieving this aim have not been documented.

Killed versus Living Biologicals. In an article of this length, it is not possible to elaborate upon the merits or otherwise of killed versus living vaccines. As a generalization, one can say that living porcine viral vaccines are considered by many to be unsafe, whereas killed viral vaccines, although safe, have often given less than desirable protection. Bacterins, however, often give adequate protection and compare favorably with living bacterial vaccines for some conditions.

Finally, there is a form of vaccination that utilizes virulent organisms to attempt to induce immunity at a time when the resultant infection causes no harm to the sow. Such a procedure could be termed *normalizing vaccination*. The feeding of feces or dead piglets, or both, to pregnant animals is of special value when new animals are added to a herd. On some occasions newly added animals will abort because they lack immunity to the resident infections to which the members of the herd are immune. Conversely, on occasion the residents of the herd may abort after introduction of new members; then the new sows or boars have introduced

TABLE 1. *Vaccination Schedules for Major Infectious Diseases Affecting Swine Reproductive Performance*

Disease	Vaccination Schedule*	Comments
1. To protect the sow:		
Erysipelas	First dose to weaned pig, second dose 1 month before first farrowing; repeat at each farrowing	Vaccines and bacterins are effective
2. To reduce abortion and stillbirth rates:		
Pseudorabies	*Live vaccines*—3 to 8 weeks of age, repeat every 6 months in breeding stock *Dead vaccines*—two doses at 14 and 28 days of age, 4 and 2 weeks prior to farrowing.	
Leptospirosis	At breeding or weaning	Bacterins are effective but should be used in conjunction with treatment during an outbreak
Erysipelas	At breeding or weaning	—
Early embryonic death associated with parvovirus infection	—	Vaccines are anticipated in near future
3. To protect piglets passively from neonatal infections:		
Transmissible gastroenteritis (TGE)	4 + 1 weeks before farrowing	The intramuscular vaccine gives only partial protection; orally administered vaccines are available in some areas and appear to give protection
Pseudorabies	See above	
Erysipelas	See above	
Enteric colibacillosis	Bacterins at least 1 month and again 1 week prior to farrowing; oral vaccines 10 to 30 days prior to farrowing for 3 consecutive days	Bacterins and oral vaccines prepared autogenously give protection
Bordetella-induced atrophic rhinitis	4 and 2 weeks before farrowing to sows and 1 and 4 weeks of age to piglets	The available autogenous and commercial vaccines should be given subcutaneously to avoid severe reaction

*In all cases the manufacturers' directions should be followed when different from those suggested here.

an infection to which they are immune but the residents were not. Feces should therefore be fed from the residents to the newcomers and vice versa.

When tissues or feces are being used, one has no control over what is being fed, as subclinical infection, for example, parvovirus or enteroviruses, could be present. However, the feeding of pure cultures of organisms at a time when there is no danger of inducing abortions or other problems lessens this danger. This procedure is often used with success in enteric colibacillosis and transmissible gastroenteritis. Its disadvantage is that an infection is established in the sow, which inevitably results in a considerably increased challenge to piglets if it is a neonatal disease, and that a carrier state may be induced in the infected sow.

Table 1 lists the major infectious diseases affecting the reproductive performance of sows and appropriate schedules for vaccination. It should be noted that in all cases the manufacturer's instructions for vaccination protocol must be followed for optimum results.

Pregnancy Diagnostic Methods for the Sow

JOHN R. DIEHL

Tuskegee Institute, Alabama

Separation of pregnant from nonpregnant females is of value to swine producers. The current estimate of the cost of maintaining a female, whether she is pregnant or not, ranges from 35 to 50 cents per day. The major portion of this cost is feed, although labor, facilities, taxes and interest on the investment are included. The more rapidly nonpregnant females are detected, the sooner they can be culled or rebred, thus reducing operating expenses.

This article will discuss the pregnancy detection methods that have been shown to be accurate in the field. A respectable degree of accuracy (90 to 95 per cent) can be achieved by several of these methods. At present it is possible to be 100 per cent accurate in diagnosing pregnancy in sows or gilts; however, clinicians should not expect such accuracy routinely.

TECHNIQUES

Estrous Detection

The oldest method is to check for the occurrence of estrus in bred females by exposing them to boars 18 to 25 days after mating. This also provides the earliest possible indication of pregnancy. The major drawback to this method is that it requires additional animal handling. Good breeding records and individual animal identification are also essential for best diagnostic accuracy. Producers who utilize hand mating can make the best use of this method.

Pen breeding makes diagnosis by estrous detection more difficult because of unknown breeding dates. Detection of estrus requires additional time and labor for daily estrous checks. The possibility of disease transmission makes it impossible for a practitioner to use this technique on a farm-to-farm basis. Moreover, a producer's records are not accurate in most instances, since producers don't always agree on the optimum time to breed.

Hormone Assays

Chemical determination of hormone levels in blood and urine has recently been developed to a high degree of reliability. Handling of the biological materials to be assayed requires specialized laboratory equipment. In addition, a good laboratory technician is essential. Hormone assays are not likely to be used as a routine and inexpensive method for pregnancy diagnosis until more highly automated techniques are available.

Vaginal Biopsy Technique

Sample Collection and Preparation. Histological evaluation of a cross section of vaginal tissue collected from 20 to 25 days after breeding is a relatively simple technique, and complete details regarding histological preparation and diagnostic procedures have been published.[1, 3] Diagnoses based on this evaluation have been shown to be 95 per cent accurate.[1] When diagnostic errors are made, nonpregnant females are more likely to be called pregnant. The major disadvantage to this technique is that breeding dates must be known for maximum accuracy, since open females in the luteal phase of the estrous cycle can be mistakenly diagnosed pregnant.

Biopsies may be taken approximately 5 cm posterior to the cervix using a good rectal biopsy forcep (see Appendix B). The forcep shaft should be at least 37 cm in length. To facilitate collection of biopsies, females can be crowded or snared. Tissue dehydration can be minimized by placing biopsies in individually labeled sample bags or vials containing saline. Biopsies should then be placed on ice until they are processed for sectioning with the aid of cryogenic techniques or by conventional histological methods.

Pregnancy Diagnosis. One to four layers of vaginal epithelial cells, 20 to 25 days postbreeding, are the necessary criteria for determining pregnancy. There is a marked difference in the appearance of vaginal epithelium observed prior to and following staining. Figure 1A shows unstained vaginal tissue as it appears under the phase contrast microscope with a brightfield light condenser. Although nuclei are not obvious, with a little experience, one can very readily count the layers of epithelial cells (above the arrows). Figure 1B shows the appearance of vaginal tissue after staining with hematoxylin and eosin.[3] Following staining, it is much easier to recognize layers of epithelium by the characteristic appearance of layers of nuclei. However, less total time

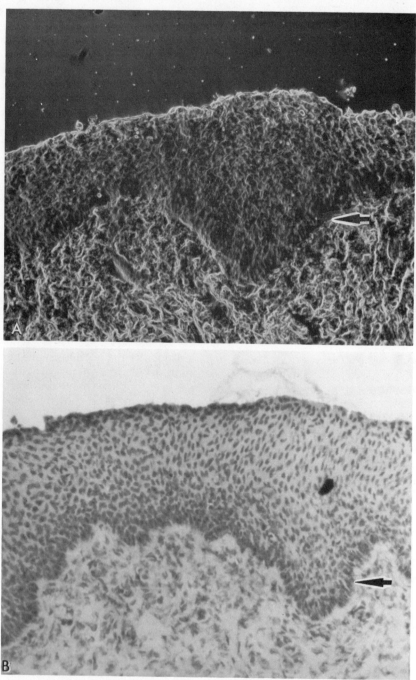

Figure 1. Sections of vaginal biopsy as they appear following sectioning on a cryostat and prior to usual histological preparation (A) and after staining (B). Note the epithelial pegs (arrows) that are typical of vaginal tissue from females in heat.

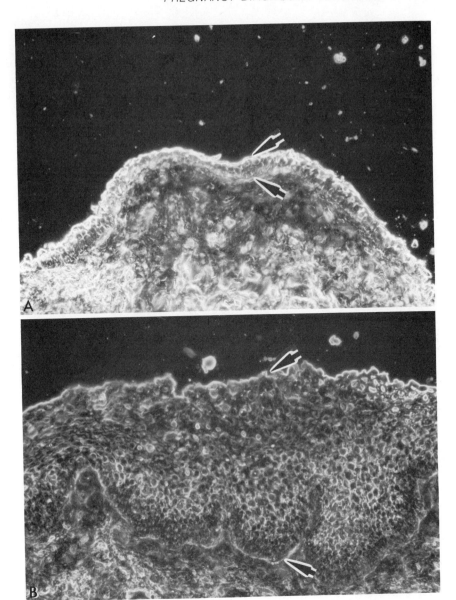

Figure 2. There are distinct differences in the appearance of unstained vaginal tissue from pregnant (*A*) and nonpregnant (*B*) females as seen through the phase contrast microscope using a brightfield objective. Note the number of layers of epithelial cells (between arrows) and the presence of epithelial pegs (*B*).

and laboratory methodology are involved with unstained sections. Figure 2 shows sections of unstained vaginal biopsies from pregnant (2*A*) and nonpregnant (2*B*) females, respectively, as seen with the aid of a phase contrast microscope. Figure 3 shows the appearance of vaginal epithelium (stained with hematoxylin and eosin) typical of pregnant (3*A*) and nonpregnant (3*B*) females, respectively. The accuracy of the biopsy technique is reduced to 65 per cent when breeding dates are unknown.[3]

ULTRASONIC PREGNANCY DETECTORS

The latest and most promising method of pregnancy detection to be developed is that using ultrasonic sound.[2] Ultrasonic detection may be compared with a ship searching for a submarine by sonar. When a submarine is spotted, a "blip" shows up on the sonar scope, which gives an indication of the submarine's distance from the ship. Ultrasonic pregnancy detection utilizes a similar

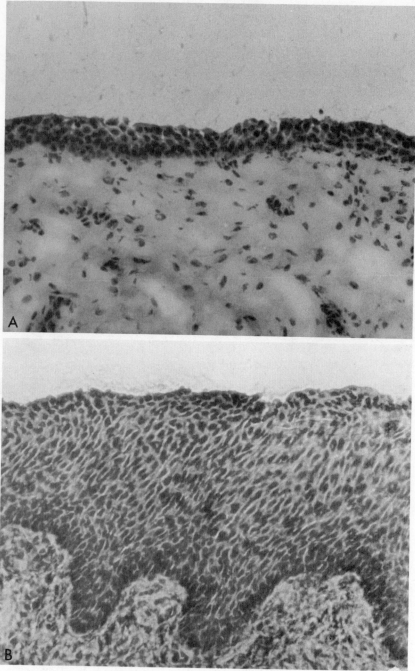

Figure 3. Stained sections of vaginal tissue from pregnant (*A*) and nonpregnant (*B*) females as seen through a brightfield microscope.

principle. Ultrasonic sound waves are emitted from a handheld sending and receiving device (transducer). When the transducer is held against an object, a blip will show up on the display screen at a point corresponding to the distance between the transducer and the interface of substances with different densities (Fig. 4).

Method. Diagnoses can be made from either side of a standing animal. The animals need not be snared. All that is necessary is to get them interested in something long enough to keep the transducer in place for a reading. Correct placement of the transducer against the sow is important if an accurate reading is to be obtained (Fig. 5). The transducer should be coated with a few drops of liquid vegetable oil (mineral oil

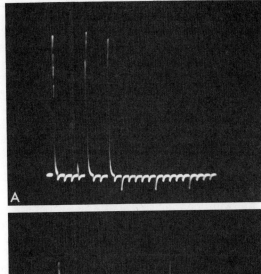

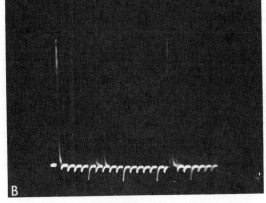

Figure 4. Ultrasonic scanning of nonpregnant female results in an oscilloscope pattern such as is seen in *A*. Note the trace or blips in the left hand portion of the screen. No major traces appear beyond the second major depth mark. Pregnant females present a pattern such as is seen in *B*, with one or more blips in the right hand half of the screen.

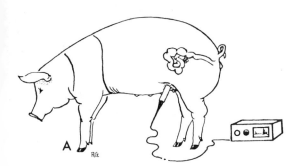

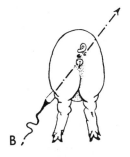

Figure 5. The correct placement of the transducer is depicted in drawings *A* and *B*. Handling the transducer in this way is correct for any type of ultrasonic detector. (The author wishes to express his gratitude to Dr. R. A. Godke for supplying the art work in this figure.)

can be detrimental to the transducer) to provide a positive contact with the skin. Place the tip of the transducer against the skin approximately 5 cm lateral to the teat line. Be sure to keep it just ahead of the stifle and behind the last rib, while pointing toward the opposite loin edge. This will allow the operator to scan the area in which the uterus is located. If the transducer is pointed outside these limits, false indications of pregnancy can result from echoes from a full bladder or other structures located at the same level anterior to the uterus.

While the transducer is in contact with the skin, look for traces on the screen of the portable console. If an echo, blip or trace (whatever you choose to call it) appears on the screen, make the diagnosis based on its location on the screen. If the trace shows only in left half, the female is nonpregnant (see Figure 4A). If the trace appears in the right half of the screen, she is pregnant (see Figure 4B). There is a second criterion that, if observed, will help minimize false readings. That is, a trace in the right half of the screen should be stable enough to be seen for at least 2 seconds and should be about as tall or as strong as the trace at the far left side, which is always on. If no traces show at all, put more vegetable oil on the transducer tip and try again; good contact may not have been established.

Pregnancy Diagnosis. As with any diagnostic method, a higher degree of accuracy can be achieved when the reproductive history of the herd in question is known. Breeding dates help minimize questionable diagnoses. When a female is diagnosed nonpregnant, use a different type mark than for a pregnant animal. After all the group have been checked, recheck those marked "nonpregnant." If "nonpregnant" is the diagnosis again, this should confirm that the animals are indeed nonpregnant. When questionable diagnoses occur, such as an oscilloscope pattern showing a blip on the midline of the screen, recheck the animal again in 1 week.

Sensitivity controls for most ultrasonic detectors are similar. When the power is turned on, the units with an oscilloscope screen (Pregnosticator, Ilis Preg-Check and Preg-Alert; see Appendix B) will have some type of depth calibration marks (Fig. 4). One brand known as the Scanoprobe has a continuous row of lights instead of a screen. There may be a buzzer or bell type of indicator on some units (Ilis Preg-Check). This theoretically makes it easier to diagnose

pregnant females. This feature, if present, appears to do little to enhance diagnostic accuracy.

In the pregnant sow, fluid concentration around the developing fetus within its amnion reaches maximum at about 30 days gestation. It is the fluid-surrounded fetus that produces the blip on the display screen, since an empty uterus produces no characteristic blip on the right half of the screen. Maximum accuracy and economic advantage with ultrasonic detectors are obtained when the instruments are used at 30 to 45 days gestation.

Most certainly the economic advantage of utilizing pregnancy diagnosis decreases for each day that passes. Accuracy also decreases as gestation age increases because as fetal weight increases, the uterus expands in volume and weight and the broad ligament stretches in response, allowing the uterus to relocate lower in the body. As the pregnant uterus expands and drops toward the abdominal wall, the corresponding echoes move closer to the center point, and diagnostic accuracy decreases significantly because structures other than the uterus can also produce echoes that show at the center line. Scanoprobe manufacturers have attempted to alleviate this problem by using a row of lights for depth calibration rather than a screen. It appears that neither machine has an advantage with regard to this problem, which occurs more often after 45 days gestation.

Of the pregnancy detection methods described, the ultrasonic technique is one of the most accurate, even when breeding dates are unknown. In addition, it is simpler and faster with regard to total amount of equipment and time involved. Although it is not possible to count the number of fetuses accurately, some users have suggested that we may be able to use ultrasonics to detect early fetal death. This may be done by checking at 30 days and again at 45 days gestation. Loss of the litter may be detected in this manner. Obviously, the only time this needs to be done is when fetal death is suspected, such as after an invasion of SMEDI, pseudorabies, or other circumstances detrimental to the fetus.

Currently, most ultrasonic detectors utilize rechargeable batteries (Scanoprobe, Ilis-Preg-Check and Preg-Alert); however, there is one instrument that also uses a 110-volt power source (Prognosticator). The battery-operated models offer greater flexibility but may cost more to purchase. As a part of the kit, some models have adjustable straps that fit around the operator's neck and another for the torso. If this is not available, something similar should be used, as this frees one hand to hold the vegetable oil bottle and the other to hold the transducer.

Trouble-Shooting. Some tips in trouble-shooting not already mentioned are in order. One tip that will help prevent the transducer cord from being broken or bitten in half is to run the cord down the sleeve of the shirt or coveralls of the operator. Since the transducer lead connector is of the twist-lock type, help keep it secure and give additional protection to the transducer by using an alligator clip insulator to cover it (Fig. 6). Polymerized vegetable oil will eventually coat the contact points between the transducer and its connector, breaking the positive contact. Clean these points with a cotton swab saturated with alcohol after every third or fourth farm visit. If oscilloscope models should show a base line that has literally hundreds of dancing blips (grass), the woven metal sheath just inside the transducer lead insulation may be broken. Since this metal sheath serves as the ground, it does not maintain constant contact if broken, hence the appearance of grass on the screen. The unit should be taken to an electronics shop or sent to the factory for repair.

Sanitization of the instrument, especially when going between farms, is not a simple problem. Some type of precautionary cleaning should be utilized. Some producers wipe the entire unit off with alcohol before and after each farm visit.

Other Uses. All types of units with continuous calibrations (oscilloscope or row of lights) can be used to estimate backfat thickness and loin-eye depth. Users must realize that the accuracy of these measurements is directly related to the experience and correct use of the probe. There is some question whether loin-eye area can be calculated from one or more depth estimates. An additional investment for a specific brand that advertises backfat and loin-eye measurements does not appear warranted, especially when a backfat probe costs less than a dollar and is much more accurate and reliable, particularly in the hands of an inexperienced user.

How many sows must a producer own or a clinician have to check to justify purchasing an ultrasonic pregnancy detector? Using the cost figures cited earlier in this article, a producer can expect to save approximately $30 per open female detected and culled at 30 days. One hundred fifty farrowings per year would pay for the lower priced models in about 2 years under the stated conditions. These figures are based on the fact that most producers seldom remove open females much before 90 days gestation, and the cost of an ultrasonic detector would average about $1300 to $1400. A clinician leasing the use of a detector could very likely pay for one in less time, especially if he practices near a high concentration of hog producers.

SUMMARY

At the present time, the vaginal biopsy technique and ultrasonic pregnancy detec-

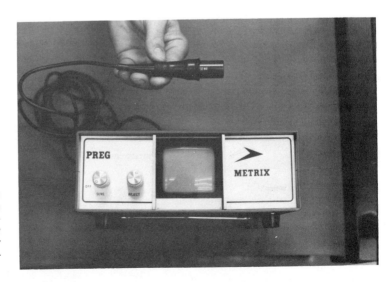

Figure 6. Additional protection against damage from dropping the transducer and maintaining a positive connection is provided by threading the twist-lock connector through a rubber alligator clip insulator, as shown above.

tors are the best choice for an accurate, inexpensive and reliable method for detecting pregnant females. The method an individual chooses depends on access to good laboratory facilities and his faith in electronic devices. Economically, either method will pay for itself, since swine producers are using increasingly more advanced equipment than ever before in their efforts to make their operation more efficient.

REFERENCES

1. Diehl, J. R. and Day, B. N.: Utilization of frozen sections with the vaginal biopsy technique for early pregnancy diagnosis in swine. J. Anim. Sci., 37:114, 1973.
2. Lindahl, I. L., Martin, P. and Dzuik, P. J.: Early diagnosis of pregnancy in sows. J. Anim. Sci., 35:1120, 1972 (Abs.).
3. Mather, E. C., Diehl, J. R. and Tumbleson, M. E.: Pregnancy diagnosis in swine utilizing the vaginal biopsy technique. J.A.V.M.A., 157:1522, 1970.

Parturition

B. N. DAY

University of Missouri, Columbia, Missouri

GESTATION AND FARROWING

Length of Gestation Period

The length of gestation is 111 to 117 days, with an average of about 115 days and a standard deviation within breeds of 1.5 days. The range in gestation length due to breed effects is 2 to 3 days, and the heritability of gestation length is about 30 per cent. Differences among sows due to litter size, proportion of living and regressing fetuses at birth or age of the sow have only minor influences on gestation length. Environmental effects on the gestation period are not well documented but also appear to be minor.

The mechanisms controlling the onset of labor and parturition are yet to be defined. Sows carrying live but decapitated fetuses have a prolonged pregnancy, as do some sows when all pigs in the litter died during late gestation. Maternally, a decrease in the circulating progesterone level appears to be a requirement for the initiation of parturition. Ovariectomy during all stages of pregnancy results in abortion.

Signs of Farrowing

Most signs of farrowing that are definite enough for predicting the precise time of parturition occur during the final 24 to 36 hours before the onset of parturition. Even then, however, there are substantial variations and telescoping of the sequence of changes leading up to the birth of the first pig. The first physical signs of pregnancy may be observed as early as the start of the last trimester. These include abdominal distention and development of the mammary glands, especially in gilts. During the last week of gestation a pronounced swelling of the vulva is usually apparent, with the coloration of the vulva becoming more reddened as parturition approaches.

There is an increasing enlargement of the mammary glands as pregnancy progresses, with individual glands becoming prominent and distended during the last 1 to 3 days of gestation. At about this same time, a few drops of clear or straw-colored mammary secretion may be expressed from the teats of some sows by manual pressure. Subsequently, milk secretion is initiated, and, typically, abundant milk can be expressed from the teats at the onset of farrowing. The interval from the initiation of milk flow to parturition provides one of the more reliable predictors of the time of farrowing. Sows will usually farrow within 6 to 12 hours after free milk flow is established, although the interval may be extended to 24 hours in some sows.

Nest-building and nervousness are behavioral characteristics exhibited by sows during the day preceding parturition. In confinement facilities the usual activity associated with the redistribution of bedding material to form a nest may be poorly expressed or may be exhibited as nervous activity including restlessness, increased respiration rate, frequent defecation and urination and chewing or biting surrounding objects. However, as labor progresses, physical activity is reduced, and during the final period before birth of the first pig, the sow becomes quiescent and settles into a recumbent position. Increased uterine contractions are indicated by abdominal and leg movements and by the flow of small amounts of fluid and meconium from the vulva.

The physical and behavioral changes preceding parturition provide useful criteria for predicting farrowing time. However, variations in the sequence of these events are not uncommon, and total reliability in their use should not be expected to time the onset of the farrowing period.

Farrowing Period

The behavior of the sow during the birth process contrasts with the beginning stages of labor, since the sow characteristically shows limited physical activity while farrowing. The pigs are usually delivered while the sow is lying on her side. This position is usually maintained, with only occasional changes to a standing or ventral position. The pigs are born with little abdominal straining by the sow. Passage of each pig through the vagina is frequently signaled by the sow switching her tail. There is only minimal fluid loss during delivery of the litter, and expulsion of the fetal membranes is usually delayed until after the birth of the last pig.

Upon delivery, the newborn pig remains immobile for a few seconds. With the onset of respiratory activity, the pig almost immediately starts to struggle to free the umbilical cord and then moves anteriorly toward the udder of the sow.

Duration of Farrowing

The duration of farrowing, as timed from the birth of the first to the last pig in the litter, may be less than 1 hour or as long as 6 to 8 hours. A great majority of the sows, however, require from 1 to 4 hours to deliver the complete litter. A tendency exists for the duration of farrowing to be longer for larger litters, but exceptions are not uncommon. Pigs are usually born singly, with an average interval between pigs of about 15 minutes. The time required for expulsion of the placental membranes after the birth of the last pig is highly variable, with a range from a few minutes to as long as 8 hours or more.

PIG CHARACTERISTICS

Pigs are delivered with ease as both anterior and posterior presentations, with slightly more than half the pigs born head first. No apparent cause-and-effect relationship has been observed between the type of presentation (anterior or posterior) and the frequency of stillbirths.

During birth, the umbilical cord remains intact and attached to the placental membranes in a majority of the pigs. However, as parturition progresses, the ratio of intact to ruptured umbilical cords nearly equalizes.

The order of birth is determined by location in the uterine horn. The pig closest to the uterine body is the first pig to be delivered from the uterine horn, and the remaining pigs follow in sequence. The order of delivery of pigs from the left and right uterine horns would appear to be a random occurrence. On occasion, one uterine horn may expel all pigs in the order of their location within the horn before any pigs are delivered from the contralateral uterine horn.

STILLBORN PATTERN

On the average, 5 to 7 per cent of all pigs farrowed are stillborn. Most stillborns represent a death that occurred during the birth process.

Stillborns may be classified into two major groups, prepartum and intrapartum deaths. Stillborns caused by prepartum deaths are recognized as pigs that show some degenerative changes, but this classification does not include mummified fetuses. The incidence of prepartum deaths may be expected to vary as the level of infectious causes of fetal deaths changes within the herd. Considerable differences may be expected among herds. Prepartum stillborns appear at random during the course of farrowing and are more frequently enclosed in the placental membranes than are intrapartum stillborns. Prepartum deaths generally represent a small percentage of the total stillborns.

Intrapartum death is the major cause of stillbirths. The interval between the birth of the first and the last pig influences the stillbirth rate, with the highest percentage of stillborns occurring when the duration of farrowing is extremely long. The interval between the birth of two live pigs within the litter is shorter than the interval prior to the birth of a stillborn pig. It is not clear, however, whether the delayed parturition causes the stillborn pig or if dead pigs are delivered more slowly. Both situations probably occur, since it has been observed that the interval to the birth of a stillborn pig caused by prepartum death is also extended.

Rupture of the umbilical cord is closely associated with the occurrence of stillbirths. In one study, the umbilical cord was still attached to the fetal membranes at birth in 61 per cent of the pigs. However, the percentage of pigs with intact umbilical cords decreased from 79 per cent during the first third of the farrowing period to 49 per cent during the last third. Also, 94 per cent of 63 stillborn pigs classified as intrapartum deaths had ruptured umbilical cords at delivery.

Of particular interest in an evaluation of causes of intrapartum deaths is the distribution of stillborn pigs during the birth of the complete litter. The first third of the birth order is characterized by a low frequency of stillbirths, and only minor increases occur during the middle third. However, a marked increase in the number of intrapartum deaths occurs during the last third of farrowing and may be as high as 10 to 20 per cent of all pigs born during this period. In one study, greater than 80 per cent of all intrapartum deaths occurred during the last third of the farrowing. Several factors may contribute to this increased loss, all of which may cause anoxia. Since pigs are delivered in sequence from the uterine horn, the last pigs born must travel the length of the uterine horn during the birth process. The incidence of ruptured umbilical cords also increases during the latter stages of the farrowing process. Therefore, it seems likely that both the general effects of a prolonged farrowing period and the intrauterine location contribute to the increased intrapartum death rate occurring in the last third of the litter to be delivered.

HORMONAL CHANGES AT PARTURITION

The corpus luteum is required for maintenance of gestation, and, it is, therefore, thought that the placental membranes fail to produce sufficient progesterone for pregnancy maintenance. In turn, a consistent hormonal change associated with the initiation of parturition in the pig is a sharp decline in the plasma progesterone level during the last 24 hours of the gestation period. At the onset of parturition, peripheral levels of progesterone are generally less than 1 to 2 ng/ml of plasma.

Plasma estrogen levels increase during the last week of gestation and then show a precipitous drop following the end of parturition. Estrogens are produced by the placental membranes. Corticoid concentrations in peripheral plasma begin to increase during the 24-hour period prior to parturition and peak on day 0. The elevation of corticoid levels would appear to be the result of the initiation of first stages of labor and parturition.

Plasma levels of relaxin also increase with the approach of parturition, peaking on day 1 prior to birth. This is followed by a decline by the day of parturition and then by a further decrease to low levels by the day following parturition. No reports are available on plasma levels of prostaglandin at parturition in the sow.

Delayed parturition can be produced by progesterone injections and by feeding a synthetic progestogen or methallibure. However, such treatments frequently increase the occurrence of stillbirths markedly.

Decapitation of the fetuses during early stages of pregnancy will also delay parturition, even though the fetuses remain alive. These observations indicate that the intact live fetus plays a major role in the initiation of parturition. Little information is available concerning fetal hormonal levels at parturition. High umbilical plasma levels of progesterone and estrogens have been reported.

INDUCED PARTURITION

Controlled parturition would provide an additional management tool for the swine producer. It is generally accepted that supervision of sows at farrowing increases the survival rate of pigs born. An induced farrowing program would reduce the labor required to accomplish this management recommendation and would likely increase the adoption rate by producers. When the farrowing period for a group of sows extends over several days or weeks, 24-hour observation of sows is much easier to recommend than to accomplish.

Controlled parturition has been accomplished by treatment of sows with prostaglandin-$F_{2\alpha}$ ($PGF_{2\alpha}$). A single intramuscular injection of 10 mg of $PGF_{2\alpha}$ on day 112 of pregnancy effectively induces the onset of parturition, with an average interval from injection to farrowing of about 28 hours. Treatment of sows at 8:00 AM results in the majority of sows farrowing the following day. In one field trial study, 141 of 149 sows farrowed wthin 48 hours following a single injection of 10 mg of $PGF_{2\alpha}$ on days 111 to 113 of pregnancy. Injections were made at 8:00 AM, and 65 per cent of the treated sows farrowed between 8:00 AM and 8:00 PM the following day. Some sows (16 per cent) farrowed within 24 hours following injection. When injections are delayed until 112 days of pregnancy or later to maximize birth weights and maturity of the offspring at the controlled farrowing, some precision in control is lost because of sows farrowing spontaneously on the day of treatment.

Typical immediate responses to $PGF_{2\alpha}$ treatment include nest-building activity by the sow, increased respiration rate, defecation and increased physical activity. Milk flow is consistently observed prior to farrowing. The average time required for farrowing (including placental expulsion) and the percentage of pigs born alive are similar for control and induced sows. Abortion at early stages of gestation can be induced by $PGF_{2\alpha}$.

Treatment of sows with prostaglandin analogues ICI 79,939 and ICI 80,996 to induce farrowing has given responses similar to treatment with $PGF_{2\alpha}$.

Premature parturition can also be induced by the administration of synthetic glucocorticoids. Sows treated with dexamethasone on days 101 to 104 of pregnancy have an average gestation period of about 109 days. Although premature delivery can be induced with dexamethasone, present treatments have limited practical application as a method for precise scheduling of the time of farrowing. Similarly, oxytocin or estrogen treatments are of limited value for the induction of parturition in a controlled farrowing program. However, oxytocin, when used with careful supervision, can be of value in the treatment of uterine inertia during the farrowing process. Parasympathomimetic drugs have been used to decrease the duration of farrowing with conflicting results. In some trials, feeding dichlorvos prior to farrowing or injecting 3 mg of carbomylcholine chloride (carbachol) subcutaneously after the birth of the first pig has reduced the time required for the completion of farrowing, with a trend toward a decrease in the rate of stillbirths.

REFERENCES

1. Randall, G. C. B.: Observations on parturition in the sow. I. Factors associated with the delivery of the piglets and their subsequent behaviour. Vet. Rec., *90*:178, 1972.
2. Randall, G. C. B.: Observations on parturition in the sow. II. Factors influencing stillbirth and perinatal mortality. Vet. Rec., *90*:183, 1972.
3. Sprecher, D. J., Leman, A. D., Dziuk, P. D., Cropper, M. and DeDecker, M.: Causes and control of swine stillbirths. J.A.V.M.A., *165*:698, 1974.

Obstetrics and Cesarean Section in Swine

LEWIS J. RUNNELS

Purdue University, West Lafayette, Indiana

Obstetrics, in relation to current development of swine production, must include the total management of parturition as well as the traditional manipulative and surgical relief of difficult parturition. Total management of parturition starts with selection of the dam and extends through gestation, lactation and weaning.

The objective of manipulative and surgical swine obstetrics is to deliver as many live, viable pigs as possible while preserving the strength and health of the sow so that she can effectively nurse and care for the live pigs. Dystocia in the gilt and sow occurs in 1 per cent or less of total farrowings[4] and is only a small part of the overall objective of swine production.

Recognition of dystocia requires supervision of farrowing in order that timely corrective measures can be effectively applied. The degree to which the objectives of obstetrics in swine can be met will depend primarily on the ability of the farrowing manager to recognize the need for obstetrical assistance as soon as possible. Therefore, good judgment must be exercised by both the manager and the veterinarian in making the decision as to the need for and the type of intervention required. Too much supervision and manipulative intervention can complicate a normal farrowing. A decision to intervene in parturition is not as easily made in swine as it is in some other species because the normal expulsive efforts of the sow are mild and there is a great variation in litter size, total delivery time and time between birth of each pig. A knowledge of the normal process of parturition in swine, experience in swine obstetrics and the availability of a good history will usually assure that beneficial actions are taken.[1,2] (See also preceding article on Parturition.)

Signs of difficult birth are prolonged gestation (more than 115 days), anorexia, appearance of blood-tinged discharge and meconium without straining or labor, straining and labor without delivery of any pigs, delivery of some pigs with subsequent cessation of labor, foul-smelling and discolored vulvar discharge and weakness and exhaustion of the gilt or sow.

The most common causes of dystocia in the pig are uterine inertia and oversized fetuses.[2-4] Positioning of the fetus is not as important in swine as in other animals, and a slightly larger number of pigs are born in anterior presentation than in posterior presentation.[3] In anterior presentation the nose and head are presented first, with the front legs extended caudally along the body. In posterior presentation the hind feet are normally presented first. If the sow is large, a pig may be born in the breech position without assistance, but this position will usually be the cause of obstructive dystocia in small sows and first litter gilts.

MANIPULATIVE TREATMENT OF DYSTOCIA

In all obstetrical manipulations in swine, it is imperative to have well-lubricated hands and instruments and to be gentle. Repeated entry into the birth canal and rough manipulation will cause contusion, bruising, swelling and infection of the maternal tissues and a resultant poor prognosis for the life of the sow. The temptation to examine the sow too frequently and the application of unnecessary assistance must be avoided.

Initially, a preliminary examination of the birth canal must be made. Strict hygiene must be practiced, and this includes washing the perineal and adjacent regions of the sow at least twice, preferably with an antiseptic soap. The hands and arms are then carefully scrubbed, and a sterile lubricating jelly is liberally applied to the hand and forearm being used in the examination. Usually it is easier to use the left hand if the sow is on her left side and the right hand when the sow is on her right side. The hand is cupped to form a cone, the lips of the vulva are gently entered and the hand is pushed gently into the birth canal. The birth canal may be so small in some gilts as to allow only the passage of one or two fingers. If dilation is complete, the vagina and uterus are confluent. When the pelvic opening is of sufficient size, the hand can be passed through the bony pelvis and then into the uterus. As the examination progresses, the birth canal should be explored for evidence of tears, bruising, a full bladder pushing against the vaginal floor, fracture of the pelvis and the presence of a fetus.

Fetuses in the birth canal can be grasped with the fingers by the nose, lower jaw, feet or head and delivered with gentle traction. Fetuses encountered cranial to the pelvic opening sometimes can be delivered with the fingers or hand in the same manner. When instruments must be used in making the delivery, they should be as simple and atraumatic as possible. An assortment of forceps, hooks and snares are available, but the pig and lamb snare has been the most useful and the least traumatic instrument. The snare consists of a rod that is 46 cm long with a handle on one end and a smooth cable terminating in a small ring slide. The cable forms a loop about 10 cm in diameter. The loop can be carefully carried or passed into the birth canal, and when the pig is encountered, it can be slipped over the nose, foot, head or hind parts, depending on which is most accessible. The loop is tightened down, and gentle traction is begun, taking care not to injure the fetus. Gentle, steady traction can be exerted for as long as 15 minutes, if necessary.

Dead fetuses that have undergone a degree of decomposition may be dry and friable. In these cases the same gentle traction must be used, along with copious lubrication of the birth canal. Sterile lubricating jelly or mineral oil is very good for this purpose. Patience and a gentle approach will allow many of these deliveries to be made. Forceful and rough traction must be avoided so that the part to which the cable is attached will not tear away, thus perhaps irretrievably losing the opportunity to make the delivery and subsequently having to resort to cesarean operation. A long forceps, such as the Knowles uterine forcep, can be used to some advantage, but this instrument is traumatic to the fetus and should be used on dead fetuses only. A small, blunt obstetrical hook can be passed into the mouth of the fetus and hooked behind the hard palate in the pharyngeal region. Traction usually results in extensive damage to the hard palate, but this is of no consequence in dead pigs. In a similar manner, two small, blunt obstetrical hooks can be placed, one in each

eye socket, and traction applied. Tissue damage will occur with this method also.

Immediately after delivery, the membranes and mucus are cleaned from the air passages of the piglet. Gentle shaking of the piglet in a head-down position will be helpful in allowing fluids to drain from the mouth and nose. Gentle rubbing and massage will help to stimulate respirations. After respirations are established, the pig should be placed next to the sow's mammary glands so that nursing can be initiated at the earliest possible moment. Routine ligation or clamping of the naval cord is not necessary but may be done if there is hemorrhage.

The birth canal should be re-examined and further deliveries made, if expedient. It is impossible to determine with certainty that parturition has been completed because the cranial tips of the horns of the uterus cannot be reached by vaginal examination. A reasonable judgment can be made, however, based on visual appraisal of the distention of the sow's abdomen, the number of piglets delivered, the quantity of placenta passed, and the character of the vaginal discharge. If the placenta is seen at the vulvar opening, it must be assumed that another piglet is present because retention of the placenta is very rare in the sow.

CESAREAN OPERATION IN THE SOW

The indications for cesarean operation in the sow are primary inertia, secondary inertia, oversized fetuses, fetal monstrosities and a small or damaged birth canal. A decision for or against cesarean operation must be based on the condition of the sow, the potential number of live fetuses remaining, the type of dystocia and the value of the sow and the pigs to be delivered. The operation is most advantageously performed on sows that are not suffering from exhaustion, with the expectation that a majority of the piglets will be delivered alive. The surgery can be performed in most modern farrowing facilities with only minor adjustments. The sow can be transported to a surgery if the farm facilities are not satisfactory, but generally it is better to avoid the additional stress and time required for transport. In the event that the sow is in a minimal disease or specific pathogen-free (SPF) herd, the surgery must be done on the premises or in a facility in which there is no contact with other swine.

The choice of anesthetic methods is optional and should suit the preference and experience of the surgeon and the conditions of surgery. One technique that has been most useful in the field is epidural anesthesia.[1] It is inexpensive, requires a minimum of equipment, needs no monitoring and causes no depression of the sow or fetuses. Anesthesia is maintained as far cranially as the umbilicus, rendering the hind parts immobile. The mobile front parts must be tied down to prevent interference with surgery.

Instruments can be sterilized by previous autoclaving or by chemical solutions just prior to initiation of surgery, and a standard preparation of the operative site is performed.

At least three different incision sites have been used, but the preferred site is 7.5 to 10 cm dorsal and parallel to the base of the mammary glands, extending 20 to 25 cm cranially from just caudal and ventral to the cranial part of the fold of the flank. The incision is made through the skin, subcutaneous tissues and muscle layers down to the peritoneum. Some of the branches of the subcutaneous abdominal vein may require ligation before entry into the abdominal cavity. After hemostasis is established, a blunt opening is made in the peritoneum, using care not to puncture the distended uterus. The final incision should be large enough to allow the uterus to be brought to the outside with minimal traction. Considerable care needs to be exercised to prevent damage or transverse tearing, because the uterus may be very friable if distended by a large number of fetuses or if decomposition has begun.

A sterile plastic or rubberized sheet is attached just below the incision. The abdominal cavity is examined, and a determination is made as to whether piglets are located in one or both horns and their approximate number. The most accessible portion of the horn containing piglets is brought through the incision and is allowed to lie on the plastic or rubber sheet. If the horn contains a large number of fetuses and if it is obvious that the contralateral horn is similarly filled with fetuses, it is best to attempt to make the incision in the uterus at a midpoint between the ovarian end and the bifurcation. Piglets can be delivered from both directions

with a minimum of manipulation. The incision is made on the side opposite the attachment of the broad ligament, avoiding as much of the vascular supply as possible. Some fetuses will have to be delivered by entering the lumen of the uterus, grasping the fetus and withdrawing it to the outside with gentle traction. Usually no attempt is made to remove the placenta unless it is free in the uterus.

After all pigs are delivered from the horn, the external surface is rinsed with warm saline and all but the incision site is replaced in the abdominal cavity. The incision is sutured with No. 1 or 2 chromic catgut with a continuous right angle Cushing pattern. A final rinse of the exposed uterus is made. It is then replaced, and the contralateral horn is withdrawn and dealt with in the same fashion.

If only a few fetuses remain in the uterus at the initial examination, an incision may be made at the bifurcation, thus delivering all pigs from both horns through one incision. Care must be exercised in locating this incision because tearing can easily occur, particularly when it is necessary to enter the uterine horns to extract pigs from the ovarian tip. A torn incision will oftentimes bleed profusely and will present difficulties in suturing. Before closure of the final uterine incision is made, both horns and the body of the uterus must be examined for any fetuses that may have been overlooked.

The abdominal incision is closed in a standard fashion using No. 2 chromic catgut. The skin incision is closed with a nonabsorbable suture that is removed in 10 days. As an alternative, a subcuticular suture may be placed for skin closure, thus eliminating the need for removing nonabsorbable sutures later.

Postoperatively, an injection of oxytocin is given to stimulate uterine contraction, and in cases in which there was a contaminating environment or decomposed pigs an antibiotic is given for 3 to 5 days. The prognosis is favorable if live pigs have been delivered and if there are no surgical complications.

The time required for the cesarean operation will depend on the availability of assistance. In most field circumstances the surgeon has no one to help other than the producer or farrowing barn manager and must perform preoperative, operative and postoperative tasks as well as administering the anesthesia, thus extending the total operative time.

REFERENCES

1. Hall, L. W.: Wright's Veterinary Anesthesia and Analgesia. 7th Ed. Baltimore, The Williams and Wilkins Co., 1971.
2. Jones, J. E. T.: Observations on parturition in the sow. Part II. Br. Vet. J., *122*:471, 1966.
3. Randall, G. C. B.: Observations on parturition in the sow. Vet. Rec., *90*:178, 1972.
4. Wrathall, A. E.: Reproductive Disorders in Pigs. Review Series No. 11 of the Commonwealth Bureau of Animal Health, Central Veterinary Laboratory, Weybridge, England, 1975, p. 216.

Surgical Procedures on Boars and Sows

W. BOLLWAHN

Tierärztliche Hochschule Hannover, Hannover, Germany

ANESTHESIA AND SEDATION IN BREEDING PIGS

Surgical procedures on the genital organs should be done under general anesthesia as a matter of principle to avoid secondary lesions caused by irritation or trauma (e.g., acute cardiac insufficiency, acute necrosis of the back muscles, injuries). The depth of the anesthesia must be adapted to the general condition of the animal. When there has been loss of blood (e.g., vulval hemorrhage, prolapsed uterus) or intoxication (e.g., emphysematous fetuses, endometritis), the general anesthesia should be as shallow as possible (stage III, 1). The required analgesic is given by local or spinal anesthesia.

Spinal anesthesia in swine is administered in the form of extra- or subdural lumbosacral anesthesia. A 2 per cent local anesthetic is injected through the foramen lumbosacrale, which is located between the two highest points of the iliac prominences (tuber sacrale) (Fig. 1). As soon as the 10- to 14-cm long mandrin cannula has penetrated into the vertebral canal (canalis vertebralis), the mandrin is removed and about 1 to 2 ml of air is injected to check the permeability of the cannula and to make sure that the tip of the cannula is in fact inside the vertebral canal. Aspiration is then attempted with the same syringe. Depending on the position of the cannular syringe, it is possible to aspirate fluid from the subdural space, blood from a vein on the floor of the spinal canal or nothing at all if the cannula is in the extradural space. If blood has been aspirated, the cannula is withdrawn slightly, and its position is checked once more.

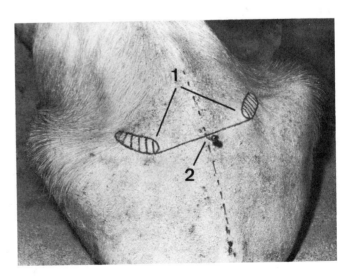

Figure 1. Spinal anesthesia. *(1)* Tuber sacrale, *(2)* position for puncture of the foramen lumbosacrale.

The dosage of the 2 per cent local anesthetic depends on the distance from the crown of the head to the base of the spine (linea nuchalis to tail root) and is 0.5 ml per 10 cm of distance for a subdural injection and 0.7 ml per 10 cm for an extradural injection. This dosage is sufficient to perform operations caudal to the costal arch. The full effects of the anesthetic develop within 4 to 10 minutes.

For general anesthesia, short-acting barbiturates or the combination of azaperone and methomidate is equally effective. Neuroleptics derived from phenothiazines (tranquilizers) should not be used to increase the potency of the barbiturate anesthesia since they have a vasodepressive effect that is difficult to control (alpha-blockade). In operations cranial to the umbilicus, spinal anesthesia can no longer be used. In such cases, e.g., amputation of claws on the forelimbs, mammectomy, a deep and long-acting anesthesia should be given, using pentobarbital that is intensified by the additional local subcutaneous application of a 2 per cent local anesthetic. In a mammectomy, a rhombic operative field is infiltrated; for a claw amputation, a circular infiltration anesthesia is applied proximal to the fetlock.

SURGICAL TREATMENT IN SOWS

Operations on gravid sows are associated with the risk of abortion or fetal damage. This risk can be avoided only by inducing anesthesia without excitation, by keeping blood losses to a minimum and by suppressing excitation conditioned by pain in the postoperative phase by means of drugs such as analgesics or neuroleptics. Maternal blood losses during the last 4 weeks of gestation lead to congenital anemia of baby pigs and should therefore be offset by iron substitution (1 to 2 g of iron per injection or ferrous fumarate orally). The barbiturates and neuroleptics that enter the fetal circulation do not reach life-threatening concentrations as long as the respiration and circulation of the brood animal are intact.

Animals with acute loss of blood, e.g., vulval hemorrhage, amputation of the uterus, mammectomy, and clinically identifiable circulatory stress, i.e., tachycardia greater than 140 beats per minute, pale conjunctiva, cyanotic snout tip, lowered body surface temperature, must be protected from circulatory failure (shock) by intravenous volume substitution (0.9 per cent NaCl solution, 6 per cent glucose solution, plasma expander) and by the application of heat (straw, infrared light). In surviving pigs, erythropoiesis should be reinforced by iron substitution.

Reposition of the Prolapsed Uterus

Definition. Inversion and prolapse of the uterus occur chiefly during parturition or up to the third day postpartum. The prolapse may have been complete (involving the corpus and cornua) or partial. In a complete prolapse, there is the danger of rupturing blood vessels in the mesovarium (artery spermatica interna, artery uterina media). Delayed involution and painful lesions in the soft birth canal that stimulate straining (labor, tenesmus) are considered to be causes of prolapse.

The attempt to perform a reposition is appropriate only when the general condition of the animal still permits the use of anesthesia. In cases of severe injuries to the uterus (contusion, rupture), extended necrosis of the mucosa and high-grade congestion, the reposition should not be attempted.

Treatment. After a general examination, the sow is anesthetized, using shallow general anesthesia and spinal anesthesia. The prolapsed uterus is cleaned with *cold* water and placed on a clean cloth. The anesthetized sow is immobilized on its right side on a plank or ladder, so that the pelvis can be kept elevated.

Every reposition, including that of a partial prolapse, should be undertaken starting from the peritoneal cavity by pulling on the tip of the horn and from the outside by pressure on the mucosa. Moreover, the opening of the peritoneal cavity makes it possible to determine if all the baby pigs have been born and if the inverted parts of the uterus have been completely everted.

If it proves impossible to reach the tip of the horn from the peritoneal cavity, the mesentery (ligamentum latum uteri) should not be pulled. Instead the prolapsed horn must be opened in the vicinity of the bifurcation by a longitudinal incision, so that the operating surgeon can grasp the tip of the horn with his right hand and pull it into the pelvis. When the reposition has been completed, this incision is positioned forward through the laparotomy incision and is sutured.

The laparotomy is done from the left flank. The surgeon places his left arm in the peritoneal cavity and locates one tip of the horn. This is carefully repositioned by pulling from the inside and exerting pressure from the outside upward as far as the bifurcation. The same procedure is followed for the second horn. The corpus uteri and the cervix are repositioned mainly by pressure from the outside. Fetuses that have not yet been expelled are extracted only when the reposition has been completed. The cavum abdominis and cavum uteri are prophylactically treated with a suspension of antibiotics. The laparotomy incision is closed either in two stages (peritoneal suture plus cutaneous-muscle suture) or three stages (peritoneal suture plus muscle suture plus cutaneous suture).

To prevent a recurrence, contraction of the uterus is stimulated by administering 20 to 30 IU of oxytocin intramuscularly, and the vagina is narrowed to an opening of approximately 4 cm by means of a Buhner closing. The Buhner closing is a deep subcutaneous suture around the

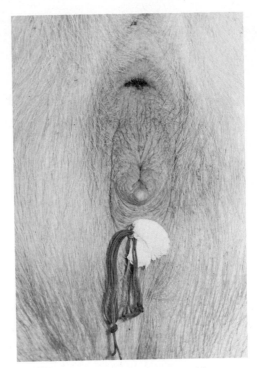

Figure 3. Closed Buhner suture with gauze.

vulva (Figs. 2 and 3). A 10-cm long needle enters the skin lateral to the distal commissure, and a strong silk or synthetic thread is drawn along the base of the labium to the dorsal commissure, at which point the skin is pierced by the needle in the medial line of the perineum. Through this exit opening, the thread is then taken along the base of the other labium to a point distal to lateral of the distal commissure, so that the beginning and end of the suture lie opposite each other here and can be tied together in a bow. The exit of the vagina is narrowed by tightly drawing the Buhner suture to approximately 2 finger breadths in order that urination and expulsion of fetal membranes can occur without interruption. Placing the Buhner suture is digitally controlled from the vagina, so that neither the mucosa nor the rectum is perforated in the process.

As of the third or fourth postoperative day, the Buhner suture can be loosened. It should not be removed before the sixth postoperative day, so that it can be closed again if the prolapse tends to recur. Following a prolapse, a catarrhal, purulent endometritis develops, which may negatively affect the chances of conception. Depending on the duration and the degree of

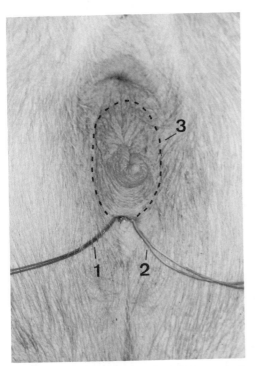

Figure 2. Buhner suture for prophylaxis against recurrence of vaginal prolapse. (*1*) Entry of needle, (*2*) exit of needle and (*3*) subcutaneous suture.

the prolapse, the success rate for this operation ranges from 30 to 80 per cent.

Reposition of the Prolapsed Vagina

Definition. Vaginal prolapse occurs predominantly during the last days of gestation. A complete prolapse in such cases is mostly associated with a severe edema of the vulva. As a result of continuous straining (labor, tenesmus), a prolapse of the rectal mucosa frequently develops as well. In addition to causing local lesions of the mucosa, this results in impeded urination and cervicitis. The latter conditions, in many cases, make it impossible to open the soft birth canal normally, so that a cesarean section is called for. Vaginal prolapse that occurs early also involves the danger of uterine infection accompanied by fetal death. Because the etiology of vaginal prolapse is unknown, only symptomatic treatment can be carried out.

Treatment. To avoid further complications such as lesions or prolapse of the rectum, the sow is anesthetized and the pelvis elevated. The prolapse is cleaned with cold water and spread with a viscous suspension of antibiotics. The prolapse must be pushed back toward the sacrum. Because of the danger of perforation, one works with the palm or fist, not with the fingertips. As soon as the prolapse has been repositioned as far as the pudendal cleft (rima vulvae), it is pushed with the fist through the opening of the pelvis (apertura pelvis) until it is in front of the pubic bone (pecten ossis pubis). The hand is then pulled back *slowly* to avoid creating a negative pressure in the vagina, for this could lead to a renewed inversion.

Before the vagina is closed to prevent a recurrence of the prolapse, the urinary bladder is emptied with a catheter. The vagina is closed with a Buhner suture, as previously described. When the farrowing begins, the Buhner suture must be opened. An imminent farrowing should be expected as soon as a continuous stream of milk comes when the sow is milked.

Repositon of the Prolapsed Rectum

Definition. Prolapse of the rectal mucosa occurs as a result of straining (tenesmus), when excretion has become difficult (solid fecal lumps, stricture) and during a bout of proctitis (diarrhea, ulcer). It also appears as a secondary disorder in vaginal prolapse. The dark red mucosa quickly becomes edematous and often shows bleeding lesions. In contrast to rectal prolapse in fattened hogs, which mostly represents an invagination of the rectal wall and must be corrected by resection, the prolapsed rectal mucosa in sows can be repositioned. The prognosis is good even for severe lesions and necroses of the mucosa.

Treatment. The reposition is performed on the anesthetized animal with the pelvis elevated. Small prolapses are pushed back *in toto* with the arched inner surface of the palm. For larger prolapses, the mucosa is rolled and pushed back with both thumbs. To prevent a renewed prolapse, the anus is narrowed by a circular purse-string suture. A strong thread of silk or synthetic is passed in and out through the skin around the anal opening at a distance of 1 cm from the rim of the anus. The ends of the thread are pulled until the anus is tightly closed. The feces that collect in the ampulla of the rectum must be removed at least once a day. To do this, the closing of the purse-string suture is opened and then is closed tightly once more. Before the suture is removed completely, it is left open for 1 or 2 days, so that it can be closed again if necessary.

To assist in the treatment, the sow should receive no solid food for the first 2 days after the rectal prolapse appears and should be given only water *ad lib.*

Amputation of the Prolapsed Uterus

Definition. In most cases, amputation of the prolapsed uterus leads to circulatory failure. Amputation is indicated when prolapses cannot be repositioned and when there are severe lesions. The procedure should be performed only if the sow still appears to be in relatively good general condition. Before the amputation, it must be ascertained that the nonprolapsed parts of the uterus contain no additional fetuses and that the urinary bladder or loops of intestine have not entered the prolapse.

Treatment. Before the amputation, the animal is anesthetized with thiobarbiturate, and the pelvis is elevated. The wall of one prolapsed horn of the uterus is opened longitudinally near the bifurcation

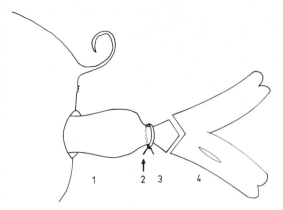

Figure 4. Amputation of the uterus. *(1)* Vaginal prolapse, *(2)* ligature, *(3)* stump of amputation and *(4)* control incision.

using a control incision, so that one hand can be placed in the pelvis to check for retained fetuses or prolapsed abdominal organs such as the urinary bladder or intestinal loops. Unborn baby pigs must first be removed by extraction or cesarean section, and the prolapsed organs must be repositioned. Next, a ligature of elastic material (rubber, synthetic) is placed around the prolapse at a distance of 10 to 15 cm from the vulva and is tied very tightly. The prolapse is then resectioned in the shape of a wedge, so that a 5- to 10-cm long stump remains (Fig. 4) and the arteries located in its center cannot be retracted. It is not necessary to suture the stump. The prolapsed vagina with the amputated stump is repositioned, and the vulva is closed with a Buhner suture, as previously described. The elastic ligature must not be removed; it will be sloughed off spontaneously after 10 to 14 days. The amputation of the uterus results in severe loss of blood, which must be replaced intra- and postoperatively by volume substitution (see previous discussion).

Treatment of Vulval Hemorrhage

Definition. As a rule, hemorrhages resulting from vulval lesions that are hard to arrest or threaten to be fatal occur only in connection with parturition. Initially, a primary vulval hematoma occurs, which increases the fragility of the labia. Lesions of the labia are then incapable of provoking spontaneously coagulating hemorrhages.

Treatment. The sow is anesthetized

and placed with the bleeding labium facing upward. Both the considerable enlargement of the labium and the fact that the tissue is saturated with blood make regulated hemostasis impossible. The bleeding is therefore arrested by means of one to three U-shaped mass ligatures at the base of the labia, i.e., the area where the labia merge into the area of the thigh and the perineum. A round (atraumatic) needle and silk or synthetic suture material are used. For each ligature, the wall of labium is pierced from the inside going outward, beginning in the dorsal commissure. The thread must be long enough (about 120 cm) so that it can be cut off on the outside after perforating the labium; thus, with each perforation, the beginning and end of a U-suture are formed (Fig. 5). To keep the thread from cutting into the skin or the mucosa of the labium, rolls of gauze are placed under it before knotting. The sutures remain in place for 2 days. To accelerate the resorption of the vulval hematoma, lead or aluminum acetate is applied to the vulva and its surrounding area twice a day.

Catheterization of the Lateroflexed Bladder

Definition. In older gravid sows in the last stage of gestation, lateroflexion of the

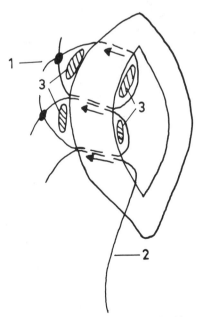

Figure 5. Mass ligature in bleeding vulval hematoma. *(1)* Beginning, *(2)* end of thread and *(3)* gauze.

urinary bladder into the space between the vagina and the pelvic wall (excavatio vesicouterina) occasionally occurs. The result is a *unilateral* forward arching of the vaginal mucosa and of the vulva that looks deceptively like a vaginal prolapse (Fig. 6). The lateroflexion obstructs urination and provokes straining (tenesmus), so that a partial or complete vulval prolapse can result.

Treatment. The reposition of the displaced urinary bladder by exerting pressure on the vulva or the perineum is usually unsuccessful. Only when the bladder is emptied by a catheter does a spontaneous reposition occur within several hours. To bring about a permanent emptying of the bladder and the retraction of the bladder wall, a self-retaining permanent catheter (Foley-type balloon catheter) is introduced and taped to the skin of the thigh (Fig. 7).

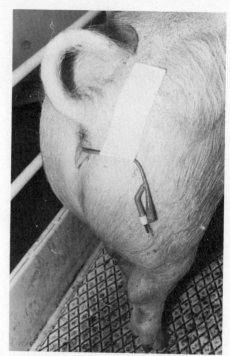

Figure 7. Catheterization of the urinary bladder.

Surgical Removal of the Mammae

Definition. Chronic infection of the mammae with *Actinomyces suis* results in the tumorous alteration of the mammary

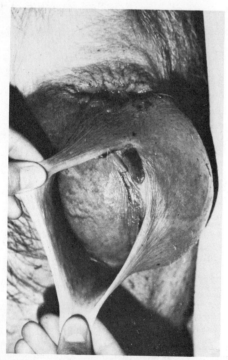

Figure 6. Lateroflexion of the urinary bladder.

parenchyma by granulomas, abscesses and fistulae. As soon as the actinomycomas have become larger than a hen's egg, their conservative treatment becomes problematic, so that a mammectomy is indicated. The operation should not be performed during the first and last 4 weeks of gestation in order to prevent the risk of abortion or of congenital anemia of baby pigs.

This operation is contraindicated if there are fewer than 12 intact mammary complexes or if problems can be expected when the incision is sutured because of the size of the actinomycoma.

Treatment. For operations caudal to the umbilicus, the combination of general and spinal anesthesia is recommended. Operations in the anterior mammary region necessitate a deep general anesthesia (pentobarbital) as well as a circular infiltration of the complex to be resected, using a 2 per cent local anesthetic *without* an adrenergic. This injection is given subcutaneously in rhombic form.

Bleeding that occurs during the operation is at first temporarily arrested with artery clamps; on the average, 12 clamps are required.

The operation begins with a circular incision in the skin at the base of the actinomycoma. The tissue that lies below the

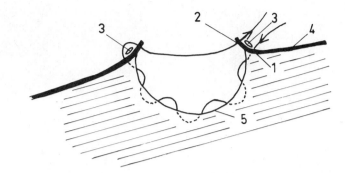

Figure 8. Suturing technique to prevent a seroma. *(1)* Entry of needle, *(2)* exit of needle, *(3)* gauze, *(4)* outside skin and *(5)* floor of incision.

tumor is separated either by blunt dissection or with a scissors in order to reduce the tendency to bleed (avoid the vena subcutanea abdominis). On the lateral side of the actinomycoma, the surgeon first penetrates at a single point into the retromammary tissue (connective and fatty tissue) and enucleates the actinomycoma from this point, proceeding medially. Before the definitive hemostasis is performed by means of vessel and mass ligatures, the floor of the incision is carefully checked for isolated microactinomycomas (as small as pea-sized nodules).

The extirpation of an actinomycotic mammary complex unavoidably causes an extensive deep incision. The closing of this wound must therefore be performed in such a way that no cavity remains, which could promote the formation of a seroma. The suture that is suitable for this purpose at first undulates through the floor of the incision and then returns in the opposite direction to catch the rims of the incision (external skin). In this way the floor of the incision and the external skin are brought into apposition when the thread is tied (Fig. 8). Gauze is placed under the extracutaneous part of the suture to protect the skin.

When the sutures have been tied, an aqueous suspension of penicillin or 5 to 10 ml of tincture of iodine is infiltrated in the area of the incision with a blunt cannula. The sutures are removed on the eighth day postoperatively.

SURGICAL TREATMENT IN BOARS

Exposure and Examination of the Penis

Definition. A passive exposure is performed on the anesthetized boar in order to examine and treat the penis. The most frequent indications for an exposure are bleeding on erection or urination, surgical treatment of injuries of the penis and collection of sperm by electroejaculation.

Technique of Exposure. The boar is placed under shallow thiobarbiturate anesthesia. For the right-handed surgeon, the animal should be placed on its right side. During the early stage of the anesthesia, there is a medium-grade intrapreputial erection that facilitates the exposure of the penis.

With the right hand, the surgeon grasps the erect shaft of the penis about 10 cm caudal to the tip of the penis. The thumb and forefinger of the left hand lie near the opening of the prepuce. While the penis is pushed cranially with the right hand, the prepuce is drawn back with the left hand. In this way, the mucosa of the prepuce is everted forward through the opening of the prepuce, so that a funnel-shaped orifice is formed, within which the tip of the penis becomes visible (Fig. 9). An assistant (wearing a cloth glove) must immobilize the penis and pull it upward.

In a complete exteriorization of the penis and retraction of the prepuce, the following should be examined primarily: the tip of the penis, the crista penis, the plica and the orificium urethrae, as well as the base of the penis. Near the base, extensive adhesions (posthitis adhaesiva) are occasionally found, and in the area of the tip, lesions and abnormalities occur.

Reposition of the Prolapsed Penis

Definition. After treatment with neuroleptics, a complete or partial prolapse of the penis and of the preputial mucosa occasionally develops (Fig. 10). Depending on the duration of the prolapse, the penis

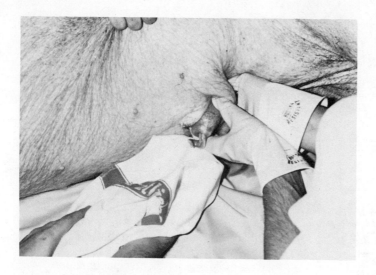

Figure 9. Exposure of the penis.

not only increases in volume because of congestion but lesions and contamination also appear. These may be significant causes of a later balanoposthitis.

Treatment. Until a veterinarian begins treatment, the prolapsed penis should be protected from injuries by being wrapped in a damp towel.

The reposition is performed on the anesthetized animal. First the mucosa is cleaned with cold water and then covered with an oily antibiotic suspension. During the reposition, the mucosa and penis must

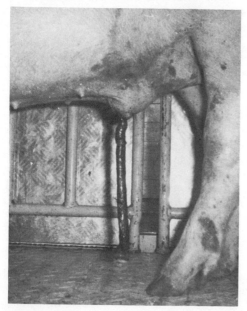

Figure 10. Prolapse of penis after injection of neuroleptic.

be pushed back through the ring-shaped opening that lies between the cranial and caudal sections of the preputial cavity (Fig. 11*d*). The closing of the preputial opening with a purse-string suture should be undertaken only if another prolapse occurs, as this provides for prophylaxis against recurrence.

To avoid sexual excitation, the boar must be isolated for the first few days after the reposition. The risk of balanoposthitis can be minimized by repeated intrapreputial instillation of an antibiotic suspension. The drug, e.g., 5 to 10 ml of chlortetracycline (Aureomycin) suspension, is given by a catheter in the caudal section of the preputial cavity and is thoroughly distributed by massage from the outside. Mating can resume 2 weeks, postoperatively.

Surgical Removal of the Prolapsed Prepuce

Definition. The prolapsed mucosa of the prepuce can develop severe swelling and rigidity as a result of injury and infection. This makes it impossible to reposition the prepuce. The resection of this part of the mucosa is possible as long as the entrance into the preputial diverticulum has remained intact (Fig. 12).

Treatment. The operation is done with the animal under general anesthesia. First the hairs at the opening of the prepuce are removed. The prolapse is pulled forward slightly, and the skin of the prepuce is pulled back somewhat, so that intact mucosa becomes visible. At this point, the pro-

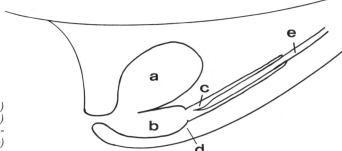

Figure 11. Preputial sac of the boar. *(a)* Preputial diverticulum, *(b)* cranial, *(c)* caudal section of preputial cavity, *(d)* ring-shaped bulge between *b* and *c* and *(e)* penis.

lapse is immobilized with a padded artery clamp or with a gauze bandage in order that the stump will not be retracted into the prepuce after the resection.

Two catgut threads (Fig. 13), each 40 cm long, are run crosswise through the prolapsed tube of mucosa. The threads are pulled tight, and the prolapse is cut off 5 mm in front of them. Now the threads are pulled upward from the middle of the tube of mucosa and are cut through so that four separate stay sutures can be tied. Between the four stay sutures, at least two more stay sutures, each with buttons, are then placed. Thus, a total of 12 stay sutures ring the edges of the stump. Now the immobilizing clamp or bandage is removed, and the stump is pushed back into the prepuce. Mating can resume 2 weeks postoperatively.

Surgical Removal of the Preputial Diverticulum

Definition. The preputial diverticulum is located dorsal to the cranial section of the preputial cavity. It consists of two indistinctly separated sacs with a common access to the preputial cavity. The physiological significance of the preputial diverticulum is not known. Occasionally, it demonstrates a high-grade dilatation with urine retention, so that the prepuce swells and the preputial opening is displaced. In some boars, the penis enters the preputial diverticulum during erection, and ejaculation subsequently takes place here. The mucosa of the diverticulum may be thickened as a result of chronic inflammation and may contain bleeding ulcers. Anomalies or diseases of the preputial diverticulum can be eliminated by its extirpation without affecting the procreative capacity of the boar.

Treatment. To remove the preputial diverticulum, a general anesthesia of about 20 minutes is necessary; thus, pentobarbital should be given. A blunt instrument, e.g., an artery clamp or catheter, is introduced into the diverticulum before the operation so that the wall of the diverticulum can be located at all times.

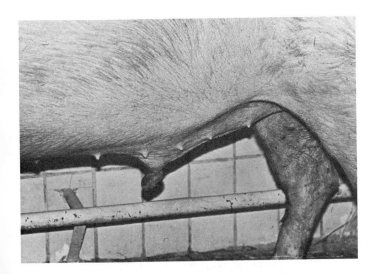

Figure 12. Prolapse of the preputial mucosa.

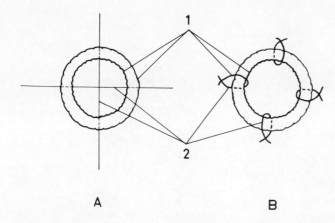

A   B

Figure 13. Suture in resection of prolapse of the preputial mucosa. *A,* Threads crossing mucosal tube. *B,* Button stay sutures made out of the threads in *A. (1)* Mucosa and *(2)* catgut. (Modified from Berge, E., and Westhues, M.: Tierärztliche Operationslehre, Berlin, Verlag P. Parey, 1969.)

The operation begins with a 10-cm incision a little above and 5 cm caudal to the preputial opening. This area has much fatty and connective tissue. The incision is carefully deepened until the preputial musculature, whose coarse fibers surround the diverticulum, is reached. To avoid injuring the very thin wall of the diverticulum, the muscle fibers are pushed apart by blunt dissection. The diverticulum that lies below the fibers is also dissected bluntly from the area surrounding it. This dissection is continued to the point at which the diverticulum merges into the preputial cavity (Fig. 14). Now both halves of the diverticulum, which are palm-sized and are linked with the preputial cavity over a short collum, can be recognized. An artery clamp is placed over this collum, and the diverticulum is cut off. The stump is closed with an inverting catgut suture (Fig. 15). The cavity that the extirpation of the diverticulum creates

between the abdominal wall and the prepuce is drawn together with a few catgut sutures. The skin incision is closed with a suture, and the epidermis and the floor of the wound are brought into close apposition (see Figure 8). The sutures are removed on the eighth postoperative day. Mating can resume 14 days, postoperatively.

Injuries to the Penis and Associated Hematuria

Definition. The most frequent injuries to the penis are abrasions on the crista penis, lacerations in the course of the plica urethralis and the loss of the tip of the penis. The injuries are caused for the most part by biting or masturbation. Acute hematuria appears after flexion of the erect penis as a result of a lesion of the corpus cavernosum or in association with urolithi-

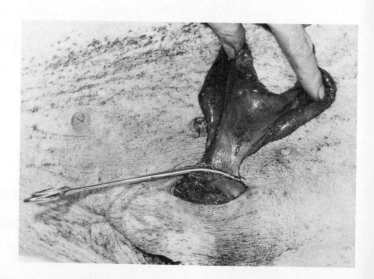

Figure 14. Resection of the preputial diverticulum. Artery clamp placed near transition to preputial cavity. Both halves of the diverticulum are exposed by dissection.

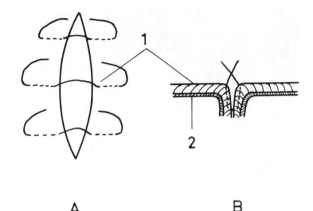

Figure 15. Inverting suture after resection of the preputial diverticulum. *A,* Dorsal view. *B,* Transverse section.

asis. The bleeding from the urethra, as well as the bleeding from the injuries, is especially intensive during ejaculation, so that the fertility of these boars decreases and disappears because of hemospermia. This type of injury-related bleeding should be distinguished by differential diagnosis from bleeding caused by ulcers of the diverticulum.

The prognosis is poor and treatment is not available for fistulae of the urethra, injuries to the tip of the penis accompanied by loss of tissue and abnormalities such as hypospadias or persistent ligamentum penis.

Treatment. If surgical treatment of the injuries (sutures, regeneration of the wound) is required, it is undertaken in connection with the examination of the passively exteriorized penis discussed previously. However, suppression of the tendency to bleed that accompanies the erection of the penis is much more important in order that the wound can form a scab and epithelialize. For this it is necessary to (1) keep the boar in isolation, (2) reduce his reflex excitability by giving neuroleptics, e.g., diazepam (Valium), with food, (3) promote the coagulation of blood by administering calcium solution and vitamin K and (4) interrupt mating for 4 weeks.

Amputation of the Claw

Definition. Infection of claw wounds caused by pyogenic bacteria often turns into a purulent arthritis of the pedal joint with osteomyelitis of the distal and middle phalanges. The disease involves primarily the outer claws of the posterior limbs and

causes an impotentia coeundi. As a rule, conservative attempts to treat this condition cause its protraction and deterioration. Therefore, amputation should be performed as soon as possible to prevent the formation of extensive necroses of the soft parts and to enable primary healing by suturing of the wound. The mating capacity of the boar returns after the amputation of the claw.

Treatment. The amputation is a very painful procedure. It necessitates general anesthesia as well as a local infiltration anesthesia (forelimbs) or a spinal anesthesia (posterior limbs). (See opening section of article.)

The preparation of the operative field (washing and shaving, removal of fat, disinfection) should reach as far as the tarsus or carpus, so that the bandage can later be attached there with tape. To suppress bleeding during the operation, an elastic ligature (Esmarch's bandage) is placed immediately distal to the tarsus or carpus.

The operation begins by making a circular incision at the edge of the horny capsule and extending it diagonally across the heel. In this way the pedal joint is opened and the distal phalanx is disarticulated. The next step is the exarticulation of the second phalanx. A 5- to 6-cm incision (Fig. 16) is made across the outside surface of the second phalanx, extending across the pastern joint into the distal region of the first phalanx. Using this incision, the second phalanx is excised from the soft parts and exarticulated in the pastern joint. The cartilage of the distal articular surface of the first phalanx is removed with a curette.

After the exarticulation of both distal

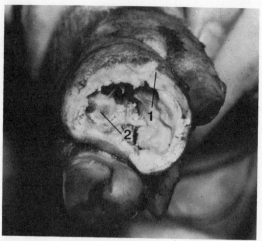

Figure 16. Amputation of the claw. *(1)* Lateral incision for exarticulation of the second phalanx and *(2)* distal end of first phalanx.

phalanges, all necrotic and discolored tissue is removed from the incision cavity and the navicular bone located in the heel is excised. With tweezers, the stumps of the sinews of the extensor tendon and of the deep flexor tendon are then pulled up from their synovial sheaths and resected as far proximally as possible. After this, the incision is ready for suturing, which is done with thick silk. The sutures should be brought into apposition with the walls of the suture cavity over the entire breadth of the surface. An oily Aureomycin suspension is instilled in the closed wound, and the stump is covered with gauze saturated with Aureomycin.

Before the bandage is put on, the accessory digits must be specially padded with cotton wool. The bandage consists of three layers: cotton wool, gauze and adhesive tape. The cotton wool should cover the stump up to the fetlock, including the accessory digits. The gauze bandage should be tight in order to have a compression effect. The adhesive tapes that are finally placed over the bandage act as mechanical protection and keep the gauze and cotton wool in place; they should reach as far as the metatarsus or metacarpus. The healthy claw remains outside the bandage. The elastic ligature is removed after the bandage has been put in place. If there is heavy bleeding from the stump, the ligature can be applied for another 20 minutes.

If the affected limb is knocked violently against the floor or wall during the awakening stage, the pig must be anesthetized or sedated once more.

The bandage is removed 8 days postoperatively under general anesthesia, the sutures are taken out and a new bandage is applied after dressing the wound. On the sixteenth postoperative day, the wound is examined again. The rims should now be epithelialized, and the center should show signs of granulation. If this is the case, a new bandage is put on. This can be removed after another 8 days without veterinary supervision. If the healing has not yet reached this stage, supervision should be continued.

Resection of the Canine Teeth

Definition. Starting with the eighth month of life, the mandibular canine teeth of the boar have grown so long that they are a dangerous weapon. The boar uses them by thrusting sideways or upwards with his head. Attacks on human beings often produce injuries in the knee (stifle joint). To make dealing with boars less dangerous, the mandibular canines are sawed off. Pinching them off makes the teeth splinter and injures the gums.

Treatment. The boar is anesthetized with a short-acting barbiturate or a combination of azaperone and methomidate and is placed on its side. With a wire saw 60 to 80 cm long, such as the one used for embryotomy, the canines are sawed off from the oral to buccal direction. The cut is made a few millimeters from the gums so that no soft parts are injured. Since the canines grow continually, they must be shortened again a few months later. The resection of the maxillary canines is usually not necessary.

REFERENCES

1. Berge, E. and Westhues, M.: Tierärztliche Operationslehre 29. Auflage. Berlin, Hamburg, Verlag P. Parey, 1969.
2. Bollwahn, W.: Die Untersuchung des Eberpenis. Dtsch. Tierärztl. Wschr., *81*:235, 1974.
3. Bühner, F.: Eine einfache chirurgische Verschluβmethode für alle Scheiden- und Uterusvorfälle Tierärztl. Umschau, *13*:183, 1958.
4. Evans, L. E. and West, J. K.: Resection of the preputial diverticulum in the boar. Proceedings 4th International Pig Veterinary Society Congress, Ames, Iowa, 1976.
5. Schulze, W. and Bollwahn, W.: Zu den Erkrankungen der Sauen vor, während und nach der Geburt. Dtsch. Tierärztl. Wschr., *69*:641;685, 1962.

Agalactia

CHARLES E. MARTIN
and RONNIE G. ELMORE
University of Missouri, Columbia, Missouri

DEFINITION

Agalactia, lactation failure or mastitis-metritis-agalactia (MMA) is an emergency disease syndrome in sows or gilts that threatens the lives of baby pigs because of starvation and neonatal diseases associated with malnutrition. Agalactia, as it is now known, occurs in the very early stages of lactation. It may be evident at the time of parturition. The incidence of the condition ranges from 0 to 100 per cent, with an average incidence of 13.1 per cent. Variations in observations by herdsmen or veterinarians have created variables in the recorded incidence because hypogalactia (reduced milk secretion) is more prevalent than agalactia (no milk secretion), and the former has often been overlooked. There is no known breed predilection, and the condtion occurs throughout the calendar year, although an increased incidence is seen during or shortly after periods of extremely high ambient temperatures.

PATHOGENESIS

Pathogenic mechanisms (cellular changes) occurring in agalactia are variable, because of different etiological agents or factors involved. Whether lactation failure is a distinct primary disease entity or more often is a secondary factor in other disease syndromes needs to be elucidated. The majority of affected animals have abnormalities within mammary gland tissues. These changes may be characteristic of mastitis or, more predominantly, of a nonfunctional lactational status when compared with normal lactating tissue in the same group of alveoli or lobules. Mastitic changes such as necrosis of parenchymal alveolar cell nuclei with cell wall degeneration may involve a single alveolus, groups of alveoli or lobules of mammary gland tissue. Lobular or more extensive involvement is less frequently observed than is small alveolar group involvement, which has prompted investigators to state that the degree of mastitis presented could not produce the clinical signs or the starvation often seen in the baby pigs.

Agalactic or hypogalactic sows often have mammary glands that have normal cellular structure with dilated, empty alveoli; dilated alveoli filled with a substance described as prelactational material; or normal collapsed alveoli. This nonfunctional status is believed to be the result of some insult to the endocrine sequence of events that allows the glandular tissue to secrete milk. Comparison of mammary gland tissues from normal control sows at similar stages of lactation with tissues from affected sows substantiates the belief. Mammary gland tissue at 3 to 4 days prepartum reveals structural similarities to the nonfunctional agalactic sow tissue. Cardiovascular changes in affected animals (physiological and pathological) are those associated with edema and hyperemia and occasionally with hemorrhage that involves tissues surrounding the mammary glands, regional and inguinal lymph glands, uterus, cervix, vagina, kidneys, synovial membranes, adrenal glands and, in some instances, the pituitary gland.

The etiology of agalactia is unknown. A triad of involvement (endotoxin, mastitis and agalactia) has been described by Nachreiner.[5] Endotoxins released within the intestinal tract as a result of individual stress susceptibility or poor management practices could be involved. Endotoxin release caused by mastitis with subsequent self-eradication of the bacteria involved is a distinct possibility. Mastitis with tissue destruction (endotoxin absence) and the resulting sequential events will produce the disease. Endocrine and metabolic disturbances can also produce agalactia; therefore, some combination of the proposed triad or a single element therein can be stated to cause agalactia. Another triad (stress, endotoxin, endocrine imbalance) could also explain the syndrome if consideration is given to the many recorded predisposing causes.

CLINICAL SIGNS

Evidence of agalactia will be present at the time of parturtion or within 72 hours postpartum. Similar signs occurring later in lactation will not be due to this disease syndrome, as presently characterized. Signs that are often observed include increased respiratory and heart rate, central nervous system depression, inappetence, elevated rectal temperature and reluctance to rise or to allow nursing, with accompanying signs of uncomfortable baby pigs. Evidence of mammary gland involvement detected by palpation may include slight-to-gross enlargement of one or more mammary glands with discoloration, excess firmness and more warmth in the affected area than in other body parts. Sensitivity reactions by the sow when handled are additional signs of involvement. A diagnosis of mastitis, assumed to be bacterial, is often made without sufficient evidence. Vaginal discharge of purulent material may be seen but is not a significant indicator of metritis. Affected sows may not reveal signs of mastitis or metritis or evidence of systemic disease. The typical affected sow will reveal one or more clinical signs that result in loss of baby pigs because of starvation or its complications. The affected sow usually recovers in 2 to 5 days, with or without re-establishment of lactation.

CLINICAL PATHOLOGY

With the present state of knowledge, the utilization of diagnostic clinical pathology testing is not economically valid except for microbiological determinations.

DIAGNOSIS

Specific clinical entities such as transmissible gastroenteritis, pseudorabies, ingestion of certain molds, metritis due to retained fetuses and certain mastitis syndromes can produce clinical signs, as previously described. A differential diagnosis must be considered in order to institute correct therapeutic or control measures, or both. Utilization of the history and clinical signs revealed and astute observations such as palpation of the mammary glands will usually permit an acceptable tentative diagnosis. Postmortem examination of one or more dead or very weak pigs will reveal additional valuable information, such as whether or not the pigs have nursed. Diagnostic efforts will be enhanced after observ-

ing results of first treatment and/or utilizing information obtained from milk cultures and sensitivity testing. The prognosis for sows or gilts is good relative to sustaining life. However, the prognosis regarding livability of the baby pigs is guarded unless lactation re-establishment is rapid or supplemental feedings are successful. Determining the prognosis must allow for factors such as chilling, diarrhea and other secondary neonatal diseases in the baby pigs.

TREATMENT

The objectives of treatment are re-establishment of milk flow as quickly as possible while sustaining the lives of the baby pigs and prevention of secondary complications in both the sow and baby pigs.

The fundamental principles of therapy on each farm or in each production unit will vary with the overall management knowledge of the associated veterinarian. This disease syndrome, with the multiplicity of stress factors that may be applicable, presents a therapeutic challenge to anyone with a distinct interest in the swine industry.

There is no single medicament superior to oxytocin. This hormone should be administered intramuscularly or intravenously. The route of administration depends on the practitioner's skill or judgments regarding excitability of the sow. Excitability and subsequent epinephrine release block the milk let-down reflex usually precipitated by oxytocin injection.

Corticosteroids should be administered at 12- to 24-hour intervals. Since cortisol (higher) and blood glucose (lower) values are significantly different in agalactic sows, there is a physiological basis for this therapy. Ringarp[6] increased baby pig livability by 7.6 per cent by the addition of prednisolone to the conventional therapy of antibiotics and oxytocin.

Antibacterials are incorporated in most therapeutic regimens since there is no immediate method of determining the presence of bacterial pathogens. Milk samples for culture and sensitivity testing should be obtained prior to initial treatments. A decision to change antibacterial therapy can be made in 24 to 48 hours, if necessary. Stock cultures of significant bacterial colonies can be obtained for future autogenous bacterin preparation. Maximum recommended dosages at the prescribed intervals for effective levels must be administered. The majority of bacterial sensitivities reveal that approved antibacterials for swine use are not generally effective.

Exogenous estradiol benzoate will produce consistently higher pituitary prolactin levels[1] and should be a part of the treatment regimen in many instances.

Phenothiazine-derivative tranquilizers are lactogenic because of an effect on hypothalamic-releasing factors in man, rabbits and rats. Although this effect is not proved in swine, there should be no hesitancy in using these products, if desired, for excitable, agalactic sows.

Drugs used for treating lactation failure in swine are summarized in Table 1.

Intravaginal or intrauterine infusions, douches or pessaries are described as successful treatments for agalactic sows. Such therapy stimulates a neurohormonal reflex action, with resultant posterior pituitary release.

In formulating therapeutic measures, one must always consider the need for supplemental dietary support for the baby pigs, as well as environmental alterations (if necessary) for the affected sow and pigs.

PREVENTION

Herd health management and nutrition counseling by the practicing veterinarian who has overall, specific swine herd knowledge is the best approach to preventing the agalactia syndrome. Full knowledge of the herd from breeding through farrowing is advantageous to initial contact at affected sow time. As flushing levels for one swine herd are maintenance levels for another, adequate nutrition is essential. This must include supplementation with selenium or other elements if the area or feedstuffs are known to be deficient. Gestational feeding of sows and gilts must be continuous and frequent enough to promote excellent health, especially late in gestation, for the "limit-fed" sow apparently cannot maintain blood glucose levels comparable with the "full-fed" sow. The level of blood glucose is extremely important to lactation and is lowered in agalactic sows.[3, 4]

Immunization procedures such as autogenous bacterins, as deemed advisable by the attending veterinarian, may assist in incidence reduction. This is especially true in those herds in which bacterial mastitis is frequent and may be the cause of agalactia or at least a secondary complicating factor.

TABLE 1. *Drugs Commonly Used in Treating Lactation Failure in Swine**

Name of Drug	Source	Dosage and Route†
Oxytocin	Most major drug companies	30–50 USP units IM or SC
Antibacterials:		
Penicillin	Most major drug companies	3000–10,000 IU/lb IM daily
Streptomycin	Most major drug companies	5–10 mg/lb IM daily
Erythromycin	Abbott Laboratories	1–3 mg/lb IM daily
Lincomycin	The Upjohn Company	5 mg/lb IM daily
Oxytetracycline	Most major drug companies	3 mg/lb IM or IU daily
Tylosin	Elanco	100–400 mg/100 lb IM daily
Corticosteroids:		
Predef 2-X	The Upjohn Company	5 mg/300 lb IM daily
Corticotropins:		
Adrenomone	Burns-Biotec	200 USP units IM at 110 days of gestation
Estrogens:		
Estradiol	Most major drug companies	1–2 mg IM within 48 hours of parturition

*This list is not exhaustive and is intended only to cite examples of available drugs for treatment of lactation failure in swine. The products listed are not recommended over any other equal product from any unlisted companies. This list is not intended to be an endorsement of only these drugs by the authors.

†The package insert of any drug should be consulted for dosages, warnings and so forth before that product is administered.

Stress reduction efforts throughout gestation are important preventive factors, especially near parturition. It has been apparent that use of new or remodeled farrowing facilities will initiate the agalactia syndrome in many sow herds. Acclimation efforts are in order, as well as acute attention to management and nutritional deficiencies.

Induction of parturition, or perhaps more correctly, the injection of prostaglandin-$F_{2\alpha}$ at day 111 to 113 has proved to be beneficial in preventing agalactia. A significant European study[2] during 1975 and 1976 revealed an incidence of agalactia of 39 per cent in treated versus a 60 per cent incidence in control sows. The physiological action of, need for and levels of prostaglandins in the preparturient and parturient sow require further attention. There are currently no commercially available prostaglandin products approved for use in food animals in the United States.

The use of corticotropin (ACTH) as an injection on day 110 has reduced clinical agalactia in some herds and should be considered, at least in those herds in which other implemented practices have failed to produce desirable effects. There are stress-susceptible and resistant lines of swine, and they do respond with an increase in ACTH levels to environmental factors such as increased humidity.

We are confronted with a complex disease syndrome that requires multifaceted considerations and efforts to produce desirable results in treatment or prevention. At this particular time, the incidence of the disease appears to be decreasing. However, there is apparently an increased understanding of the disease syndrome among swine herdsmen, and they may be making the adjustments and treatments that allow for reports of a decrease by veterinarians. Research efforts are few and slowly productive, but continuing.

REFERENCES

1. Anderson, L. L., Peters, J. B., Melampy, R. M. and Cox, D. F.: Changes in adenohypophysial cells and levels of somatotrophin and prolactin at different reproductive stages in the pig. J. Reprod. Fertil., 28:55, 1972.
2. Backstrom, L., Einarsson, S., Gustafsson, B. and Larsson, K.: Prostaglandin F_2 alpha-induced parturition for prevention of the agalactia syndrome in sows. Proceedings of International Pig Veterinary Congress, Ames, Iowa, 1976.
3. Martin, C. and McDowell, W.: Lactation failure. *In* Dunne, H. W. and Leman, A. D. (eds.): Diseases of Swine. 4th Ed. Ames, Iowa, Iowa State University Press, 1976.
4. Merck Veterinary Manual. 4th Ed. Rahway, New Jersey, Merck & Co., Inc., 1973.
5. Nachreiner, R. F.: Report NCR64. Tech. Comm., Lincoln, Nebr., 1973.
6. Ringarp, N.: Clinical and experimental investigation into a post-parturient syndrome with agalactia in sows. Acta Agr. Scand., Suppl. 7, 1960.

Porcine Pediatrics

STANLEY E. CURTIS
University of Illinois, Urbana, Illinois

KEITH W. KELLEY
Washington State University, Pullman, Washington

Preweaning deaths take a huge toll and greatly hinder improvement of reproductive efficiency in swine production. Fifteen to thirty per cent of all liveborn piglets die before they are weaned. Over half of these succumb during the first few days after birth. Neonatal morbidity leads to further waste. Major causes of death are chilling, starvation, overlay by the sow and infectious diseases.

Piglets that are heavier at birth are less prone to die neonatally. Half of all preweaning casualties weighed less than 2 pounds at birth, although there is no reason why most such piglets — if provided proper care — should not survive. Nutriture of the gestating dam can be managed so as to increase the birth weight of the piglets to a certain extent, but gestation nutriture and lactational performance are complexly related. Sows fed a specific diet during gestation in order to deliver piglets weighing more than 2 3/4 pounds or so on average tend to perform less well during lactation. Furthermore, heritability of birth weight in swine is practically nil. Reductions in neonatal morbidity and mortality must therefore be achieved primarily by improved management of smaller, weaker piglets. It follows that such care would support the life of their heavier, stronger littermates as well.

Birth is an abrupt and profound environmental change. The critical sequence of perinatal tasks facing the piglet makes the fact that any survive more remarkable than the fact that many do not.

INTRAPARTAL STRESS

Prenatal asphyxia is normal in all species, but it is especially severe in the pig. Fetal blood O_2 tension falls and blood CO_2 tension rises during parturition, mainly caused by reduced fetoplacental respiratory gas exchange.

Respiratory acidosis occurs when blood CO_2 tension rises without a simultaneous drop in renal bicarbonate excretion. Randall has compared blood CO_2 tension and blood pH (both measured just after delivery, but before the first breath) with subsequent viability in piglets. He developed a composite viability score for five traits — breathing quality, heart rate, muscle tone, time until standing was attempted and color. Piglets with lower viability scores had higher blood CO_2 tension and lower blood pH; respiratory acidosis was associated with both low viability and stillbirth.

Asphyxia causes increased peristalsis, anal sphincter relaxation and deep breathing. Meconium is found in the respiratory tract of most stillborn piglets, apparently having been inhaled with amniotic fluid when breathing movements were initiated prematurely in response to prenatal asphyxia. Attendance at farrowings to insure that each piglet's airway is clear has been found to increase neonatal survival.

Most stillborn piglets are lighter than liveborn littermates and are delivered toward the end of the birth order within a litter. The umbilical cord is ruptured before delivery in about 20 per cent of the piglets in the first third of the birth order, but in about 50 per cent in the last third. The umbilical cord has ruptured prematurely in almost all intrapartally stillborn piglets, and thus premature umbilical rupture probably contributes greatly to the severe perinatal asphyxiation that leads to stillbirth or low neonatal viability. It is not known whether the incidence of premature umbilical rupture can be reduced.

Although the duration of farrowing and the between-piglet interval tend to be directly related to stillbirth and to low viability of liveborns, there is considerable variation in these relations. Indeed, weak or stillborn piglets are sometimes delivered at the same time as strong, liveborn littermates. There is no evidence that shortening farrowing time by using drugs either decreases stillbirth or increases the viability of liveborn piglets.

TEMPERATURE STRESS

Chilling may be the underlying factor in death from any of the major direct causes. The chilled piglet is less likely to nurse and to get out of the sow's way. It is also more likely to develop an infectious disease. Of course, chilling may also directly cause the piglet to die.

The environment that the neonatal piglet finds itself in determines to a great extent how well body temperature can be controlled. The cooler the environment, the faster body heat will flow from the warm piglet to the relatively cool environment and thus the more trouble the piglet will have keeping its body temperature elevated.

Roughly 10 per cent of the neonatal piglet's body heat is lost during the normal evaporation of water from its upper respiratory tract and skin. Another 15 per cent of body heat flows to the floor by conduction when the piglet is lying down. Floor temperature and floor material affect this, but heat loss by conduction to the floor is relatively small in any case.

At least 75 per cent of the baby pig's heat flows to the environment by radiation or convection. The ratio between these two depends on environmental conditions. Certainly, environmental factors that affect either radiant or convective heat loss are important.

Wall and ceiling temperatures are the main factors determining radiant heat loss, while air temperature and air speed affect convective heat loss. Dropping wall and ceiling temperatures — even when air temperature remains the same — greatly increases heat loss from the piglets. Thus, farrowing houses should be well insulated to insure warm walls and ceiling.

When air, wall and ceiling temperatures all drop, for example, from 29°C to 21°C, the piglet's heat loss is two-thirds greater, meaning that it needs to consume about two-thirds more milk so as to be able to produce two-thirds more "make-up" body heat in the cooler environment.

The major effect of air speed on heat loss by convection occurs at very small departures from stillness. If any draft at all is present, the effect is almost as great as that of a large draft. The piglet is sensitive to drafts that the human hand can hardly feel.

Straw bedding is still probably the most effective means of providing baby pigs with a comfortable thermal environment. It permits the piglet to alter its own surrroundings to suit its needs. The piglet will make itself comfortable if given the opportunity. Covering the floor with 4 inches of straw in a 10°C environment has the same effect as does raising environmental temperature to 18.5°C. Furthermore, when the pig burrows in the straw, both radiation and convection are reduced. The straw then serves as a radiant shield between the pig and the wall and ceiling, as well as a protection against drafts.

Temperature, as measured by a standard thermometer, gives a very incomplete assessment of the environment that the piglet is experiencing. Also, if such a temperature measurement is to be of any use at all, it must be made in the piglet's immediate environment, not on a wall 5 feet up and 30 feet away. Air temperature at pig level may be as much as 8C° lower than at human eye level. Furthermore, the common wall thermometer gives almost no information about air speed at piglet level or about wall and ceiling temperatures. The piglet itself, by its behavioral reactions to the thermal environment, is still the best thermometer.

The newborn piglet is at an extreme disadvantage with regard to thermal insulation. It has neither much hair nor much subcutaneous fat. This is why its critical temperature of 35°C is so high. What this means is that the neonatal piglet must increase its metabolic rate in attempting to offset heat loss any time that the environmental temperatures fall below 35°C under draft-free conditions.

Any time a piglet is scrunched, lies in a tense position or is huddled, it is not as comfortable as it should be. General farrowing-house temperature should be between 21°C and 27°C at piglet level even when supplemental radiant heat is provided. Floor drafts should be prevented by solid partitions at least 1 foot high between farrowing stalls. The piglets ought to have more choice of environment than simply being under a radiant heat source or not. The means of providing a wider choice may involve placing a little box, which can serve as a radiation shield and heat retainer, in the stall so piglets can retreat to it if necessary, or it may involve placing some straw on the floor so the piglets have some burrowing material if they want it.

The piglet knows better than we do when it needs to have more environmental protection. Given a choice of effective environmental temperatures ranging from about 24°C to about 36°C, piglets in groups choose on average to reside at about 29.5°C. Not many farrowing houses consistently provide this warm an effective temperature.

Age has much to do with the piglet's ability to control body temperature. During the first 24 hours after birth there is an amazing improvement in its resistance to cold stress. This is mostly because its ability to increase its metabolic rate is greater at 1 day of age than at birth.

Many more neonatal piglets could be saved if they had warmer environments at their disposal. This is especially so during the first 12 hours after farrowing.

IMMUNITY

It is now clear that piglets already have immunoglobulins in their blood at birth, but the concentrations are too low to afford significant protection against infections. Absorption of colostral immunoglobulins (mostly IgG) by enterocytic pinocytosis is the main way piglets achieve passive humoral immunity. Of course, the "open gut" is nonselective — permitting direct access to the blood for certain environmental contaminants — and thus it is a mixed blessing.

Early-born piglets may have an advantage over later-born littermates because they have more time to consume colostrum. After 4 hours of nursing the concentration of immunoglobulins in colostrum is halved, and piglets deprived of early access to colostrum have significantly lower serum immunoglobulin concentrations than earlier-born littermates. One remedy might be to remove all piglets from the sow as they are delivered and return all littermates simultaneously after farrowing is completed. In this way, all piglets in the litter would have an equal opportunity to compete for colostrum. The fasted piglet's gut remains "open" to macromolecules for several hours after birth.

Sow's milk also contains immunoglobulins (mostly IgA) and this provides local protection in the intestinal tract. Hence, continual bathing of the neonatal piglet's intestinal lining by milk immunoglobulins is crucial to defenses against enteric pathogens.

Stress, in general, reduces the piglet's defenses against a variety of microbial pathogens. Because the neonatal piglet is particularly susceptible to cold stress in practical environments, chilling often predisposes the piglet to infectious disease.

BEHAVIOR

Within a litter, earlier-born piglets tend to have a greater chance for neonatal survival than those coming later in the birth order. In addition to reduced access to colostral immunoglobulins, the findings of more intrapartal stress and lighter birth weights in later-born piglets have already been noted. All of these may be related to differences in neonatal mortality.

Piglets that are heavier or less stressed at birth are generally more vigorous. Thus, they are more successful in fighting with littermates as teat order is established and consequently have earlier and more fre- quent access to the colostrum, even when all in the litter are put to the udder at the same time. Such piglets would then be expected to be better able to defend themselves against infections, such as those that commonly occur in the umbilicus, and against foot and leg abrasions.

ARTIFICIAL REARING

Most small or weak piglets are capable of surviving if cared for appropriately. One possible means of increasing their chances for survival is to wean piglets after as little as 12 hours of nursing the colostrum and then rearing them artificially. If consistent, favorable results are to be expected, however, strict management regimens must be followed: the piglets' environment must be comfortable and sanitary, and a special, sanitary diet must be provided at frequent intervals.

REFERENCES

1. Curtis, S. E.: Responses of the piglet to perinatal stressors. J. Anim. Sci., *38*:1031, 1974.
2. England, D. C.: Husbandry components in prenatal and perinatal development in swine. J. Anim. Sci., *38*:1045, 1974.
3. Hartsock, T. G. and Graves, H. B.: Neonatal behavior and nutrition-related mortality in domestic swine. J. Anim. Sci., *42*:235, 1976.
4. Lecce, J. G.: Rearing piglets artificially in a farm environment: A promise unfulfilled. J. Anim. Sci., *41*:659, 1975.
5. Randall, G. C. B.: The relationship of arterial blood pH and pCO_2 to the viability of the newborn piglet. Can. J. Comp. Med. Vet. Sci., *35*:141, 1971.
6. Wilson, M. R.: Immunologic development of the neonatal pig. J. Anim. Sci., *38*:1018, 1974.

Reducing Preweaning Mortality

JØRGEN SVENDSEN

The Swedish University of Agricultural
Sciences, Lund, Sweden

NILS BILLE

Royal Veterinary and Agricultural University,
Copenhagen, Denmark

During the past 15 to 20 years, the swine industry has undergone remarkable structural changes in most countries. The very small herds with only a few sows and gilts are rapidly disappearing, larger sow herds with a specialized production of weaner pigs are becoming increasingly common and large, highly mechanized feeding-finishing units are having an ever-growing share of the hog market. Structural changes within sow production and the application of new techniques by highly educated and capable producers may have increased the profitability of the entire production but have not, in general, led to a decline in death losses during the suckling period. Available statistics from many different countries show rather unanimously that 20 to 25 per cent of the total number of pigs born die before weaning, and this high mortality rate does not appear to have changed significantly during the past 15 to 20 years.

This article will discuss some of the economically important causes of preweaning mortality and the factors influencing these losses. Such general information is important for the successful introduction and implementation of relevant measures, which at the herd level aim at reducing the losses that are of major significance in the particular herd.

FACTORS INFLUENCING PREWEANING MORTALITY

Most of the death losses before weaning occur during parturition or in the early neonatal period. This is illustrated in Figure 1, which shows that almost 80 per cent of the total preweaning mortality occurs during the first week of life. This indicates that particular attention should be given to the perinatal period when attempts are made to reduce the preweaning mortality. When looking at the age distribution of the losses during the suckling period, it is also relevant to point out that the losses incurred during the first week of life, i.e., during the neonatal period, by and large are due to *noninfectious* causes. This means that noninfectious losses account for a significant proportion of the total preweaning mortality. Losses due to *infectious* diseases occur during the entire suckling period (Fig. 1). Again, most losses occur during the first week of life and may be a very serious problem in the individual herd. Only such diseases leading to death losses are considered. Total losses due to infectious diseases may be considerably higher.

The total preweaning mortality in a herd will be influenced by litter size at birth and by the age of the sow. Thus, it was observed that an average of 2.5 pigs, or 14.3 per cent, were lost before weaning in litters having 8 pigs born,[4] while 4.8 pigs, or 32 per cent, were lost from litters with 14 pigs born. However, the large litter with the higher mortality will still wean more pigs than the small litter, and this serves to illustrate that "preweaning mortality" may not by itself be used as a parameter of productivity but must be viewed in the context of the particular herd. The age of the sow also influences the death losses during the suckling period, in that old sows that have had eight or more litters have a considerably higher preweaning mortality rate than younger sows.

There is considerable herd-to-herd variation in the incidence of preweaning mortality. A consistently low level of preweaning losses in a herd over a longer period of time and a correspondingly higher average number of pigs weaned per litter is, to a great extent, a reflection of superiority with regard to management and husbandry in the herd and is also an indication of what may be achieved in commercial hog operations.

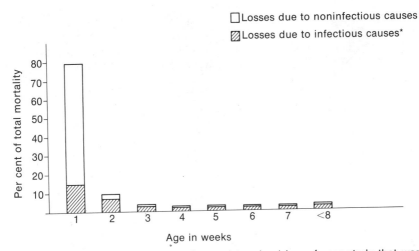

Figure 1. Age distribution of preweaning mortality as determined by a 4-year study that was conducted by the Laboratory of Swine Disease, Tåstrup, Denmark. The study involved 17 sow herds with a total of 5678 litters. Coworkers in the project were Drs. N. Bille, N. C. Nielsen, H. J. Riising and J. Svendsen.
*Infectious diseases such as TGE, hog cholera, brucellosis and leptospirosis do not occur in Denmark.

CAUSES OF PREWEANING MORTALITY

The main causes of preweaning mortality in pigs are presented in Table 1. The figures are derived from a 4-year study, involving 5678 litters, that was conducted in Denmark. The total preweaning mortality observed in this study was 22.3 per cent. Although it is realized that the figures may vary somewhat from country to country, it is believed that the relative distribution of the main groups of losses will prove to be similar, as will the factors influencing the losses.

Preweaning Mortality Due to Noninfectious Causes

From Table 1 it is apparent that losses due to death before or during parturition, starving or undersized pigs and trauma account for a very significant proportion of the total preweaning mortality. These losses occur almost exclusively within the first week of life, i.e., in the perinatal period, and most of them are due to noninfectious causes. Losses in the perinatal period and the herd and husbandry factors that influence these losses will be discussed in the following paragraphs.

Classification of Losses

Antepartum Deaths. Such deaths occur at a certain low level in all herds and may show considerable herd-to-herd variation. They occur with approximately the same frequency in small litters as in large litters, but the number increases with increased parturition time and is significantly higher in litters having a parturition time that exceeds 6 hours, than in litters that have a parturition time of less than 6 hours. In addition, there is a higher incidence of antepartum deaths among offspring from sows that have been strictly confined during the gestation period than in litters from sows that have been confined in pens.[2]

TABLE 1. *Classification of Death Losses before Weaning on Preweaning Mortality in Pigs**

Cause	Per Cent of Total Number of Pigs Born	Herd Variation
Death antepartum	1.6	(0.5– 5.6)
Death intrapartum	4.5	(3.0– 6.4)
Starvation/undersized	3.5	(0.6– 5.0)
Trauma	4.0	(1.3– 7.1)
Gastrointestinal diseases	2.0	(0.5– 3.9)
Pneumonias	0.6	(0.0– 1.3)
Acute generalized infections	0.9	(0.4– 1.7)
Malformations	1.1	(0.4– 2.1)
Arthritis/polyarthritis	1.1	(0.2– 1.7)
Miscellaneous	2.4	(0.6– 3.6)
No cause found	0.5	(0.0– 1.2)
Total Preweaning Mortality	22.2	(15.2–26.9)

*Data from a study on preweaning mortality conducted by the Laboratory of Swine Diseases, Tåstrup, Denmark.

A multitude of factors may be involved, and it has been estimated that approximately 70 to 75 per cent of the antepartum mortality is due to noninfectious causes, while 25 to 30 per cent of deaths are considered to be caused by viral or bacterial infections. Fully developed pigs that die antepartum have characteristic pathological anatomical changes. The skin is grayish-brown, connective tissues are dark red and edematous and the liver, lungs and spleen have an identical reddish-brown color. These discolorations are due to hemolysis, autolysis and a certain degree of resorption.

Intrapartum Deaths. Deaths during the intrapartum period account for a very significant proportion of the total preweaning mortality (see Table 1). These animals are normal-sized, normally developed pigs that are born to term. Some of the pigs die during parturition, but approximately 70 per cent are born alive, although only the heart is beating and the pigs die immediately after birth.[5] However, many of these pigs may be saved by using some form of artificial respiration.

The main cause of death is intrapartal asphyxia due to premature rupture of the umbilical cord, impeded umbilical blood flow or tenuous connections between the placenta and uterus. Asphyxia during parturition is normal in many species. However, species such as the pig, which at birth are relatively mature, are only able to withstand asphyxia and the resultant hypercapnia for a very short period of time.

For this reason intrapartal asphyxia is associated not only with perinatal mortality but also with postnatal morbidity, and liveborn piglets that suffer asphyxia during delivery may often show lower viability for several hours postpartum, which endangers their ability to survive throughout the entire neonatal period. Most intrapartal death losses occur during the last third of the birth order. They increase significantly with increased litter size and increased length of parturition.

The housing of the dam during the period of gestation also significantly influences losses due to intrapartal death, in that sows that are tied up in pens or confined in crates during the period of gestation give birth to a significantly higher proportion of intrapartal dead pigs than sows that are allowed exercise.[2]

Intrapartal dead pigs appear fresh when examined postmortem. They often show discoloration of the skin caused by meconium, their lungs are totally or partially atelectatic and they often have gastric contents consisting of amniotic fluid. Some of the pigs are wrapped in the placenta.

Starving or Undersized Pigs. Such pigs comprise another important mortality group (see Table 1). Starving pigs are defined here as normal-sized pigs that have not received sufficient feed because of agalactia of the dam or because the number of piglets in the litter is larger than the number of functional teats. Thus they are a particular problem in herds with a high incidence of mastitis-metritis-agalactia (MMA).

Undersized pigs are liveborn pigs that, because of their size, are judged unable to survive in an ordinary litter under standard husbandry conditions. Some of the undersized pigs are developmentally immature at birth or have decreased vigor caused by intrapartal asphyxia, but, in general, they are viable. However, they are underprivileged compared with their littermates because they are smaller and physically weaker. Thus, they are not always successful in fighting for a teat and maintaining suckling during the first 24 to 48 hours when the social order and sucking behavior of the litter are established. Small pigs are also at a disadvantage in reaching teats that are placed too high or are covered by the dam's body,[3] and they may have an inadequate capacity to nurse vigorously and rapidly during the time that milk is available.

The losses due to undersized and weak pigs increase with increasing litter size at birth, especially when the litter size exceeds 12 pigs. Part of the explanation may be that not all sections of the uterus are equally suited for providing sufficient nutrients for the fetus and that the intrauterine order of the fetuses may be important.

The starving and undersized pigs quickly become weak and chilled because of a relatively large surface area and because they do not receive an adequate supply of colostrum and milk. In addition, their own energy reserves are very limited and quickly become exhausted. They die as a result of hypoglycemia, trauma or secondary infections. At postmortem examination, these pigs appear emaciated and often are dehydrated. The striated musculature has a characteristic mahogany brown color, which is almost pathognomonic for pigs dying of starvation. The stomach may contain pieces of straw or other foreign material, and the stomach and intestines are extended by air. Excoriations, scratches and wounds are often present, as an indication of fighting with littermates in competition for the teats.

Trauma. Death losses caused by crushing by the dam and other fatal traumatic lesions constitute the highest mortality group among liveborn pigs and contribute significantly to the noninfectious losses (see Table 1). There is considerable herd-to-herd variation in the incidence of fatal traumatic injuries. This is particularly due to differences in farrowing accommodations and management procedures. Thus, a significantly higher incidence of death losses due to trauma is seen in herds in which the farrowing unit consists of pens without fenders or creep area and in which the sow is allowed to move freely, as compared with herds in which the farrowing units are equipped with crates so that the farrowing sow is confined during the first week after parturition or is housed in pens that have fenders and creep area to prevent crushing. Attendance at farrowing also decreases losses due to trauma in these herds.[1] Postparturient diseases of the sow (MMA) also influence losses due to trauma, in that offspring from sows suffering from MMA have a significantly higher incidence of trauma.

Most fatal cases of crushing occur in the perinatal period, and pigs that are born weak because of prenatal asphyxia or that have a physical disadvantage due to size, malformation, arthritis, septicemia or other infections are frequently traumatized by the sow. The majority of pigs that succumb because of traumatic injuries show exsanguination to the serous cavities. Liver rupture frequently occurs, whereas rupture of the spleen is rarely seen. Hemothorax is frequently caused by perforation of the lungs in connection with multiple rib fractures. Many pigs appear to die because of choking. They are slightly cyanotic, the head and neck areas are congested and edematous and intramuscular hemorrhages are frequently present. The lungs are usually edematous and petechial hemorrhages in the upper part of the respiratory tract may occasionally be present.

Umbilical Cord Bleeding. Over a period of time, bleeding from the umbilical cord may be a very important cause of perinatal mortality in certain herds. In general, the mortality due to umbilical cord bleeding is less than 0.1 per cent of the pigs born and does not occur in all herds. However, in some herds mortality rates of more than 2 per cent of the pigs born have been recorded. The etiology is unknown, and the pigs do not show other bleeding abnormalities.

At postmortem examination the pigs appear well developed and large but are pale and have bloodstained skin. The umbilical cord is black, wet and frayed at the end. The lungs are extremely pale. Many of the pigs die shortly after their first suckle, and their stomach is filled with clotted milk.

Reducing Mortality Due to Noninfectious Causes

The housing, husbandry and management factors that are known to influence perinatal mortality due to noninfectious reasons have just been discussed. Attempts to reduce the death losses must be directed toward correction of these factors. The following summarizes important components for a perinatal care program:

1. Modification of the farrowing pens by providing for correctly adjusted fenders and creep area in order to minimize losses due to trauma and starvation.

2. Provision for proper exercise of the sows during gestation, thus reducing losses due to antepartal and intrapartal deaths.

3. Proper treatment of sows that show signs of prolonged parturition time, thus reducing intrapartal death losses.

4. Prevention or immediate treatment of diseases of the sow that cause agalactia, thus reducing death losses due to starvation, chilling and traumatic injuries.

5. Attendance at farrowing, making it possible to (a) limit the death losses due to asphyxiation, using some form of artificial respiration; (b) give proper care to the liveborn but hypoxic pigs during their first period of extrauterine life when they are still very weak; (c) secure colostrum for each piglet; (d) reduce losses due to trauma and (e) provide for artificial feeding and special care of weak and undersized animals.

6. Application of a ligature or a clamp to the umbilical cord immediately after birth

in herds in which this is indicated, thus reducing losses due to umbilical bleeding.

Attempts to reduce the neonatal mortality would, in particular, prove economically advantageous if fitted into a production program in which sows farrow in batches, thus making it possible to:

1. Form uniform litters with one functional teat per pig.
2. Secure an adequate supply of colostrum and milk for each animal.
3. Give special attention to weak and underprivileged but viable piglets by raising them in a special box under optimal conditions.

It has been stressed that most of the preweaning losses occur within the first week of life and that the majority are due to noninfectious causes. Attempts to reduce these very significant losses require a concerted effort of technical and biological expertise. Such efforts will prove rewarding because one pig saved during the first week of life means one more pig at weaning. Good stockmanship and sound application of the suggested husbandry and management procedures will prove important tools in reducing the losses.

Preweaning Mortality Due to Infectious Causes

The main losses due to infectious diseases during the suckling period may be associated with gastrointestinal diseases, respiratory diseases, acute septicemia and arthritis/polyarthritis. Death losses that result from these diseases are presented in Table 1. Only mortality figures are shown, whereas the very significant losses that may occur from nonfatal infectious diseases are not included. For the purpose of this presentation, some of the husbandry and herd factors that have been shown to influence death losses due to infectious diseases will be discussed, and general suggestions will be made for reduction of these losses. For information concerning the multitude of various infectious diseases and their specific treatment, the reader is referred to standard textbooks on the subject.

Husbandry and Herd Factors that Influence Losses

Closed versus Open Herds. Closed herds are herds that, as far as practically possible, are operated without contact with other swine-producing units. Generally, such herds have a lower incidence of the preweaning losses that are caused by infectious agents than have herds that have had contacts with other sow herds (e.g., by the purchase of female and male breeding stock on a regular basis). The closed herd is usually not free from disease-causing agents, but the animals are in balance with these agents because of the build-up of an adequate immunity. Such herd immunity is very difficult to maintain in open herds because of a regular introduction, via animals and man, of infectious agents foreign to the herd and because the newly introduced animals have a resistance pattern to diseases that may be different from that of the established animals in the herd.

A completely closed herd, in which all contacts with pig pathogens foreign to the herd are avoided, while all pigs within the herd are systematically exposed to existing pathogens, would probably have a very low level of losses due to infectious diseases. Such a system, however, is difficult to maintain and is impossible to implement for the producer who wishes to take advantage of progress in hybrid breeding and genetics.

Climate Control. Herds having stables with considerable fluctuations in the indoor temperature and humidity, high concentrations of noxious gases and very dusty air have a significantly higher incidence of respiratory diseases and losses due to acute generalized infections than herds having stables with an adequate control of the indoor climate. Possible reasons for this are that the abrupt and sudden changes in the indoor climate, in particular problems with draft, that may occur in such stables may possibly lower the nonspecific resistance of the animals, thus making them more susceptible to infectious agents.

Hygiene. The level of hygiene exerts a pronounced influence on the incidence of gastrointestinal diseases. Thus, herds in which there is a systematic and thorough cleaning of the farrowing pens before the introduction of clean sows and in which a higher day-to-day hygiene level is maintained have significantly lower mortality due to gastrointestinal diseases than have herds in which such cleaning procedures are not consistently being maintained. A high level of hygiene is particularly efficient in reducing losses due to nonspecific intestinal infections but is also an integral part of all programs and attempts to reduce losses caused by specific gastrointestinal diseases.[6]

Health Status of the Dam. The offspring of sows suffering from postparturient diseases (MMA) have a significantly higher incidence of fatal gastrointestinal diseases and acute generalized infections. This probably occurs because diseased sows do not produce adequate amounts of colostrum and milk at a time when their offspring are entirely dependent on the milk antibodies of their dam for protection against infectious agents.

Breeding. There has been conflicting evidence in regard to the extent to which heredity plays a role in determining the average number of pigs weaned per litter per sow. However, it is now generally accepted that crossbred pigs exhibit more vigor than purebreds, and considerable improvement with regard to the number of pigs weaned per litter may be expected in an organized and systematic three-breed cross program. The exact nature of the hybrid vigor is not elucidated. However, the pigs are claimed to be more resistant to infectious diseases, and a lower perinatal mortality has also been recorded.

Reducing Preweaning Losses Due to Infectious Causes

The following recommendations will be of importance on the herd level for reducing losses due to infectious causes:

1. Keep the herd closed. Reduce contacts with other hog operations to a minimum and limit the introduction of new breeding stock as much as is practically possible. Only breeding animals from herds with known health status should be introduced, and only after a period of quarantine. Persons who regularly are in contact with other swine herds should be admitted to the herd only if proper measures for preventing diseases are taken. Animals that are to be removed from the herd should be placed in a separate room so that the truck driver does not enter the stables. Within the herd it is essential to maintain a high level of immunity against existing pathogens by providing for a management system by which the pigs are gradually exposed to the pathogens of the herd.

2. When introducing new breeding stock, be systematic and careful. Animals that are introduced to a herd should be brought in as weaners and kept isolated from the rest of the animals. These pigs should be observed daily for signs of disease. After a period of 8 to 12 days, one or more older sows that were to be culled from the herd are placed adjacent to the new animals in the quarantine unit, in order to provide for a gradual and broad exposure to the microflora of the herd. Manure from the farrowing unit may also be transferred to the animals in the quarantine unit after some time. In order to be certain that the newly introduced animals are not carriers of pathogens such as SMEDI (entero) viruses; transmissible gastroenteritis (TGE) virus; *Clostridium perfringens,* type C; *Hemophilus parahemolyticus* and other agents against which the animals of the herd are not protected, it may be advisable to admit to the quarantine unit pregnant gilts that, in general, are most susceptible to infectious diseases. All animals in quarantine should receive prophylactic treatment against swine dysentery and antiparasitic treatment upon admittance to the gestation unit of the herd.

3. Maintain a high level of hygiene in the farrowing unit, thus minimizing the number of pathogens in the environment. This includes a systematic and thorough cleaning of the farrowing pens between each farrowing, washing of the pregnant animals before introduction into the cleaned farrowing unit, daily and careful removal of manure from each pen and prevention of manure from one pen being brought into contact with the animals of another pen.

4. Maintain an acceptable control of the indoor climate, thus reducing losses due to respiratory diseases and to acute generalized infections. Draught problems and sudden changes in indoor temperature should be avoided. The relative humidity should be kept between 50 and 80 per cent, and the average room temperature in the farrowing unit should never be less than 19 to 22°C. The level of noxious gases and the

dust content should permanently be kept low.

5. Reduce and prevent postparturient diseases of the dam, thus assuring an adequate supply of colostrum and milk to the offspring.

6. Select breeding animals from older sows that have consistently weaned litters that are above average for the herd in number, size and performance. If a hybrid breeding program is being considered in order to improve performance of the herd, it should be emphasized that such programs always entail frequent introduction of new breeding stock to the herd and hence increase the risk of a higher incidence of infectious diseases. Therefore, an integral part of all management systems that call for regular introduction of breeding stock to the herd is use of proper introduction procedures, which involve a period of quarantine.

In most instances it will be necessary to combine the recommended husbandry and management procedures for reducing infectious losses with strategic chemotherapeutic and prophylactic measures. It should be remembered, however, that advice and implementation of specific husbandry and management procedures that aim at reducing an infectious disease on the herd level and render the animals more resistant to infections should be an integral part of all prophylactic and therapeutic treatment with chemotherapeutics.

REFERENCES

1. Bille, N., Nielsen, N. C. and Svendsen, J.: Preweaning mortality in pigs. 3. Traumatic injuries. Nord. Vet. Med., 26:617, 1974.
2. Bille, N., Nielsen, N. C., Larsen, J. L. and Svendsen, J.: Preweaning mortality in pigs. 2. The perinatal period. Nord. Vet. Med., 26:294, 1974.
3. English, P. R. and Smith, W. J.: Some causes of death in neonatal piglets. Vet. Ann., 50:95, 1974.
4. Nielsen, N. C., Christensen, K., Bille, N. and Larsen, J. L.: Preweaning mortality in pigs. 1. Herd investigations. Nord. Vet. Med., 26:137, 1974.
5. Randall, G. C. B.: Observations on parturition in the sow. II. Factors influencing stillbirth and perinatal mortality. Vet. Rec., 90:183, 1972.
6. Svendsen, J., Bille, N., Nielsen, N. C., Larsen, J. L. and Riising, H. J.: Preweaning mortality in pigs. 4. Diseases of the gastrointestinal tract in pigs. Nord. Vet. Med., 27:85, 1975.

Postpartum Sow Management for Maximum Reproductive Performance

HAROLD H. HODSON, Jr.
Southern Illinois University, Carbondale, Illinois

INTRODUCTION

Reproductive performance of the sow herd is a key factor, if not the major factor, in controlling the efficiency of the swine production unit. Recent research indicates that an increase of 0.25 litter per sow per year reduces the cost of producing each pig by approximately $1.50, while an increase of one pig weaned per litter reduces the production cost by approximately $2.00 per pig. This article discusses sow breeding systems that maximize the number of litters produced per sow per year. These systems are also designed to facilitate farrowing and baby pig management, which should aid in increasing the number of pigs weaned per litter.

EARLY WEANING AND REBREEDING AT FIRST ESTRUS

Lactational anestrus represents a major limitation that must be overcome if the interval between farrowings is to be decreased. Early weaning of piglets and rebreeding at the first estrus is one means of overcoming this problem and decreasing the farrowing interval.

From the standpoint of baby pig performance, early weaning has been practical for more than 20 years, owing to the development of highly palatable and nutritionally adequate baby pig starters. It is also more efficient to feed the 3-week old pig directly rather than through the sow's conversion of feed to milk. Of course, early weaned pigs must be provided an ideal environment, but this problem is being alleviated by the rapid conversion to environmentally controlled confinement systems.

From the standpoint of reproductive efficiency, the full potential of early weaning rarely has been realized in swine production units in the United States. The resultant inefficiency has been due either to routine breeding at the second estrus following early weaning or to improper management, which results in low conception or farrowing rates. Extensive studies conducted by V. C. Speer[5, 6] at Iowa State University have indicated that maximum sow productivity can be obtained with an early weaning-first estrus breeding system. From both Speer's studies and the experiences of commercial producers, the following recommendations are offered.

1. Lactation length should be approximately 3 weeks. Litter size may be substantially reduced if sows are bred at the first estrus following a lactation of much less than 3 weeks duration. Although the number of pigs born may be slightly lower for sows bred at the first estrus following a 3-week weaning than for sows bred at the second estrus, the number of pigs weaned per litter will be essentially equal.

2. Hand mating should be utilized to insure acceptable conception or farrowing rates. If pen mating is utilized, sow groups should be kept as small as possible, with a minimum of one boar for every five to six sows.

3. Housing weaned sows in individual crates or stalls may be desirable. Fighting and other stresses that result from mixing sows can reduce conception rates.

4. Withholding feed for the first 2 to 3 days after weaning may aid in reduction of milk flow, which is reaching its peak at this time.

Speer estimated annual production figures with first estrus mating after weaning at 3 weeks and compared these with production figures for second estrus mating or 6 weeks weaning. These estimations are shown in Table 1. Even though the expected conception and farrowing rate of sows mated at the first estrus would be reduced, there would be an increase in the number of litters per sow per year with a resultant increase in the number of pigs weaned per sow per year. This projection assumes that sows that fail to settle on first mating are rebred at the second estrus and that the final farrowing rate is 90 per cent. Such a repeat mating system would abolish any attempt to establish a specific farrowing schedule; however, most large confinement units utilize a continuous farrowing schedule to maximize the use of facilities.

USE OF GONADOTROPINS WITH EARLY WEANING

The interval between weaning and estrus is usually longer and more variable when sows are weaned at 3 weeks than when they are weaned later in the lactation period. Gonadotropin injections can be utilized to shorten and synchronize the onset of estrus after early weaning. Although several dosages and time schedules have been utilized, the following sequence is recommended for the most consistent results:

1. Subcutaneous injection of 1000 IU of pregnant mare serum gonadotropin (PMSG) at the time of weaning. This initiates immediate follicular development.

TABLE 1. *Estimated Number of Pigs Produced per Sow per Year for Different Lactation Lengths and Mating Systems*

Lactation Length (wks)	3		6	
ESTRUS MATED	1st	2nd	1st	2nd
Farrowing rate based on first exposure to boar	65%	75%	70%	85%
Final farrowing rate with repeated mating	90%	90%	90%	90%
Avg. number days from farrowing to farrowing	163	184	185	205
Litters/sow/year	2.24	1.98	1.97	1.78
Number pigs/sow/year*	15.7	13.9	13.8	12.5

*Based upon seven pigs weaned per litter farrowed for all systems.

2. Intramuscular injection of 500 IU of human chorionic gonadotropin (HCG) 96 hours after PMSG treatment. Injection of HCG at 72 hours after PMSG treatment instead of 96 hours has been successful in some studies. Eliminating the HCG and mating as the sow exhibits standing heat will result in a less precise ovulation time and incomplete synchronization of the weaned sows.

3. Breeding of sows 28 hours after HCG injection. Most sows can be artificially inseminated successfully even when there is no detectable estrus. If double mating is used, breeding at 24 and 36 hours post-HCG treatment is recommended.

This technique of breeding at a fixed time facilitates the use of artificial insemination because estrous detection is not required. It also groups farrowing more closely, which results in more efficient utilization of existing housing and labor and facilitates baby pig management. In addition, the superovulatory effect of PMSG should eliminate the smaller litter size at birth, which is normally encountered with first estrus breeding after early weaning. Based on limited studies, the use of gonadotropins to induce estrus will allow weaning as early as 15 days postpartum. However, this may be too early for proper perinatal care in most operations.

INDUCTION OF PREGNANCY DURING LACTATION

Although some sows exhibit estrus 3 to 5 days following parturition, this is usually an infertile estrus. In addition, sows often will exhibit estrus during the seventh week of lactation or later, but breeding at this time will reduce the number of litters per sow per year when compared with early weaning and rebreeding at first estrus. It is possible to induce estrus, ovulation and pregnancy during the fourth week of lactation by separating the sow and the litter for 12 hours per day for 3 consecutive days and then injecting gonadotropin. However, this method involves additional labor and facilities and would be objectionable to most producers.

The following system has been developed at Southern Illinois University (SIU) to induce pregnancy in lactating sows:

1. Subcutaneous injection of 1000 to 1500 IU of PMSG.

2. Intramuscular injection of 500 to 1000 IU of HCG at 96 hours post-PMSG treatment.

3. Insemination at 24 and again at 36 to 42 hours post-HCG injection.

A level of 1500 IU of PMSG has resulted in an average of 30 ovulations and 14 viable embryos at 35 to 45 days postbreeding in the SIU crossbred herd. However, in a purebred Chester White herd in which this technique was utilized, ovulation of 40 to 50 ova often occurred and resulted in poor embryonic survival and conception rates. In the Chester White herd, 1000 IU of PMSG and 500 IU of HCG appeared to be adequate. Therefore, the ranges of 1000 to 1500 IU of PMSG and 500 to 1000 IU of HCG are suggested at the present time until more definitive information is obtained on the most feasible dosage of PMSG and HCG.

It appears that a high percentage of the sows exhibit estrus and could be bred naturally. However, artificial insemination is recommended for those sows not exhibiting a standing heat, because ovulation occurs spontaneously after the PMSG/HCG regimen.

Acceptable conception rates and litter size can be obtained when the PMSG treatment is started as early as 15 days postpartum. With sows started on the PMSG treatment at day 15 of lactation or after, a 70 to 80 per cent conception rate and an average litter size at birth of 12 pigs can be expected.

The majority of the sows treated to date in the SIU studies have been weaned within 3 to 4 days after breeding. Even though sows often go off feed for a short time at the initiation of the PMSG/HCG treatment, limited results indicate no substantial effect on the performance of the nursing litter up to the thirty-fifth day of lactation when sows received the PMSG treatment as early as 15 days postpartum. In addition, preliminary results indicate that the technique can be used during several successive lactations with no complications.

Although the development of this technique is based on limited work, the following benefits deem it worthy of consideration for certain commercial or seedstock operations:

1. It would reduce farrowing intervals, resulting in more pigs produced per sow per year without early weaning.

2. It would synchronize estrus and facili-

tate multiple farrowings, resulting in a more uniform pig crop and a more efficient use of labor and facilities.

3. In combination with induced farrowing by the injection of 5 mg of prostaglandin-$F_{a\alpha}$ at 111 to 115 days postbreeding, it would greatly facilitate baby pig management by having all litters from a particular farrowing group born in a span of a few hours.

4. It would facilitate the use of artificial insemination because heat detection is not necessary at the time of breeding and the sows are confined in the farrowing crate. This would allow greater use of superior sires, facilitate the introduction of new genetic material and reduce the spread of costly diseases.

5. It would allow synchronization of ovulation time and control of ovulation rate in donor and receptor sows for ova transplants. From limited work, it appears that it is possible to obtain 25 to 35 embryos from donor sows with this technique. These embryos could be transferred into three synchronized receptor sows. Ova trans-

plants would allow greater use of superior sows and provide a technique whereby new genetic material could be introduced into a herd with less chance of introducing disease organisms.

REFERENCES

1. Christenson, R. K. and Teague, H. S.: Synchronization of ovulation and artificial insemination of sows after lactation. J. Anim. Sci., *41*:560, 1975.
2. Crighton, D. B.: The introduction of pregnancy during lactation in the sow: The effects of a treatment imposed at 21 days of lactation. Anim. Prod., *12*:615, 1970.
3. Kuo, D., Hodson, H. H., Jr. and Hausler, C. L.: Induction of ovulation, artificial insemination and conception in lactating sows. Proceedings International Pig Veterinary Society. College of Veterinary Medicine, Iowa State University. 1976, p. D-23.
4. Longenecker, D. E. and Day, D. N.: Fertility level of sows superovulated at post-weaning estrus. J. Anim. Sci., *27*:709, 1968.
5. Speer, V. C.: Reducing farrowing intervals. Cooperative Extension Service Leaflet AS 353B. Iowa State University, 1970.
6. Speer, V. C.: Reducing the farrowing intervals of sows. Feedstuffs. Feb. 4, 1974, p. 30.

Testicular and Ovarian Pathology in Swine

BORJE K. GUSTAFSSON
University of Illinois, Urbana, Illinois

TESTICULAR AND EPIDIDYMAL ABNORMALITIES

Intersexuality and Cryptorchidism

Intersexuality and cryptorchidism are common abnormalities of genetic origin. Although some affected animals may be able to reproduce, it is strongly recommended that these animals not be kept for breeding purposes. The clinical diagnosis is usually easy in cases of cryptorchidism. In cases of intersexuality, however, the external appearance of the genitalia may vary from slight to severe modification. Most hermaphrodites have female external characteristics with overdevelopment of the clitoris. There is usually a narrowed opening to the vulva, small labia and a narrow vestibule of the vagina. A definite diagnosis must frequently await postmortem examination.

Testicular Hypoplasia

This is an inherited congenital underdevelopment of the testicles. It occurs less frequently in the boar than in the bull. Testicular hypoplasia can be classified as unilateral or bilateral and as total or partial. In cases of bilateral total hypoplasia, the seminiferous tubules lack germinal epithelium, and, therefore, sperm production does not occur. These boars are sterile. In unilateral total or partial hypoplasia or bilateral partial hypoplasia, sperm production is reduced but fertility rates may be acceptable, which leads to a wide spread of this heritable defect. Total hypoplasia is characterized by reduced size of the affected testicle. Testicle shape is usually round rather than oval. The epididymal tail on the affected side is small and flaccid. In partial hypoplasia, the reduction of testicular size is usually less pronounced than in the total defect. The disorder may, therefore, be difficult to detect — especially in bilateral cases in which relatively few seminiferous tubules are affected.

The ejaculate from boars with bilateral total hypoplasia is characterized by aspermia. In other types of hypoplasia, semen evaluation usually reveals a reduced sperm concentration. The sperm motility is often reduced, and the incidence of pathological spermatozoa is frequently increased. A striking feature in partial hypoplasia seems to be an increased incidence of spermatozoa with proximal cytoplasmic droplets (immature spermatozoa). Furthermore, there is an increased frequency of abnormal sperm heads. An increased number of round cells from the spermatogenic epithelium (spermatid-like cells) may occur.

The clinical diagnosis of testicular hypoplasia is based on breeding history, palpation of the testicles and epididymides and semen evaluation. Affected boars usually have normal libido and mating behavior. Testicular degeneration should be considered in the differential diagnosis. There is no treatment for testicular hypoplasia. Because of the hereditary nature of the condition, affected boars should be culled.

Histological examination, either postmortem or of biopsy specimens, reveals small seminiferous tubules without spermatogenic epithelium in cases of total testicular hypoplasia. The Sertoli cells are normal, as is the intertubular tissue. In boars with partial hypoplasia, there are varying numbers of seminiferous tubules without spermatogenic epithelium, while other tubules have a normal epithelium or an epithelium with varying degrees of degeneration.

Testicular Degeneration

This condition is probably the most common cause of infertility or sterility in the boar. It is an acquired disorder. The cause of testicular degeneration is often complex and difficult to establish in the individual boar. Factors causing testicular degeneration include systemic disease, fever, chronic diseases, traumatic injury, endogenous or exogenous toxins, nutritional factors, high ambient temperature, hormonal imbalance and stress. Furthermore, local irritation or inflammation caused by insect bites, disinfectants or certain insecticides can result in testicular degeneration.

In general, clinical examination does not reveal systemic disease. Sexual behavior is usually normal. The size of one or both testicles may be somewhat smaller or larger than normal. Testicular consistency may be increased and localized indurations occasionally palpated. In advanced cases, testicular atrophy develops.

Affected boars usually produce a normal volume of semen. Sperm concentration may be normal or reduced. Different degrees of reduced sperm motility are a major finding. A variety of morphological alterations of the sperm head, acrosome, midpiece or sperm tail may occur. A very striking defect seems to be the high frequency of spermatozoa with proximal cytoplasmic droplets and midpiece defects. An excessive degeneration of the germinal epithelium often results in a clinical picture similar to cases of testicular hypoplasia. Boars with testicular degeneration usually have had prior normal fertility or semen quality.

If the causative agent is eliminated, a regeneration of the germinal epithelium may occur. Complete recovery is dependent upon the cause and duration of the disease. Reevaluation of boars in about 2 months will usually aid in establishing a definite diagnosis and prognosis. Effective medical treatment for testicular generation is unknown.

Degenerative changes of the spermatogenic epithelium are observed on histological examination. The changes may affect all spermatogenic layers or may be limited to one or several cell types, e.g., spermatid, spermiocytic or spermiogonial layers. In excessive degeneration, there is usually a complete cessation of spermatogenesis resulting in almost empty seminiferous tubules containing only Sertoli cells. The interstitial fibrous tissue is usually increased, and thickening of the basement membrane occurs in varying degrees. In infectious cases, inflammatory cell infiltration of the testicular and epididymal interstitium is frequently observed.

Inflammation

Orchitis or epididymitis, or both, rarely occurs in swine. The causes may be bacterial, mycoplasmal or viral. A common cause is traumatic injury. The inflammation may be unilateral or bilateral. Pain, edema, heat and testicular enlargement are usually observed at the onset of orchitis. In cases of unilateral orchitis, the contralateral testicle is frequently affected by increased local temperature, resulting in alterations in its sperm production. Treatment of orchitis-epididymitis should be directed at the etiological agent, or agents, involved. Systemic administration of antibiotics, unilateral castration and local administration of cold may be beneficial. The prognosis depends on whether only one or both testicles are affected, the severity of injury, duration and the causative agent and must be guarded because the inflammation may result in chronic degenerative changes of the testes or epididymides, or both. Orchitis frequently results in severe testicular fibrosis. Semen evaluation at 6- to 8-week intervals will assist in establishing the prognosis. Bacteriological culture of semen may be beneficial in establishing the etiology.

Brucellosis must be considered in all cases of orchitis-epididymitis. *Brucella suis* orchitis results in a purulent, necrotizing orchitis-epididymitis. Brucellosis may also affect the locomotor system and result in lameness (arthritis, tenosynovitis) and serving inability. The disease may be venereally transmitted and cause early embryonic death and abortion.

There is no effective treatment for brucellosis. The control of the disease is based on various types of eradication programs.

Epididymal Disorders

Epididymal disorders are not common in the boar, although, as discussed, epididymitis is common in cases of orchitis. Segmental aplasia of the vas deferens or the epididymal duct is rare. Occasionally, aplasia of the tail of the epididymis may be diagnosed by palpation. If other parts of the excurrent ducts are involved, the diagnosis is more difficult. In certain cases of segmental aplasia, spermiostasis (sperm granuloma, spermatocele) develops and can be palpated.

Functional disturbances of the epididymis may result in abnormal composition of the epididymal plasma, with subsequent lowered sperm motility and increased frequency of sperm tail changes (bent tails, coiled tails). The incidence of proximal cytoplasmic droplets may be increased. Repeated ejaculations within a short time period may result in improved sperm motility and sperm morphology, These exhaustion tests are used to differentiate between disorders of epididymal and testicular origin. The cause of the epididymal dysfunctions is not known. Varying degrees of infertility have been found in similar cases in bulls. In boars, the

relationship between epididymal dysfunction and fertility has not been well established.

OVARIAN PATHOLOGY

Developmental Abnormalities

Developmental abnormalities affecting the ovaries seem to be extremely rare (the exception being hermaphroditism, see previous discussion). However, such abnormalities are common in other structures close to the ovaries, mostly in the form of so-called parovarian cysts in the mesosalpinx and in the infundibulum of the oviduct. These cysts, which are thin-walled and distended by a clear fluid, are remnants of wolffian duct system. Most of these cysts apparently do not affect fertility. However, when they are localized to the infundibulum and its fimbria, they might adversely affect the fertility. In one postmortem survey, more than 8 per cent of the gilts had parovarian cysts localized in the infundibulum.

Ovarian Subfunction

The primary cause of ovarian subfunction is usually not located in the ovaries. The inactive status of the ovaries merely reflects an endocrine dysfunction, which often has a very complex background. The lack of normal follicular development or ovulation, or both, results in anestrus. The anestrous condition occurs both in gilts and sows. The most common anestrous problem in swine breeding in gilts is associated with delayed puberty. The cause of delayed puberty is complex. Hereditary, as well as environmental factors, may be involved (see article on puberty in gilts and boars, page 1107). Since the genital tract is not available for palpation, the clinical diagnosis of ovarian dysfunction is difficult to make. Analysis of blood progesterone concentrations at 7- to 10-day intervals may be valuable in evaluating the ovarian function. Low progesterone values on both occasions indicate inactive ovaries. A change from a low to high or from a high to low value indicates that the ovaries are undergoing cyclic changes. The examination may assist in predicting the subsequent estrus.

The treatment of anestrus in gilts can be handled in different ways. Several management techniques have been used to induce puberty in gilts (see article on puberty in gilts and boars). The techniques comprise various changes of the environment. The gilts that do not respond to these external stimuli should probably be culled because of the suspected genetic predisposition. Another form of treatment includes administration of hormones, with or without environmental changes. Pregnant mare's serum gonadotropin (PMSG) in doses of 400 to 800 IU intramuscularly has been used with varying success alone or in combination with 200 to 500 IU of human chorionic gonodotropin (HCG) injected simultaneously or 3 to 4 days after the PSMG injection. Combinations of gonodotropins (PMSG and HCG) and estrogens (for .example, 2 to 3 mg of estradiol benzoate) have shown good effect in cases of delayed puberty. The risk in using estrogen-containing preparations is that they may cause prolongation of the luteal function in gilts that happen to be injected during midcycle. A correct diagnosis of the ovarian status by progesterone determination would be helpful before the hormones are given.

A number of factors influence the cyclic activity following weaning. Very early weaning (2 to 10 days lactation) may result in ovarian dysfunction. Weaning-to-service interval has been shown to be inversely related to lactation length. Furthermore, anestrus appears to be more common in sows that lose weight excessively during lactation. Weight loss is natural, but adverse effects on reproduction may result if the loss exceeds the net pregnancy weight gain. Anestrus is most common after the first litter. A seasonal pattern regarding the occurrence of postweaning anestrus has been observed in some countries. It appears that the anestrus is associated with high ambient temperature. Various other environmental factors, identical to those involved in the etiology of delayed puberty, are also involved in the sows. Genetic predisposition may occur but does not appear to be as common as in the gilts.

A clinical diagnosis of the ovarian status is possible by determination of blood progesterone levels.

The treatment of the condition should preferably be directed toward preventive measures, the most important probably being to provide adequate nutrition during lactation, especially in sows with their first litter. Other environmental and management fac-

tors that should be considered include heat detection methods, sows' exposure to boars, housing system, ventilation, light and temperature. A kind of flushing is practiced in several countries and generally involves an increase of the amount fed by 50 to 100 per cent over maintenance levels during the period from weaning to ovulation. The regimen is considered to be beneficial, especially for sows in poor condition after lactation. Hormones may be the treatment of choice in certain cases. When hormones are used, the same regimen applies as for gilts regarding hormones, doses and so on. It should be pointed out that in the case of a herd problem, a herd investigation would be preferable before hormone treatment is used.

Ovarian Cysts

Cystic ovarian disease appears to be responsible for a substantial percentage of infertility, especially in older sows. Both follicular and lutein cysts occur, although the lutein cysts seem to predominate. The follicular cysts usually occur as single cysts, i.e., one or two thin-walled 2- to 3-cm cysts together with solid corpora lutea during the lutein cysts seem to predominate. The follicular cysts usually occur as single cysts, many as 20 small, multiple follicular cysts of about 1 cm in diameter may appear in each ovary, but the condition is much less common than single follicular cysts. Usually there are no corpora lutea present, and the condition has been associated with irregularities of the estrous cycle and infertility.

Multiple lutein cysts are considered to be associated with infertility. The most common form seems to be the large, multiple luteal cysts, which usually measure 2 to 10 cm in diameter. The walls of the cysts are luteinized to various degrees. Solid corpora lutea or cystic corpora lutea may occur at the same time. The clinical symptoms vary from complete anestrus (most common) to estrus at very frequent intervals.

It has been suggested that sows may be affected gradually by cystic ovarian disease. The disease may start from a point at which only one or two follicles fail to ovulate and become cystic. In these sows, the cycles continue normally, and the fertility is probably only slightly affected. At a transitional stage of the disease, some luteinization can still occur, resulting in luteinized cysts. Finally, it appears that the luteinizing hormone (LH) is blocked completely, which results in multiple follicular cysts and a complete inhibition of the ovarian function.

The cause of the cystic ovarian disease is not known. An LH insufficiency is very likely involved. Whether there is a genetic predisposition for the disease is not known. Since the pathogenesis is unknown and the clinical diagnosis is difficult, established methods for treatment are not available. However, gonadotropins or gonadotropin-releasing hormone (GnRH) may be effective in treatment.

REFERENCES

1. Einarsson, S. and Gustafsson, B.: Developmental abnormalities of female sexual organs in swine. Acta Vet. Scand., *11*:427, 1970.
2. Einarsson, S., Linde, C. and Settergren, I.: Studies of the genital organs of gilts culled for anestrus. Theriogenology, *2*(5):109, 1974.
3. Holst, S.: Sterility in boars. Nord. Vet. Med., *1*:87, 1949.
4. Roberts, S. J.: Veterinary Obstetrics and Genital Diseases. Ithaca, New York, 1971 (Distr. Edwards Brothers, Inc., Ann Arbor, Michigan).
5. Wrathall, A. E.: Reproductive disorders in pigs. Review Series No. 11 of the Commonwealth Bureau of Animal Health, Farnham Royal, Slough SL2 3 BN, England, 1975.

Effects of Heat, Light and Housing on Reproduction

ALDON H. JENSEN
University of Illinois, Urbana, Illinois

Although confinement rearing of pigs from birth to market weight is commonly practiced, only a relatively small percentage of the breeding herds are continuously confined. As used in this article, confinement implies a relatively small area per animal on nondirt floors in either partially or completely enclosed buildings. Problems generally associated with confinement, in comparison with field rearing, include later sexual maturity and breeding age and lower conception rates in gilts and lower rebreeding efficiency in sows. With both gilts (and sows) and boars, longevity of production is shortened because of foot and leg problems.

External stress of any kind may alter body functions sufficiently to cause a decrease in production efficiency. Frequently, however, the effect is sufficiently subtle that it cannot readily be defined or quantified. Thus, environmental factors in confinement housing for the breeding animals may adversely affect physiological function but escape specific identity. The environmental factors considered here are temperature, light and housing.

TEMPERATURE

In order to maintain a rather constant temperature, the animal adjusts its body functions to meet the stress from an environmental factor. The degree of diversionary activity necessary to compensate for the stress factor determines the modification of normal, i.e., reproductive, bodily processes.

Effects on Sexual Maturity.   High ambient temperature stress affects sexual development. Data from several stations show that it can affect development and reproduction in gilts. Results indicate that exposure to high temperature can result in irregular estrous behavior and reduced growth rate with an associated increase in the age at puberty and possibly in a lower ovulation rate. In the young boar, high ambient temperature can reduce sperm motility, total sperm ejaculate and fertility. Raising the testicular temperature to 40.5°C by local heating of the scrotum can severely damage the germinal epithelium.

Effects on Breeding and Gestation.   Stresses from high ambient temperature affect reproduction. Matings during summer months frequently result in poorer reproductive performance than matings in cool seasons. In an Illinois study, littermate gilts were assigned to tether or groups of five in a slotted-floor building with normal temperature variation or to 1.5 m × 1.5 m individual slotted-floor pens in a room with an ambient temperature of 33 to 36°C. The gilts in the high temperature environment responded by markedly reducing feed intake and activity, and no evidence of estrus was detected in these gilts, although this was checked daily, using a boar. After 100 days, these gilts were moved to a room with normal diurnal temperature fluctuations. Within 14 days, all gilts evidenced estrus and were mated. Only two of these ten gilts, however, were pregnant at 25 days postmating, and the number of live embryos was significantly lower than in the gilts in the other treatment environments. In an earlier test, exposure to a continuous 32°C environment from 14 days postmating to day 109 of gestation did not significantly affect reproductive performance of gilts and sows.

Heat stress directly after mating appears to lower the ovulation rate and to adversely affect embryonic survival. High ambient temperature stress will cause the death of gilts and sows pregnant 20 or more days before it adversely affects embryo survival. Thus, the adverse effects of heat stress are greatest both during and two weeks after mating and again both immediately preceding and during parturition.

Boars are also adversely affected by high temperature stress. During summer months, boars housed in outside pens with maximum temperatures of 30 to 39°C had a lower conception rate than similar boars housed in a temperature-controlled (18 to 24°C) piggery. Litters sired by boars in outside pens during the summer were significantly smaller than in other seasons; however, no significant seasonal variation was observed in the temperature-controlled piggery.

LIGHT

Research concerning the role of light or darkness on reproductive performance has been less than conclusive. Canadian workers compared continuous darkness and 12 hours light:12 hours darkness for gilts from birth to breeding. Gilts in the 12:12 cycle of light and darkness reached first estrus an average of 9 days sooner than the continuous darkness gilts. This was in contrast to a previous report that indicated that continuous darkness, except for 1 hour per day, resulted in the onset of puberty at an earlier age compared with normal diurnal light:darkness. In a recent study, the effects of schedules of 18:6 and 6:18 light:dark hours were evaluated from birth. The gilts on 18 hours of daily light reached puberty about 30 days earlier than the gilts that had 6 hours of light daily. All gilts were artificially inseminated during the second estrus. The 18-hour-light gilts had lower ovulation

rates and fewer fetuses than the 6-hour-light gilts. Also, the conception rate at first mating was lower for the 18-hour-light gilts. Examination of the pineal gland indicated its involvement in the response to the light:dark schedules. Thus the effect of artificial light, including duration and intensity, on the reproductive performance of swine needs clarification. At this time, controlled lighting schemes for swine do not seem of primary concern in commercial production.

HOUSING

Little research information concerning the specific effects of confinement *per se* is available. However, in the housing environment, in addition to climatic effects, there are several other factors of management concern. Two of these are social and structural environmental factors. Social factors deal with the animals' response to one another, and structural aspects relate to the effect of items such as floor type, design, surface, equipment and so on.

Space and Restriction. Restriction of mobility and movement of young gilts may interfere with normal sexual development. When littermate gilts were randomly assigned to either individual tether (confined by a neck collar to an area approximately 0.43 × 1.77 m) or to groups of five to seven in a totally enclosed building with a slotted floor, first observed estrus was on the average 4 days earlier in the grouped gilts. The occurrence of quiet estrus (no observed estrus but positive evidence of ovulation at slaughter) was significantly higher in the tethered than in the grouped gilts.

Commercial producers have observed more erratic estrous behavior in tethered than in grouped gilts. There is some, although limited, evidence that gilts penned in individual stalls (0.3 m × 2.0 m) showed a higher incidence of irregular estrus and mating behavior than similar gilts in groups. However, conception rates at first service were not significantly different. The performance during second and subsequent parities was similar in individually and group penned sows.

Feeding Management. Many methods of providing adequate nutrients for breeding animals are used. The larger the number of animals per group and the greater the range in body weight, the less will be the herdsman's control of the individual animal's condition. A maximum efficiency of feed utilization will be realized with individual feeding when the animals are in a comfortable environment.

Floor Material and Design. Although very little published data are available, observations suggest that several structural factors can materially affect behavioral patterns and reproductive performance. Nebraska workers have reported on the relationship of foot and leg injuries of growing-finishing swine to floor design and materials. Significant differences in the number of injuries were noted for different floor arrangements (partially slotted, totally slotted, different slat materials). Although comparable data are not available, breeding animals have frequently been culled because of immobility due to lameness. Rough and slick floors discourage, if not permanently ruin, normal sexual behavior of boars and gilts. Large groups, crowded conditions and inadequate feeding space can all adversely affect reproductive performance.

Facility Design. In general, available information would indicate that for breeding and gestation, facilities varying from very simple to very elaborate designs that provide a suitably comfortable environment are satisfactory. A dry sleeping area that is free of draft conditions is essential. The use of totally slotted floors minimizes labor and enhances maintenance of a sanitary environment. It must be recognized, however, that environmental control is more exacting than for partially slotted or totally solid floor units.

RECOMMENDATIONS

Confinement housing for breeding and gestating animals must provide at least the following: (1) a suitable environment for the animal, (2) minimal requirements for routine labor and (3) a comfortable environment and convenient arrangements for the herder.

Floor Space. Floor space allowance should reflect the minimum area per animal unit that allows maximum productive expression. The values shown in Table 1 represent "free-floor" area. Additional area will be necessary for feeders, waterers, aisles ad so forth.

Flooring Materials. Carefully select the kind, size and design of slats or slotted material. Concrete is the most durable and is easily cleaned. Soft woods are unsatisfactory because of rapid wear and warping. Animals also chew through unprotected soft wood slats and boards. When possible, avoid use of materials that become very slippery when wet or that have rough or sharp edges or other characteristics that might injure the animal's feet and legs. The slat surface should be smooth.

Variable spacing as a result of warping or of careless installation due to insecurely fas-

TABLE 1. *Floor Space per Animal Unit and Number of Animals per Pen**

Animal Unit	Weight (kg)	SOLID FLOOR	PARTIALLY SLOTTED FLOOR	SLOTTED FLOOR	No. of Animals per Pen
Boars	–	6.5	5.0	5.0	1–3†
Breeding females					
Gilt	114–136	1.4	1.1	1.1	12–15
Sow	136–225	1.7	1.4	1.4	10–12
Gestating females‡					
Gilt	114–180	1.6	1.3	1.3	12–15
Sow	136–225	1.7	1.4	1.4	12–15

Minimum Space per Animal Unit (m²)

*Recommendations are based on research results and management observations of intensive swine-rearing programs.
†If possible, pen boars individually. When it is necessary to have more than one boar in a pen, put the boars together when they are young. Mixing mature boars that are strangers to one another may result in vigorous fighting and subsequent injury.
‡Individual pens should be about 56 cm wide and 1.8 m long for gilts and 60 cm wide and 2.1 m long for sows. Tethered animals require essentially the same amount of space.

tened slats and uneven heights of slats also have an adverse effect on the behavior of animals on completely slotted floors. On partially slotted floors, these factors will be of less effect, since the animals spend only a fraction of their time on the slat sections. Less environmental control is needed in partially slotted-floor buildings than in totally slotted-floor buildings. Also, on-floor feeding is easily accomplished on partially slotted floors. Suggested slat widths and spacings are shown in Table 2.

Environmental Control. Table 3 lists recommended ambient temperatures for maximum efficiency of performance, based on available research information.

SUMMARY

The effect of confinement *per se* has not been clearly defined, but several relevant factors have been studied. High environmental temperatures can adversely affect sexual maturity of females and reproductive capacities of both females and males. Management practices (individual versus group) may modify behavior and reproductive efficiency. A structural environment (floor design, material and condition) that inhibits natural mobility and behavior can result in ineffective boars and unresponsive gilts. There is suggestive evidence that a controlled daily light:dark cycle, compared

TABLE 2. *Suggested Slat Widths and Spacing for Flooring Material for Swine Housing*

Width (cm)	Space between Slats (cm)
10 to 15	2.5
18 to 20	3.2

TABLE 3. *Recommended Ambient Temperature for Maximum Swine Performance*

Animal	Ambient Temperature (°C)
Young boars and replacement gilts	15
Gestating gilts, sows and mature boars:	
With bedding	10
Without bedding or on slotted floors	15

with normal diurnal variation, may affect female sexual maturity and reproductive potential, but additional research is needed to clarify this.

To insure maximum reproductive performance from a breeding herd in confinement, the facility design and management must provide an environment suited to optimum physiological function.

REFERENCES

1. Hacker, R. R., King, G. J. and Bears, W. H.: Effects of complete darkness on growth and reproduction in gilts. J. Anim. Sci., *39*:155, 1974.
2. Jensen, A. H., Yen, J. T., Gehring, M. M., Baker, D. H., Becker, D. E. and Harmon, B. G.: Effects of space restriction and manaagement on pre- and post-puberal response of female swine. J. Anim. Sci., *31*:745, 1970.
3. Sigornet, J. P. and Du Nesnil du Brusson, F.: Influence of the housing conditions of boars on farrowing rate after artificial insemination. 6th International Congress on Animal Reproduction A. I. Paris, 1968, p. 74.
4. Teague, H. S.: Effect of temperature and humidity on reproduction. Proceedings NPPC Symposium on Effect of Disease and Stress on Reproductive Efficiency in Swine: 70-2-C. Des Moines, Iowa, 1970.
5. Wettemen, R. P., Wells, M. E., Omtuedt, I. T., Pope, C. E. and Turman, E. J.: Influence of elevated ambient temperature on reproductive performance of boars. J. Anim. Sci., *42*:664, 1976.

Normal and Abnormal Development and Puberty in Gilts and Boars

G. W. DYCK

Agriculture Canada, Research Station, Brandon, Manitoba, Canada

The changes that occur in the reproductive system of the pig from birth to puberty are set on a definite time schedule of events that is basically dependent upon the physiological maturation of the animal. The development of the hypothalamic-hypophysial axis that results in sexual differentiation is accomplished prior to birth. Thus, both sexes can be treated separately in respect to sexual maturation. The boar, exclusive of diurnal variation and modulating hormone secretion, has a stable hormone picture. By contrast, the female develops a cyclic hormone secretory pattern that is repeated at approximately a 21-day interval. This basic difference becomes increasingly important when we look at the developmental process that results in sexual maturity.

With adequate management, the changes that occur can be related directly to age and environment. Extremes in feed quality and quantity can produce divergence from the mean or normal development pattern. The effects of the proximity of the opposite sex and of climate on development also are of considerable importance. This article deals with the normal animal, while pointing out the effects of extreme treatments on reproductive organ development and puberty and the consequence of anatomical abnormalities.

THE GILT

Ovaries

Oogenesis (germ cell formation) in the embryo commences about 30 days after conception and continues until approximately 35 days postpartum. Following parturition, the number of egg cords and nests decreases as a result of separation by layers of granulosa cells. Ovarian weight changes and follicular growth from birth to puberty are shown in

Figure 1. Ovaries show a definite pattern of development, increasing rapidly in weight from about 0.3 gm (two ovaries) at 70 days of age to 5.5 gm at 112 days of age. At puberty, ovarian weight is still about 5.5 gm. The first vesicular follicles appear on the surface of the ovaries at about 70 days of age. Within 6 weeks the number of small (<3 mm in diameter) vesicular follicles reaches its maximum, then gradually declines in number until relative stability is reached 4 weeks later (140 days of age). Concomitantly, a few larger (>3 mm in diameter) follicles are present on the ovaries and reach a maximum at 140 days. A further reduction in the number of ovarian follicles occurs at puberty, after which follicular growth and regression, or ovulation and luteal tissue formation, occur in a regularly defined cyclic pattern. Following puberty, ovarian weight changes become cyclic and follow the pattern of follicle growth and luteal tissue formation.

Uterus

Uterine weight changes from birth to puberty are shown graphically in Figure 2. During the first 70 days of life, uterine growth is slow. Uterine weight increases from 0.3 gm to 3 gm and length from 10 cm to 14 cm per uterine horn. There is a gradual increase in the thickness of the uterine wall and endometrium and initiation of development of the uterine glands. Between 70 and 84 days of age, there is an initial rapid increase in uterine weight (20 gm) and uterine horn length (29 cm) followed by a continual slower growth until just prior to puberty. During this period of prepuberal growth, uterine wall thickness increases from 1500 μ to 5000 μ and the endometrium increases from 1000 μ to 3700 μ. At the same time, the uterine glands complete their development through the endometrium to the myometrium. Uterine gland development is completed by 120 days of age. At puberty, uterine weight increases rapidly from 60 gm to 180 gm. Further increases in uterine weight are observed during subsequent estrous cycles and pregnancy. The most dramatic increase, however, occurs at puberty.

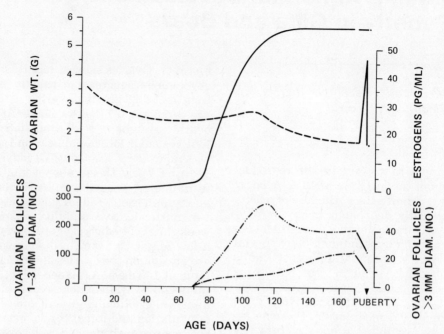

Figure 1. Age changes in total ovarian weight ———, the number of ovarian follicles 1 to 3 mm in diameter —·——·—, and >3 mm in diameter —·—·—, and total free plasma estrogens ---- from birth to puberty. The puberal change is identified by a solid line. (Dyck, G. W., unpublished data.)

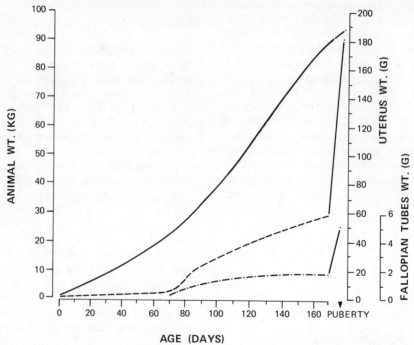

Figure 2. Age changes in gilt weight ———, uterine weight --- and total fallopian tube weight —·—·— from birth to puberty. The puberal change is identified by a solid line. (Dyck, G. W., unpublished data.)

Fallopian Tubes

The fallopian tubes also show a specific growth pattern that can be observed visually only after 70 days of age and is completed by 112 days of age (Fig. 2). This growth represents an increase in mean tubal length from 6 cm to 16 cm and an increase in mean weight from 0.1 gm to 0.8 gm. At puberty there is a dramatic increase in mean length to 22 cm and weight to 2.5 gm.

Endocrine Glands

The growth of the thyroid, adrenal and pituitary glands from birth to puberty is shown in Figure 3. The thyroid gland has a rapid increase in weight between 70 and 112 days (3.0 gm to 7.5 gm) and then remains constant to puberty. Although this growth curve resembles that of the ovary, the significance is unknown. In contrast to the thyroid gland, total adrenal and pituitary weights show linear increases from birth to puberty (0.25 gm to 3.8 gm and 0.03 gm to 0.27 gm, respectively).

Hormone Levels

During prepuberal development, as shown in Figure 1, the concentration of free estrogens in the plasma declines gradually from birth (36 pg/ml) to 12 weeks of age (23 pg/ml).

Subsequently there is an increase in the concentration of free estrogens (27 pg/ml), followed by a gradual decline to puberty (<20 pg/ml). At or immediately prior to puberty, there is a rapid rise in estrogen concentration (50 to 60 pg/ml). Urinary estrogen excretion has been observed to increase at the beginning of the formation of tertiary follicles (70 to 112 days of age) and then decline up to the time of puberty, when the preovulatory peak is observed. In contrast to estrogens, progesterone is not detectable (concentration <2 ng/ml) in plasma before 13 weeks of age. As the gilt approaches puberty, progesterone concentrations of 2 to 4 ng/ml are found in the plasma.

General Considerations

The data discussed here suggest that the basic prepuberal development in the gilt is accomplished over a minimum period of 6 weeks but may require as long as 10 weeks. Puberty could occur at any time after the developmental process is completed. The beginning of puberal development may be observed as early as 8 weeks of age or perhaps even earlier in some breeds of swine. Conversely, the initiation of puberal development could commence considerably later. This assumption is based on the relatively wide variation in age at puberty actually observed between breeds of swine and sire families and as a result of animal manage-

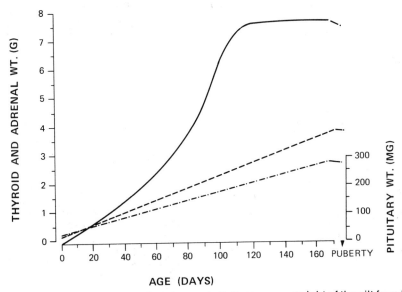

Figure 3. Age changes in thyroid ———, adrenal --- and pituitary –·–·– weight of the gilt from birth to puberty. The puberal change is identified by a solid line. (Dyck, G. W., unpublished data.)

ment, level of feeding, season and environment. Age at puberty, although averaging about 200 days, has been observed earlier than 100 days for individual gilts, whereas others have not cycled when marketed at 10 months. In a herd of 100 gilts, a range in age at puberty of 100 days can be expected.

Induction of Puberty

Several management techniques effectively induce puberty in many gilts. Housing gilts away from boars from weaning to at least 135 days of age will reduce age at puberty by 30 days. Short-term stress situations such as transportation, changes in housing conditions, short (24 to 48 hour) periods of starvation and checking for estrus with a different boar also are known to stimulate puberty. Hormone injections have distinct effects on puberty. Estrogens stimulate earlier puberty, whereas estrogens and progesterone or testosterone delay the onset of puberty. Gonadotropins are effective in inducing ovulation when vesicular follicles are present on the ovaries. However, pregnancy is not maintained, owing to failure of the corpora lutea, unless ovulation is stimulated late in the prepuberal period.

THE BOAR

Spermatogenesis

The development of puberty in the boar is based on the process of spermatogenesis, which requires 34.5 days for completion. Spermatogenesis commences with the division of the gonadocytes (spermatogonia), at which time three basic types of spermatogonia may be found along the basement membrane of the seminiferous tubules: dark type A, pale type A and type B. Type A spermatogonia are always present. Type B spermatogonia eventually give rise to the spermatozoa and are first observed on day 4 of spermatogenesis. On day 8 the type B spermatogonia are transformed to primary spermatocytes. On day 20 primary spermatocytes become secondary spermatocytes and form spermatids with round nuclei within 10 hours. By day 27 the spermatids have elongated nuclei, and on day 28 they become spermatozoa. The spermatozoa stay in the seminiferous tubules to day 34.5. This sequence of development is repeated at an interval of 8.6 days in any one location in a seminiferous tubule. Thus, in the mature boar there are four cycles in progress at all times.

Spermatogenesis commences at about 70 days of age. There is considerable variation in the onset of spermatogenesis, with initiation being observed as early as 60 days of age and as late as 90 days. It is conceivable that breed or line differences could result in greater variation in the onset of spermatogenesis than is presently observed. Although spermatogenesis does not begin in all tubules at the same time, the proliferation of spermatogenic activity throughout the seminiferous tubules appears to be very rapid. Within 25 days of the appearance of spermatozoa in the caudae epididymides, there are sufficient spermatozoa present (2.5 $\times$ 10^9 motile sperm at 140 days of age) to impregnate sows.

Testes

The typical testes growth curve and the appearance of spermatozoa in the epididymides is show in Figure 4. From birth to the beginning of spermatogenesis, the testes grow slowly. The seminiferous tubules remain relatively constant (55 μ in diameter) and contain two types of cells along the basement membrane: the supporting cells with irregular nuclei and gonadocytes with round nuclei. At birth the supporting cells form an almost continuous layer next to the basement membrane. By 42 days the supporting cells are also present more centrally in the tubules. There are approximately 800 m of tubules at this time.

Following the initiation of spermatogenesis (day 70), testes growth rate increases to about day 140. During this period of rapid puberal testes growth, the concentration of spermatozoa in the caudae epididymides follows the testes growth curve, with a delay of 44 days. This is the time required for spermatogenesis plus transit through the capita and corpora epididymides. By 140 days there are sufficient spermatozoa present in the caudae epididymides to impregnate sows. By 154 days the concentration of spermatozoa in the caudae epididymides has increased to 21 $\times$ 10^9 spermatozoa. Testes growth continues in the mature boar, and by 255 days of age the testes weigh 875 gm. The spermatozoal content of the capita-corpora and caudae epididymides is 96 $\times$ 10^9 and

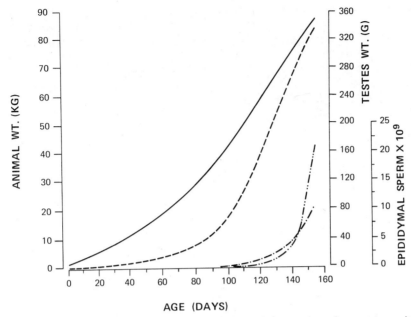

Figure 4. Age changes in boar weight ———. testes weight ---- and the number of spermatozoa in the capita and corpora —·—·— and caudae —··—··— epididymides from birth to puberty. (Adapted from Swierstra, E. E.: Proceeding International Pig Veterinary Society, Ames, Iowa, 1976.)

90×10^9, respectively (24 hours after ejaculation). These mature boars have 6000 to 8000 m of seminiferous tubules and an average daily production of 17.5×10^9 spermatozoa.

General Considerations

Along with the observed variation in age when spermatogenesis begins, there is also variation in age when sufficient sperm are present to impregnate sows. Some boars are able to impregnate sows at 125 days of age, whereas others must be 175 days of age or older. By 8 to 9 months of age, spermatozoa production should be similar for most boars. Furthermore, there are several factors that may affect spermatozoa production and quality (percentage of progressively motile sperm) and the ability of the boar to mate. Both high ambient temperatures and low levels of feed consumption will slow puberal development and may affect sperm quality. Short periods of illness also will affect the quality of sperm. These effects are not immediate but occur 10 to 40 days later, owing to the duration of spermatogenesis and epididymal transit time. Thus, it is very difficult to accurately diagnose a reproductive problem in the boar.

The management of the young boar is also of considerable importance. If boars are housed in isolation of gilts from weaning to puberty, they may lack all interest in the mating process. A similar effect may occur when a strange boar is placed with a group of gilts and the gilts commence fighting with him. Some breeds and lines normally have a low libido, and care must be taken in the handling of these boars. Locomotor defects and the inability to attain normal erection, protrusion and intromission of the penis are problems that can be detected only after puberty.

GENETIC DEFECTS

Genetic disorders that affect normal puberal development are basically of anatomical origin and include intersexuality, gonadal hypoplasia and various other abnormalities (see also Testicular and Ovarian Pathology in Swine, page 1099). Intersex pigs constitute up to 0.5 per cent of the population and have been identified as true hermaphrodites and male pseudohermaphrodites. True hermaphrodites are female and contain both ovarian and testicular tissue, either separately or together. Reproduction is often possible, although litter size may be reduced. This condition can only be detected at slaughter. Male pseudohermaphrodites are genetically female with female external and internal genitalia, except that testes are present in place of ovaries. This condition is detectable at puberty when a masculine type of behavior develops. Gonadal hypoplasia is not common and may affect only part of one gonad. Sperm production is reduced, even though testes size may be normal. Cryptorchidism, in which normal testicular descent has not occurred, is easily detected early in life. Reproduction is possible in these animals provided that one of the testes is in the scrotum.

There are numerous other defects that may occur, such as female pseudohermaphrodites, genetically male pseudohermaphrodites, freemartins, XXY karyotypes and anatomical abnormalities in the reproductive tract. Although the number of types of genetic defects in growing pigs is numerous, the incidence in the population is low and may affect no more than 1 to 2 per cent of the population. However, most of the defects are not detected until failure of the normal reproductive process is observed.

REFERENCES

1. Bal, H. S. and Getty, R.: Postnatal growth of the swine uterus from birth to six months. Growth, *34*:15, 1970.
2. Casida, L. E.: Prepuberal development of the pig ovary and its relation to stimulation with gonadotropic hormones. Anat. Rec., *61*:389, 1935.
3. Swierstra, E. E.: Cytology and duration of the cycle of the seminiferous epithelium of the boar; duration of spermatozoan transit through the epididymis. Anat. Rec., *61*:171, 1968.
4. Swierstra, E. E.: Testicular development and establishment of spermatogenesis in the boar. Proceedings International Pig Veterinary Society. Ames, Iowa, 1976.
5. Wrathall, A. E.: Reproductive disorders in pigs. Commonwealth Agricultural Bureaux (Review No. 11) Slough, England, 1975.

section **XIII**

LABORATORY AND ZOO ANIMALS

Consulting Editor

S. W. J. SEAGER

Reproduction of Wild Ungulates

B. BOEVER
St. Louis Zoo, St. Louis, Missouri

Ungulates are four-legged mammals with digits that are more or less fused. The ends of the digits are protected with a horny coating or hoof. These hooved mammals belong to two orders, Perissodactyla and Artiodactyla. The domestic horse is a member of the order Perissodactyla, and the domestic ruminants (cattle, sheep and goats) are all members of the order Artiodactyla. Hence, the domestic counterparts to these wild ungulates serve as a model in which we derive most of our knowledge about reproduction of the wild hooved animals.

These animals are in great demand in zoos and various game parks. They make excellent displays. Many are extremely rare or are even becoming extinct in the wild. It is of utmost importance that we are able to reproduce these species in captivity to insure the continued existence of these animals and possibly to release them back into the wild. Other ungulates, although not threatened by extinction, are kept in great numbers in deer parks and by private individuals. Bison, elk and various small deer are on the increase in small private preserves.

The diseases and reproductive problems of the wild ungulates are very similar to those of the domestic hooved mammals. There are, of course, some differences that are due to different anatomical structures, differences in susceptibility and different means of treatment. However, the basic concepts are the same. The clinical signs, pathogenesis, transmission and etiology of the different disease entities are usually the same in the zoological species as in the domestic species. The difficulty and challenge of zoo animal medicine are to devise ways and means to utilize these routine diagnostic methods and to modify treatment techniques so that they are applicable to the wild animals.

RESTRAINT

Obviously, the means of restraint is of utmost importance and will be discussed in detail. Once the animal is restrained, the diagnostic workup is the same as for domestic livestock. Blood samples are drawn for hematology and blood chemistry studies; auscultation, percussion and palpation are carried out; cultures are obtained for bacterial or viral isolation and radiographs are taken. In addition, once the animal is restrained, surgery is easily carried out and treatments are performed. I cannot emphasize enough the fact that the animals are exotic, not the diseases. The diseases and reproductive problems are the same ones found in domestic livestock.

Manual and Mechanical Restraint

Of the many methods of restraint the oldest is probably brute force. Manual restraint is sometimes helpful and in the smaller ungulates is the method of choice. Many of the smaller deer, gazelles, wild sheep and goats can be caught by hand and restrained for examination and short treatments. It requires a knowledgeable person to catch the animal because many of these species are very delicate and can be stressed very easily. Care must be taken to avoid injury to the animal and to the handler. Some of the sturdier hooved stock can be worked with ropes, but in general this is not desirable.

Catching chutes and squeeze chutes that are used for cattle may be helpful for some hooved mammals, but most chutes have to be modified. The typical head catchers do not work, and only certain species can withstand this type of stress. The bison and some of the exotic cattle can be worked in this manner, but often the squeeze chute must be reinforced. Again, I must emphasize that many of the Artiodactyla and Perissodactyla will not tolerate any type of manual restraint. Injuries such as fractures, concussions and abrasions may result for both the handlers and the animals. The legs, horns, antlers and head of the animals may be caught in crates, chutes or fences used for manual restraint. Serious concussions occur if the head is not padded, and the animal will continue to struggle until death.

Chemical Restraint

Chemical restraint and immobilization also have their shortcomings. Normally,

TABLE 1. *Etorphine (M99) Dosages for Ungulates*

Family	Species	Total Adult Dose (mg)	Total Juvenile Dose— Approx. 6 mo–2 yr (mg)
Order Perissodactyla:			
Equidae	Przevalsky's horse	2.0–4.0	1.0–3.0
	Onager	2.0–4.0	1.0–3.0
	African wild ass	1.0–3.0	1.0–2.0
	Grévy zebra	2.0–4.0	1.5–3.0
	Burchell's zebra	1.5–3.0	1.0–2.0
	Mountain zebra	1.5–3.0	1.0–2.0
Tapiridae	Brazilian tapir	1.0–3.0	0.5–2.0
	Baird's tapir	1.0–3.0	0.5–2.0
	Mountain or wooly tapir	1.0–3.0	0.5–2.0
	Malayan tapir	1.0–3.0	0.5–2.0
Rhinocerotidae	Indian rhinoceros	3.0–5.0	1.0–4.0
	Square lipped (white) Rhinoceros	2.0–5.0	1.0–4.0
	Black rhinoceros	3.0–5.0	1.0–4.0
Order Artiodactyla:			
Suidae	Wild boar	3.0–6.0	1.0–4.0
	Domestic pig	3.0–6.0	1.0–4.0
Tayassuidae	Peccary	1.0–2.0	0.5–1.0
Hippopotamidae	River hippopotamus	5.0–8.0	3.0–6.0
	Pygmy hippopotamus	4.0–7.0	2.0–5.0
Camelidae	Bactrian camel	2.0–4.0	0.5–2.0
	Dromedary camel	2.0–4.0	0.5–2.0
	Guanaco	1.0–3.0	0.5–2.0
	Llama	1.0–3.0	0.5–2.0
Cervidae	Muntjac deer	1.0–3.0	0.5–2.0
	Fallow deer	2.0–4.0	1.0–3.0
	Hog deer	1.5–3.0	0.5–2.0
	Barasingha deer	3.0–5.0	2.0–4.0
	Axis deer	3.0–6.0	1.5–3.0
	Sika deer	2.0–4.0	1.0–3.0
	European red deer	2.0–5.0	1.0–3.0
	Wapiti (American elk)	3.0–6.0	1.0–3.0
	Pere David's deer	2.0–5.0	1.0–3.0
	Roe deer	2.0–5.0	0.5–2.0
	White tailed deer	3.0–6.0	1.5–3.0
	Mule deer	2.0–4.0	1.0–3.0
	Caribou (reindeer)	2.0–5.0	1.0–3.0
	Moose	4.0–8.0	2.0–5.0
Giraffidae	Giraffe	3.0–8.0	2.0–5.0
	Okapi	3.0–5.0	2.0–4.0
Antilocapridae	Pronghorn	2.0–5.0	1.0–3.0
Bovidae	Greater kudu	4.0–7.0	1.0–4.0
	Lesser kudu	3.0–6.0	2.0–3.0
	Sitatunga	3.0–6.0	1.0–3.0
	Nyala	1.5–3.0	0.5–1.5
	Eland	5.0–10.0	4.0–6.0
	Nilgai	4.0–6.0	1.0–4.0
	Buffalo	6.0–10.0	2.0–6.0
	Bison	6.0–10.0	2.0–6.0
	Wisent	4.0–8.0	2.0–4.0

TABLE 1. *Etorphine (M99) Dosages for Ungulates—Continued*

Family	Species	Total Adult Dose (mg)	Total Juvenile Dose— Approx. 6 mo–2 yr (mg)
	Yak	3.0–8.0	2.0–4.0
	Domestic cattle	6.0–10.0	2.0–6.0
	Hartebeest	2.0–3.0	1.0–2.0
	Blesbok	2.0–3.0	1.0–2.0
	White tailed gnu	3.0–5.0	2.0–4.0
	Brindled gnu	3.0–5.0	2.0–4.0
	Roan antelope	1.5–3.0	1.0–2.0
	Sable antelope	3.0–6.0	2.0–4.0
	Oryx	5.0–10.0	3.0–7.0
	Addax	5.0–8.0	2.5–5.0
	Waterbuck	3.0–5.0	1.5–3.0
	Gazelles	2.0–3.0	1.0–2.0
	Blackbuck	2.0–3.0	1.0–2.0
	Impala	2.0–5.0	1.5–2.0
	Springbok	1.5–3.0	1.0–2.0
	Musk ox	1.5–4.0	1.0–2.0
	Ibex	1.0–3.0	0.5–2.0
	Tahr	2.0–4.0	1.0–2.0
	Aoudad	2.0–4.0	1.0–2.0
	Wild sheep	1.0–3.0	1.0–2.0
	Red sheep	1.0–3.0	0.5–1.5
	Bighorn sheep	2.0–4.0	1.0–2.0
	Mouflon	1.0–2.0	0.5–1.5

there is a species variation in reaction to the drug used. Usually the animal's weight and physical condition are unknown prior to immobilization. In addition, it is frequently difficult to administer the drug with a hand syringe. All of these complications go along with the normal hazards of chemical restraint.

The cap-chur gun is usually used to administer drugs to the wild ungulates. This equipment makes use of an automatic syringe propelled by a gas- or powder-powered projector. A person may propel 1 to 15 ml of any liquid to an animal and have the syringe inject the liquid into the animal upon contact. Various sized syringes and various sized needles are available, depending upon the use. Antibiotics, vaccines and anesthetics can be administered in this way.

Chemical agents used most frequently to immobilize ungulates for reproductive work include etorphine (M99), diprenorphine (M5050) and xylazine. Etorphine is a highly potent analgesic. Diprenorphine is an antagonist to etorphine for complete reversal of drug effect. Following the administration of etorphine, the onset of action is about 4 minutes. This is evident when the animal begins to circle and high step. Peak effect is reached in 15 to 30 minutes. Additional doses are usually necessary after approximately 1 hour. Little or no muscle relaxation is obtained with etorphine alone. Complete reversal is accomplished in 2 to 5 minutes by the intravenous administration of diprenorphine at twice the milligram dosage of the administered etorphine. Fifteen to 30 minutes are necessary for reversal with intramuscular administration of diprenorphine. Etorphine is often used in combination with tranquilizers such as acepromazine and xylazine. When using etorphine, it has been my experience that dosages in the higher range are safer than the dosages in the lower range. The antagonist is always available if toxic effects are evident. Most problems that result from a low dosage of etorphine are due to the addition of manual restraint to achieve adequate immobilization. If complete immobilization is not obtained with the dose, either administer additional etorphine or an accompanying tranquilizer or reverse the animal and attempt the procedure on a different day. Dosages for etorphine are species specific, ranging from 1 mg/200 kg of body weight to 1 mg/2000 kg of body weight. Excited animals usually require a heavier dosage, whereas sick and depressed animals require a lighter dosage. Dosages that I use for administration of etorphine are listed in Table 1.

Xylazine (Rompun) is a thiazine derivative with marked sedative and central muscle relaxant effect. Induction time from intramuscular injection is between 1 and 15 minutes, with peak effect at 15 to 60 minutes. Complete recovery takes several hours. Xylazine has a wide margin of safety. Most Artiodactyla require approximately 1 mg/kg of body weight for sedation and 2 mg/kg of body weight for immobilization. Often the animal appears to be immobilized but when approached may become aroused so that it will stand up and run away from the veterinarian. Although xylazine can be used alone, its greatest use is in combination with etorphine, at 0.05 mg/kg of body weight (Table 2).

REPRODUCTIVE CYCLES AND REPRODUCTIVE MANAGEMENT

The Artiodactyla and Perissodactyla in most zoos reproduce with success, and dystocias are the most common reproductive problem. However, recently more emphasis has been given to artificial breeding and herd management. With the number of animals decreasing in the wild, it has become more and more important to obtain maximum reproduction from these species in captivity. For many of these species, very little or nothing is known about their reproductive cycles and the physiology involved. Even less is known about the artificial means of reproducing these animals.

Female

Physical examination of most of these wild ungulates requires restraint of some type. Prior to any restraint measures, one must observe the animal — how it walks, its disposition, overall condition, position in the herd and so forth. Only then is the means of restraint chosen. Once the animal has been immobilized, a complete physical examination can be carried out similar to that performed for domestic livestock, including rectal palpation if the species is large enough.

Puberty and the Estrous Cycle

Onset of puberty is different for each species (Table 3). Behavior plays an important role in this, and the breeding season or the herd structure will also affect the onset of

TABLE 2. *Xylazine (Rompun) Dosages for Ungulates**

Species	For Sedation (mg/kg)	For Immobilization (mg/kg)
Equidae:		
Zebra	3.0–5.0	Not possible
Ass	3.0–5.0	Not possible
Onager	3.0–5.0	Not possible
Przevalsky's horse	3.0–5.0	Not possible
Camelidae:		
Camel	0.1–0.5	1.0–2.0
Guanaco	0.3–1.0	2.0
Llama	0.2–0.5	1.0–2.0
Cervidae:		
Fallow deer	1.0–2.0	5.0–8.0
Hog deer	1.0–2.0	3.0–4.0
Axis deer	1.0–2.0	3.0–4.0
Sika deer	2.0	3.0–4.0
Red deer	1.0–2.0	3.0–4.0
Wapiti (American elk)	1.0–2.0	3.0–4.0
Roe deer	0.5–1.0	1.5–3.0
White tailed deer	0.5–1.0	3.0–4.0
Moose (American)	0.5	1.5
Reindeer	0.5	2.0
Bovidae:		
Maxwell's duiker	1.0	2.0
Greater kudu	1.0	3.0
Nyala	1.0	3.0(?)
Sitatunga	1.5	3.0
Bushbuck	1.0	
Eland	1.0	3.0
Nilgai	1.0	3.0
Hartebeest		2.0(?)
Blesbok		4.0(?)
White tailed gnu	1.0	1.5–3.0
Brindled gnu	1.0	1.5–3.0
Roan antelope	1.5	3.0
Sable antelope	1.5	3.0
Oryx	1.5	3.0
Addax		0.5(?)
Waterbuck		2.0–3.0
Kob		1.0(?)
Gazelles	1.0	2.0–4.0
Blackbuck	1.0	3.0
Springbuck	1.0	1.0–3.0
Impala	1.0	3.0
Domestic buffalo	0.05–0.15	0.2–0.5
Cape buffalo		1.0(?)
Gayal		1.0–1.5(?)
Banteng		0.5–1.5
Domestic ox	0.05–0.2	0.2–0.6
Wild ox	0.1–0.3	0.3–1.0 (2.0)
Yak	0.3	0.6–1.0
American bison	0.1–0.3	0.6–1.0 (2.0)
European bison	0.5	2.0–3.0
Chamois		2.0–3.0
Ibex	0.5–1.0	3.0–4.0
Goat	0.05–0.3	0.3–0.5
Aoudad	0.3–0.5	0.5–2.0
European mouflon	2.0	3.0–6.0
Kara tau sheep	1.0–1.5	
Wild sheep	0.05–0.3	0.3–0.6
Musk ox	0.5	0.5–1.5

*From Bauditz, R.: Sedation, immobilization, and anesthesia with Rompun in captive and free-living wild animals. Vet. Med. Rev. 3:204, 1972.

puberty. An animal may be sexually mature physically, yet it does not breed until the psychological needs are met and the proper season has arrived.

The estrous period of various species is classified in Table 3. For some species the estrous period, duration of cycles and so forth have been mapped out. With other rare animals little is known. Often there are no visible signs of estrus in the exotic stock. There is very little riding by females and little or no discharge. One of the few external signs of estrus is a mounting by the male of the species. Some studies are now being conducted on estrous stimulation and synchronization with human chorionic gonadotropin (HCG) and prostaglandins.

Pregnancy

Infertility problems are sometimes very difficult to diagnose with the wild ungulates. Often there are more than physical reasons for infertility. The behavioral and environmental conditions must be considered. Territory, herd structure and season affect breeding, and each species has its own peculiarities. Field research and behavioral data are available on many of the species. Infertility problems of a physiological nature in wild ungulates are diagnosed and treated similar to problems in their domestic counterparts.

Pregnancy examination is seldom carried out on the wild ungulates. The usual method is to record the breeding date and observe the animal. Pregnancy examination would require chemical or manual restraint, which might affect the fetus. If pregnancy diagnosis is necessary, rectal examinations can be done on the larger hooved stock, and radiography has been used in the later stages of gestation for some of the smaller hooved stock. The Cuboni urine test has been used successfully on some of the wild ungulates, and hormonal assays of the blood are being attempted.

Parturition is variable, depending upon the species. Some species deliver at night, others in daylight. Some isolate themselves from the herd to deliver, others do not. Some have quick births, some lie down and others deliver while standing. Space prevents listing the various differences. In general, parturition in wild ungulates proceeds similar to parturition in domestic ungulates.

Obstetrical procedures for wild ungulates have not presented too many difficulties when approached similar to procedures for domestic animals. One of the common faults with wild animals is waiting too long to offer assistance with the delivery. Our present policy is to offer assistance if the calf is not delivered after the cow has been in heavy labor for 2 hours. When giving assistance either to pull the calf or for cesarean section, I normally use etorphine as the general anesthetic, although manual restraint is sometimes used. When etorphine is used, some of the diprenorphine antagonist has to be given to the calf after it is delivered. Usually I will administer the full dose of antagonist to the mother and 25 per cent of the antagonist dose to the calf.

Surgical procedures for reproductive problems are seldom carried out on wild animals, although routine methods would be used if necessary.

Postpartum and Neonatal Care

Postpartum care varies with the species. Almost all animals require greater attention to their nutritional needs during lactation. Some are kept isolated with their offspring for several weeks after delivering. Other are left with the herd of females without the male. Still others are reintroduced back into the herd with the male. Again, the species variations dictate the methods used.

Normally little extra care is given to the offspring. The umbilicus is usually treated with iodine. Occasionally antibiotics or serum is administered to the offspring if navel disorders have been a problem in the herd. Usually we try to have the female care for her youngster. However, it is occasionally necessary to hand-raise the offspring (Table 4).

Male

Physical examination should proceed as in the female, with much observation of the animal prior to immobilization. Once the animal is immobilized, the complete examination can be carried out. Again, rectal palpation is possible only in the larger species.

Onset of puberty in the male is very dependent upon behavior. Even though a male may have reached sexual maturity, he can psychologically be kept from breeding by an older bull until he is several years of age (see Table 3).

Semen Collection and Evaluation

Similar methods of semen collection have been attempted with wild animals as with domestic animals. The only method that is

Text continued on page 1125

TABLE 3. *Reproductive Data for Ungulates*

Common Name	Breeding Season	Sexual Maturity (months)	Gestation Period (days)	No. of Young	Normal Adult Weight (kg)	Life Expectancy (years)	Herd Size	Comments
Order Perissodactyla:								
Equidae:								
Przevalsky's horse	All year (especially April and May)	36–60	330–360	1	250–300	25–30	Small groups (up to 20)	
Onager	All year	36–48	330	1	200–250	20–25	Singly, small groups or large groups	
African wild ass	All year (especially April and May)	24–60	360	1	250	25–30	10–15	
Grévy zebra	April–Sept.	36–60	350–390	1	400	20–30	10–15 (in large groups during migration)	
Burchell's zebra	April–May	24–48	350–390	1	350	20–30	10–15 (in large groups during migration)	
Mountain zebra	April–Sept.	24–48	300–375	1	350	20–30	Small groups (7–12)	
Tapiridae:								
Brazilian tapir	All year	36–48	390–400	1	225–300	25–30	Alone or in pairs	All tapirs have striped offspring and cycle every 50–80 days with a 2-day heat
Baird's tapir	All year	36–48	390–400	1	225–300	25–30	Alone or in pairs	
Mountain tapir	All year	36–48	390–400	1	225–250	25–30	Alone or in pairs	
Malayan tapir	All year	36–48	390–400	1	225–300	25–30	Alone or in pairs	
Rhinocerotidae:								
Indian rhinoceros	March and April	48–60	510–570	1	2000–4000	50	Solitary	Heat every 46–48 days for 24 hours
Square lipped (white) rhinoceros	July–Sept.	48–60	530–550	1	2000–3000	30	Small groups up to 18	
Black rhinoceros	All year	48–60	530–550	1	1000–1800	30	Singly or in small groups (1–5)	
Order Artiodactyla								
Suidae:								
River hog	Aug. and Sept.	8–10		2–8	75–130	10		Striped offspring
Wild boar	Dec.–Jan. (highest), all year	8–10	115	4–8	150	15		Striped offspring, female cycle every 21 days estrous period 2–3 days
Wart hog	June–July	12	171–175	3	100	15	Small groups	Striped offspring
Forest hog		8–10	125	2–6	200	2	20	Striped offspring
Babirussa		8–10	125–150	2	100	10		
Tyassuidae:								
Collared peccary	All year	10	142–149	2–3	30	20	5–15	
White lipped peccary	All year	10	142–149	2–3	35	13	50–100	

Species	Breeding season		Gestation	Young			Grouping	Remarks
Hippopotamidae:								
Nile hippopotamus	All year	36	227–240	1	1300–2000	40–45	Singly or in pairs	Nurse in water 35-day cycle with 3-day estrous period; wean at 4 months, 38-day cycle with 1–2 day estrous
Pygmy hippopotamus	All year	48	206–210	1	200–250	35		
Camelidae:								
Dromedary camel	Feb.–March (especially)	24	315–360	1	500	20	Small groups (5–10)	
Bactrian camel	March	30	389–406	1	700	20	6–20	
Llama	All year	24	330	1	100	15–20	Small groups	
Guanaco	Nov.–Feb.	24	330	1	100	15–20	Small groups	
Vicuna	Aug.–Sept.	24	300	1	50	15–20	Small groups	
Alpaca		24	330	1	70	15–20	Small groups	
Cervidae:								
Chevrotain	June and July	18	120–180	1–2	2–5	1–2	Singly	Postpartum estrus 1 day after parturition; no antlers—penis has thread-like extension
Musk deer	Jan.	18	160	1–2	7–17	10	Singly or in pairs	
Muntjac	Jan.–Feb.	18	180	1	15–35	16	Singly or in pairs	
Tufted deer	April–May	18	180	1	40–50	7	Small herds (2–3)	
Fallow deer	Sept.–Oct.	18	230	1	35–80	20	Small groups (2–3)	
Axis deer	All year	18	210–225	2	75–100	15–20	Small groups (2–3)	
Sanbar deer	All year	18	249–284	1	60–150	10–25	Small groups (2–3)	
Barasingha deer	Oct.–Nov.	18	250	1	230–283	20	Small groups	
Elk deer	March–May	18	180	1	80–150	20	Large herds	
Sika deer	Sept.–Oct.	18	222–246	1	25–110	20	Large herds	
Red deer	July–Sept.	24	225–262	1	125–350	15–20	"	
American elk	"	"	"	"	"	"	12–15	
Pere David deer	June–July	30	250–270	1–2	150–200	20	Singly or in small groups (5)	
White tailed deer	Nov.	7	201	1–2	50–150	10	Singly or in small groups (5)	
Mule deer	Nov.–Dec.	7	210–260	1–2	50–150	10	Singly or in pairs	Difficult to keep in captivity
Moose	Sept.–Oct.	18	240–250	1	80–150	25		
Reindeer	Sept.–Oct.	18	240	1–2		15	5–40	
Roe deer	July–Aug.	15	240	1–3		10	Small groups (2–3)	
Giraffidae:								
Giraffe	All year	42	420–468	1	500–800	25	Singly or in small groups	14-day estrous cycle, 24-hour estrus period, wean 6–9 months
Okapi	June–July	30	426–457	1		15–20	Singly	
Antilocapridae:								
Pronghorn		16	230–240	2	50	7–10	Small to large groups	

Table continued on the following page

TABLE 3. Reproductive Data for Ungulates—Continued

Common Name	Breeding Season	Sexual Maturity (months)	Gestation Period (days)	No. of Young	Normal Adult Weight (kg)	Life Expectancy (years)	Herd Size	Comments
Order Artiodactyla (Continued)								
Bovidae:								
Greater kudu	All year	30	210–240	1	200–250	15	6–20 in herd	
Lesser kudu	All year	24	210	1	100	12–15	6 in group	
Sitatunga	Jan.–Feb.	24	210–225	1–2	100	17		
Nyala		30	210	1	100–125	15	Singly or in pairs	
Bushbuck	All year	24	225	1	100	12	Small groups	
Eland		30	255–270	1	1000	25	Singly or in pairs	
Bongo		30	225	1	200	20	Small groups	
Nilgai	End of March	30		1 first year, 2 thereafter	200	15		
Four horned antelope	June–July	24	225–240	1–3	15–25	10	Singly or in pairs	
Anda	All year (especially May)	30	275–315		150–300	28	Singly or in pairs	
Water buffalo	All year	30	300–340	1	1000	20–25	Herds (10–20)	
African buffalo	All year	18	300–330	1	300–800	25	Herds (30–60)	
Gaur	July–Aug.	24	270–280	1	700–1000	25	Groups (8–12)	Wean 6 months
Banteng	April–May	24	270–280	1	500–900	15	Small groups	Wean at 9 months
Kouprey	Aug.–Sept.	60	270	1	900	12	Small groups (8–11)	
Yak	May–Sept.	24	258	1	1000	25	Large herds 100+	Wean at 12 months
Bison	Aug.–Sept.	24	270–285	1	1000	20–25	Herds (20–30)	
Wisent			260–270	1	1000	25	Large and small herds	
Duiker			120	1	25	10	Singly or in pairs	
Hartebeest	Dec.–March		240	1	120–215	15	5–30 in group	
Sassaby		24	210–240	1	125	15	Small groups	
Blesbok			225–240	1	100	15	Small groups (8–10)	
White tailed gnu	June	30	240	1	145–270	20	Small groups (8–10)	
Brindled gnu	June	30	240–270	1	150–300	15	Large herds	
Roan antelope	All year	24	270–280	1	150–250	15–20	Small groups (3–15)	
Sable antelope	All year	24	270–281	1	100–200	18	Small groups (20)	
Oryx	All year	24	270	1			Small herds, up to 20	
Addax	March–May (especially), all year	24	300–360	1	50–100		5–20	
Waterbuck	All year	24	240–270	1	170–250	15	Up to 30	
Lechne waterbuck	Oct.–Jan.	24	210	1	60–120	15	Group, up to 50	
Kob	All year	24	240–270	1	50–120	15	Small groups	
Reedbuck	All year	20	180–210	1	25–75	12	Small groups, up to 20	
Dik-dik	All year	6	180	1	2–6	7	Pairs	
Klipspringer		15	210	1	15	15	Singly and pairs	
Steinbok			210	1	20	12	Singly or pairs	
Gazelles	All year	12	150–180	1–2	15–25	10	5–20, herds	
Blackbuck	All year	12	180	1	25–45	15	6–10, herds	
Impala	Feb.–April	12	190–200	1	40–90	10	6–60	

Gerenuk	May	15	210	1	35–52	7–8	Pairs or small groups	
Springbok	Nov.–Dec.	15	180	1	18–45	10	Small to large groups	
Tibetan antelope	Nov.		180	1–2	25–35		10–20	
Saiga antelope	Sept.–Oct.	8	150	1	23–40	4	2–50	
Goral			180	1	25–35	11	Small groups	
Serow			210–240	1	55–140		Small groups	
Takin		24	210–240		350		Small herds	
Chamois	Oct.–Jan.	18	80	1	14–62	5–10	Small groups, up to 10	
Rocky mountain goat			180		150	8	Small groups, up to 10	
Musk ox	July–Aug.	24	255	1	200–300	10	15	
Ibex	Dec.–Jan.	18	150–180	1–3	35–150	15–20	Small herds, up to 20	
Markhor	Nov.–Jan.	18	180		32–40	10		
Wild goat	Nov.–Jan.	18	180	1–3	25–40	10		
Tahr	Dec. (especially), all year	18	150–180	1–3	100	15–20	30–40	
Blue sheep	Oct.–Nov.	18	160	1	25–80	15	Small and large herds	
Aoudad (Barbary sheep)	Nov.	18	150–165	1–3	40–140	15	Singly or in small groups	Wean in 6 months
Moufflon	Oct.–Dec.	18	150	1–2	35–50	15–20	Small groups	
Red sheep (Marco Polo)		18	147–188			5–10	Large groups	
Big horn sheep		18	180	1	150		Large groups	

TABLE 4. *Criteria For Hand-Raising Ungulates*

Name	Weight at Birth (kg)	Type of Nipple	Birth to 2 Weeks FEEDINGS/DAY	Birth to 2 Weeks AMOUNT/FEEDING	2 Weeks FEEDINGS/DAY	2 Weeks AMOUNT/FEEDING	Formula Recommended
Zebra	30–50	Albers' calf nipple	4–5	300–500 ml	4–5	500 ml–1 liter	1 part evaporated milk, 1 part distilled water
Tapir	3–10	Lamb or calf nipple	4–5	300–500 ml	4–15	500 ml–1 liter	1 part evaporated milk, 1 part distilled water
Rhinoceros	25–75						
Peccary	0.5–1.0		4–5	15–60 ml	4–5	30–120 ml	1 part evaporated milk, 1 part water
Nile hippopotamus	30–50						
Pygmy hippopotamus	3–5						
Dromedary camel	30–45	Albers' calf nipple (small cross-cut)	4–6	0.5 liter	4	1.5 liters	3 parts evaporated milk, 3 parts distilled water, 1 part lime water
Llama	7–15	Regular Evenflow nipple (small cross-cut)	4–5	120–240 ml	4	240 ml	1 part evaporated milk, 1 part water
White tailed deer		Evenflow	4–5	60–120 ml	3–5	120–240 ml	Straight evaporated milk
Bison	24–27	Albers' calf nipple	4–6	300 ml–1 liter	4–5	0.5–1 liter	1 part evaporated milk, 1 part distilled water
Eland	31	Albers' calf nipple	3–5	180 ml–1 liter	3–5	240 ml–2 liters	1 part evaporated milk, 1 part water
Springbok	3	Evenflow	4–5	90–150 ml	3–4	150–240 ml	1 part evaporated milk, 1 part water
Impala		Evenflow	2–3	30–180 ml	3	150–240 ml	1 part evaporated milk, 1 part water
Kudu		Lamb or calf nipple	2–6	240–360 ml	4–6	100–240 ml	1 part evaporated milk, 1 part water
Aoudad	2.5–5.0	Evenflow	4–6	60–120 ml	4–5	120–180 ml	1–1.5 parts evaporated milk, 1 part water
Mouflon	2.5–5.0	Preemie large pinhole, small cross-cut	4–6	60–150 ml	4	120–240 ml	1–1.5 parts evaporated milk, 1 part water
Artiodactyla in general			5	Depends on size, approximately 20 ml/kg	5	Depends on size, approximately 20 ml/kg	1 part evaporated milk, 1 part water

consistently effective is electroejaculation, which is usually carried out under chemical immobilization with either etorphine or xylazine. Again, the techniques used are basically the same.

Evaluation of wild animal semen is the same as for domestic stock except that only a small number of samples are available for comparison. Often the semen has some peculiarities, and it is not known whether these are abnormalities or if this is normal for that species.

Artificial Insemination

Artificial insemination of wild ungulates has not been used to any great extent, although I feel it will be an important factor in the future. However, there are certain problems that are not as yet worked out for all species. Estrous detection is extremely difficult at this point. Semen freezing, although successful with some species, does not work with all species. Again, these problems will be worked out in the future as more knowledge is gained of these species.

With a few exceptions, natural service is the only method of breeding used in zoos and game parks.

Infertility Problems

Infertility problems in males are often a serious setback to a breeding program in a zoo that usually has only one male of a species. Physical examination and semen evaluation are used to diagnose these problems. However, many of the species do not produce sperm all year round, and spermatogenesis peaks at certain times of the year. This makes semen evaluation particularly confusing. Nevertheless, a fertile male should have at least a slight amount of spermatogenesis, even when it is not the breeding season. Again, behavior plays an important role, with territory and harem size being factors. It is important to study the behavioral traits of the male of a particular species, along with the physical examination, to determine the animal's breeding capabilities.

Surgical procedures are seldom carried out on wild animals, although castrations and vasectomies are sometimes performed in a manner similar to that for domestic animals.

GENERAL CONSIDERATIONS

Factors Affecting Reproduction

Not enough is known at this time about hereditary problems of wild animals. Various birth defects are seen from time to time, and a high percentage of the offspring of wild ungulates are weak at birth. In the captive environment there is a high incidence of inbreeding as a result of shipping difficulties and gene pool restrictions. Hopefully, artificial reproduction will help to eliminate some of these problems.

The diseases affecting reproduction in domestic ungulates also affect the exotic ungulates. Diagnosis and treatment are the same as in domestic stock.

Immunization programs for wild ungulates are rather limited. The difficulty of administering the vaccine plus the fact that most zoos are isolated from other livestock by the metropolitan area has reduced the importance of immunization procedures.

Behavior is very closely related to reproduction, as has been mentioned numerous times earlier. Territoriality, herd size, sex ratio and even mating behaviors of wild animals are all important. Different species have different characteristics. Some of these needs have to be duplicated to allow for successful reproduction.

Nutrition is important, as with all species. If adequate nutrition is not provided, spermatogenesis suffers and often females do not cycle or are unable to carry a fetus to term. Sufficient nutrition must therefore be provided.

An effective approach to diagnosing a herd infertility problem starts with (1) physical examination and semen evaluation of the herd bull, (2) physical examination of the females and (3) accurate records and close observation for behavioral problems or difficulties.

Reproductive Management Programs

The goal of a reproductive management program in a zoo setting is usually aimed at high reproduction, with each female reproducing to her maximum efficiency. To accomplish this it is important to have the proper facilities and a well-trained staff. The female hooved animals are usually kept in herds with one herd sire. If the females are separated for calving, it is important to reintroduce them to the herd as quickly as possible so they are not open for too long a period. Care must be taken not to overwork the females, and occasionally they should be kept separate from the herd bull for a while longer after parturition to rebuild their condition. One management approach is to sell male offspring and keep a few female offspring for replacement of older females. Every 5 years the herd sire is replaced by purchasing a new bull from an unrelated herd. Other management techniques are possible, depending upon the goals. Breeding season and other behavioral characteristics will have to be taken into consideration when planning a program.

Records are necessary for wild animals, just as for domestic stock. Each individual animal is tagged, and an accurate record is kept for each animal, including its lineage, medical problems, diagnosis and treatment. Breeding date, estrous period and reproductive performance records are kept for each animal.

In summary, reproduction of wild ungulates is very similar to that of domestic cattle and horses. There are some peculiarities and some major differences in behavior and restraint, but basically wild ruminant reproduction should be approached in a manner similar to that for domestic stock.

The Effect of Nutrition on Reproduction in Zoo Animals

R. S. PATTON

Deht Company, Los Angeles, California

Day to day, little else is of greater concern to those involved in zoo husbandry than nutrition and reproduction. This is also true for people involved in animal agriculture, but the zoo professional brings more anxiety to the problem. The main thing he is certain about is how little is known. Definitive studies of reproduction in exotic species are rare, and studies investigating the effect of nutrition on reproduction are even more uncommon.

OBTAINING NUTRITIONAL DATA

There is a great potential for generating much of the lacking data. Zoo personnel are successfully reproducing endangered species at an impressive rate in some quarters, in spite of a suboptimum diet. This unfortunately leads them to believe the diet is adequate; however, if a trained investigator could simply quantify conditions extant during each successful reproduction, a great body of useful data could be collected. Likewise, a trained researcher could greatly increase the useful information so gleaned by eliminating confounding effects that nonre-search-oriented zoo personnel unknowingly impose. Usually, adequate controls are not possible when dealing with rare animal collections, but normal experimental procedures such as standardization of conditions throughout the time period studied could still be followed. Anyone turning to the literature for aid in approaching a reproduction problem will be discouraged by the lack of data. This should, in turn, arouse a determination to learn as much as possible from his own efforts. Eventually a researcher will collect data pertaining to the entire reproductive cycle, and regardless of its outcome, these will be of great value to others, if carefully noted.

Admittedly, this approach can only accomplish so much. Hormonal blood titers, especially serially, are difficult to obtain in a 400-pound tiger. Obtaining them, with the concomitant anesthetizing of the cat, would greatly alter conditions from normal. Veterinarians and reproductive physiologists must bear in mind that the agricultural animals they trained on, while by no means tame, have been highly selected for compatibility with man and his management systems. Zoo animals are wild, in the strictest sense of the word, and will kill themselves while avoiding restraint, whereas a domestic sheep or hog will merely struggle violently. There is thus a distinct difference between zoo and domestic animals.

EXTRAPOLATING NUTRITIONAL DATA

Given the perplexities of finding or obtaining data about nutrition and zoo reproduction, the procedure of choice is one of extrapolation. The basic rules of nutrition apply regardless of species, but on a more specialized level, the data from the domestic bovine can serve as a good guide for the exotic bovine, humans are the best model available for higher primates, the domestic cat tends to parallel the large cats and so on. Of course, the snow leopard is not a house cat, and a Holstein calf is not a musk ox, but in the absence of exact information, these domestic models provide a safer starting point than a wild guess or intuition.

In the late 1960's, the Topeka Zoo (Gage Park, Topeka, Kansas) started feeding a pair of Bengal tigers a balanced prepared diet, formulated primarily on known needs of domestic cats. In conjunction with proper management, this approach enabled this pair of tigers to set two world records in exotic animal reproduction — the highest number of cubs raised by a single pair of tigers in captivity and the highest number of cubs born in one litter. A similar "back to basics" approach to the nutrition of birds of prey enabled the Topeka Zoo to be the first to hatch and rear golden eagles in captivity.

Regardless if gestation time is a mystery or if the last picogram of prostaglandin is unequivocally delineated, the rules of nutrition for reproduction are exactly the same: *adequate intake of an adequate diet.* This obviously is merely the cardinal rule of nutrition, reproduction notwithstanding. Hence, the following, although it appears to address nutrition in general to the exclusion of reproduction, is the approach to be taken, not because it is the only information available but because it happens to be the correct one for optimum reproduction.

Defining and obtaining an adequate diet are not that difficult and will be discussed directly. Achieving adequate intake is less easily accomplished, mainly because people are involved. This primary problem of zoo animal nutrition, i.e., people, will be discussed subsequently.

PROVIDING AN ADEQUATE DIET

For a diet to be adequate, it needs to contain the needed nutrients in proper ratio, balanced against the energy content of the diet. An organism's foremost nutrient need (other than water) is energy. There is a pervasive attitude among laypeople to consider protein or some of the vitamins as the crucial entity in nutrition. Granted, lack of protein will cause death, but not nearly as rapidly as lack of energy. A normal wild animal population contains no fat animals. This is because an animal in its natural environs tends to eat to meet its energy needs. The main trigger for the hunger mechanism (with a possible exception in reptiles and amphibians) is low blood sugar level, with gut distention acting as a secondary stimulus. Therefore, it is imperative for all animals consuming a meal that provides energy to the point of satiety (and thus terminates feeding) that all other needed nutrients have also been consumed in the needed amounts *and ratios.*

The importance of a ratio is depicted, for example, by the feeding of all-meat diets. Calcium and phosphorus are needed in a ratio of about 1.2:1 to 2:1, depending on the species. Muscle meat not only contains a highly inverse calcium-to-phosphorus level, with phosphorus being ten- to fifteen-fold more than calcium, but the phosphorus is still only one-fifth the level required for normal maintenance. In years past, it was not an uncommon practice to feed deboned meat to exotic cat collections, with a resultant high incidence of secondary nutritional hyperparathyroidism. The problem is easily ameliorated by providing the bone, joint and associated connective tissue along with the meat.

There are a number of resources available as a frame of reference to help determine what constitutes an adequate diet. The National Research Council publishes a series of booklets in which a committee of professionals reviews all the literature for a given species and summarizes in table form the recommended intakes for each nutrient, both macro and micro. The pamphlets are available for dairy cattle, beef cattle, horses, swine, poultry (chicken, turkey, duck, quail, pheasant) sheep, dogs, lab animals (cat, monkey, hamster, rat, mouse), fish (catfish, trout, salmon), rabbits, mink and foxes. These are available for a nominal fee from the Printing and Publishing Office, National Academy of Sciences, 2101 Constitution Avenue, N.W., Washington, D.C. 20418.

From these pamphlets it is possible to determine quite closely the relative profile that a diet should have for just about any exotic animal. The problem then becomes one of knowing the composition of what is being offered to the animals. Laboratory analysis is the best approach, but as this is often unattainable, there is a very useful publication referred to as Handbook No. 8. It is put out by the United States Department of Agriculture (USDA) and lists several thousand foods with the chemical analysis in raw, processed and table-ready forms. The major vitamins and minerals are also included (available from the Superintendent of Documents, United States Government Printing Office, Washington, D.C. 20402). Professional nutritionists consider themselves ill-prepared without these resources, and anyone addressing a nutrition issue, be it for reproduction or not, is well advised to make use of these booklets.

The larger pet food companies produce well-balanced nutritional products, and between diets made for growing pets and those for mature pets, there is a wide selection of quality feeds. All contain the required macro and micro nutrients, are balanced for energy content and are usually fairly palatable. The unique aspect about pet foods, as well as many feed store agricultural products, is inclusion of the micro nutrients. A swine growing ration produced by a well-known firm can be an ideal feed for certain zoo animals. One can use this product knowing that it has been designed to nourish and grow young monogastrics and that the agribusiness community would not long tolerate its poor performance. One concept to be kept in mind however is that zoo animals differ from agricultural animals in a very important way: they are to be kept alive for as long as 20 to 40 years in some cases. Rapid growth and slaughter goals of agribusiness can therefore cause diets to have a slightly different emphasis than is best for zoo animals. Finally, from the standpoint of prepared diets, there are reputable firms that cater exclusively to zoos. Use of such firms should be considered if they have proven products that offer intelligent alternatives.

PROVIDING ADEQUATE INTAKE

Management in a zoo has a great deal of difficulty achieving adequate intake for the animals in some situations because people are involved. The vast majority of nutrition problems in zoos are people problems. Zoo keepers are highly motivated and concerned for the well-being of their charges. Consequently, they are easily manipulated by the animals. For example, the primates are presented a collection of food that includes both assorted fruit and produce and a balanced primate diet. Naturally, monkeys will consume the succulent fruit and produce first and then turn to the balanced, completely nutritious manufactured diet. If they have satisfied their hunger on produce and fruit, the biscuit simply becomes a missile to fling at the keeper. The keeper incorrectly assumes the monkey doesn't like the biscuit and won't eat it and starts to increase the fruit offered and to decrease the balanced diet. The facts are that the monkey prefers the fruit but if presented the balanced diet alone may well eat it with relish if hungry. Fruit and produce, very poor nutrition on the whole, should be offered as a reward for consuming the proper amount of the balanced diet.

Fruit and produce are poor nutrition because they are 90 per cent (or greater) water. Because of their bulk, they appear to be a voluminous meal to the keeper. Often, it is the practice to offer produce (lettuce, celery, carrots, potatoes, apples and so forth) to elephants. Ten 2-gallon buckets of produce may seem ample supplement to a keeper also feeding hay and grain. It is true that an elephant subsists solely on fresh forage in the wild but does so only by consuming incredible quantities, up to 700 pounds per day. On a *dry matter basis,* the keeper is feeding only one bucket of nutrients when he provides 10 buckets of produce.

This concept of dry matter is rarely appreciated by laypeople, but it is indispensable to understanding and achieving proper nutrition. Food is consumed for the dry matter nutrients in it. Water is easily obtained by itself, and when in a food, it simply takes up room otherwise used for useful dry matter. Comparing two feedstuffs or evaluating a given diet's nutritional worth must always be done on a dry matter basis (which is done by dividing the "as is" weight of the feedstuff by the dry matter percentage of that same feedstuff).

The approximate levels of the various trace minerals and vitamins to use are available (Tables 1 and 2), with the possible exception of selenium. This element has been the object of attention in the zoo business because of its known involvement in white muscle disease and the conflicting rec-

TABLE 1. *Approximate Mineral Levels for Zoo Animals**

Mineral	Dietary Level	Common Source	Comment
Calcium	1.0%	Steamed bone meal, calcium carbonate, dicalcium phosphate	Ca:P ratio – 1.2:1
Phosphorus	0.8%	Steamed bone meal, dicalcium phosphate	Ca:P ratio – 1.2:1
Sodium	0.25%	Salt	
Potassium	0.8%	Potassium chloride	
Magnesium	0.1%	Magnesium oxide	
Iron	60 mg/kg	Iron oxide, iron sulfate	Needed in production of hemoglobin
Manganese	5 mg/kg	Manganous oxide, manganous carbonate, manganous sulfate	
Copper	7 mg/kg	Copper oxide, copper sulfate, copper carbonate	Needed for iron absorption
Cobalt	7 mg/kg	Cobalt carbonate	Part of vitamin B_{12}, used for red blood cell integrity
Zinc	50 mg/kg	Zinc oxide	
Iodine	1 mg/kg	Iodized salt, potassium iodide	Thyroid function
Selenium	0.5 mg/kg	Sodium selenate	Involved in white muscle disease

*To be used as a frame of reference in the absence of specific data.

TABLE 2. *Approximate Vitamin Levels for Zoo Animals**

Vitamin	Dry Matter Basis Dietary Level	Representative Function	Deficiency Symptoms	Source	Comment
A	5–20,000 IU/kg	Sight, reproduction	Nosebleed, anorexia	Fish liver oils, fruits, vegetables	Beta-carotene is precursor
C	?	Collagen synthesis	Scurvy	Fresh fruit	Sickness may alter need
D	500–4000 IU/kg	Absorption of calcium from the gut	Demineralized bone, rickets	Fish liver oils	Sunlight on skin is source
E	50–200 mg/kg	Antioxidant	White muscle disease	Plant oils	
K	1.0 mg/kg	Antihemorrhagic	Bleeding	Liver	Produced by gut
Thiamin (B₁)	1.5 mg/kg	Transketolase reaction	Beriberi	Plant seeds, lean pork	Heat destroys quickly
Riboflavin (B₂)	5 mg/kg	Flavin adenine dinucleotide (coenzyme)		All green plants	
Niacin	15 mg/kg	Nicotinamide adenine dinucleotide (coenzyme)	Pellagra (blacktongue)	Liver	Domestic cat needs total supplementation
Pyridoxine (B₆)	1 mg/kg	Protein metabolism		Liver	
Pantothenic acid	10 mg/kg	Fat metabolism		Yeast, eggs, liver	
Biotin	0.1 mg/kg	Carboxylase (enzyme)	Very hard to establish	Peanuts, eggs, chocolate, liver, yeast	Avidin (egg white) binds biotin
Folic acid	0.2 mg/kg	Deoxyribonucleic acid synthesis	Hard to establish	Widely found in animals and plants	
B₁₂	20 ppb	Coenzyme	Anemia	Soil microbes, manure	Plants and animals cannot manufacture
Inositol	?	Bone metabolism		Heart muscle, seeds	
Choline	2 gm/kg	Fat metabolism		Soy oil, glandular tissue	

*To be used as a frame of reference in the absence of specific data.

ommendations of various regulatory agencies. Zoo ruminants should have selenium in their diets, but at the level of no more than 0.5 ppm. Some investigators feel it may require up to 2 years or two reproductive cycles to replenish a seleinium-depleted dam to the point at which she bears viable offspring.

Generally speaking, no special measures need be taken for exotic mammals during the first two trimesters of pregnancy. A diet sufficient to provide for maintenance (or growth if the mother is still growing) can meet the slight, if any, increase in needs by being consumed in larger quantities. During the third trimester, and especially during lactation, a two- to three-fold increase in food intake can be observed in some species. There is a tendency to oversupplement the dam. Although one certainly would not knowingly provide a deficient diet to a pregnant animal, normal diets are usually very close to, if not totally, adequate, and increased needs are met by increasing con-

sumption. Remember that in the natural situation all members of a species (except suckling young) consume exactly the same fare. The only variable that they control is the amount they consume.

SUMMARY

In conclusion, because of the lack of reliable data, exotic animal investigators are obligated to make scientific observations of all their work concerning nutrition's effect on reproduction. Government publications are a useful guide for extrapolation to exotic animal nutrient needs, and the pet food and agribusiness industries offer a wide variety of nutritionally complete diets that often meet these needs closely. Well-intentioned but naive zoo personnel often cause nutritional problems because of their poor understanding of the basics involved.

Reproduction in the Mink *(Mustela vison)*

With Particular Reference to Current Breeding Practices

C. E. ADAMS

A.R.C. Institute of Animal Physiology, Animal Research Station, Cambridge, England

For a comprehensive account of reproduction in the mink reference should be made to Enders[3] and Hansson[4] and for a more recent review to Venge.[7] In this article, emphasis will be placed on those aspects of mink reproduction that affect current breeding practices.

THE FEMALE

The breeding season is restricted to the period from late February through March, the onset and duration varying slightly according to color phase and season. According

to Venge[7] female mink usually come into heat, i.e., are receptive, two to three times in one season. Mink are not normally examined for signs of heat, although some breeders claim to be able to detect changes in the external genitalia. The changes, however, are never pronounced, as in the ferret. The usual procedure is to place a female with a male and observe her behavior.

Ovulation is induced by mating and takes place after about 48 hours,[3] with a range of 33 to 72 hours.[7] It seems to be easily triggered and may follow pairing without mating, or it can be reliably induced by the subcutaneous injection of 50 IU of human chorionic gonadotropin (HCG).

Mating Systems

Females mated early in the season, i.e., before mid-March, are, if willing, remated after an interval of 7 or 8 days, referred to as

1 + 7 or 1 + 8. Those mated for the first time after mid-March are remated the following day (1 + 1). Some breeders attempt to get up to four matings, as 1 + 1 + 7 +1. In the 1 + 7 system about 90 per cent of the kitts come from the final mating, which also yields the majority (70 per cent) in the 1 + 1 combination. Females that refuse to mate should be retried the following day and thereafter at weekly intervals on consecutive days. A female may refuse to mate with one male but accept another. Overall about 1 to 2 per cent of females fail to mate, even after 10 to 12 tries; such animals are pelted out toward the end of March.

Pregnancy

No examination is made for pregnancy; all mated females are assumed to be pregnant and treated accordingly. About mid-April they are given nesting material, and the cages are fitted with "false" bottoms to prevent the young from falling through the mesh.

Most births occur during the first week of May. The presence of young can be detected from their squeaking. Another sign of parturition is the change that occurs in the excreta, which become dark colored and "tarlike."

Gestation

Because of the phenomenon of delayed implantation, the length of gestation may vary from 39 to 76 days or more, with an average of 50 days. The postimplantation period is 30 days ± 1 day. No experimental procedure has yet been developed for inducing implantation. Early matings tend to result in longer gestations, smaller litters and significantly more barren females. Normally, about 80 to 85 per cent of mated females produce litters.

The average litter size is approximately four (with a range of 1 to 12). The repeatability and heritability of litter size are very low. Neonatal mortality is comparatively high, averaging 15 to 16 per cent; about 50 per cent of young found dead on day 1 are stillborn. Many farmers do not count the young until day 10 or even later and therefore underestimate the number born. Experiments are in progress to test whether long-acting progestogens, e.g., Primolut, injected on day 10 postcoitum, can reduce the level of kitt mortality.

Composition of the Herd

Typically, about 50 to 60 per cent of the herd is composed of first-year (kitt) females. This is accounted for by heavy culling, especially of barren and low-producing animals (less than three young). Few females are retained beyond their fourth year. The ratio of males to females is normally 1 to 3.5 or 1 to 4.0.

THE MALE

Immediately before the onset of the breeding season, i.e., late February, males should be examined, as described by Onstad,[6] to insure that they have well-developed, descended testes; small testes and cryptorchidism are quite common in mink. Ishikawa *et al.*[5] have estimated that about 10 per cent of males suffer from anomalies of the genitalia, copulation problems, lack of libido, or aggressive temperament at mating. Sperm production may be checked by taking a vaginal flushing immediately after mating; the best results are obtained when mating is broken after 12 to 15 minutes. For details of the technique and semen evaluation, see Onstad.[6]

Copulation is prolonged, lasting on average 60 minutes; it becomes longer as the season advances. To insure maximal fertility, copulation should last at least 15 minutes, after which a pair may be separated. The practice of "breaking matings" is quite common, as it enables males to be more fully exploited. The average number of matings per male in a season is about 10, but exceptional males may cover 40 or 50 females.

Semen Collection

Semen cannot be collected with an artificial vagina but can be obtained by electroejaculation. However, the yield is low, averaging only 3.75×10^6 spermatozoa (range 0.5 to 12.5×10^6 sperm).[2] Much larger yields, 100×10^6 spermatozoa, can be obtained from the caudal epididymides postmortem. Such sperm have been stored successfully by deep freezing in liquid N_2.[1] Samples frozen in 1974 have proved fertile when used in the 1977 breeding season. As it is standard practice to pelt out males at the end of each breeding season, banks of epididymal sperm are easily obtained.

Artificial Insemination

The production of a few litters following artificial insemination (AI) has been reported, but the rate of success was very low and recent attempts to repeat this work have failed. However, if the sperm are deposited directly into the uterus at laparotomy, highly satisfactory results can be obtained, provided sufficient spermatozoa are used. With deep-frozen samples, as many as 3×10^6 spermatozoa per uterine horn may be required; 0.5×10^6 sperm per uterine horn gave much less satisfactory results. Ovulation is induced by treatment with HCG given 24 hours before insemination. The failure of conventional AI is due to lack of a means of sperm transport through the cervix. If this barrier could be overcome, AI would be widely used.

CURRENT BREEDING PRACTICES

Use of Hormones

In the past the use of hormones has met with little or no success in mink, and it is only recently that the new approaches have been tried. One promising innovation is to replace the initial mating, or matings, with an injection of HCG. Subsequently, mating takes place after 7 or 8 days in the usual way. This system saves time and also enables a considerable degree of planning, as the majority of females mate to order as if "synchronized." The proportion of unmated females is slightly higher than normal, but fertility and fecundity equal that of controls. In 1978 more than 6000 females were so treated on one United States ranch.

Experimentally, it has proved possible to produce litters out of season by treating "barren" females with pregnant mare serum gonadotropin (PMSG) and inseminating them with deep-frozen sperm. This approach is being further developed.

Use of Light

Sometimes mink are exposed to extra light, either to stimulate the onset of sexual activity in males (from mid-January) or to facilitate implantation (from about March 20th). Great care is needed in changing the normal pattern of daylight, as mink are particularly light sensitive. Reproductive function can be easily disturbed by unsatisfactory lighting.

Herd Infertility

When considering the diagnosis of herd infertility problems, nutrition and disease aspects are particularly important. The special problems caused by diethylstilbestrol in capon offal and, more recently, by fish obtained from polluted waters are well recognized. Female mink should be slimmed down before the breeding season; certain color phases are more difficult to slim than others and, therefore, require special attention. Males should be in good breeding condition and not too slim at the start of the season; otherwise, they become increasingly emaciated and vicious.

Of the diseases that may affect reproduction, Aleutian mink disease (plasmacytosis) is by far the most serious. It is diagnosed by the iodine agglutination test (IAT), but unfortunately this test is not sufficiently sensitive to permit eradication. A new, more sensitive test, using counterelectrophoresis (CEP), is currently being developed.

Anesthesia

Excellent results have been obtained with halothane (Fluothane) delivered in oxygen via a pediatric face mask. Induction is particularly rapid. Before anesthesia, mink should be handled as quietly as possible. If the animals are frightened and agitated during catching, the risk of death increases.

CONCLUSION

Recent economic pressures have forced many of the smaller mink farmers out of business. Conversely, the bigger enterprises have tended to expand and have become increasingly professional in outlook. They are ready to seek expert guidance and adopt new techniques. Undoubtedly, the industry will undergo significant changes in the next decade.

REFERENCES

1. Adams, C.E.: Artificial insemination in the mink, *Mustela vison*. U.K. Fur Breeders' Gazette, *25*:19, 1976.
2. Aulerich, R.J., Ringer, R. K. and Sloan, C.: Electroejaculation of mink (*Mustela vison*). J. Anim. Sci., *34*:230, 1972.
3. Enders, R. K.: Reproduction in the mink (*Mustela vison*). Proc. Am. Phil Soc., *96*:691, 1952.

4. Hansson, A.: The physiology of reproduction in mink (*Mustela vison,* Shreb) with particular reference to delayed implantation. Acta Zool., *28*:1, 1947.
5. Ishikawa, I., Tiba, T., Kagota, K., Kawabe, K. and Kinoshita, S.: Étude experimentale sur l'insemination artificielle chez les minks. Jap. J. Vet. Res., *13*:1, 1965.
6. Onstad, O.: Studies on post-natal testicular changes, semen quality and anomalies of reproductive organs in the mink: A clinical, histological and histochemical study. Acta Endocr. Supp., *117*:1, 1967.
7. Venge, O.: Reproduction in the Mink. Roy. Vet. & Agric. Univs. Yearbook, Copenhagen, 1973, p. 95.

Artificial Insemination of Nonhuman Primates

D. C. KRAEMER and T. J. KUEHL

Texas A & M University, College Station, Texas

Artificial insemination (AI) has been successfully applied to only three genera of nonhuman primates; squirrel monkeys, macaque monkeys and baboons, but there are no published reports of successful inseminations with frozen semen. Only with the rhesus monkey (*Macaca mulatta*) have enough inseminations been done to establish what conception rates can be expected. Dede and Plentl[3] obtained a 12.1 per cent conception rate in macaques using AI, which was similar to the 13.7 per cent conception rate obtained by natural mating. Czaja *et al.*[2] obtained a 39.9 per cent conception rate from 218 artificial inseminations of *M. mulatta*. Valerio and Dalgard[8] obtained 4, 19, 20 and 18 per cent conception rates from vaginal, intrauterine and intracervical insemination and natural mating, respectively, in *M. mulatta*. Thus, in *M. mulatta*, although the conception rates obtained by AI vary considerably among investigators, in each case the results of AI are similar to those obtained from natural matings. The only other nonhuman primate species in which pregnancies have been produced by AI are the squirrel monkey (*Saimiri sciureus*)[1] and the baboon (*Papio cynocephalus.*)[5]

Much remains to be learned about AI in nonhuman primates, such as the minimum number of cells required for conception, total volume required and methods of semen preservation. Nevertheless, the general principles can be discussed under four topic headings: (1) semen collection, (2) semen dilution and storage, (3) determination of optimal breeding time and (4) insemination.

Semen Collection. Nonhuman primate semen is usually collected by electroejaculation. Procedural details will be described in the following article.

Semen Dilution and Storage. Two diluents have been used successfully for AI in *M. mulatta* — the first, 25 per cent egg yolk, 0.20 M TRIS-buffered glucose, streptomycin-sulfate, penicillin G and buffered potassium[2] and the second, lactated Ringer's solution.[8] Pregnancies were obtained with 7.5×10^6 motile cells delivered intracervically in a 0.1-ml volume.

Several groups have frozen nonhuman primate semen, with approximately 50 per cent survival. The diluents used include 20 per cent egg yolk, 3 per cent glutamate with 14 per cent glycerol[5, 6] and 25 per cent egg yolk in 0.20 M TRIS-buffered glucose.[4] However, no nonhuman primate pregnancies have been reported to date with frozen semen.

Determination of Optimal Breeding Time. The optimum time to artificially inseminate the various species appears to be similar to the optimum time for natural breeding. Several methods may be used for determination of optimal breeding time, including (1) cycle day, (2) plasma or urinary estrogen peak, (3) vaginal smears and (4) sex skin patterns.

Insemination. For those species in which the female can be handled by manual restraint (squirrel monkey and rhesus monkey) the vagina is opened using a nasal speculum, and the semen is placed within the cervix using a blunted 18-gauge needle.[2, 8] The larger species must be restrained in a squeeze cage, in which case the semen is deposited into the vagina using a syringe.

The effects of chemical restraining agents on ovulation and sperm transport must be determined in the larger species before intracervical insemination can be recommended.

REFERENCES

1. Bennett, J.P.: Artificial insemination of the squirrel monkey. J. Endocrinol., *37*:473, 1967.
2. Czaja, J.A., Eisele, S.G. and Goy, R.W.: Cyclical changes in the sexual skin of female rhesus; relationships to mating behavior and successful artificial insemination. Fed. Proc. *34*:168, 1975.
3. Dede, J.A. and Plentl. A.A.: Induced ovulation in a rhesus colony. Fertil. Steril., *17*:757, 1966.
4. Eisle, S.: Artificial insemination techniques aid breeding of nonhuman primates. Primate Rec., *3*:7, 1972.
5. Kraemer, D.C. and Vera Cruz, N.C.: Collection, gross characteristics and freezing of baboon semen. J. Reprod. Fertil., *20*:345, 1969.
6. Roussel, J.D. and Austin, C.R.: Preservation of primate spermatozoa by freezing of baboon semen. J. Reprod. Fertil., *20*:345, 1969.
7. Settlage, D.S.F., Swan, S. and Hendrickx, A.G.: Comparison of artificial insemination with natural mating techniques in rhesus monkeys; *Macaca mulatta*. J. Reprod. Fertil., *32*:129, 1973.
8. Valerio, D.A. and Dalgard, D.W.: Experiences in the laboratory breeding of nonhuman primates. Lab. Anim. Handbooks, *6*:49, 1975.

Semen Collection and Evaluation of Breeding Soundness in Nonhuman Primates

D. C. KRAEMER and T. J. KUEHL

Texas A & M University, College Station, Texas

COLLECTION OF SEMEN

Electroejaculation

The most commonly used method of semen collection in nonhuman primates is electroejaculation. The two basic approaches to electroejaculation of these species are (1) direct stimulation, first introduced by Mastroianni and Manson,[3] and (2) stimulation of the internal reproductive organs via rectal electrodes, first reported by Weisbroth and Young.[7]

The larger animals may be chemically restrained with either phencyclidine hydrochloride or ketamine hydrochloride. Atropine should be avoided, as it may block ejaculation. Males of the smaller species may be held by physical restraint.

The equipment for penile stimulation consists of a stimulator such as a Model S-5 stimulator and two metal strip electrodes that can be made of either woven mesh or aluminum foil. The penis is washed with a mild detergent, rinsed thoroughly with sterile distilled water and dried with sterile cloth or parchment. The electrodes are moistened with saline. One electrode is placed around the base of the penis and held in place with a clamp electrode. The other is held with a gloved hand around the base of the glans penis.

Several different levels of stimulation have been used successfully in macaque species. Stimulation consists of intermittent charges increased at 10-volt increments to 40 to 45 volts of monophasic alternating current delivered at a frequency of 20 impulses per second and a duration of 25 to 50 milliseconds. The voltage should not exceed 45 volts, or burning of the penis might occur.[6] Ejaculation should occur within 5 minutes of stimulation in approximately 90 per cent of the cases. There is evidence that animals can be conditioned to respond more readily by frequent collection during a 2- to 3-week period.

Rectal probes for delivering the ejaculatory stimulus may be constructed with either horizontal rings[1] or longitudinal metal strips (Fig. 1). The appropriate diameters of rectal probes for various nonhuman primate species are given in Table 1. In addition, there are several commercially available electronic ejaculators that are effective. Circuit diagrams of stimulators have also been published.[7]

Semen is collected in tubes or small beakers that have been warmed to body temperature. Care must be taken to avoid contact of semen with water. The rectum should be cleared of feces before insertion of the electrodes. An electrolytic lubricant such as K-Y jelly is placed on the electrode before insertion to avoid irritation of the rectum and to facilitate conduction of the current. The appropriate depth of insertion of the rectal probe varies among the species, but generally the probes are placed

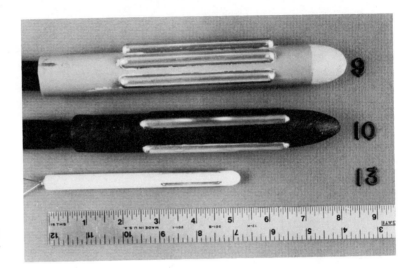

Figure 1. Rectal probes used for electroejaculation of nonhuman primates.

TABLE 1. *Rectal Probe Diameters and Approximate Voltage Required for Semen Collection from Nonhuman Primates*

Species	Common Name	Diameter (cm)	Approximate Voltage Required	Reference
Gorilla gorilla	Lowland gorilla	2.5	—	4
Pongo pygmaeus	Orangutan	2.5	—	4
Pan troglodytes	Chimpanzee	2.6	7	5
Hylobates lar	Gibbon	1.3	—	5
Papio cynocephalus	Baboon	3.0	13.5	2
Macaca mulatta	Rhesus macaque	1.3	4.5	5
Macaca irus	Crab-eating macaque	1.3	4.5	5
Macaca speciosa	Stumptail macaque	1.3	5.6	5
Macaca nemestrina	Pigtail macaque	1.3	4.5	5
Cercopithecus aethiops	African green monkey	1.3	2	5
Theropithecus gelada	Gelada baboon	1.3	4.5	5
Erythrocebus patas	Patas	1.3	4.5	5
Cercocebus galeritus	Mangabey	1.3	4.5	5
Cebus apella	Capuchin	1.3	4.5	5
Ateles fusciceps	Spider monkey	1.0	—	4
Colobus colobus	Colobus monkey	1.0	—	4
Saimiri sciureus	Squirrel monkey	0.7	4.5	5
Saguinus nigricollis	Tamarin	0.6	—	4
Callithrix jacchus	Marmoset	0.6	—	4
Cacajao rubicundus	Red nakari monkey	0.6	—	4
Tupaia glis	Tree shrew	0.7	4.5	5

TABLE 2. *Semen Volume and Sperm Concentration in Ejaculates from Nonhuman Primates*

Species	Semen Volume (ml)		Sperm Concentration per ml ($\times 10^6$)		Reference
	MEAN	RANGE	MEAN	RANGE	
Gorilla gorilla	0.4	—	153.5	—	4
Pongo pygmaeus	2.5	—	14.5	—	4
Pan troglodytes	1.9	0.5–6.2	608.8	230.9–1268.9	5
Hylobates lar	1.3	0.5–4.0	152.4	51.0–350.4	5
Papio cynocephalus	3.6	SD 1.4	71.2	SD 58.8	2
Macaca mulatta	1.1	0.2–4.5	1069.1	100.2–3600.2	5
Macaca irus	1.2	0.5–3.0	458.2	160.5–830.1	5
Macaca speciosa	1.6	0.4–4.0	468.2	214.1–1268.1	5
Cercopithecus aethiops	0.9	0.3–2.0	439.6	165.8–810.8	5
Theropithecus gelada	1.0	0.5–2.0	502.9	350.8–650.6	5
Erythrocebus patas	0.6	0.4–1.0	1153.4	250.6–3600.0	5
Cerocebus galeritus	1.3	1.1–1.5	575.5	541.8–609.2	5
Cebus apella	0.6	0.3–1.0	161.1	56.0–740.2	5
Ateles fusciceps	0.7	—	17.2	—	4
Colobus colobus	0.06	—	20.0	—	4
Saimiri sciureus	0.4	0.2–1.5	205.9	80.8–310.9	5
Saguinus nigricollis	0.03	—	833.3	—	4
Tupaia glis	0.1	0.1–0.1	103.2	90.1–116.8	5

TABLE 3. *Size and Weight of Testes in Nonhuman Primates**

Species	Size (cm)	Weight (gm)	% of Body Weight
Galago demidovii	1.1 × 0.7		
Galago elegantulus	1.5 × 0.5		
Perodicticus potto	2.0 × 1.7		
Loris tardigradus		1.7	0.65 (138)
Avahi laniger	1.5 × 1.1		
Lemur macaco fulvus	3.0 × 1.5		
Microcebus murinis (active)	1.5 × 1.2		
Microcebus murinis (inactive)	0.75 × 0.6		
Callithrix geoffroyi		1.8	0.32
Aolus trivirgatus		1.2	0.12
Alouatta villosa palliata		25.0 (8)	0.34 (8)
Lagothrix lagothricha		11.2	0.22
Ateles geoffroyi		13.4	0.17
Macaca fascicularis		30.8 (12)	0.67
Macaca radiata		57.6	0.69
Macaca nemestrina		66.7	0.67
Macaca mulatta		76.0 (2)	0.73 (2)
Papio sphinx		88.9	0.28
Papio anubis		114.5 (4)	0.42 (4)
Papio hamadryas		30.1 (6)	0.14 (6)
Theropithecus gelada		21.5	0.10
Cercopithecus aethiops		18.5 (6)	0.36 (6)
Colobus polykomos		13.7 (3)	0.14 (3)
Presbytis cristatus		5.5 (14)	0.09 (14)
Presbytis rubicundus		3.6 (12)	0.06 (12)
Nasalis larvatus		11.9 (8)	0.06 (8)
Hylobates moloch		4.6 (7)	0.08 (7)
Hylobates agilis	2.8 × 1.4		
Pongo pygmaeus	3.9 × 3.0	35.3 (2)	0.05 (2)
Pan troglodytes		118.8 (3)	0.27 (3)
Pan paniscus		250.0	0.55
Gorilla g. berengei	5.5 × 3.5	36.0	0.017

*The number in parentheses indicates the number of animals, if more than one. (From Kinzey, W. G.: Male reproductive system and spermatogenesis. *In* Hafez, E. S. E. (ed.): Comparative Reproduction of Nonhuman Primates. Springfield, Ill., Charles C Thomas, Publisher, 1971.)

over the prostate gland. Insertion of the electrode too deeply will generally result in contamination of the semen with urine. The electrical stimulus is delivered in 2- to 3-second impulses at 1- to 2-second intervals. The voltage is increased stepwise until ejaculation is obtained. The appropriate stimuli for various species are given in Table 1. Oftentimes, ejaculation will occur spontaneously after 1- to 2-minute intermittent stimulation.

Other Methods

There are several other methods for obtaining semen for evaluation. Semen can be aspirated from the vagina of a female immediately after mating. If a gauze sponge or other absorbant material is placed in the vagina prior to mating, it can be removed and rinsed with saline after copulation, and some sperm cells can be recovered. Such samples yield qualitative, but not quantitative, information about the sperm production of a male. The artificial vagina has not been generally useful for semen collection in nonhuman primates. However, with extensive individual training, these animals could very likely be trained to serve an artificial vagina.

SEMEN EVALUATION

The semen characteristics of various nonhuman primate species are given in Table 2. Semen evaluation procedures for

nonhuman primates are basically similar to those used for other mammalian species. Most ejaculates will contain some coagulum. Portions of the coagulum will liquefy spontaneously within 10 to 14 minutes, but other portions remain firm unless treated with enzymes such as trypsin or chymotrypsin and lipase.

A fertility examination of a male nonhuman primate should include palpation of the testes, epididymis and prostate gland. The size and tone of these structures should be compared with those of known fertile animals of the same species. Testis measurements for some of the nonhuman primate species are given in Table 3.

REFERENCES

1. Hendrickx, A.G., and Kraemer, D.C.: Primates. *In* Hafez, E.S.E. (ed.): Reproduction and Breeding Techniques for Laboratory Animals. Philadelphia, Lea & Febiger, 1970, pp. 316–337.
2. Kraemer, D.C. and Vera Cruz, N.C.: Collection, gross characteristics and freezing of baboon semen. J. Reprod. Fertil., *20*:345, 1969.
3. Mastroianni, L. and Manson, W.A., Jr.: Collection of monkey semen by electroejaculation. Proc. Soc. Exp. Biol. Med., *221*:1025, 1963.
4. Platz, C. and Seager, S.W.J.: Personal communication.
5. Roussel, J.D. and Austin, C.R.: Improved electroejaculation of primates. J. Inst. Anim. Tech., *19*: 22, 1968.
6. Settlage, D.S.F. and Hendrickx, A.G.: Electroejaculation technique in *Macaca mulatta* (rhesus monkeys). Fertil. Steril., *25*:157, 1974.
7. Weisbroth, S. and Young, F.A.: The collection of primate semen by electroejaculation. Fertil. Steril., *16*:229, 1965.

Noninfectious Conditions Affecting Reproduction in Nonhuman Primates

B. FLOW and D. C. KRAEMER
Texas A & M University, College Station, Texas

There are many noninfectious factors that can affect reproduction in the nonhuman primates, and many are related to management. Stress is such a factor, as female rhesus monkeys caged in groups have been shown to have lower conception rates than those housed individually. Similarly, workers reduced abortions and stillbirths in another group of rhesus monkeys by avoiding restraint during early pregnancy, avoiding caging changes and improving the environment for reproduction.

Certain species also have seasonal breeding patterns. In the rhesus monkey, breeding decreases during the hot summer months and increases again with cooler weather during the fall months. There are also reports of structural changes in the male reproductive tract associated with these seasonal changes.

Sexual incompatibility may exist between certain animals and may be overcome by mating the female with a different male — preferably one more appealing to her tastes.

Nutrition is a significant management-related factor, especially in species such as *Saimiri sciureus* whose infants weigh more in proportion to their mothers' weight than do infants of some of the other primate species. There are also reports of megaloblastic anemia in the squirrel monkey neonate related to low rates of absorption of folic acid.[1] Fetal losses can be reduced, but not completely eliminated, by maternal dietary supplementation with folic acid during the last 9 weeks of pregnancy. There are also reports of a hemolytic disease in marmosets similar to erythroblastosis fetalis.

The young primates also need to observe the adults to learn proper mating methods. The male rhesus mounts the female by standing on her hocks. Young animals isolated from the adults do not exhibit the proper mounting procedure and have reduced conception rates. Proper maternal traits are also learned by observation. Many young zoo primates have been lost to cannibalism by males as well as to agalactia by females. It has also been reported that early fetal death losses were reduced in squirrel monkeys by waiting until 48 hours after parturition before handling the mother to examine the infant.

Reproductive problems can also be encountered during parturition.[1] Dystocia may occur due to fetal structure. Uterine inertia may result and could lead to the performance of a cesarean section. Endometriosis may occur following a cesarean section, but this disorder has also been reported following abdominal irradiation studies in animals that had no previous history of surgery. Endometriosis, or ectopic endometrium, is a condition in which tissue resembling the endometrium occurs aberrantly in various locations in the abdominal cavity (endometriosis externa). Some authors have suggested that frequent pregnancies may prevent the development of endometriosis following hysterotomy. It has also been suggested that endometriosis may develop if pregnancy does not occur within a certain critical period. There is also evidence that endometriosis externa in the human may result from hyperestrinism and from the failure of formation of corpora lutea.[2]

REFERENCES

1. Hendricks, A.G. and Giles-Nelson, V.: Reproductive failure. *In* Hafez E.S.E. (ed.): Comparative Reproduction of Nonhuman Primates. Springfield, Ill., Charles C Thomas, Publisher, 1971, pp. 403–425.
2. Kraemer, D.C. and Vera Cruz, N.C.: The female reproductive system. *In* Fiennes, R.N. (ed.): Pathology of Simian Primates. Part I. Basel, Karger, 1972, pp. 841–877.

Infectious Diseases Affecting Reproduction in Nonhuman Primates

B. FLOW and D. C. KRAEMER
Texas A & M University, College Station, Texas

Viral, bacterial, mycotic and parasitic agents have been associated with reproductive disorders in nonhuman primates. In man, transplacental infection of the fetus with rubella virus during the first trimester produces developmental abnormalities of the heart, eyes, brain, bone and ears in 40 per cent of the cases without interrupting pregnancy.[2] In nonhuman primates, the rubella virus has been shown to produce fetal abnormalities, fetal death and abortions. Abortions are more frequent if exposure occurs early in pregnancy. In addition to the rubella virus, the adenovirus type 12 has been shown to produce abortions in the baboon *(Papio cynocephalus)* when given by amnioinjection.[3] Mumps, herpes simplex, rubeola, vaccina, western equine encephalitis, chickenpox and coxsackie virus have been implicated in reproductive failure in the nonhuman primate. Parenteral infection with the mumps virus during early pregnancy has resulted in late fetal and postnatal growth retardation in rhesus monkeys *(Macaca mulatta)*.[6] The cytomegalovirus has been shown to produce increased deaths *in utero* and reproductive failure in man; however, an attempt to produce cytomegalovirus infections in pregnant *M. mulatta* was unsuccessful. Focal necrosis of the testes has also been associated with viral infections, particularly monkeypox.[5]

In addition to the viral agents, the bacterial agents have also been studied in reproductive failure of nonhuman primates.[7] Although a direct relationship between mycoplasmas and nonhuman primate abortions may be questioned, the isolation of *Mycoplasma* species from two aborted chimpanzee fetuses deserves attention. This should be noted particularly because the agent has been isolated from the blood and cervical discharge of a human mother and also from the liver and lungs of a stillborn human infant. Mycoplasmas have also been isolated from the genital tracts of talapoins, patas and crab-eating macaques. The talapoins had not reproduced successfully over a 2-year period.[4] Fertility in the patas had been reduced, and there had been a high incidence of stillbirths and abortions. T-strain mycoplasma has also been reported as being sexually transmitted in a chimpanzee. However, the chimp became pregnant and had a normal delivery.[1]

Although positive serological tests have been reported, brucellosis does not appear to be a serious problem of nonhuman primates. *Leptospira ballum* has been serologically associated with a rise in abortions and stillbirths among baboons. However, the organism could not be isolated from the aborted fetuses. *L. pomona* has been associated with reproductive failure in domestic animals but has not been linked to nonhuman primates and man. In addition to these agents, staphylococci, streptococci, actinomyces and other bacterial and mycotic agents have been isolated from cases of pyometra and of puerperal sepsis.

The nonhuman primates do not appear to be naturally infected with the agent of syphilis, *Treponema pallidum;* however, experimental infections can be produced. Skin lesions, uveitis and the isolation of spirochetes from the aqueous humor have been reported in an owl monkey, which indicates a generalized syphilitic involvement. Likewise, naturally occurring gonorrheal infections have not been reported, but experimental infections have been produced using exudate from human males.

Leukocytosis has been reported from the semen of one male baboon. Culture yielded a diphtheroid bacteria, and treatment with chloromycetin quickly cleared the leukocytosis. Orchitis has also been reported in cases of disseminated tuberculosis.

The protozoa also play a role in reproductive failure. Although trichomoniasis is able to infect a large number of mammals, the vagina of the common laboratory monkeys appears inhospitable to *Trichomonas foetus*. *T. vaginalis* will infect nonhuman primates but the condition produced appears to be a self-limiting disease. The schistosomes are another parasite that can affect reproduction. The heavy deposition of schistosome eggs in the reproductive organs can impair fertility. The filarid worm *(Tetrapetalonema digitata)* has been isolated from the ovaries of two gibbons. Animals from areas where these parasites are endemic could have related reproductive disorders.

Nonhuman primates can be infected with many different mycotic agents. However, in a study conducted with *P. cynocephalus,* *Candida* was the most frequently occurring yeast in the vagina. Balanitis (infection of the glans penis) has also been reported in a male *M. mulatta*.[3]

There is still much to be learned about infectious causes of reproductive failure in nonhuman primates as well as the treatment of these conditions.

REFERENCES

1. Brown, W. J., Jacobs, N. F., Arum, E. S. and Arko, R. J.: T-strain mycoplasma in the chimpanzee. Lab. Anim. Sci., *26*:81, 1976.
2. Dorland's Illustrated Medical Dictionary. 25th Ed. Philadelphia, W. B. Saunders Co., 1974.
3. Kraemer, D. C. and Vera Cruz, N. C.: Infectious diseases influencing reproduction. *In* Hafez, E. (ed.): Comparative Reproduction of Nonhuman Primates. Springfield, Ill., Charles C Thomas Publisher, 1971.
4. Kundsin, R. B., Rowell, T., Shepard, M. C., Parreno, A. and Lunceford, C. D.: T-strain mycoplasmas and reproductive failure in monkeys. Lab. Anim. Sci., *25*:221, 1975.
5. McNutty, W. P.: Pox diseases in primates, pathology of simian primates. *In* Fiennes, N. (ed.): Pathology of Simian Primates (Part II). White Plains, N.Y., S. Karger, 1972, pp. 612–645.
6. St. Geme, J. W. and Van Pelt, L. F.: Fetal and postnatal growth retardation associated with gestational mumps virus infection of the rhesus monkey. Lab. Anim. Sci., *24*:895, 1974.
7. Valerio, D. A., Miller, R. L., Innes, J. B. N., Courtney, D. A., Pallotta, A. J. and Guttmacher, R. M.: *Macacca mulatta.* Management of a Laboratory Breeding Colony. New York, Academic Press, 1969, p. 68.

Reproductive and Sexual Cycles in Nonhuman Primates

D. C. KRAEMER

Texas A & M University, College Station, Texas

The age at puberty, breeding season, duration of sexual cycle, gestation period and numbers of young per gestation of the common nonhuman primates are listed in Table 1.

The general endocrine pattern of nonhuman primates during the menstrual cycle is shown in Figure 1. The endocrine events around the time of ovulation are very similar. There are, however, differences in the lengths of the follicular and luteal phases of the cycle, as one would expect from the differences in sexual cycle. Although the ideal comparative study, in which all of the species of nonhuman primates are studied by the same laboratory, has not been done, it is apparent that the peripheral steroid hormone levels in the marmoset are markedly higher than in the other nonhuman primates

studied to date. Four species show marked changes in perineal skin during the menstrual cycle: chimpanzees, baboons, talapoins and pigtail macaques. The rhesus macaque also exhibits sexual skin changes during the menstrual cycle; however, this skin is located in the thigh region rather than perineally, as in the other four species. Cyclic changes in vaginal smears and endometrium have been identified for chimpanzees, rhesus monkeys and baboons; however, the changes are not as precise as in man and therefore have not been as useful for monitoring the sexual cycle in nonhuman primates as they have been in man.

REFERENCES

1. Hearn, J.P. and Lunn, S.F.: The reproductive biology of the marmoset monkey, *Callithrix jacchus*. Lab. Anim. Handbook, *6*:191, 1975.
2. Hendrickx, A.G.: *Embryology of the Baboon*. Chicago, University of Chicago Press, 1971, pp. 6–18.

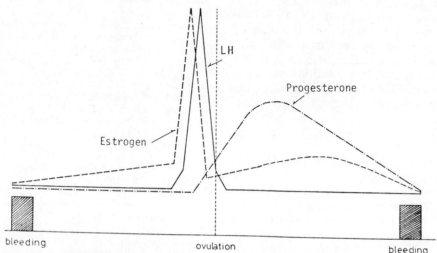

Figure 1. Schematic representation of the general endocrine pattern of the nonhuman primate menstrual cycle. (From Nomura, T. and Ohsawa, N.: The use and problems associated with nonhuman primates in the study of reproduction. *In* Antikatzides, T., Erichsen, S. and Spiegel, A. (eds.): Proceedings of 6th ICLA Symposium, Thessaloniki, 1975, Gustav Fischer Verlag, 1976, p. 3.)

TABLE 1. *Age at Puberty, Breeding Season, Sexual Cycle Duration, Gestation Period and Young per Litter for Commonly Used Primates**

	Age at Puberty (years)	Breeding Season	Sexual Cycle Duration (days)	Gestation Period (days)	Young per Litter
Prosimians					
Tree shrew	–	All year	–	46–50	1–2
Lemur	–	Once or twice a year		120–150†	1–2
Loris (*Loris* sp.)	–	Twice a year	–	180†	1–2
Nycticebus spp.	–	All year	–	90†	1
Potto	–	–	–	–	–
Galago (Bush baby)	1.5	April–October	42	110–120	1–2
Tarsier	–	All year	23–24	–	1
New World Monkeys					
Tamarin	1.5	February	–	120†	1–2
Marmoset	1.5	–	–	142–150	1–3
Squirrel monkey	–	–	24–25	140–180	1
Night or owl monkey	–	–	–	140–180	1
Titi monkey	–	All year	–	–	1
Ringtail or capuchin monkey	–	–	16–20	180†	1
Spider monkey	–	–	24–27	139	1
Wooly monkey	–	–	–	130–150†	1
Howler monkey	–	–	–	140†	1
Old World Monkeys					
Vervet or African green monkey	–	–	31	150–210	1
Syke's monkey	–	–	–	–	–
Talapoin monkey	–	All year	–	150–210	1
Mangabey	–	–	–	–	–
Patas monkey	3–4	All year	–	150–270	1–2
Macaques					
Barbary ape	–	–	27–33	210†	–
Carb-eating macaque or cynomolgus monkey	–	All year	25–39	160–170	–
Japanese macaque	–	–	–	–	–
Rhesus macaque	3–4 (male) 1.5–2.5 (female)	All year	28	144–197	1
Pig-tailed macaque	4	All year	32	172–210	1
Bonnet macaque	–	–	30	–	–
Stump-tailed macaque	–	–	–	–	–
Celebes-crested macaque	–	–	–	–	–
Silvered langur or leaf monkey	–	–	–	–	–
Hanuman langur	6–7	April–August	30	196†	1–2
Baboons					
Gelada	5	All year	–	–	1
Mandrill	–	–	–	220–270	–
Savannah	3–4	All year	32–36	164–186	1
The Great Apes					
Gorilla	5–8	–	45	270	1
Chimpanzee					
Typical	8–9	All year	34–35	216–260	1
Pygmy	–	–	–	–	–
Orangutan	–	–	29	240–270	1
Gibbon					
Hylobates hoolock	7	–	–	210†	1
Siamang	–	–	–	210†	1

*From Hendrickx, A. G. and Kraemer, D. C.: Primates. *In* Hafez, E. S. E. (ed.): Reproduction and Breeding Techniques for Laboratory Animals, Philadelphia, Lea & Febiger, 1970, p. 321.

†Approximate gestation period.

Captive Breeding and Laparoscopy in Nonhuman Primates

W. R. DUKELOW

Michigan State University, East Lansing, Michigan

More than 25 years ago the production of poliomyelitis vaccine from rhesus monkeys caused the government of India to place an embargo upon the exportation of this species. This action reflected concern by that government of a high incidence of transit losses and the decimation of the native population of rhesus monkeys. The embargo placed a severe strain upon the availability of these primates for research.

Similar concerns existed with regard to the use of nonhuman primates as pets. Despite obvious disadvantages, nonhuman primates have been kept as pets for centuries, and, until recently, a great many animals were imported annually for this purpose, especially South American species. The natural death rate of nonhuman primates in home situations is very high. Common problems have been parasitism, malnutrition and exposure to an adverse environment after escape from the home. These concerns caused several South American governments to restrict or ban exportation of nonhuman primates in the last 10 years, and recent action by the United States government places severe restrictions on the importation and sale of nonhuman primates as pets. It is anticipated that in the future, veterinary contacts with nonhuman primates will be restricted to animals housed in research laboratories or in zoos.

The objectives of this article are to provide background information on a variety of nonhuman primates that a veterinarian might encounter in research and zoo situations and to provide information on clinical techniques applicable to those species. This report outlines patterns of reproductive management that have been successful in the past and details the relationship of basic physiological principles to a successful breeding program.

ADAPTATION OF ESTROUS CYCLICITY TO CAPTIVE CONDITIONS

Normal purchases of feral primates from dealers fall into three major classifications: (1) pregnant females; (2) adult, proven animals, normally several years postpuberal and (3) adult animals of young age. Primates in the first category are normally characterized as having an abnormally high incidence of abortion and have the disadvantages of an unknown time of mating and an unknown sire. Mature adult primates are often selected because of their proven ability to sire young, yet have the disadvantage of being removed from a pre-established social structure for placement in another environment.

Young puberal adults are the animals of choice for the establishment of a breeding colony. Valerio[29] has observed a tendency for rhesus monkeys under laboratory conditions to mimic their natural cyclic patterns for the first year in captivity (mating from November through January), but subsequently the breeding cyclicity is attenuated and conceptions can occur during every month of the year.

In the squirrel monkey living in a semi-natural environment, a distinct seasonality of cycling occurs, as in the wild state. With confinement there is a very definite shift in the time of year of the mating and birth seasons. In one report[9] the birth peak shifted from March to July-August over a 3-year period. The birth season then remained constant in later years.

In northern climates the squirrel monkey can expect to adapt to normal cyclicity in 8 to 9 months but will continue to show a seasonal pattern even in environmentally controlled conditions.[11] The exact mechanism controlling this seasonality is unknown. It does not appear to relate to photoperiod since, in the Amazon, the difference between the longest and shortest day of the year is only 11 minutes. Some have suggested a relationship between rainfall and humidity as a controlling factor. The start of the breeding season does correlate with the dry season whether the monkeys are in the Amazon or in Florida, and in controlled environments, there is evidence for maximal response to an ovulation induction regimen to occur during those months when relative humidity is lowest.

In menstruating species (generally the "Old World" primates and apes) the regularity of the cycle is easier to ascertain, and these species will generally adapt to captivity within a year. Some animals that show a distinct birth season in the wild (such as the crab-eating macaque) will actually produce offspring throughout the year in captivity. In other species, such as the rhesus monkey, a distinct seasonality remains, and a large percentage of these animals will show anovulatory cycles during the summer months in captivity. There are, of course, exceptions to these phenomena, and some rhesus monkeys will continue to cycle throughout the year.

In dealing with any new species, it is necessary to have a base knowledge of reproductive parameters of that species. Unfortunately, such information for primates is often difficult to find. Table 1 lists some of the known reproductive parameters of the primate families. With the exception of the macaques, squirrel monkeys, baboons, galagos and the chimpanzee (all species used in research environments), reproductive characteristics of the other species are relatively unknown. Information that is available usually reflects a limited number of animals in zoos or private collections.

PHYSIOLOGICAL PRINCIPLES APPLIED TO CAPTIVE BREEDING

Assuming the presence of fertile and mutually compatible animals (a major assumption in primates!) there are four basic parameters that, if known, greatly enhance the breeding efficiency: (1) the starting date of either menstruation or estrus; (2) the exact time of ovulation, whether naturally or artificially induced, relative to the start of estrus or the time of mating; (3) the time requirement for sperm capacitation and (4) the fertilizable life of the ovum. It is unfortunate that the only species in the animal kingdom in which all of these facets are known is the rabbit. One must know the start of menstruation (if it occurs) or the period of sexual receptivity (estrus) in order to predict the approximate day or time of

ovulation. Spermatozoa capacitation, the phenomenon that occurs in the female reproductive tract and by which spermatozoa attain the ability to fertilize the ovum, normally is measured in hours and ideally occurs prior to ovulation. The fertilizable life of the ovum is short in most species (12 to 20 hours) and is the most critical parameter. The fertilizable life of the sperm can also be of importance if mating occurs a long time before ovulation. However, since the fertilizable life of the sperm of most species appears to be between 24 and 72 hours and since the period of maximum receptivity in the female usually occurs near the time of ovulation, this factor is of less importance. Ideally, for maximum conception, mating should precede ovulation by the period of time necessary for capacitation to occur.

For the highest conception rate, especially with the rarer species, one should allow mating, capacitation and ovulation to occur naturally. Occasionally, however, it becomes necessary to superimpose an artificial regimen upon the animal to bring about pregnancy. Techniques such as ovulation induction, superovulation, steroid treatments to control estrus or enhance fertilization and artificial insemination are accomplished facts in many nonprimate species. In the nonhuman primate these techniques have been used with some success.

OVULATION INDUCTION

As early as 1935, Hisaw, Greep and Fevold,[15] using crude ovine anterior pituitary extracts, reported ovulation induction in three out of four macaques. Hartman[12] reported a total of seven ovulations out of 104 cycles in anovulatory adult rhesus monkeys. In 1942, he reported an additional six ovulations out of 46 cycles.[13] Pfeiffer[24] attempted to prevent ovulation in rhesus monkeys with administration of 0.5 mg of progesterone daily from the tenth to the fourteenth day of the cycle. Four ovulations were obtained from 11 monkeys after the final treatment.

Most of the work on the induction of ovulation in nonhuman primates has been carried out by van Wagenen[31] and her colleagues. Beginning in 1935, she unsuccessfully attempted to induce ovulation in macaques with pregnant mare serum gonadotropin (PMSG). Later work with purified follicle-stimulating hormone (FSH) and interstitial cell-stimulating hormone

TABLE 1. *Reproductive Parameters of Nonhuman Primates*

Taxonomic Name	Common Name	Age of Maturation (yrs)	Menstrual (Estrual) Cycle (days)	Menses (Estrus) Length (days)	Gestation Length (days)	Season of Birth*
PROSIMII						
Tupaiidae:						
Tupaia	Tree shrews	0.5	9–12	Conti.	41–56	All Year
Lemuridae:						
Lemur	Lemurs	1.5	39.3	4.7	120–135	Mar.–June
Lepilemur	Sportive lemurs	1.5			120–150	Sep.–Nov.
Hapalemur	Gentle lemurs					Dec.–Jan.
Cheirogaleus	Dwarf lemurs		30–50	3.0	70	
Microcebus	Mouse lemurs	0.8	45–55	3.0	59–62	Dec.–Mar.
Indriidae:						
Indri	Indrises				60	
Propithecus	Sifakas	2.5			150	June–Jul.
Avahi	Avahis					Aug.
Lorisidae:						
Loris	Slender lorises				160–174	Apr.–May & Nov.–Dec.
Nyciticebus	Slow lorises		42.3		193	All year
Arctocebus	Angwantibos		38–45		131	
Perodicticus	Pottos	1.0			170	
Galago	Greater galago (*G. crassicaudatus*)		50.3		128	May–June Oct.–Nov.
	Lesser galago (*G. senegalensis*)		30–37	4–6	121–124	Aug.–Sep. Apr.–May
	Allen's galago (*G. alleni*)		47.0			
	Demidoff's galago (*G. demidovii*)		38.0	3.0		
Tarsiidae:						
Tarsius	Tarsiers		24.0	1.0	180	All year
ANTROPOIDEA:						
Callithrichidae:						
Callithrix	Marmosets	1.2			130–140	
Saguinus	Tamarins				140	All year
Leontideus	Golden lion tamarins				132–134	
Cebidae:						
Cebus	Capuchins	3–4	18.0		180	All year
Saimiri	Squirrel monkeys	3.0	8–12		163	Jul.–Aug.
Aotus	Owl monkeys				120–140	June
Cercopithecidae:						
Cercopithecus	Grivet, green (*C. aethiops*)		30.9–33.0	3.7	163	
	Syke's monkey (*C. albogularis*)		30.0			Nov.–Mar.
	Talapoins (*Miopithecus talapoin*)		33.0	2–6	195	
Erythrocebus	Patas monkey		30.0		170	Dec.–Feb.
Mandrillus	Drill		32.6		245	
Cercocebus	Gray-cheeked mangabey (*C. albigena*)		29.0		175	
	Black mangabey (*C. atterrimus*)		31.0			
	White-collared mangabey (*C. torquatus*)		33.4	4–5		
Papio	Chacma baboon (*P. ursinus*)	4–6	35.6	4–9		
	Yellow baboon (*P. cynocephalus*)		33.3	3.0		
	Olive baboon (*P. anubis*)	3.5–4	34.7		184	
	Hamadryas baboon (*P. hamadryas*)		31.4			

TABLE 1. *Reproductive Parameters of Nonhuman Primates—Continued*

Taxonomic Name	Common Name	Age of Maturation (yrs)	Menstrual (Estrual) Cycle (days)	Menses (Estrus) Length (days)	Gestation Length (days)	Season of Birth*
Theropithecus	Gelada baboon		32–36			Feb.–Apr.
Macaca	Formosan macaque		29.9	3.3		
	(*M. cyclopsis*)					
	Japanese macaque	4.0	24.4	3.5		Mar.–May
	(*M. fuscata*)					
	Cynomolgus macaque	3.3	30.8	2.8	164.4	Apr.–Jul.
	(*M. fascicularis*)					
	Rhesus macaque	3.5–4.5	27.4	4–6	168	
	(*M. mulatta*)					
	Stump-tailed macaque		30.5		180	
	(*M. arctoides*)					
	Pig-tailed macaque		32.1			
	(*M. nemestrina*)					
	Bonnet macaque		29.5		162	
	(*M. radiata*)					
	Lion-tailed macaque		39.6	2.5		
	(*M. silenus*)					
	Toque monkey		29.0	1–4		
	(*M. sinica*)					
	Barbary ape		27–33	3–4		May–Sep.
	(*M. sylvana*)					
	Celebes macaque	4.5	30–40		155–175	June
	(*M. manurus*)					
Colobus	Guerezas					All year
Presbytis	Entellus		21–26	2–4		
	(*P. entellus*)					
	Purple-faced leaf monkey	4.0			194–217	May–Aug.
	(*P. senex*)					
Nasalis	Proboscis monkey				166	All year
Hylobatidae:						
Hylobates	Gibbons	5–8	29.8	2–5	210	All year
Symphalangus	Siamangs				230–235	
Pongidae:						
Pongo	Orangutans	6–9	29–32	3–4	233	
Pan	Chimpanzees	7–10	37.0	2–3	227–242	All year
Gorilla	Gorillas	6–7	31.0	8.0	265	All year

*Season of birth: In Northern hemisphere if known, otherwise in native habitat.

(ICSH) of ovine origin was ineffective in inducing ovulation. In 1956, Knobil, Morse and Greep[20] reported the importance of species-specificity in some primate pituitary hormones. This led to the important observation that in a significant number of cases, multiple ovulation was obtained with gonadotropins of primate origin. Subsequently, Knobil, Kostyo and Greep[19] induced ovulation in hypophysectomized macaques by treatment with porcine FSH and human chorionic gonadotropin (HCG).

In the intervening years, various ovulation-inducing agents have been studied for their effect on ovulation in rhesus monkeys. Dede and Plentl[4] used injections of Pergonal (human menopausal gonadotropin, HMG) for 8 to 10 days followed by 2-day injections of HMG and HCG. The animals were then mated or artificially inseminated, and pregnancies were obtained.

Wan and Balin[32] used HMG and HCG, clomiphene citrate, and DL-18-methyl estriol to induce ovulation in macaques and were successful in 60, 59 and 32 per cent of the treated cycles, respectively. They were also successful in obtaining high incidences of single ovulations, in contrast to Simpson and van Wagenen,[28] who reported multiple ovulation on each ovary.

Bennett[1, 2] induced multiple ovulation in the squirrel monkey with various regimens of PMSG and HCG. He demonstrated that ova can be recovered from the oviducts and suggested that, probably because of the elevated level of estrogens from the ovary, tubal transport could be speeded up by the high level of PMSG employed. Bennett began injections without reference to the stage of the cycle.

In our own studies,[5] we found that ovulation obtained in this species by a single pretreatment regimen of 5 days of progesterone (5 mg/day) mimicked the luteal phase of the cycle. This was followed by four daily IM injections of follicle-stimulating hormone (1 mg/day) and a single IM injection of human chorionic gonadotropin (500 IU) on the evening of the fourth day of FSH administration. This regimen results in single or double ovulations in 60 per cent of the animals within 12 hours. During the summer months the regimen becomes less effective because of a decreased sensitivity to the FSH, and the level of FSH must be increased to 2 mg daily or given for 5 days, rather than 4. This regimen results in ovulation, and the ova recovered are capable of fertilization either *in vivo*[17] or *in vitro*.[6, 21, 22] The regimen has also been used in the crab-eating macaque with a 50 per cent incidence of ovulation.[34] With macaques the progesterone pretreatment was omitted, and the FSH-HCG regimen was given beginning 3 to 4 days after menstruation. This results in ovulation on about day 9 or 10.

So-called "superovulation" regimens are available, usually using greatly increased levels of FSH and HCG or PMSG. This induction of ovulation is not difficult, but it should be emphasized that although this research technique is useful in the laboratory, it has less application in the area of breeding management. In primates the problem is often merely to obtain a pregnancy, not to alter litter size to astronomical proportions.

OVULATION DETECTION AND LAPAROSCOPY

Obviously, determination of the time of ovulation is important in mating regimens, especially those associated with "timed mating" in which male-female exposure is limited to only a few hours. Although classic methods of ovulation detection (vaginal cytological changes, discrete changes in blood hormone levels and so forth) are useful in the research situation, they are of little help in large-scale breeding operations. For practical purposes, only two ovulation detection techniques are widely used. The first of

these is the occurrence of deturgescence of the perineum (sex skin) in some species (notably the baboon[14] but also some macaque species, talapoins and others). In baboons, ideal mating time is 2 to 3 days prior to deturgescence, as sex skin swelling reaches its maximum. Obviously, the use of this criterion requires a strong knowledge of individual animals and a record of previous swelling characteristics.

A second method for determination of ovulation is by the use of the laparoscope. In recent years the use of laparoscopy (also termed endoscopy or pelviscopy) in breeding programs has greatly increased. Application of this technique from the area of human gynecology to animal research situations[7, 8] allows rapid inspection of the internal organs without the stress of major abdominal surgery. Graham *et al.*[10] have described the technique for laparoscopy of the chimpanzee, and Wildt *et al.*[35] have described the use of laparoscopy in studying follicular development in the baboon.

For most laparoscopy examinations the animal is prepared for normal surgery and placed on a sloped table (Fig. 1). A 5-mm pediatric laparoscope is adequate for all but the larger primates and is inserted in a dorsal-posterior position in such a manner that, upon removal, the skin and abdominal entry punctures are not aligned. This prevents herniation and reduces the chance of abdominal infection.

The two most popular anesthetic agents used with nonhuman primates in recent years have been phencyclidine hydrochloride and ketamine hydrochloride. The former is usually administered intramuscularly at a dose of from 0.5 to 3.0 mg/kg to macaques and South American species. The baboon and chimpanzee require lower doses of 0.5 to 1.0 mg/kg. Ketamine hydrochloride is usually given intramuscularly at a dose of 5 to 10 mg/kg for rhesus monkeys. Slightly higher levels (12 to 15 mg/kg) are recommended for cebus, squirrel, cynomolgus and bonnet monkeys. For complete anesthesia in chimpanzees, Graham *et al.*[10] followed administration of phencyclidine or ketamine with intubation and a mixture of 1 to 2 per cent halothane, 60 per cent nitrous oxide and 40 per cent oxygen.

The basic procedure for the examination is as follows:

1. Anesthetize the animal and place in dorsal recumbency, head down, sloped position.

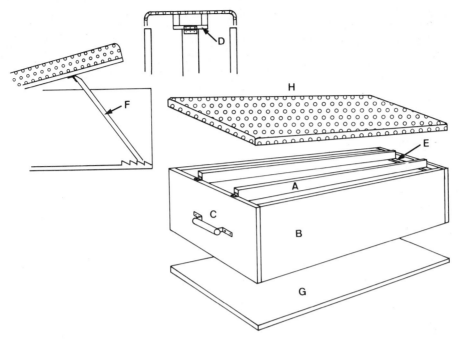

Figure 1. Laparoscopic examination stage. *A*, Support braces; *B*, body; *C*, carrying handle; *D*, hinge support; *E*, support brace stop; *F*, elevation by support; *G*, base; and *H*, perforated metal surgery stage.

2. Clip the abdominal area and scrub with surgical soap. Rinse and swab with iodine solution or equivalent.

3. Using a scalpel, make a small midline skin incision (not through the abdominal wall) near the umbilicus.

4. Slowly push the trocar-cannula slightly under the skin and then downward (dorsally) through the abdominal wall. This allows a nonalignment of skin and abdominal wall when the instruments are removed, precluding the need for suturing. With the animal restrained head down on a 45° sloped surface, the same effect is accomplished by inserting the trocar-cannula at a dorsal-posterior angle.

5. Attach the gas line to the cannula and slightly insufflate the abdomen. Alternatively, you can insert the Verres cannula first and attach the gas line for insufflation before trocar-cannula insertion. The latter technique is routinely used in human laparoscopic examination.

6. Slowly withdraw the trocar (too rapid withdrawal will result in a suction action, pulling the abdominal contents against, or into, the cannula).

7. Insert the telescope and attach it to the light source.

8. Insert the ancillary probe (Verres or larger, depending on the species) of the tele-

scope several centimeters to the right (left, if you are left-handed).

9. Manipulate the organ you wish to view into position while observing through the telescope.

10. If an ancillary port is needed for the insertion of biopsy or surgical instruments, insert the smaller trocar-cannula lateral to the telescope. The chance of damage to internal organs and blood vessels is greater than on the midline, and the abdomen should be distended with gas.

11. At the conclusion of the procedure all instruments are slowly withdrawn; a suture is used to close the wound, if desired; and the animal receives a prophylactic injection of penicillin. The entry site is dusted with nitrofurazone (Furacin) powder.

The stress involved with laparoscopy is minimal. In our colony of cynomolgus macaques, nearly 50 per cent of all cycles have been studied by laparoscopy over an 8-year period. An average cycle in which laparoscopy is carried out entails two to three laparoscopic examinations for a 3-day period near the time of ovulation. No effect has been noted on ovulation, menstrual cycle length or gestation. In fact, the procedure has been used to predict ovulation time for timed-mating studies.[18] Some animals in our colony have been laparoscoped as many as 83 times without apparent ill effects, and macaques laparoscoped as many as 49 times have subsequently become pregnant and borne normal young.

SEMEN COLLECTION AND ARTIFICIAL INSEMINATION

Many techniques commonly used in other domestic animals have been applied to primates as a means of semen collection. The commonly used techniques with primates involve electrical stimulation of either the penis or the accessory sexual glands. As with other domestic animals, certain criteria must be used in selecting the males that will be utilized for semen collection, and it is a well-recognized phenomenon that not all males are capable of artificial ejaculation. The proper choice of males is of prime importance. They should be in a strong physical state and of proven fertility as determined by use in natural mating schemes. Since larger animals can be quite dangerous and because of the close working relationship of the male and the animal technician, the canine teeth should be removed from all experimental subjects before they are used. The penile electrode technique[23] has been widely used in many laboratories, including our own. In some species that lack a distinct glans penis, such as chimpanzees, this technique is not possible because of the inability to keep the electrodes on the penile shaft. To improve this, workers at the Yerkes Regional Primate Research Center, Atlanta, Georgia, have developed a sheath with brass ring electrodes imbedded in the inner surface. Placing this over the penis eliminates the necessity for the foil strips. Another form of electroejaculation frequently used is the rectal probe. This was first described for use with monkeys in 1965. This type of electroejaculation consists of placing the probe electrodes within the rectum in the vicinity of the male accessory glands and eliciting ejaculation by stimulation of the glands. This type of probe[26] has also been used for semen collection from chimpanzees, gibbons, baboons, macaques, patas monkeys, cebus monkeys, squirrel monkeys and tree shrews.

Primate semen coagulates but will liquefy to a small degree by incubation at 37°C. The coagula are not affected by compounds capable of dissolving fibrin such as Evans blue, cysteinamine, N-acetyl cysteine and bromsulphalein. Many enzyme preparations have been used in attempts to liquefy the coagulum. Varizyme (streptokinase-human plasminogen-streptodornase) was used without success.[33]

Collagenase, α-amylase and β-amylase are ineffective. The best results have been obtained with 1 per cent solutions of Pronase, α-chymotrypsin and trypsin (bovine pancreas, type 1).[25] Lipase also has a dissolving effect on the coagula at a concentration of 1 per cent in a 3 per cent sodium glutamate solution. In our laboratory a 2 per cent lipase solution dissolved the squirrel monkey coagulum, but the time requirement for this incubation precludes the recovery of motile sperm.

One interesting approach to the prevention of the formation of the coagulum is the collection of semen directly into a 2 per cent chymotrypsin solution.[16] By this procedure, complete dissolution was obtained within 5 minutes.

Several workers have successfully frozen and thawed nonhuman primate semen, but no fertilization has occurred using semen that has been frozen. The semen of rhesus, stumptailed macaques, patas and green monkeys, as well as chimpanzees, have been frozen and thawed, with recoveries of motile sperm ranging from 50 to 54 per cent. The semen was frozen in an extender consisting of 20 per cent egg yolk, 64 per cent of a 3.0 per cent w/v sodium glutamate solution and 14 per cent glycerol. Semen was added to the extender in a ratio of 1:10 and equilibrated for 30 minutes at room temperature. The semen was ampuled (0.5 ml in 1.2-ml glass ampules) and lowered into the nitrogen refrigerator for deep-freezing.

The best semen extenders reported for freezing chimpanzee semen were: (1) egg yolk — 2.9 per cent sodium citrate with 10 per cent glycerol, (2) milk-egg with 10 per cent glycerol and (3) glucose-egg yolk with 7 per cent glycerol.[27]

Baboon semen has been frozen by the nitrogen vapor technique just described with the semen extended in the sodium glutamate-egg yolk solution containing 500 IU of penicillin and 500 mg of streptomycin per ml.[20a] Generally speaking, attempts at artificial insemination in nonhuman primates have involved placement of the coagulum into the vagina without dilution of the semen. This is normally done with the unanesthetized female held in an inverted position while the liquefied semen is sprayed onto the cervix with a syringe. The coagulum is then inserted into the vagina, and the female is held in the inverted position for 15 to 20 minutes. In the squirrel monkey, three females were inseminated, and 72 hours later ova were recovered up to the 4-cell stage.[2]

It is possible to inseminate rhesus monkeys intraperitoneally.[30] In eight animals so treated three became pregnant on the first cycle. Two of these pregnancies were terminated by cesarean section in the eighth week, and one pregnancy went full term. The semen was collected by the penile electrode technique, diluted and washed and injected intraperitoneally in volumes varying from 22 to 183 ml.

MATING STRATEGIES

The method of male-female exposure for mating varies with the requirement of the research project or zoo. Traditionally, zoo animals have been housed continuously in pairs or in harem groups. This provides maximum opportunity for mating and pregnancy while at the same time providing a "family group" display for the public. The same approach relates to the establishment of large troops of animals in compounds for either the large-scale production of primates or research studies on behavior and aggression. In the large-compound approach to mating, the social structure of the group assumes major importance, and occasionally there will be fighting between rivals and rearrangement of the social structure. Removal of an animal for treatment for several days will often create problems concerning the reintroduction of the animal.

In the caged environment, females are housed singly or in small groups of up to 10 animals. The male is then introduced to the group for periods of 4 to 5 days and then removed. This type of mating assures knowledge of the parentage of all offspring and also allows a reasonable estimate of gestation length. If animals are caged individually, it allows maximum utilization of the male. In these situations (in macaques) the male should be introduced about the tenth or eleventh day of the cycle and allowed to remain with the female for 4 or 5 days.

A third strategy frequently used in laboratory breeding situations is termed "timed mating" and refers to male-female exposure of less than 48 hours. This procedure is used when an accurate date of conception is needed for studies relating to pregnancy, tera-

tology or fetal development. The term "timed mating" has been used with varying connotations, ranging from exposure of only a few minutes to females continuously housed with males but subjected to frequent rectal palpation of the uterus for a temporal estimation of the date of conception. The latter is of questionable accuracy for most studies requiring precisely known conception dates.

For practical purposes male-female exposure for 24 to 48 hours provides sufficient accuracy for most specialized studies and, at the same time, allows a reasonable rate of conception. Pregnancies have been obtained in crab-eating macaques and stumptailed macaques with as little as 20- to 30-minute exposure to the male[3, 18] with a resultant conception rate of approximately 15 per cent. Such an approach is essential for some types of studies. However, for estimating the exact date of conception this procedure probably is no more accurate than 24-hour male-female exposure because of variation in the time of ovulation, sperm capacitation time required and an estimated fertilizable life of the sperm of several days.

In an extensive recent analysis of pregnancies resulting from 20- to 30-minute male-female exposure in the crab-eating macaque and stumptailed macaque, the time of mating was designated by the DB/CL ratio (day of breeding/previous cycle length). The values for the two macaque species were 0.45 and 0.41, respectively.[5a] These values would indicate that an animal should be mated on a day approximately 40 per cent through the cycle. In other words, a female showing a 30-day cycle should be mated about day 12 of the next cycle for optimal opportunity for pregnancy. A similar calculation can be made for cycles of varying duration.

SUMMARY

The captive mating of any wild-caught animal is always difficult, especially if basic data on the reproductive physiology of the animal are lacking. By the careful observation of cycle characteristics, assessment of ovulatory status and the application of known breeding strategies, a reasonable reproduction rate can be achieved in the laboratory or zoo environment with nonhuman primates.

REFERENCES

1. Bennett, J. P.: The induction of ovulation in the squirrel monkey (*Saimiri sciureus*) with pregnant mares serum (PMS) and human chorionic gonadotropin (HCG). J. Reprod. Fertil., *13*:357, 1967.
2. Bennett, J. P.: Artificial insemination of the squirrel monkey. J. Endocrinol., *37*:473, 1967.
3. Brüggemann, S. and Grauwiler, J.: Breeding results from an experimental colony of *Macaca arctoides*. Med. Primat., *1*:216, 1972.
4. Dede, J. A. and Plentl, A. A.: Induced ovulation and artificial insemination in a rhesus colony. Fertil. Steril., *17*:757, 1966.
5. Dukelow, W. R.: Induction and timing of single and multiple ovulation in the squirrel monkey (*Saimiri sciureus*). J. Reprod. Fertil., *22*:303, 1970.
5a. Dukelow, W. R.: Ovulation detection and control relative to optimal time of mating in nonhuman primates. Symp. Zool. Soc. London *43*:195, 1978.
6. Dukelow, W. R., and Kuehl, T. J.: *In vitro* fertilization of nonhuman primates. La Fécondation (Colloque de la Société Nationale pour L'Étude de la Stérilité et de la Fécondité). Masson et Cie, editeurs, Paris, 1975, pp. 67–80.
7. Dukelow, W. R. and Ariga, S.: Laparoscopic techniques for biomedical research. J. Med. Primat., *5*:82, 1976.
8. Dukelow, W. R., Jarosz, S. J., Jewett, D. A. and Harrison, R. M.: Laparoscopic examination of the ovaries in goats and primates. Lab. Anim. Sci., *21*:594, 1971.
9. Dumond, F. V.: The squirrel monkey in a seminatural environment. *In* Rosenblum, L. A. and Cooper, R. W. (eds.): The Squirrel Monkey. New York, Academic Press, 1968, p. 88.
10. Graham, C. E., Keeling, M., Chapman, C., Cummins, L. B., and Haynie, J.: Method of endoscopy in the chimpanzee: Relations of ovarian anatomy, endometrial histology, and sexual swelling. Am. J. Phys. Anthrop., *38*:211, 1973.
11. Harrison, R. M. and Dukelow, W. R.: Seasonal adaptation of laboratory maintained squirrel monkeys (*Saimiri sciureus*). J. Med. Primat., *2*:277, 1973.
12. Hartman, C. G.: The use of gonadotropic hormones in the adult rhesus monkey. Bull. Johns Hopkins Hosp., *63*:351, 1938.
13. Hartman, C. G.: Further attempts to cause ovulation by means of gonadotropes in the adult rhesus monkey. Carnegie Inst., Wash. Contrib. Embryol., *30*:113, 1942.
14. Hendrickx, A. G. and Kraemer, D. C.: Observations on the menstrual cycle, optimal mating time and preimplantation embryos of the baboon, *Papio anubis* and *Papio cynocephalus*. J. Reprod. Fertil. (Suppl.), *6*:119, 1969.
15. Hisaw, F. L., Greep, R. O. and Fevold, H. L.: Experimental ovulation of Macacus rhesus monkeys. Anat. Rec. (Suppl.), *61*:24, 1935.
16. Hoskins, D. D. and Patterson, D. L.: Prevention of coagulum formation with recovery of motile spermatozoa from rhesus monkey semen. J. Reprod. Fertil., *13*:337, 1967.
17. Jarosz, S. J., Kuehl, T. J. and Dukelow, W. R.: Vaginal cytology, induced ovulation and gestation in the squirrel monkey (*Saimiri sciureus*). Biol. Reprod., *16*:97, 1977.
18. Jewett, D. A. and Dukelow, W. R.: Laparoscopy and precise mating techniques to determine gestation length in *Macaca fascicularis*. Lab. Primat. Newsletter, *10*:16, 1971.
19. Knobil, E., Kostyo, J. L. and Greep, R. O.: Production of ovulation in the hypophysectomized rhesus monkey. Endocrinology, *65*:487, 1959.
20. Knobil, E., Morse, A. and Greep, R. O.: The effects of beef and monkey pituitary growth hormone on the costochondral junction in the hypophysectomized rhesus monkey. Anat. Rec., *124*:320, 1956.
20a. Kraemer, D. C. and Vera Cruz, N. C.: Collection, gross characteristics and freezing of baboon semen. J. Reprod. Fertil., *20*:345, 1969.
21. Kuehl, T. J. and Dukelow, W. R.: Ovulation induction during the anovulatory season in *Saimiri sciureus*. J. Med. Primat., *4*:23, 1975.
22. Kuehl, T. J. and Dukelow, W. R.: Fertilization *in vitro* of *Saimiri sciureus* follicular oocytes. J. Med. Primat., *4*:209, 1975.
23. Mastroianni, L. and Manson, W. A.: Collection of monkey semen by electroejaculation. Proc. Soc. Expt. Biol. Med., *112*:1025, 1963.
24. Pfeiffer, C. A.: Effects of progesterone upon ovulation in the rhesus monkey. Proc. Soc. Expt. Biol. Med., *75*:455, 1950.
25. Roussel, J. D. and Austin, C. R.: Enzymatic liquefaction of primate semen. Int. J. Fertil., *12*:288, 1967.
26. Roussel, J. D. and Austin, C. R.: Improved electroejaculation of primates. J. Inst. Anim. Tech., *19*:22, 1968.
27. Sadleir, R. M. F. S.: The preservation of mammalian spermatozoa by freezing. Lab. Pract., *15*:413, 1966.
28. Simpson, M. E. and van Wagenen, G.: Induction of ovulation with human urinary gonadotrophins in the monkey. Fertil. Steril., *13*:140, 1962.
29. Valerio, D. A.: Breeding *Macaca mulatta* in a laboratory environment. Lab. Anim. Handb., *4*:223, 1970.
30. van Pelt, L. F.: Intraperitoneal insemination of *Macaca mulatta*. Fertil. Steril., *21*:159, 1970.
31. van Wagenen, G.: Induction of ovulation in *Macaca mulatta*. Fertil. Steril., *19*:15, 1968.
32. Wan, L. S. and Balin, H.: Induction of ovulation in rhesus monkeys. A comparative study. Fertil. Steril., *20*:111, 1969.
33. Weisbroth, S. and Young, F. A.: The collection of primate semen by electroejaculation. Fertil. Steril., *19*:229, 1965.
34. Werbinski, J. and Dukelow, W. R.: Unpublished data.
35. Wildt, D. E., Doyle, L. L., Stone, S. and Harrison, R. M.: Correlation of laparoscopy, perineal swelling, and serum hormone levels during the baboon menstrual cycle. Primates *18*:261, 1977.

Artificial Breeding in Captive Wild Mammals and Its Possible Future Use

S. W. J. SEAGER, D. E. WILDT, JR. and C. C. PLATZ, JR.

Texas A & M University, College Station, Texas

To date, development of programs for artificial means of semen collection and insemination in the captive wild mammal population has been, for the most part, negligible. These methods have been developed to a high degree of proficiency in many domestic mammals, such as the bovine, ovine, porcine and avian species. In our laboratory, attempts are being made to adapt systems from domestic species, as well as develop new procedures and technical approaches, to provide a means of solving many of the breeding problems associated with the captive wild populations in zoos and game parks.

We have collected semen by electrical and manual stimulation in a number of species. Also, data from our laboratory have shown that artificial induction of estrus and ovulation can be achieved routinely in the domestic feline with the aid of laparoscopy for direct observation of reproductive activity. We have obtained a number of viable progeny from the use of frozen semen in the domestic dog, cat and timber wolf *(Canis lupus)*.[3, 6, 7]

SEMEN COLLECTION

Anesthesia is generally required for electroejaculation. This process has been performed successfully in the squirrel monkey *(Saimiri sciureus)* and rhesus macaque *(Macaca mulatta)* without anesthetic; however, this may be traumatic to the animal. Drugs used either singularly or in combination for electroejaculation in the various species are ketamine hydrochloride, phencyclidine hydrochloride, thiamylal sodium, C1744, xylazine, acepromazine, promazine, and M-99.

A deep surgical plane of anesthesia is desirable for electroejaculation. Successful ejaculates have been collected, however, in animals in light to medium anesthetic planes. A list of the species that have undergone electroejaculation is shown in Table 1.

The procedure for electroejaculation is similar to that reported in the domestic cat.[2, 4] A rectal probe is used with either an AC or a DC power source for the electroejaculation procedure. It is rarely possible to collect semen from any of the captive wild mammals using manual stimulation and an artificial vagina. In a few instances, successful collections have been obtained from timber wolves, Siberian tigers, ocelots and cheetahs; however, great precautions must be taken.

After the semen is obtained, it is evaluated both macro- and microscopically if freezing is desired. The semen sample is then equilibrated at 5° C, pelleted on dry ice and deposited into liquid nitrogen for storage. It can be inseminated immediately or, if of good quality, held for 2 to 3 days at 5° C in proper extenders until used for insemination.

Semen stored in liquid nitrogen for more than 6 years is capable of fertilization in the dog. Cattle have been produced from artificial insemination of semen that had been stored 30 years. Based on these data, we assume that a similar result would be possible in the captive wild mammals.

LAPAROSCOPY

Laparoscopy has been a valuable technique for monitoring reproductive cyclicity in both domestic and wild mammals. It has been used successfully to monitor the effects of exogenous hormones on follicle development and ovulation in the domestic cat. In our laboratory successful pregnancies have been produced in the domestic cat from the artificial induction of estrus and ovulation followed by artificial insemination with previously frozen semen. Future attempts at obtaining pregnancies in wild animals will be based on these successful procedures developed in the domestic cat and dog.[9]

Table 2 illustrates the species in which laparoscopy has been performed.

TABLE 1. *Species Electroejaculated to Date in Program for Artificial Insemination of Nondomestic Animals (Institute of Comparative Medicine)*

Golden marmoset	*Leontideus rosalia**
Lowland gorilla	*Gorilla gorilla gorilla**
Baboon, hamadryas	*Papio hamadryas**
Squirrel monkey	*Saimiri sciuresus**
White handed gibbon	*Hylobates lar*
Red Uakari monkey	*Cacajao rubicundus*
Grey gibbon	*Hylobates moloch*
Orangutan	*Pongo pygmaeus**
Spider monkey	*Ateles fusciceps**
Black and white Colobus monkey	*Colobus colobus*
Black and red Tamarin	*Saguinus nigricollis*
Hamlyn guenon	*Cercopithecus hamlyni*
Assamese macaque	*Macaca assamenses*
Lion tailed macaque	*Macaca silenus*
Moor macaque	*Macaca maurus*
Mandrill	*Papio sphinx*
Owl monkey	*Aotus trivirgatus**
Chimpanzee	*Pongo pygmaeus*
Yellow baboon	*Papio cyanocephalus*
Greater kudu	*Tragelaphus strepsiceros*
Fallow deer	*Dama dama*
Black rhinoceros	*Diceros bicornis*
Bactrian camel	*Camelus bactrianus**
Pere David deer	*Elaphuras davidianus*
Blesbok	*Damaliscus albifrons*
Muntjac	*Muntiacus reevesi**
South American tapir	*Tapirus terrestris*
Axis deer	*Axis axis*
Sitatunga	*Tragelaphus spekei*
Arabian oryx	*Oryx leucoryx**
Red sheep	*Ovis orientalis*
Red Lechwe	*Kobus leche*
Slender horned gazelle	*Gazella leptoceros*
Eld's deer	*Cervus eldii eldii**
Speke's gazelle	*Gazella spekei*
Yellow backed duiker	*Cephalophus sylvicultor*
Dik-dik	*Madoqua kirki*
Brocket deer	*Mazama americana temama**
Pygmy hippopotomus	*Choeropsis liberiensis*
Onager	*Equus heminonus onager*
White or square lipped rhinoceros	*Ceratotherium simum*
Dorcus gazelle	*Gazella dorcus**
South American llama	*Llama peruana*
Binturong	*Arctictis binturong**
Tree kangaroo	*Dendrolagus matschiei*
Meerkat	*Suricata suricata**
Egyptian mongoose	*Herpestes ichneumon**
Palm civet	*Paradoxurus hermaphroditus**
Spotted hyena	*Crocuta crocuta**
Lesser panda	*Ailurus fulgens*
Polar bear	*Thalarctos maritimus**
American black bear	*Ursus americanus**
Bush dog	*Speothos venaticus**
North American red fox	*Vulpes fulva*
Canadian timber wolf	*Canis lupus canadensis**
Kodiak bear	*Ursus arctos middendorffi*
Sloth bear	*Melursus ursinus*
European brown bear	*Ursus arctos arctos*
Spectacled bear	*Tremarctos ornatos**
African water mongoose	*Atilax paludinosis*
Cougar	*Felis concolor**
North Chinese leopard	*Panthera pardus japonensis*
Canadian lynx	*Felis lynx canadensis**
Bobcat	*Felis rufa**
Temminck's golden cat	*Felis temminckii**
Ocelot	*Felis pardalis**
Geoffroy's cat	*Felis geoffroyi**
Clouded leopard	*Neofelis nebulosa**

TABLE 1. *Species Electroejaculated to Date in Program for Artificial Insemination of Nondomestic Animals (Institute of Comparative Medicine) Continued*

Lion	*Panthera leo**
Bengal tiger	*Panthera tigris tigris**
Siberian tiger	*Panthera tigris altaica**
Leopard	*Panthera pardus*
Sand cat	*Felis margarita*
Amur leopard cat	*Felis bengalensis euptilura*
Jaguar	*Panthera onca**
African cheetah	*Acinonyx jubatus**
Leopard cat	*Felis bengalensis*
Margay	*Felis wiedii*
Crab eating fox	*Cerdocyon thous**
Bull snake	*Pituophis melanoleucus*
Angolan python	*Python anchietae**
Green sea turtle	*Chelonia mydas**
Galapagos tortoise	*Testudo elephantopus**
Hog nose snake	*Heterodon platyrhinus platyrhinus*
Red eared pond turtle	*Pseudemys scripta elegans*
Degu	*Octodon degus**
Patagonian cavy	*Dolichotis patagona*
White rat	*Mus norvegicus albinus*
Sugar glider	*Petaurus breviceps**
Mexican fruit eating bat	*Artibeus jamaicensis**
Giant panda	*Ailuropoda melanoleuca**

*Denotes more than one ejaculation obtained from the species by electroejaculation.

DISCUSSION

Our program for semen collection and freezing has been very successful in most species. The artificial insemination, estrus and ovulation induction program is currently being investigated in several of the large species of felines and other captive animal species.[5, 8]

The eventual goal of this project is to establish a program of artificial breeding in nondomesticated animals for the following reasons:

1. To establish reproductive physiological parameters.

2. To develop and refine methods:

TABLE 2. *Species in Which Laparoscopy Has Been Utilized*

Man	Dog	Lion
Mouse	Nonhuman primates	Tiger
Rat	Birds	Cheetah
Guinea pig	Sheep	Leopard
Hamster	Pig	Jaguar
Rabbit	Cow	Polar bear
Cat	Horse	Reptiles
		Fish

a. Of physical restraint for artificial insemination and semen collection.

b. Of electroejaculation, semen freezing and artificial insemination.

c. Of estrus and ovulation induction and detection and pregnancy diagnosis.

3. To improve breeding and preservation of common and endangered zoo animals.

4. To preserve valuable cells for future breeding and research study.

5. To establish a national and eventually an international semen bank.

The advantages of a frozen semen artificial breeding program are:

1. To eliminate the risk and expense of shipping captive wild animals for breeding.

2. To inseminate the female without the male being present or to eliminate the problem of incompatible pairs.

3. To prevent possible disease transmission from outside animals brought in for breeding.

4. To introduce new bloodlines into the gene pool from the wild animal game parks and reserves and zoos.

5. To help eliminate complicated legal procedures and animal shipments involved with breeding loans.

6. To improve bloodlines with possible reduction or elimination of undesirable genetic traits.

7. To make available the possibility of progeny testing males.

The authors advocate the use of an artificial breeding program only as a part or an aid in an overall breeding program. We believe that animals given ideal situations and habitat need little help from man to reproduce. It is when man has put such constraints on the "ideal" situation, whether it be disease, caging, diet or other stress, that we suggest artificial insemination can play a vital role in wild animal reproduction. The success thus far observed leads us to believe that the capability for breeding many captive wild mammals, including some of the endangered species, can be brought about using artificial methods.

REFERENCES

1. Bush, M., Wildt, D. E., Kennedy, S. and Seager, S.: Laparoscopy in zoological medicine. J.A.V.M.A., *173*:1081, 1978.
2. Hammer, C. E.: *In* Hafez, E. S. E. (ed.): The Semen Reproduction and Breeding Techniques for Laboratory Animals. Philadelphia, Lea and Febiger, 1970, pp. 56–73.
3. Platz, C., Wildt, D. E. and Seager, S. W. J.: Pregnancy in the domestic cat after artificial insemination with previously frozen spermatozoa. J. Reprod. Fertil. *52*:279, 1978.
4. Seager, S. W. J.: Electroejaculation of cats. *In* Klemm, W. R. (ed.): Electronics in Veterinary Medicine. Springfield, Ill., Charles C Thomas, Publisher, 1975.
5. Seager, S. W. J. and Demorest, C. N.: Reproduction of captive wild carnivores. *In* Fowler, M. E. (ed.): Zoo and Wild Animal Medicine. Philadelphia, W. B. Saunders Company, 1978, pp. 667–706.
6. Seager, S. W. J., Platz, C. and Fletcher, W.: Conception rates and related data using frozen dog semen. J. Reprod. Fertil. *45*:189, 1975.
7. Seager, S. W. J., Platz, C. and Hodge, W.: Successful pregnancy using frozen semen in the wolf. Int. Zoo Yrbk. *15*:140, 1975.
8. Seager, S. W. J., Wildt, D. E. and Platz, C.: Artificial breeding of non-primates. Symp. Zool. Soc. Lond. *43*:207, 1978.
9. Wildt, D. E., Bush, M., Whitlock, B. and Seager, S. W. J.: Laparoscopy: a method for direct examination of internal organs in zoo veterinary medicine and research. Int. Zoo Yrbk. *15*:192, 1978.

section XIV

DIAGNOSTIC PROCEDURES

Consulting Editor

R. B. MILLER

Necropsy Procedures for the Reproductive System

P. W. LADDS

James Cook University of North Queensland, Queensland, Australia

Detailed examination of the genitalia is often neglected in routine necropsy procedures; the ovary or testis receives little attention in comparison with organs such as the liver, kidney or brain so that even experienced pathologists may have difficulty in assessing pathological changes in these structures.

Changes associated with aging tend to be more pronounced in the genitalia than in other organs, and in the female, knowledge of morphological changes associated with pregnancy and the ovarian cycle is essential before detailed interpretation of pathological change can be attempted.

Time spent examining the genitalia of all animals necropsied will therefore be rewarding since it will provide the practitioner with a clear idea of the range of "normality" and familiarize him with the more common lesions.

FEMALE GENITALIA

Removal

Satisfactory examination of the pelvic organs can be achieved only after removal of a portion of the bony pelvis.

Most necropsy procedures involve placing the animal on its side, disarticulation of the uppermost hip joint, reflection of both legs and the skin on one side, removal of the abdominal and thoracic walls and examination *in situ*, followed by removal of the thoracic viscera and the abdominal viscera other than the kidneys.

After completion of these steps, removal of part of the bony pelvis can be achieved by cutting (with saw or garden pruning shears) along the symphysis pubis and through the shaft of the ilium on the uppermost side. A knife is then used to cut adjacent fibrous and muscular tissue, and a complete segment of pelvis is removed.

Because of their close association, it is frequently desirable to examine and remove the entire genital and urinary systems, including the kidneys, simultaneously. This is accomplished by dissecting the kidneys and ureters free by cutting attachments on their *lateral* aspects. In order to achieve complete removal of the ovaries and related structures, the ovarian ligaments should also be cut at their lateral extremities, as close to the body wall as possible.

In small animals it is possible to hold the kidneys, ovaries and attached ductular structures in one hand and use the other hand to dissect free the remaining intrapelvic structures. Inclusion of a generous amount of contiguous adipose and fibrous tissue with the urogenital organs will insure complete removal. These organs are lifted through the opening made on the ventrolateral aspect of the pelvis, and removal is completed by incising the skin around the vulva and anus — a small portion of rectum then being removed with the genitalia.

With large animals, genitalia are frequently collected after slaughter rather than at necropsy. In such cases it is customary for the genitalia to be removed from the carcass along with other viscera. Prior discussion with the slaughterman will result in more suitable specimens; little extra effort is required to achieve removal of the entire genital tract, and delays in abattoir procedure are unlikely.

Gross Examination

The urinary organs should first be examined, and the occurrence of conditions that might involve both the genital and urinary systems (e.g., congenital malformations, endometritis-pyelonephritis) should be noted.

The *ovaries* should next be exposed, and particular attention should be paid to whether any cysts that may be present are located in the ovary or in the paraovarian tissues. Adhesions between these tissues or between genital and extragenital organs should also be noted.

Ovarian size, weight, surface characteristics, color and internal appearance after sagittal midline sectioning can all be used to ascertain the presence of congenital defects (e.g., ovarian hypoplasia), ovarian activity or inactivity, inflammation, intraovarian cysts and neoplasia.

Patency of the *oviducts* can then be checked by carefully inserting a blunted hypodermic needle (with syringe containing saline attached) into the ovarian extremity of the oviduct. Insertion of the needle into the minute opening (the abdominal ostium) is facilitated by stretching the delicate ovarian and oviduct membranes over one forefinger, with the funnel-shaped dilation of the oviduct lumen (infundibulum) uppermost. Gentle pressure on the syringe will force saline into the oviduct, which becomes visibly dilated as the saline progresses downward. Small incisions into the tips of the uterine horns permit visualization of the entry of saline from the oviducts. Size of the needle will depend on the species, and 22-SWG and 18-SWG needles are suitable for small and large animals, respectively. For fixation the oviduct is dissected away from the mesosalpinx, wrapped around cardboard and placed in Bouin's fixative.

The remaining genitalia should initially be palpated and examined externally for the presence of congenital defects such as segmental aplasia (in which a distinct segment is absent) or incomplete fusion (especially caudally) of the tubular organs. Using blunt pointed Mayo scissors, both uterine horns, the uterine body, cervix, vagina and vulva are then opened on the dorsal aspect. Patency of the cervix should be recorded.

Attention should first be directed toward the uterine contents, particularly fetal or embryonic remnants that may be present. Such remnants may easily be overlooked if present in a large volume of exudate.

The color, viscosity, volume and odor of any intrauterine exudate should be noted. The underlying endometrium is then examined for the presence of inflammation and/or hyperplastic and cystic changes.

In the cervix, vagina and vulva, the color, viscosity and volume of mucus should again be noted and a search made to detect vesicles, pustules, erosions or ulcerations of epithelium and neoplasms such as transmissible venereal tumor. Other abnormalities that may be observed after opening the genitalia in this location include cystic Gartner's ducts (cattle), imperforate hymen, fusion defects as previously indicated and incomplete

separation of the vagina and rectum, resulting in a form of cloaca.

Specimen Collection

Samples obtained at necropsy for microbiological study are best acquired before dissection of the genitalia is commenced.

The surface of the uterus is seared with a heated spatula, and a disposable sterile needle and syringe are used to aspirate the contained exudate. A drop of the aspirate may be placed on a glass slide, coverslipped and examined directly (e.g., for trichomoniasis in cattle), or smears may be prepared for fixation, Gram-staining and bacteriological identification.

The syringe is then sealed (using a plastic needle cover) and dispatched for culture and other laboratory examinations (e.g., darkground study).

Specimens for histopathological study should be placed in fixative as soon as possible. Bouin's fluid (containing picric acid)* is preferable to formalin for fixation of genital tissues. Tissue to be fixed should be cut to a thickness of less than 1 cm, and the ratio of tissue to fixative should be about 1 to 20. These tissues must be removed from the fixative after 24 to 48 hours and stored in 10 per cent formalin.

Interpretation

Interpretation of necropsy, microscopic and microbiological findings must in most instances be based on a complete history involving factors such as breeding records, therapy (e.g., hormone administration), nutrition and the presence of intercurrent disease. Of primary importance is the differentiation of conditions occurring spontaneously and involving only one animal (e.g., uterine leiomyoma) from conditions that may involve other animals (e.g., brucellosis, vibriosis) or their progeny (e.g., ovarian hypoplasia).

MALE GENITALIA

Removal

As in the female, removal of pelvic organs in the male again necessitates removal of

---

*Saturated aqueous picric acid 75 ml, formalin 25 ml and acetic acid glacial 5 ml.

portions of the bony pelvis (as previously described). Before cutting along the symphysis pubis in the male, it is necessary to carefully dissect free the fibrous attachments of the root of the penis to the ischium.

The urogenital organs can then be removed as in the female, the vas deferens being cut near the internal inguinal rings. If care is taken, the penis can be freed from its ischial attachments and dissected anteriorly to include the prepuce.

When it is necessary to collect male genitalia after slaughter in an abattoir, it is convenient to obtain the accessory sex glands, urinary bladder and urethra by dissecting these organs free from the rectum after the animal has been eviscerated. Care should be taken to obtain the small bulbourethral (Cowper's) glands, which (in the bull) are located posteriorly, associated with the bulbocavernosus muscle. The remainder of the genitalia can then be readily obtained by taking the root of the penis plus the scrotum and its contents and dissecting these free by cutting forward to the anterior aspect of the prepuce.

Gross Examination

Dissection of the male genitalia involves three areas: the external genitalia, the testes and epididymides and the accessory sex glands. Examination of the *external genitalia* should commence with the scrotal skin. Lesions here that may impair fertility include dermatitis, varicose dilation of scrotal veins and neoplasia — e.g., mastocytoma in the dog.

The skin of the prepuce, especially the preputial orifice, should be examined, and the *penis* should then be extruded to permit visualization. Conditions to be noted in this location include preputial eversion or prolapse, persistent penile frenulum, congenital short penis, duplicated penis (diphallia), hypospadias, phimosis or paraphimosis, inflammation, traumatic lesions or neoplasms such as papillomatosis, squamous cell carcinoma or transmissible venereal tumor.

Ulceration of the preputial diverticulum in the boar is quite common and appears to be of little significance in regard to fertility.

In the bull the sigmoid flexure should be palpated to detect the presence of hematomas, and the rectractor penis muscle should

be examined in its midportion for evidence of degeneration and calcification.

When indicated, the penis should be opened by cutting along the urethra; predilection sites for urinary obstruction are the caudal end of the os penis in the dog and the vermiform penile appendage in the ram.

On removal of the *testes* and *epididymides* from the scrotum, the attached spermatic cord should be exmained, and the presence and type (fibrous or fibrinous) of any tunic adhesions should be noted. After checking the completeness and continuity of the epididymides and attached vas deferens (to detect segmental aplasia), the epididymides are then separated from the testes; it is advisable to weigh and measure these organs.

The testes are next dissected by a longitudinal (midsagittal) cut to expose the mediastinum, and the testicular parenchyma is then examined to detect the presence of calcified foci (occasional small foci are of no significance), fibrosis, orchitis or neoplasms.

Testicular "halves" are then cut transversely with a sharp knife, making slices no more than 1 cm in thickness.

The epididymides are examined for the presence of cysts, and the size, location and content of these should be recorded. Sperm granulomas and larger foci of epididymitis will be detected at this time, especially in the ram. Occlusion and dilation of more proximal epididymal ducts result from these conditions. On gross examination it is to be remembered that accumulated sperm resemble purulent exudate and that microscopic examination of a smear of the exudate will clarify its composition.

The *accessory sex glands* comprise the seminal vesicles, prostate, bulbourethral (Cowper's) glands and the ampullae (dilations of the proximal extremities of the vas deferens). Among the domestic species there is considerable variability in the morphology and pathological involvement of these glands. In the bull the seminal vesicles are most often affected, whereas in the dog the prostate is more frequently involved.

After examination of the urinary bladder, a cut in the neck of the bladder on its dorsal aspect is extended along the urethra to the root of the penis. Size and symmetry of the prostate (dog) should be noted at this time.

The accessory sex glands should be examined for the presence of congenital defects and should be palpated to detect cysts, foci of inflammation, fibrosis, hyperplasia or neoplasia. Any adhesions to adjacent structures should be noted.

After collection of specimens for microbiological examination, all glands are opened by multiple incisions. The type of exudate present in each gland should be recorded, but again there is marked species variation (e.g., seminal vesicle secretion in the boar is copious and extremely tenacious).

It is often convenient to collect samples of spermatozoa at this time. In the bull, spermatozoa for morphological examination can usually be obtained by incising the ampullae with a sharp scalpel and aspirating the contents into a Pasteur pipette. This sample can be washed into saline or formal saline or used to prepare fresh smears. Spermatozoa collected in this way can be identified with either the right or the left gonad, and this may be helpful in evaluating other findings in the testis or epididymis on a particular side.

Specimen Collection

For microbiological sampling of the preputial cavity, the penis is held with rat-tooth forceps and drawn from the prepuce. The moist preputial and penile epithelium are then gently scraped with a sterile scalpel blade. Preputial contents so obtained may be placed directly into tissue culture medium for virological studies (e.g., to detect infectious pustular vulvovaginitis, IPV, in cattle), incubated in special media for the detection of trichomoniasis (in cattle) or used for bacterial (e.g., vibriosis) isolation. Samples for microbiological examination from lesions in the remaining genitalia are collected using sterile procedures as previously described for the uterus.

For satisfactory histopathological evaluation of the testis and epididymis, fixation within a short time after collection is necessary. As for the female genitalia, Bouin's fluid is again the preferred fixative. It is best to fix thin transverse slices of testicular tissue (previously discussed) taken from three locations — the dorsal pole in the area of attachment of the epididymal head, the central region and near the ventral pole. If a sharp knife is used, it is possible to cut slices less than 1 cm (in the bull), which include both the tunica albuginea laterally and the mediastinum centrally. After the epididy-

mis has been grossly examined and cut by multiple sections, it is best fixed *in toto*. Representative portions of the remaining genitalia and tissue from any lesions that may be present are fixed as indicated.

Interpretation

Particularly difficult in many cases is the differentiation of testicular degeneration from hypoplasia. Even after histological studies, differentiation without adequate history may not be possible.

CONCEPTUS AND NEONATE

The conceptus comprises the embryo or fetus plus the embryonic or fetal membranes. Perhaps too frequently in the diagnosis of abortion emphasis is placed on fetal examination while the membranes are overlooked.

Gross Examination

When available, the *chorioallantois* should be stretched on a flat surface with the detached cotyledonary surfaces uppermost. Samples for microbiological examination should be selected from affected cotyledons at this time and impression smears made for direct examination.

Particular matter (dirt, straw and so forth) should then be removed and the tissue cleaned by gentle washing with tap water. A good assessment can then be made of any pathological changes in the cotyledons and the number of cotyledons affected. These changes may include focal or more extensive necrosis, granulomatous proliferation, calcification, suppuration or hemorrhage.

The intercotyledonary area should also be closely examined for changes such as edema, fibrin exudation, hemorrhage, loss of translucency, marked thickening and formation of plaques.

Specimens of lesions, preferably including some adjacent "normal" tissue, should be fixed in Bouin's fluid for histopathological study.

Before discarding the membranes, they should be turned so that the smooth (allantoic) side is uppermost. This surface and the *amnion* should then be examined for the features just mentioned.

Note, however, that small, pale foci of calcium deposition and amniotic plaques (or concrescences) of squamous epithelium are normal findings in many species. The latter are most common at the point at which the amnion envelops the umbilical cord.

Examination of the *embryo* or *fetus* should commence by tape measuring the crown-rump length (base or tail); this permits a reasonably accurate determination of age.

Next, the extent of intrauterine autolysis should be assessed. Cloudiness of the cornea, color changes and degree of slipping or sloughing of skin and color and amount of fluid in the subcutis are good indications of this.

External appraisal for lesions such as congenital defects (e.g., failure of closure of the cranium or spinal canal), hemorrhages or cutaneous plaques (e.g., mycotic dermatitis) should then be made. Absence of thrombosis of the umbilical vessels indicates preparturient death. In the case of farm animals that die in the neonatal period, examination of the feet will indicate whether or not the animal ever walked.

Necropsy procedures for the fetus or neonate are the same as those for adult animals. Special attention is, however, directed toward the amount and type of fluid in body cavities, the *lungs* (aerated or otherwise, presence of edema or hemorrhage), *liver* (size, presence of pale foci of necrosis), *stomach* (content) and *brain* (cerebellar hypoplasia, dilation of ventricles with excessive fluid).

Specimen Collection

For bacteriological examination, specimens should include amniotic fluid (when available), ascitic or thoracic fluid and lung, liver and brain tissue. The fluids should be aspirated into a sterile syringe before the respective cavities are opened. Smears prepared from stomach contents sometimes suggest a diagnosis (e.g., mycotic abortion). Tissue (e.g., brain, lung, liver, kidney) for virological culture or fluorescent antibody examination should be collected using a sterile technique and be either processed immediately or frozen.

Fetal fluids, serum or plasma should be collected for serological study.

As previously indicated, specimens for histopathological study should be fixed in Bouin's fluid. Fetal tissues are softer and more friable than adult tissues, and longer fixation times are necessary.

Interpretation

Diagnosis of the cause of abortion or neonatal death is frequently difficult, and it is desirable to obtain a detailed history and a complete range of specimens from the dam, the placenta and the fetus or neonate. Microbiological findings may be meaningless if gross and microscopic changes in the conceptus cannot be demonstrated.

REFERENCES

1. Bloom, F.: Pathology of the Dog and Cat. The Genitourinary System, with Clinical Considerations. Evanston, Ill., American Veterinary Publications, 1954.
2. Dennis, S. M.: Laboratory diagnosis of infectious bovine abortion. J.A.V.M.A., *155*:1913, 1969.
3. Dillman, R. C.: Sequential sterile autolysis in the ovine fetus: Macroscopic changes. Am. J. Vet. Red., *37*:403, 1976.
4. Dunn, R. B.: Aging the merino foetus, Aust. Vet. J., *31*:153, 1955.
5. Hubbert, W. T.: Recommendations for standardizing bovine reproductive terms. Cornell Vet., *61*:216, 1971.
6. Jubb, K. V. and Kennedy, P. C.: Pathology of Domestic Animals. Vol. I. New York, Academic Press, 1970.
7. Marrable, A. W. and Ashdown, R. R.: Quantitative observations on pig embryos of known ages. J. Agric. Sci., Cambridge, *69*:443, 1967.
8. McFarlane, D.: Perinatal lamb losses. I. An autopsy method for the investigation of perinatal losses. New Zealand Vet. J., *13*:116, 1965.
9. Rooney, J. R.: Autopsy of the Horse — Technique and Interpretation. Baltimore, The Williams & Wilkins Co., 1970.

Serological Testing

D. W. JOHNSON

University of Minnesota, St. Paul, Minnesota

INTRODUCTION

Serological testing can be an important tool in the diagnosis of abortion or reproductive disease. Such testing can be used to determine the presence of specific antibodies in the serum of the dam or sire or may be used to detect antibodies in the serum or body fluids of the aborted fetus or newborn prior to nursing. The presence of antibodies in an animal's serum may be indicative of an active infection or of postinfection, depending upon the titer obtained against a particular antigen. In some diseases, a titer is considered indicative of active infection; in others, the same titer may be meaningless because the animal has been previously immunized or comes from an area where the disease is endemic. If possible, serological testing should always be done by testing two samples taken at at least 3-week intervals. A four-fold or more increase in titer can then be taken as indicative of active infection. The exception to this is a fetus or a term neonate prior to nursing, in which single sample with antibody titer is indicative of infection by specific agent that likely caused the disease or abortion.

SEROLOGICAL TESTS

Five serological tests are commonly used in the laboratory diagnosis of bacterial, viral and fungal reproductive diseases. They are (1) the agglutination test, (2) the hemagglutination-inhibition (H-I) test, (3) the neutralization (N) test, (4) the complement fixation (CF) test and (5) the precipitin tests. Several variations of each of these tests are in use, and the conditions under which they may be conducted vary. The test and test conditions selected will depend primarily upon established procedure or upon the antigen used.

Agglutination Test

In general, agglutination tests are quite simple to perform. The term agglutination describes the aggregation or clumping of particles due to complexing of antigen and antibody. The various ways by which agglutination reactions can be observed (e.g., plate, tube, card, slide and ring test) will not be described here, as the main point of this article is to set forth which serological tests are available and how results are interpreted.

The most common agglutination test used in the diagnosis of reproductive disease is the plate and tube agglutination test for the diagnosis of brucellosis.

Agglutination is the principal serological test for the diagnosis of most bacterial, fungal and parasitic diseases. Specific diseases for which agglutination tests are available are presented in Table 1.

The test can be performed on any body fluid that contains antibodies. Blood serum is used most frequently, but milk, semen plasma, vaginal mucus, or thoracic fluid from fetuses may be used under certain circumstances. Samples for agglutination tests should be fresh and free of chemicals but need not be sterile.

Hemagglutination-Inhibition (H-I) Test

The basis for the hemagglutination-inhibition test lies in the fact that certain viruses possess the capacity to agglutinate red blood cells and that specific antibody prevents or inhibits hemagglutination. This reaction therefore can be utilized for antibody assay or for virus identification. This test is used primarily in the diagnosis of myxoviruses (parainfluenza-3, PI-3), enterovirus (or picornavirus) and parvovirus infections that may be associated with reproductive diseases.

Serum for this test must be free of bacterial contamination, as bacteria may cause either lysis or false agglutination of the red blood cells, thus making it impossible to obtain interpretable results.

Neutralization (N) Test

The neutralization test is based on the principle that when a specific immune serum is added to its corresponding virus, the virus is rendered noninfective or is "neutralized." Since demonstration of infectivity requires the use of living tissues, the host system employed in most diagnostic laboratories is an *in vitro* cell culture system. Thus, if the serum being tested has antibodies to the virus added, it is "neutralized," and when this neutralized virus is placed into cell cultures, it will no longer produce cytopathological findings. This test is used in the diagnosis of several viral diseases including infectious bovine rhinotracheitis (IBR), bovine viral diarrhea (BVD), equine rhinopneumonitis (ERV) and pseudorabies (PRV). Sera for the neutralization test must be sterile and must not be contaminated with toxic substances. Cell cultures are very susceptible to infection with live bacteria and to the endotoxin or exotoxins produced by them. They are also destroyed by very small amounts of detergents, alcohol, heavy metals from nondistilled water and anything that may cause a drastic change in culture pH.

Complement Fixation (CF) Test

The complement fixation test consists of two antigen-antibody reactions — the non-hemolytic or primary reaction and the hemolytic or secondary reaction. The former consists of an antigen and its homologous antiserum, the latter of red blood cells and an antierythrocytic serum referred to as hemolysin. The presence of complement in the hemolytic system permits lysis of the red blood cells to occur when they have been sensitized by their homologous antibodies, and test results are based on the extent of hemolysis.

Complement also enters into the reaction of the nonhemolytic system when an antigen reacts with a homologous antiserum. This latter reaction is referred to as complement fixation because the complement is removed from the nonhemolytic system and therefore is not available to react with the hemolytic system, thus preventing hemolysis of the red blood cells. This test is used in the serological diagnosis of blue tongue, anaplasmosis and chlamydial infections. Sera for the CF test must be free of bacterial and chemical contaminants, as they can cause anticomplementary action. Anticomplementary chemicals include alcohol, detergents, anticoagulants and preservatives.

Precipitin Tests

One of two precipitin tests may be employed: either the tube or capillary tube test or the agar gel immunodiffusion test. In the tube test, a soluble antigen is mixed with the unknown antiserum, and if antibodies to the antigen are present, a precipitate forms. All components in this test must be perfectly unclouded, otherwise weak reactions may be obscured. In the agar gel immunodiffusion test, the soluble antigen is added to an agar gel mixture, and this is placed on a glass slide or in a plastic plate. Wells are formed in the agar, and unknown sera are added. If antibody to the antigen is present, a white precipitin band forms around the well.

The immunodiffusion precipitin test is used in the diagnosis of mycotic reproductive diseases.

Samples for the precipitin test should be free of any chemicals, agents causing hemolysis or bacterial contaminants, as these substances may interfere with the tests.

COLLECTION AND HANDLING OF SPECIMENS FOR SEROLOGICAL TESTS

Collection

A serological diagnosis is based on the appearance or increase in titer of humoral antibodies during the course of an illness. Consequently, at least two, and sometimes more, specimens of blood taken during various stages of the illness are required. The first specimen of blood should be taken early in the acute phase of the illness or when a viral infection is suspected; this first specimen cannot be taken too early. In general, the second specimen of blood should be taken from 21 to 30 days after the first. In some diseases, antibody is relatively late in appearing, and, hence, additional specimens are desirable. These should be collected 10 to 14 days later or as indicated by clinical findings and other laboratory results. In the case of reproductive disease, it may be desirable

Text continued on page 1168

TABLE 1. Serological Tests for the Diagnosis of Reproductive Diseases

Species	Disease and Agent	Sample to Submit to Laboratory	Serological Tests	Comments on Interpretation of Results
Bovine	Brucellosis (Br. abortus)	Blood serum, rarely semen plasma	Agglutination (plate, tube, card)	Diagnosis directed by state and federal regulations governing control of brucellosis; however, agglutination titer of 1:25 is considered positive if animal not officially vaccinated
		Milk	Ring test, brucella ring test (BRT)	Screening test to determine herd infection with Brucella
		Blood serum	Mercaptoethanol acidified plate test, heat inactivated test, Rivanol test, complement fixation test	Supplemental tests to differentiate classes of antibody; used in problem herds
	Trichomoniasis (T. foetus)	Cervical mucus	Agglutination	Rarely used
	Vibriosis (Campylobacter fetus)	Blood serum	Agglutination	Serological test not considered reliable
		Cervical mucus	Agglutination	Titer of 1:25 considered suspicious, 1:50 considered positive
	Leptospirosis (L. pomona L. grippotyphosa L. hardjo)	Blood serum	Agglutination-lysis	Titer > 1:100 considered positive
	Listeriosis (L. monocytogenes)	Blood serum	Agglutination	Titers > 1:400 considered positive; limited value because many animals have high titers
	Aspergillosis (A. spp.)	Blood serum	Immunodiffusion	Serology is an aid in diagnosis of abortion caused by Aspergillus spp. and A. boydii
	Bovine viral diarrhea (BVD)	Blood serum from dam and serum or thoracic fluid from fetus	Neutralization test	Acute and convalescent sample needed with at least four-fold rise; positive titer considered > 1:4; fetus can be diagnosed positive on one sample
	Infectious bovine rhinotracheitis (IBR)	Same as BVD	Neutralization test	Same as BVD
	Chlamydiosis	Blood serum	Complement fixation	Titers > 1:2 considered positive; acute and convalescent samples needed with at least four-fold rise in titer

Animal	Disease	Sample	Test	Interpretation
	Parainfluenza-3 (PI-3)	Blood serum	Hemagglutination-inhibition	Titers > 1:20 considered positive; acute and convalescent samples needed with at least four-fold rise in titer; fetus positive on one sample.
	Malignant catarrhal fever (MCF)	Blood serum	Complement fixation and neutralization	Tests conducted only at Plum Island Animal Disease Center, ARS, USDA, Greensport, Long Island, NY
	Blue tongue	Blood serum	Complement fixation and immunodiffusion	Acute and convalescent samples needed and at least a four-fold rise in titer considered positive
	Anaplasmosis	Blood serum	Complement fixation and agglutination (card, capillary)	Rarely causes abortion or reproductive diseases
Equine	Several bacterial causes of abortion, no serological tests available (*Streptococcus zooepidemicus Escherichia coli Pseudomonas aeruginosa Corynebacterium equi Streptococcus equi Staphylococcus aureus Sarcina Klebsiella pneumoniae var. genitalium*)		No serological test; bacterial culture of fetus and placenta best diagnostic approach	Presence of organism in pure culture and pathological lesions indicates agent is cause of disease
	Salmonella abortus equi	Blood serum	Agglutination	Titers of 1:500 to 1:5000 considered positive; titers of 1:300 are considered nonspecific
	Leptospirosis (5 species of *Leptospira*)	Blood serum	Agglutination	Titers > 1:100 considered positive
	Rhinopneumonitis	Blood serum	Neutralization	Acute and convalescent samples needed and must have four-fold rise in titer
	Equine arteritis	Blood serum	Neutralization	Not commonly used
Swine	Leptospirosis (5 species)	Blood serum	Agglutination-lysis	Titers > 1:100—aborting sows may have titers 1:800 to 1:3200 or higher
	Brucellosis (*Brucella suis*, rarely *Br. abortus*)	Blood serum	Agglutination	Nonspecific antibody titers up to 1:50 common; titers of 1:100 or greater indicate presence of infection in herd

Table continued on the following page

TABLE 1. *Serological Tests for the Diagnosis of Reproductive Diseases (Continued)*

Species	Disease and Agent	Sample to Submit to Laboratory	Serological Tests	Comments on Interpretation of Results
	Miscellaneous bacterial causes without serological tests (*Staphylococcus aureus* *Mycobacterium avium* *Escherichia coli* *Corynebacterium pyogenes* *Pseudomonas* *Salmonella enteritis*)	—	No serological tests	—
	Pseudorabies	Blood serum from dam, thoracic fluid and serum from fetus	Neutralization	Acute and convalescent samples required for diagnosis with four-fold increase in titer; titers considered positive when > 1:2; fetal serology valuable in diagnosis
	Picornaviruses (SMEDI)	Blood serum from dam, thoracic fluid and serum from fetus	Neutralization	Serology as diagnostic test limited to testing paired samples (acute-convalescent) or fetal fluids; most breeding swine have low to moderate titers, 1:16 to 1:32
	Parvovirus	Blood serum from dam, thoracic fluid and serum from fetus	Hemagglutination	—
	Aspergillosis (*Aspergillus* spp.)	Blood serum	Immunodiffusion	See section on Bovine spp.
Sheep and goats	Vibrionic abortion (*Campylobacter fetus,* *C. intestinalis* and others)	Vaginal mucus	Agglutination	Titer of 1:50 considered positive in cattle
	Listeriosis (*L. monocytogenes*)	Blood serum	Agglutination	Limited value because many animals have high titers; titers > 1:400 considered positive
	Brucellosis (*Br. ovis*)	Blood serum	Agglutination and complement fixation	If any animal in the herd has a titer of 1:100, all animals reacting at 1:50 or 1:25 should be considered infected
	Leptospirosis (5 species of *Leptospira*)	Blood serum	Agglutination-lysis	Same as in cattle and swine
	Pasteurella spp.	Blood serum	Agglutination	Unreliable, as crossreacts with other organisms; bacterial culture best
	Bacterial causes of abortion (*Corynebacterium* spp., *E. coli* and others)	—	No serological tests; bacterial culture best diagnostic approach	—

	Enzootic abortion of ewes (EAE)	Blood serum	Complement fixation	Many animals have a low titer to CF test; serological findings, to be specific, must have four-fold rise in titer between acute and convalescent samples
	Toxoplasmosis (*T. gondii*)	Blood serum	Complement fixation	Limited value
	Aspergillosis (*A. fumigatus*)	Blood serum	Immunodiffusion	See Bovine section (rarely found in sheep)
Canine	Brucellosis (*Br. canis*)	Blood serum	Agglutination	Some dogs give nonspecific agglutination reactions; high titers seen for long period of time after infection
	Distemper	Blood serum	Neutralization	Rarely cause of abortion
Feline	Panleukopenia	Blood serum	Neutralization	Rarely cause of abortion
Canine/ feline	Toxoplasmosis (*T. gondii*)	Blood serum	Complement fixation and Sabin-Feldman dye test	Not a common cause of abortion
Canine/ feline	—	—	As in other species, bacterial organisms are frequently associated with sporadic abortions and there are no routine serological tests; bacterial culture is the main laboratory diagnostic test	—

to collect an initial sample at the time of breeding. This could then be paired with a sample collected at the time the animal aborts or shows indication of fetal resorption.

It must be emphasized that the blood specimens for serological tests for viral and chlamydial diseases must be obtained with aseptic precautions. This can best be done with the Vacutainer Evacuated Tube System. No anticoagulants, preservatives or other chemicals such as disinfectants should be used or in any way come in contact with the blood, as these may affect serological test results or make it impossible to obtain results. These substances may kill or so alter the live cells in the neutralization test system that one cannot determine the presence of specific antibody.

Shipping and Storage

To be certain that the sample collected remains usable for serological tests, it should be shipped to the laboratory with minimal handling and as rapidly as possible. If the serum is to be removed from the clot, it should be done using aseptic techniques and transferred to an aseptic container. Each tube should be properly labeled to indicate the corresponding veterinarian, animal's identity and date the sample was collected.

Whole blood should never be frozen, since freezing will result in total hemolysis of the specimen. For purposes of *in vitro* serological testing, serum, or the serum on the blood clot, may be shipped at refrigeration temperatures (4° C). When prolonged storage is required, the *serum samples* (blood clot removed) should be stored at −20°C.

Most diagnostic laboratories provide spe-cial mailing cartons for blood or serum tubes, and these greatly facilitate and simplify the task of the practitioner in submitting samples to the laboratory.

INTERPRETATION OF SEROLOGICAL RESULTS

The interpretation of serological results, the various tests currently available and the sample or samples that may be submitted to a laboratory to obtain serological information for the diagnoses of infectious reproductive disorders are presented in Table 1. The table is intended to be complete. Therefore, some tests mentioned may not be available at all diagnostic laboratories but only in specialized laboratories in which some research may currently be conducted on some of the diseases presented.

SUPPLEMENTAL READINGS AND FILMS

1. Bodily, H. L., Updyke, E. L. and Mason, J. O. (eds.): Diagnostic Procedures for Bacterial, Mycotic and Parasitic Infections. 5th Ed. New York, Am. Pub. Health Assn., 1970.
2. Lennette, E. H. and Schmidt, N. J. (eds.): Diagnostic Procedures for Viral and Rickettsial Infections. 4th Ed. New York, Am. Pub. Health Assn., 1969.
3. Sound 16-mm film and 35-mm slides with tape cassettes: Milestones in Veterinary Medicine. Produced by Scientificon for Becton-Dickinson Co.
   a. Perman, V., Osborne, C. A., Stevens, J. B. and Johnson, D. W.: Part I: The Purpose of Blood Sampling in Veterinary Medicine. 1976.
   b. Osborne, C. A., Perman, V., Johnson, D. W. and Stevens, J. B.: Part II: The Collection of Blood Samples in Small Animals. 1976.
   c. Johnson, D. W., Stevens, J. B., Perman, V., and Osborne, C. A.: Part III: The Collection of Blood Samples in Large Animals. 1976.
   d. Stevens, J. B., Johnson, D. W., Osborne, C. A. and Perman, V.: Part IV: The Management of Blood Samples in Veterinary Medicine. 1976.

Uterine Cultures

STEVEN D. VAN CAMP

University of Georgia, Athens, Georgia

INTRODUCTION

Cultures from the reproductive tract can be a valuable tool to diagnose infertility, to determine the drug of choice when treating infections of the reproductive tract and to be used as part of a prebreeding health examination. Several points must be kept in mind when culturing. (1) Asceptic technique is essential to assure a valid sample. (2) Sterile equipment and proper restraint are required for aseptic technique. (3) The sample must be handled properly to prevent false results. (4) Sensitivity determinations should be done on all cultures.

The interpretation of the results and the decision to initiate therapy can be difficult problems. One must understand which organisms are likely to be pathogens and which are normal microflora or probable contaminants. The decision to treat is based on the reasons for culturing, clinical examination of the reproductive tract, history of the animal or herd and the quantity and quality of the growth on the culture plate.

"Uterine cultures" are routinely done only in horses and cattle. Sheep, goats, swine and small animals are usually cultured from the vagina.

SAMPLING

Sampling Mares

Mares should be in estrus when they are cultured. Some organisms that are present in the diestrous phase of the cycle are cleared by the bactericidal effects of the mare's estral fluids, leaving the organisms that are more likely pathogenic to be cultured.

The mare must be restrained effectively in stocks or with a twitch and a leg held up. The tail should be wrapped with sterile gauze and tied out of the way. The vulva should be washed with a mild detergent and moist cotton, being careful not to force water into the vestibule of the vagina. Some practitioners prefer to wipe the vulva with an antiseptic cream or lotion instead of using water. A sterile speculum is lubricated with a clear nonbactericidal lubricant and is introduced into the vagina through the parted vulvar lips.

A guarded "tiegland" type of uterine swab is exposed after the guard is inside the uterus. Care should be taken to be sure that the swab tip touches the wall of the endometrium. The tip is withdrawn into the guard before removing the swab from the uterus. An alternative method is to introduce the swab through the cervix by guarding it in the palm of a sterile gloved hand and arm, which are passed through the vulva.

The sample should be kept cool and moist until it is plated. Transport medium is recommended to insure that the sample does not dessicate. In addition, transport medium keeps the organism from drying and does not allow one organism to overgrow another. The sample should be sent to a laboratory in which personnel are familiar with veterinary pathogens; otherwise, inaccurate interpretation of the identity of the organism may result. If mycoplasmal or viral agents are suspected, be sure that the laboratory is capable of identifying these organisms. Check with lab personnel for use of special media. A direct smear and sensitivity can be done in a veterinarian's private laboratory, if properly equipped. When doing your own sensitivity determinations, be sure that you know how to interpret the zones of inhibition properly. The largest is not always the best.

Recently, endometrial biopsies have become a valuable tool for determining the causes of infertility in the mare. The biopsy specimen can also be cultured before putting it in preservative. The biopsy instrument can also be cultured if care is used in introducing and withdrawing it.

Sampling Cows

Cows can be cultured during any stage of the estrous cycle. Passing the culture swab through the cervix is more difficult than with the mare. The cow should be restrained. The tail should be wrapped with a sterile

1169

gauze and the vulva washed thoroughly. A guarded swab is inserted through a sterile speculum that has been passed through the vulva. With one hand in the rectum and the other holding the end of the swab, the swab is worked through the cervix, as if passing an insemination pipette. The culture tip of the swab is not exposed until the swab is through the cervix, and the tip is withdrawn into the guard before the swab is removed.

Another method that has been used successfully in cattle is aspiration of mucus from the anterior cervix or body of the uterus. An insemination rod with a sterile syringe attached can be used for this purpose, or a glass tube with cotton-plugged rubber aspiration tubing attached may be used. The preparation is the same as for the other methods, and a bimanual technique is used to pass the rod. The aspirated mucus is then transferred to a sterile vial or transport medium for culture.

Endometrial biopsies have also been used for cattle.

Sampling Ewes, Does and Sows

Ewes, does and sows are usually cultured from the vagina. Ewes can be restrained in a grooming stand, in lateral recumbency or by elevating the rear legs. Does can be restrained in a breeding stock, in a milking stand, in lateral recumbency or with the rear legs elevated. Sows can be restrained with a snout snare or a crush board, or if they are in heat, they may stand well enough by pressing the hand in the middle of the back.

The vulva is washed, and for ewes and long-haired goats the hair around the perineum is moistened to hold it out of the way. The tail should be held out of the way also.

Various objects have been used for speculums — otoscope cones, plastic tubes, disposable syringe cases with the ends cut off or true vaginal speculums. A guarded swab is usually not used to culture from the vagina. The swab should be taken from the anterior part of the vagina as near the cervix as possible. Vaginal biopsies may also be cultured.

Sampling Bitches and Queens

Small animals are usually cultured from the vagina. They can be sampled at any time. Proper restraint for dogs usually means immobilization of the head, stabilization and support of the rear quarters and restraint of the tail. Cats should be held by the back of the neck and have both the front and rear legs and the tail immobilized. Long-haired animals should have the hair around the perineum moistened to keep it out of the way. A vaginal speculum should be used. However, some bitches and most queens resent this.

Otoscope cones, human nasal speculums, syringe cases or true vaginal speculums can be used. With dogs, the vulva is washed thoroughly, and the lips of the vulva may then be everted to introduce the speculum. The swab is taken from the anterior vagina near the cervix. Speed is important with queens (remember how fast they will turn on the tom even when they are in heat). Try to take the swab from near the cervix. If vaginal cytological studies are being done on the bitch or queen during the same examination, the first swab is used for culturing. A vaginal douche using sterile water can be recovered and cultured in some cases.

INTERPRETATION OF THE RESULTS OF CULTURES

Vaginal and uterine cultures lend themselves to invalid results because of contaminants. Pathologically significant organisms are often cultured in low numbers from the reproductive tract. Culture results should show pure cultures of one or two specific organisms, and these organisms should be demonstrable on repeated samples. Repeated cultures are especially important for accurate interpretation when no pathological findings are seen or expected but positive results of a few colonies are found on a prebreeding examination.

REFERENCES

1. Greenhoff, G. R. and Kenney, R. M.: Evaluation of the reproductive status of nonpregnant mares. J.A.V.M.A., *167*:449, 1976.
2. Lieux, P., Baker, J., DeGroot, A., Leskey, H., Raynor, R., Simpson, J. and Tobler, E.: Results of a survey on bacteriologic culturing of broodmares. J.A.V.M.A., *157*:1460, 1970.
3. Osbaldison, G. W., Nurn, S. and Mosier, J. E.: Vaginal cytology and microflora of infertile bitches. J.A.A.H.A., *8*:39, March, 1972.

4. Scott, P., Daley, P., Baird, G., Sturgess, S. and Frost, A.: The aerobic bacterial flora of the reproductive tract of the mare. Vet. Rec., 88:58, 1971.

5. Zemjanis, R.: Diagnostic and Therapeutic Techniques in Animal Reproduction. 2nd Ed. Baltimore, The Williams & Wilkins Co., 1970.

Endometrial Biopsy

PAUL A. DOIG

University of Guelph, Guelph, Ontario, Canada

INTRODUCTION

Endometrial biopsy is a relatively easy and safe technique to perform and can be easily utilized by the practicing veterinarian with a minimum of equipment. When used in conjunction with a detailed history, rectal examination, vaginoscopy and uterine culture, the technique can add a considerable amount of valuable information needed by the clinician to accurately evaluate the reproductive capabilities of the mare and cow.

In the smaller domestic animals, endometrial or uterine biopsy necessitates a laparotomy, and for this reason the technique has not been used as a routine diagnostic procedure.

INDICATIONS

Endometrial biopsy has been shown to be of value in a number of types of subfertile mares. These can include any mare found barren to the previous breeding season, "repeat breeder" mares during the breeding season, mares with a history of early embryonic death and mares with clinical endometritis, pyometra or mucometra. In addition, the biopsy may be of value as a prognostic aid prior to the surgical correction of genital abnormalities such as urovagina, cervical adhesions or lacerations. It may also be used as an additional criterion for fertility evaluation.[4]

In the cow, endometrial biopsy has been used primarily to evaluate the infertile animal.

TECHNIQUE

A number of biopsy instruments have been used to obtain acceptable endometrial samples. Proper instrumentation and handling of the specimen are important to minimize the development of artifacts that may make interpretation difficult.

Mares

One instrument used for the mare is a punch with a 20 × 4-mm basket that obtains a larger and more suitable specimen than most other instruments. In the absence of palpable abnormalities, a single biopsy has been found to be representative of the endometrium as a whole.

Because of the ease of dilating the equine cervix, the procedure may be performed during estrus or diestrus. The rectum is emptied, and a detailed internal examination is performed. A tail bandage is then applied, and the vulva and perineum are thoroughly washed and dried. The vagina and cervix are examined by vaginoscopy, and a uterine culture is taken prior to biopsy. A sterile gloved hand, lubricated with sterile surgical jelly, is used to carry the closed punch through the vagina to the cervix. The tip of the punch is passed by the index finger through the cervix and into the body of the uterus. The gloved hand is then withdrawn from the vagina and is inserted into the rectum. Any pneumovagina resulting from the previous vaginoscopy is relieved, and the tip of the punch is located and directed to a point just inside either the left or right uterine horn. The punch is then rotated in order to approach the endometrium on its side. The jaws are opened, and the endometrium is pushed between the jaws and pinched off. A sharp pull completes the biopsy. If indicated, a uterine infusion with an appropriate antibiotic may be carried out to complete the procedure.

To date, no adverse effects have been noted following more than 600 biopsies in our laboratory. Others have also reported the technique to be safe, and the procedure may even by performed during estrus after breeding without interfering with the subsequent pregnancy.

Cow

Because of the smaller diameter and the inability to dilate the bovine cervix, a smaller punch is used with a basket approximately 4 × 5-mm.

Although a biopsy on some older cows is possible during diestrus, the technique is much easier and probably less traumatic to the cervix in the estral animal. As in the mare, the biopsy is taken following a detailed rectal examination and vaginoscopy. If indicated, cervical or uterine cultures can be taken prior to the biopsy.

The vulva and perineum are thoroughly cleaned, and the closed punch is introduced through the parted vulvar lips to the anterior vagina. The punch is then gently threaded through the cervix by rectal manipulation and the biopsy taken from the intercornual area to avoid uterine rupture.

Tissue Preparation

The biopsy specimen is removed from the jaws of the punch with a fine hypodermic needle and dropped in Bouin's solution. Bouin's solution tends to produce a firmer specimen with less tissue distortion on sectioning. Following 1 to 3 hours in Bouin's fluid, the specimen is placed in 70 per cent alcohol or 10 per cent formalin, which may be used by practitioners as the transport medium from the field to the laboratory.

Routine histopathological procedures follow, and the sections are routinely stained with hematoxylin-eosin.

INTERPRETATION

Mare

The normal variation that occurs in the endometrial architecture during the estrous cycle and anestrus has been well documented and should be appreciated prior to interpreting the biopsy specimen.[1, 6]

A number of arbitrary classifications have been used to describe the endometrial changes that occur. The most common changes noted are varying degrees of cellu-lar infiltration and stromal or periglandular fibrosis. The cellular infiltrations may be combinations of either polymorphonuclear and mononuclear cells (acute infiltrative endometritis) or mononuclear and plasma cells (chronic infiltrative endometritis).[6] Endometrial fibrosis (chronic degenerative endometritis) should be graded as to severity and extent. Periglandular fibrosis is often associated with glandular nesting and cystic glandular degeneration. If severe and diffuse, endometrial fibrosis necessitates a poor prognosis for the future breeding potential of the mare.[4]

A high correlation between subfertility and demonstrable endometrial histopathology has been noted. Approximately 94 per cent of more than 130 subfertile mares had evidence of endometrial change in each of two studies. Chronic infiltrative endometritis, chronic degenerative endometritis, or a combination of both, accounted for approximately 70 per cent of the changes observed.[2, 6]

Less common abnormalities observed include acute infiltrative endometritis, endometrial atrophy, hypoplasia or hyperplasia. Lymphatic lacunae and endometrial lymphatic cysts have also been reported.[5]

A grading system categorizing the degree and extent of endometrial changes has been used as a promising prognostic indicator of a mare's ability to carry a foal to term.[4] Mares with minimal changes have been found to have acceptable foaling rates that reflect the type of management practices used. Mares with demonstrable endometrial changes judged to be neither severe nor permanent can be expected to have lower foaling rates but may be assisted with treatment or improved management practices. Very poor foaling rates and a higher incidence of early embryonic death have been demonstrated in mares with severe and usually permanent endometrial changes.

Additional data on the correlation between the severity of endometrial changes and subsequent foaling rates may further improve the value of endometrial biopsy as a prognostic aid in evaluating subfertile mares.

Cow

As in the mare, the bovine endometrium may be evaluated for degrees of cellular infiltration, cystic glandular change and stromal or periglandular fibrosis. Endometrial biopsy has been used to confirm and quantitate the clinical diagnosis of endometritis. A correlation between the severity of the endometritis and the resulting infertility has been noted.

In the clinically normal "repeat breeder" cow, however, there has not been a high percentage of animals with demonstrable histopathology. Endometritis severe enough to cause infertility or sterility has been reported to occur in a low percentage of clinically normal repeat breeders.[3] The presence of nonspecific infection or endometritis around the time of service does not appear to be an important cause of infertility in cows free from clinically detectable disease.

Additional studies are needed to adequately document the role of the endometrium in clinically normal infertile cows. Although the incidence of endometrial change may be low, the technique of endometrial biopsy should be considered in the individual infertile dairy cow as further aid in achieving a diagnosis.

REFERENCES

1. Brandt, G. W.: The significance and interpretation of uterine biopsy in the mare. Proceedings 16th Convention American Association of Equine Practitioners, 1970, pp. 279–285.
2. Doig, P. A. and Miller, R. B.: Unpublished data.
3. Hartigan, P. J., Murphy, J. A., Nunn, W. R. and Griffin, J. F.: An investigation into the causes of reproductive failure in dairy cows. II. Uterine infection and endometrial histopathology in clinically normal repeat breeder cows. Irish Vet. J., *26*:245, 1972.
4. Kenny, R. M.: Endometrial biopsy in the mare: A diagnostic aid in fertility evaluation and prognostication. Proceedings Annual Meeting Society for Theriogenology, 1976, pp. 14–25.
5. Kenny, R. M.: Cyclic and pathologic changes of the mare endometrium as detected by biopsy, with a note on early embryonic death. J.A.V.M.A., *172*:241, 1978.
6. Ricketts, S. W.: The technique and clinical application of endometrial biopsy on the mare. Equine Vet. J., 7:102, 1975.

Laboratory Diagnosis of Viral and Chlamydial Infections

DAVID E. REED
Iowa State University, Ames, Iowa

VIRAL INFECTIONS

Laboratory examinations available for identifying viral agents associated with abortion and congenital infections include virus isolation, fluorescent antibody examinations and serological tests.

Virus Isolation

Isolation of viruses causing abortions and congenital infections generally requires inoculation of homogenized fetal or placental tissues or vaginal swab material from dams onto cell cultures of the homologous species. Agents isolated in cell cultures are usually identified by fluorescent antibody tests. Identification of less commonly encountered viruses may require extensive physical, chemical and serological testing. The time required for obtaining results of positive virus isolation ranges from 1 to 4 days for viruses such as infectious bovine rhinotracheitis virus and pseudorabies virus to several weeks for slower viruses such as adenoviruses.

Samples for virus isolation should be packed in ice and rapidly transported to a diagnostic virology laboratory. Freezing of tissues should be avoided since it causes distortion, which hinders fluorescent antibody and histological examinations. Interpretation of results of virus isolation is complicated in some instances because abortion or stillbirths may occur several weeks or months after the initial infection. In these cases, attempts at virus isolation may provide meaningless negative results, and diagnosis can be suggested only after herd histories are considered along with clinical and serological findings at the times of abortion or parturition.

Attempts to isolate viruses from fresh unextended semen samples from males involved in reproductive disease outbreaks may also be worthwhile.

Fluorescent Antibody Procedures

Fetal and placental tissues for fluorescent antibody (FA) examinations should be packed in ice for transportation to the laboratory. In viral infections of the fetus, the best FA results are often obtained using sections of lung and kidney because nonspecific fluorescence, as well as autofluorescence is less common in these tissues than in liver and spleen. The placenta (cotyledon and intercotyledonary tissue) can be used for FA examinations, but autofluorescence often interferes with interpretation of the results.

A FA procedure that has been used successfully for rapid diagnosis of infectious bovine rhinotracheitis (IBR) virus, equine rhinopneumonitis (ERP) virus, pseudorabies virus (PRV), and porcine parvovirus-induced abortions is as follows: Lung or kidney tissues (approximately 1 cm^3) are frozen (-20°C to -70°C) on sectioning blocks, and sections are cut 6 to 10 microns thick with a freezing microtome. Sections are picked up on glass slides and fixed in -20°C acetone. Slides may be stained immediately or stored frozen for staining later. Fluorescein isothiocyanate-labeled antiserum is spread over the sectioned tissue, and the slides are incubated 20 to 30 minutes in a humid chamber at 37°C. The stained slides are rinsed twice (5 minutes per rinse) in 0.01 M phosphate-buffered saline (PBS) (pH 7.2) and once in distilled water. Coverslips are applied with a mounting medium of buffered glycerin (pH 7.2), and the slides are examined with a fluorescence microscope. Sections of known positive and negative tissue should be stained to test the FA conjugate. A further control using fluorescein conjugated negative antiserum to check for nonspecific fluorescence is advisable.

Virus Serological Testing

Serum neutralization (SN), hemagglutination-inhibition (H-I), complement fixation (CF) and agar gel precipitin tests are available (see also article on Serological Testing, page 1162). Paired serum samples may be useful because reinfection of the dam can occur at the time of abortion. For example, a 4- to 16-fold increase in IBR virus SN antibody titer is often found in the second sample of paired serums drawn at the time of abortion and 2 to 3 weeks after IBR virus-induced abortion. This anamnestic response is presumably caused by virus liberated from the placenta during abortion.

Virus serological testing is helpful in indicating the absence of specific virus infections in dams or sires. This is particularly useful with herpesviruses such as IBR, ERP, and PRV when a negative SN test on serum from a sire suggests the absence of the virus in the semen. There may be, however, some question regarding exactly what constitutes a serologically negative animal. For example, animals probably can be considered to be free of herpesvirus infections such as IBR or PRV if negative results are obtained using undiluted serum (1:2 final dilution) in the SN test or, even better, in the plaque reduction test. Because occasional nonspecific reactions may be encountered using undiluted serum, some laboratories have adopted less stringent standards such as requiring negative results at 1:4 serum dilutions.

Serological tests on fetal or precolostral serums have been used to detect intrauterine infections with parainfluenza-3 (PI-3) virus, enteroviruses, bovine viral diarrhea (BVD) virus and parvoviruses. This technique is valuable as long as results are carefully interpreted. For example, the presence of high levels of BVD virus antibody in serum from an aborted fetus cannot be considered diagnostic for BVD virus-induced abortion. However, the presence of fetal BVD virus antibodies in conjunction with typical BVD lesions in the fetus would be strong evidence of BVD virus-induced abortion.

Analysis of immunoglobulins in fetal serums has potential diagnostic application. The presence of immunoglobulin-G (IgG) in fetal serum at 6 to 9 months gestation is presumptive evidence of antigenic stimulation. The problem then becomes one of determining which infectious or noninfectious antigen caused the IgG response.

Diagnostic Methods for Specific Viruses

Herpesvirus

Examples of herpesvirus include infectious bovine rhinotracheitis virus, pseudorabies virus, equine rhinopneumonitis, feline herpesvirus and canine herpesvirus.

The fluorescent antibody test on lung or kidney tissue is the preferred method for diagnosing IBR and ERP abortions. The technique is not as consistently successful in diagnosing PRV abortions in swine. Prominent focal areas of fluorescence are present in FA-positive sections. Virus isolation from fetal and placental tissues is frequently successful although the severe autolysis that often occurs in aborted fetuses may inactivate the virus. Four-fold or greater increases in antibody levels may be found in the second sample of paired serums collected from dams at the time of abortion and 2 to 3 weeks after abortion. The presence of distinctive fetal lesions aids diagnosis.

Bovine Viral Diarrhea

There are three biotypes of BVD virus of which the cytopathic types (NADL and Oregon) are most frequently associated with clinically apparent BVD in mature cattle and the noncytopathic type (e.g., New York-1) is most frequently associated with fetal infections and inapparent infections of adults. Diagnosis of congenital BVD infections in cattle, sheep or pigs may be accomplished by isolating the virus from fetal or placental tissue or demonstrating BVD virus neutralizing (SN) antibodies in fetal fluids or precolostral serum. Since congenital BVD infection may be inapparent and may not lead to abortion or the development of fetal lesions, demonstration of a congenital infection does not necessarily indicate the cause of abortion.

Diagnosis of BVD virus-induced reproductive disease may be suggested by (1) finding BVD virus or BVD virus antibodies in a fetus that has typical BVD lesions or (2) finding abortions or fetuses with typical BVD lesions as sequelae to clinically apparent BVD in the dams. Diagnosing BVD in cows requires isolation of the virus from whole blood, feces or nasal swabs or demonstration of four-fold or greater increases in serum antibody levels in the second of paired acute and convalescent serums.

Hog Cholera

Laboratory detection of congenital hog cholera (HC) infection is most often accomplished by demonstrating the presence of the infection in sows. Diagnosis is by virus isola-tion from tissues, FA examination of tonsil sections or serological tests, each supported by the presence of compatible gross and histological lesions. Interpretation of serological results (SN tests) is complicated by cross reactions between the antigenically related HC and BVD viruses.

Parvovirus

Examples are infectious feline enteritis virus (congenital cerebellar ataxia) and porcine parvovirus.

Diagnosing parvovirus-induced cerebellar hypoplasia in kittens is possible by isolating the virus from newborn to 4-week-old kittens or demonstrating infectious feline enteritis infection in queens several weeks before parturition. More practically, diagnosis can be based upon persistent ataxia in kittens and the presence of distinctive cerebellar lesions.

Porcine parvovirus that produces abortions can be detected by FA examination of fetal lung sections or isolation of the virus from fetal tissues. Porcine parvovirus may infect pig fetuses and produce no clinical signs or lesions.

Orbivirus

Blue tongue virus (BT) of cattle and sheep is an example of orbivirus. Blue tongue virus-induced abortions are usually diagnosed by isolating the virus from whole blood of infected dams or demonstrating BT antibodies (CF test or agar gel precipitin test) in serums of dams. The serological methods provide only presumptive evidence and require support from other procedures to establish a firm diagnosis.

Enteroviruses

Example of enteroviruses include porcine SMEDI viruses and bovine enteroviruses. The collection of syndromes under the acronym SMEDI, for *S*tillbirth, *M*ummification, *E*mbryonic *D*eath and *I*nfertility is easily diagnosed clinically but is very difficult to ascribe to a specific viral agent. At least four serotypes of porcine enteroviruses are capable of causing the SMEDI syndrome, but the viruses are rarely isolated from aborted fetuses, even under experimental conditions. Serological tests are also of little use because of the existence of numerous serotypes and the ubiquitous nature of enteroviruses. The most successful methods of diagnosis involve virus isolation attempts from numerous sows (vaginal swabs) and their aborted or stillborn fetuses. The SMEDI syndrome was originally ascribed to enteroviruses but parvoviruses, adenoviruses and reoviruses are also associated with SMEDI. Enteroviruses have been isolated from fetal and placental tissues from bovine abortions, but these organisms have not been proved capable of causing abortions in cows.

Other Viruses

Poorly documented or less common are congenital infections and/or abortions associated with adenovirus (cattle and pigs), rhinovirus (foot and mouth disease virus), reovirus (pigs and mice), paramyxovirus (PI-3 of cattle), orthomyxovirus (swine flu) and bovine syncytial virus.

CHLAMYDIAL INFECTIONS

Chlamydial abortion refers to abortion as a result of infection with bacterial agents of the genus *Chlamydia*. These bacteria previously have been named *Bedsonia, Miyagawanella* or psittacosis-lymphogranuloma venereum-trachoma (PLT) agents. Although naturally occurring chlamydial abortion has been reported in cattle, goats, domestic rabbits, pigs and humans, it is most commonly recognized in sheep.

The clinical syndrome in sheep is described as enzootic abortion in ewes (EAE). The incidence of abortion in a flock generally ranges from 1 to 5 per cent but may be considerably higher when the flock is exposed to the agent for the first time. Abortions usually occur in the last third of gestation, and no impaired fertility is seen in subsequent breedings.

In cattle, some cases of the epizootic bovine abortion (EBA) syndrome or "foothill abortion" are apparently of chlamydial etiology. However, there is considerable doubt that the clinical syndrome can be attributed entirely to chlamydiae. Abortions usually occur from the seventh to ninth month of gestation, and infection may result in the birth of weak or stillborn term calves.

Placental edema and necrosis are consistently present in chlamydial abortion. Aborted fetuses often contain excessive pleural and peritoneal fluid. Petechiation of the skin, thymus, salivary glands and mucous membranes is reported with the EBA syndrome. Microscopic lesions seen in both EBA and EAE are primarily reticuloendothelial hyperplasia in the liver, spleen, heart, thymus, kidney and lung and a nonsuppurative choriomeningitis.

Diagnosis of chlamydial abortion can be accomplished by isolating the agent from infected placentae or, more rarely, from aborted fetuses. Most isolates have been recovered by yolk sac inoculation of 7-day developing chick embryos. Isolates are identified as chlamydiae by the complement fixation test and by demonstrating the presence of distinctive 0.4- to 0.5-micron elementary bodies in stained yolk sac impression smears. Rapid diagnosis of ovine chlamydial abortion can often be accomplished by identifying the elementary bodies in Gimenez-stained impression smears from infected placentae.

Intracytoplasmic inclusions of chlamydial organisms may be seen in histological sections of trophoblastic epithelium stained with hematoxylin-eosin or Gimenez stains. A diagnosis of chlamydial abortion can also be based upon a four-fold or greater increase in complement fixation antibody titer in paired serum samples taken from the dam at the time of abortion and 2 to 3 weeks after abortion.

A diagnosis of EBA can be made based upon the clinical picture and gross and microscopic lesions. Assigning a chlamydial etiology to the abortion, however, is rarely accomplished.

Genital infections with chlamydiae have also been reported in rams and bulls with seminal vesiculitis, epididymitis and orchitis. This rarely recognized infection is associated with poor semen quality and may be diagnosed by isolating chlamydiae from the semen, epididymides or testicles.

REFERENCES

1. Braun, R. K., Osburn, B. I. and Kendrick, J. W.: Immunologic response of bovine fetus to bovine viral diarrhea virus. Am. J. Vet. Res., *34*:1127, 1973.
2. Hubbert, W. T., Bryner, J. H., Fernelius, A. L., Frank, G. H. and Estes, P. C.: Viral infection of the bovine fetus and its environment. Arch. ges. Virus-Forsch., *41*:86, 1973.
3. Leman, A. D., Cropper, M. and Rodeffer, H. E.: Infec-

tious swine reproductive diseases. Theriogenology, 2:149, 1974.
4. McAdaragh, J. P., Anderson, G. A. and Leslie, P. F.: A five year summary of virus isolations from swine fetuses. Proceedings 18th Ann. Meeting Amer. Assoc. Vet. Lab. Diag., 1975, pp. 187–191.
5. Reed, D. E., Bicknell, E. J., Larson, C. A., Knudtson, W. W. and Kirkbride, C. A.: Infectious bovine rhinotracheitis virus-induced abortion: Rapid

diagnosis by fluorescent antibody technique. Am. J. Vet. Res., 32:1423, 1971.
6. Ruth, G. R., Kirkbride, C. A. and Langpap, T. J.: Fetal serology as an aid to diagnosis of bovine abortion. Proceedings 17th Ann. Meeting Amer. Assoc. Vet. Lab. Diag., 1974, pp. 9–18.
7. Storz, J. S.: Chlamydia and Chlamydia-Induced Diseases. Springfield, Ill., Charles C Thomas, Publisher, 1971.

Animal Blood Typing

RUTH SAISON

University of Guelph, Guelph, Ontario, Canada

INTRODUCTION

Apart from sporadic work in a few centers, no significant work was done on animal blood groups until the research of Ferguson, Irwin and Stormout[5] on cattle blood groups. At that time, the potential for a practical application of these groups as genetic markers stimulated an interest in further research on animal blood groups.

In the subsequent years many species were investigated, and a wealth of knowledge on animal blood groups exists. These studies of the blood groups of domestic animals have been proved to be of value, not only in assessing the genetic make-up of the individual animal but as markers for identification and as possible markers for associations between blood groups and disease. In addition, with the increased sophistication of veterinary practice, a knowledge of blood groups is necessary for transfusions and transplantations.

Animals to be used as models for certain conditions occurring in or procedures performed on humans must be clearly defined genetically. The dog, in particular, is an excellent medical and surgical model and is frequently used for experimental surgery related to transplantation in humans. This has subsequently stimulated extensive investigation of the histocompatibility (transplantation) antigens in the dog.

The blood groups of cattle, sheep, pigs and horses and the systems that they form are well understood, and extensive work on these species has produced a sizable contribution to the general knowledge of blood groups. In addition to the work in this field, other genetically controlled systems in the blood, i.e., serum protein and enzyme systems of serum, red blood cells and white blood cells, have added significantly to the number of genetic markers now recognized in many species. These genetic markers in blood have an important practical application for identifying individual animals, parentage testing, recognizing freemartins and preventing hemolytic disease of the newborn, in addition to the applications just referred to.

Blood group antigens may be either simple (of single specificity) or complex (possessing several specificities or factors). They are detected by either heteroimmune or isoimmune sera containing antibodies, some of which are agglutinins and others hemolysins.

These antigens are the products of genes coding for certain specificities or factors. They are under simple mendelian inheritance and with few exceptions are dominant in character, i.e., any factor possessed by a parent and passed on to the progeny will be expressed in the progeny.

The same type of inheritance holds for the serum protein and enzyme systems. These systems are identified by electrophoresis. This technique requires (1) starch, acrylic, agarose or similar gels as supporting media; (2) electrophoresis, using suitable buffers, to separate the components of different electrophoretic mobilities and (3) biochemical staining to observe these components, which appear as bands that have migrated various distances from the line of insertion. Components of different mobilities inherited from each parent will have codominant expression in the progeny, i.e., each component will be expressed.

SOLUBLE ANTIGEN SYSTEMS IN CATTLE, SHEEP AND PIGS

Cattle, sheep and pigs have blood group systems resembling the ABO system of man. The antigens of these systems are present as soluble substances in the serum of the individuals and are adsorbed onto the cell surfaces at varying periods after birth.

The antigen system of cattle is known as the J system. The J antigen is similar, but not identical, to the A antigen of man, the R antigen of sheep and the A antigen of pigs. It may be present both on the cells and in the serum or in the serum but not on the cells.[18] The J antigen of cattle is recognized by naturally occurring anti-J present in the sera of animals lacking the J antigen.

The R-O system of sheep has two alleles, the R and O.[10] These two antigens are also soluble serum substances adsorbed onto the sheep red blood cells after birth. Anti-R is present in the sera of O-positive sheep. The O antigen can be detected by naturally occurring anti-O (hemolysin) present in the sera of some cattle (Hereford) and goats and very rarely in sheep. When ovine red cells are of the groups RO, only the R antigen can be detected. Therefore in this case one blood group gene (R) has dominant expression and the other (O) is recessive.

A genetic system at another locus controls the expression of the R-O antigens.[10, 13] This is the I system. It is composed of two alleles, I and i. I is dominant to i, and if present in the homozygous (II) or heterozygous (Ii) form, the antigens of the R system will be expressed (dominance). If an animal inherits an i allele from each parent (homozygous ii), the production of the soluble form of the R and O antigens is inhibited. These sheep are designated "i," as no antigens of this system can be detected on the red cells.

The A system of pigs is not unlike that of the R system of sheep. The A and O antigens of this system are also present in the sera of pigs and are acquired by the red cells during the first week of life.[1,15] The sera of O pigs contains naturally occurring anti-A. The O

antigen on pig cells may be detected by anti-O sera of cattle, as may that of sheep. When A and O antigen are both inherited, only the A antigen can be detected, indicating that A is dominant to O in this species.

A suppressor gene is present in pigs that controls the manifestation of the A and O antigens on pig red cells. This suppressor system, S, has dominant (S) and recessive (s) alleles. When the recessive gene, s, is present in the homozygous state, the antigens of the A and O systems are not present on the cells. They may, however, be present in sera, saliva and stomach mucin. The reason that they do not appear on the cells may be due to a difference in the sequence of terminal surgars of the antigen molecule, which interferes with adsorption of the antigens to the red cells.

Pigs lacking the A and O antigens because the double dose of s alleles are designated "–" (Table 1).

If sheep and pigs are not tested for O as well as R and A antigens, confusion in blood types of progeny may result. The example given in Table 1 illustrates the possibilities of the types of progeny possible from a mating in which one parent is "–". Without the use of anti-O sera, this parent might be assumed an O type and the mating deemed incompatible. The same type of mating applies to sheep.

Mink have also been shown to have a soluble form of the A antigen, which is similar, but not identical, to that of A antigen of pigs[14] and is acquired by the cells during the first 2 weeks of life. It has been detected with very high titered pig anti-A.

The cattle J, sheep R, pig A and mink Å systems all have "A-like" antigens that resemble the human A antigen of the ABO system.

BLOOD GROUPS

Cattle

The most extensive use of animal blood typing is provided for cattle. Blood typing

TABLE 1. *Porcine Progeny from a Mating with One " – " Parent*

Parents				Possible Types of Progeny			
Phenotypes	O	x	" – "	A	O	" – "	
Genotypes	OOSs	x	AOss	AOSs	OOSs	AOss	OOss

laboratories have been set up in many countries having a significant cattle industry. All registered bulls must be blood typed. This insures that the blood types of all herd sires is available not only throughout a bull's life but as long as artificial insemination (AI) units are using his semen. As semen may be used long after the donor died, a record of the bull's blood type is of prime importance if cases of disputed parentage arise. The various aspects of this and other uses of bovine blood groups are dealt with in a later section of this article.

Blood group systems at 12 loci have been identified in cattle. More than 100 reagents are now available for recognition of the antigens and factors of these systems. With the exception of the J system, immune sera are used. These sera are mostly isoimmune, although in some instances heteroimmune sera, produced in rabbits, may be employed.

The B blood group system itself is an excellent source for identification. It is comprised of almost 40 factors that, in various combinations, form many alleles and more than 1000 genotypes. Although all the alleles of the B system are considered as one blood group system, it is probably composed of a number of genes, closely linked, which are inherited as a unit. Some of the antigens are doubtless complex and some simple. The C system is also complex, having 10 factors that form more than 50 alleles and are probably the products of closely linked genes. The remaining systems consist of from one to seven factors, making the number of permutations of possible combinations of all factors in all systems astronomical.

As cattle blood group reagents contain hemolysins, a large number of tests can be done in one day. A hemolytic test is used that requires individual cell suspensions, reagents and the addition of rabbit complement. The degree of lysis can be read macroscopically, and consistent results are obtained.

In addition to red cell typing, systems of serum proteins and enzymes at 11 loci have been shown to be polymorphic by their electrophoretic mobilities.

The combined use of all these systems and methods produces a blood type pattern that is unique for each animal. The likelihood of identical blood types in unrelated animals is remote.

All reagents are not necessarily used in service laboratories, but a sufficient number

are available for dependable results. The International Society for Animal Blood Group Research (ISABR) organizes comparison tests between laboratories of many countries at frequent intervals for the standardization of reagents and the recognition of new specificities. These tests insure the uniformity of bovine blood typing, which is not only desirable but necessary, as animals are frequently imported and exported between countries, as is semen.

Sheep

There are eight blood group systems in sheep, six of which are recognized by immune sera. As described previously, anti-R is naturally occurring in O-positive sheep, and the I system is concerned with the expression or inhibition of the R and O antigens. Six of the blood group systems are recognized by hemolysins, and the seventh, the D system, is recognized by agglutinins. The B and C systems are similar, although not identical, to the B and C systems of cattle.

The M system of sheep is of special interest in that the antigens of this system are the only blood group antigens known to exhibit a functional effect. The red cell potassium levels of sheep are directly controlled by the M antigens present.[11, 12, 20, 21]

This system has three alleles, M^a, M^{ac} and M^b. All sheep of the phenotypes M^a and M^{ac} have low red cell potassium levels, and all those possessing M^b, whether in the homozygous or heterozygous state, have high potassium levels. Although these alleles are codominant in their expression on the red cells, the M^b allele is dominant for potassium levels.

Eleven red cell and serum polymorphic systems have been recognized in sheep. These include serum protein and enzyme systems.

Pigs

Reported cases of hemolytic disease in newborn pigs stimulated the early work on blood groups of pigs. Blood group investigations of this species have been extensive in a number of laboratories in Europe and on the North American continent.

As in cattle and sheep, some systems are complex and others simple. Although some antisera contain hemolysins, the majority of antigens and the factors of these antigens are recognized by agglutination. Identification requires the saline agglutination test or the antiglobulin (indirect Coombs') tests.

With the exception of the A-O system, all other porcine blood types are identified by immune, usually isoimmune, sera.

Because of the necessity to use several serological methods for porcine blood typing, routine testing is much more cumbersome and time-consuming than it is for cattle or sheep. Certain sera requiring the antiglobulin test method contain antibodies that can be demonstrated by the capillary-papain method. This test requires minute quantities of reagents and can be completed and read in a matter of minutes, in comparison to the hours required for the antiglobulin test. However, the ability to react with papain is peculiar to only a few specific antisera. The capillary method can also be used for certain strong saline-agglutinating antibodies.

Systems at 15 loci have been recognized in pigs. The most complex are the E and L systems, both of which are comprised of many factors, which in various combinations form many alleles. Twelve polymorphic serum protein and enzyme systems have also been identified. Along with the antigens on red cells, they play an important role in identifying individual animals.

Horses

Blood groups of horses have gained importance as genetic markers, both for identification of sires and for preventing hemolytic disease of the newborn. Laboratories in several countries, mainly the United States, France, Sweden and Great Britain, have contributed significantly to the knowledge of equine blood group systems.

Nine blood group systems in horses are currently recognized, almost all of which form open systems. An open system may contribute one or more factors to the individual animal, or an animal may lack all known factors of this system. This apparent absence of factors may be the result of incomplete knowledge of the system. Antigens or alleles may exist that have not yet been identified. As new specificities are recognized, it is likely that most blood groups would form closed systems, i.e., some factor would always be present. Antibodies to horse cells occur as agglutinins or hemoly-

sins, or both. Most reagents are iso- or heteroimmune in nature.

Serum proteins and enzymes form known polymorphic systems at 13 loci in the horse. Some of these are complex, having a number of alleles of various electrophoretic mobilities. Used in conjunction with red cell antigens, these genetic markers are reliable tools for identification.

Dogs

The early work on canine blood groups by Swisher et al.[19] reported eight blood group antigens, seven of which were independently inherited. Later one additional specificity was described by Bull. The early studies were concerned with the mechanism involved in the destruction of incompatible cells by antibodies induced by foreign antigens of transfused cells. The antigens were recognized by the immune antibodies produced in the recipients to the incompatible blood.

Later Bowdler et al.[2] described an additional specificity that was recognized by naturally occurring antibodies in the serum of dogs lacking the specific antigen. Several new antigens were reported at the Second International Workshop on Canine Immunogenetics. Six new groups have been established by Colling and Saison,[3] five of which are inherited independently. The sixth is an allele to the Tr antigen, recognized on red cells by Bowdler, and on tissues by Zweibaum et al.[23]

PRACTICAL APPLICATION OF BLOOD GROUPS

Cattle

Genetic markers in blood provide a useful and dependable tool for the identification of individual animals. In the case of cattle the blood type is almost as unique as a human fingerprint because of the many systems involved and the complexity of those systems. Blood typing offers by far the greatest service to cattle breeders than to any other group because of the economic importance of the cattle industry.

Paternity or Parentage Testing

From time to time the question of paternity arises when a breeder suspects that a

TABLE 2. *Bovine Sire Verification*

Ani-mal	Blood Group Systems										
	A	B	C	F-V	J	L	M	N	S	Z	R'-S'
Bull	A_1/D	BG_2O_1/O_1D'	C_1WX_2/RW	F_1/V	J	L/–	–/–	–/–	U_1H'	Z/	R'/
Dam	D/D	BOY_2D'/I	C_1E/WX_2	F_1/F_1	J	L/–	–/–	N/	–/–	–/–	R'/S'
Calf	A_1/D	BOY_2D'/O_1D'	RW/WX_2	F_1/F_1	J	–/–	–/–	N/	–/–	Z/	S'/

The calf has no blood type that is incompatible with either parental type; therefore, this bull may be presumed to be the sire. It can be stated that he is eligible, or qualifies, as sire.

cow has not been bred to a chosen sire or that the wrong semen sample was used for insemination. The latter reason is the most likely one, since artificial breeding has become the most commonly used breeding method. In some instances the parentage of a calf may be suspect, and both sire and dam may come under question.

In order to be qualified for registration, all purebred bulls on the North American continent and in other countries must be blood typed. This is a necessary measure, particularly since the advent of artificial insemination, as the semen of a good herd sire may be used long after his death. Should paternity of a calf come under question the records of the bull are available.

For a paternity test the dam and calf are blood typed, and the blood type of the calf is compared with those of the dam and sire. Should a second bull be implicated, his blood type also must be available. If the calf's blood type is compatible with those of the dam and the sire of the intended mating, the validity of the mating would be verified (Table 2). The compatibility may be referred to as sire verification. However, as it is possible that another bull might have the same blood type, discretion would dictate that the report state that the intended bull *qualifies* as the sire, rather than that he *is* the sire.

The latter statement would not stand up in a court of law, and lawyers are capable of becoming experts on blood groups overnight when such a loophole occurs.

In the case of two putative sires (Table 3), one can usually be excluded. In this case the first sire is compatible and the second constitutes an exclusion. Sire exclusion can result in a firm statement because the calf possesses factors that were not inherited from the dam and that could not possibly have been inherited from the second bull, as bull 2 does not possess them. Bull 1, however, does have these alleles and so can be assumed to be the sire of the calf.

Therefore, sire verification establishes the compatibility of the mating without definite proof, as another bull could conceivably have contributed the same blood factors. Sire exclusion states that a certain bull could not have sired this particular calf as a firm conclusion. The same circumstances apply in cases of doubtful maternity or maternity and paternity.

Recognition of Freemartins

When cattle twins of unlike sex are born, it is desirable to know whether or not the female twin is a freemartin. In cases of freemartins the female is probably sterile, and it

TABLE 3. *Bovine Sire Exclusion*

Ani-mal	Blood Groups										
	A	B	C	F-V	J	L	M	N	S	Z	R'-S'
Bull 1	A_1/A_1	$BGKO_XE'_2F'$/I_2	C_1WX_2/RW	FV	J/	–/–	–/–	N/	–/–	–/–	S'/R'
Bull 2	A_1/D	B_1Y_1B'/I'O'	C_1W/X_1	FF	–/–	L/–	M/	–/–	–/–	–/–	S'/
Dam	D/D	BO_1/I	RW/X_1	FF	J/	L/–	–/–	–/–	–/–	Z/–	S'/
Calf	D/A_1	I/I_2	RW/C_1WX_2	FV	J/	L/–	–/–	N/–	–/–	Z/–	S'/

Based on the B system, Bull 2 is excluded, as the calf has alleles from his sire that Bull 2 does not possess. They are compatible with those of Bull 1, who qualifies as sire.

is of economic importance to eliminate these animals from the breeding herd.

In cattle twins, anastomosis of the circulatory vessels of the embryos frequently occurs, establishing a common circulation. The hormones produced by the testes of the male fetus are thus circulated through the female fetus. These hormones have a modifying effect on the developing female's reproductive tract, resulting in pseudohermaphroditism. These intersex females are infertile. In twins of like sex no problems arise, whether the twins are mono- or dizygotic.

To ascertain whether or not the female co-twin of a bull calf is a freemartin the twins are blood typed for chimerism. If anastomosis of blood vessels does occur in prenatal life, primordial cells will pass freely from one twin to the other. As the fetuses are not immunologically competent at this stage of their development, the germ cells take root in the hematopoietic tissue of each recipient and are accepted as "self." The precursor cells then develop, and two populations of blood cells are produced and maintained by each twin. The twins are then chimeras.

If there has been an exchange of cells, both twins appear to have identical blood types upon testing. In the hemolytic test, a good reagent will cause 100 per cent hemolysis of antigen-positive cells. When chimerism is present, only the cells of the twin possessing the antigen under test will lyse. If the cells of the co-twin are negative for this antigen, the second population of cells in the sample will remain intact and will form a button of cells on the bottom of the tube or well. These cells are then removed from the test specimen, washed and retested. By this method the genetic type of each twin can be determined. When two populations of cells exist, the female twin is diagnosed as a freemartin. A twin may have a greater percentage of cells from the co-twin than from its own hematopoietic tissue.

Additional markers are available if the twins possess different alleles for a red or white cell enzyme system or hemoglobin (Hb) variants. The cells may be separated by differential hemolysis and tested electrophoretically. As an example, if one twin has HbA and the other twin HbB, unseparated cells will type as HbAB. After separation, one cell population would be type HbA and the other HbB.

Hemolytic disease of the newborn does not occur in cattle.

Pigs

Sire Verification

As mentioned previously, testing services may develop for the identification and verification of herd sires and breeding stock in swine, particularly as frozen boar semen is now being exported and imported between several countries.

Double mating programs have been used for testing herd sires, using both natural and AI breeding.[16] By choosing a boar that is homozygous for a factor lacking in both the second boar and the dam, the sire of each of the progeny from such a mating can be identified. Double matings eliminate one set of genes (that of a second sow) and insure an identical environment for the progeny of both boars from conception to marketing age.

Nutritional and Genetic Studies

Nutritional studies have also been done by this method to determine the utilization of energy by purebred and crossbred pigs.[17] In this case one sire and the dam were of the same breed, and the second sire was of a different breed. The crossbred and purebred progeny from a single litter could then be idenitifed by blood types and their utilization of energy under certain nutritional programs evaluated.

In Scandinavia, blood typing is done routinely for genetic studies to evaluate market pigs. Four pigs are chosen randomly from a litter, and growth, development, back fat and other factors are recorded. These pigs and their parents are blood typed to insure their breeding. The quality of pigs from each breeding indicates the performance of the breeding stock.

Hemolytic Disease of the Newborn

Hemolytic disease of newborn pigs has been reported that was shown to be the result of vaccinating for hog cholera.[7] The crystal violet vaccine used was made from a pool of porcine whole blood. The sow's immune mechanism was stimulated by the presence of foreign antigens, and antibodies to these antigens were produced. Litters were affected after sucking, receiving the antibodies from the colostrum and milk. If kept from the sow for up to 36 hours, at which time the gut had become impermeable, the piglets were unaffected.

Since the use of this vaccine was discontinued, some cases of naturally occurring hemolytic disease have been reported.[8, 9] The incidence of naturally occurring hemolytic disease of newborn pigs was probably masked previously by the immune antibodies present in vaccinated sows. The incidence of naturally occurring hemolytic disease of clinical importance is very rare.

Horses

Sire Verification

The importance of individual blood group patterns for identification is evident when mares are shipped, sometimes a great distance, to be bred to a particular stallion. Stud fees can be high, and if any doubt arises as to the sire of a foal, blood typing is the only means for clarifying the breeding. There are far fewer antigen markers recognized in horses than in cattle, but with the number of transferrin and albumin markers available, the likelihood of discriminating between putative sires is good.

Hemolytic Disease of the Newborn

Hemolytic disease of newborn foals is not uncommon.[6] The exact method of sensitization of the mare is not known, but it is probably the result of fetal blood entering the maternal circulation at parturition. This disease can have serious consequences if a valuable foal is lost because of this condition.

As a preventive measure, the cells of the stallion should be tested with the serum of the mare before mating to see if there are antibodies present to any antigens on his cells. If this should prove to be the case and if it is a particularly desirable mating, the foal should be kept from the mare for the first few days after birth to avoid sensitization of its red cells, resulting in hemolytic disease. If such a mating is made, it must be remembered that this mare's blood contains antibodies and that in producing an incompatible foal the titer to the foreign antigens may have risen significantly. Crossmatches should be done with all sires used in subsequent matings. Even in the presence of incompatible matings the incidence of harmful isoimmunization is not high.

Chimerism and Freemartins

Chimerism has been reported in equine twins of unlike sex, but the reproductive tract of the female twin may be unaffected. The occurrence of freemartins in horses is probably very rare.[22]

Dogs

No routine service is offered for parentage testings of dogs, although breeders often request such a service. The cost of maintaining a bank of antisera for occasional tests is uneconomical, and such a service is unlikely to pay for itself.

TRANSFUSIONS

The most frequently transfused animal is probably the dog. Only one antigen is important in causing transfusion reactions. The A antigen is very antigenic, and if A-positive blood is administered to an A-negative dog, antibodies to the antigen are almost invariably produced. Clinics practicing transfusion should have an A-negative donor available, as this blood type may be successfully administered to either A-positive or A-negative dogs.

Cats are also transfused, blood being obtained randomly from any available donor. Feline blood groups have not been investigated to any extent. However, the response of this species to incompatible blood seems negligible under normal circumstances, and if carefully watched, no undesirable effects result from these transfusions.

Large animals may also be transfused at times if serious blood loss occurs. A single transfusion may be successful, but if additional transfusions are necesary, the administration of plasma is desirable. This will avoid sensitization of the recipient and the resultant danger of reactions from multiple transfusions. In addition, sensitization is critical for brood mares because of the resulting effects on the foal if antibodies are produced and go undetected.

Crossmatching Blood for Transfusions

To avoid transfusion reactions, particularly in an animal that has already been transfused, donor and recipient blood should be crossmatched. This practice is also indicated as a precautionary measure for a first transfusion if naturally occurring antibodies are present in the serum of the recipient.

The crossmatch must be adapted to the type of antibody present in the species to be transfused. A hemolytic test would be required for cattle.

Crossmatches for horses may be done by direct agglutination, but care must be taken in interpreting results, as rouleaux formation is common and may be mistaken for agglutination.

Crossmatches for canine transfusions require both direct agglutination and indirect (Coombs') test. For this test a canine antiglobulin serum is required. Washed cells are sensitized with test serum, washed four times in saline and resuspended, and a drop of antiglobulin serum at the appropriate dilution is added. The test is then incubated for 1 hour and read macroscopically and microscopically. This test should be used for any species when the type of antibody that may be present is not known. High titered antisera containing IgG antibodies will appear negative by the direct agglutination method.

DIAGNOSTIC TESTS FOR AUTOIMMUNE HEMOLYTIC ANEMIAS AND HEMOLYTIC DISEASE OF THE NEWBORN

Certain hemolytic anemias may be caused by the presence of antibodies on red cells. These antibodies may be directly attached to the cells (truly "auto" immune) or be part of an antigen/antibody complex that is fixed to the red cells. In order to detect this red cell sensitization, a direct antiglobulin test may be performed. The cells of the patient are washed four times in saline in order to remove all residual globulin from the cells. The cells are suspended in saline, and the appropriate antiglobulin serum is added (species-specific). If the cells are sensitized, agglutination will occur. This test is an important diagnostic tool in cases of rheumatoid arthritis, lupus erythematosus and similar conditions of an autoimmune nature.

When cases of hemolytic disease of the newborn are suspected, the same procedure is used. The cells of piglets and foals can be shown to be unsensitized at birth if cord blood samples are tested. However, if antibodies have been produced in the dams and the young are allowed to suck, the antibodies are ingested in the colostrum and milk, and hemolytic disease may ensue.

To prevent the occurrence of hemolytic disease of the newborn in species in which sensitization occurs after birth, the cells of the sire can be tested with the serum of the dam. If agglutination occurs, the young should be artifically fed for the first few days of life and put back on the dam after the gut has become impermeable.

REFERENCES

1. Andresen, E.: Blood groups of pigs. Ann. N. Y. Acad. Sci., *97*:205, 1962.
2. Bowdler, A. J., Bull, R. W., Slating, R. and Swisher, S. N.: A canine red cell antigen related to the A-antigen of human red cells. Vox Sang., *24*:242, 1971.
3. Colling, D. and Saison, R.: Unpublished data.
4. Ferguson, L. C.: Heritable antigens in cattle. J. Immunol., *40*:213, 1941.
5. Ferguson, L. C., Stormont, C. and Irwin, M. R.: On additional antigens in the erythrocytes of cattle. J. Immunol., *44*:147, 1942.
6. Franks, D.: Horse blood groups. Ann. N. Y. Acad. Sci., *97*:235, 1962.
7. Goodwin, R. F. W., Saison, R. and Coombs, R. R. A.: The blood groups of the pig. II. Red cell isoantibodies in the sera of pigs injected with crystal violet vaccine. J. Comp. Path., *65*:79, 1955.
8. Linklater, K. A.: Iso-antibodies to red cell antigens in pig sera. II. The incidence of iso-antibodies to red cell antigens in the sera of adult pigs. Anim. Blood Grps. Biochem. Genet., *2*:215, 1971.
9. Linklater, K. A.: Iso-immunization in the parturient sow by foetal red cells. Vet. Rec., *83*:203, 1978.
10. Rasmusen, B. A.: Blood groups of sheep. Ann. N. Y. Acad. Sci., *97*:306, 1962.
11. Rasmusen, B. A. and Hall, J. G.: Association between potassium concentration and serological type of sheep red blood cells. Science, N. Y., *151*:1551, 1966.
12. Rasmusen, B. A. and Hall, J. G.: An investigation into the association between potassium levels and blood types in sheep and goats. Polymorphismes biochimiques des animaux. 10th Eur. Conf. Animal Blood Groups and Biochemical Polymorphisms. Paris, Institut National de la Recherche Agronomique, 1966, pp. 453–457.
13. Rendel J., Neimann-Sørensen, A. and Irwin, M. R.: Evidence for epistatic action of genes for antigenic substances in sheep. Genetics, *39*:396, 1954.
14. Saison, R.: The blood groups of mink. II. The detection of an A-like antigen on the red blood cells of mink by the use of pig anti-A serum. J. Immunol., *93*:20, 1964.
15. Saison, R. and Ingram, D. G.: A report on blood groups in pigs. Ann. N. Y. Acad. Sci., *97*:226, 1962.
16. Saison, R. and Moxley, J. E.: The use of blood

groups as markers in a double mating program in swine and evidence for preferential fertilization. Xe Congres Européen sur les Groupes Sanguins et le Polymorphisme Biochemique des Animaux. Paris, 1966, pp. 171–174.

17. Sharma, V. D., Young, L. G., Smith, G. C. and Saison, R.: Effects of cross-breeding and sex on energy requirements and utilization by young pigs. Can. J. Anim. Sci., *52*:751, 1973.
18. Sprague, L. M.: On the recognition and inheritance of the soluble blood group property "Oc" of cattle. Genetics, *43*:906, 1958.
19. Swisher, S. N. and Young, L. E.: The inheritance of blood types in the dog. J. Hered. *44*:225, 1961.
20. Tucker, E. M.: The development of adult potassium types and the appearance of antigen M on the red cells of lambs. Proc. Phys. Soc. J. Phys., *198*:33, 1968.
21. Tucker, E. M.: Genetic variation in the sheep red blood cell. Biol. Rev., *46*:341, 1971.
22. Vanderplassche, M. and Podliachuk, L.: Chimerism in horses. 11th European Conference of Animal Blood Groups and Biochemical Polymorphism Proceedings. 1968, pp. 459–462.
23. Zweibaum, A. and Steudler, V.: Cresence chez le chien d'un system d'isoanticorps naturels specifiques d'antigenes de groupe des secretions digestives. Ann. Past., *177*:839, 1969.

Amniocentesis for Prenatal Detection of Sex and Cytogenetic Defects in Cattle

PARVATHI K. BASRUR
and A. T. BONGSO

University of Guelph, Guelph, Ontario, Canada

INTRODUCTION

Amniocentesis (the aspiration of amniotic fluid from the pregnant uterus) is a well-known procedure that is currently being used in human medicine for the early detection of sex, as well as for the diagnosis of chromosomal anomalies and biochemical disorders in the fetus of parents who are carriers of such inherited defects.

The method involves the transabdominal aspiration of fetal fluid from the amniotic cavity, generally after the fourth month of gestation, and the *in vitro* cultivation of the amniotic fluid cells for 3 to 4 weeks prior to the preparation of cultured cells for karyotype or enzyme analysis, or both. Since the anatomy of the reproductive system and the conditions prevailing in a pregnant cow are not identical to those in a pregnant woman, the method used for cattle differs in aspects such as the route of approach to the fetal sac, the instruments used for aspiration and the method of cultivation of amniotic cells.

ASPIRATION OF FETAL FLUID

The most practical approach for collection of fetal fluid is through the transvaginal route between 80 and 120 days of gestation. Aspiration of fetal fluid through the vagina is impractical when the bovine uterus becomes gradually drawn forward and downward into the abdominal cavity. Since the uterus rests on the abdominal floor beneath the intestine on the right side, after the fourth month of gestation, rectal manipulation of the uterus and localization of the fetal compartments will be difficult.

The unit most suitable for aspirating amniotic fluid includes a sterile plastic tubing obtained from a Plexitron blood collection set fitted with a 60-ml syringe on one end and a 12-inch needle (18 gauge), partially encased in a 6-inch artificial insemination pipette on the other (Fig. 1).

In preparation for fetal fluid aspiration, the rectum is first evacuated by hand, and the uterus is palpated *per rectum,* as for pregnancy diagnosis. The anogenital region is rinsed with a soap solution and scrubbed with a surgical scrub brush to insure that the area is free of contamination. The needle is then carried in the lubricated left palm of the operator and inserted into the vagina while the syringe end of the tubing is held by an assistant. On approaching the cervix, the needle is thrust forward through the adhesive tape wrapping and through the dorsal fornix (Fig. 2) to enter the pelvic cavity. By palpation, the interplacentomal area is located, and by rectal manipulation of the pregnant uterus with the right hand, the needle is inserted into the amniotic sac. Fifteen to 20 ml of amniotic fluid is drawn into

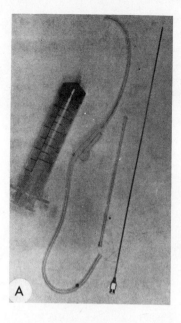
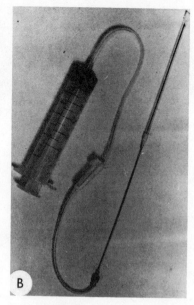

Figure 1. Instrument used for the aspiration of bovine fetal fluid. *A,* Components of the instrument: a 6-inch artificial insemination pipette, a 12-inch needle (18 gauge), an 18-inch Plexitron blood collection tubing and a 60-ml B-D Plastipak syringe. *B,* The assembled unit. The Plexitron tubing is fitted with the syringe at one end and the needle at the other. The needle is encased in the pipette and sealed securely with adhesive tape prior to gas sterilization of the unit in ethylene oxide for 24 hours.

the syringe by the assistant by gently withdrawing the plunger. The volume of the fluid aspirated is controlled by the "Flo-trol" clamp on the Plexitron tubing and by the removal of the needle from the fetal sac. The syringe is capped and brought to the laboratory for culture.

FETAL FLUID CELLS

There is a progressive increase in total fetal fluid volume, and a shift in the proportion of allantoic to amniotic fluid throughout the trimesters of pregnancy in cattle. The allantoic fluid is more abundant than the amniotic fluid during the early part of the first trimester, and the amniotic fluid is pro-

portionately more during the greater part of the second trimester. Between 80 and 120 days, when fetal fluid aspiration is relatively easy, the volume of amniotic fluid rises from 150 to 1125 ml, whereas the allantoic fluid increases from 250 to 500 ml. Therefore, amniotic fluid is more accessible during this period of gestation in cattle, and the aspiration of 20 to 25 ml of amniotic fluid is not harmful to the fetus.

The total amniotic fluid cell count ranges from 12,000 to 31,000 cells per ml during this stage of gestation. Of these, the viable cells range from 11,000 to 21,000 cells per ml, a majority of which originate from different surface layers of the fetus and the amniotic and allantoic epithelium.

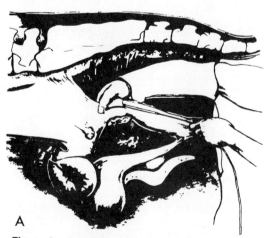
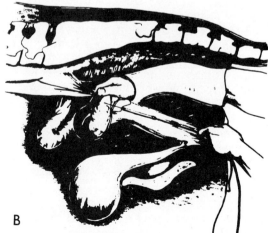

Figure 2. Aspiration of amniotic fluid. *A,* The needle is held in the dorsal fornix of vagina while the cervix is held in position *per rectum. B,* The needle is inserted into the amniotic sac while the uterus is held in position *per rectum.*

Cultivation of Fetal Fluid Cells. The fetal fluid sample is centrifuged at 1250 g for 10 minutes in a clinical centrifuge, and the cell pellet is suspended in Hanks' balanced salt solution (HBSS). After recentrifugation at 1250 g, the cell button is dispersed by gentle aspiration with a sterile Pasteur pipette and suspended in a growth medium containing 40 per cent Eagle's minimum essential medium (EMEM) and 40 per cent HBSS supplemented with 20 per cent calf serum, 100 IU/ml of potassium penicillin G and 100 μg/ml of streptomycin. Two-ml aliquots of the suspension containing approximately 10,000 cells are seeded in Leighton tubes and incubated at 37° C.

The medium is changed 48 hours after the initiation of culture in order to remove the dead cells and to replenish the growing cells with fresh medium.

CHROMOSOME PREPARATION

Sufficient cell growth is detected in the cultures between 5 and 10 days after the initiation of cultures. The cells that are most prolific *in vitro* are the nucleated cyanophilic cells originating from the amniotic membrane, and therefore these cells can be considered representations of "fetal biopsies." When adequate mitotic activity is confirmed by a cursory examination of the culture under a phase contrast microscope, 0.2 ml of colcemid solution (10 μg/ml in HBSS) is added to the medium in each Leighton tube, and after a further 3-hour incubation, the culture is terminated and 6 ml of prewarmed (37° C) distilled water is introduced into the Leighton tube to render the medium hypotonic and to allow osmotic swelling of cells. After 10 minutes of osmotic treatment, the hypotonic medium is decanted, and 6 ml of fresh fixative (3:1 absolute ethanol: glacial acetic acid, by volume) is introduced into each tube. The ethanol-acetic acid fixative is decanted after 10 minutes, and the cells are exposed to 50 per cent acetic acid for 30 seconds in order to allow the cells to swell further prior to air-drying and staining the coverslips with aceto-orcein.

DETECTION OF SEX AND CHROMOSOME ANOMALIES

The detection of the genetic sex of cattle is relatively easy since the sex complements are easy to distinguish from the autosomes. Thus, the cells that exhibit two medium-sized submetacentric chromosomes (XX) are identified as female cells and those carrying a medium-sized submetacentric chromosome and a small submetacentric chromosome (XY) are male cells. Identification of sex, sex chromosome anomalies and reciprocal translocations including Gustavsson's anomaly detected in various breeds (Fig. 3), as well as the other less widely distributed translocations, can be accomplished without recourse to karyotyping since the sex chromosomes and translocated chromosomes are distinguished from bovine autosomes because of being biarmed.

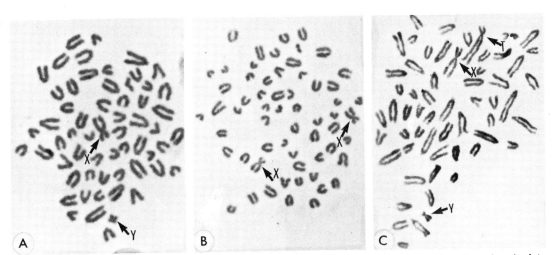

Figure 3. Metaphase plates from bovine amniotic cell cultures. *A,* Chromosomes of a normal male fetus, *B,* chromosomes of a normal female fetus and *C,* chromosomes of a male fetus carrying the 1/29 translocation. Note that the sex chromosomes and the translocation chromosome 1/29 are readily distinguished from the bovine autosomes, all of which are acrocentric.

SEX PREDICTION BASED ON TESTOSTERONE LEVELS IN FETAL FLUIDS

The concentration of testosterone in bovine allantoic fluid exhibits a sex-associated dimorphism, whereas this feature is not as clearcut in amniotic fluid (Table 1). The values expressed are based on the results of radioimmunoassay on fetal fluids at various stages of gestation and represent testosterone equivalents (Table 1). During 91 to 120 days of gestation, the mean testosterone level in allantoic fluid is 458 pg/ml ±32 when the fetus is a male and 199 pg/ml ±11 when the fetus is a female. The period at which these testosterone levels were detected in allantoic fluid overlaps the time best suited for aspiration of fetal fluid for sex prediction. Based on a double blind study of a large number of samples from pregnant uteri, it is considered that an arbitrary testosterone value of 320 pg/ml at 100 days gestation can be used as a cut-off level for the prediction of fetal sex. The fetus is likely to be a male if the testosterone level is above 320 pg/ml, and if it is below 240 pg/ml, the fetus is a female. Since the testosterone level that is considered the arbitrary limit for the prediction of a male fetus is well below the mean value detected in male pregnancies and that of a female fetus is well above the level detected in female pregnancies, the chance of erroneous fetal sex prediction is low.

For the estimation of testosterone level, the allantoic fluid is centrifuged at 1250 g for 10 minutes, and the supernatant is decanted in 1-ml aliquots into a test vial for storage for routine radioimmunoassay.

STORAGE OF FETAL FLUID SAMPLE

Fetal fluid samples can be refrigerated for 2 to 4 hours or kept cool during short transit without damaging their ability to grow *in vitro*. Testosterone assay, however, can be carried out on fetal fluid samples stored at −20° C for several weeks. Furthermore, the amount of allantoic fluid required for the estimation of testosterone concentration is very small (1.0 ml), which further emphasizes the value of this test for the prediction of fetal sex during the period from 91 to 120 days of gestation.

DISCUSSION

Prenatal diagnosis of genetic disorders by amniocentesis has become an area of great importance in human medicine during the past two decades. The major stimulus for technological advancement in this area has been the public and medical awareness of the familial nature of many disorders and of the role of genetic counseling in the detection of birth defects. Amniocentesis has only limited application with regard to litter-bearing (polytocous) animals. This procedure, however, is advantageous to the livestock industry for the prenatal detection of sex in cattle and for the diagnosis of chromosomal or genetic anomalies in other monotocous animals, including horses. This is especially true when the mare is a known carrier of a sex-linked disorder.

Early detection of the fetal sex in cattle either by chromosome analysis on amniotic cells or by testosterone assay on allantoic

TABLE 1. *Testosterone Levels (pg/ml) in Amniotic and Allantoic Fluid Samples from Cows at Various Stages of Gestation*

Stage of Gestation	Amniotic Fluid		Allantoic Fluid	
	MALES	FEMALES	MALES	FEMALES
< 60	120.7 ± 7.2* (3)†	62.0 ± 6.98 (4)	114.0 ± 13.3 (3)	77.5 ± 8.7 (4)
61–90	155.5 ± 3.5 (2)	111.7 ± 10.7 (3)	190.0 ± 30.0 (2)	129.0 ± 19.2 (3)
91–120	237.0 ± 16.1 (9)	169.6 ± 16.7 (9)	457.8 ± 32.3 (9)	199.0 ± 11.4 (9)‡
121–150	217.3 ± 15.5 (9)	191.8 ± 13.7 (10)	426.7 ± 27.3 (9)	229.4 ± 11.4 (10)‡

*Standard error of mean.
†Numbers in parentheses indicate the number of samples examined.
‡(p < 0.001).

fluid may contribute significantly to better planning and management and to the establishment of a dairy or beef herd in a relatively short time. The advent of embryo transfer as a routine commercial practice adds further impetus to adopting amniocentesis not only for the detection of fetal sex but also for the diagnosis of cytogenetic defects in the fetus in order to assess the success rate with various recipient cows.

A variety of chromosome rearrangements, including translocations and pericentric inversions causing low fertility, have been reported in cattle. Chromosome analysis on cultured amniotic cells would facilitate the detection of these defects in the fetus. The information obtained could be used as the basis for deciding the further course of action with regard to the early elimination of such calves by induced abortion.

REFERENCES

1. Arthur, G. H.: Fetal fluids of domestic animals. J. Reprod. Fertil. (Suppl.), *9*:45, 1969.
2. Bongso, T. A. and Basrur, P. K.: Prenatal diagnosis of sex in cattle by amniocentesis. Vet. Rec., *96*:124, 1975.
3. Bongso, T. A. and Basrur, P. K.: Bovine fetal fluid cells: *In vitro* fate and fetal sex prediction. *In Vitro, 13*:769, 1977.
4. Nadler, H. L.: Indications for amniocentesis in the early prenatal detection of genetic disorders. *In* Bergsma, D. (ed.): Intrauterine Diagnosis of Birth Defects, Original Article, Series. The National Foundation March of Dimes, 1971, pp 5–9.

Appendices

APPENDIX A
Drug List

APPENDIX B
Equipment and Materials List

APPENDIX C
Karin L. Harter
Consulting Editor

Appendix A

Drug List*

Drug	Supplier
Absolute alcohol (200 proof)	IMC Chemical Group, Inc. Terre Haute, IN
Acepromazine maleate, acetylpromazine (Plegicil)	Ayerst Laboratories, Inc. New York, NY 10011
Acriflavine hydrochloride	City Chemical Corp. New York, NY 10011
Alevaire mucolytic solution	Breon Laboratories, Inc. New York, NY 10016
Ampicillin (Polyflex)	Bristol Laboratories Syracuse, NY 10022
Anhydrous sodium sulfite	J. T. Baker Chemical Company Phillipsburg, NY 08865
	Mallinckrodt, Inc. St. Louis, MO 63147
Atropine sulfate, injectable	Med-Tech, Inc. Elwood, KS 66024
	Evans Medical, Ltd. Speek, Liverpool, England
Benzyl procaine and benethamine penicillin (Trilopen)	Glaxo Laboratories Palmerston North, New Zealand
Betadine Scrub	Purdue Frederick Company Norwalk, CN 06856
Bethanechol chloride (Urecholine)	Merck Animal Health Rahway, NJ 07065
Biosol solution	The Upjohn Company Kalamazoo, MI 49001
Bovoflavin Salve	Farbwerke Hoechst. AG Frankfurt, Germany
Boric acid ointment, 10%	Day-Baldwin, Inc. Hillside, NJ 48232

*As more than one manufacturer may supply the same product, drug companies cited are used as examples and are not intended as recommendations.

Table continued on the following page

Drug	Supplier
CI744—tiletamine or zolazepam (Tilazd)	Parke, Davis & Company Detroit, MI 48232
Calcium borogluconate	May & Baker, Ltd. Essex, England
Calcium chloride, 10%, intravenous ampules	The Upjohn Company Kalamazoo, MI 49001
Calcium gluconate, injectable	Vitarine Company, Inc. New York, NY 11413
Calcium glycerophosphate and calcium lactate (Calphosan)	The Carlton Corporation Tenafly, NJ 07670
Calf serum	Grand Island Biological Company Grand Island, NY 14072
Carboxymethylcellulose (sodium salt)	Hercules, Inc. San Francisco, CA
Chlorambucil (Leukeran)	Burroughs Wellcome Company Research Triangle Park, NC 27709
Chloramphenicol sodium succinate (Chloromycetin)	Parke, Davis & Company Detroit, MI 48232
Chlortetracycline	American Cyanamid Company Princeton, NJ 08540
Cloprostenol (Estrumate)	Imperial Chemical Industries (ICI), Ltd. Macclesfield, Cheshire, England
	ICI United States, Inc. Wilmington, DE 19897
Cloxacillin (Orbenin)	Beecham Veterinary Products Bristol, TN 37620
Cortisone acetate	Merck Sharp & Dohme West Point, PA 19486
Cyclophosphamide (Cytoxan)	Mead Johnson Laboratories Evansville, IN 47721
Cytarabine (Cytosar)	The Upjohn Company Kalamazoo, MI 49001
Demecolcine (Colcemid)	Grand Island Biological Corporation Grand Island, NY 14072
Dexamethasone	Schering Corporation Kenilworth, NY 07033
Dexamethasone trimethylacetate (Opticortenol)	CIBA-Geigy Corporation Ardsley, NY 19502
Diazepam (Valium)	Roche Laboratories Nutley, NJ 07110
Diethylstilbestrol (Stilbestrol)	Chemvet Laboratories, Inc. Kansas City, MO 64108
	Eli Lilly & Company Indianapolis, IN 46206
Digoxin (Lanoxin)	Burroughs Wellcome Company Research Triangle Park, NC 27709

Drug	Supplier
Dihydrostreptomycin (Streptomycin)	Eli Lilly & Company Indianapolis, IN 46206
	Sussex Drug Products Edison, NJ 08817
Dimetridazole (Emtryl)	Salsbury Laboratories Charles City, IA 50616
Diminazene aceturate (Berenil)	Farbwerke Hoechst. AG Frankfurt, Germany
Diprenorphine (M5050)	DM Pharmaceuticals Rockville, MD 20850
Doxapram hydrochloride (Dopram-V, injectable)	A. H. Robins Company, Inc. Richmond, VA 23220
Epinephrine, injectable	Haver-Lockhart Laboratories Shawnee Mission, KS 66201
Ergonovine maleate	Affiliated Laboratories Myerstown, PA 17067
	Eli Lilly & Company Indianapolis, IN 46206
Ergotamine maleate	Elanco Products Indianapolis, IN 46208
Erythromycin	Abbott Laboratories North Chicago, IL 60064
	E. R. Squibb & Sons Princeton, NJ 08540
17β-estradiol	Steraloids, Inc. Wilton, NH 03085
Estradiol cypionate (ECP)	The Upjohn Company Kalamazoo, MI 49001
Estradiol valerate	Wolins Pharmaceutical Corporation Farmingdale, NY 11735
Estrone (V-estrovarin)	Affiliate Laboratories Myerstown, PA 17067
Etorphine (M99)	DM Pharmaceuticals Rockville, MD 20850
Flumethasone	Eli Lilly & Company Indianapolis, IN 46206
	Syntex Corporation Palo Alto, CA 94302
Fluorouracil	Roche Laboratories Nutley, NJ 07100
Fluprostenol (Equimate)	Imperial Chemical Industries (ICI), Ltd. Macclesfield, Cheshire, England
	ICI United States, Inc. Wilmington, DE 19897
Flurogestone acetate (Synchro-mate)	Searle Laboratories Chicago, IL 60680

Table continued on the following page

Drug	Supplier
Follicle-stimulating hormone	Burns-Biotec Oakland, CA 94621
	The Upjohn Company Kalamazoo, MI 49001
Follicle-stimulating hormone-pituitary (FSH-P)	Burns-Biotec Oakland, CA 94621
Furazolidone (Topazone)	Eaton Laboratories Norwich, NY 13815
Gonadotropin, equine pituitary (Pitropin)	Biological Specialties Middletown, WI 53562
Gonadotropin-releasing hormone, GNRH (Cystorelin, Gonadorelin)	Abbott Laboratories North Chicago, IL 60064
Halothane (Fluothane)	Halocarbon Laboratories, Inc. Hackensack, NJ 07601
	Imperial Chemical Industries (ICI), Ltd. Macclesfield, Cheshire, England
Hank's balanced salt solution	Grand Island Biological Company Grand Island, NY 14072
Human chorionic gonadotropin (HCG)	Ayerst Laboratories New York, NY 10017
	Paines & Byrne, Ltd. Greenfield, England
	E. R. Squibb & Sons Princeton, NJ 08540
Hydrocortisone acetate	Merck Sharp & Dohme West Point, PA 19486
Insulin (Lente Iletin)	Eli Lilly & Company Indianapolis, IN 46206
Iodine (tamed iodine wound aerosol)	A. A. Satterthwaite & Company, Ltd. Christchurch, New Zealand
Ketamine hydrochloride (Ketaset, Vetalar)	Bristol Laboratories Syracuse, NY 13201
	Parke, Davis & Company Detroit, MI 48232
K-Y Lubricating Jelly	Johnson & Johnson New Brunswick, NJ 08903
Lidocaine hydrochloride (Xylocaine hydrochloride)	Astra Pharmaceutical Products, Inc. Worcester, MA 01606
Lugol's solution	Humco Laboratory Texarkana, TX 75501
Luteinizing hormone	Burns-Biotec Oakland, CA 94621
	Reheis Chemical Company Phoenix, AZ 37620
Massengill Powder	Beecham Laboratories Bristol, TN 37620
Medroxyprogesterone acetate (Depo-Provera)	The Upjohn Company Kalamazoo, MI 49001

Drug	Supplier
Megestrol acetate (Ovaban)	The Schering Corporation Kenilworth, NJ 07033
Meperidine hydrochloride (Demerol)	Winthrop Laboratories New York, NY 10016
Methohexital sodium (Brevital)	Eli Lilly & Company Indianapolis, IN 46206
Methotrexate	Lederle Laboratories Pearl River, NY 19065
Methoxyflurane (Penthrane)	Abbott Laboratories North Chicago, IL 60064
Methoxyflurane (Metofane)	Pitman-Moore, Inc. Washington Crossing, NJ 08560
Methyl-acetoxyprogesterone (MAP) (Provera)	The Upjohn Company Kalamazoo, MI 49001
Methylprednisolone acetate (Depo-Medrol)	The Upjohn Company Kalamazoo, MI 49001
Metronidazole (Flagyl)	Searle Laboratories Chicago, IL 60680
Mibolerone (Cheque)	The Upjohn Company Kalamazoo, MI 49001
Minocycline hydrochloride (Vetrin)	Parke, Davis & Company Detroit, MI 48232
Neomycin sulfate (Biosol)	The Upjohn Company Kalamazoo, MI 49001
Nikethamide (Coramine)	CIBA Pharmaceutical Company Summit, NJ 07901
Nitrofurazone (Furacin)	Eaton Laboratories Norwich, NY 13815
Norgestomet	Abbott Laboratories North Chicago, IL 60064
Oxytetracycline (Liquamycin 100)	Pfizer, Inc. New York, NY 10017
Oxytocin	Parke, Davis & Company Detroit, MI 48232
	Sussex Drug Products, Inc. Edison, NJ 08817
Penicillin-streptomycin (Combiotic)	Pfizer Laboratories New York, NY 10017
Pentazocine (Talwin)	Winthrop Laboratories New York, NY 10017
Pentylenetetrazol (Metrazol sterile solution, 10%)	Summitt Hill Laboratories Avalon, NJ 08202
Phencyclidine hydrochloride (Sernylan)	Parke, Davis & Company Detroit, MI 48232
Phenytoin (Dilantin)	Parke, Davis & Company Detroit, MI 48232

Table continued on the following page

Drug	Supplier
Pituitary luteinizing hormone	Abbott Laboratories North Chicago, IL 60064
	Burns-Biotec Oakland, CA 94621
Potassium penicillin G	E. R. Squibb & Sons Princeton, NJ 08540
Polyglycolic acid (Sexon synthetic absorbable solution)	American Cyanamid Company Princeton, NJ 08540
Povidone-iodine (Betadine solution)	Purdue Frederick Company Norwalk, CN 06856
Pregnant mare serum gonadotropin (PMSG)	Abbott Laboratories North Chicago, IL 60064
	Colorado Serum Company Denver, CO 80216
	Organon West Orange, NJ 07052
Procaine (2%) with ephedrine (epidural solution)	Haver-Lockhart Laboratories Shawnee Mission, KS 66201
Progesterone, injectable	Interstate Drug Exchange Long Island, NY 11808
Progesterone, repository	Haver-Lockhart Laboratories Shawnee Mission, KS 66201
	Pitman-Moore, Inc. Washington Crossing, NJ 08860
Progesterone in oil	Wolins Pharmaceutical Corporation Farmingdale, NY 11735
Progesterone-releasing intravaginal device (PRID)	CEVA Neuilly-sur-Seine, France
Promazine hydrochloride (Sparine)	Wyeth Laboratories Philadelphia, PA 19101
Prostaglandin-$F_{2\alpha}$ (Lutalyse)	The Upjohn Company Kalamazoo, MI 49001
Prostalene (Synchrocept)	Diamond Laboratories, Inc. Palo Alto, CA 94304
Reserpine injectable	Eli Lilly & Company Indianapolis, IN 46206
Saffan (steroidal anesthetic)	Glaxo Laboratories Palmerston North, New Zealand
	Schering Corporation Kenilworth, NJ 07033
Scarlet (Turkol) solution	Norden Laboratories Lincoln, NB 68501
Sodium thiamylal (Surital)	Parke, Davis & Company Detroit, MI 48232
Sodium thiopental (Pentothal)	Abbott Laboratories North Chicago, IL 60064
Streptomycin sulfate	Eli Lilly & Company Indianapolis, IN 46206

Drug	Supplier
Sulfamethazine Oblets	American Cyanamid Company Princeton, NJ 08540
Testosterone enanthate	Med-Tech Elwood, KA 66024
	E. R. Squibb & Sons Princeton, NJ 08540
Testosterone propionate	Sigma Chemical Company St. Louis, MO 63178
Testosterone suspension, aq.	Far-Vet Company St. Paul, MN 55104
Tetracycline hydrochloride	American Cyanamid Company Princeton, NJ 08540
Thibendazole (Equizole)	Merck Animal Health Rahway, NJ 07065
Thiomersol (Merthiolate)	Sigma Chemical Company St. Louis, MO 63178
Tramisole (Levasole)	Pitman-Moore, Inc. Washington Crossing, NJ 08560
Trimethoprim-sulfadiazine (Tribressin)	Burroughs Wellcome Company Research Triangle Park, NC 27709
Trypticase peptone	BBL Division of BioQuest Cockeysville, MD 21030
Tylosin (Tylan)	Eli Lilly & Company Indianapolis, IN 46206
Vaccines: Bovine rhinotracheitis-parainfluenza intranasal vaccine (Rhivin)	Glaxo Laboratories Palmerston North, New Zealand
Bovine rhinotracheitis vaccine (Respacine)	Diamond Laboratories, Inc. Palo Alto, CA 94304
Bovine rhinotracheitis-parainfluenza-3 vaccine (Nasalgen, IP)	Jensen-Salsbery Laboratories Kansas City, MO 64141
Bovine rhinotracheitis-parainfluenza-3 vaccine (inactivated)	Fort Dodge Laboratories Fort Dodge, IA 50561
Bovine rhinotracheitis-virus diarrhea vaccine (Rhivax 2, IM)	Pitman-Moore, Inc. Washington Crossing, NJ 08860
Bovine rhinotracheitis-virus diarrhea- parainfluenza-3 vaccine (Rhivax 3, IM)	Pitman-Moore, Inc. Washington Crossing, NJ 08860
Bovine virus diarrhea vaccine, MLV	Diamond Laboratories, Inc. Palo Alto, CA 94304
Scourvax II	Norden Laboratories, Inc. Lincoln, NB 68501
Tetanus antitoxin vaccine	Norden Laboratories, Inc. Lincoln, NB 68501
Tetanus toxoid enterotoxemia vaccine (Clostrid DT)	Fort Dodge Laboratories Fort Dodge, IA 50561
Vatspen 500 (hypodermic penicillin)	Glaxo Laboratories Palmerston North, New Zealand

Table continued on the following page

Drug	Supplier
Vincristine sulfate (Velban)	Eli Lilly & Company Indianapolis, IN 46206
Vincristine sulfate (Oncovin)	Eli Lilly & Company Indianapolis, IN 46206
Vitamin E-selenium (Bo-Se)	Burns-Biotec Oakland, CA 94621
Vitamin K (Konakion)	Roche Laboratories Nutley, NJ 07710
Xylazine (Rompun)	Haver-Lockhart Laboratories Shawnee Mission, KS 66201

Appendix B

Equipment and Materials List*

Product	Supplier
Allard V601 pregnancy detector	Allard International, Ltd. England
All Weather Paint Stik	Lake Chemical Company Chicago, IL 60612
Artificial vagina	Schack Rubber Mills, Ltd. Auckland, New Zealand
Barn Breeding Chart	Various artificial insemination organizations
Biopsy forceps	Storz Instrument Company St. Louis, MO 63122
	Welch Allyn, Inc. Skaneateles Falls, NY 13153
Boar probe	Dr. Tracy Clark Iowa State University Ames, IA 50011 (special order)
Bottles (for serum, 100-ml capacity)	Fisher Scientific Company Cleveland, OH 44123
Bozeman uterine forceps	Arista Surgical Supply Company, Inc. New York, NY 10010
Buhner suture needle	Haver-Lockhart Laboratories Shawnee Mission, KS 66201
Buhner suture tape	Haver-Lockhart Laboratories Shawnee Mission, KS 66201
Bull-Point Marker	Ag-Tronic, Inc. Hastings, NB 68901
Burdizzo Bloodless Castrator	Arnolds Veterinary Products, Ltd. Reading, England
Burdizzo Emasculatome	Haver-Lockhart Laboratories Shawnee Mission, KS 66201

*As more than one manufacturer may supply the same product, suppliers cited are used as examples and are not intended as recommendations.

Table continued on the following page

Product	Supplier
Cassou AI gun	Cassou Paris, France
	United Breeders, Inc. RR 5, Guelph, Ontario, Canada
Castrating knife	Arista Surgical Supply Company, Inc. New York, NY 10010
Chin-Ball Mating Device	Frank Paviour, Ltd. Hamilton, New Zealand
	NASCO Fort Atkinson, WI 53538
Collection dishes	Wesley Coe (Cambridge) Ltd. Cambridge, England
Conray (intravascular angiography material)	Mallinckrodt Inc. St. Louis, MO 63147
Cowculator	Raytec Manufacturing Company Ephrata, PA 17522
CTA medium	BBL Division of BioQuest Cockeysville, MD 21030
Culture transport medium	BBL Division of BioQuest Cockeysville, MD 21030
Cylinders, graduated	Fisher Scientific Company Cleveland, OH 44123
Dairy Herd Monitor	Ozland Enterprises Vicksburg, MI 49097
Eagle's minimum essential medium	Grand Island Biological Company Grand Island, NY 14072
Elastikon (elastic tape)	Johnson & Johnson New Brunswick, NJ 08903
Electronic ejaculator	Standard Precision Electronics Denver, CO
Embryo transfer medium	Fisher Scientific Company Cleveland, OH 44126
	Grand Island Biological Company Grand Island, NY 14072
Embryotomy knife	Jorgensen Laboratory Loveland, CO 80537
Endometrial biopsy punch with basket (for mares)	Pillings Surgical Instrument Company Fort Washington, PA 19034
Endometrial biopsy punch with basket (for cows)	Rogar/S.T.B. London 12, Ontario, Canada
Eosin-nigrosin (live/dead) stain	Haver-Lockhart Laboratories Shawnee Mission, KS 66201
	Society of Theriogenology Hastings, NB 68901
Estrous Expectancy Chart	Various artificial insemination organizations
Fetatome (Utrecht model or Danish model)	Jorgensen Laboratory Loveland, CO 80537

Product	Supplier
Fibre Optic Light Projector	R. Wolfe Medical Instruments Corp. Rosemont, IL 60018
Filters (cellulose acetate, millipore)	Fisher Scientific Company Cleveland, OH 44128
Foley catheter	American Hospital Supply Company Edison, NJ 08817
Funnels	Fisher Scientific Company Cleveland, OH 44128
Gerlach suture needle	Jorgensen Laboratory Loveland, CO 80530
Guarded culture system	Albion Laboratories Clearfield, UT 84105
	Kaylayjian Industries, Inc. 6050 Appian Way Long Beach, CA 90803
Ilis Preg-Check	International Livestock Improvement Service Corporation Ames, IA 50010
Individual Cow Lifetime Health Record and Barn Sheets	David A. Morrow, D.V.M. 2148 Belding Court Okemos, MI 44864
KaMar Patches	KaMar, Inc. Steamboat Springs, CO 80477
Laparoscope (adult and pediatric)	R. Wolfe Medical Instruments Corp. Rosemont, IL 60017
Laboratory animal feeding needles	Pepper & Sons, Inc. New Hyde Park, NY 10040
Leighton tube	Wheaton Laboratories Millville, NJ 08332
Lumina telescope (10 mm, 130°)	R. Wolfe Medical Instruments Corp. Rosemont, IL 60018
Mare Immunological Test (MIP)	Diamond Laboratories Des Moines, IA 50304
Marking ink	NASCO Fort Atkinson, WI 53538
Model S-5 penile stimulator	Grass Instrument Company Qunicy, MA
Nicholson transistorized electroejaculator	Nicholson Manufacturing, Inc. Denver, CO 80222
Obstetrical forceps	Arnolds Veterinary Products, Ltd. Reading, Berkshire, England
Pasteur pipettes	Fisher Scientific Company Cleveland, OH 44128
Penrose drainage tubes	American Hospital Supplies Edison, NJ 08817
Planar R202 Mark II freezing unit	Planar Products, Ltd. Sunbury-on-Thames, England
Plexitron blood collection tubing	Baxter Laboratories Marlton, Canada
Preg-Alert	American Lifestock Corporation West Laurens, IA 50554

Table continued on the following page

Product	Supplier
Pregnosticator	Animark, Inc. Aurora, CO 80011
	P. Dzuik Champaign, IL 61820
Pulsator II electronic ejaculator	Lane Manufacturing, Inc. Denver, CO 80222
Ram harness and crayon (Fergus Ram Harness)	Manning Division of Merck Sharp & Dohme (NZ), Ltd. New Zealand
Rusch urethral catheter	American Hospital Supply Company Edison, NJ 08817
Scanoprobe (pregnancy detector)	Ithaco 735 W. Clinton Street Ithaca, NY 14850
Securline-MH-100 culture system	Precision Dynamics Corporation Burbank, CA 91504
Septum, sleeve type	Fisher Scientific Company Cleveland, OH 44128
Spray Mark	Vetco Products Auckland, New Zealand
Stereomicroscope	American Optical Company Buffalo, NY 14215
	Nikon Garden City, NY 11530
	Olympus Corporation of America New Hyde Park, NY 11040
Synthofil suture	R. Braun Melsungen AG, West Germany
Syringes, single use, 3 ml	Fisher Scientific Company Cleveland, OH 44128
Technoviz (hoof acrylic)	Jorgensen Laboratory Loveland, CO 80537
Thiogel culture medium	BBL Division of BioQuest Cockeysville, MD 21030
Thioglycollate fluid medium	Difco Laboratories Detroit, MI 48232
Tomac (tubular stockinette)	American Hospital Supplies Edison, NJ 08817
Trichosel culture broth	BBL Division of BioQuest Cockeysville, MD 21030
Trocar sleeves (6 and 10 mm)	R. Wolfe Medical Instruments Corp. Rosemont, IL 60018
Trypticase soy agar	BBL Division of BioQuest Cockeysville, MD 21030
Ultrasound pregnancy detector	Foss America, Inc. Fishkill, NY 12525

Product	Supplier
Umbilical cotton tape	Ethicon, Inc. Somerville, NJ 08876
Union Carbide CRF-1 freezing unit	Union Carbide Corporation New York, NY 10017
Vacutainer (evacuated type system)	Becton-Dickenson Rutherford, NJ 07070
Veal infusion culture broth	Difco Laboratories Detroit, MI 48232
Venotube	Abbott Laboratories North Chicago, IL 60064
Verres needles	R. Wolfe Medical Instruments Corp. Rosemont, IL 60018
Vetafil (synthetic polyamide nonabsorbable polyfilament)	S. Jackson, Inc. Washington, DC 20014
Vicryl synthetic absorbable suture	Ethicon, Inc. Somerville, NJ 08876
Yale needles	Fisher Scientific Company Cleveland, OH 44128
Yoeman biopsy instrument	Lawton Instruments New Haven, CT 06503

Appendix C

TABLE 1. *Unit Equivalents within the Metric System*

1 gm (gram)	=	10^3 mg (milligram)	=	10^6 μg (microgram)	=	10^9 ng (nanogram)	=	10^{12} pg (picogram)

TABLE 2. *Metric-English Conversion Factors*

Length

Metric to English:
Centimeters (cm) $\times$ 0.394 = inches (in)
Meters (m) $\times$ 39.4 = inches
Meters $\times$ 3.28 = feet (ft)
Meters $\times$ 1.09 = yards (yd)

English to Metric:
Inches $\times$ 2.54 = centimeters
Feet $\times$ 30.5 = centimeters
Feet $\times$ 0.305 = meters
Yards $\times$ 0.914 = meters

Capacity

Metric to English:
Milliliters (ml) $\times$ 0.0338 = fluid ounces (fl oz)
Liters $\times$ 33.8 = fluid ounces
Liters $\times$ 2.11 = pints
Liters $\times$ 1.057 = quarts
Liters $\times$ 0.264 = gallons

English to Metric:
Fluid ounces $\times$ 29.6 = milliliters
Pints $\times$ 473 = milliliters
Quarts $\times$ 946 = milliliters
Quarts $\times$ 0.946 = liters
Gallons $\times$ 3.79 = liters

Weight

Metric to English:
Grams (gm) $\times$ 0.0353 = ounces
Kilograms (kg) $\times$ 35.3 = ounces
Kilograms $\times$ 2.2 = pounds (lb)

English to Metric:
Ounces $\times$ 28.3 = grams
Pounds $\times$ 454 = grams
Pounds $\times$ 0.454 = kilograms

Temperature

Centigrade to Fahrenheit:
($^\circ$C $\times$ 9/5) + 32 = $^\circ$F

Fahrenheit to Centigrade:
($^\circ$F − 32) $\times$ 5/9 = $^\circ$C

TABLE 3. *Commonly Used Names for Breeding Animals and Their Young*

Species	Bovine	Equine	Ovine	Caprine	Porcine	Canine	Feline
Common name	Cattle	Horse	Sheep	Goat	Pig	Dog	Cat
Male	Bull	Stallion	Ram	Buck	Boar	Dog	Tom
Female	Cow	Mare	Ewe	Doe	Sow	Bitch	Queen
Parturition	Calve	Foal	Lamb	Kid	Farrow	Whelp	Queen, kindle
Name of young	Calf	Foal	Lamb	Kid	Pig (litter)	Puppy (litter)	Kitten (litter)
Young male	Bull	Colt	Ram lamb	Buckling	Boar	—	—
Young female	Heifer	Filly	Ewe lamb	Doeling	Gilt	—	—
Castrated male	Steer	Gelding	Wether	Wether	Barrow	—	—

TABLE 4. *Male Reproductive Parameters in Domestic Animals**

	Bull	Stallion	Ram	Buck	Boar	Dog	Tom
Age of puberty (months)	10–12	18–24	6–10	3–6	5–6	6–12	8–12
Age of sexual maturity (effective sire)	3–4 yrs	3–4 yrs	18–20 mos	8–12 mos	8–9 mos	8 mos	5–7 mos
Testicle location	Scrotal	Scrotal	Scrotal	Scrotal	Scrotal	Scrotal	Scrotal
Accessory glands†	P, B, VG	P, B, VG	P, B, VG	P, B, VG	P, B, VG	P	P, B
Techniques of semen collection‡	AV, EE	AV	AV, EE	AV, EE	AV	AV	AV, EE
Time required for spermatogenesis (days)	60–70	38–42	59–73	Unknown	50–60	55–70	Unknown
Season	Nonseasonal	Seasonal fluctuation in semen components	Somewhat seasonal; low in summer, highest in fall	Seasonal variation in volume, cell number and quality	Nonseasonal	Nonseasonal	Nonseasonal, depressed somewhat in fall

*Adapted from Mather, E. C. and Rushmer, R. A.: In Alexander, N. J. (ed.): Animal Models for Research on Contraception and Fertility. Hagerstown, Md., Harper & Row, 1979, p. 567.
†P = prostate, B = bulbourethral gland, VG = vesicular gland.
‡AV = artificial vagina, EE = electroejaculation.

TABLE 5. *Averages of Semen Characteristics of Domestic Animals**

	Bull	Stallion	Ram	Buck	Boar	Dog	Tom
Volume (ml)	5	60	1	0.8	225	5	.04
Total sperm/ejaculation ($\times 10^9$)	7	9	3	2.0	45	1.5	.057
Sperm concentration (10^9/ml)	1.2	0.15	3.0	2.4	0.2	0.3	1.7
Motile sperm (%)	70	70	75	80	60	85	78
Normal morphology (%)	80	70	90	90	60	80	90
Ejaculates/week	6–10	3–10	6–24	20	4–10	2–6	2–3

*The editor acknowledges Brian Gerloff, D.V.M., for preparing this table.

TABLE 6. *Number of Females per Male during the Breeding Season (year)*
in Domestic Animals*

Type of Breeding	Bull	Stallion	Ram	Buck	Boar	Dog	Tom
Pasture:							
Immature male	10–25	10–15	20–30	20–30	10–20	20–40	Unknown
Mature male	40–60	20–40	40–80	40–80	20–40	30–80	Unknown
Hand (services/week):							
Immature male	2–4	2–5	6–12	6–12	2–4	1–2	3–5
Mature male	4–12	3–12	6–24	6–24	4–10	2–6	7–10

*Adapted from Roberts, S. J.: Veterinary Obstetrics and Genital Diseases. 2nd ed., p. 625. Published by the author, Ithaca, N.Y., 1971. Distributed by Edwards Brothers, Inc., Ann Arbor, Mich.

TABLE 7. *Female Reproductive Parameters in Domestic Animals**

	Cow	Mare	Ewe	Doe	Sow	Bitch	Queen
Age of puberty (months)	10–12 (breed differences)	15–24 (seasonal effects)	7–10	6–8	5–8	6–12	5–12
Age of sexual maturity (months)	30	36	10	8 (if born early in year)	10	5–12	6–12
Type uterus	Bipartite	Bipartite	Bipartite	Bipartite	Bicornuate	Bicornuate	Bicornuate
Type placenta, gross	Cotyledonary	Diffuse	Cotyledonary	Cotyledonary	Diffuse	Zonary	Zonary
Type placenta, histologic	Epitheliochorial	Epitheliochorial	Controversial	Controversial	Epitheliochorial	Endotheliochorial	Endotheliochorial
Breeding season	All year	April–Sept., easily maintained all year with lights	Breed variation from autumn to all year	Sept.–Jan. in northern latitudes	All year, slight seasonal influence	All year	Jan.–Oct.
Type estrous cycle	Polyestrous	Seasonally polyestrous	Seasonally polyestrous	Seasonally polyestrous	Polyestrous	Monestrous	Polyestrous
Length estrous cycle	21 days	21 days	17 days (range, 14–19)	21 days	21 days	16–56 weeks	2–3 weeks (if not mated)
Duration of estrus	12–18 hours	4–7 days	36 hours (range, 24–48)	18–36 hours	48–72 hours	9–10 days	3–6 days
Optimal breeding time (hours after onset of estrus)	10–16	48–72	18–24	24–36	12–30	48–96	During estrus
Mechanism of ovulation	Spontaneous	Spontaneous	Spontaneous	Spontaneous	Spontaneous	Spontaneous	Induced
Time of ovulation	4–16 hours after estrus	24–48 hours before end of estrus	24 hours after onset of estrus	12–36 hours after onset of estrus	24–42 hours after beginning of estrus	1–3 days after onset of estrus	25–50 hours after coitus
Ovulation rate (number of ova)	1	1	1–2	2–3	10–20	6–8	4
Transit time of ovum in oviduct (days)	3–4	4	3–4	3–4	2–3	6–8	4–8

Implantation (days)	10–12	25–56†	14–18	10–11	11–16	17–21	11–14
Pseudopregnancy	Not reported	Occasionally	Not reported	Frequent	Rare	Common (60 days)	Uncommon (6 weeks)
Gestation length (days)	278–293	330–345	144–151	146–151	112–115	59–68	58–65
Birth numbers	1	1	1–2	1–3	6–12	1–12	1–8
Birth weight	18–45 kg	9–40 kg, breed variation	4–5 kg	3–5 kg	1–1.5 kg	100–300 gm	~100 gm
Weaning weight	20–180 kg	70–300 kg, pony to draft horse variation	10–20 kg	14–16.5 kg	4.5–13 kg	~1400 gm	750–800 gm (8 weeks)
Weaning age	3–205 days (variable management)	4–6 months (variable management)	30–180 days (variable management)	8–10 weeks (variable management)	14–56 days	3–8 weeks	3–8 weeks
Return to cyclic activity postpartum	20–30 days ovulation; conception poor at less than 60 days	4–16 days postpartum estrus; conception slightly lower	Artificially next season unless induction in nonbreeding season	Artificial induction in nonbreeding season	Nonovulatory estrus at 1–3 days; lactational anestrus; estrus 4–9 days post-weaning	5–6 months	1–6 weeks
Time to rebreed	45–90 days postpartum	25–30 days postpartum	First estrus	First estrus	First estrus	First estrus	First estrus

*Adapted from Mather, E. C. and Rushmer, R. A.: *In* Alexander, N. J. (ed.): Animal Models for Research on Contraception and Fertility. Hagerstown, Md., Harper & Row, 1979, pp. 568–569.

TABLE 8. *Signs of Estrous Behavior in Domestic Animals**

Species	Signs
Cow	Restlessness, bellowing, mucous discharge and swollen vulva. Stands to be mounted and may mount other cows.
Mare	Association of mare with stallion, elevation of tail to one side when stallion present, squatting or urinating in front of stallion and winking of clitoris. Stands to be mounted by stallion.
Ewe	Restlessness, switching of tail and standing to be mounted. May see cervical mucus and vulvar erythema.
Doe	Rapid side-to-side or up-and-down tail movement is often detected. External genitalia may be swollen, reddened and moist. Restlessness, increased vocalization, increased urination, decreased milk production and decreased appetite may also be observed. Will stand for buck.
Sow	Reduced appetite, restlessness, salivation, frequent grunting and swollen, congested vulvar lips. Sawhorse-like stance to be mounted, which can be induced by boar or pressure of hand on back. Whitish mucous discharge present in late estrus.
Bitch	Follows period of hemorrhagic discharge. Soft vulvar swelling, yellow discharge. Female receptive, "flags" male.
Queen	Crouching, raising and extension of pelvis, treading, lateral deflection of tail, lordosis, crying out and rolling, acceptance of male.

*The editor acknowledges Brian Gerloff, D.V.M., for preparing this table.

TABLE 9. *Characteristics of Gametes within the Female Reproductive Tract in Domestic Animals**

Species	Capacitation Time (hours)	Retention of Sperm Motility (hours)	Retention of Sperm Fertility (hours)	Retention of Ovum Fertility (hours)
Cow	4	15–56	30–48	8–12
Mare	Unknown	70–140	70–140	6–8
Ewe	1.5	48	~24	10–25
Sow	3–6	50	24–48	8–10
Bitch	7†	144–264	150–240	>96
Queen	2–24	48	24–48	26

*The editor acknowledges Brian Gerloff, D.V.M., for preparing this table.
†In vitro.

TABLE 10. *Gestation Length of Domestic Breeds*

Species	Breed	Gestation Length (Days)
Cattle		
(Dairy)	Ayrshire	277–279
	Shorthorn	275–292
	Brown Swiss	288–291
	Holstein	278–282
	Guernsey	282–285
	Jersey	277–280
(Beef)	Angus	273–282
	Brahman	271–310
	Hereford	283–286
	Simmental	285–287
	Charolais	285–287
	Limousin	287–290
Horse	Arabian	335–339
	Morgan	342–346
	Thoroughbred	336–340
	Belgian	333–337
	Clydesdale	334
	Percheron	321–345
Ass		365–375
Hinny	(Stallion × Ass)	348–350
Mule	(Jack × Mare)	355
Sheep	Southdown	143–145
	Dorset	143–145
	Hampshire	144–146
	Shropshire	145–147
	Cornedale	148–150
	Rambouillet	149–151
	Merino	147–155
Goat		146–155
Pig		111–116
Dog		59–68
Cat		56–65
Siamese		63–69

*The editor acknowledges Brian Gerloff, D.V.M., for preparing this table.

TABLE 11. *Characteristics of Milk in Domestic Animals*

	Cow	Mare	Ewe	Doe	Sow	Bitch	Queen
Water (gm/L)	873	890	837	866	788	790	820
Lipid (gm/L)	37	16	53	41	96	85	50
Total protein (gm/L)	33	27	55	33	61	75	70
Calcium (mg/L)	1250	1020	1930	1300	2100	2300	350
Lactose (gm/L)	48	61	46	47	46	37	50
Phosphorus (mg/L)	960	630	1000	1060	1500	1600	700

*The author acknowledges Brian Gerloff, D.V.M., for preparing this table.

TABLE 12. *Male Reproductive Parameters of Representative Nonhuman Primates**

	New World Monkeys		Old World Monkeys				Anthropoid Ape
	MARMOSET	SQUIRREL MONKEY	BABOON	BONNET MACAQUE	CRAB-EATING MACAQUE	RHESUS MACAQUE	CHIMPANZEE
Age puberty (appearance of spermatozoa) (years)	1.2–1.7	3–5	3–4	3–4	4	2.5–3.5	7–8
Age sexual maturity (effective sire) (years)	1.2–1.7	3–5	4–6	3–4	4	4.5	7–8
Testicle location	Scrotal, parapenile	Scrotal	Scrotal	Scrotal	Scrotal	Scrotal	Scrotal
Accessory glands†	SV, P, B	SV, P, B	SV, P, B	SV, P, B	SV, P, B	SV, P, B	SV, P, B
Techniques of semen collection		Electro-ejaculation	Electro-ejaculation	Electro-ejaculation	Electro-ejaculation	Electro-ejaculation	Electro-ejaculation
Volume of ejaculate, ml, mean (range)		0.4(0.2–1.5)	1(0.5–2.0)		1.2(0.6–3.0)	1.1(0.2–4.5)	1.9(0.5–6.2)
Sperm concentration no. × 10^8/ml, mean (range)		2.1(0.8–3.1)	5(3.5–6.5)		4.6(1.6–8.3)	1.1(1.0–3.6)	6.1(2.3–12.7)

*Adapted from Mather, E. C. and Rushmer, R. A.: In Alexander, N. J. (ed.): Animal Models for Research on Contraception and Fertility. Hagerstown, Md., Harper & Row, 1979, p. 562.
†SV = seminal vesicles, P = prostate, B = bulbourethral gland.

TABLE 13. *Female Reproductive Parameters of Representative Nonhuman Primates**

	New World Monkeys		Old World Monkeys				Anthropoid Ape
	MARMOSET	SQUIRREL MONKEY	BABOON	BONNET MACAQUE	CRAB-EATING MACAQUE	RHESUS MACAQUE	CHIMPANZEE
Age puberty (years)	1.5	3	3–4	3–4	4	2–3.5	6–8.5
Age sexual maturity (years)	1.5	3	5–6	3–4	4	3–5	8–11
Type uterus	Bicornuate	Simplex	Simplex	Simplex	Simplex	Simplex	Simplex

	1	2	3	4	5	6	7
Type placenta, gross	Zonary, monodiscoid	Zonary, bidiscoid	Zonary, bidiscoid	Zonary, bidiscoid	Zonary, monodiscoid	Zonary, monodiscoid	Zonary, mono-discoid
Type placenta, histologic	Hemochorial	Hemochorial	Hemochorial	Hemochorial	Hemochorial	Hemochorial	Hemo-chorial
Breeding season	All year	All year cycling, conception fluctuates, max. Jan.–Mar.	All year, decrease in winter	All year	All year	Restricted, depends on location	All year
Length sexual cycle, days, mean (range)	35(33–38)	28(23–33)	28(25–39)	30(25–36)	31–32	9	
Menstrual flow	3 days	2–7 days	2–7 days	10 days	3 days	None	None
Mechanism of ovulation	Spontaneous	Spontaneous	Spontaneous	Spontaneous	Spontaneous	Spontaneous?	Spontaneous
Time of ovulation	22–28 days after onset menses	11–14 days after onset menses	11–14 days after onset menses		2–3 days prior to onset of marked sex skin deturgescence		
Ovulation rate (number of ova)	1	1	1	1		1	1–3
Pseudopregnancy	None	None	None	None	None	None	None
Gestation length, days, mean (range)	228(216–260)	165(156–180)	160–170	153–169	175(164–186)	155(140–180)	142–150
Birth numbers	1	1	1	1	1	1	2(1–3)
Birth weight	1–2 kg	0.5–0.7 kg	230–470 gm	330–370 gm	650–800 gm	96 gm	
Weaning weight	4–5 kg	750–900 gm			2–4 kg	300–500 gm	
Weaning age (months)	12–24	3–6			5–7	4	6
Return to cyclic activity postpartum	After weaning	3 months or after weaning			4–8 months		

*Adapted from Mather, E. C. and Rushmer, R. A.: In Alexander, N. J. (ed.): Animal Models for Research on Contraception and Fertility. Hagerstown, Md., Harper & Row, 1979, p. 564.

TABLE 14. *Male Reproductive Parameters of Representative Laboratory Animals**

	Chinchilla	Ferret	Gerbil
Age puberty (appearance of spermatozoa)	2–3 months		
Age sexual maturity (effective sire)	8 months	9–12 months	10–12 weeks
Testicle location	No scrotum, testes inguinal or subcutaneous	Perianal	
Accessory glands†			VG, P, CG, B, A
Techniques of semen collection	Manual manipulation, electroejaculation, cauda epididymides maceration		Epididymal maceration
Volume ejaculate	0.01–0.02 ml		
Sperm/ejaculate	$1–100 \times 10^6$		
Season			

TABLE 14. *Male Reproductive Parameters of Representative Laboratory Animals* (Continued)

Guinea Pig	Hamster	Mouse	Rabbit	Rat
7–8 weeks	4–6 weeks	4–6 weeks	4 months	6 weeks
8–10 weeks	6–7 weeks	6–8 weeks	6–9 months	10–11 weeks
Perianal			Scrotal	Scrotal
VG, P, CG, B	VG, P, CG, B, A	VG, P, CG, B, A	VG, P, CG, B, A	VG, P, CG, B, A
Epididymal maceration, electroejaculation	Epididymal maceration, electroejaculation	Flush female tract, epididymal maceration	Artificial vagina	Flush female tract, epididymal maceration
0.5 ml	0.01–0.02 ml		0.5–1.5 ml	1–2 drops
2–160 × 10^6	1.8–2.8 × 10^3		10–1000 × 10^6	50–60 × 10^6
	Decreased testicular weight Nov.–Jan.		Decreased sperm production in summer	

*Adapted from Mather, E. C. and Rushmer, R. A.: *In* Alexander, N. J. (ed.): Animal Models for Research on Contraception and Fertility. Hagerstown, MD., Harper & Row, 1979, p. 572.
†VG = vesicular gland, P = prostate, CG = coagulating gland, B = bulbourethral gland, A = ampullae.

TABLE 15. *Female Reproductive Parameters of Representative Laboratory Animals**

	Chinchilla	Ferret	Gerbil
Age puberty	7–12 months		9 weeks
Age sexual maturity	7–12 months	Bred 1 year from birth	10–12 weeks
Type uterus	2 horns, 2 cervices		
Type placenta, gross		Zonary	
Type placenta, histologic	Hemoendothelial	Endotheliochorial	
Breeding season	Nov.–May	Mar.–Aug.	All year
Type estrous cycle	Polyestrous	Polyestrous	Polyestrous
Length estrous cycle	41 days (variable)	No regular cycle, in heat until bred	4–6 days
Duration of estrus	2 days	Prolonged	12–18 hours
Mechanism of ovulation	Spontaneous	Induced	Spontaneous
Time of ovulation		30–40 hours postcoitus	
Ovulation rate (number of ova)	4	5–13	7 (4–9)
Pseudopregnancy		41–42 days	13–18 days
Gestation length	111 days (105–118)	41–44 days	24–26 days
Birth numbers	3 (1–5)	8 (5–15)	4 (1–12)
Birth weight (gm)	43 (30–50)	10 (6–12)	3 (4–8)
Weaning weight (gm)		300–450	11–18
Weaning age (weeks)	6–8	6–8	3
Return to cyclic activity postpartum	Estrus 2–48 hours, conception common	After weaning or next season	Estrus 3 days

TABLE 15. *Female Reproductive Parameters of Representative Laboratory Animals* (Continued)

Guinea Pig	Hamster	Mouse	Rabbit	Rat
2 months	4–6 weeks	4–6 weeks	5–9 months	50–72 days
3–4 months	6–8 weeks	6–8 weeks	5–9 months	60–100 days
2 horns, single external cervical os	2 horns, 2 cervices, single external os	2 horns, 2 cervices, 2 external ora	2 horns, 2 cervices,	2 horns, 2 cervices, 1 external cervical os
Discoidal		Discoidal	Discoidal	Discoidal
Hemochorial		Endotheliochorial	Hemoendothelial	Hemochorial
All year	All year, some decrease Oct.–Feb.	All year	All year, decrease in summer	All year
Polyestrous	Polyestrous	Polyestrous	Polyestrous	Polyestrous
16 days 6 hours	4 days	4–6 days	No regular cycle	4–5 days
8 hours	12–20 hours	10–20 hours	Prolonged	10–20 hours
Spontaneous	Spontaneous	Spontaneous	Induced	Spontaneous
10 hours after onset estrus	8–12 hours after onset estrus	2–3 hours after onset estrus	10–13 hours postcoitus	8–11 hours after onset estrus
3–4	10	10	7 (6–10)	10
None	9–10 days	12 days	14–18 days	12 days
63 days (59–72)	16 days	19–21 days	30–32 days	21–23 days
3 (1–6)	7 (5–10)	8 (6–12)	10 (8–12)	9 (7–14)
90 (60–110)	2	1–3	30–70	5–6
180–240	35–40	10–12	800–1500	40–50
3	3	3	6–8	3
Postpartum estrus, then regular cycles	Postpartum estrus, regular cycles after lactation ends	Postpartum estrus, regular cycles after lactations	Postpartum estrus, resume cycling 4th week lactation	Postpartum estrus, regular cycle after end of lactation

*Adapted from Mather, E. C. and Rushmer, R. A.: *In* Alexander, N. J. (ed.): Animal Models for Research on Contraception and Fertility. Hagerstown, Md., Harper & Row, 1979, pp. 573–574.

TABLE 16. *Breeding Data for Felidae**

Species	Age of Puberty	Characteristics of Cyclicity	Duration of Heat	Duration and Frequency of Copulation	Gestation
African lion	Usually 3 years female and 4–6 years male; can be as early as 2 years	Polyestrous all year with peaks in April and Oct. in some areas	4–16 days	21 second avg. duration; 157 times within 55 hours	98–114 days
Tiger	3½–5 years	Polyestrous all year	3–10 days, avg.: 7.1	0.5–3 (avg. 2) minute duration; 3–23 copulations daily for from 3 to 21 days; 100 observed in 6 days	98–110 days
Leopard		Polyestrous all year in most ranges. Peak births occur in April in India. In Manchuria and eastern Siberia mating is seasonal, i.e., Jan. and Feb.	3–14 days, avg.: 6–9		98–105 days
Jaguar	2½–3 years	Polyestrous all year; may be seasonal in some northern ranges (spring)	6–17 days, avg.: 12.9	2–35 second duration; avg.: 9; in excess of 20 times daily	93–110 days
Snow leopard	2–3 years	Seasonal; usually breed during winter months every second year but have been reported breeding as frequently as twice within a single year and as late as May	4–8 days	10–20 pairings/day have been observed	93–105 days
Clouded leopard	About 2–3 years	2 litters born at Frankfurt Zoo and 1 at Dallas Zoo were born in the spring			86–92 days
Cheetah	14–16 months; 9 months possible for 1 female at Whipsnade Zoo	Seasonally polyestrous; Jan.–April appears to be the peak mating period in East Africa	Approx. 10–14 days	1 minute duration; mating usually 1–8 hours apart	Approx. 90–95 days
European wild cat	Females about 1 year, sometimes as early 10 months. Males 9–10 months	Seasonally polyestrous. Males become sexually active in Jan. Occasionally females have more than 1 litter/year. Females usually do not conceive until 2 years but have done so at 1 year	Up to 8 days, 5–6 avg.	Males will continue copulation even when females are pregnant and after parturition	63–69 days
African wild cat or kaffir cat		Polyestrous, with peak litters, 2–3 in summer. Calls a harsh "mwa, mwa" during mating; very vocal	2–3 days		About 56 days
Jungle cat		Probably polyestrous all year. May is the chief mating season in India and Feb.–March in Russian Central Asia			About 66 days

*From Seager, S. W. J. and Demorest, C. N.: Reproduction of captive wild carnivores. *In* Fowler, M. E. (ed.): Zoo and Wild Animal Medicine. Philadelphia, W. B. Saunders Company, 1978, pp. 668–673.

TABLE 16. *Breeding Data for Felidae (Continued)*

Litter Size	Weaning Age	Captive Birth Recorded	Young Reared by Mother in Captivity	Second Generation Young Produced in Captivity	Remarks
1–6 mean: 3.04. A litter of 7 has been reported	Approx. 3 months+	Yes	Yes	Yes	Complex social order and reproductive processes interrelated
1–6; avg.: 2–3	3–5 months	Yes	Yes	Yes	Male should have avenue for escape after mating. Complete isolation for mother and kittens
1–5; avg.: 2	6 weeks	Yes	Yes	Yes	Males should be removed after mating. Pairs often not compatible
1–4; usually 1–2		Yes	Yes	Yes	Males should be removed after mating. Pairs often not compatible
1–4	8–12 weeks	Yes	Yes	Yes	Estrous females may not eat about one third of their usual ration
1–4; avg.: 2	5 months	Yes	Yes	Yes	Males notorious for killing females. Females may kill cubs. Young born in tree hollow.
Avg.: about 4 in wild, with high infant mortality. Usually smaller litters in captivity	About 3 months	Yes	Yes	Yes	Large enclosure with view. Live food may stimulate. Various sex ratios are being tried as well as anestral isolation. View of prey species may be helpful. Denning area for female
1–8; avg.: 3 (Prague Zoo), 4 (Berne Zoo)	6–7 weeks	Yes	Yes, but female has been known to kill young	Yes	Young have been raised without removing male, even though in nature these are very solitary cats. Provision of hiding places considered very important for breeding
1–5; avg.: 3		Yes		Yes	
Usually 3–4, up to 5		Yes	Yes		

Table continued on the following page

TABLE 16. *Breeding Data for Felidae* (Continued)

Species	Age of Puberty	Characteristics of Cyclicity	Duration of Heat	Duration and Frequency of Copulation	Gestation
Sand cat		Birth recorded in Transcapia from first of April onward			59–63 days
Black-footed cat	21 months (one report of 8 months for first heat)	Mating is in Feb.–March	36 hours, male only accepted by female for 5–10 hours	Males lose interest sooner than domestic toms. Usually no more than 6 couplings with more time between the earlier and later matings	68 days
Serval cat		Polyestrous all year with peaks in Dec. and March. Have produced 2 litters in a single year	Usually 1 day, sometimes 3–4 days		67–77 days; avg.: 74
Leopard cat or Bengal cat	About 2 years	May is chief mating season in India. Have been recorded as producing more than one litter within a year	4–7 days		63–66 days after last copulation
Rusty spotted cat		Young born in spring in India			
Fishing cat		Assumed to be polyestrous all year. Characteristic mating call heard mainly at night			63 days
Iromote cat		Not discovered until 1967; nothing known about reproductive biology			
Flat-headed cat		A young one was found in the wild in Jan.			
Pallas' cat		Mating occurs during April and May in Transbaikalia			
Marbled cat		Scant literature about reproductive biology			
Bay cat		Scant literature about reproductive biology			
Temminck's golden cat		In wild likes to den in hollow trees			
African golden cat		Scant literature about reproductive biology			
Caracal	Less than 2 years	Polyestrous all year with peaks possibly in Feb., March and Aug.		Has been observed to last approx. 10 minutes/copulation	69–78 days
Puma or mountain lion	2–3 years	Polyestrous all year with birth peaks in June–Sept. in the western U.S. Cycle length averages 22.8 days. Most females litter every 2 years	4–9 days		Approx. 3 months
Pampas cat					

TABLE 16. *Breeding Data for Felidae* (Continued)

Litter Size	Weaning Age	Captive Birth Recorded	Young Reared by Mother in Captivity	Second Generation Young Produced in Captivity	Remarks
2–4		Yes			
		Yes	Yes		Smallest member of Felidae, very shy and antisocial; lowered humidity associated with breeding success
1–4; avg.: 2.35		Yes	Yes		Adapt well to captivity. Need a fairly large enclosure
2–3 avg.		Yes	Yes	Yes	Success in rearing has been had with male and female left in enclosure at same time
2–3					
1–4; usually 2	Greater than 6 months	Yes	Yes		Male and female may need to be separated after mating. A quiet denning area is essential for the female
					Very rare
		Yes			Very rare
5–6		Yes	?		Mating call said to resemble a cross between the bark of a small dog and an owl's hoot
		Yes			
1–3		Yes		Yes	Very nervous
		Yes			
1–6; avg.: 2–3		Yes		Yes	Loud calling at mating. Male should be removed after mating. Increased appetite, with anorexia noted the day before parturition
1–5; rarely 6 (usually 2–3)	about 3	Yes	Yes	Yes	Pregnant females should be isolated. Young stay with mother about 1 year in wild
1–3		Yes			

Table continued on the following page

TABLE 16. *Breeding Data for Felidae* (Continued)

Species	Age of Puberty	Characteristics of Cyclicity	Duration of Heat	Duration and Frequency of Copulation	Gestation
Mountain cat or Andean highland cat		Nothing known about the reproductive biology			63–70 days
Jaguarundi		Probably polyestrous all year. Peak mating season in Mexico is Nov. and Dec. Solitary at other times. Two litters (March and Aug.) may be produced			63–70 days
Lynx or northern lynx or European lynx	2–3 years	Seasonal: March is primary mating season and May secondary; usually mate at night; females failing to become pregnant probably return to heat in secondary season. Males vocal	7–10 days		63–74 days
Spanish lynx	1 year for females, to 21 months; male, 33 months	Seasonal: Nov.–Feb. Very vocal during mating season	1–4 days		
Bobcat	1–2 years	Seasonal: From Jan.–July depending on locale. Peak is always in March–April. Animals not pregnant from primary mating period may come in heat again in summer and/or early fall. Mating is a series of running encounters	Approx. 1 week	Fewer copulations than most felids	Approx. 63 days
Ocelot	First heat as early as 8 months, usually do not conceive until 2 years	Polyestrous all year with peak mating activity in Dec. and Jan.	7–10 days, can be out if conceives		89 ± 2 days once cat conceives
Brazilian ocelot-cat or tiger ocelot	About 1 year	Mating peak in Dec.–June	Several days		74–76 days
Margay or tree ocelot					83 days
Geoffroy's cat					71–76 days
Kod Kod or Guina					

TABLE 16. *Breeding Data for Felidae* (Continued)

Litter Size	Weaning Age	Captive Birth Recorded	Young Reared by Mother in Captivity	Second Generation Young Produced in Captivity	Remarks
2–4					
2–4		Yes			
1–3	12 weeks	Yes	Yes	?	Postpartum aggressiveness and anorexia observed in female. Male may or may not have to be removed. One tom has bred two females in same cage
	About 2 months	Yes			Bear young in a rocky ledge, natural cavity or thicket
1–6; avg.: 3.5		Yes	Yes		Some bobcats may produce 2 litters/year
1–3; avg.: 1–2		Yes			Often mates are not compatible and males have been known to kill females. It is recommended that females in heat not be presented to strange males. Rather poor overall reproductive success, but as many as 3 litters within a year have been reported
1–2		Yes	Yes		Males have been noted to be very aggressive toward females
1–2		Yes	Yes		Estrous females should not be presented to strange males
2–3		Yes			Mate and kitten slaying have been recorded. Rotating males can increase breeding
					Little known of behavior, but some believe this species may be quite social

Index

Umbilical cord, equine, abnormalities of, and abortion, 750
  porcine, bleeding from, and preweaning mortality, 1093
  rupture of, and stillbirth, 1066, 1087, 1092
Umbilical hernia, bovine congenital, 430(t)
Underlines, porcine, examination of, 1028–1029, *1029*
Undernutrition. See *Malnutrition.*
Undersized pigs, 1092–1093
Undescended testis. See *Cryptorchidism.*
Ungulates, wild. See *Wild ungulates.*
United States straws, for frozen bull semen. See *Continental straws.*
Urea, and bovine endocrine function, 476
  and bovine infertility, 451
  and bovine reproduction, 474–479
  bovine tolerance to, 474
  breakdown of, 474
  in bovine feed, guidelines for, 476–478, 477(t)
Urea toxicity, bovine, and abortion, 475
Urethra, bovine, male, *316, 317*
  congenital defects of, 435(t)
  canine, rupture of, 615–616
  caprine, obstruction of, 999–1000
Urethral cultures, for equine breeding soundness examination, 700
Urethral fistulae, bovine, 384–385, *385*
Urethral-penile adhesions, ovine, pubertal breakdown of, 929
Urethral process, penile, ovine, shearing injury of, 938
Urethritis, bacterial, equine, and hemospermia, 699
Urethroplasty, equine, 812
Urinary bladder, caprine, rupture of, 1000
  equine, patent, in newborn, vs. meconium coli, 757(t), 762
  prolapse of, surgery for, 814–815
  ruptured, in newborn, first signs of, incidence of appearance of, 757(t)
  porcine, lateroflexed, catheterization of, 1075–1076, *1076*
Urinary calculi, feline, and dietary ash, 858
Urinary catheterization, equine, for penile injuries, 785
  porcine, for lateroflexed bladder, 1075–1076, *1076*
Urination posture, canine, sexual dimorphism in, 567, 568
Urine, abnormal, in newborn foal, 763
  vaginal pooling of, bovine, 263–264, *263, 264*
Urine reflux, equine, episioplasty for, 805–806
  urethroplasty for, 812
Urogenital sinus, canine, abnormal development of, 586–587
Urolithiasis, caprine, male, 999–1000
  feline, and dietary ash, 858
Urovagina, bovine, 263–264, *263, 264*
Uterine artery, middle, bovine, changes in during pregnancy, 234(t)
  palpation of, and duration of pregnancy, 233, 233(t)

Uterine caruncles, caprine, 971, *971*
Uterine cultures, 1169–1171. See also under *Uterus, bovine, cultures of,* etc.
Uterine horn(s), caprine, 971, *971*
  equine, diameter of, during pregnancy, 738(t)
  enlargement of, in pregnancy, 738(t), 743
  feline, morphology of, during estrous cycle, 828–829, *828*
  porcine, blind, 1031, *1031*
  missing, 1031
Uterine tubes, caprine, 971, *971*
Uterus, bovine, abscess of, and repeat-breeding, 211
  antibiotic perfusion in, 32
  atony, of and retained placenta, 184
  bacteria isolated from, 26
  bacterial defense mechanisms of, 25–26
  birth injuries of, 273
  blood flow in, and uterine temperature, 447–448, *447*
  cultures of, 1169–1170
    postpartum, histological evaluation of, 223–226
  disorders of, and repeat-breeding, 208–211
  endocrine support to, inadequate, 210–211
  gravid, changes in, 234(t)
    protein and energy deposition in, 466(t)
    size of, and duration of pregnancy, 233
    weight of, 466(t)
  inflammatory changes in, physical findings in, 163
  infusion of. See *Intrauterine infusion.*
  leptospirosis lesions in, 490
  manual retraction of, 229–230, *230*
  postpartum, drug absorption by, 41–42, 42(t)
    evaluation of, 289–291, 289(t)
  rectal palpation of, for pregnancy, diagnosis, 229–232, *230, 231, 232*
  ruptured, as indication for cesarean section, 269
  temperature of, and blood flow, 447–448, *447*
    and fertility, 442, 447–448
  torsion of, prolonged, as indication for cesarean section, 269
  tumors of, and repeat-breeding, 211
  canine, examination of, 580
    gravid, *592*, 593
    inertia of, primary, 599–601, 601(t)
      medicinal treatment of, 602–603
    postpartum, diseases of, 608–611
      involution of, 573
    prolapse of, 617
    pyometrial lesions of, 624–625
    subinvolution of, 609–610
    tumors of, 644
      epidemiological aspects of, 638, 639(t)
  caprine, 971
    postpartum involution of, 981
    prolapse of, 981
    torsion of, and dystocia, 980